Nuclear cardiac imaging

NUCLEAR CARDIAC IMAGING
PRINCIPLES AND APPLICATIONS

Third Edition

Edited by

AMI E. ISKANDRIAN, M.D., F.A.C.C., F.A.H.A.

MARIO S. VERANI, M.D., F.A.C.C., F.A.H.A.

OXFORD
UNIVERSITY PRESS
2003

OXFORD
UNIVERSITY PRESS

Oxford   New York
Auckland   Bangkok   Buenos Aires   Cape Town   Chennai
Dar es Salaam   Delhi   Hong Kong   Istanbul   Karachi   Kolkata
Kuala Lumpur   Madrid   Melbourne   Mexico City   Mumbai
Nairobi   São Paulo   Shanghai   Taipei   Tokyo   Toronto

Published by Oxford University Press, Inc.
198 Madison Avenue, New York, New York, 10016
http://www.oup-usa.org

Oxford is a registered trademark of Oxford University Press

Iskandrian, Abdulmassih S., 1941–
Nuclear cardiac imaging : principles & applications /
by Ami S. Iskandrian and Mario S. Verani.—3rd ed.
p. ; cm.   Includes bibliographical references and index.
ISBN 0-19-514351-5
1. Heart—Radionuclide imaging.
I. Verani, Mario S. II. Title.
[DNLM: 1. Heart—radionuclide imaging. WG 141.5.R2 I8ln 2003]
RC683.5.R33 I85 2003   616.1′207575—dc21   2002017076

9 8 7 6 5 4 3 2 1

Printed in the United States of America
on acid-free paper

Be like the bird, who
Halting in flight
On limb too slight
Feels it give way beneath him,
Yet sings
Knowing he hath wings.
                                                    VICTOR HUGO

This book is dedicated to my coeditor and best friend, Mario S. Verani, who lost his fight with pancreatic cancer on October 30, 2001. Mario spent many of the last months of his life reviewing and editing the chapters contained herein and collaborating with the contributors of our book. It is with much love and respect that I dedicate this third edition of *Nuclear Cardiac Imaging: Principles and Applications* to his memory. Rest in peace, my friend.

Ami E. Iskandrian
Birmingham, Alabama
November 2001

Preface

It is a sure sign of the rapid pace of scientific advancement that a book printed barely 5 years ago already needs revisions. Thus this third edition. Contrary to the first two editions of this book, which were essentially the work of one person (AEI, first edition), and two persons (AEI and MSV), the original authors have opted for a multi-authored book.

We wished to edit a book that would remain for some years as a comprehensive, detailed source of information in the field of nuclear cardiology. At the same time, we wanted to take advantage of the personal knowledge and opinions of many of the leaders in the field. Although not all of the leaders in the field have contributed to this volume, because of overcommitment or other reasons, the contributors are all prominent investigators and practitioners of nuclear cardiology. In fact, the authors of each of the chapters in the book were handpicked for their particular expertise and focused contribution to the field.

The editors are delighted the contributors to this volume provided us not only with a rich, comprehensive review of the state-of-the-art of their respective topics but also with their personal insight and "bottom-line" messages. Because myocardial perfusion imaging today accounts for perhaps 90% of all nuclear cardiology imaging procedures done in the United States, great emphasis is given to the instrumental, technical, and clinical aspects of perfusion imaging. However, other important areas such as radionuclide angiography, metabolic and receptor imaging, and positron emission tomography are also comprehensively assessed by our team of experts.

The editors felt it would be important to have a brief description of nonnuclear techniques that may compete with nuclear cardiac procedures and how they compare with one another. Also discussed in separate, new chapters are the cost-effectiveness of nuclear cardiac imaging, the special considerations of applying nuclear techniques to female subjects, and imaging in the Emergency Department. In addition, because of its great practical importance, a whole chapter has been dedicated to the nitty-gritty of interpreting and reporting nuclear cardiac procedures and another to NRC regulations, certification in nuclear cardiology, and laboratory accreditation. The most current ACC/AHA/ASNC guidelines are included as an appendix.

As expected in any multi-authored textbook dealing with topics that are often interrelated, some degree of overlap is unavoidable. The editors worked with the authors to eliminate any excessive or superfluous amount of thematic duplication. However, to the extent that different experts often have different perspectives on the same topic, some degree of overlap was allowed. The editors are grateful to each of the contributors to this textbook for their superb chapters, to the staff of Oxford University Press for their patience and editorial advice, and to Ms. Rose Perry and Ms. Jo Ann Rabb for their secretarial skills.

A. E. I.
M. S. V.

Contents

Contributors

STEPHEN L. BACHARACH, PH.D.
Head, Imaging Science Group
Medical Physicist, the Clinical Center
National Institutes of Health
Bethesda, Maryland

TIMOTHY M. BATEMAN, M.D.
Director, Cardiac and Vascular Radiologic Imaging
Mid-America Heart Institute
Professor of Medicine
University of Missouri—Kansas City
Kansas City, Missouri

JEROEN J. BAX, M.D., PH.D.
Professor, Department of Cardiology
Leiden University Medical Center
The Netherlands

DANIEL S. BERMAN, M.D., F.A.C.C.
Director, Nuclear Cardiology
Cedars-Sinai Medical Center
Professor of Medicine
UCLA School of Medicine
Los Angeles, California

JEFFREY S. BORER, M.D.
Gladys and Roland Harriman Professor of Cardiovascular
  Medicine
Chief, Division of Cardiovascular Pathophysiology
Director, the Howard Gilman Institute for Valvular Heart
  Diseases
Weill Medical College of Cornell University
New York, New York

KENNETH A. BROWN, M.D., F.A.C.C.
Professor of Medicine
Director, Cardiac Stress and Nuclear Cardiology
  Laboratories
University of Vermont College of Medicine
Burlington, Vermont

IGNASI CARRIÓ, M.D., PH.D.
Professor of Nuclear Medicine
Autonomous University of Barcelona
Director, Department of Nuclear Medicine
Hospital Sant Pau
Barcelona, Spain

JAMES A. CASE, PH.D.
Director, Physics and Reserach
Cardiovascular Imaging Technologies
Kansas City, Missouri

MANUEL D. CERQUEIRA, M.D.
Professor of Medicine and Radiology
Director of Nuclear Cardiology
Georgetown University Hospital
Associate Chief of Cardiology
Georgetown University Hospital
Washington, D.C.

S. JAMES CULLOM, PH.D.
Director, Research and Development
Cardiovascular Imaging Technologies
Kansas City, Missouri

MICHAEL W. DAE, M.D., MBA
Professor of Radiology and Medicine
University of California at San Francisco
San Francisco, California

E. GORDON DePUEY, M.D.
Director of Nuclear Medicine
Department of Radiology, St. Luke's—Roosevelt Hospital
Professor of Radiology
Columbia University College of Physicians and Surgeons
New York, New York

ALBERT FLOTATS, M.D.
Associate Professor of Nuclear Medicine
Autonomous University of Barcelona
Nuclear Medicine Department
Hospital Sant Pau
Barcelona, Spain

GAVIN I.W. GALASKO, M.D.
Department of Cardiology
Northwick Park Hospital
Harrow, Middlesex
United Kingdom

GUIDO GERMANO, PH.D.
Director, Nuclear Medicine Physics
Cedars-Sinai Medical Center
Professor of Radiological Sciences
UCLA School of Medicine
Los Angeles, California

AMI E. ISKANDRIAN, M.D., F.A.C.C., F.A.H.A.
Distinguished Professor of Medicine and Radiology
Director, Nuclear Cardiology
University of Alabama at Birmingham
Birmingham, Alabama

LYNNE L. JOHNSON, M.D.
Director, Nuclear Cardiology
Professor of Medicine
Brown University
Providence, Rhode Island

AVIJIT LAHIRI, M.B.B.S.
Department of Cardiology
Northwick Park Hospital
United Kingdom

JEFFREY LEPPO, M.D.
Professor of Medicine and Radiology
Interim Chairman, Department of Radiology
University of Massachusetts Medical Center
Worcester, Massachusetts

ROBERTO MAASS-MORENO, PH.D.
Physicist, Department of Nuclear Medicine
National Institutes of Health
Bethesda, Maryland

JOHN J. MAHMARIAN, M.D.
Associate Professor of Medicine
Baylor College of Medicine
Medical Director, Nuclear Cardiology
The Methodist Hospital
Houston, Texas

PAUL H. MURPHY, PH.D.
Professor, Department of Radiology
Baylor College of Medicine
St. Luke's Episcopal Hospital
Houston, Texas

JAGAT NARULA, M.D., PH.D.
Thomas J. Vischer Professor of Medicine
Vice-Chairman (Research), Department of Medicine
Director, Heart Failure—Transplant Center
Hahnemann University School of Medicine
Philadelphia, Pennsylvania

ADRIAN D. NUNN, PH.D.
International Area Head Discovery Biology
Bracco Research USA, Inc.
Princeton, New Jersey

HEINRICH R. SCHELBERT, M.D., PH.D.
Professor of Pharmacology and Radiological Sciences
Department of Molecular and Medical Pharmacology
UCLA School of Medicine
Los Angeles, California

COLIN SHAFER M.D.
Fellow in Cardiology
Tufts-New England Medical Center
Clinical Instructor in Medicine
Tufts University School of Medicine
Boston, Massachusetts

LESLEE J. SHAW, PH.D.
Director, Outcomes Research
Atlanta Cardiovascular Research Institute
Atlanta, Georgia

ALBERT J. SINUSAS, M.D.
Associate Professor of Medicine and Diagnostic Radiology
Yale University School of Medicine
Director, Animal Research Laboratories
Section of Cardiovascular Medicine
Associate Director, Cardiovascular Nuclear Imaging
  and Stress Laboratory
Yale New Haven Hospital
New Haven, Connecticut

PHYLLIS G. SUPINO, ED.D.
Research Associate Professor of Public Health
Medical Division of Cardiovascular Pathophysiology
Weill Medical College of Cornell University
New York, New York

RAYMOND TAILLEFER, M.D., F.R.C.P (C), A.B.N.M.
Director, Department of Nuclear Medicine
Centre Hospitalier de l'Université de Montréal
Professor of Nuclear Medicine
Department of Radiology
Université de Montréal
Montreal, Canada

NAGARA TAMAKI, M.D., PH.D.
Professor and Chairman
Department of Nuclear Medicine
Hokkaido University Graduate School of Medicine
Sapporo, Japan

JAMES E. UDELSON, M.D.
Associate Chief, Division of Cardiology
New England Medical Center Hospitals
Associate Professor of Medicine and Radiology
Tufts University School of Medicine
Boston, Massachusetts

ERNST E. VAN DER WALL, M.D., PH.D.
Professor, Department of Cardiology
Leiden University Medical Center
The Netherlands

DAVID M. VENESY, M.D.
Assistant Professor of Medicine
Tufts University School of Medicine
Associate Director, Cardiovascular Imaging Laboratory
Associate Director, Advanced Heart Failure Center
Lahey Clinic Medical Center
Department of Cardiovascular Medicine
Burlington, Massachusetts

MARIO S. VERANI, M.D., F.A.C.C., F.A.H.A.*
Professor of Medicine
Baylor College of Medicine
Director, Nuclear Cardiology
The Methodist Hospital
Houston, Texas

FRANS J. TH. WACKERS, M.D.
Yale University School of Medicine
Professor of Diagnostic Radiology and Medicine
Cardiovascular Medicine
Nuclear Cardiology Laboratory
New Haven, Connecticut

FATHY F. WAHBA, M.D., PH.D.
Research Fellow
Department of Cardiology
Leiden University Medical Center
The Netherlands

DENNY D. WATSON, PH.D.
Professor of Radiology
Nuclear Cardiology
University of Virginia Health System
Charlottesville, Virginia

KIM A. WILLIAMS, M.D.
Associate Professor of Clinical Medicine and Radiology
University of Chicago School of Medicine
Director of Nuclear Cardiology
Chicago, Illinois

BARRY L. ZARET, M.D.
Robert W. Berliner Professor of Medicine
Chief, Section of Cardiovascular Medicine
Associate Chair for Clinical Affairs
Medical Director, YNH Heart Center
Department of Internal Medicine
Yale University School of Medicine
New Haven, Connecticut

*Deceased.

Nuclear cardiac imaging

1 | A brief historical perspective on nuclear cardiology

BARRY L. ZARET

Nuclear cardiology is generally considered a clinical phenomenon of the past two decades. However, the field has its roots in earlier times. This chapter focuses on these historical roots as they have evolved. Space constraints mandate focusing solely on the highlights. My apologies to the many highly productive investigators and laboratories whose contributions helped the field grow to its current level but who could not be included.

The initial application of radioisotopes to the study of the circulation occurred in the mid-1920s. The famous cardiologic investigator of that era, Hermann Blumgart, in an elegant series of studies employing radon gas dissolved in saline as the radionuclide marker and a modified Wilson cloud chamber as the radiation detector, measured central circulation transit times in man [1]. These studies, which were well ahead of their time, resulted in substantial improvement in the general understanding of cardiovascular function in a variety of disease states. They were early forerunners of the studies of the 1950s and 1960s in which substantial attention was given to hemodynamic characterization in both health and human disease states. Blumgart's laboratory in Boston also served as fertile ground for training the next generation of cardiovascular investigators.

It was not until the 1940s that Myron Prinzmetal built upon this concept for potential clinical use, employing a simple sodium iodide probe to record transit of radiolabeled albumin through the central circulation. Prinzmetal, a practicing cardiologist, made important clinical observations utilizing nonimaging Geiger tubes and scintillation detectors in a procedure termed "radiocardiography" to define cardiac output, pulmonary blood volume, and pulmonary transit time [2].

However, the major impetus for the development of nuclear medicine technology occurred when Hal O. Anger, working in Berkeley, California, developed the first practical widely utilized high-resolution dynamic imaging device, the gamma (Anger) camera [3]. Utilizing this device, early pioneers in the field such as Joseph Kriss demonstrated the ability to visualize cardiac structures from rapid sequential radionuclide images obtained with the gamma camera following injection of a radioactive bolus of technetium-99m (Tc-99m) labeled radioactive tracers [4,5]. From these serial images a number of inferences could be made concerning cardiac pathophysiology and cardiac chamber and great vessel size. Following these qualitative studies, quantitative techniques were developed for assessing left and right ventricular ejection fraction as well as the degree of left:right intracardiac shunting [6,7]. For over a decade, first-pass approaches to ejection fraction were widely utilized. Extensive studies were subsequently performed by many laboratories, particularly at Duke and Yale, establishing efficacy and clinical utility [8–11].

In 1971 the principle of electrocardiographic gating of the stable labeled (equilibrium) blood pool to evaluate cardiac performance was first proposed by Zaret and Strauss [12,13]. This forerunner of current equilibrium radionuclide angiocardiography required separate manual gating of end-systole and end-diastole for subsequent measurement of left ventricular ejection fraction and assessment of regional function. This was a cumbersome and time-consuming procedure. However, once efficacy had been established, it was only a short time before automation of this technique occurred, and, using relatively simple computerized techniques, the entire cardiac cycle could be visualized in an endless loop display with automated calculation of ejection fraction and visualization of the entire ventricle volume curve. For over a decade this technique was the standard for measuring ventricular function noninvasively. In large part, echocardiography now has superseded equilibrium radionuclide angiocardiography in this context. However, for precise measurements of ejection fraction made serially, such as in the situation involving the monitoring of cardiotoxicity in patients receiving cancer chemotherapy, the radionuclide technique still remains the procedure of choice [14].

Newer evolutionary advances in ventricle function assessment involve single-photon emission computed tomography (SPECT) studies of the cardiac blood pool. This allows a more comprehensive assessment of right and left ventricular regional function [15]. At present, with the marked advances in gated SPECT perfusion studies, ventricular function is often evaluated concomitantly with assessment of myocardial perfusion, and this has often obviated the need for separate studies [16].

MYOCARDIAL PERFUSION IMAGING

In the early 1960s, Carr, in a pioneering set of experiments, demonstrated the localization of radioactive potassium and other radioactive potassium analogs, such as cesium and rubidium, in the myocardium of experimental animals [17]. He also demonstrated that under conditions of acute coronary ligation there was a decreased accumulation of these radioactive tracers in the evolving infarct zone. However, it was not until 1973 that the ability to image the site and extent of myocardial ischemia was first demonstrated by combining physiologic stress with static cardiac imaging. In these initial studies, performed directly in humans, Zaret and Strauss and colleagues working at Travis Air Force Base in California established the paradigm of imaging ischemia induced by treadmill exercise stress, utilizing potassium-43 (K-43) as the tracer and the rectilinear scanner as the imaging device [18]. This relatively simple observation formed the clinical and physiologic basis of nuclear cardiology and stress imaging as practiced today. These investigators were able to demonstrate a pattern of relatively decreased perfusion in an ischemic area only under conditions of stress, with homogeneous radioactive tracer uptake under resting conditions. The kinetics of K-43 mandated separate injections for rest and stress studies. The authors were also able to establish direct relationships between perfusion patterns and coronary stenosis as demonstrated by coronary angiography. Following that initial demonstration, subsequent clinical studies demonstrated the utility of this approach, again using K-43 and the rectilinear scanner, in assessing the patency of bypass grafts following cardiac surgery [19] and in assessing the presence of false positive exercise tests [20]. These studies, which set the stage for the rapid development of the field, clearly employed a suboptimal radioactive tracer in the form of K-43. Its high-energy spectrum, which was not a problem for the rectilinear scanner, was a significant problem for the gamma camera. Of note, this same group, in the early 1970s, also demonstrated that with appropriate pinhole collimation and shielding, one could obtain acceptable planar cardiac images utilizing these high-energy, positron-emitting agents, using a conventional gamma camera [21]. This study was a forerunner of current hybrid gamma camera technologies.

Thereafter Lebowitz et al. introduced thallium-201 (Tl-201) for imaging [22]. The ease of using the lower-energy Tl-201 with the gamma camera heralded a major breakthrough in the development of nuclear cardiology as a clinically viable discipline. In 1975 Pohost et al. defined the phenomenon of "redistribution" on thallium imaging [23]. This allowed the use of a single radionuclide injection and sequential imaging to assess transient ischemia or heterogeneity of blood flow that was normalized in a subsequent resting state several hours later. In the mid-1970s, Gould, who had already made important contributions to understanding the pathophysiologic basis of perfusion imaging, developed the concept of detection of heterogeneity of coronary perfusion in the presence of stenosis by utilizing vasodilator pharmacologic stress as opposed to exercise stress [24]. This was first performed utilizing dipyridamole. This advance established the utility of the field of perfusion imaging for individuals incapable of exercising. In the same decade, Wackers et al., in Amsterdam, demonstrated the potential utility of thallium imaging for detecting acute infarction [25]. This study was a forerunner to current imaging approaches to emergency department imaging.

The late 1980s and 1990s saw the development of technetium-99m (Tc-99m) perfusion agents as important new radiopharmaceuticals for identifying ischemia and infarction. The initial two agents were Tc-99m labeled sestamibi and teboroxime [26,27]. While sestamibi has survived and remains a major tracer today, teboroxime currently is not employed. The reason for this resides in the very rapid transit of teboroxime from the myocardium. Consequently, for purposes of imaging ischemia it remains a suboptimal agent. In the mid-1990s, tetrofosmin became available as an alternative to sestamibi for perfusion imaging [28]. The technetium labeled perfusion agents have provided a more optimal situation for tomographic imaging employing SPECT. The more optimal energy and ability to use higher doses have led to substantial improvement in resolution. However, it must be noted that the optimal perfusion imaging agent has not as yet been defined. Such an agent would, while utilizing Tc-99m as the radionuclide, provide better myocardial uptake and kinetic characteristics and not have excessive subdiaphragmatic tracer accumulation.

PROGNOSIS

In the 1970s, as the field was developing, it focused primarily on diagnostic issues. This could be called the "decade of discovery." The subsequent decades have focused increased attention on functional assessment and prognosis in patients with already identified cardiovascular disease. The field entered an important new area that demonstrated in elegant and meticulous detail the prognostic value of nuclear cardiology. In 1983 Gibson and Beller first established the prognostic value of thallium imaging following myocardial infarction [29]. Thereafter numerous studies by major laboratories have defined prognostic value in both and acute chronic coronary artery disease [30]. While the number of investigators involved in this field of research is large, the seminal contributions of Berman and Hachomovitch and their colleagues at Cedars-Sinai [31,32] and Iskandrian and his colleagues in Philadelphia [33,34] are particularly noteworthy. No discipline has demonstrated the same rigorous and comprehensive approach to the assessment of noninvasive risk stratification that has been displayed by nuclear cardiology.

INFARCT IMAGING

In parallel with the development of perfusion imaging, there developed great interest in identifying areas of acute necrosis with radioactive tracers that would be incorporated into the infarct zone. Much as with perfusion imaging, these advances were heralded by earlier experimental work, once again by Carr and colleagues [35]. The first important studies in humans were by Holman et al. who utilized technetium labeled tetracycline to define zones of acute myocardial infarction [36]. This particular radioactive tracer, however, was complex in preparation with significant limitations. Shortly thereafter, Willerson, Parkey, and Bonte in Dallas, Texas, reported the utility of imaging acute myocardial infarction with Tc-99m labeled stannous pyrophosphate [37]. There then developed great interest in defining acute myocardial infarction of both right and left ventricles. However, it became clear that there were time constraints involving how one could utilize this technique in a clinically meaningful sense. For the most part, this

technique has not survived. In the late 1970s, Khaw and Haber demonstrated for the first time that a radiolabeled specific antibody against cardiac myosin could be used to define acute myocardial necrosis and infarction [38]. These studies were designed initially based upon biologic rather than clinical principles. Elegant in vitro and subsequent experimental studies preceded application to humans. Thereafter antimyosin imaging, utilizing indium-111 (In-111) as the radioactive marker, was employed in the study of myocardial infarction, myocarditis, and cardiac transplant rejection [39]. Regrettably, at the present time antimyosin imaging also is no longer utilized.

More recently, technetium labeled annexin-V has been developed for defining varying states of myocyte death, including apoptosis as well as necrosis [40]. This agent has been demonstrated in zones of acute infarction as well as in experimental and clinical situations where apoptosis is an expected pathophysiologic event [41].

VIABILITY

Nuclear cardiology was the first field to focus intensively on the definition and identification of viable but nevertheless dysfunctional myocardium in coronary artery disease. This work proceeded using a variety of radioactive tracers and technologies. In the 1980s, the UCLA group under the leadership of Schelbert utilized the glucose analog fluorine-18 (F-18)-fluorodeoxyglucose (FDG) to identify viable myocardium [42]. Thereafter, numerous investigations demonstrated the phenomenon of increased glucose accumulation in dysfunctional yet viable myocardium. This imaging approach has predominately involved positron emission tomography (PET). However, work with new cameras that allow imaging of positron agents with SPECT and coincidence detectors may substantially broaden this area of investigation in the future. In 1988 Kiat, Berman, and colleagues at Cedars-Sinai Medical Center in Los Angeles suggested that 24 hour delayed thallium imaging also could be used to define viability [43]. Thereafter, the 1990s saw an explosion of studies evaluating thallium imaging for the definition of viable myocardium in states such as hibernation [44]. Both the PET approach with FDG and the SPECT approach with thallium often have been utilized as gold-standards for assessing viable myocardium. However, additional work has demonstrated, based upon quantitative techniques, that the Tc-99m labeled agents, sestamibi and tetrofosmin, also may be employed for defining viable myocardium [45].

INSTRUMENTATION

Many of the current and future advances in perfusion imaging have and will be dependent upon advanced instrumentation. The field has moved dramatically from the ancient rectilinear scanner, through an era of planar imaging, and now into an era of advanced SPECT imaging. The advances in SPECT imaging have involved both instrumentation development and computation. The multiheaded SPECT systems have been a substantial improvement. The recognition that there is substantial degradation in SPECT images due to both attenuation and scatter has led to the development of substantial new correction approaches to address both of these issues [46]. While there is no consensus now as to the best technique for attenuation and scatter correction, it is clear that one will be developed soon.

Whereas the initial techniques involved a visual assessment of images, we have now entered an era of substantial quantification. Programs have been developed at Cedars-Sinai, Emory University, and Yale University that are being employed widely for direct quantification [47–49]. Such quantification forms an important basis for the future of the field. In addition, the combination of perfusion imaging with ECG gating has allowed attainment of the long established goal of definition of perfusion and function from a single study. Finally, the utilization of new instrumentation such as hybrid cameras that can be used for imaging for both single-photon and positron-emitting radionuclides also should lead to major advances for the field [50].

METABOLIC IMAGING

Whereas metabolic imaging has been associated primarily with FDG imaging of viable myocardium, other specific radioactive tracers involving both PET and SPECT have been employed. Particularly in Japan, SPECT imaging utilizing radioiodinated fatty acids has been employed for over a decade [51]. These agents have been used to define viable myocardium and ischemic myocardium. As yet, predominately because of reasons surrounding the widespread availability of iodine-123 (I-123), this set of approaches has not been widely used throughout the world. Nevertheless, fatty acid imaging utilizing both fatty acid analogs that are relatively trapped within the myocardium to allow optimum imaging and other agents whose period of residence within the myocardium is somewhat limited, may find use in the field [52].

PET imaging of metabolism, in addition to FDG, has involved radioactive acetate and free fatty acids. However, FDG appears to be the agent that has and will continue to be used most widely. In addition, its widespread use in the field of oncology imaging will ensure its continued availability.

FUTURE IMAGING AGENTS

Any historical perspective that attempts to define the development of the field should also look to the future of the field. With respect to nuclear cardiology, we are about to embark upon a new era that will be based on paradigms of molecular biology and cell biology, as opposed to the paradigms of physiology and pathophysiology that have dominated the thinking of the field over the past three decades [53]. Use of these new paradigms will lead to the development of a host of new radiopharmaceuticals that can address issues relating to the biology of the myocyte and the biology and pathobiology of the vascular wall.

RECOGNITION AS A SUBSPECIALTY

As nuclear cardiology developed, there was an intense and at time acrimonious interaction between the fields of nuclear medicine and cardiology, both of which claimed paternal primacy. In 1993 the American Society of Nuclear Cardiology (ASNC) was formed and formally incorporated. ASNC provided the field with the stature of a significant professional society and also established its advocacy role for nuclear cardiology on an international basis. Shortly thereafter national and international meetings were established that focused solely on nuclear cardiology. In January 1994 the *Journal of Nuclear Cardiology* (JNC) was first published. Now into its ninth volume, the journal has provided an additional focused vehicle for the dissemination of experimental and clinical nuclear cardiology and has been a further stimulus for development of the field.

REFERENCES

1. Blumgart HL, Weiss S. Studies on the velocity of blood flow. VII. The pulmonary circulation time in normal resting individuals. J Clin Invest 1927; 4:399.
2. Prinzmetal M, Corday E, Sprizler RJ. Radiocardiography and its clinical applications. JAMA 1949;139:617.
3. Anger HO, Van Dyke DC, Gottschalk A, et al. The scintillation camera in diagnosis and research. Nucleonics 1965;23:57.
4. Kriss JP, Yeh SH, Farrer PA, et al. Radioisotope angiocardiography. J Nucl Med 1966;7:367.
5. Kriss JP, Enright LP, Hayden WG, et al. Radioisotopic angiocardiography: wide scope of applicability in diagnosis and evaluation of therapy in diseases of the heart and great vessels. Circulation 1971;43:792.

6. Schelbert HR, Verba JW, Johnson AD, et al. Nontraumatic determination of left ventricular ejection fraction by radionuclide angiocardiography. Circulation 1975; 51:902.

7. Askenazi J, Ahnberg DS, Korngold E, et al. Quantitative radionuclide angiocardiography: detection and quantitation of left to right shunts. Am J Cardiol 1976;37:382.

8. Jones RH, Floyd RD, Austin EH, et al. The role of radionuclide angiocardiography in the preoperative prediction of pain relief and prolonged survival following coronary artery bypass grafting. Ann Surg 1983;187:743.

9. Pryor DD, Harrell FE, Lee KI, et al. Prognostic indicators from radionuclide angiography in medically treated patients with coronary artery disease. Am J Cardiol 1984;53:18.

10. Marshall RC, Berger HJ, Costin JC, et al. Assessment of cardiac performance with quantitative radionuclide angiocardiography: sequential left ventricular ejection fraction, normalized left ventricular ejection rate, and regional wall motion. Circulation 1977;56:820.

11. Reduto LA, Berger HJ, Cohen LS, et al. Sequential radionuclide assessment of left and right ventricular performance following acute transmural myocardial infarction. Ann Intern Med 1978;89:441.

12. Strauss HW, Zaret BL, Hurley PJ, et al. A scintiphotographic method for measuring left ventricular ejection fraction in man without cardiac catheterization. Am J Cardiol 1971;28:575.

13. Zaret BL, Strauss HW, Hurley PJ, et al. A noninvasive scintiphotographic method for detecting regional ventricular dysfunction in man. N Engl J Med 1971;284:1165.

14. Schwartz RG, McKenzie WB, Alexander J, et al. Congestive heart failure and left ventricular dysfunction complicating doxorubicin therapy: a seven year experience using serial radionuclide angiocardiography. Am J Med 1987;82:1109.

15. Corbett JR. Tomographic radionuclide ventriculography: opportunity ignored? J Nucl Cardiol 1994;1:567.

16. Sharir T, Germano G, Kavanagh PB, et al. Incremental prognostic value of post-stress left ventricular ejection fraction and volume by gated myocardial perfusion single photon emission computed tomography. Circulation 1999;100:1035.

17. Carr EA, Walker BJ, Bartlett J. The diagnosis of myocardial infarct by photo scanning after administration of cesium-131. J Clin Invest 1963;42:922.

18. Zaret BL, Strauss HW, Martin MD, et al. Noninvasive regional myocardial perfusion with radioactive potassium: study of patients at rest with exercise and during angina pectoris. N Engl J Med 1973;288:809.

19. Zaret BL, Martin ND, McGowan RL, et al. Rest and exercise potassium-43 myocardial perfusion imaging for the noninvasive evaluation of aortocoronary bypass surgery. Circulation 1974;40:688.

20. Zaret BL, Stenson RE, Martin ND, et al. Potassium-43 myocardial perfusion scanning for the noninvasive evaluation of patients with false-positive exercise tests. Circulation 1973;48:1234.

21. Martin ND, Zaret BL, Strauss HW, et al. Myocardial imaging using 43K and the gamma camera. Radiology 1974;112:446.

22. Lebowitz E, Greene MW, Bradley-Moore P, et al. ^{201}Tl for medical use. J Nucl Med 1973;14:421.

23. Pohost GM, Zirl M, Moore RH, et al. Differentiation of transiently ischemic from infarcted myocardium by serial imaging after a single dose of thallium-201. Circulation 1977;55:294.

24. Gould KL. Noninvasive assessment of coronary stenosis by myocardial perfusion imaging during pharmacological vasodilation. I. Physiologic basis and experimental validation. Am J Cardiol 1987;41:267.

25. Wackers FJ, Sokole EB, Samson G, et al. Value and limitations of thallium-201 scintigraphy in the acute phase of myocardial infarction. N Engl J Med 1976;295:1.

26. Holman BL, Jones AG, Lister-James J, et al. A new Tc-99m-labeled myocardial imaging agent, hexakis(t-Butylisonitrile)-Technetium(I) [Tc-99m TBI]: initial experience in the human. J Nucl Med 1984;25:1350.

27. Seldin DW, Johnson LL, Blood D, et al. Myocardial perfusion imaging with technetium-99m SQ30217: comparison with thallium-201 and coronary anatomy. J Nucl Med 1989;30:312.

28. Zaret BL, Rigo P, Wackers FJ, et al. Myocardial perfusion imaging with 99m-Tc Tetrofosmin: comparison to 201TL imaging and coronary angiography in a phase III multicenter trial. Circulation 1995;91:313.

29. Gibson RS, Watson DD, Craddock GB, et al. Prediction of cardiac events after uncomplicated myocardial infarction: a prospective study comparing predischarge exercise thallium-201 scintigraphy in coronary angiography. Circulation 1983;68:321.

30. Brown KA. Prognostic value of myocardial perfusion imaging: state-of-the-art and new developments. J Nucl Cardiol 1996;3:516.

31. Hachamovitch R, Berman DS, Kiat H, et al. Exercise myocardial perfusion SPECT in patients without known coronary artery disease: incremental prognostic value and use in risk stratification. Circulation 1996;93:905.

32. Berman DS, Hachamovitch RH, Kiat H, et al. Incremental value of prognostic testing in patients with known or suspected ischemic heart disease: a basis for optimal utilization of single-photon emission computed tomography. J Am Coll Cardiol 1993;6:665.

33. Iskandrian AS, Chae SC, Heo J, et al. Independent and incremental prognostic value of exercise single-photon emission computed tomographic (SPECT) thallium imaging in coronary artery disease. J Am Coll Cardiol 1993;22:665.

34. Iskander S, Iskandrian AE. Risk assessment using single-photon emission computed tomographic technetium-99m sestamibi imaging. J Am Coll Cardiol 1998;32:57.

35. Carr EA Jr, Beierwaltes WH, Patno ME, et al . The detection of experimental myocardial infarcts by photoscanning. Am Heart J 1962;64:650.

36. Holman BL, Lesch M, Zweiman FG, et al. Detection and sizing of acute myocardial infarcts with ^{99m}Tc (Sn) tetracycline. N Engl J Med 1974;291:159.

37. Parkey RW, Bonte FJ, Meyer SL, et al. A new method for radionuclide imaging with acute myocardial infarction in humans. Circulation 1974;50:540.

38. Khaw BA, Beller GA, Haber E, et al. Localization of cardiac myosin-specific antibody in myocardial infarction. J Clin Invest 1976;58:439.

39. Carrio I, Berna L, Ballester M, et al. Indium-111 antimyosin scintigraphy to assess myocardial damage in patients with suspected myocarditis and cardiac rejection. J Nucl Med 1988;29:1893.

40. Blankenberg FG, Katsikis PD, Tait JF, et al. In vivo detection and imaging of phosphatidylserine expression during programmed cell death. Proc Natl Acad Sci USA 1998; 95:6349.

41. Hofstra L, Liem IH, Dumont EA, et al. Visualisation of cell death in vivo in patients with acute myocardial infarction. Lancet 2000;356:209.

42. Tillisch J, Brunken R, Marshall R, et al. Reversibility of cardiac wall-motion abnormalities predicted by positron tomography. N Engl J Med 1986;314:884.

43. Kiat HK, Berman DS, Maddahi J, et al. Late reversibility of to-

mographic myocardial thallium-201 defects: an accurate marker of myocardial viability. J Am Coll Cardiol 1998;12:1456.

44. Dilsizian V, Rocco TP, Freedman NMT, et al. Enhanced detection of ischemic but viable myocardium by the reinjection of thallium after stress-redistribution imaging. N Engl J Med 1990;323:141.

45. Udelson JE, Coleman PS, Metherall J, et al. Predicting recovery of severe regional ventricular dysfunction: comparison of resting scintigraphy with 201-Tl and 99m-Tc-sestamibi. Circulation 1994;89:2552.

46. King MA, Tsui BMW, Pan T. Correction of attenuation and scatter for single-photon emission computed tomography. In: *Nuclear Cardiology: State-of-the-Art and Future Directions*, 2nd edition, edited by BL Zaret and GA Beller. St. Louis: Mosby, Inc. 1999, pp. 125–36.

47. Sharir T, Germano G, Waechter PB, et al. A new algorithm for the quantitation of myocardial perfusion SPECT. II. Validation and diagnostic yield. J Nucl Med 2000;41:720.

48. Faber TL, Cooke CD, Folks RD, et al. Left ventricular function and perfusion from gated SPECT perfusion images: an integrated method. J Nucl Med 1999; 40:650.

49. Liu YH, Sinusas AJ, DeMan P, et al. Quantification of SPECT myocardial perfusion images: methodology and validation of the Yale-CQ method. J Nucl Cardiol 1999;6:190.

50. Dilsizian V, Bacharach SL, Khin MM, et al. Fluorine-18-deoxyglucose SPECT and coincidence imaging for myocardial viability: clinical and technologic issues. J Nucl Cardiol 2001;8:75.

51. Nishimura T. Fatty acid analogs. In: *Nuclear Cardiology: State-of-the-Art and Future Directions*, 2nd edition, edited by BL Zaret and GA Beller. St. Louis: Mosby, 1999, pp. 72–87.

52. Tamaki N, Kudoh T, Tadamura E. Fatty acid imaging. In: *Nuclear Cardiology: State-of-the-Art and Future Directions*, 2nd edition, edited by BL Zaret and GA Beller. St. Louis: Mosby, 1999, pp. 573–586.

53. Zaret BL. Call to molecular arms. J Nucl Cardiol 1997; 4:347.

2 | Radiation physics and radiation safety

PAUL H. MURPHY

ATOMIC AND NUCLEAR STRUCTURE

To understand the emission of radiation from atoms, both atomic and nuclear, requires an understanding of atomic and nuclear structure and forces. The simplest description of the atom is that proposed by Bohr (Fig. 2.1). In this atomic model constructed of fundamental particles (Table 2.1), the nucleus, consisting of protons and neutrons, is surrounded by electrons in discrete energy states, each described by a unique set of quantum numbers. The quantum numbers and the allowed values are shown in Table 2.2. The number of electrons is equal to the number of protons for a neutral atom. The electrons are arranged in energy states designated as shells and subshells as illustrated in Table 2.3. The energy states of electrons in atoms are specific, discrete, and defined by a set of four quantum numbers per electron. The atom is most stable when the electrons reside in the lowest energy states. This observation and the Pauli exclusion principle allow a description of the electron state of an atom and thus the structure of the periodic table of the elements. The Pauli exclusion principle states that in a given atom no two electrons can have the same values for the set of quantum numbers and therefore exist in the same energy state. Note that the maximum number of electrons in a shell is $2n^2$ and the outermost shell always has eight or fewer electrons. Examples of electron configurations are illustrated in Table 2.4 and the shorthand designation in Table 2.5. Transitions between energy states in an atom are discrete, corresponding to the difference between the two states. These transitions result in the absorption and emission spectra observed in the visible region of the electromagnetic spectrum for low-energy transitions, as in low atomic number (Z) materials, or outer shell transitions in high Z elements. Inner shell transitions produce the characteristic X-rays observed in higher Z elements (Fig. 2.2).

In general the electrons reside in the lowest energy states, so that as a whole, the atom is in its lowest and therefore most stable energy state. When electrons are raised to higher allowable energy states they spontaneously return to a lower energy state with the emission of energy corresponding to the difference between the higher and lower energy states. Similarly, electrons can be raised to higher energy states by the addition of energy equal in magnitude to that corresponding to the difference between energy states.

When sufficient energy is transferred to an electron to remove it from the atom, a process called *ionization*, the vacancy created in the electron structure will eventually be filled by another electron and the resulting energy difference between the initial and final energies of the electron can be emitted as a photon. For a given element, and therefore a specified atomic number, the energy states are characteristics of that element. Therefore, the absorption and emission energy corresponding to transitions in electron states are characteristic of that element. These energies, referred to as the *binding energies*, are listed for several elements in Table 2.6 [1]. Characteristic X-ray emission is the result of the filling of inner shell vacancies in high atomic elements. For example, the $K_{\alpha 1}$ characteristic X-ray of lead is 72.1 keV. This process is also important in some modes of radioactive decay.

In the Bohr model of the atom the nucleus consists of nucleons, either protons or neutrons, held together by strong nuclear forces that act only over very small distances, that is, the dimensions of the nucleus. The dimension of the nucleus is about 10^{-23} cm and that of the atom about 10^{-8} cm. To completely describe a particular nuclide requires knowledge of the number of protons, thus the element, and the number of neutrons, thus the mass number. The conventional designation is the chemical symbol, which implies the atomic number (Z), and the mass number (A) as superscript. The neutron number (N) is the difference between the mass number and the atomic number, $N = A - Z$. Isotopes are nuclides that have the same number of protons, thus the same element, but different number of neutrons, thus different mass numbers. Isotones are nuclides having the same number of neutrons. Isobars are nuclides having the same mass number but different numbers of protons. We will see that many of the nuclear transformation

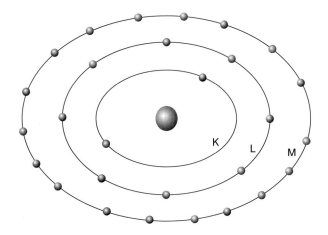

FIGURE 2.1 Schematic diagram of an atom illustrating the nucleus and surrounding electron energy shells.

TABLE 2.1 *Properties of Some Fundamental Particles*

Particle	Symbol	Mass (kg)	m_0c^2 (MeV)	Charge
Electron	e^-, β^-	9.11×10^{-31}	0.511	−1
Positron	e^+, β^+	9.11×10^{-31}	0.511	+1
Proton	p	1.672×10^{-27}	938.3	+1
Neutron	n	1.675×10^{-27}	939.6	0
Neutrino	v	0	0	0
Antineutrino	$\hat{v}$	0	0	0
Gamma ray	γ	0	0	0

TABLE 2.2 *Orbital Electron Quantum Numbers*

Quantum No.	Symbol	Allowed Values
Principle	n	$1,2,3,\ldots$
Orbital	l	$0,1,2,\ldots(n-1)$
Magnetic	m_l	$(-l),(-l+1),\ldots,0,1,2,\ldots,(l-1),l$
Spin	s	$+1/2, -1/2$

TABLE 2.3 *Energy State Designation and Maximum Numbers of Electrons in Shells and Subshells*

Shell	Subshell	Maximum Electrons	$2n^2$
K	s	2	2
L	s	2	
	p	6	8
M	s	2	
	p	6	
	d	10	18
N	s	2	
	p	6	
	d	10	
	f	14	32

TABLE 2.4 *Examples of Electron Configurations*

		K	L		M			N
Element	Z	1s	2s	2p	3s	3p	3d	4s
Carbon	6	2	2	2				
Oxygen	8	2	2	4				
Phosphorus	15	2	2	6	2	3		
Potassium	19	2	2	6	2	6		1
Chromium	24	2	2	6	2	6	5	1

TABLE 2.5 *Shorthand Notations for Electron Configurations*

Element		Electron Configuration
Carbon	6	$1s^2 2s^2 2p^2$
Oxygen	8	$1s^2 2s^2 2p^4$
Phosphorus	15	$1s^2 2s^2 2p^6 3s^2 3p^3$
Potassium	19	$1s^2 2s^2 2p^6 3s^2 3p^6 4s^1$
Chromium	24	$1s^2 2s^2 2p^6 3s^2 3p^6 3d^5 4s^1$

modes of interest in gamma ray imaging are isobaric transitions. Isomers are nuclides having the same number of protons and the same number of neutrons, but different nuclear energy states. To designate an excited energy state of a nucleus that has a measurable lifetime, a meta-stable state, a lower case m is appended to the mass number, for example Tc-99m. An isomeric transition is one type of gamma ray emission (Table 2.7).

Several models to explain nuclear forces have been proposed, often relying upon a sharing of fundamental particles, such as mesons, resulting in strong attractive forces between pairs of nucleons. This is analogous to the sharing of electrons between atoms to form molecules. Pairing of nucleons, implying stability, is observed in the 249 known stable nuclear configurations [2]. Of these known stable nuclear configurations only four have an odd number of protons and an odd number of neutrons. These are H = 2, Li = 6, B = 10, and N = 14, the four smallest, odd Z, elements. All others either have even numbers of both protons and neutrons, or even numbers of neutrons, or even numbers of protons. In addition to this pairing observation for nucleus stability, another descriptive characteristic is the relationship between the number of neutrons and protons that yield stable configurations. For the lower atomic numbered stable nuclei the proton to neutron ratio is approximately one. For the more massive, high atomic number, stable nuclei this ratio approaches 1.5. A plot of this relationship, shown in Figure 2.3, is referred to as the *line of stability*. The 249 data points define a narrow range for the neutron to proton ratio over the range of elements observed in nature. Any other nuclear configuration will be unstable, meaning it will undergo transformation by the process of radioactive decay to eventually arrive at a stable nu-

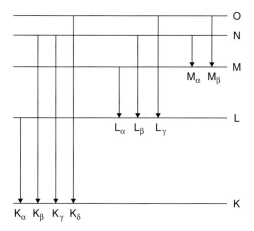

FIGURE 2.2 Characteristic X-rays are produced by electron transitions in high atomic number elements. For example, a K_α X-ray results from an electron transition from the L shell to the K shell.

TABLE 2.6 *Electron Binding Energies (keV)*

Atomic No.	Element	K Shell	L Shell s Subshell	L Shell p Subshell	L Shell d Subshell
6	Carbon	0.3			
8	Oxygen	0.5			
53	Iodine	33.2	5.2	4.9	4.6
74	Tungsten	69.5	12.1	11.5	10.2
82	Lead	88.0	15.9	15.2	13.0
92	Uranium	115.6	21.8	20.9	17.2

clear configuration. If a nucleus has a higher neutron to proton ratio than its neighboring stable nuclei, it will undergo a nuclear transformation so that the neutron to proton ratio will decrease. This will generally be in the form of beta (β^-) decay. Conversely, if the unstable nucleus has a neutron to proton ratio that is lower than its neighboring stable nuclei, then the mode of radioactive decay will result in an increase in the neutron to proton distribution, which can occur by means of either positron (β^+) emission or electron capture (EC). Thus, it is often possible to predict the mechanisms of radioactive decay for a given unstable nucleus by comparing the neutron to proton distribution to that of the stable isotopes. There can be more than one stable isotope of an element. Elements with "magic numbers" (2,8,20,50,82,126) of protons or neutrons tend to have multiple stable configurations. For example, calcium, with $Z = 20$, has 5 stable isotopes and tin, with $Z = 50$, has 10 stable isotopes.

RADIOACTIVITY

Modes of Radioactive Decay

If the nucleus is unstable it is radioactive. Unstable nuclei rearrange through one of several mechanisms to arrive at a stable configuration, that is, lowest energy state. The rearrangement processes are referred to as the *modes of radioactive decay*. These include alpha decay (α), beta (β^-) particle emission, positron (β^+) emission, electron capture (EC), gamma (γ) ray emission or isomeric transmission (IT), and internal conversion (IC). During these processes there could also be emission of characteristic X-rays from the electron orbits surrounding the nucleus and emission of discrete energy orbital electrons, either internal conversion electrons or Auger electrons. By all of these mechanisms energy is released and the nucleus and entire atom end up in a lower total energy state.

An alpha particle is the nucleus of a He-4 atom. It consists of two neutrons and two protons. Alpha decay usually occurs only for high atomic number nuclei. They are emitted in one or more discrete energies and the resulting daughter nucleus has an atomic number two less than the parent and a mass number four less.

$$^A X_Z \rightarrow {}^{A-4} Y_{Z-2} + \alpha + Q$$

Q is the disintegration energy and includes the alpha particle energy, any recoil energy of the nucleus, and any gamma ray energy.

Because an alpha particle is such a massive, doubly charged, ionizing particle, its range in solid material is small, typically microns. This high ionization density results in large amounts of energy deposited in a small volume around the atom. The high radiation dose from alpha emitters precludes their use in diagnostic radiopharmaceuticals although there is increasing interest in their use in radiation therapy.

The following modes of radioactive decay are more

TABLE 2.7 *Nuclide Notations*

Name	Definition	Examples
Isotopes	Same Z, different N	O-15, O-16, O-17, O-18
Isotones	Same N, different Z	B-12, C-13, N-14, O-15
Isobars	Same A, different Z	Fe-59, Co-59, Ni-59, Cu-59
Isomers	Same Z, same N, different energy	Kr-81m-Kr-81, Sr-87m-Sr-87, Tc-99m-Tc-99, In-113m-In-113

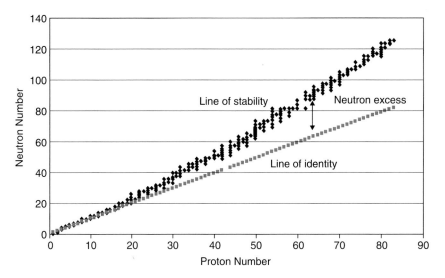

FIGURE 2.3 The relationship between the number of neutrons and protons for the stable nuclear configurations.

commonly encountered in radionuclides used for diagnostic imaging. Beta decay, the emission of a high-energy electron and an antineutrino from a nucleus, results in the transformation of the parent element to a different element having an atomic number one larger than that of the parent (Fig. 2.4). The mass number of the parent and daughter nuclei remains unchanged.

$$^{A}X_{Z} \rightarrow {}^{A}Y_{Z+1} + \beta^{-} + \acute{\nu} + Q$$

The transformation is equivalent to the conversion, within the nucleus, of a neutron to a proton plus the electron and an antineutrino, with the emission from the nucleus of the electron and the antineutrino. The

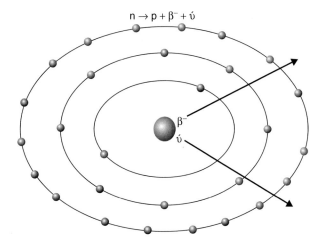

FIGURE 2.4 In beta decay, the beta particle and an antineutrino are emitted from the nucleus.

effect on the neutron to proton ratio is the loss of one neutron and the gain of one proton, resulting in a decrease in the ratio from parent to daughter. Thus one would predict that unstable nuclei with excess neutrons would decay by beta emission. The neutrino and antineutrino are chargeless, essentially massless particles traveling at a velocity approaching the speed of light (see Table 2.1). Their existence was predicted many years before experimental verification in order to explain the continuum of beta particle energies that was observed from beta emitting radionuclides. The sum of the energy of the beta particle and the antineutrino is a constant for a given beta transition and is characteristic of the nuclear transformation. This energy is shared by the beta particle and the antineutrino so the beta particle can have an energy ranging from zero up to that maximum.

A positron is a positive electron, the antiparticle to an electron. Positron decay is equivalent to the transformation within the nucleus of a proton to a neutron plus a positron and a neutrino. The positron and the neutrino are ejected from the nucleus (Fig. 2.5).

$$^{A}X_{Z} \rightarrow {}^{A}Y_{Z-1} + \beta^{+} + \nu + Q$$

The result of this transformation is an increase in the neutron to proton ratio from the parent to the daughter. Thus one would predict that unstable nuclei with neutron deficits might decay by positron emission. Being an antiparticle to an electron, the positron, after losing most of its kinetic energy, will encounter an electron, combine, and annihilate. To satisfy the principle of conservation of energy the two electron masses upon

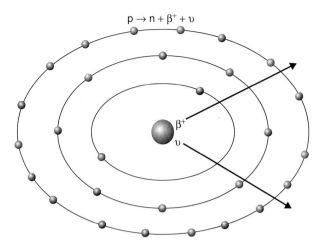

FIGURE 2.5 In positron decay the positron and a neutrino are emitted from the nucleus.

annihilation are converted into photons with total energy of 1.022 MeV, 0.511 MeV for each particle. From $E = mc^2$, the energy equivalence of an electron mass of 9.11×10^{-31} kg is 0.511 MeV (see Table 2.1). These two 0.511 MeV photons are emitted at approximately 180° to each other to satisfy conservation of linear momentum, that is, the net linear momentum of the two particles before the annihilation equals the net linear momentum of the two photons after the annihilation. The simultaneous emission and fixed spatial orientation and energy of these two photons are the basis of positron emission tomography (PET) imaging.

Electron capture is another mechanism whereby the nucleus can undergo a transformation that results in a higher neutron to proton ratio. An orbital electron, typically a K shell electron, combines with a proton in the nucleus to produce a neutron and a neutrino. The neutrino is ejected from the nucleus (Fig. 2.6). The resulting daughter nucleus has an atomic number one less than the parent nucleus.

$$^{A}X_Z + e^- \rightarrow \,^{A}Y_{Z-1} + v + Q$$

Because a neutrino is virtually undetectable, if there are no other energy transitions, the electron capture would be undetectable. However, the capture of the electron results in a vacancy in typically the K shell of the atom, which is now the daughter element, Y, and therefore there is the potential for the emission of a characteristic X-ray. Characteristic X-ray emission following orbital electron capture can be a major photon contributor from some medically useful radionuclides. Tl-201 is an example of a radionuclide in which the most abundant photon emissions are the characteristic X-rays of

the daughter Hg-201 following the capture of an orbital electron by the Tl-201 nucleus.

Following any of the modes of nuclear transformation described above, the nucleus may still have excess energy over that of the stable configuration. Under these circumstances a photon, a gamma ray, may be emitted, carrying away some or all of this excess energy. These gamma ray emissions are either instantaneous at the time of the nuclear transformation or delayed. If delayed, such that there is a measurable lifetime to the exited energy state, the emission is called an *isomeric transition*. These excited or metastable energy states are designated with an m following the mass number, as in Tc-99m (see Table 2.7).

An alternative to the emission of the gamma ray from the nucleus is a transfer of the gamma ray energy directly to an orbital electron of that atom, with the ejection of the electron from the atom. The gamma ray energy must exceed the binding energy of the electron for this to occur. The most probable electron is one from the shell that has a binding energy closest to, but less than, the gamma ray energy. This process, called *internal conversion*, results in a discrete energy electron and a vacancy in an electron shell of the atom. Subsequent electron filling of the vacant shell can result in either a characteristic X-ray or an Auger electron.

Auger electron emission is an alternative to characteristic X-ray emission and the process is analogous to internal conversion electron emission instead of the gamma ray. Auger electrons originate from a lower energy state than that of the original electron shell vacancy, with the emission producing another electron shell vacancy. This process can occur several times in

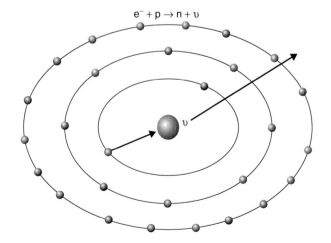

FIGURE 2.6 In electron capture an orbital electron combines with a nuclear proton to produce a neutron and a neutrino. The neutrino is emitted from the nucleus and the daughter atom has an electron vacancy in one of the inner shells.

a single atom, resulting in the emission of a number of ionizing electrons. This cascading effect of Auger electrons can produce relatively high energy deposition within very small volumes and is of some interest in the development of therapeutic radiopharmaceuticals.

The probability that a gamma ray will be internally converted is designated by the internal conversion coefficient, α. It is defined as the number of internal conversion electrons emitted divided by the number of gamma rays emitted. It is typically designated for each of the electronic shells and therefore the individual shell internal conversion coefficients add to give the total conversion coefficient.

$$\alpha = (\text{\# IC e's})/(\text{\# gammas})$$

$$\alpha = \alpha_k + \alpha_l + \alpha_m + \ldots$$

The probability that a characteristic X-ray will be emitted when a vacancy occurs in an electronic shell is described by the fluorescent yield. It is a probability that ranges from 0 to 1.0. The Auger electron yield is 1 minus the fluorescent yield. These parameters are important in describing and developing diagnostic and therapeutic radiopharmaceuticals, since they impact directly on patient radiation absorbed dose.

An energy level diagram, also referred to as a decay scheme, can illustrate the possible mechanisms by which a radionuclide may undergo transformation. In these schematic presentations, nuclear energy levels are represented as horizontal lines and energy transitions by arrows originating at one energy level and terminating at another, lower level. The horizontal axis represents the atomic number, so that a transformation resulting in an increase in the atomic number from parent to daughter nuclide, such as β^- decay, is diagramed by an arrow pointing downward to the right. A decrease in atomic number, such as β^+ or EC, is diagramed as an arrow pointing downward to the left. A vertical ar-

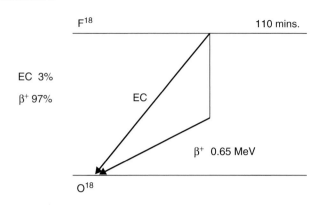

FIGURE 2.8 Decay scheme for F-18.

row represents no change in atomic number, such as gamma emission. The parent radionuclide with half-life is represented by the top horizontal line and the daughter by the bottom line.

In the most simple decay scheme, only one energy transition is allowed, as illustrated by the β^- emission from P-32 (Fig. 2.7). More often there are multiple possible transitions of defined frequency, subsequently followed by gamma emission (Figs. 2.8–2.10) [3].

The decay schemes illustrate the allowed transitions, but generally do not indicate information on any internal conversion of the gamma emissions or emission of X-rays or Auger electrons. A table of all transitions and emissions usually accompanies the decay scheme to provide additional information on IC electrons, Auger electrons, and characteristic X-rays.

Math of Radioactive Decay

Radioactive decay is a spontaneous, random process, meaning that the probability that a nucleus will undergo decay over a specified time period can be pre-

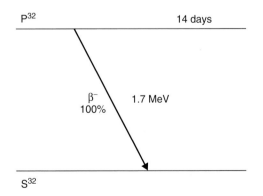

FIGURE 2.7 Decay scheme for P-32.

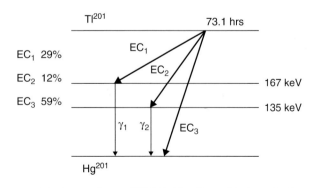

FIGURE 2.9 Decay scheme of Tl-201. Not discernible from the decay scheme is an abundance of Hg-201 X-rays from vacancies created by the electron capture and internal conversion of the gamma rays.

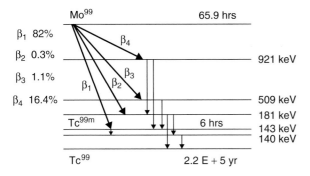

FIGURE 2.10 The decay of Mo-99 results in an isomeric state of Tc-99, enabling the Tc-99m generator.

dicted or the fraction of a number of unstable nuclei that will undergo decay per unit time can be defined, but not the exact time of any individual transformation. The number of nuclei undergoing transformation per unit time, dN/dt, is directly proportional to the total number of nuclei present, N. The constant relationship between the disintegration rate and the number of atoms present is expressed by the decay constant, λ, which is characteristic of the radionuclide.

$$dN/dt = -\lambda N$$

The decay constant is the probability per unit time that a given nucleus will undergo decay, or equivalently, the fraction of the nuclei present that will undergo decay per unit time. The number undergoing decay per unit time, the number of transformations per second, is defined as the activity. The International Standard Unit for activity is the becquerel (Bq.). One becquerel is one disintegration per second. The traditional unit is the curie, which is equal to 3.7×10^{10} disintegrations per second. This relationship between the activity and the decay constant and the number of atoms present is referred to as the differential form of the decay equation. It can be expressed in the integral form,

$$N(t) = N_0 e^{-\lambda t}$$

and because activity, A, equals λN, it can also be expressed as

$$A(t) = A_0 e^{-\lambda t}$$

$N(t)$ = the number of atoms at time = t

N_0 = the number of atoms at time = 0

$A(t)$ = the activity at time = t

A_0 = the activity at time = 0

The exponential relationship indicates that the activity will change by the same fraction for equal time intervals. It is convenient to express the fractional change of 1/2 and therefore the associated time interval is referred to as the half-life, $T_{1/2}$. Substituting in the above equation

$$A = A_0/2 \text{ when } t = T_{1/2}$$

$$T_{1/2} = (\ln 2)/\lambda = 0.693/\lambda$$

where ln2 is the Naperian or natural logarithm of 2.

Another useful measure of the change in activity of a radioactive material is the mean life, or average life, T_{aver}. It is equal to the reciprocal of the decay constant,

$$T_{aver} = 1/\lambda$$

When a radiopharmaceutical is administered to a patient, the decrease in activity with time is a combination of radioactive decay and biological elimination. If the biological removal is exponential, that is, a constant fraction per unit time, then the total removal fraction per unit time is the sum of the individual rate constants,

$$\lambda_T = \lambda p + \lambda_b$$

where

λ_T is the total removal rate,

λp is the physical removal rate (the decay constant), and

λ_b is the biological removal rate.

The effective half-life (T_{eff}) reflects both mechanisms of removal and is obtained from the relationship between the half-life and decay constant.

$$T_{eff} = (T_p \times T_b)/(T_p + T_b)$$

where

T_p is the physical half-life, and

T_b is the biological half-life.

Half-lives and photon emission energies of the principal radionuclides encountered in a nuclear cardiology laboratory are shown in Table 2.8 [4,5].

Examples of the application of the decay equations are shown in Tables 2.9 and 2.10.

Not all nuclear transformations result in stable daughter nuclides. If the daughter is also radioactive it

TABLE 2.8 *Characteristics of Radionuclides Used in Gamma Ray Imaging*

Nuclide	Half-life	Photon Energies (keV)	Γ^*_{20} (R/(hr-mc)@1 cm)	HVL (mm Pb)	HVL (cm tissue)
F-18	110 min	511	5.7	3.9	7.0
Co-57	271 days	123	0.56	0.2	4.0
Tc-99m	6 hr	140	0.59	0.3	4.5
Cs-137	30 yr	662	3.26	6.5	7.5
Tl-201	73.1 hr	68-80, 135, 167	0.45	0.2	3.5

*For photons greater than 20 keV.
Γ, specific gamma constant; HVL, half value layer.

will undergo decay to a subsequent decay product, which may also be radioactive. If the daughter in a radioactive series has a half-life less than that of the parent, an equilibrium relationship between the activities of the two will become established after a period of time. Under the circumstances where the parent's half-life is much longer than that of the radioactive daughter, after a buildup period of several half-lives of the daughter, there will be a constant relationship between the activity of the parent and that of the daughter in a closed system. This is the basis for radionuclide generators. The Mo-99 to Tc-99m transformation is the basis for the most widely used radionuclide generator in diagnostic imaging. The extraction of the inert gas Rn-222, a 3.8 day half-life daughter of Ra-226 ($T_{1/2}$ = 1620 years), was the first medical applications of radionuclide generators soon after the discovery of radioactivity by Becquerel in 1896.

PRODUCTION OF RADIONUCLIDES

The earth and its atmosphere contain many naturally occurring radioactive elements. In addition to several radioactive decay series originating from parent radionuclides that have half-lives of billions of years, there is constant production of radioactive materials in the earth's atmosphere from the interaction of cosmic rays with the elements of the atmosphere. In particular these interactions produce large quantities of C-14 and H-3. Another notable long life, naturally occurring radionuclide is K-40. This radioisotope of potassium is incorporated in living organisms in proportion to the total potassium of the organism. In humans it is the major contributor to radiation dose from naturally occurring, internally deposited, radioactive materials. Most radionuclides used in medicine are not naturally occurring but are created, produced by intentional transformations of a stable nuclide to an unstable configuration usually employing nuclear reactors or charge particle accelerators.

A nuclear reactor is a device in which a controlled chain reaction of a fissionable fuel material, such as U-235, is initiated and maintained. The fission of an atom of U-235 results in the breakup of the nucleus into two fission products (FP) and several high-energy neutrons.

$$U\text{-}235 + n^1 \rightarrow U\text{-}236 \rightarrow FP_1 + FP_2 + neutrons + gammas$$

Maintaining a chain reaction with U-235 requires slowing down these neutrons and ensuring that at least one initiates another fission of a U-235 nucleus. The rate

TABLE 2.9 *Examples of Radioactive Decay Calculations*

A 200 mCi vial of Tc-99m in 5 ml was received at 8:00 AM, calibrated for 10:00 AM. What was the concentration at 8:00 AM? At 3:00 PM that afternoon?

At 8:00 AM
2 hr/6 hr = 0.333 $T_{1/2}$
$(0.5)^{0.333} = 0.794$
(40 mCi/ml)/0.794 = 50.4 mCi/ml

At 3:00 PM
5 hr/6 hr = 0.8333 $T_{1/2}$
$(0.5)^{0.8333} = 0.561$
(40 mCi/ml)(0.561) = 22.4 mCi/ml

TABLE 2.10 *Radioactive Decay Calculation*

If a 100 mCi source of Tc-99m is stored for complete decay of the Tc-99m, what is the resulting Tc-99 activity? Must the Tc-99 be treated as radioactive waste?

$A = \lambda N$
For Tc-99m, $A = 3.7 \times 10^9$ dps
$N = (3.7 \times 10^9 \text{ dps})/\lambda_{99m}$

For Tc-99, $A = \lambda_{99}N$
$A = (\lambda_{99}/\lambda_{99m})(3.7 \times 10^9 \text{ dps})$
Since $(\lambda_{99}/\lambda_{99m}) = T_{99m}/T_{99}$
$A = (6 \text{ hr})(3.7 \times 10^9 \text{dps})/\{(2.1 \times 10^5 \text{yr})(365 \text{ days/yr})(24 \text{ hr/day})\}$
$A = 12.1 \text{ dps} = 0.33 \text{ nanoCi}$

This level of activity would not be distinguishable from background and could be treated as nonradioactive waste.

of fission determines the rate of energy released and thus the power level of the reactor. The power can be adjusted by competing for the fission neutrons with a material that absorbs neutrons but does not fission. This is the function of the control rods in the reactor. Control rods commonly contain cadmium, which has a high probability of interaction, high cross section, for thermal neutrons. The fission products are usually radioactive and at the time of the fission high-energy gamma rays are commonly emitted. Thus the environment around the reactor core has very high radiation levels and requires massive protective shielding. The majority of the energy released in fission results in heating of the coolant, which is typically water or heavy water. In a reactor designed to produce electricity from this heat, the reactor vessel is usually sealed and pressurized to produce the steam to drive turbines. In experimental reactors the vessel is often open and contains a large volume of water as the coolant, the neutron moderator, and as a radiation shield. There are also other reactor fuels besides uranium enriched in U-235 that rely upon high-energy neutrons for fission.

In a reactor, a radionuclide with a higher than stable neutron to proton ratio can be produced by either neutron bombardment of a stable target nucleus to add a neutron or by splitting a large nucleus into two smaller unstable nuclei. The resultant radionuclides, with neutron excesses are most likely to decay by beta emission. An example of a neutron capture reaction is the production of Mo-99 by the neutron irradiation of Mo-98 with the emission of the gamma ray at the time of the capture of the neutron. This gamma ray is referred to as a prompt gamma, and is not from the subsequent radioactive decay of the Mo-99.

$$Mo\text{-}98 + n \rightarrow Mo\text{-}99 + \gamma$$

Nuclear reactions are often abbreviated with the target material to the left, the product to the right, and the incident particle and output particle in parentheses.

$$Mo\text{-}98 \ (n,\gamma) \ Mo\text{-}99$$

Another mechanism to produce Mo-99 is by fission of U-235. The fission products resulting from the U-235 breaking into two smaller nuclides are not uniformly distributed over the atom mass scale but have a bipolar distribution resulting in relatively high yields for mass numbers around 100 and 130. Thus Mo-99 can be produced with fairly high yield from the fission of U-235. This "fission product" Mo-99 has a much higher specific activity, activity/gm, than that produced by neutron irradiation of stable Mo-98. The higher spe-

TABLE 2.11 *Reactor-Produced Radionuclides*

Radionuclide	Half-life	Reaction
P-32	14.3 days	S-32 (n,p) P-32
Co-60	5.2 yr	Co-59 (n,γ) Co-60
Mo-99	66 hr	U-235 (n, fission) Mo-99
		Mo-98 (n,γ) Mo-99
I-125	60 days	Xe-124 (n,γ) Xe-125,
		Xe-125 → I-125
I-131	8.1 days	Te-130 (n,γ) Te-131,
		Te-131 → I-131
		U-235 (n, fission) I-131
Cs-137	30.0 yr	U-235 (n, fission) Cs-137

cific activity produces higher Tc-99m concentrations when used in Mo-99-Tc-99m generators. Other examples of reactor-produced radionuclides are shown in Table 2.11 [1,4].

A cyclotron is a device used to accelerate charged particles to very high energies for the purpose of bombarding a target to produce a nuclear transformation in the target element. Most often the bombarding particle is a proton or a deuteron and early cyclotrons were designed to accelerate positive charged particles. Modern cyclotrons still bombard the targets with positive charged particles but attach excess electrons to the particles to render them negative ions during the acceleration phase. Just prior to striking the target the electrons are stripped off to yield the high-energy positive charged particle. In either case the operation principles are the same. An ion source is at the center of an evacuated chamber that contains two hollow conductive shells, called *dees*, separated by a gap across which an electric field is applied. The chamber is between the poles of a high field strength magnet. The charged particle acquires an incremental increase in kinetic energy when accelerated by the electric field between the two dees. Upon entering one of these hollow conductive dees, the particle no longer experiences the effects of the electric field, but is affected by the magnetic field, which causes it to move in a circular path within the dee. As it emerges from the dee, the polarity of the electric field has been switched so the particle again receives an incremental boost in kinetic energy as it crosses the gap between the two dees. Once inside the second dee it moves in a circular path of larger radius than previously because of the higher energy. This process of incremental boosts in energy at each gap crossing repeats until the particle is at desired energy to be projected into the target. The resulting radionuclide usually has a low neutron to proton ratio and therefore accelerator-produced radionuclides typically decay by either positron emission or electron capture. Tl-201 and F-18 are two accelerator-produced ra-

TABLE 2.12 *Accelerator-Produced Radionuclides*

Radionuclide	Half-life	Reaction
O-15	2 min	N-14 (d,n) O-15
		N-15 (p,n) O-15
F-18	110 min	O-18 (p,n) F-18
Co-57	271 days	Fe-56 (d,n) Co-57
Ga-67	78.2 hr	Zn-68 (p,2n) Ga-67
I-123	13.2 hr	Sb-121 (α,2n) I-123
Tl-201	73 hr	Tl-203 (p,3n) Pb-201,
		Pb-201 $\rightarrow$ Tl-201

dionuclides that are important in cardiac imaging. These and other accelerator-produced radionuclides important for gamma ray imaging are shown in Table 2.12 [1,4]. Other types of particle accelerators besides cyclotrons can be used for radionuclide production, but the cyclotron is the most common.

INTERACTION OF RADIATION WITH MATTER

Ionization is the process of separating an electron from an atom thereby producing an ion pair, a free electron and a positive charged atom. Ionizing radiations are those with sufficient energy to produce ion pairs. Directly ionizing radiations are charged particles. Indirectly ionizing radiations include photons and uncharged particles such as neutrons. The interaction of indirectly ionizing radiation results in energetic charged particles, and subsequent interactions of these charged particles transfer energy to the surrounding medium.

Charged Particle Interactions

Because indirectly ionizing X-ray and gamma rays results in the production of high-energy electrons, a discussion of these interactions with matter reverts back to one of interaction of charged particles with matter after the initial photon interaction. Charged particles transfer energy to matter by one of three processes: excitation, ionization, Bremsstrahlung.

Excitation is the transfer of sufficient energy from a charged particle to an orbital electron of an atom to raise it to a higher, or an excited, energy state of that atom. The electron is still attached to the atom but in a higher energy state and therefore energy has been transferred from the incoming charged particle to the atom of the medium through which the particle is passing. The excited atom will eventually return to the lower energy, ground, state with the transferred energy ultimately dissipated in the form of heat.

Ionization is the process whereby the incoming charged particle transfers sufficient energy to an orbital electron to completely remove it from the atom. This requires an energy transfer greater than the binding energy of the orbital election (see Table 2.6). The result is an ion pair, a positive charged atom and a free electron. The electron may have sufficient energy to be a secondary ionizing particle. In a gas such as the air used in ionization chambers, the expenditure of approximately 34 electron volts of energy is required to produce a single ion pair. This is the amount of energy on the average expended by an incoming charge particle through the processes of both excitation and ionization to produces a single ion pair. The accurate determination of this quantity is necessary to specify the exposure rate and subsequently to calculate the dose rate from an ionization measurement from an X-ray or gamma ray source.

Another mechanism by which high-energy charged particles can lose energy to the surroundings is in the emission of photons caused by a change in acceleration of the charged particle in the vicinity of a nucleus. The deceleration of charged particles by the strong electrostatic force between the positive charged nucleus and the negative charged electron can result in the emission of photons with a continuum of energies. This mechanism is the basis for the production of the majority of the X-ray photons emitted from typical diagnostic X-ray tubes. This radiative process, named *Bremsstrahlung*, meaning breaking radiation, becomes more probable as the energy of the charged particle increases and as the atomic number of the medium increases. For example, the percentage energy loss by Bremsstrahlung of 1 MeV beta particles in tissue is negligible, whereas in lead it is about 1%–2%.

Photon Interactions

X-rays and gamma rays transfer energy to matter by several processes, the most important being photoelectric absorption, Compton scattering, and pair production. In a photoelectric interaction a high-energy photon transfers all of the energy to a tightly bound orbital electron, most probable with an electron of a high atomic numbered element (Fig. 2.11*a*). The energy of the photon, hν, where h is Planck's constant and ν is the photon frequency, must exceed the binding energy of the electron for the transfer to occur. The electron is ejected from the atom with kinetic energy equal to the initial gamma ray energy minus the binding energy for that electron (Fig. 2.11*b*).

$$KE_e = h\nu - BE$$

The photon no longer exists and in its place is a high-energy electron and a vacancy in one of the shells of

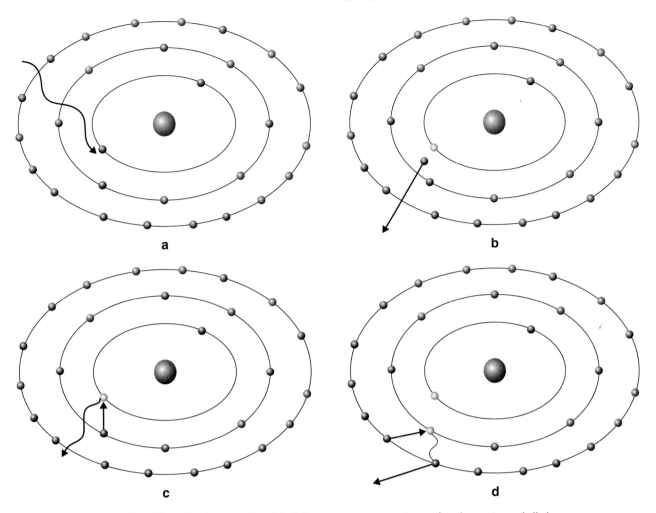

FIGURE 2.11 Photoelectric interaction. (*a*) all the gamma ray energy is transferred to an inner shell electron; (*b*) this photoelectron is ejected from the atom leaving a vacancy in the shell; (*c*) the vacancy is filled by an outer shell electron with the emission of a characteristic x-ray; (*d*) an Auger electron may be emitted instead of a characteristic X-ray.

the atom. The electron, referred to as a photoelectron, subsequently transfers energy to the surroundings by the mechanisms described previously, that is, ionization, excitation, and Bremsstrahlung. An outer shell electron fills the vacancy in the electron shell of the atom with the energy difference emitted as a characteristic X-ray (Fig. 2.11*c*) or an Auger electron (Fig. 2.11*d*). However, since the photoelectric interaction is most probable with high atomic numbered materials, and since the fluorescent yield is highest for high atomic numbered materials, typically the characteristic X-ray will be emitted. Since the charged electron has a relatively short range in solid matter, and with the assumption that the characteristic X-ray is also locally absorbed, the photoelectric process is usually considered to be an absorption process, all of the photon energy is deposited locally. The probability of photoelec-

tric interaction, τ, increases rapidly as the atomic number of the absorber increases and decreases rapidly as the energy of the gamma ray increases.

Another method of energy transfer from a high-energy photon to an orbital electron is Compton scattering. Typically this is an interaction with a loosely bound, essentially free electron with the result that a fraction of the incoming photon energy is transferred to the electron, and the photon is scattered with a lower energy in a different direction than the incident photon (Fig. 2.12). The scattering angle is predictable from the magnitude of the energy transfer. The relationship between the incoming and scattered gamma ray energies and angle of scattering is described by the Compton equation.

$$h\nu' = h\nu/[(1 + h\nu/m_0c^2)\,(1 - \cos\theta)]$$

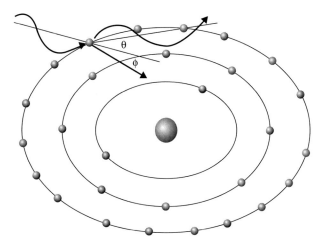

FIGURE 2.12 Compton scattering. The gamma ray is scattered at reduced energy at angle θ from the original direction. Energy is transferred to the Compton electron, which is propelled at the angle θ.

where

$h\nu'$ is the scattered gamma ray energy,

$h\nu$ is the incoming, unscattered gamma ray energy,

m_0c^2 is the rest mass energy equivalence of an electron, and

θ is the gamma ray scattering angle.

In terms of local energy deposition, it is the energy transferred to the electron that is relevant. The probability for Compton's scattering, σ, is usually expressed as the sum of two probabilities, one relating to the fractional energy transferred to the electron and therefore absorption, σ_a, and one relating to the fraction of the incident energy carried away by the scattered gamma ray, σ_s.

$$\sigma = \sigma_a + \sigma_s$$

A third mechanism of photon interaction that occurs only at very high photon energies is pair production. The pair produced is an electron and a positron by the transformation of the photon energy into the two electron masses (Fig. 2.13). Because the energy equivalence of two electron rest masses is 1.022 MeV, this interaction can only occur for gamma ray energies higher than that. However, it is only likely to occur at much higher photon energies. The probability of occurrence, κ, increases as the energy of the photon increases and as the atomic number of the absorber increases. The difference between the photon energy and 1.022 MeV is the total kinetic energy of the two particles.

$$KE(e^- + e^+) = h\nu - 1.022 \text{ MeV}$$

The positron will subsequently undergo annihilation with an electron resulting in two annihilation photons emitted at 180°, the same process described previously under positron radioactive decay (Fig. 2.14).

The likelihood of a gamma ray interacting by one of these three mechanisms in a specified material depends upon the energy of the gamma ray and the atomic number of the material. Photoelectric absorption is the dominant mode of interaction in high atomic numbered materials in the relatively low gamma ray energy range. For higher energies and for low atomic numbered ma-

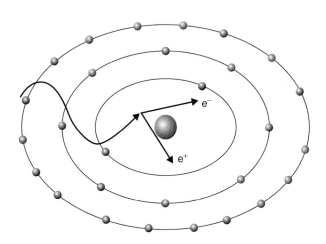

FIGURE 2.13 Pair production. The gamma ray energy, minus 1.022 MeV, is shared by the two electrons.

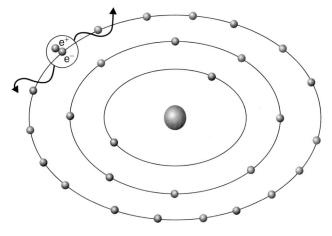

FIGURE 2.14 The positron created in a pair production interaction or from positron decay combines with an electron, producing two 0.511 MeV photons which are emitted at 180°.

terials, Compton scattering is the primary mode of interaction. Pair production is not important for radionuclides used in gamma ray imaging, since the gamma ray energies are less than 1.022 MeV.

An understanding of the probability of photoelectric versus Compton scattering in gamma ray imaging is important. Collimators and radiation shields are designed with high atomic numbered materials to maximize the probability of photoelectric interaction and minimize the probability of Compton scatter. On the other hand, the interaction of gamma rays in tissue is dominated by Compton scattering. The abundance of scattered photons coming from a patient administered a radiopharmaceutical has a significant detrimental impact on gamma ray image quality. Scatter removal or compensation in gamma ray imaging is one of the major challenges in attempts to improve image quality. The probability of interaction by each of these mechanisms is specified by an attenuation or absorption coefficient, μ. Since each mechanism is independent, the total probability of interaction is the sum of the coefficients of the individual mechanisms.

$$\mu = \tau + \sigma + \kappa$$

The energy and atomic number dependence of photon interaction are illustrated in Figure 2.15.

Math of Charged Particle Interactions

When a high-energy charged particle transfers energy to the surrounding medium by ionization, excitation, or Bremsstrahlung, the density of energy deposition is defined by the specific ionization, which is the number of ion pairs produced per unit distance along the track of the charged particle. The linear energy transfer (LET)

TABLE 2.13 *Linear Energy Transfer and Quality Factors of Ionizing Particles*

	LET (keV/micron)	Q
Electron	15	1
Proton	200	20
Alpha	2000	20
Neutron	200	20

LET, linear energy transfer; Q, quality factors.

is the energy deposition per unit distance along the charged particle track, typically several keV per micron (Table 2.13) [5,6]. The magnitude of the LET for beta-particles, and electrons produced by interactions of X-rays and gamma rays are classified as low LET radiation. Much higher energy density is produced by more massive charged particles such as protons and alpha particles. The density of energy deposition is a major factor in producing radiation effects on cells and thus in describing radiation detriment and quantifying radiation risk.

The range of a charged particle is the linear distance from its origin to where it has lost sufficient kinetic energy to no longer be an ionizing particle. For electrons and positrons in air the range can be several meters. In solid matter, such as tissues, it is typically millimeters. Because the probability of Bremsstrahlung production is proportional to the energy of the electron and the atomic number of the medium through which it is passing, it is essentially zero in tissue. Whereas in high atomic numbered material such as lead, it can be 1%–2% for high-energy beta particles. For this reason, high-energy beta emitters are usually shielded with a low atomic number material closest to the source followed by a layer of lead.

Math of Photon Interactions

For a monoenergetic narrow beam of gamma rays incident upon an absorber of thickness x, a fraction of the photons will be transmitted through the absorber. If the thickness of the absorber is doubled, the same fraction of the initially transmitted beam will be transmitted through the second layer, that is, the process is exponential. The fraction attenuated per unit thickness of the absorber is a characteristic of the material and varies with the energy of the gamma ray. The intensity of a monoenergetic narrow gamma ray beam transmitted through an attenuator of thickness x is described by

$$dI/I = -\mu x \, dx$$

$$I = I_0 \, e^{-\mu x}$$

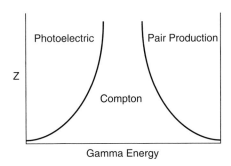

FIGURE 2.15 The likelihood of photon interactions is determined by the photon energy and the atomic number of the absorber. Photoelectric is dominant at low energies and high Z, Compton at higher energies and low Z, and pair production only for energies above 1.022 MeV.

where

I is the transmitted intensity,

I_0 is the incident intensity,

x is the thickness, and

μ is the linear attenuation coefficient.

The linear attenuation coefficient is the probability per unit thickness of the photon interacting by any of the photon interaction modes described previously. It is the sum of the probabilities for each of the possible modes of interaction. There is a difference between the attenuation coefficient and the absorption coefficient. Attenuation refers to the removal of photons from a narrow beam by either absorption or scattering. Therefore the attenuation coefficient includes the total Compton coefficient, σ, both the absorption portion, σ_a, and the scattering portion, σ_s. Absorption implies energy deposition and therefore the energy transferred to the electron in either the photoelectric or Compton interactions, thus the absorption portion only of the Compton coefficient.

The exponential nature of monoenergetic photon attenuation applies only to narrow beams, where gamma rays scattered in the media do not contribute to the measurement of the photons transmitted. For a broad beam, the scattering in the media can contribute to the measurement of transmitted photons and therefore this simple exponential function is no longer applicable. Typically a buildup factor is added to account for this scatter contribution. The buildup factor, B, is a function of the energy of the gamma ray, the area of the absorber exposed, the thickness of the absorber, and the material of the absorber.

$$I = I_0 B e^{-\mu x}$$

In high atomic numbered materials, such as lead and tungsten used for shielding gamma rays, there is relatively little Compton scattering over the range of gamma ray energies used in diagnostic imaging. Thus the buildup factor is approximately 1.0. However, in tissue Compton scattering is dominant and the buildup factor can be very significant.

For exponential attenuation of a photon beam, it is convenient to describe the attenuating properties of a material by the thickness needed to attenuate to a specified fraction of the incident intensity. The fraction 1/2 is commonly used, and the corresponding thickness is the half-value thickness (HVT) or half-value layer (HVL). From

$$I = I_0 e^{-\mu x}$$

$$\text{for } I/I_0 = 1/2$$

$$\text{HVT} = (\ln 2)/\mu = 0.693/\mu$$

where ln2 is the Naperian or natural logarithm of 2.

The attenuating property of a material for high-energy photons is primarily determined by the atomic number of the material and the number of electrons along the path of the photon in the material, since photoelectric absorption and Compton scattering are the two relevant interactions. The atomic number defines the number of electrons per atom and the binding energy of the electrons. The electron binding energy is the major factor determining the probability of photoelectric interaction. With the exception of hydrogen, the electron density, in electrons/gm, of different elements varies over a relatively small range. Because of this and also to more easily measure very thin absorbers, it is often more convenient to specify an absorber thickness as a density thickness, ρx, that is, mass per unit area such as gm/cm^2. The corresponding interaction probability coefficient becomes the mass absorption or attenuation coefficient, μ/ρ, instead of the linear coefficient, μ. The units of μ/ρ are cm^2/gm. The corresponding attenuation equation is

$$I = I_0 \, e^{-(\mu/\rho)(\rho x)}$$

The atomic number and the density determine the effectiveness of shielding materials for X-rays and gamma rays. Most frequently lead is used because of a reasonable density, high atomic number, and low cost. For high-energy photons, such as the 511keV annihilation photons from positron emitters, higher density materials become desirable to minimize the bulk of the shield. This is the reason tungsten is often used instead of lead for shielding positron emitters. If cost were not an issue, uranium and gold would be the shielding materials of choice for high-energy photons (Table 2.14) [7].

DOSIMETRY

Dosimetry is the measurement or calculation of radiation absorbed dose. Special quantities and units are defined to describe dose and its relationship to the biologic effects of ionizing radiation and radiation safety regulations (Table 2.15).

Radiation exposure is a measure of the amount of ionization produced by X-rays or gamma rays in air. It only applies to air and only for X-rays or gamma rays within a defined energy range, a range that encompasses that encountered in X-ray and gamma ray

TABLE 2.14 *Absorption Properties of Several Materials of Interest in Gamma Ray Imaging*

Material	Z	Density (gm/cm³)	K-edge (keV)	HVL @ 80 keV (mm)	HVL @ 140 keV(mm)	HVL @ 511 keV (mm)
H₂O	8(O)	1.00	0.54(O)	39.6	46.2	72.9
NaI	53(I)	3.67	33.16(I)	0.66	2.36	21.0
W	74	19.30	69.69	0.05	0.17	3.0
Au	79	19.32	80.96	0.16	0.14	2.39
Pb	82	11.35	88.29	0.29	0.27	3.82
U	92	18.95	116.11	0.11	0.12	1.92

imaging. The traditional unit for radiation exposure is the roentgen and is equal to 2.58×10^{-4} coulombs per kilogram of air at standard temperature and atmospheric pressure. The International Standard (SI) unit is one coulomb per kilogram. A related quantity is the air kerma. Kerma is an acronym for <u>k</u>inetic <u>e</u>nergy <u>r</u>eleased in <u>ma</u>terial by transfer of energy to electrons from X-rays or gamma rays. It is essentially a measure of the absorbed dose to the air if Bremsstrahlung is negligible and electronic equilibrium in the air is established.

Radiation absorbed dose is the amount of energy absorbed per unit mass by any material. The traditional unit is the rad equal to 100 ergs per gram. The SI unit is the gray, equal to one joule per kilogram.

$$1 \text{ gray} = 100 \text{ rad, since}$$
$$1 \text{ joule} = 10^7 \text{ erg}$$
$$1 \text{ kg} = 10^3 \text{ gm}$$
$$1 \text{ gray} = 1 \text{ joule/kg} = 10^7 \text{ erg}/10^3 \text{ gm}$$
$$= 10^4 \text{ erg/gm} = 100 \text{ rad}$$

For a specified tissue there may be different biologic responses for the same amount of energy absorbed per unit mass by different types of ionizing radiation, primarily because of different LETs. The quantity *dose equivalent* is used to express this response. It is the absorbed dose multiplied by a quality factor that reflects ranges of the ionization density or linear energy transfer of the specific type of radiation (see Table 2.13). A

TABLE 2.15 *Quantities and Units in Dosimetry*

Quantity	Traditional Unit	International Standard Unit
Exposure	Roentgen	Coulombs/kilogram
Absorbed dose	Rad	Gray
Dose equivalent	Rem	Sievert
Equivalent dose	Rem	Sievert
Effective dose equivalent	Rem	Sievert
Effective dose	Rem	Sievert
Activity	Curie	Becquerel

related quantity, the *equivalent dose*, is defined as the average absorbed dose over an organ or tissue multiplied by a radiation weighting factor. These radiation weighting factors in general are the same as the quality factors used for the dose equivalent. For most of the radiation encountered in diagnostic medicine the quality factors and weighting factors equal one and therefore the dose and the dose equivalent are equal in magnitude. The traditional unit of dose equivalent and equivalent dose is the rem. The SI unit is the sievert, where 1 sievert equals 100 rem.

In addition to different types of radiation having different biologic effects for the same absorbed dose, different tissues have different radiation sensitivities for the same dose equivalent. To specify the total radiation risk when multiple tissues are exposed, a weighted average dose equivalent is used in which the weighting factors relate to the radiation risk for that particular organ or tissue. The International Commission on Radiological Protection (ICRP) in 1977 initially defined this quantity, the *effective dose equivalent*. The weighting factors were related to the lifetime risk per unit dose equivalent of the production of a fatal cancer or significant genetic defects in the subsequent two generations. More recently a refinement of this concept has resulted in the *effective dose*, which is also a weighted average dose equivalent. Here the weighting factors relate to detriment, which takes into account in addition to the lifetime risk of a fatal cancer, nonfatal cancers, potential years of life lost, and other factors that more directly relate to the quality of life. The weighting factors of the effective dose equivalent and the effective dose are shown in Table 2.16 [8].

This average tissue weighted dose approach is helpful in comparing the radiation risks or detriment of nonuniform exposure or radiation exposure by different modalities such as radiopharmaceuticals compared to diagnostic X-rays. Uniform whole body exposure at this magnitude should produce the same total risk or detriment.

Since radiation risks are related to radiation dose it is important to understand how to calculate and meas-

TABLE 2.16 *Weighting Factors for the Effective Dose Equivalent and the Effective Dose*

Tissue	Effective Dose Equivalent w_T	Effective Dose w_T
Gonads	0.25	0.20
Red marrow	0.12	0.12
Colon		0.12
Lung	0.12	0.12
Stomach		0.12
Bladder		0.05
Breast	0.15	0.05
Liver		0.05
Esophagus		0.05
Thyroid	0.03	0.05
Skin		0.01
Bone surface	0.03	0.01
Remainder*	0.30	0.05

*One-fifth for each of the remaining five highest dose tissues.

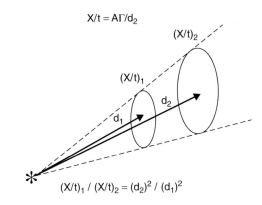

FIGURE 2.16 The exposure rate (X/t) from a point source of gamma rays varies inversely as the square of the distance (d). It is the product of the activity (A), and the exposure rate constant (Γ) divided by the distance squared.

ure radiation absorbed doses. Any radionuclide that emits gamma rays or X-rays has an associated exposure rate constant, or if only gamma rays are emitted, a specific gamma constant. This quantity indicates the exposure rate at a specified distance from a point source of that radionuclide per unit activity. Traditionally the units employed are roentgens per hour per millicurie at 1 centimeter or roentgens per hour per curie at 1 meter. This quantity is a characteristic of the radionuclide and can be either calculated or obtained from published tables. Some examples are shown in Table 2.8. With this quantity the exposure rate in air can be calculated at any distance from a point source of the radionuclide for any activity. A *point source* is defined as one that has dimensions that are small compared to the distance from the source to the location at which the exposure rate is to be calculated. For example, a syringe can be considered a point source at a distance of about 1 meter, whereas a radioactive patient is not. When it is assumed to be a point source the inverse square relationship applies; the intensity and therefore the exposure rate varies inversely as the square of the distance from the source (Fig. 2.16). By this method calculating the exposure rate at a location from a gamma ray source allows one to then calculate the absorbed dose rate to a small volume of material at that location by multiplying the exposure rate by the ratio of the mass energy absorption coefficients for the material in question and air times 0.87. This is referred to as the f-factor or the roentgen-to-rad conversion factor.

$$f = 0.87[(\mu_{en}/\rho)_{material}/(\mu_{en}/\rho)_{air}]$$

An alternative method to calculate the dose rate to a small mass of a material at a distance from a ra-

dioactive source is to measure the exposure rate and then convert to absorbed dose, again using the appropriate mass energy absorption coefficients. An example of the use of the exposure rate constant, inverse square relationship, and attenuation is shown in Table 2.17. The measurement of exposure rate to calculate absorbed dose rate is typically performed with a calibrated ionization chamber. The reverse process, the calculation of the activity of a radioactive source from a measurement with a radiation detector, can be accomplished if one measures the exposure rate or the count rate and knows the detection efficiency of the detector for the gamma ray or X-ray energy emitted from the radioactive source. The measured count rate is related to the disintegration rate of the source, which is the activity, by the intrinsic and geometric detection effi-

TABLE 2.17 *Example of Exposure Rate and Attenuation Calculations*

What is the exposure rate at 20 cm from a 30 mCi point source of Tc-99m in air?

What would it be if the source were shielded by 1/16" of lead?

For Γ = 0.59 R/hr/mCi @ 1 cm

$$\text{Exposure rate, } X/t = A \times \Gamma/d^2$$
$$X/t = (30 \text{ mCi})(0.59 \text{ R/hr/mCi @ 1 cm})/(20)^2$$
$$X/t = 44.25 \text{ mR/hr}$$

With 1/16" of lead shielding

$$1/16" = (25.4 \text{ mm/in})(1/16 \text{ in}) = 1.59 \text{ mm}$$

For HVL = 0.27 mm

$$1/16" = 1.59 \text{ mm}/0.27 \text{ mm} = 5.9 \text{ HVL}$$

Transmission factor = $(0.5)^{5.9}$ = 0.017

With shield, X/t = (44.25 mR/hr)(0.017) = 0.8 mR/hr

TABLE 2.18 *Calculation of Activity from a Count Rate Measurement*

A thyroid uptake probe has a 2.5 cm diameter, 2.5 cm thick NaI(Tl) detector for which the intrinsic efficiency for the 159 keV gammas from I-123 is 90%. If the I-123 source is measured at 25 cm from the detector, and a net count rate of 1000 cps is observed, what is the activity of the I-123 source? The 159 keV gamma rays are emitted in 83% of the disintegrations.

$$A(dps) = CR(cps)/(\varepsilon_i \times \varepsilon_g \times f)$$

$A(dps)$ = activity in disintegrations per sec(Bq)

$CR(cps)$ = net count rate in counts per second

ε_i = intrinsic detection efficiency

ε_g = geometric detection efficiency = area of detector/surface area of sphere with radius = 25cm

f = photon yield

$$\varepsilon_g = \pi(1.25)^2/[4\pi(25)^2] = 6.25 \times 10^{-4}$$
$$A = (1000)/[(0.9)(6.25 \times 10^{-4})(0.83)$$
$$A = 2.14 \times 10^6 \text{ dps} = 2.14 \text{ MBq} = 57.8 \ \mu Ci$$

ciencies, and the photon yield, the number of photons emitted per disintegration, from the source for the radiation being detected. An example of this application is shown in Table 2.18.

When a radiopharmaceutical is administered to a patient, it is not possible or at best very difficult to measure directly the dose to any specific organ or tissue. Generally a calculation is performed that is based upon a computer model of the human patient. The scheme that is universally used is that developed by the Medical Internal Radiation Dose committee of the Society of Nuclear Medicine, referred to as the MIRD scheme [9]. This approach relies upon knowledge of the decay scheme of the radionuclide, the dynamics and the distribution of the radiopharmaceutical in the patient, and the fraction of the energy emitted from a source organ or tissue that has taken up the radiopharmaceutical, that is absorbed in the target organ or tissue. The target organ or tissue is that for which the dose is being calculated. The dose equation and definitions of parameters are described in Table 2.19.

The *equilibrium dose constant* is the amount of energy emitted in the form of the ith type of radiation per disintegration. The *absorbed fraction* is the fraction of the energy of ith type of radiation that is absorbed in the target organ from the source organ. The *cumulated activity* is the total number of disintegrations that have occurred over the time for which the dose is being calculated. The product of these factors divided by the mass of the target organ is the dose to that organ from the ith type of radiation. The product of these is summed for all the different types of emissions, and all source

organs or tissues, to yield an average energy absorbed per unit mass in the target organ, therefore radiation absorbed dose. Tables of equilibrium dose constants and absorbed fractions are provided in the MIRD publications [3]. Also a computer program is available that includes several human models and many radionuclides. A simplification of this process uses S factors, where an S factor is the absorbed dose per unit cumulated activity, for example, rads per microcurie-hour or gray per Bq-hour. S factors are provided for each radionuclide and each combination of source and target organs for the human computer models that are available in the MIRD program. These human models include males and females of different ages and several stages of pregnancy. Radiation absorbed doses for organs and tissues and the effective doses for F-18-FDG, Tl-201, and Tc-99m MIBI are shown in Table 2.20 [10,11].

RADIATION SAFETY

The biological effects of ionizing radiation begin with the transfer of energy from the radiation to an electron of an atom of the organism. The atom may be associated with a significant organic molecule of the organism or it may be an atom of a molecule of water in the cell or extracellular fluid. The energy transferred can produce biochemical changes by production of reactive free radicals in the water or by direct interaction, altering the chemical bonds of biochemically important molecules. By either mechanism, depending upon the type of cell, either somatic or genetic effects may be manifest. Biologic effects of radiation are classified as either stochastic or deterministic. Occasionally the

TABLE 2.19 *MIRD Scheme for Internal Dose Calculation*

For a single source region

$$D = \bar{A} \ \Sigma_i[(\Delta_i)(\phi_i)]/m$$

where

D = absorbed dose to the target organ from radioactivity in the source region

$\bar{A}$ = the cumulated activity in the source region over the time period for which the dose is calculated

Δ_i = the equilibrium dose constant for the ith type of emitted radiation

ϕ_i = the absorbed fraction of the energy of the ith type emitted from the source region and absorbed in the target organ

m = the mass of the target organ

If there is more than one source region, which is usually the case, the dose contributions from each are summed.

TABLE 2.20 *Absorbed Dose per Unit Activity Administered to an Adult (mGy/MBq)*

Organ	FDG	Tl-201	MIBI-rest	MIBI-stress
Adrenals	1.2E-02	5.7E-02	7.5E-03	6.6E-03
Bladder	1.6E-01	4.0E-02	1.1E-02	9.8E-03
Bone surfaces	1.1E-02	3.4E-01	8.2E-03	7.8E-03
Brain	2.8E-02	2.2E-02	5.2E-03	4.4E-03
Breast	8.6E-03	2.4E-02	3.8E-03	3.4E-03
Esophagus	1.1E-02	3.6E-02	4.1E-03	4.0E-03
Gall bladder	1.2E-02	6.5E-02	3.9E-02	3.3E-02
GI-tract				
Stomach	1.1E-02	9.9E-02	6.5E-03	5.9E-03
SI	1.3E-02	1.4E-01	1.5E-02	1.2E-02
Colon	1.3E-02	2.3E-01	2.4E-02	1.9E-02
ULI	1.2E-02	1.7E-01	2.7E-02	2.2E-02
LLI	1.5E-02	3.2E-01	1.9E-02	1.6E-02
Heart	6.2E-02	2.0E-01	6.3E-03	7.2E-03
Kidneys	2.1E-02	4.8E-01	3.6E-02	2.6E-02
Liver	1.1E-02	1.5E-01	1.1E-02	9.2E-03
Lungs	1.0E-02	1.1E-01	4.6E-03	4.4E-03
Muscles	1.1E-02	5.2E-02	2.9E-03	3.2E-03
Ovaries	1.5E-02	7.3E-01	9.1E-03	8.1E-03
Pancreas	1.2E-02	5.7E-02	7.7E-03	6.9E-03
Red marrow	1.1E-02	1.6E-01	5.5E-03	5.0E-03
Salivary glands			1.4E-02	9.2E-03
Skin	8.0E-03	2.2E-02	3.1E-03	2.9E-03
Spleen	1.1E-02	1.2E-01	6.5E-03	5.8E-03
Testes	1.2E-02	4.5E-01	3.8E-03	3.7E-03
Thymus	1.1E-02	3.6E-02	4.1E-03	4.0E-03
Thyroid	1.0E-02	2.2E-02	5.3E-03	4.4E-03
Uterus	2.1E-02	5.1E-02	7.8E-03	7.2E-03
Remaining organs	1.1E-02	5.8E-02	3.1E-03	3.3E-03
Effective dose (mSv/MBq)	1.9E-02	2.2E-01	9.0E-03	7.9E-03

equivalent terms of probabilistic or nonstochastic are encountered.

The *stochastic effects* are those for which the probability of occurrence increases with the radiation dose. The effect either occurs or it does not occur. The severity is not related to the magnitude of the dose. Stochastic effects are usually assumed to occur without a dose threshold. Therefore, any dose, no matter how small, is assumed to have some risk. Also, the risk–dose relationship is assumed to be linear. This linear, nonthreshold dose response assumption has been a point of contention for decades, since it gets to the heart of the issue of radiation risk estimates at low doses, for example less than 0.1 gray, the dose range of interest for occupational radiation exposures and diagnostic testing. Examples of stochastic effects are genetic abnormalities and radiation induced cancers.

Deterministic effects are those that occur only above a dose threshold. Above the threshold the severity of the effect increases with increasing dose. Examples of this type of effect are skin injury from high doses of an external beam of X-rays and radiation-induced cataracts. These effects generally are only observed at doses above several gray.

Early in the application of radiation in medicine it was the deterministic effects that were first observed. Radiation safety guidelines were based upon minimizing or eliminating the occurrence of these deterministic effects. The concept initially used was that of a tolerance dose, which often related to the observation of erythema. Since these early years of radiation medicine many consensus groups, regulatory agencies, and scientific organizations have studied and reported on topics of radiation risks and regulations. Some of the most prominent ones are listed in Table 2.21.

In subsequent years, as it became appreciated that there was also the potential of stochastic effects, the need to define the magnitude of radiation risk in the low-dose range became more important. The assumption of a linear relationship between risk and dose for stochastic effects eventually became the working assumption for regulations on occupational dose limits. The linear dose response model implies that any exposure has some risk and therefore the regulations are

TABLE 2.21 *Organizations Providing Radiation Guidance and Regulations*

Abbreviation	Organization
NRC	Nuclear Regulatory Commission
NCRP	National Council on Radiation Protection and Measurements
ICRP	International Commission on Radiological Protection
UNSCEAR	United Nations Scientific Committee on the Effects of Atomic Radiation
BEIR	Biological Effects of Ionizing Radiation Committee of the National Research Council, National Academy of Sciences
CRCPD	Conference of Radiation Control Program Directors
OAS	Organization of Agreement States
ICRU	International Commission on Radiation Units and Measurements

based on the concept of acceptable risk. It was recognized that there are other occupational risks besides radiation exposure and the magnitude of the radiation risk in relationship to total occupational risk was considered. Over the years the occupational dose limits have decreased as refinements have occurred in the estimates of risk per unit dose [12]. The occupational dose limits and dose limits to members of the public from the use of radiation sources in the United States are summarized in Table 2.22. Dose limits apply to occupational exposure and members of the public who are exposed as a consequence of the use of ionizing radiation by licensed sources. They do not include natural background radiation exposure or personal medical exposure. There are no regulatory dose limits for the patient, either diagnostic or therapeutic, although there are some attempts for diagnostic X-rays to define reference doses that set the standards for typical diagnostic tests and the package inserts of radiopharmaceuticals give guidance on the recommended dosage. Table 2.23 illustrates the enormous radiation dose range that an individual might encounter.

TABLE 2.22 *Annual Regulatory Dose Limits in USA*

Radiation worker	50 mSv total effective dose equivalent*
	150 mSv lens of eye
	500 mSv skin
	500 mSv any organ or extremities
Member of the public	1 mSv total effective dose equivalent*
	0.02 mSv in any one hour
Fetal dose of declared pregnant worker	5 mSv over term of pregnancy
	<0.5 mSv /month recommended

*Sum of the external and internal dose equivalents.

TABLE 2.23 *A Range of Doses*

Radiation Exposure	
PA chest film-entrance skin dose	0.3 mSv
Average USA background	3 mSv
Declared pregnancy dose limit	5 mSv
KUB-entrance skin dose	5.5 mSv
Tc^{99m} MIBI effective dose (30 mCi)	8.8 mSv
Tl^{201} effective dose (5 mCi)	41 mSv
CT of the body	20–40 mSv
Occupational TEDE*	50 mSv/year
Occupational eye dose limit	0.15 Sv
Occupational extremity dose limit	0.5 Sv
Erythema	2 Sv
LD_{50} man	4.5 Sv
Tumor treatment dose	60 Sv

*Total effective dose equivalent.

In addition to the regulatory occupational and members-of –the-public dose limits, there is a guiding principle of an operational radiation safety program that doses, both to individuals and collectively, should be kept as low as reasonably achievable (ALARA), social and economic factors being taken into account [13]. The ALARA principle does not suggest that efforts should be made to keep doses as low as possible, since at some point of added protection the deleterious effects of the radiation exposure become vanishingly small and the cost-to-benefit tradeoff of further reductions becomes inappropriate. A typical application of the ALARA principle is to establish investigational dose levels that are below the regulatory levels and customized to each exposed group. For example, the investigational levels for the workers in a nuclear cardiology department should be higher than those for individuals performing in vitro testing with small quantities of P-32 or I-125. Tracking exposures above the investigational levels focuses the attention of the radiation safety officer on the frequency and appropriateness of occupational exposures below the regulatory limits.

Since occupational exposures are regulated there must be a mechanism to document that the workers are within the allowable dose limits. Usually a personnel radiation monitor is worn, which can consist of either X-ray film in a special holder or other radiation sensitive devices that can be processed after exposure to the radiation to emit light, which can be related to the original radiation exposure. The two commonly used in the latter category are thermoluminescence dosimeters and optically stimulated luminescence dosimeters. There are also electronic devices that can be used for personnel monitoring. These personnel monitors are usually worn on the trunk as an indicator of the effective dose equivalent. If individuals handle substantial quantities of radioactive materials then generally it is also required that they wear extremity monitors to estimate the exposure to the hands to ensure compliance with the extremity dose limits. Also, if the potential for internal contamination is significant then a bioassay program must be established.

The pregnant worker requires special consideration because of the higher radiation sensitivity of the embryo/fetus. In the United States the pregnant worker has the option of declaring that she is pregnant. If she does so, then lower dose limits become applicable to the embryo/fetus. Generally a separate radiation monitor is worn on the abdomen, under any protective apparel if any is worn, in order to get the best estimate of dose to the embryo/fetus. The limits to the embryo/fetus are 5 mSv during the pregnancy with a recommendation that the dose be kept below 0.5 mSv in any one month. In some cases, particularly in a busy cardiovascular nuclear medicine laboratory using Tc-99m myocardial perfusion agents, it can be a challenge to keep the occupational exposure below 0.5 mSv per month. Under these circumstances one should consider alternative work assignments for pregnant technologists if that is practical, or recommend having the technologists wear a lead apron skirt. A 0.5 mm lead apron will attenuate approximately 70% of the 140 keV gamma rays from Tc-99m (Table 2.24). If a lead apron is worn it is important to determine that it is one of the traditional lead aprons containing lead, and not the newer lightweight composite aprons that are now commonly used in diagnostic radiology departments and cardiac catheterization laboratories. These do not attenuate the 140 keV gamma rays nearly as effectively as the true lead aprons.

The staff doses in a nuclear cardiology laboratory occur primarily from preparation of the radiopharmaceutical, measurement of the dosage, injection into the patient, and being in close proximity to the patient during the stress and imaging procedures. Additional exposure is received from the daily quality control testing of the gamma cameras. The exposure rates, and therefore staff occupational doses, are much higher when Tc-99m myocardial perfusion agents are used than with Tl-201. The exposure rates from patients for stress/rest Tc-99m myocardial perfusion studies are 2 to 3 mR/hr at a meter. Staff in a busy laboratory can be exposed at this level for much of their workday. It is not uncommon to have personnel monitor readings that are higher than 0.5mSV per month under these circumstances. The patient's effective dose with Tc-99m myocardial perfusion agents is less than with Tl-201, even though the activity administered may be much higher, but the staff doses are higher. For example, an adult patient's effective dose for 5 mCi of Tl-201 is 40.7 mSv, whereas for 30 mCi of Tc-99m MIBI during stress it is 8.8 mSv, one-fifth the dose with six times the activity [11].

Radiation workers must be constantly aware of the mechanisms to minimize their radiation exposure. The primary methods involve optimizing the influences of time, distance, and shielding. The time factor relates to the time in proximity of the radiation sources, either the patient or preparation of the dose for injection. The distance factor pertains primarily to maintaining a significant distance from the patient during imaging and using tongs when handling multidose vials or other unshielded sources. Shielding relates primarily to syringe shields during the administration of the radiopharmaceutical and working behind appropriate body and face shields when doses are being prepared for injection. Nurses and EKG technologists who might have to monitor the patients' vital signs during and after pharmacological or treadmill stress tests using Tc-99m agents might consider draping the patient with a lead apron, if feasible, to minimize their exposure during the recovery period after the stress. Also, if positron-emitting radiopharmaceuticals are used, such as F-18-FDG, staff dose will usually increase. The high-energy photons resulting from positron annihilations require substantially more shielding for the radioactive sources and the exposure rates from patients are higher.

TABLE 2.24 *Effectiveness of Lead Aprons in Pregnancy*

A nuclear medicine technologist works full time in a nuclear cardiology lab where only Tc-99m imaging agents are used. Her occupational exposure monitor averages 100 mrem/month, worn at the waist. She has recently become pregnant. How much would a 0.5 mm lead apron reduce the monthly exposure to her abdomen?

$$\text{For HVL} = 0.27 \text{ mm}$$
$$0.5 \text{ mm}/0.27 \text{ mm} = 1.85 \text{ HVL}$$
$$\text{Transmission factor} = (0.5)^{1.85} = 0.28$$

Thus her abdomen exposure under the apron should be approximately 28 mrem/month, below the recommended maximum for pregnancy of 50 mrem/month to the embryo/fetus.

REFERENCES

1. *Medical Physics Data Book, National Bureau of Standards Handbook 138.* Washington, D.C.: U.S. Government Printing Office, 1982.
2. Brucer M. Trilinear Chart of the Nuclides. St Louis: Mallinckrodt, Inc, 1979.
3. Weber DA, Eckerman KF, Dillman LT, et al. *MIRD: Radionuclide Data and Decay Schemes,* The Society of Nuclear Medicine, 1989.

4. Saha GP. *Fundamentals of Nuclear Pharmacy*, 4th edition. New York: Springer-Verlag, 1998.

5. Shapiro J. *Radiation Protection A Guide for Scientists and Physicians*, 3rd edition. Boston: Harvard University Press, 1990.

6. NCRP Report No. 91. *Recommendations on Limits for Exposure to Ionizing Radiation*. Bethesda: National Council on Radiation Protection and Measurements, 1987.

7. Shleien B. *The Health Physics and Radiological Health Handbook*, Revised Edition. Silver Spring, MD. Scinta, Inc, 1992.

8. NCRP Report No. 122. *Use of Personal Monitors to Estimate Effective Dose Equivalent and Effective Dose to Workers for External Exposure to Low-Let Radiation*. Bethesda: National Council on Radiation Protection and Measurements, 1995.

9. Loevinger R, Budinger TF, Watson EE. *MIRD Primer for Absorbed Dose Calculations*, Revised Edition. The Society of Nuclear Medicine, 1991.

10. ICRP Publication 53. Annals of the ICRP. *Radiation Dose to Patients from Radiopharmaceuticals*. New York: Pergamon Press, 1988.

11. Valentin, J. Annals of the ICRP. *Radiation Dose to Patients from Radiopharmaceuticals*. New York: Pergamon Press, 1999.

12. National Research Council. *Health Effects of Exposure to Low Levels of Ionizing Radiation, BEIR V*. National Academy Press, 1990.

13. NCRP Report No. 127. *Operational Radiation Safety Program*. Bethesda: National Council on Radiation Protection and Measurements, 1998.

3 | Imaging instrumentation

ROBERTO MAASS-MORENO AND STEPHEN L. BACHARACH

Nuclear medicine images trace the activity of radiolabeled biochemical compounds by representing, in two or three dimensions, the distribution of their concentration in space. These images can be snapshots representing static or steady-state physiological processes, or dynamic, time-dependent processes represented by a sequence of images that could be displayed in movie format. One key feature of nuclear medicine images is that a proportional relationship is always sought between the concentration of radioactivity in any given volume within the scanned object and its corresponding representation in the image (e.g., its brightness). While this may not be a requirement for other imaging modalities where the emphasis is image contrast and resolution rather than quantification, it is the basis for the quantitative nature of nuclear images. The ability to quantify nuclear medicine images is crucial for many cardiologic applications and it is therefore advantageous to examine nuclear cardiology instrumentation from the perspective of imaging as a measurement process.

Meeting the requirements necessary to produce quantitatively accurate images is not easy. Nuclear imaging depends on physical phenomena and instrumentation characteristics that are often nonlinear. Many technical innovations have been required to at least partially overcome these limitations and to establish the current basis of quantitative nuclear imaging. Much more research will be needed before truly quantitative imaging is a reality. Therefore it is necessary to acquire and to read nuclear medicine images with a sound understanding of the imaging process. The aim of this chapter is to assist in this understanding.

The first sections of this chapter discuss the instrumentation required to perform planar imaging. Planar imaging, using a gamma camera, is the most common imaging technique in nuclear medicine and is the basis for single-photon emission computed tomography (SPECT) and single-photon positron imaging. Each of the basic components of a gamma camera is described by tracing the fate of a gamma ray from the time it is emitted from within the body until it produces a count in the image. Subsequent sections describe the instrumentation considerations necessary to understand and perform cardiac SPECT imaging. Finally, the challenges of imaging positron emitters using single-photon SPECT methods (511 keV SPECT) are discussed. Overall, the chapter emphasizes the technical aspects of imaging instrumentation that affect clinical efficacy. The references given should provide further detail or derivations from fundamental principles.

PLANAR IMAGING—AN OVERVIEW

The planar large-crystal gamma camera conceived by H.O. Anger is probably the most successful nuclear medicine device of the last 50 years. Its aim is to detect the invisible penetrating photons (gamma rays, X-rays, and annihilation radiation) emanating from the patient and produce a visible image. In traditional planar imaging, the images produced are representations of volumes as two-dimensional projections. For SPECT the images are series of tomographic slices representing the object that was imaged. These can be displayed as pseudo three-dimensional volumes (the word "pseudo" is used because video displays are only two dimensional) or as slices at any selected plane through the object, or even as projected images, in which the tomographic data are reprojected to give a planar view from any angle.

The main component of the gamma camera is the detector assembly shown schematically in Figure 3.1. It comprises a large collimator facing the patient (*a*), which acts as the "lens" of the system. This figure shows the most common type of collimator, called a parallel-hole collimator, consisting of a large array of parallel holes in a thick (1 cm to several) sheet of lead. The parallel-hole collimator prevents any photons from reaching the detector unless they travel parallel to the holes (and therefore perpendicular to the camera face). The collimator is placed against the radiation detector comprising a large (e.g., 23" × 17" × 3/8") NaI scintillation crystal (*b*), and, behind it, a closely packed array of light-sensitive detectors, called photomultipliers

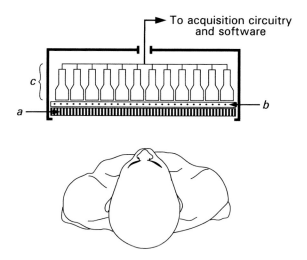

FIGURE 3.1 Cross-sectional view of the three basic components of a gamma camera head. (*a*) collimator; (*b*) scintillation crystal; and (*c*) photomultiplier array.

(*c*). The operation of the gamma camera can be summarized as follows: Photons are emitted from the patient's body in all directions. Only those photons heading straight for the camera (i.e., perpendicular to the camera's face) will be able to pass through the collimator. When the photons strike and interact in the crystal they produce a flash of visible light. This flash of light is detected by the photomultipliers, each of which produces an electrical signal proportional to the amount of light it detected. All these electrical signals can be combined to determine the precise location of the flash of light in the *x,y* plane. Determining the location of the flash of light allows the direction from which the gamma ray came to be deduced. As this description suggests, this photon detection process occurs one photon at a time. Even though many thousands of photons may strike the camera each second, in the microsecond scale of the processing electronics, the arrival of photons can be discerned as single events.

In addition to the detector assembly, a gamma camera includes a gantry with circuitry, digitizers, and software necessary to control and position the detector assembly, and the circuitry, computers, and software necessary to acquire, process, and display the data.

The word "camera" was likely inspired by its photographic counterpart and one may, from time to time, pursue this analogy to understand the role of the different components in the gamma camera. A good optical camera needs a high-quality lens and high-quality film and must have at least three important properties: (*1*) the lens must form a two-dimensional image; (*2*) the lens must also allow as much light emitted by the object as possible to reach the film; and (*3*) the film

must be sensitive enough to record that light and ensure that the amount of light recorded by the film is proportional to the brightness of the object being imaged. In the gamma camera the first and second requirements are met by the collimator and the third by the combined action of the scintillation crystal and the photodetectors. The ability of a camera to meet the first requirement influences the *spatial linearity* and the *spatial resolution* of the device. Requirements (*2*) and (*3*) determine the sensitivity of the camera—how dim the intensity of light emanating from the object can be (for an optical camera) or how few gamma rays can be emitted by the patient (for a gamma camera), and yet still produce a good image. The third requirement determines the correspondence or proportionality between the brightness pattern of the image and the brightness pattern of the object.

The visible light imaged by a conventional optical camera consists of photons of very low energy (and therefore long wavelengths). Such photons can employ standard optical lenses. Photons from nuclear or atomic transitions (called gamma rays and X-rays, respectively) are identical to visible photons, but with much higher energy (and comparably shorter wavelengths). Because of their higher energy, gamma rays are not refracted by conventional, visible light lenses. In addition, the photons from nuclear and atomic transitions penetrate most objects rather than reflecting from them. Although this makes conventional lenses useless for gamma rays, the relative transparency of biological materials to high-energy photons has the desirable effect of allowing the detection of photons arising both from the surface and from inside the body, so that deep structures can be visualized. However, like visible light going through a cloud, gamma rays and X-rays can be dispersed or *scattered* when passing through matter. These scattered photons can degrade the image.

The following sections examine these processes in detail by following the fate of a gamma ray as it is emitted by the patient, passes through the collimator, strikes the crystal, and eventually adds to the information in the image.

THE PATH THROUGH THE PATIENT'S BODY TO THE DETECTOR

As the radioactive molecules that have been injected into the patient decay, photons (e.g., gamma or X-rays) are emitted in all directions. Only some will be emitted in the direction of the detector. Of those, some will preserve their image-forming capability by following a straight path from their point of origin to the crystal.

Others will go astray as they encounter atoms in their transit through the tissue (mostly water) and interact with them. These interactions are of two very different types (see Chapter 2). They may collide with electrons and scatter off of them, losing part of their energy in the process (a Compton scattering event), or they may disappear altogether transferring their energy to electrons and nuclei as kinetic energy in what is called a photoelectric event. The probability of these two events occurring depends on the energy of the photon and on the type of tissue. In soft tissue, and at the photon energies of the isotopes most commonly employed in radiopharmaceuticals, almost all the interactions are Compton scattering. In bone, at low energies (e.g., Tl-201) some of the interactions may also be photoelectric.

Figure 3.2 summarizes the possible fates of a photon traveling from the tissue to the crystal. Photon *a* follows the ideal path: it travels unscattered, reaches the detector, and contributes to the image. Photon *b* also has the desired initial path but loses all its energy through a photoelectric collision and disappears. Photon *c* also has the desired initial trajectory, but scatters away from the detector. Photon *d*, on the other hand, is not initially headed for the detector, but instead travels in another direction, and then scatters toward the detector. This photon will contribute to the image but will degrade it. It will appear to the camera as though the photon emanated from a radioactive molecule somewhere along

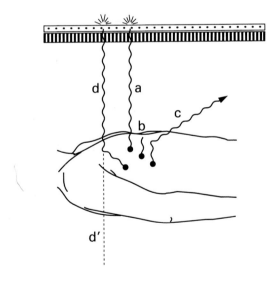

FIGURE 3.2 Possible fates of photons emanating from an organ perfused with a labeled compound: (*a*) an image-forming unscattered photon reaching the scintillation crystal; (*b*) a photon that has suffered complete (photoelectric) absorption before leaving the body; (*c*) a photon initially headed to the camera with an image-forming trajectory but that is then scattered away from the camera; (*d*) a photon that is scattered toward the detector and distorts the image by masquerading as having originated along trajectory *d'*.

line *d-d'* when in reality this was the line along which the scatter took place and not the point of decay.

Events such as those depicted in *b* and *c* of Figure 3.2 reduce the number of photons reaching the detector. As the thickness of tissue through which the photons must travel increases, the number of photons proceeding in the direction of the detector decreases due to the correspondingly greater opportunity for interactions. This attrition, called *attenuation*, is due to both Compton scattering and, much less likely in the body, photoelectric absorption. While attenuation is the basis of contrast in X-ray imaging, in nuclear medicine it detracts from the quality of the image primarily because it decreases the amount of radiation reaching the detector, thereby increasing image noise. In addition, the image is distorted, because concentrations of activity deeper in the tissue will appear less intense than the same concentrations nearer to the detector.

In materials with roughly uniform density and composition (e.g., the soft tissue of the body), the effects of attenuation can be predicted, because under these circumstances attenuation causes a simple exponential decrease in the number of photons as a function of distance. That is, if one measures the number of photons at a point in the tissue that are headed in the direction of the detector, then the number of those photons still headed in that direction after travelling x cm in tissue will decrease by a factor $e^{-\mu x}$ where μ is called the *linear attenuation coefficient* or just the attenuation coefficient for short. The attenuation coefficient depends on the energy of the photon and the type of material. It is higher—that is, there is more attenuation—for low-energy photons, and lower (less attenuation) for high-energy photons. A more practical measure of attenuation is the half-value-thickness (HVT), describing that thickness of material which reduces the number of photons by half. HVT can be derived from the attenuation coefficient (HVT = $0.693/\mu$). A selected sample of μ values and HVTs is shown in Table 3.1 for commonly encountered photon energies and materials. As an illustration of the effects of attenuation consider two equally perfused regions, one in the posterior and one in the anterior wall of the left ventricle. The posterior region might be 5 cm further from the chest wall than the anterior region during diastole. With 140 keV photons, less than half as many of the photons from the posterior wall will reach the camera compared to the anterior wall (using the HVT (water) = 4.5 cm in Table 3.1). With 511 keV photons the situation is somewhat improved, while for Tl-201 it is even worse (see Table 3.1 for the corresponding HTV values).

In contrast to the events depicted in Figure 3.2 *b* and *c* that resulted in loss of photons, the events depicted

TABLE 3.1 *Attenuation Values in Water (~Tissue), Lead (Collimator), and NaI (Crystal) for Isotopes Commonly Used in Nuclear Cardiology*

Nuclide	Energy (keV)	μ (water) (1/cm)	μ (lead) (1/cm)	μ (NaI) (1/cm)	HVT (water) (cm)	HVT (lead) (cm)	HVT (NaI) (cm)
Tl-201	71	0.18	20.38	14.44	3.85	0.034	0.048
Tc-99m	140	0.15	24.75	2.62	4.50	0.028	0.265
Fl-18 (β+)	511	0.10	1.69	0.34	7.10	0.410	2.050

μ, coefficient of linear attenuation; HVT, half-value thickness.

in *d* result in image distortion due to scattering. By understanding a little more about how Compton scattering works, it is possible to see how one might reduce this distortion. In Compton scattering the gamma ray interacts with one of the electrons that surround the nuclei of the atoms in the medium. Usually the interaction is with an outer shell electron. When the gamma ray strikes the electron the impact causes the gamma ray to be deflected in a new direction, with reduced energy. The larger the angle of deflection, the greater is the energy lost by the incident gamma ray [1]. The top half of Table 3.2 shows the energy loss (ΔE) resulting from a photon scattering through 30° (top three rows) for three different incident energies. The more energetic the incident photon, the larger the fraction of its energy (ΔE%) it loses in a collision for a given angle. As will be described in more detail later, this energy loss provides a way to discriminate those photons that have *not* scattered (those with all their energy) from those that *have* scattered (those with reduced energy). This discrimination is performed with an "energy window" that rejects those photons whose energy has been reduced by more than 10% (typically). The bottom three rows in Table 3.2 show how big a scattering angle is required for a photon to lose 10% of its energy. Low-energy photons (e.g., Tl-201) must scatter through a

very large angle (78°) before losing more than 10% of their energy. High-energy photons such as those from F-18 have to scatter only 27° to suffer a 10% reduction in energy. In addition, the probability of scattering in tissue increases with decreasing energy. For both these reasons scatter is a worse problem at low energies (e.g., for Tl-201) than for higher energies (e.g., Tc-99m) and a still smaller problem for the positron annihilation photons (e.g., F-18 FDG). Because scattering involves interaction with electrons, the higher the number of electrons in the material (e.g., higher density or more total volume), the more scatter will be incurred. Therefore bone scatters more than soft tissue and obese subjects produce more scattered radiation than thin subjects.

An example of the effects of scattering in an image is seen in Figure 3.3. It shows an image of two line-shaped sources of radioactivity contained in two plastic tubes. The square pattern around the sources is not radioactivity; it is scattered radiation from the Plexiglas frame holding the line sources.

TABLE 3.2 *Energy Loss and Scattering Angle of Selected Photons*

Nuclide	Initial Photon Energy (keV)	Energy Loss (ΔE in keV)	ΔE (%)	Scattering Angle
Same angle				
Tl-201	71	1.3	1.8	30°
Tc-99m	140	5.0	3.6	30°
Fl-18 (β+)	511	60.7	11.9	30°
Same %ΔE				
Tl-201	71	7.1	10.0	78°
Tc-99m	140	14.0	10.0	54°
Fl-18 (β+)	511	51.1	10.0	27°

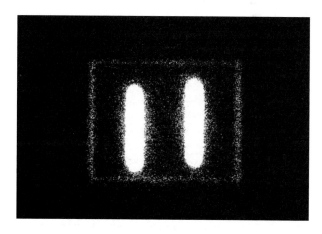

FIGURE 3.3 Image of two line sources of Tc-99m showing scattered radiation from the nonradioactive plastic holder (squared shadow around the sources). (The intensity of the scattered radiation is relatively small compared to the intensity of the line sources. To show both scattered radiation and line sources in the same image, the brightness range was set to allow visualization of the scattered counts and therefore the line sources appear saturated.)

In summary, gamma cameras are designed to make an accurate image representing the number of photons leaving the body. It is assumed that the number of photons leaving the body represents the distribution of the radiopharmaceutical within the body. This assumption is true only if the photons travel from their origin in the body to the detector without interactions. However, attenuation and scatter violate this assumption and prevent the image produced by the gamma camera from reflecting the distribution of radioactivity within the body. One must be aware of these effects and must provide methods (to be described later) for correction or compensation if one intends to preserve the proportionality between tissue activity and its representation in the image.

COLLIMATION

After emerging from the patient's body, the photons must pass through the collimator. To understand why a collimator is necessary, consider a gamma camera without a collimator, as shown in Figure 3.4A. Imagine that an incident gamma ray has just produced a flash of light in the crystal, as shown. The photomultiplier tubes can tell quite accurately where in the crystal the flash of light occurred. Unfortunately, this piece of information tells us nothing about where the gamma ray came from. Since there is no collimator, the gamma ray producing the flash of light could have come from almost any direction, as shown by lines *a*, *b*, and *c* in Figure 3.4A. The collimator limits the photons striking the detector to only those coming from a certain direction—for example, blocking all photons except those perpendicular to the crystal face. The collimator in Figure 3.4B does exactly this. It is made of lead, and it is clear that now photons *a* and *c* will be excluded, while photon *b* will be accepted. When the position of the flash of light is computed by the photomultiplier tubes one can deduce that the radioactive source must lie somewhere on a line perpendicular to the camera face and passing through the point at which the flash of light was detected (Fig. 3.4B, photon *b* and dotted line).

As mentioned, the collimator shown in Figure 3.4B is the most common collimator type for nuclear cardiology, a "parallel-hole" collimator [2]. It is usually made in the form of a honeycomb of parallel holes with hexagonal, square, or circular cross section. The accepted photon trajectories are only those closely parallel to the holes. The image produced by this collimator has the same dimensions as the object; it preserves its orientation and does not introduce any image size changes or geometric distortion. Figure 3.5 shows a

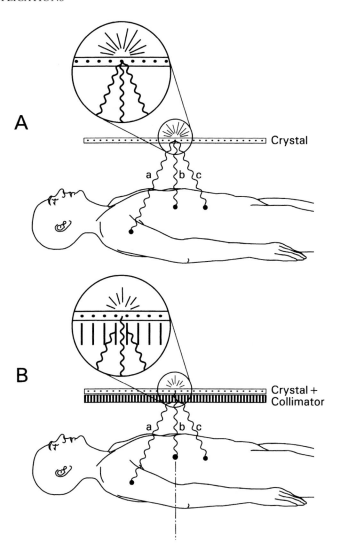

FIGURE 3.4 Effect of a collimator. (*A*) Without collimator, photons incident on a given point in the crystal will cause scintillations regardless of their trajectory and no image is formed. (*B*) The presence of a parallel-hole collimator excludes non-image-forming photons (*a* and *c*) from the imaging process while the image-forming photon (*b*) is allowed to reach the crystal (inset).

more detailed view of several of the collimator holes. Any gamma rays traveling within the cone shown will pass through the collimator and strike the crystal. The conical shape of this volume has fundamental consequences on the two most important attributes of a collimator, namely, its resolution and its sensitivity.

Resolution describes how well the camera is able to distinguish two closely spaced objects as separate entities. The resolution of the gamma camera is the combination of two parts: the resolution of the collimator and the resolution of the crystal/photomultiplier (PM) tube assembly. That is, the gamma camera resolution

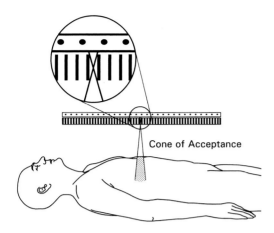

FIGURE 3.5 A detailed view of a collimator hole showing the conical shape of the photon-accepting region. Any photon with all its trajectory within that cone will be considered image-forming and will reach the crystal. The width of the cone, therefore, represents the inherent uncertainty in the direction of a photon passing through a collimator hole. The larger the distance from the collimator, the wider is the cone, the more uncertain is the direction. The cone shown is exaggerated in size for illustrative purposes.

is determined by how accurately the collimator selects the direction of the photons, and how accurately the crystal/PM combination is able to locate the flash of light produced when the gamma ray interacts in the crystal. The ability of the crystal/PM tube combination to determine the position of the flash of light is called the *intrinsic resolution* of the camera. When the intrinsic resolution is combined with the collimator resolution the resultant total resolution is called the *extrinsic resolution*. The resolution of a gamma camera is often measured by imaging a small point source of radioactive material, or a thin line source of radioactivity, as shown in Figure 3.6A. The plot of image intensity versus distance across the point or line (shown at the top in Figure 3.6A) is used to compute the resolution. Resolution is usually defined as the width of this plot at half its maximum height (shown by the arrows in Figure 3.6A). This full width at half maximum height (FWHM) is expressed in distance units (typically millimeters). When one says that a camera has a resolution of, for example, 9 mm, it is understood that the FWHM of the plot shown in Figure 3.6A is 9 mm. The bigger the value the more difficult it will be to distinguish two closely spaced objects as being separate (Fig. 3.6B). Usually the collimator, rather than the crystal and PM tubes, is the dominant factor determining camera resolution.

The *sensitivity* of a gamma camera determines the fraction of photons emitted by a radioactive source (with no attenuation or scatter) that are able to pass through the

collimator and be detected by the crystal/PM tubes. Just as with resolution, the gamma camera sensitivity is the combination of the collimator sensitivity and the crystal sensitivity. Usual units for sensitivity are counts per second per becquerel. It is often measured by placing a source of known activity in front of the gamma camera and then measuring the resultant count rate of the camera. Or, for SPECT or PET cameras, by placing a standard shaped phantom (often a 20 cm diameter cylinder filled with water and radioactivity) in front of the camera and measuring the resultant total count rate. In this case the units of sensitivity are counts $\cdot$ sec^{-1} $\cdot$ Bq^{-1} $\cdot$ cc,

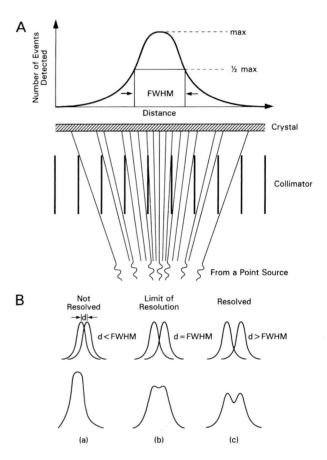

FIGURE 3.6 (A) A plot of count rate vs. position obtained by exposing the camera head to a point source. At any given distance this plot is Gaussian shaped. Ideally, a point source should be 'seen' by only one collimator hole. Instead overlap in the acceptance cones of neighboring holes causes some spillover of counts, affecting the maximum achievable resolution. The distance encompassing count rates larger than half the maximum, or full width at half maximum (FWHM), is a measure of the camera resolution. (B) The count profile of two point sources at three different separations. The two point sources are considered detectable as two separate sources only when they are separated by at least one FWHM (b and c). If the sources are closer than a FWHM, their combined profiles (curves at the bottom) become difficult to distinguish as having arisen from two separate sources.

i.e. counts/sec per activity concentration. For Tc and Tl pharmaceuticals it is the collimator, not the crystal/PM tubes, which plays the dominant role in determining gamma camera sensitivity.

As explained, the collimator is the determining factor of overall gamma camera sensitivity and resolution. Since the nuclear cardiologist or technologist can choose among several types of collimators when performing a study, it is necessary to understand how these choices can influence resolution and sensitivity. Ordinarily one would seek to maximize both sensitivity and resolution. However, the conical shape of the acceptance region for each collimator hole (see Fig. 3.5) creates a conflict between sensitivity and resolution so that one can be improved only at the expense of the other. To see how this happens, one must examine the separate effect of three collimator dimensions: the diameter of the holes, their depth (i.e., the collimator thickness), and the distance between holes or, equivalently, wall thickness (also known as septal thickness). The interplay between these three parameters is illustrated in Figure 3.7 where one can see the effect of depth and diameter on the size and overlap of acceptance cones. For a given depth (Fig. 3.7A), the width of the acceptance cone defines the range of directions that photons may travel and still be able to enter the hole. The narrower this range of possible directions is, the more accurately the collimator can determine from which direction the photons have come. This cone can be regarded as the range of uncertainty about the point of origin of any photon entering a given hole. A narrow cone decreases that uncertainty and hence produces better resolution but at the cost of decreased angle of acceptance and hence lesser sensitivity. The converse would be true for wide cones. With this understanding one can now characterize the collimator designs in Figure 3.7. In Figure 3.7A the collimators both have the same hole depth. The one with the widest hole diameter has the highest sensitivity (and lowest resolution), while the collimator with the smallest diameter has the highest resolution (and lowest sensitivity). In Figure 3.7B the two collimators have different hole depths and diameters, adjusted so that the two collimators have comparable resolution and sensitivity.

Figure 3.7A also reveals a clinically important relationship between collimator–object distance and resolution. Because the cross section of the acceptance cone increases with distance, the region of uncertainty increases. Therefore, the resolution degrades with increasing distance from the collimator and the best resolution is obtained when the patient is as close as possible to the collimator.

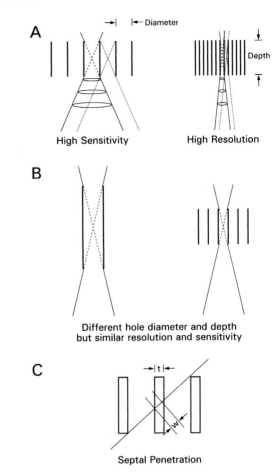

FIGURE 3.7 Effect of collimator hole diameter and depth: (A) Two collimators with same depth but different diameter. The wider holes on the left-hand side provide higher sensitivity as they accept a wider range of trajectory angles but at the cost of poorer resolution. The collimator with narrower holes, to the right, has cones of acceptance that overlap less, has less uncertainty about the point of origination of the photons, and therefore has better resolution than the one on the left. However, the increased resolution comes at the cost of reduced sensitivity. (B) These two collimators have similar sensitivity and resolution by combining different diameter and depths. (C) A third parameter of collimator design is the septal thickness, t. The distance w indicates a possible path for septal penetration by the photon.

For patient to collimator distances typical in cardiac imaging, there is no similar degradation of sensitivity with distance. This may appear surprising, if not counterintuitive, but the reason is simple. Imagine that a certain number of photons are emitted per second from some small region of the heart. When the patient is close to the collimator, a certain number of these photons will go through a particular hole in the collimator. They cannot go through other holes, because the collimator blocks them. As the patient moves further and further from the collimator, fewer and fewer of the photons from this small region of the heart will pass through that particular collimator hole (in fact, as described in Chapter 2, the number will fall off roughly as the square of the distance to the collimator). This one hole will therefore receive fewer photons from this small region of the myocardium as collimator–patient distance increases. However, the cones of neighboring holes will widen at increasing distances, enabling these neighboring holes to accept photons from the same region of the myocardium. The loss of photons in any particular hole with increasing distance is almost exactly compensated for by an ever increasing number of holes able to accept photons (this increasing number of holes is what causes deterioration of resolution with distance). Total sensitivity therefore stays almost constant with increasing patient–collimator distance. Thus resolution degradation, not loss of sensitivity, is the primary concern when increasing the distance between the imaged object and the collimator.

The effects of distance on resolution are shown in the plots in Figure 3.8. This plot highlights the importance of keeping the patient close to the collimator. It is especially important to do so for so-called high sensitivity collimators, since their resolution (by virtue of their large angle cones) falls off most dramatically with collimator–patient distance. Also note from Figure 3.8 that as the imaged plane gets closer to the face of the collimator there is less difference in resolution between the various collimator designs shown. Thus, inasmuch as their resolution deteriorates steeply with distance,

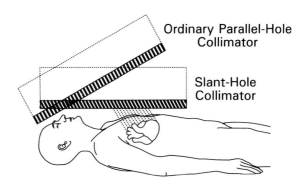

FIGURE 3.9 The slant-hole collimator allows the required tilt for an unobstructed heart view during gated blood pool studies while keeping the face of the collimator close to the patient to preserve resolution.

high-sensitivity collimators are effective only when placed very close to the patient.

One collimator design guided by the above relationships is the *slant-hole parallel collimator* occasionally used for nuclear cardiology applications (Fig. 3.9). A caudal tilt is sometimes desired in planar imaging in order to best separate the left ventricle from the atrium, especially for blood pool scintigraphy. Tilting the camera caudally, however, usually necessitates moving the camera off the chest wall, with a corresponding decrease in resolution. By slanting the holes at an appropriate angle, the face of the collimator can be placed close against the patient's body and yet achieve the caudal tilt desired.

There is an additional collimator dimension to consider in collimator design, namely, the thickness of the wall between holes or septal thickness. Because the septal wall is the point through which undesired photons can penetrate the collimator, its width is an important design consideration. The diagonal dotted line across the two neighboring holes in Figure 3.7C represents a possible path of septal penetration. A reasonable design criterion therefore is to require photon penetration through such a path to be small (e.g., < 5%). Because collimators are made of lead (a high atomic number material), attenuation in collimators is almost entirely due to the photoelectric effect at Tc and Tl energies (Chapter 2). Even for annihilation photons (511 keV) the photoelectric effect dominates. Because the attenuation depends strongly on the energy of the incoming photon, optimal septal thickness will also depend on the energy range for which the collimator will be used.

Septal thickness requirements constrain even further the degree to which depth and diameter can be manipulated to achieve specific imaging needs: the thicker the wall, the smaller the hole diameter (or the larger the hole spacing) and therefore the lower the sensitivity. To meet

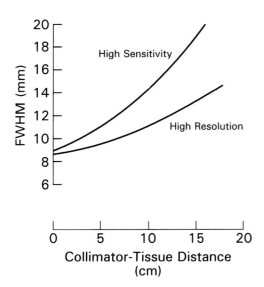

FIGURE 3.8 The effect of distance from the collimator on the resolution of a high sensitivity and a high resolution collimator. Note that although the two collimators have comparable resolution at the collimator surface, the high sensitivity collimator's resolution falls off more rapidly with distance from the collimator face.

the 5% criterion above, the distance w in Figure 3.7C would have to be less than 0.5 mm for the 71 keV Tl-201 emission but 17.3 mm for a 511 keV photon.

Although the discussion has focused on parallel-hole collimators, other types of collimators, such as converging, diverging, and pin-hole collimators, are also used in nuclear imaging. Many of the general concepts described for the parallel-hole collimator can also be applied to other collimator types. The pin-hole collimator, however, is somewhat unique. Pin-hole collimators have the same simple design as their optical counterpart, and their magnifying capabilities are often useful to image the heart in small animals. Converging, diverging, and other similarly modified designs have had, to date, very few applications in clinical cardiac studies.

In summary, the collimator allows only photons traveling from certain directions to reach the detecting crystal. The collimator is usually the most important determinant of image quality. Three critical attributes of a collimator are its spatial resolution, its sensitivity, and its septal penetration. All three characteristics can be adjusted by altering the hole depth, diameter, and the distance between neighboring holes. Except for the slant-hole collimator occasionally used in blood pool studies, nearly all cardiac applications employ only the parallel-hole collimator. When using parallel-hole collimators, it is important to keep in mind that the distance between the surface of the collimator and the patient has important effects on resolution—although not on sensitivity—and this distance should be minimized to obtain optimal resolution.

THE SCINTILLATION CRYSTAL

If a film existed that was sufficiently sensitive to the radiation emitted by Tc-99m or Tl-201 an image could be made simply by placing a sheet of this film behind the collimator. Even if such a film existed, employing it would have numerous significant disadvantages. Instead, the location of the gamma rays emerging from the collimator are detected electronically, with a scintillation crystal and an array of photomultiplier tubes (i.e., an Anger camera).

The role of the scintillation detector is to convert the invisible, elusive gamma rays into more easily manageable visible light radiation. The scintillation crystal is usually a large circular or rectangular crystal of NaI (many tens of centimeters in diameter or length), which has been treated with trace amounts of an impurity (usually non-radioactive thallium). This impurity gives the crystal its desired "scintillation" properties—that is, the crystal emits a flash of visible light whenever radiation of suf-

ficient energy (e.g., a photon from Tl-201 or Tc-99m) interacts in the crystal. Photons striking the crystal may interact through either Compton scattering or by photoelectric effect, just as in the case of tissue. Unlike tissue, however, the most common interaction in the crystal for Tl-201 or Tc-99m radiation is the photoelectric effect. Compton scatter within the crystal plays only a minor role. Thus, most of the gamma or X-rays that strike the crystal disappear and deposit all their energy in the crystal. The energy deposited by the Tl-201 or Tc-99m photons is partially converted by the crystal to a flash of visible light in the blue end of the spectrum (peak emission = 410 nm)—hence the name "scintillation" crystal. The intensity of the flash of light produced by each Tc gamma ray, for example, is directly proportional to the energy deposited by the gamma ray in the crystal. For a photoelectric interaction (the most probable situation) the intensity of the flash of light is directly proportional to the energy of the incident gamma ray: the higher the energy, the brighter the flash. The 140 keV gamma rays from Tc-99m, then, will produce a flash of light that is about twice as bright as the flash produced when a Tl-201 71 keV photon strikes the crystal.

In gamma cameras, the scintillator of choice is a thallium-activated sodium iodide crystal [NaI(Tl)], but other crystals may have similar and in some respects even better properties. NaI(Tl) is chosen because of its high scintillation efficiency (i.e., relative brightness of the flash of light produced per energy deposited by the gamma or X-ray) and its high probability of photoelectric events for 140 keV photons (by virtue of the high atomic number iodine atoms present in the crystal—see Chapter 2), and good stopping power. These attributes are valuable because (1) the quality of an image increases with the total amount of light generated per gamma ray, as will be seen later, and (2) the higher the photoelectric probability the higher the probability that a gamma ray will deposit all of its energy in a single interaction in the crystal, thereby guaranteeing that the flash of light will be produced exactly behind the corresponding collimator hole. One disadvantage of NaI is that it is hydroscopic—that is, if left exposed to the air, the crystal absorbs moisture and quickly deteriorates. Therefore all NaI crystals must be encapsulated in a sealed container (often a thin "can" of aluminum).

THE PHOTOMULTIPLIER ARRAY: EVENT LOCALIZATION AND SPATIAL RESOLUTION

The scintillation crystal converts the collimator-projected gamma ray image into a visible image. By standing in a dark room behind the crystal it would in theory be possible to actually see the flashes of light produced when each gamma ray interacted in the crystal, and in principle to see the image of the distribution of the photons emitted by the body (although each flash of light is exceedingly faint). Instead, an array of light-sensitive detectors is placed behind the scintillation crystal. The particular kind of photodetectors used in most gamma cameras are called photomultiplier (or PM) tubes. They are not the only type of photodetectors and not even the most modern, yet they continue to best combine three crucial properties: sensitivity, speed, and low cost. Photomultiplier tubes produce an electronic pulse each time they are exposed to a flash of light. The magnitude (e.g., voltage) of this electronic pulse is proportional to the intensity of the flash and therefore to the energy deposited in the crystal (which, in turn, for photoelectric interactions, is proportional to the energy of the incident gamma ray). In this way, each photomultiplier produces one electrical pulse for each gamma ray that interacts in the crystal, and the size of that pulse is proportional to the amount of light seen by the PM tube.

Gamma cameras typically use many tens of photomultiplier tubes (often 50 or more depending on the field of view and manufacturer) arranged in a close-packed array (e.g., hexagonal). The output of all the photomultiplier tubes is used to determine the location of the flash of light in the crystal. The tube seeing the most light must be closest to the location of the scintillation. By examining (electronically) the relative amount of light seen by each PM tube, an accurate determination of the position of the light flash can be made. To increase the probability that each flash in the crystal is exposed to as many photomultipliers as possible, these latter are placed at a slight distance from the scintillation crystal through an optically coupled glass plate known as *light pipe*. The thickness of the light pipe must be carefully chosen—if it is too thick all the PM tubes will see nearly the same amount of light. It may seem surprising that this relatively small number of photomultipliers is sufficient to precisely locate the flash of light produced in the scintillation crystal. The localization process is one of the fundamental ideas behind Anger's invention of the gamma camera. This process is illustrated in Figure 3.10. In panel *A* the flash has occurred exactly in front of photomultiplier #5, so, photomultiplier #5 produces the largest pulse. Photomultipliers #4 and #6 also receive light, in lesser amount as they are farther away from the flash, but they receive it in equal amounts as they are equally far from the flash. Similarly for PMs #3 and #7. Since PM #5 sees the largest amount of light, and each symmetric pair of PM tubes surrounding PM #5 sees exactly

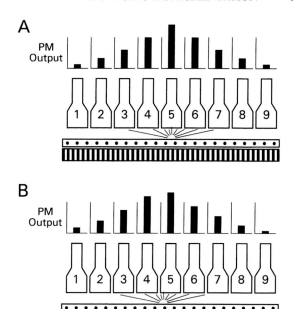

FIGURE 3.10 One-dimensional illustration of the event localization process. (*A*) Symmetric response of neighboring photomultipliers as a photon strikes the crystal at a point exactly centered under photomultiplier #5. (*B*) Asymmetric photomultiplier response as the photon strikes slightly to the left of photomultiplier #5. A weighted, spatial average of the photomultiplier outputs determines the exact location of the event in either case.

the same amount of light, then the Anger positioning circuitry is able to tell that the light flash (and therefore the gamma ray interaction) occurred in a position exactly centered on PM #5. Similarly for the other rows of PM tubes. If the flash of light occurred just a few millimeters to the left of the center of PM #5 (Fig. 3.10*B*) then PM #5 would still see the most light, but now PM #4 would see slightly more light than PM #6, indicating that the flash occurred slightly closer to PM #4 than to PM #6. The positioning circuits in the Anger camera compute this new position based on the relative inequality of light seen by PMs #4 and #6, as well as all other surrounding PM tubes. Although the localization process has been illustrated in one dimension, one may visualize the exact same process applied to the entire two-dimensional array of photomultipliers in order to obtain the position (coordinates) of the event along both the *x* and the *y* axes.

The accuracy with which the Anger arithmetic can determine the position of the flash of light (and hence the position of the gamma ray interaction) is referred to as the "intrinsic" resolution of the camera. Typically this resolution might be 3–6 mm FWHM—clearly much better than the resolution of the collimator. The total resolution of the camera (crystal, PM tubes, and collimator), i.e., the "extrinsic" resolution, can be computed as:

Total Extrinsic Resolution (FWHM)

$$= \sqrt{FWHM^2_{CRYSTAL\ and\ PM's} + FWHM^2_{COLLIMATOR}}$$

ENERGY DETECTION

For a given flash of light, the amount of light seen by any one phototube will depend on where the flash occurred. However, by summing all the outputs of the PM tubes, an electronic pulse can be produced whose size is proportional to the total amount of light present in the flash, independent of where the flash occurred (there are some difficulties near the crystal edge, and for this reason reflective coatings are often applied to the crystal edges). This total amount of light is proportional to the energy of the gamma ray (providing it had a photoelectric interaction and therefore deposited all its energy in the crystal). Ideally, every time a 140 keV gamma ray struck the crystal (and had a photoelectric interaction) it would produce an equally bright flash of light and therefore the same size "total summed" electronic pulse. In reality, imperfections in the whole system (mostly the PM tubes) cause the size of the electronic pulse to vary slightly from one 140 keV gamma ray to the next.

Consider 10,000 140 keV gamma rays striking the crystal and all having photoelectric interactions. If a plot were made showing the number of electronic pulses seen by the PM tubes (i.e., the number of light flashes) versus the size of the electronic pulse (i.e., the total summed amount of light produced) it would look as shown in Figure 3.11. Figure 3.11A shows the ideal case—all 10,000 electronic pulses are measured to be exactly the same size (i.e., all 10,000 flashes of light are measured to be exactly the same brightness). Figure 3.11B depicts the more realistic case—each flash is detected as having a slightly different total brightness, giving the approximately Gaussian appearance shown, with the location of the peak corresponding on average to the amount of light detected for 140 keV photons. This peak is often called the "photopeak," since it arises from the 140 keV gamma rays that have had photoelectric interactions in the crystal. The histogram plots of number of events versus "energy" (i.e., size of signal) shown in Figure 3.11 are called an "energy spectrum." The full width at half maximum of the photopeak is called the "energy resolution" (not to be confused with the spatial resolution) of the camera. The energy resolution is a measure of the ability of the camera to distinguish different energy

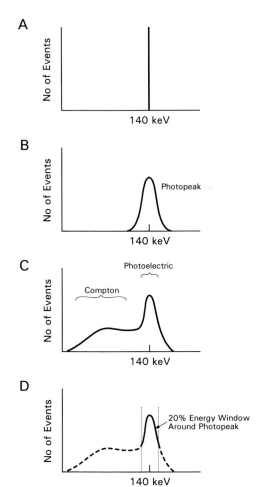

FIGURE 3.11 (A) Ideal spectrum of a Tc-99m emitter (no scattering and perfect energy resolution). (B) Same as A but showing the effects of the finite energy resolution of the crystal/PM tube array. (C) Approximate appearance of an actual spectrum from a patient, showing Gaussian smear due to instrumental uncertainties plus the spectral component of Compton scattering to the left of the photopeak. (D) Part of the spectrum selected electronically by an energy window with a width of approximately 20% of the photopeak.

gamma rays. If the peaks corresponding to two different gamma ray energies are closer together than a distance related to the energy-FWHM then they merge with each other and it becomes impossible to ascertain if one gamma ray is more energetic than the other. In current gamma cameras energy resolutions vary between 10% and 15% at 140 keV [3]. Figure 3.11C shows an even more realistic situation. This energy spectrum is typical of one that might arise from a camera viewing a patient who has been injected with a Tc-99m radiopharmaceutical. It has the characteristic photopeak, but also contains many pulses of smaller size. These smaller size pulses (i.e., the low energy part of the spectrum) correspond mostly to photons that have scattered and therefore have lowered their energy before striking the crystal. The scattering occurs primarily in the patient, but (with a very much smaller probability) can also occur in the detector.

The ability to measure the energy of the photons provides a tool to exclude scattered radiation from the image. By electronically rejecting those pulses that do not occur within the photopeak, scattered, low-energy photons are rejected. To accomplish this, the energy signal (the summed outputs of all the PM tubes) is passed through a narrow *energy window* centered around the peak, as shown in Figure 3.11*D*. This energy window is also sometimes called a single-channel analyzer or pulse height analyzer. Ideally one would make this window as narrow as possible, because photons can scatter at fairly large angles and still lose only a small percentage of their energy (see Table 3.2). Figure 3.11*D* makes it clear that by using such a narrow energy window not only are scattered photons eliminated but also, because of the finite energy resolution of the system, unscattered photons are eliminated. Therefore there is a cost in reduced sensitivity to "good" (unscattered) photons when narrowing the window. A good compromise is to set the energy window to accept all pulses within a 20% window. That is, to accept all pulses whose energy is within ± 10% of the maximum of the photopeak. For Tc-99m this corresponds to accepting only those pulses corresponding to energies between 140 −

14 = 126 keV to 140 + 14 = 154 keV. Again, as noted previously in Table 3.2, this is a compromise. This window still accepts 140 keV photons that have been scattered by as much as 54°. For the lower energy photons emitted by Tl-201, the situation is even worse, and a larger fraction still of scattered photons is accepted with a 20% window. This additional scatter is one of the reasons that myocardial images acquired using Tl-201 appear poorer in quality than those acquired with Tc-MIBI. Despite the above limitations, an appropriate energy window is the first line of defense against the effects of scattering in planar and SPECT imaging.

Once the pulse has passed successfully through the energy window, it is a valid "count"—that is, it represents a valid photon that should be added to the other photons forming the image. The image is represented in the computer as a matrix of points called "pixels" (picture elements). The "intensity" of each point in the image is determined by how many photons were detected at that point. When a pulse is accepted, and the coordinates of the corresponding photon have been computed, the value of the matrix at those coordinates is incremented by one. In cameras with persistence scopes, the passage of the pulse through the energy window causes the scope to be "triggered" on, and the corresponding coordinates on the screen are increased in brightness.

The complete process of forming a planar image is summarized in Figure 3.12. An arbitrary pixel *a* in the

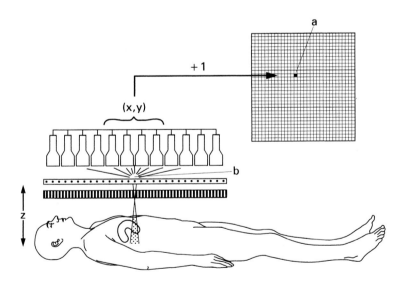

FIGURE 3.12 Summary of the imaging process of a gamma camera. A count contributing to pixel *a* in the image is the result of the photomultiplier arithmetic indicating that a scintillation event was localized at the corresponding *x,y* coordinates in the crystal and that the pulse amplitude fell within the energy window selected. The scintillation, in turn, was the result of a gamma ray originating in the body somewhere in the shaded cone (width exaggerated) with a trajectory fully contained in that cone. Because its energy fell within the window around the photopeak, that photon suffered no (or minimal) scatter as it traveled between the tissue and the crystal.

image is incremented by one whenever a flash occurs in its corresponding region *b* in the crystal. The size of region *b* is determined by the intrinsic resolution of the crystal/photomulitiplier assembly—which is a measure of the uncertainty with which this assembly can locate the flash of light in the crystal. The photons that reach *b* are only those with trajectories within the cone of acceptance of the corresponding hole in the collimator and that end within area *b*. Therefore, the accumulated value of our arbitrary pixel *a* is an indicator of the activity occurring within the entire cross-hatched conical volume depicted in Figure 3.12. Recall that planar images record a two-dimensional projection of a three-dimensional distribution of radioactivity. As such, they delineate the boundaries of the distribution of radioactivity in the *x,y* plane parallel to the collimator but have no geometric information about the *z* or depth dimension. Although the two-dimensional projection can never reveal the full three-dimensional information present in the object, it often contains sufficient information for diagnostic purposes. However, when interpreting planar images one must always keep in mind that they represent a superposition of many planes of varying activity, and that any single planar image provides no information about the depth at which the radioactivity is located.

IMAGE UNIFORMITY AND LINEARITY

Two other gamma camera performance measures, aside from spatial resolution and energy resolution, are important. The first of these is *spatial uniformity*. Spatial uniformity measures the ability of the camera to respond equally over its field of view—that is, whether an image of a uniform distribution of activity appears uniform. Spatial uniformity is important for planar imaging, but it is even more critical for SPECT imaging, as will be seen later (nonuniformities are one of the key causes of SPECT artifacts). The "extrinsic" spatial uniformity (the spatial uniformity with the collimator in place) is often measured by exposing the camera and collimator to a uniform flood of gamma rays. Often a thin, flat sheet of Co-57 imbedded in plastic, slightly bigger than the face of the camera, is used. Alternatively, a shallow, cylindrical plastic container (with diameter greater than that of the camera) is filled with a uniform solution of water and Tc-99m and placed on the surface of the collimator (although it is often awkward to fill and mix such phantoms). The "intrinsic" spatial uniformity (i.e., the uniformity of the crystal/PM tube array alone, without the collimator) can be measured by taking the collimator off and placing a point

source at a large distance (at least five gamma camera diameters) distant from the face of the camera. There are considerable precautions that must be taken to make accurate measurements of intrinsic or extrinsic uniformity, and these are discussed in greater detail elsewhere [4,5]. Intrinsic nonuniformities arise primarily from the inherent problems associated with using an array of photomultipliers to determine the location of each light flash, as will be discussed later. Extrinsic uniformity includes the additional effects of imperfections in the collimator. These imperfections may be inherent to the collimator manufacture or produced inadvertently by, for example, slightly denting the thin array of holes forming the collimator. This is easier to do than one might imagine, as lead is a soft material, and the lead septa are often quite thin.

To quantify uniformity one calculates the maximum difference between any two pixels (after appropriate processing [4]) in the entire field or, more regionally, within small neighborhoods around each pixel in the horizontal or vertical direction. These values, known as integral or differential uniformity, respectively, are expressed as a percentage of the average number of counts. Again, the details of performing these measurements are described in the NEMA [4] and AAPM [5] documents.

There are several factors that influence the intrinsic spatial uniformity of a gamma camera. First, not all the PM tubes will produce the same size output signal when exposed to the same intensity flash of light (although this problem can, in principle, be corrected for by proper gain adjustments of the PM tubes). Even if the response of each tube were identical, if one focused a narrow beam of 140 keV photons at one particular location in the crystal, the resulting photopeak (produced by the sum of all the outputs from all the PM tubes) might not be at exactly the same apparent energy as would be obtained if the narrow beam of radiation were aimed at another location in the crystal. This problem is caused in part by the slightly nonuniform optical response of the PM tube array (e.g., the total light detected by all the PM tubes may be different for a flash produced between two tubes, compared to the same flash produced in the center of a tube, or at the edge of the crystal).

First consider the effect of the energy window on this nonuniformity. Since each region of the crystal produces an energy spectrum whose peak is slightly shifted from every other region, the total energy spectrum produced by a flood source (irradiating the entire crystal) will be the sum of all these individual spectra (Fig. 3.13). If only a single energy window is placed around this total photopeak, as shown in Figure 3.13, this win-

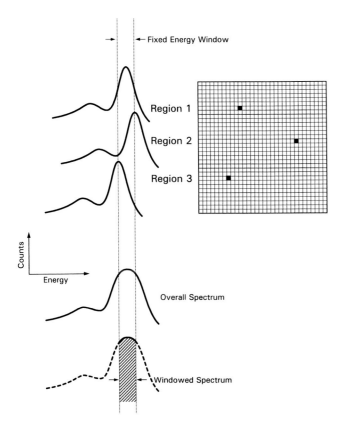

FIGURE 3.13 Effect of nonuniformities in the energy response of the photomultipliers. The energy spectrum at three different locations in the field of view, although from the same isotope, show offset due to gain differences in the corresponding group of photomultipliers. If one single energy window is used the offsets will result in differing numbers of counts at each region, producing intensity nonuniformities in the image. The overall (summed up) spectrum smears out the details present in the local energy spectra and the energy resolution is degraded.

topeaks (or alternatively repositions the photopeaks to fit the window). In this manner, the nonuniformity due to energy response may be nearly eliminated. Depending on the camera, it may be desirable to have a separate energy correction table stored for each isotope, and another still for situations in which it is desired to place an asymmetric window around the photopeak (occasionally done to reduce scatter).

After the energy correction has been performed, there is a second source of nonuniformity that must be corrected for. This nonuniformity is caused by spatial nonlinearities in the camera. That is, if one images a line, the image of the line may not be perfectly straight, and instead may have small curves in it. A nonlinearity by itself would not be that critical to nuclear cardiac imaging—it would produce only small distortions in the image. Unfortunately, these nonlinearities also cause nonuniformities. If a large number of parallel line sources were imaged, the image of each line would have a small wavelike pattern in it. Depending on where the lines are in relation to the PM tubes, the waves in the lines may bunch together (forming erroneously hot regions) or bow away from each other (forming cold regions). Thus the nonlinearity (which by itself may be tolerable) results in nonuniformities which are not acceptable. Again, a computer can be used to correct for this effect. A special phantom (often a so-called orthogonal hole phantom) is imaged. This phantom may have a matrix, for example, of holes lined up in straight lines. The computer measures how the image of the position of these hole deviates from the known (straight) position of the holes in the phantom, and stores the pattern of this deviation. During clinical imaging, when a gamma ray is detected and its position determined, the computer adjusts this position using the known deviations at that location. The photons from what would be erroneously hot regions are not removed; they are just repositioned back to where they belong.

Finally, a third correction table is often used to compensate for nonuniformities introduced by the collimator (one table for each collimator). First, the above-mentioned energy and linearity corrections must be made. Then, with the collimator in place, a uniform source of activity, commonly a flat sheet of Co-57, is used to acquire a flood image. A carefully acquired image of a flood with adequate total counts is itself an inverse map of the correction factors to be used to achieve spatial uniformity for a given collimator: if one pixel appears systematically brighter in a flood image, then the values of that pixel in any other image using the same collimator must be dimmed in the same proportion. The resulting table is sometimes called the collimator uniformity table. This collimator flood correc-

dow will not be uniformly positioned about many of the individual photopeaks making up the total. This means that in some regions of the crystal a larger fraction of the photopeak will be accepted than in others—causing the resultant image to be erroneously brighter or dimmer in certain regions (i.e., to be spatially nonuniform). To correct for this, manufacturers often build into their cameras a so-called energy correction. One way this correction might work is by having the user place a point source at a distance from the camera face (with no collimator). A computer then acquires an energy spectrum at many different locations across the crystal. The location of each of the regional photopeaks is recorded as well as the overall summed photopeak. Although the user may still place a single energy window around the overall summed photopeak, the computer repositions that window to be properly centered around each of the individual regional photion should only be performed after it is assured that the intrinsic uniformity is within specified limits (i.e., after proper energy and nonlinearity corrections have been made). Because an energy uniformity calibration would affect the linearity and the collimator uniformity tables, calibration must respect this order of precedence: energy, linearity, and collimator.

Daily images of flat, uniform sources, such as Co-57 foil floods, are used as quality control for camera uniformity. They would reveal any major departure from uniformity. They can be read visually but, preferably, they should be quantified as described earlier.

COUNT RATE AND DEAD TIME

A gamma camera detects one gamma ray at a time. Therefore, an indicator of gamma camera performance that must be considered is the ability of the camera to perform at high count rates. This ability is usually described by a parameter known as *dead time*. After any photon strikes the crystal there is a small period of time (called the dead time) during which the system will be unable to properly process another photon. Dead time can be caused by many factors. For example, if two photons were to strike the crystal at nearly the same time, the two flashes of light they produce might not be distinguishable by the PM tubes and associated electronics as two separate flashes of light, but rather as one large flash of light. Such an event might be rejected by the energy window. Similarly, if two distinguishable flashes of light both produce very closely spaced (in time) electrical pulses, it is possible that the electronics (e.g., the energy window) might be busy processing the first pulse and therefore miss the second pulse. For these and similar reasons, a plot of activity versus count rate, as shown in Figure 3.14, is not linear at high-activity levels. The camera can behave in one of two general ways as it is exposed to increasing activity levels. The observed count rate may simply flatten out (as shown by the solid line in Figure 3.14), so that further increases in injected activity produce no further increase in count rate. A camera system that exhibits this behavior is often called a "nonparalyzable" system. Alternatively, as shown by the dashed line in Figure 3.14, the measured count rate may reach a peak and then actually *fall* with increasing activity. A system showing this behavior is referred to as "paralyzable." In either case it is important to know at what observed count rates the camera begins to function nonlinearly, as this will adversely affect its clinical performance. Detailed information about how to determine dead time can be found in the appropriate NEMA [4] and AAPM [5] documents. One

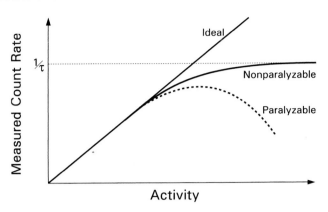

FIGURE 3.14 Effects of a finite dead time (τ) on the measured count rate from a paralyzable and a nonparalyzable system.

rough but quick way to make the measurement, and which demonstrates the concept of dead time, is called the *two source* method. A source is placed near the detector and the count rate determined (CR1). Then a second source is placed near the first and the count rate determined with both sources in place (CR12). Finally, the first source is removed and the count rate of the second source alone is measured (CR2) (making the measurements in this order minimizes the effects of source positioning). In a system with no dead time, the sum of the count rates from the two individual sources would exactly equal the count rate obtained with both sources. In fact, the count rate when both sources are present will be slightly less than the sum of the individual sources due to dead time. After correcting the values for decay, dead time (τ) can be estimated as*:

$$\tau = \frac{CR1 + CR2 - CR12}{CR12^2 - CR1^2 - CR2^2}$$

The source strengths are best chosen roughly equal, and such that there are around 10%–30% losses.

Dead time is usually specified in μsec. Three to 10 μsec might be typical (the smaller the better). If the measured count rate during a cardiac study is known, the percentage counts that are being lost to dead time can be roughly estimated as:

$$\% \text{ of counts lost} \approx 100^* \text{ CR} * \tau$$

where CR is the measured count rate and τ is the dead time defined above.

Note that this approximate formula should be used only when the counting losses are roughly 20% or less.

*For a nonparalyzable system. For paralyzable systems alternative expressions are available (see Sorenson and Phelps [1]).

As an example, if the count rate of a MIBI study is 20,000/sec, and the camera dead time is 6 μsec (quite a typical value), then

% counts lost
$$= 100 * (20{,}000/\text{sec}) * (6*10^{-6} \text{ seconds}) = 12\%$$

This means that 12% of the radioisotope given to the patient is producing radiation exposure to the patient, but not producing any counts. For a SPECT study the losses may vary at different angles around the patient, which as will be seen in the section which follows, may produce artifacts. For first-pass studies count rates can be much higher, and dead time effects can be quite severe. As seen in Chapter 18, dead time may be the limiting factor in being able to use a gamma camera to perform coincident positron emission tomography (PET) imaging.

TOMOGRAPHY WITH SINGLE-PHOTON EMITTERS (SPECT): INSTRUMENTATION

The term *tomography* refers to the process of producing a three-dimensional cross section (i.e., a "slice") of an object. In single-photon emission computed tomography (SPECT), as well as in positron emission tomography (PET), computed tomography (CT), and to some extent magnetic resonance (MR), this process is based on the use of multiple planar projection images acquired at various angles around the object. It is intuitively evident that one way to gain knowledge about the three-dimensional structure of an object is to view it from different angles. This is how the human eye–brain combination creates three-dimensional views of the world. Even with a limited number of angles (two—one from each eye) humans are able to "reconstruct" in their brains a partial three-dimensional representation of an object from this pair of two-dimensional views ("projections"). Less intuitive but also true is the fact that, with penetrating radiation, one can achieve a numerically accurate representation of a tomographic slice from a finite collection of projections or views taken along planar orbits around the object. The gamma camera can obtain such planar views. Therefore, in an effort to gain the advantages of three-dimensional imaging compared to two-dimensional planar imaging (no superimposition of organs, improved contrast, etc.) gamma cameras are mounted on a gantry capable of moving the detector around the patient.

There are three basic motivations for pursuing tomography. First, it allows the three-dimensional localization and visualization that is lacking in planar images. Second, by allowing the three-dimensional delineation of anatomically distinct volumes (i.e., avoiding the problems of superimposed structures) it becomes possible to pursue quantification of activity in absolute terms, that is, in units such as μCi/ml. Third, and perhaps most important, tomography produces increased image contrast, one of the most important factors in diagnostic sensitivity. This last advantage can be understood with the help of Figure 3.15. Consider the large cube of 20 cm on each side shown in this figure as a crude model of a thin patient's chest. For simplicity, attenuation effects will be ignored. The small 1 cm cube inside the patient can be thought of as a tumor, or a small region of the myocardium. Imagine that this "patient" is injected with a new radiopharmaceutical that localizes to the tumor (or myocardium) with a 10 to 1 ratio of myocardium/background. Very few real radiopharmaceuticals are able to achieve such a high target to nontarget ratio. The uptake of the compound in the 1 cm tumor or myocardium might then be 10 μCi/cc while in the rest of the tissue it is only 1 μCi/cc—a 10 to 1 uptake ratio. The image produced by the gamma camera indicated in the figure, is shown at the left. One can easily deduce that a pixel representing the activity from the background area surrounding the "hot" spot reflects the counts produced by 20 cm thick patient $\times$ 1 μCi/cm^3 or 20 μCi/cm^2. A pixel from the "hot" area will, on the other hand, reflect the activity of the superimposed overlying and underlying background (19 cm $\times$ 1 μCi/cm^3 = 19 μCi/cm^2) plus the piece of myocardium itself (1 cm $\times$ 10 μCi/cm^3 = 10 μCi/cm^2) or a total of 19 + 10 = 29 μCi/cm^{-2}. Thus, the image contrast between the hot and the surrounding tissue is 29/20. Despite the fact that the uptake ratio was 10 to 1, the two-dimensional planar image does not even achieve a 1.5 to 1 contrast! If instead one were able to eliminate the superimposed background volumes in front of and behind the hot spot by creating a *tomographic* slice through this hot spot (bottom, Fig. 3.15) then the image contrast would match the 10 to 1 ratio of the pharmaceutical uptake.

Image reconstruction is the name of the process one uses to generate the three-dimensional representations (i.e., the slices) of activity from multiple two-dimensional projections. A later chapter deals more extensively with this topic, but the basics are discussed here because the reconstruction process interacts strongly with issues related to instrumentation. Reconstruction is typically performed using one of two approaches, both based on the mathematical fact that an infinite number of two-dimensional projections around an object (e.g., around an axis through the body running from head to feet) can be combined to synthesize any

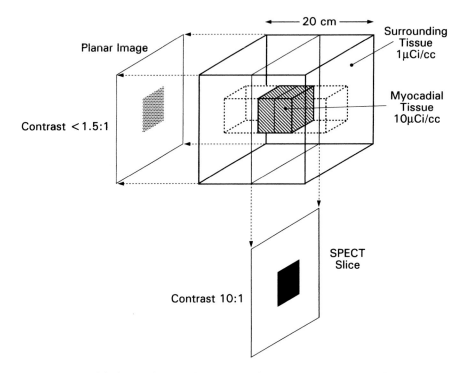

FIGURE 3.15 This model of tissue illustrates how tomography improves contrast. The planar image shown at the top left superimposes on the 'hot' area the background activity in front and behind (prism outlined with a dotted line) reducing the relative difference between hot and surrounding areas and therefore the contrast. In the tomographic slice shown below the hot area does not include background and thus the true, local difference in uptake is translated into actual image contrast. (For clarity, the small 1 cm per side cube representing the heart tissue is not drawn to scale.)

view of that object. The situation is more complicated when attenuation is present (which it always is), so for the moment the effects of attenuation will be ignored. The first method of tomographic reconstruction is an analytic method—that is, a formula allows the gamma camera views taken around the body (i.e., the projections) to be used to compute the intensity values of every pixel in the tomographic slice. The second method attempts to determine the intensity values of every pixel in the tomographic slice, using an iterative approach. Iterative methods are based on making a series of educated guesses as to what the slice might look like. Each successive guess is then designed to be a slight refinement of the previous guess, so that ultimately the guesses approach the true solution.

The idea behind the reconstruction process is illustrated in Figure 3.16, in which a number of gamma camera images (i.e., projections) of four spherical objects are shown. Two of the objects have intensity of 150 and two have intensity of 50. If one had taken only a lateral and anterior projection image (e.g., the 0° and 90° projections in Figure 3.16), it would not even be clear that there were four objects—there equally well could have been only two objects of intensity 200 each,

for example. Nor would it be clear what the intensity of the objects actually is, even if it were somehow known in advance that there were four objects. The intensities could, for example, be 100 in each object, or 75 in one pair and 125 in the other or any of a number of other possibilities. Obviously there are an infinite number of possible solutions if one takes only two views. When the additional 45° oblique view is taken (Fig. 3.16), the situation becomes a little clearer. From all three views in Figure 3.16 it is now certain that there are at least three objects. Clearly the more views (i.e., the more projections), the more information will be available to understand what the distribution of activity in the object really is. A computer is used to take this information and reconstruct the tomographic slice.

The most widely used analytic solution to the reconstruction problem is based on a concept known as *backprojection*. Consider again the anterior projection from Figure 3.16 reproduced in Figure 3.17*A* without the corresponding images. In the anterior and lateral views, the camera "sees" two spots of 200 counts each as shown by the count profile. As described before, these 200 counts could have come from the superposition of four 50 count objects, or two 100 count objects, or one hun-

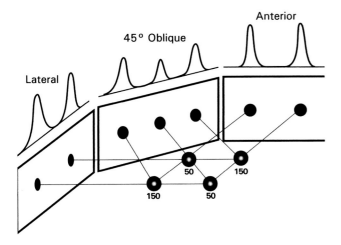

FIGURE 3.16 Rationale of tomographic reconstruction: individually, each of the three planar projections shown gives only an incomplete version of the real objects. The three projections together, while still not sufficient to reconstruct a view of the four objects, indicate that there are at least three objects and give a better idea of their activity. Additional projections will provide additional information necessary to reconstruct a slice view of the objects.

dred 2 count objects, etc. It is totally unknown where these 200 counts come from, except that they come from somewhere along the line of sight of the collimator holes. Lacking any other information, one assumes that the 200 counts are equally likely to have come from anywhere along the path shown in Figure 3.17A. In Figure 3.17B, using the information in the count profiles (total counts and projection angle), shaded lines have been traced into a blank area. The intensity of each shaded line is set proportional to the corresponding total counts seen along this path—200 for the bright areas in the anterior and lateral projections and the corresponding values for the other two views. Each of these shaded lines is called a back-projection line, and the process of producing the lines is called back-projection. In Figure 3.17B it is seen that the back-projection lines all intersect at the location of the hot objects. In general, the hotter lines intersect where the hotter objects were located, and the dimmer lines where the colder objects were located. The superposition of these back-projected lines starts to reconstitute the appearance of the original objects imaged, four objects in this case. This back-projection process could actually be performed (somewhat tediously) with paper and pencil, taking care to shade the lines with intensities proportional to the counts seen at the corresponding position. In practice, of course, a computer performs this task.

The image formed in Figure 3.17B is similar to the original one but is not exactly the same. First, if one examined the relative brightness of the image formed

by the back-projection, the intensities might be inaccurate (although they would be roughly correct). In addition, the presence of all the back-projection lines that do not intersect at the points of activity form a sort of background of streaks. If sufficient angles are taken the streaks will blend together and produce a spatially varying background fog of counts in the image—a background that was not present in the original object. These two problems occur because the reconstruction process described so far is not yet complete. Mathematically it can be shown [6] that the reconstruction process requires two steps. First, the data must be back-projected as described, and second the data must be "filtered" with what is known as a "ramp-filter" (hence the name *filtered back-projection*). A filter is simply a

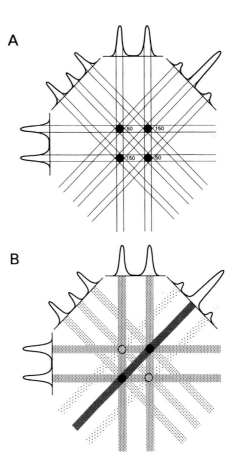

FIGURE 3.17 (A) Same "data" as in Figure 3.16 with an additional view showing only the count profiles. (B) The information in the count profiles (height and projection angle) is used to back-project beams of intensity proportional to the activity in the count profile onto a blank area. The superposition of these beams creates a tomographic view of the objects recorded by the projections. It also leaves a background of streaks to be removed by digitally filtering the image. The larger the number of projections the better the detail (in-plane resolution) and the more homogeneous the background of streaks.

method of averaging neighboring pixels together. Certain pixels may be weighted more heavily than others in the averaging process. A ramp-filter is a pixel averaging scheme that uses certain specified weighting factors (some of which are negative). The process is described in more detail in Chapter 5. After the filtering is done, the background fog is, on the average, removed, and the relative brightness in the image becomes quantitatively accurate. Unfortunately, the weighting factors used to perform the pixel averaging in the ramp-filter (unlike most of the "smoothing" filters used in nuclear medicine) tend to emphasize high-frequency, pixel to pixel, noise. Because of this, additional smoothing filters are also often applied. Because "good" data are mixed with the noise that this last filter seeks to eliminate, use of the smoothing filter trades off quantitative accuracy for a more pleasing, less noisy image. Determining the optimal trade-off between smoothing and noise is not easy, because it depends on the particular features one is interested in preserving in the images. The details of this process are further discussed in Chapter 5 and are important to understand in order to be able to optimize image quality and diagnostic efficacy with SPECT (or PET).

The second method of image reconstruction is the iterative method mentioned earlier. This method seems more empirical, but it has been shown that after sufficient properly modified "guesses," the process will converge to the correct reconstructed slice. The first guess for the reconstructed image is usually that the total activity is uniformly distributed everywhere in the image (this at least is an unbiased guess). The projection data that would be obtained from this first guess are then computed, and these projections are compared to those from the measured data. The difference between the projections from the guessed image and the original projections is obtained. Based on this difference a modified set of images is produced. The improved image is again projected, repeating the process as necessary in the hope that the consecutive images will gradually converge to the true image data. One difficulty with the method is knowing when to stop. If one stops too early in the process, the final guess will not have converged to the true image. On the other hand, each new guess takes additional computer time (and, under some circumstances, may produce images with increased noise). The iterative method is attractive because there are methods of including within the reconstruction process the effects of scatter, attenuation (see Chapters 5 and 7), and other imperfections in the imaging system. Such corrections are often crucial to efficacious SPECT imaging. The downside of iterative reconstruction is that it is computationally lengthy.

With this elementary explanation of the reconstruction process, it is now possible to explain how problems with instrumentation can affect the reconstruction process. Unfortunately, the reconstruction process often tends to amplify what were only small imperfections in the planar projection images, producing far more severe artifacts in the reconstructed SPECT slices. For this reason several aspects of the instrumentation require increased attention in SPECT. These include spatial uniformity of the camera, collimator selection, axis of rotation errors (which of course are unique to SPECT), and the effects of scatter and attenuation.

Nearly all the common artifacts observed in SPECT are due to a phenomenon known as *inconsistent projections*. For example, if two projection images both view the same object from two different angles (and if we continue to assume there is no attenuation), the two images should have the same total counts. If they do not, the projections are inconsistent. An example of inconsistent projections in visual imaging would be if when looking at a person, your left eye saw a person with a large nose while your right eye (a view which is at a slightly different projection angle) saw a person with a small nose. The two views are inconsistent, and our eye–brain computer could not make a meaningful "reconstruction" of the three-dimensional appearance of such a person. One (of many) common artifacts that inconsistent projections produce are "ring" artifacts. These are often caused by nonuniformities in the planar gamma camera response.

In planar imaging detector uniformity is important to preserve the proportionality between measured activity and brightness in the image but these nonuniformities are often only barely detectable by visual examination of a flood image, and generally do not have a significant impact on nonquantitative clinical planar images. In SPECT, however, these same small nonuniformites are amplified by the filtered back-projection process, producing significant artifacts. Figure 3.18 illustrates schematically how this happens. In this figure, the gamma camera is assumed to have perfectly uniform response, except for one small area of increased response, as shown. In a planar image this very small erroneously hot region, while detectable, would probably be lost in the image noise. However, in acquiring a SPECT study, one rotates the camera around the patient. Assume the rotation is circular about a fixed center of rotation, as shown in the figure. Then each of the large number of projection images of the uniform cylinder being imaged in the figure will have this same slightly hot spot in exactly the same location, forming a ring of slightly (erroneously) hot activity. If this hot ring of activity were really present in the object, then

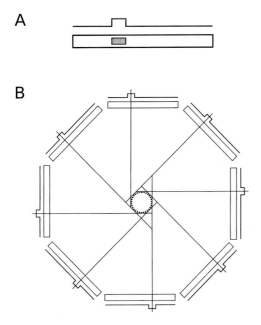

FIGURE 3.18 (*A*) Count profile across a uniform flood (shown in two dimensions only). The camera has a small region of nonuniformity (an overresponsive area). (*B*) When the overresponsive activity is back-projected, it forms a ring of erroneously hot activity in the reconstructed slice.

all the other projections would see the activity from this ring at many locations in the projection data (over a region as wide as the diameter of the ring). Since the hot ring is not really present in the object, the projection images do not see its activity over its diameter, and so the data are inconsistent. The net result is that the nonuniformity is much more apparent in the reconstructed image than it is in the planar image and manifests itself not as a small hot spot, but as a very noticeable, artifactual ring of activity.

The appearance of these telltale artifacts can be seen in the example shown in Figure 3.19. If the planar nonuniformity is near the center, the ring diameter will be small (and its intensity brighter), while if the nonuniformity is nearer the detector edge, the diameter will be larger. Even if the camera is capable of producing quite uniform images, if the correction flood (e.g., the extrinsic flood) has insufficient counts, the noise in the resulting correction factors can also produce ring artifacts in exactly the same manner as described above. For this reason, great care must be taken to follow established guidelines on the acquisition of such floods.

Another source of instrument-produced artifacts results from improper center of rotation correction in the SPECT camera. The detectors can rotate about the patient in either a circular orbit an elliptical orbit, or an even more complex orbit with the radius of rotation

changing to keep the collimator as close as possible to the patient. In all of these cases it is essential that the computer know the exact center of rotation (or its equivalent), and that this center not drift from its predicted position due to mechanical imperfections. Consider the simple case of a gantry that rotates the camera in an orbit with fixed or varying radius. The center of rotation (COR) can be determined by imaging a small source placed so that it appears near the center in all projections. If an anterior view of the source produces an image with the hot spot at pixel 120, and a posterior view produces a hot spot at pixel 136, then the center of rotation must be located midway between the two values: (120 + 136)/2 = 128. This center of rotation should be constant for all projection angles. If the gantry is not in perfect mechanical condition, the weight of the heads may cause them to droop at certain angles, and a left lateral and right lateral view of the same object may not predict the center to be at 128. This center of rotation shift will produce inconsistent projections, resulting in characteristic artifacts in the reconstructed images—point sources, for example, may appear as slightly distorted donuts. Departures of even a pixel could produce visible artifacts. It is necessary both that the COR be constant and that it be precisely known by the computer software. Each manufacturer provides a method to determine the COR and ensure its constancy, usually based on taking views of a slightly off center source from all angles. In a well-aligned detector/gantry, the projected (not reconstructed) images should show the test object moving across the field in a perfectly sinusoidal pattern centered around a line across the center of the image.

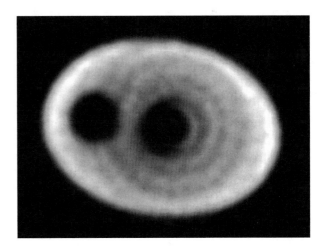

FIGURE 3.19 Ring artifact caused by nonuniformity on an ellipsoidal-shaped phantom with uniform activity and two cylindrical cold inserts. The projections were obtained with a single detector and thus form complete rings. Such rings are centered on the axis of rotation of the detector head.

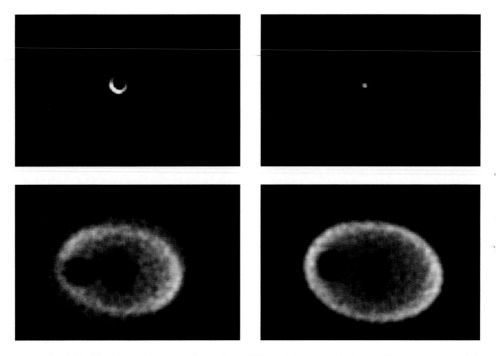

FIGURE 3.20 (A) The effects of center of rotation (COR) misalignment (1.4 cm off) on a tomographic slice of a line source (top) and of a uniform phantom with two 'cold' cylinders (bottom). (B) The images represent the same objects after realigning the COR.

An example of how a center of rotation artifact would appear in a reconstructed image is shown in Figure 3.20 Most cameras allow limited software-based corrections based on the user's regular monitoring of the constancy of the axis of rotation.

Apart from the instrumentation problems described above, the biggest source of inconsistent projections is attenuation. A view of the heart from the left anterior oblique position will obviously result in far more counts from the heart than a view from, for example, a right posterior oblique position. Such inconsistent projections produce artifacts. Similarly, breast attenuation can cause certain views to have more counts than other views, resulting in characteristic artifacts. Nuclear cardiologists have learned over the years how to "read around" most of these artifacts, but obviously their presence will reduce sensitivity and specificity for the detection of disease. Methods to correct for attenuation have recently been developed, and despite initial difficulties bringing these methods into clinical practice they show much promise, and are discussed in detail in Chapter 7.

As described in Chapter 7, these attenuation correction methods effectively correct the projection counts along a particular projection line for the depth at which the radioactivity lies. For example, in a view in which a particular region of the myocardium lies deep within the soft tissue, the attenuation correction program must increase the counts from that region by $e^{+\mu x}$, where μ is the effective attenuation coefficient of the overlying tissue, and x is the path length traveled by the photon. However, if there are a significant number of scattered photons arriving along this line, these scattered counts will also be amplified by the attenuation correction. Thus even the small number of scattered photons that are accepted by the typical 20% energy window may be considerably amplified by the attenuation correction. For these reasons, instrumentation has been developed to make additional corrections for scattered radiation, above and beyond use of the usual ±10% energy window.

SPECT AND PLANAR IMAGING USING 511 KEV EMITTERS

The positron-emitting compound F-18-deoxyglucose (FDG) has become increasingly available with the development of regional distribution centers (it has a 2 hour half-life). FDG is of great value in the measurement of myocardial viability. Usually this pharmaceutical can only be imaged with a dedicated (and quite expensive) PET system. In recent years, however, it has become possible to image FDG with conventional, or slightly modified gamma camera systems. This can be done in one of two ways. First, the coincident nature of the two photons emitted by F-18 can be ignored, and the compound can be imaged using conventional SPECT techniques, with slightly modified instrumentation to account for the high energy of F-18. Second, two cameras (often facing each other) with their collimators removed, can be used to detect the coincident radiation. Such systems are usually called coincident gamma camera PET (or just gamma camera PET), or sometimes "hybrid" PET. Coincident systems are discussed further in Chapter 18. Here we discuss the instrumentation difficulties of performing FDG SPECT.

Conventional cameras are often optimized to operate with gamma rays in the ~50–350 keV range. Extending their capabilities to higher energy imaging often requires hardware modifications and it is important that the physician understand the impact these modifications may have on the quality of the images.

Positron emitters result in the formation of an annihilation photon pair when the positron interacts with an electron. The two resulting photons travel in almost exactly opposite directions, each with the energy equivalent of the annihilated electron (or positron). That energy is 511 keV and is the same for all positron emitters. Such high-energy photons have much greater penetration in both soft tissue and especially in lead, compared to the 140 keV or 70–80 keV photons used in Tc or Tl imaging, as shown in Table 3.1. On the patient side, this is an advantage because it implies reduced attenuation effects. Also, as was shown in Table 3.2, a larger fraction of the incident energy is lost when a 511 keV photon scatters compared to a 70 or 140 keV photon, for the same scattering angle. In 511 keV single-photon imaging, therefore, there is generally less image degradation due to attenuation and scattering.

SPECT at 511 keV actually has considerably less attenuation than does coincidence imaging (either dedicated PET or gamma camera coincidence PET). This is because for SPECT a single photon has to travel only from the myocardium to the detector, while for coincidence imaging each of the two photons must reach both detectors—an attenuation path equal to the entire thickness of the patient's body.

The high-energy photon causes several problems in the detector and collimator. Collimating 511 keV radiation requires significant increases in septal thickness, which, in addition to imposing substantial weight demands on the gantry, also results in reduced sensitivity and resolution. Conventional "high-energy" collimators such as used for I-131 imaging do not in general have sufficient septal thickness to produce adequate FDG images. Instead one must use ultra high energy collimators that have been specially designed for 511 keV photons, and even these collimators may have significant septal penetration (recall from Collimation that it would take a septal width (w) of more than 17 mm to stop 95% of 511 keV emissions.)

Figure 3.21 shows how septal penetration affects the image of a point source. The count profile on the right shows that the star-shaped halo around the point although extended, contributes relatively few counts to each pixel in the image. The consequences in an actual image are increased background and loss of some contrast but the overall effect is not so severe as to prevent acquiring interpretable images. Typical values of resolution using 511 keV collimators are on the order of 12–18 mm (FWHM) at 10 cm from the camera [7]. Clearly from Figure 3.21 FWHM is probably not an

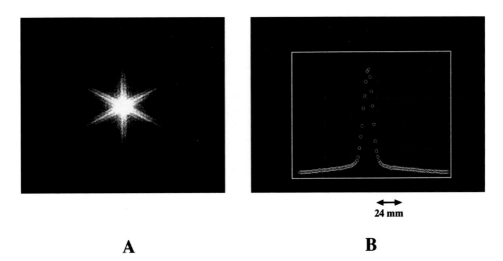

A   **B**

24 mm

FIGURE 3.21 (A) Appearance of a point source with a collimator allowing substantial septal penetration. (B) Count profile showing the relative magnitude of the halo around the point source image caused by septal penetration. This count profile follows a line through the center of the source and along one of the three lines shown in (A) where septal penetration is maximal.

adequate measure of collimator performance. Often resolution is sacrificed for sensitivity in ultra high energy collimator design, especially for cardiac applications. It is argued that because cardiac defects tend to be large, trading resolution for increased sensitivity may be an acceptable practice in cardiac studies [8].

NaI is a nearly ideal material for detection of the 140 keV photons from Tc-99m, and for detection of other low-energy photons used in nuclear medicine. However, the attenuation coefficient of NaI at 511 keV is greatly reduced compared to 140 keV, and while nearly all the interactions in the crystal at 140 keV are photoelectric interactions, many interactions at 511 keV are Compton scattering events. About 75% of 511 keV photons will pass through a conventional 3/8 inch thick crystal without interacting at all (vs. around 9% for a 140 keV Tc-99m photon). Of those 511 keV photons that do interact with the crystal, only about 1 in 20 will be fully absorbed in photoelectric events (compared to nearly all of the 140 keV photons). The large fraction of 511 keV photons that interact through Compton scattering in the crystal means that many photons will deposit less than their full energy at the point of interaction in the crystal (and therefore produce only a weak flash of light at that point). In addition, the photons that have scattered in the crystal have reduced energy, and so have an increased probability for interacting a second or even a third time, producing additional flashes of light at the wrong location. The location assigned to that event will be the average of the position of those simultaneous flashes of light causing degraded resolution. This factor must be considered when deciding to purchase a crystal with increased thickness in order to stop more of the 511 keV photons. Nonetheless, it is often beneficial to increase crystal thickness, although beyond a certain thickness low-energy image resolution also begins to degrade [9].

One instrumentation advantage of imaging the 511 keV annihilation photons is that their higher energy will produce brighter flashes in the crystal, resulting in better intrinsic resolution and better energy resolution. As mentioned previously, this better energy resolution translates into increased scatter rejection. A second important advantage of FDG SPECT (compared to either gamma camera or dedicated coincidence imaging) is that two different isotopes can be imaged simultaneously, since they can be distinguished by their respective energies. Therefore, simultaneous perfusion and metabolic imaging (e.g., with F-18 FDG and Tc-99 MIBI) can be performed, provided that a suitable correction is made for the 511 keV photons that down scatter into the 140 keV window. Of course the requirement to use an ultra high energy collimator results in reduced sensitivity and resolution at 140 keV, compared to what could be obtained with a low-energy–high-resolution collimator. Still, the technique shows much promise [10] and may prove to be an important advantage over coincidence imaging techniques.

Because of the interest in using gamma cameras to image 511 keV photons, other crystal compositions have recently been investigated. Several promising compounds have been developed based on lutetium (Lu), such as lutetium ortho silicate (LSO). This material produces a little less light per unit of energy deposited than NaI, but its high effective atomic number and density gives it a considerably increased stopping power for high-energy photons. Because of its high effective Z, a larger percentage of high-energy photons that interact in LSO do so by the photoelectric effect, compared to NaI. In addition, the crystal produces a faster flash of light (i.e., one that does not "glow" for any substantial period of time) than does NaI, allowing for higher count rates. One drawback of this substance is that Lu is itself slightly radioactive, and so large crystals based on lutetium produce an inherent background of counts that may be deleterious in certain applications. Despite this disadvantage lutetium-based crystals show great promise in both positron tomographs and gamma cameras meant to be used for both low and high energies.

REFERENCES

1. Sorenson J, Phelps ME. *Physics in Nuclear Medicine*, 2nd Edition. Orlando: Grune and Stratton, Inc., 1987.
2. Anger HO. Scintillation camera with multichannel collimators. J Nucl Med 1964; 5:515.
3. Green M, Seidel J. *Single photon imaging.* In: *Nuclear Medicine: Diagnosis and Therapy*, edited by JC Harbert, WC Eckelman, RD Neumann. New York: Thieme Medical Publishers, Inc., 1995.
4. NEMA. *Performance Measurements of Scintillation Cameras.* Nema publication no. 1-1994. Washington, D.C.: National Electrical Manufacturers Association, 1994.
5. Siegel JA, Benedetto AR, Jaszczak RJ, et al. *Rotating Scintillation Camera SPECT Acceptance Testing and Quality Control.* New York: American Association of Physicists in Medicine, 1987.
6. Parker JA. *Image Reconstruction in Radiology.* Boca Raton: CRC Press, Inc., 1990.
7. Dilsizian V, Bacharach SL, Khin MM, et al. Fluorine-18-deoxyglucose SPECT and coincidence imaging for myocardial viability: clinical and technologic issues. J Nucl Cardiol 2001;8:75.
8. Links JM. Advances in nuclear medicine instrumentation: considerations in the design and selection of an imaging system. Eur J Nucl Med 1998; 25:1453.
9. Turkington TG, Laymon CM, Coleman RE, et al. Imaging properties of a half-inch sodium iodide gamma camera. IEEE Trans Nucl Sci, 1997; 44:1262.
10. Delbeke D, Videlefsky S, Patton JA, et al. Rest myocardial perfusion/metabolism imaging using simultaneous dual-isotope acquisition SPECT with technetium-99m-MIBI/Fluorine-18-FDG. J Nucl Med 1995; 36:2110.

4 | Kinetics of myocardial perfusion imaging radiotracers

RAYMOND TAILLEFER

Since its introduction more than two decades ago, myocardial perfusion scintigraphy has significantly evolved. Two major factors have more specifically contributed to this evolution: technical improvements in scintigraphic data acquisition and analysis and introduction of new Tc-99m labeled myocardial perfusion imaging radiopharmaceuticals with different properties. This chapter reviews the most important characteristics of the various radionuclide myocardial perfusion imaging agents that are currently commercially available (thallium-201, Tc-99m-sestamibi, Tc-99m-tetrofosmin, and Tc-99m-teboroxime) or are likely to be available soon, (Tc-99m-N-NOET). Since numerous extensive studies and reviews on Tl-201 imaging have been previously reported, this chapter focuses mostly on Tc-99m labeled perfusion imaging agents. Furthermore, although many articles have been published on Tc-99m-furifosmin, this radiotracer is not discussed here, since its developmental program has been canceled and, therefore, it is very unlikely that this agent will be used for clinical purposes.

THALLIUM-201

In the mid-1950s, Sapirstein [1] elaborated the criteria necessary for a radiopharmaceutical to be used to determine regional perfusion. As described by the Sapirstein principle, a given type of radiopharmaceutical will be distributed in proportion to regional perfusion if its extraction by the organ of interest is high and if its clearance from the blood is rapid. One of the first class of radiopharmaceuticals used to image myocardial perfusion was the potassium analogs, a group of monovalent cations of potassium, cesium, rubidium, and thallium, which enter the myocardium by the sodium-potassium-ATPase pump mechanism [2]. Although different radioisotopes of these cations have been evaluated, Tl-201 was found to have the best physical and biological characteristics for imaging in humans. Since the mid-1970s, and for more than two decades, Tl-201 has been the most popular radionuclide myocardial perfusion imaging agent used in noninvasive detection and evaluation of patients with known or suspected coronary artery disease.

Chemistry and Constituents

Tl-201 is a metallic element in group IIIA of the periodic table with a crystal radius of 1.44 A (between that of potassium and rubidium). Tl-201 is a cyclotron-produced monovalent cation with a physical half-life of 73.1 hours. It decays by electron capture to mercury Hg-201. Tl-201 is a low-energy gamma emitter with principal photo-peaks at 135.3 keV (2.7% abundance) and 167.4 keV (10% abundance) and X-rays emitted from the mercury daughter at 68 to 80.3 keV (95% abundance). Some contaminants such as Tl-200 ($< 0.3\%$), Tl-202 ($< 1.2\%$), and Pb-202 ($< 0.2\%$) can be present but that usually represents less than 2% of the total Tl-201 activity at the time of calibration. Contrary to the Tc-99m labeled myocardial perfusion imaging agents, there is no in-house preparation and no quality control procedure required before injection in humans.

Physiologic Characteristics

Basic characteristics of myocardial perfusion imaging radiotracers

Although many different classes of radioactive myocardial perfusion imaging agents exist, they should all present a minimum of common basic characteristics [3]. The myocardial uptake of the radiotracer must be proportional to the regional myocardial blood flow over a relatively wide range of blood flows. The myocardial uptake should be high enough to allow for detection of regional inhomogeneity by external gamma scintigraphy. The initial myocardial distribution of the radiotracer at the time of injection must remain stable during the acquisition time of the images. The effect of blood flow on myocardial transport of the radiotracer must be predominant to the effect of metabolic cellular alterations. Finally, the agent should be labeled to a radionuclide having adequate physical characteristics in order to provide high photon flux and optimal counting statistics.

Information on basic properties of radionuclide myocardial perfusion imaging agents is generally obtained from cultured myocardial cells, isolated perfused hearts, or in vivo animal models [4]. Precise measurements of cellular or capillary-tissue tracer kinetics are usually obtained from cell cultures and isolated perfused heart models, whereas regional tracer distribution and uptake in other organs are studied in in vivo animal models.

The two most important physiologic factors that affect the myocardial uptake of a myocardial perfusion imaging agent are the variations in regional myocardial blood flow and the myocardial extraction of the radiotracer. Three major parameters (Enet, Emax, and PS cap) can be determined using indicator–dilution techniques and radiolabeled albumin used as an intravascular reference. The difference between the intravascular albumin reference and the radiopharmaceutical that is evaluated (i.e., a diffusible perfusion agent) on a venous dilution curve is used to calculate its instantaneous cardiac extraction. The early peak of the curve, or Emax, represents the maximum fractional tissue extraction of the diffusible agent. This value is used to calculate the capillary permeability-surface area product, or PS cap. The net extraction (Enet) is the integral of the curve and is used as a measure of myocardial radiotracer retention, including both initial extraction and subsequent back-diffusion. A high value for Emax and PS cap indicates a rapid blood–tissue exchange and suggests that the diffusible radiotracer will be able to assess high levels of hyperemic flow accurately. The my-

ocardial transmicrovascular transport of Tl-201 was evaluated by Leppo and Meerdink [5] in a blood-perfused, isolated rabbit heart model. The averaged myocardial extraction (Emax) of Tl-201 was 0.73 ± 0.10. The net myocardial extraction measured over a 2 to 5 minute period was 0.57 ± 0.13. The mean capillary permeability-surface area product of Tl-201 was 1.30 ± 0.45 ml/g/min. Table 4.1 summarizes and compares these values, as a reference, to those of the four Tc-99m labeled perfusion imaging agents.

Although Tl-201 is considered biologically similar to potassium, its myocardial uptake Tl-201 is greater than that of potassium. The myocardial extraction fraction of Tl-201 in in vivo model is approximately 87% at normal flow rates [6]. Studies on the relationship of myocardial uptake of Tl-201 to regional coronary blood flow as determined by radiolabeled microspheres showed that there is a nearly linear correlation over a wide range of coronary blood flows (Fig. 4.1). However, at high flow rates (at approximately 2.5 ml/min/g), there is a diffusion limitation and a fall in tracer extraction fraction and also an increased cellular washout, resulting in a plateau in myocardial uptake. This results in an overall underestimation of higher levels of coronary blood flows. Conversely, at very low flow rates (usually less than 10% of the baseline blood flow), there is an increased myocardial extraction fraction of Tl-201 relative to blood flow, resulting in an overestimation of coronary blood flow. This phenomenon has been described with all other Tc-99m labeled myocardial perfusion imaging agents, at various degrees.

One of the most clinically important characteristics of Tl-201 is its myocardial redistribution. Myocardial uptake of Tl-201 is not static over time. This property forms the basis of the stress-redistribution imaging protocol currently used to diagnose the presence of coronary artery disease with Tl-201. The redistribution or the filling in of a myocardial perfusion defect occurring a few (generally between 3 and 5 hours) hours after the

TABLE 4.1 *Comparative Characteristics of Radiopharmaceuticals for Myocardial Perfusion Imaging*

	Thallium-201	Tc-99m-Sestamibi	Tc-99m-Teboroxime	Tc-99m-Tetrofosmin	Tc-99m-N-NOEt
Class	Element	Isonitrile	BATO	Diphosphine	Nitrodo
Charge	Cation	Cation	Neutral	Cation	Neutral
E max	0.73 ± 0.10	0.38 ± 0.09	0.72 ± 0.09	0.32 ± 0.07	0.48 ± 0.10
E net	0.57 ± 0.13	0.41 ± 0.15	0.55 ± 0.18	0.23	0.24 ± 0.08
PScap (mL/μg)	1.30 ± 0.45	0.44 ± 0.23	1.10 ± 0.40	0.40	1.02 ± 0.32
Myocardial redistribution	Yes	Partial	Yes	No	Yes
Myocardial uptake (%ID)	3.0–4.0	1.4 ± 0.3	3.0–4.0	1.0–1.2	3.0–3.5
Labeling	Ready	100°C × 10 min	100°C × 15 min	15°C–25°C × 15 min	15°C–25°C × 20 min
IV Imaging interval	5–10 min	15–60 min	< 2 min	15 min	10–15 min
Target organ	Kidney	Upper large intestine	Upper large intestine	Gallbladder wall	Kidneys

E max, maximum radiotracer extraction; E net, net radiotracer extraction; PScap, radiotracer permeability-surface area product.

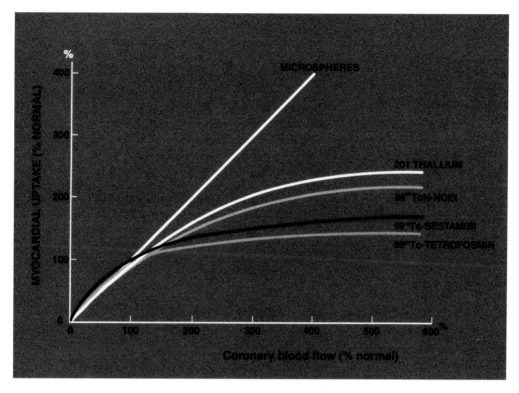

FIGURE 4.1 Schematic representation of the relationship between coronary blood flow and myocardial uptake of various perfusion imaging radiotracers. (Adapted from Glover et al. Circulation 1995–1997.)

injection of Tl-201 at peak stress is related to two factors: the rate of influx of Tl-201 into the myocardium from whole-body blood pool activity and the rate of clearance or washout of Tl-201 from the myocardium. A myocardial perfusion defect related to ischemic disease will show a normalization of the Tl-201 uptake at 3–4 hours after the injection at stress because of a delayed accumulation into the ischemic segment and a more rapid washout from normal myocardial segments than from hypoperfused segments. Two Tc-99m labeled perfusion imaging agents also demonstrate some degree of myocardial redistribution, similar to that of Tl-201: Tc-99m-teboroxime and Tc-99m-N-NOET.

Biodistribution and Dosimetry

The greatest concentration of Tl-201 is found in kidneys, heart, and liver. The activity in these organs remains high for few hours after the injection. Maximal myocardial uptake, which is approximately 3.7%–4.0% of the injected dose, is achieved by 10–15 minutes after the administration of the radiopharmaceutical. Tl-201 myocardial uptake has two components: an early component with a half-life of approximately 4 hours (80%)

and a delayed component with a half-life of 40 hours (20%). Disappearance of Tl-201 from the blood compartment is rapid with two components: 92% of the blood activity disappears with a half-life of 5 minutes and the other 8% will be cleared from the blood with a half-life of approximately 40 hours. This rapid clearance of Tl-201 from the blood results in a decreased blood pool background when myocardial perfusion imaging is performed. Table 4.2 summarizes the radiation dose estimates for Tl-201 and all other Tc-99m labeled myocardial perfusion imaging agents. Data on Tl-201 were obtained in humans [7], assuming a bladder voiding interval of 4.8 hours. Kidneys are the target organs. Based on the dosimetric data, the recommended adult dose of intravenous Tl-201 for SPECT myocardial perfusion imaging is 74 to 111 MBq (2–3 mCi), although several authors are using doses up to 4.0 mCi.

Tc-99m-SESTAMIBI

Although hundreds of studies have demonstrated the clinical value of Tl-201 myocardial perfusion scintigraphy since its first use in 1975, the physical charac-

TABLE 4.2 *Radiation Dose Estimate for Myocardial Perfusion Imaging Agents (Rads/30 mCi)*

	THALLIUM-201 Stress (Rads/3mCi)	TC-99M-SESTAMIBI Rest	Stress	TC-99M-TEBOROXIME Rest	TC-99M-TETROFOSMIN Rest	Stress	TC-99M-N-NOET Rest	Stress
Adrenals	0.7	—	—	—	0.5	0.5	—	—
Brain	0.7	—	—	0.4	0.2	0.3	—	—
Breasts	0.4	0.2	0.2	—	0.2	0.2	—	—
Gallbladder wall	0.9	2.0	2.8	2.9	5.4	3.7	—	—
LLI	1.60	3.9	3.3	2.6	2.5	1.7	—	—
ULI	0.80	5.4	4.5	3.7	3.4	2.2	1.9	1.4
Small intestine	0.20	3.0	2.4	2.0	1.9	1.3	—	—
Stomach	0.3	0.6	0.5	—	0.5	0.5	—	—
Heart wall	0.3	0.5	0.5	0.6	0.4	0.5	0.7	0.8
Kidneys	5.1	2.0	1.7	0.6	1.4	1.2	1.8	2.0
Liver	1.1	0.6	0.4	1.9	0.5	0.4	1.3	1.2
Lungs	0.5	0.3	0.3	0.8	0.2	0.2	0.5	0.6
Muscles	0.5	—	—	—	0.4	0.4	—	—
Ovaries	1.1	1.5	1.2	1.1	1.1	0.9	1.1	1.0
Pancreas	0.8	—	—	—	0.5	0.6	—	—
Red marrow	0.6	0.5	0.5	0.5	0.4	0.5	0.4	0.4
Bone surface	1.0	0.7	0.6	—	0.6	0.7	—	—
Spleen	2.0	—	—	0.4	0.4	0.5	0.6	0.5
Testes	0.9	0.3	0.3	0.3	0.3	0.4	0.3	0.3
Thymus	0.5	—	—	—	0.3	0.3	—	—
Thyroid	3.0	0.7	0.3	0.3	0.6	0.5	0.6	0.6
Bladder wall	0.6	2.0	1.5	0.8	2.1	1.7	—	—
Uterus	1.0	—	—	—	0.9	0.2	—	—
Total body	—	0.5	0.4	0.5	0.4	0.4	0.5	0.4
Effective dose equivalent (rem/30 mCi)	3.9 (rem/3mCi)	1.5	1.3	1.1	1.0	0.8	0.8	0.8

LLI, lower large intestine; ULI, upper large intestine.

teristics of this radionuclide are suboptimal for scintillation camera imaging. Therefore, in the late 1970s and early 1980s, many investigators attempted to develop a myocardial perfusion imaging agent labeled with Tc-99m in order to circumvent the physical limitations of Tl-201. The potential advantages of a Tc-99m labeled agent over Tl-201 are significant and include the following: (1) The 140 keV photon energy of Tc-99m, which is optimal for standard gamma camera imaging, results in an improved resolution due to less Compton scatter and less tissue attenuation in the patient (in comparison to the low photon energy of 68–80 keV for Tl-201). (2) The much shorter physical half-life of Tc-99m (6 hours vs 73 hours for Tl-201) and the better radiation dosimetry permit the administration of a 10-times higher dose of a Tc-99m labeled compound than Tl-201. This yields better image quality and images can be performed in a shorter time period. (3) The resulting overall better counting statistics of Tc-99m allows for the perfusion images to be optimally obtained in a gated mode. Simultaneous assessment of perfusion and function (global and regional wall motion) can thus

be obtained. (4) It is also possible to perform first-pass function studies (if the initial lung transit is rapid enough) with a Tc-99m labeled radiopharmaceutical agent. (5) Since Tc-99m is constantly available from a molybdenum generator in a nuclear medicine laboratory, special deliveries from a distribution center or a commercial radiopharmacy are not required. A Tc-99m labeled myocardial perfusion imaging agent can thus be available almost 24 hours a day.

For all the above mentioned reasons and although Tl-201 has excellent physiologic characteristics for myocardial perfusion imaging, it was obvious that a Tc-99m labeled agent able to assess myocardial perfusion could be very useful clinically [8–10]. Significant developments were finally seen in the early 1980s with the initial article published in 1984 by Jones et al. [11] on a new group of Tc-99m labeled myocardial perfusion radiotracers, the Tc-99m-isonitriles. Initial animal studies showed that the myocardial uptake of Tc-99m-isonitriles was proportional to the regional myocardial blood flow. The first member of the Tc-99m-isonitrile family to be evaluated in humans was the hexakis (t-butyl-isonitrile)-technetium (I) also known as Tc-99m-TBI [12,13]. Although the myocardial uptake of Tc-99m-TBI was proportional to myocardial blood flow and was satisfactory for imaging purposes, its routine clinical use was limited by an increased lung uptake and prominent and persistent liver uptake, which frequently masked defects in myocardial walls adjacent to the hepatic parenchyma. The initial lung uptake and subsequent washout of Tc-99m-TBI from the lungs also created significant imaging problems. Then, a second Tc-99m-isonitrile compound was synthesized and evaluated in humans: the carboxyisopropyl isonitrile, or Tc-99m-CPI [14]. Like Tc-99m-TBI, Tc-99m-CPI showed an excellent myocardial uptake proportional to blood flow but a relatively rapid washout from the myocardium and a significant progressive accumulation in the liver over time. A third Tc-99m-isonitrile compound has emerged from this intensive search [15]. Initially known by the coded name of RP-30A (nonlyophilized form) or RP-30 (lyophilized form), and then as either Tc-99m-hexakis 2-methoxyisobutyl isonitrile, Tc-99m-hexakis-2-methoxy-2-methylpropyl-isonitrile, Tc-99m-

hexamibi, or Tc-99m-MIBI. DuPont Pharmaceutical commercially developed Tc-99m-sestamibi (generic name) or Cardiolite (trademark name). In comparison to its two isonitrile predecessors, Tc-99m-sestamibi had the most favorable biologic characteristics for clinical applications. Unlike Tc-99m-TBI and Tc-99m-CPI, which showed a poor myocardial-to-background activity ratio, Tc-99m-sestamibi showed a transient liver uptake and subsequent rapid hepatobiliary excretion. Furthermore, the lung uptake was minimal in comparison to the other two isonitrile agents. Tc-99m-sestamibi was approved by the Food and Drug Administration (in the United States) for clinical application in December 1990.

Chemistry and Constituents

Tc-99m-sestamibi or hexakis (2-methoxyisobutyl isonitrile) technetium is a monovalent cation with a central Tc (I) core that is octahedrally surrounded by six identical lipophilic ligands coordinated through the isonitrile carbon (Fig. 4.2). A 5 ml vial of Tc-99m-sestamibi

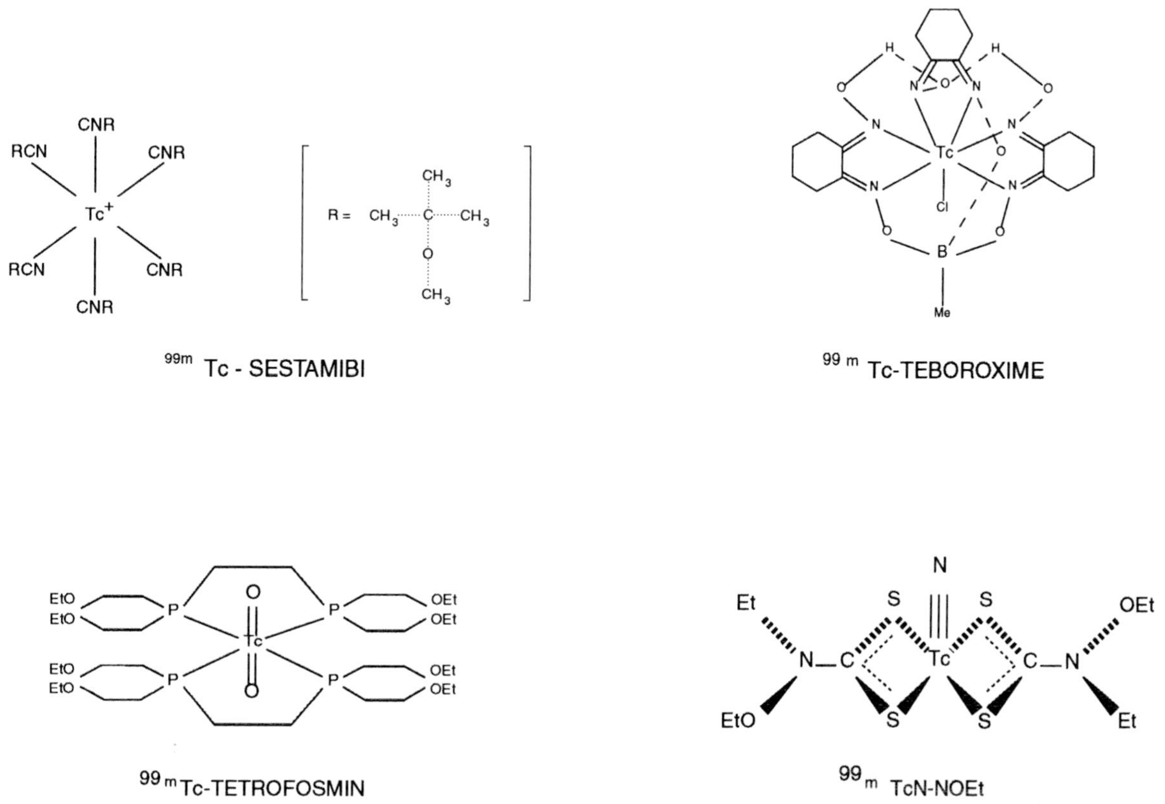

FIGURE 4.2 Schematic chemical structures of the four Tc-99m labeled perfusion imaging agents.

or Cardiolite supplied by DuPont Merck Pharmaceutical Co. (Billerica, Massachusetts, USA) contains a sterile, nonpyrogenic, lyophilized mixture of: 1.0 mg of tetrakis (2-methoxy isobutyl isonitrile) copper tetrafluoroborate, 0.025 mg (minimum) of dihydrate stannous chloride, 2.6 mg of sodium citrate dihydrate, 0.086 mg (maximum) of total tin, 1.0 mg of L-cysteine hydrochloride monohydrate, and 20 mg of mannitol. The contents of the vial (pH = 5.3–5.9) are lyophilized and stored under nitrogen. After reconstitution with oxidant-free sodium pertechnetate Tc-99m, the pH of the product to be injected is 5.5 (5.0 to 6.0). There is no bacteriostatic preservative. The final structure of the technetium complex is Tc-99m-(MIBI)6+ where MIBI is 2-methoxy isobutyl isonitrile. Intravenous injections of Tc-99m-sestamibi has been associated with very few adverse reactions. According to the product monograph, during clinical trials (Phase III study) approximately 5% to 10% of patients experienced transient parosmia and/or taste perversion (metallic or bitter taste) occurring a few seconds after the injection. Usually, this side effect disappears within 15 to 30 seconds. This parosmia and/or taste perversion seems to be related to the presence of the copper salt in the kit formulation, and its incidence may be related to the concentration of Tc-99m-sestamibi used.

Physiologic Characteristics

Initial myocardial uptake of Tc-99m-sestamibi

Among the Tc-99m labeled myocardial perfusion imaging agents, Tc-99m-sestamibi has probably been the most extensively studied one with the different previously mentioned research models. Tc-99m-sestamibi is a cationic complex that is taken up by myocytes in proportion to regional myocardial blood flow. The cationic charge of the compound provides hydrophilic properties, while the six isonitrile groups allow hydrophobic interaction with cell membranes. The myocardial uptake of Tc-99m-sestamibi is known to be dependent on mitochondrial derived membrane electrochemical gradient, cellular pH, and intact energy production pathways. Piwnica-Worms et al. [16] studied the net myocardial uptake and retention of Tc-99m-sestamibi using a cultured chick embryo ventricular myocytes model. They showed that when mitochondrial and plasma membrane potentials are hyperpolarized, there is an increase in cellular uptake and retention of Tc-99m-sestamibi. Conversely, when mitochondrial and plasma membrane potentials are depolarized, there is inhibition of net myocardial uptake and retention of the radiotracer. Tc-99m-sestamibi, which is retained

within cells because of the negative charge generated on the mitochondria, has a high affinity for the cytoplasm and shows very little extracellular exchange. Thus, metabolic derangements affecting myocytes' viability would also result in decreased Tc-99m-sestamibi uptake, independently of myocardial blood flow. Using aerobic metabolic blockade (with sodium cyanide) and a sarcolemmal detergent (Triton X-100), which directly disrupts the membrane integrity, Beanlands et al. [17] showed that an irreversible cellular injury resulted in a marked increase in Tc-99m-sestamibi clearance rate. They concluded that the accumulation and clearance kinetics of Tc-99m-sestamibi were dependent on sarcolemmal integrity and on aerobic metabolism and were significantly affected by cell viability.

Okada et al. [18] investigated the myocardial kinetics of Tc-99m-sestamibi in dogs undergoing a partial occlusion of the left circumflex coronary artery. They showed that Tc-99m-sestamibi was rapidly taken up by nonischemic and ischemic myocardium at rest in proportion to regional myocardial blood flow. There was a good correlation between the initial myocardial flow at normal resting flow rates and the Tc-99m-sestamibi myocardial distribution (linear relationship with an r value of 0.92). Another study from the same group of investigators [19] using the same animal model evaluated the myocardial kinetics of Tc-99m-sestamibi after pharmacologic vasodilation with dipyridamole. They showed that Tc-99m-sestamibi was rapidly taken up by nonischemic, mild-to-moderate, and severe ischemic myocardium and that the initial myocardial uptake of Tc-99m-sestamibi was linearly related (r value of 0.97) to the regional myocardial blood flow at rates up to approximately 2.0 ml/min/gr. However, at higher flow rates, there is a plateau in the myocardial distribution versus flow curve, resulting in an underestimation of coronary blood flow. Similar findings have been reported by Mousa et al. [20], who demonstrated in swine a linear distribution of both Tl-201 and Tc-99m-sestamibi with myocardial blood flow at rates up to 2.4 ml/min/gr. Above this level, there was a leveling off of the distribution versus flow curve for both radiotracers. Furthermore, myocardial uptake of Tc-99m-sestamibi in low flow regions is higher relative to nonischemic uptake than in the regional blood flow determined with radiolabeled microspheres. This overestimation of myocardial blood flow at low flows (as previously discussed with Tl-201) is probably related to an increased extraction seen with diffusible indicators. Other studies [21] have confirmed that myocardial uptake of Tc-99m-sestamibi, as with Tl-201, is proportional to regional myocardial blood flow over the physiological flow range with decreased extraction at hyperemic flows and increased extraction at low flows.

The myocardial transmicrovascular transport of Tc-99m-sestamibi was evaluated and compared to that of Tl-201 by Leppo and Meerdink [22] in a blood-perfused, isolated rabbit heart model. The averaged myocardial extraction (Emax) of Tc-99m-sestamibi (0.38 ± 0.09) was significantly less ($p < .001$) than that of Tl-201 (0.73 ± 0.10). The net myocardial extraction measured over a 2 to 5 minute period was also significantly ($p < 0.001$) less for Tc-99m-sestamibi (0.41 ± 0.15) than for Tl-201 (0.57 ± 0.13). Although the mean capillary permeability-surface area product of Tl-201 (1.30 ± 0.45 ml/g/min) is significantly greater ($p < 0.001$) than that of Tc-99m-sestamibi (0.44 ± 0.13 ml/g/min), the parenchymal cell permeability and volume distribution of Tc-99m-sestamibi are much greater than that of Tl-201, resulting in a longer residence time within the myocardium for Tc-99m-sestamibi. The net result of these differences in myocellular kinetics of the two radiopharmaceuticals is that very little difference is observed in the initial myocardial accumulation when both are imaged in vivo.

Myocardial redistribution

In contrast to Tl-201, Tc-99m-sestamibi shows a very slow myocardial clearance after its initial myocardial uptake. A fractional Tc-99m-sestamibi clearance of 10%–15% over a period of 4 hours has been measured by Okada et al. [18] in a canine model of partial coronary occlusion. The clearance was similar in the hypoperfused and normal zones. Animal studies have shown that after injection during brief periods (6–15 minutes) of coronary occlusion in dogs, the occluded zone shows a continued myocardial uptake of Tc-99m-sestamibi during the reperfusion phase, resulting in a slight increase in the ischemic/normal wall Tc-99m-sestamibi activity ratio during 2–3 hours. Thus, following transient ischemia and reperfusion, there is some degree of myocardial redistribution of Tc-99m-sestamibi, although it is slower and less complete than Tl-201 [23,24].

Myocardial cell viability

Sinusas et al. [25] studied the myocardial uptake of Tc-99m-sestamibi and Tl-201 in a canine model of transient occlusion and reperfusion and in a chronic low flow state. They showed that as long as myocardial cells were still viable, the myocardial uptake of Tl-201 and Tc-99m-sestamibi was not affected by an ischemia producing profound systolic dysfunction. They did not observe a flow-independent inhibition of Tc-99m-sestamibi myocardial uptake in the stunned or in the chronically ischemic myocardial tissue. Thus,

data in experimental models of coronary occlusion and reperfusion and studies of isolated, perfused heart models showed that as long as myocyte membrane integrity is intact and blood flow persists, Tc-99m-sestamibi is extracted by myocardial cells. These data suggest that Tc-99m-sestamibi can also be an agent able to assess myocardial viability. Tc-99m-Sestamibi uptake is maintained in viable myocardium but reduced in necrotic tissue. Using a dog model with coronary occlusion and reperfusion, Verani et al. [26] demonstrated that the size of the perfusion defect during occlusion as detected by scintigraphic images correlated with the amount of myocardium supplied by the occluded vessel, the area at risk. A smaller perfusion defect was detected on Tc-99m-sestamibi imaging during reperfusion. This defect correlated with the amount of infarcted myocardium. The area showing improved perfusion pattern after reflow represented the salvaged myocardium.

Biodistribution and Dosimetry

The results of multicenter Phase I and Phase II studies on blood clearance, biodistribution, dosimetry, and safety of Tc-99m-sestamibi after injection at rest or during exercise were initially reported by Wackers et al. in 1989 [15]. The Phase I study involved a total of 17 normal volunteers. Both rest and stress blood clearance curves approximate a dual exponential curve with an initial fast and later slow component. The maximal activity at rest was noted at 1 minute after injection ($36 \pm 18\%$ of injected dose) while the maximal activity after injection during exercise was measured at 0.5 minute. At 1 hour after the intravenous injection of Tc-99m-sestamibi, the blood pool activity progressively decreased to $1.10 \pm 0.01\%$ and $0.7 \pm 0.1\%$ of the injected dose at rest and after stress, respectively. At 60 minutes after the injection of Tc-99m-sestamibi at rest, the uptake in the heart was $1.0 \pm 0.4\%$ of injected dose. The 24-hour urinary excretion was 29.5% of injected dose, whereas the 48-hour fecal excretion was 36.9% of injected dose. The study of the upper-body organ distribution showed that the highest initial Tc-99m-sestamibi concentration (counts/pixel) is found in gallbladder and liver followed (in decreasing order) by heart, spleen, and lungs. The myocardial activity remained relatively stable over time ($27 \pm 4\%$ of initial activity has cleared from the heart at 3 hours), whereas activity in the spleen and lung decreased gradually. The maximal accumulation in the gallbladder occurred approximately at 60 minutes after the injection.

The uptake in the heart was $1.4 \pm 0.3\%$ of injected dose at 60 minutes after the injection of Tc-99m-sestamibi during exercise. The 24-hour urinary excretion was 24.1% of injected dose, whereas the 48-hour fecal excretion was 29.1% of injected dose. The upper-body organ distribution evaluation showed that immediately after the injection, the highest concentration of Tc-99m-sestamibi was also found in the gallbladder, followed by heart, liver, spleen, and lungs. As for the rest study, by 3 hours after injection, 26 + 12% of initial cardiac activity had cleared.

Radiation dose estimates for Tc-99m-sestamibi have been evaluated from whole body images obtained in the Phase I study [15]. The estimated radiation absorbed dose at rest and at stress, assuming a 2.0 hour void, are summarized in Table 4.2. The uptake in the heart is $1.0 \pm 0.4\%$ of injected dose at 60 minutes after injection at rest and $1.4 \pm 0.3\%$ at 60 minutes for the stress study. The upper large intestine wall receives the highest dose of radioactivity, both at rest and at stress. In order to decrease dosimetry to the urinary bladder, increasing voiding frequency should be encouraged. If patients are administered a total dose of 30 mCi of Tc-99m-sestamibi, no individual organ dose will exceed 5 rads (50 mGy). Although there is accumulation of Tc-99m-sestamibi in the mammary glands, there is a minimal transfer into milk: approximately 0.01% to 0.03% of the injected Tc-99m-sestamibi activity can be excreted in human breast milk of a breastfeeding female patient [27].

Technical Aspects

Preparation

Preparation of the Tc-99m-sestamibi from the kit supplied by the manufacturer is a relatively simple procedure. Under aseptic and radiation safety regular conditions, a recommended maximum dose of 150 mCi (5.6 GBq) of additive-free, sterile, nonpyrogenic Tc-99m sodium pertechnetate in approximately 1–3 ml of solution is added into the 5 ml vial in a lead shield. An equal volume (1–3 ml) of headspace is removed in order to maintain atmospheric pressure within the vial. The contents of the vial are swirled for a few seconds. Then the vial containing Tc-99m-sestamibi is placed upright in a boiling water bath for 10 minutes. After this time period, the vial is removed from the water bath, placed in a lead shield, and another period of approximately 15 minutes is needed to allow the vial to cool before the intravenous injection. The reconstituted vial should be stored at 15°–25°C and Tc-99m-sestamibi doses should be aseptically withdrawn within 6 hours. The total preparation time, including the recommended quality control step (described in the next section) usually takes between 30 and 40 minutes. In some acute clinical conditions where a dose of Tc-99m-sestamibi must be rapidly available to permit administration without any delay, this period of 30–40 minutes is too long and would limit the availability of Tc-99m-sestamibi on an emergency basis. Gagnon et al. [28] and Hung et al. [29] have proposed a method of rapid preparation of Tc-99m-sestamibi using a microwave oven heating method for labeling Tc-99m-sestamibi instead of the boiling water bath method. The "heating" time was reduced from 10 minutes with the recommended "standard" method to 13 seconds with the microwave oven method. These authors have emphasized that users of the microwave oven method for the labeling of Tc-99m-sestamibi must follow the specifications that are published, otherwise the user must test the labeling procedure with the user's own microwave oven if the technical specifications differ. Those technical specifications of any commercial microwave oven used are very important, since the power output, microwave frequency, cavity dimensions, and cavity volume may differ and thus may have a different impact on the labeling procedure. Labeling Tc-99m-sestamibi with the microwave oven method has been shown to be safe and reliable. Radiochromatographic quality control methods showed that both boiling water bath and microwave oven methods gave similar values with a very high labeling efficiency of Tc-99m-sestamibi. However, it is important to note that the use of the microwave oven method is not the one specified in the package insert. Another method for rapid labeling of Tc-99m-sestamibi has also been recently described [30].

Quality control

The verification of radiochemical purity of Tc-99m-sestamibi is not always required prior to its administration to a patient. However, it is considered to be good radiopharmacy practice to ensure an injection with a radiopharmaceutical of the highest purity, safety, and efficacy. The recommended radiochromatographic procedure for the determination of radiochemical purity of Tc-99m-sestamibi involves the use of an aluminum oxide–coated (Baker-flex) plastic thin-layer chromatography plate with absolute ethanol as developing agent. One drop of ethanol is applied at 1.5 cm from the bottom of a dry plate and two drops of Tc-99m-sestamibi solution are added on top of the ethanol spot. Only the Tc-99m-sestamibi migrates with ethanol to the solvent front. It is not recommended to use Tc-99m-sestamibi if the radiochemical purity is less than 90%.

Like the recommended labeling preparation procedure, the recommended quality control is time-consuming and needs to be significantly reduced in order to use Tc-99m-sestamibi for emergency purposes. Hung et al. [29] proposed the use of a mini-paper chromatography method. They compared the two methods and showed that the average time for drying and developing the aluminum oxide–coated thin-layer chromatography plates was 35 minutes, whereas the average time for developing the mini-paper chromatogaphy strip was 2.3 minutes. The results of the two methods were similar. Using alternative methods [31–33], it is thus possible to rapidly prepare and perform the quality control of Tc-99m-sestamibi. However, the legal considerations of using these alternative methods should be judged and decided by each individual institution, based on local or federal regulations.

Tc-99m-TEBOROXIME

Tc-99m-teboroxime became commercially available in December 1990, when it was approved by the Food and Drug Administration in the United States. However, Tc-99m-teboroxime has rapidly become far less commonly used than Tc-99m-sestamibi, mainly because the peculiar pharmacokinetic properties of Tc-99m-teboroxime have challenged the users of this radiopharmaceutical. Despite the technical constraints related to its use, Tc-99m-teboroxime remains one of the best myocardial blood flow radiotracers available for planar or tomographic perfusion imaging. The unique pharmacodynamic characteristics of Tc-99m-teboroxime offer an interesting niche with specific potential clinical applications for myocardial perfusion imaging [34–43]. Although not clinically used anymore because of the technical limitations, it is not impossible for Tc-99m-teboroxime to be used again, especially if high-quality ultrafast SPECT acquisition imaging becomes available.

Chemistry and Constituents

Tc-99m-teboroxime, a cationic compound, is chemically very different from Tc-99m-sestamibi or Tl-201. It has a smaller molecular size than sestamibi but it is larger than thallium. Tc-99m-teboroxime, a neutral and highly lipophilic compound, is a member of the boronic acid adducts of technetium dioxime complexes (BATO). These complexes are neutral seven coordinate technetium vicinal dioxime complexes which have a boron group at one end. Tc-99m-teboroxime is the generic name for [Bis[1,2-cyclohexanedione dioximato (1-)-O]-[1,2-cyclohexane-dione-ioximato (2-)-O] methylborato(2-)-N,N',N'',N''',N'''',N''''']-chloro-technetium,

also referred as SQ30217 (developmental name) or Cardiotec (trademark name from Squibb Diagnostics, Princeton, NJ).

According to the product monograph, a 5 ml vial of Tc-99m-teboroxime, or Cardiotec supplied by Squibb Diagnostics (Princeton, NJ), contains a sterile, nonpyrogenic, lyophilized formulation of: 2.0 mg of cyclohexanedione dioxime, 2.0 mg of methyl boronic acid, 2.0 mg of pentetic acid, 9.0 mg of citric acid anhydrous, 100 mg of sodium chloride, 50 mg of gamma cyclodextrin, and 0.020 mg–0.058 mg of total tin expressed as stannous chloride ($SnCl_2$). The contents of the vial are lyophilized after pH adjustment (3.3–4.1) and then sealed under nitrogen. There is no bacteriostatic preservative. Tc-99m-teboroxime differs from other Tc-99m labeled radiopharmaceuticals in that the ligand is not present in the vial before addition of Tc-99m-pertechnetate, since it is formed by template synthesis around the technetium atom.

There are no known contraindications to the administration of Tc-99m-teboroxime and no known pharmacologic action at the recommended doses. Uncommon adverse reactions have been reported in clinical trials. These include metallic taste in mouth, hypotension, nausea, burning at injection site, facial swelling, and numbness of hand and arm.

Physiologic Characteristics

Myocardial uptake

Because of its neutral, lipophilic properties Tc-99m-teboroxime comes close to being a freely diffusible radiotracer similar to Xe-133. The extraction fraction of Tc-99m-teboroxime is very high over a wide range of blood flow rates [44], higher than Tc-99m-sestamibi or Tl-201. Leppo and Meerdink [45,46] studied the transcapillary exchange of Tc-99m-teboroxime and Tl-201 in isolated, blood-perfused rabbit heart model. Using different blood flows varying from 0.15 to 2.44 ml/min/gr, the mean peak extraction (Emax) of Tc-99m-teboroxime was 0.72 ± 0.09, the mean net extraction (Enet) was 0.55 ± 0.18, and the mean capillary permeability-surface area product (PS cap) was 1.1 ± 0.4 ml/min/gr. All these values are higher than those obtained with Tl-201: 0.57 ± 0.10 ($p < .03$), 0.46 ± 0.17 ($p < .03$), and 0.7 ± 0.3 ($p < .001$), respectively. Subsequent studies performed by Marshall et al. [47] using a similar in vitro model showed slightly different results with a better extraction for Tl-201. However, the authors concluded that Tc-99m-teboroxime and Tl-201 appear to be comparable radiotracers of myocardial perfusion for up to 10 minutes after injection under the single-pass conditions used in their study.

The myocardial uptake of Tc-99m-teboroxime has been shown to be slightly higher than that of Tl-201 in rat heart. Narra et al. [48] reported that the myocardial uptake at 1 minute postinjection was 3.44% of injected dose for Tc-99m-teboroxime and 3.03% of injected dose for Tl-201. Other studies [44,49] showed that myocardial uptake of Tc-99m-teboroxime parallels myocardial blood flow in a linear fashion, even when blood flow is increased to four times the level of resting blood flow, without the "roll-off" seen at high flow levels with Tl-201 or Tc-99m-sestamibi. Beanlands et al. [44] showed that at 1 minute after injection, the relationship of Tc-99m-teboroxime retention to blood flow was linear over a wide flow range, up to 4.5 ml/min/gr. However, after 5 minutes the retention–flow relationship was linear only to 2.5 ml/min/gr. Stewart et al. [50] injected Tc-99m-teboroxime intracoronarily in open-chested dogs under baseline conditions and after the administration of intravenous dipyridamole. The first-pass myocardial retention fraction averaged 0.90 ± 0.04 in this animal model. However, they found a rapid clearance of the radiotracer soon after myocardial uptake was complete. Myocardial clearance of the radionuclide occurred in a biexponential manner, suggesting that the kinetics of Tc-99m-teboroxime represent both blood flow as well as non-flow-related cellular binding. Sixty-seven percent of retained activity cleared with a half-time of 2.3 ± 0.6 min, while the residual activity demonstrated slow clearance. Myocardial clearance rate determined by dynamic imaging with tomography averaged 21 ± 4 min and dropped to 13 ± 4 min following dipyridamole administration.

Pieri et al. [51] studied sequential changes in the regional distribution of Tc-99m-teboroxime in nine dogs with graded coronary artery stenosis. Coronary blood flow was measured by Doppler, and regional myocardial perfusion was assessed by microspheres. A linear relationship between the Tc-99m-teboroxime abnormal/normal activity ratio and coronary blood flow (r = 0.96) and regional myocardial perfusion (r = 0.99) was found. Their results also showed that the myocardial clearance half-times at 100%, 75%, and 50% flow were not significantly different, while clearance half-time at total occlusion was significantly faster (p < .01). The effects of metabolic inhibition on the uptake of Tc-99m-teboroxime, Tc-99m-sestamibi, and Tl-201 were assessed in cultured myocardial cells by Maublant et al. [52]. Overall, Tc-99m-teboroxime showed the lowest sensitivity to metabolic impairment. The uptake of Tc-99m-teboroxime was significantly decreased at low temperature (approximately 30% at 0°C), while osmotic lysis or metabolic inhibition with either cyanide (a blocker of the mitochondrial respiratory chain), iodoacetate (an inhibitor of the glycolytic pathway), and ouabain (an inhibitor of Na-K sarcolemmal ATPase) had no definite effect. However, the uptake of Tl-201 and Tc-99m-sestamibi was severely diminished by metabolic impairment or in the presence of dead cells. Since Tc-99m-teboroxime myocardial uptake is largely independent of the metabolic status of the cells, it should be particularly suitable as a myocardial blood flow imaging agent in situations such as in the postischemic phase where there is discrepancy between coronary blood flow and metabolic activity of the myocardial tissue. The differential uptake of Tc-99m-teboroxime, Tc-99m-sestamibi, and Tl-201 was assessed in normal, hypoperfused, and border-zone rabbit myocardium by quantitative dual-radioisotope autoradiography. Based on this technique, Weinstein et al. [53] concluded that Tc-99m-teboroxime and, to a lesser extent, Tc-99m-sestamibi, can better delineate hypoperfused myocardium in comparison to Tl-201. Since Tc-99m-teboroxime detected the largest area of hypoperfusion, the authors suggested that Tc-99m-teboroxime may provide the most accurate assessment of myo-cardium-at-risk distal to coronary stenosis.

Differential myocardial washout

Stewart et al. [54] studied the clearance kinetics of Tc-99m-teboroxime in poststenotic and normal myocardium in response to occlusive, rapid pacing and pharmacologic stress in the intact preinstrumented canine experimental model. They showed that the Tc-99m-teboroxime clearance was accelerated in normal myocardium by adenosine and by dipyridamole compared to the control state. The myocardial clearance half-time was 11.9 ± 1.8 min in the control state and 8.9 ± 1.1 min and 9.3 ± 1.9 min after adenosine and dipyridamole, respectively (p < .05). Using adenosine stress test, the poststenotic clearance half-time was significantly prolonged (11.2 ± 3.7 min.) compared to nonoccluded contralateral perfusion zones (6.3 ± 1.5 min., p < .05). These results indicate that Tc-99m-teboroxime myocardial washout is flow dependent and that myocardial regions with reduced blood flow exhibit delayed clearance in comparison with regions with enhanced myocardial perfusion. This differential myocardial washout of Tc-99m-teboroxime was also shown in human studies [55–57]. This reflects differences in regional myocardial flow reserve as well as ongoing differences in regional blood flow during imaging.

While most of the animal studies have reported a decreased Tc-99m-teboroxime clearance from flow-restricted myocardium following either pharmacologic stress test or atrial pacing, Tc-99m-teboroxime kinetics in flow-restricted myocardium at rest were not well defined until Johnson et al. [58] studied Tc-99m-teboroxime clearance kinetics at rest in normal and flow-restricted myocardium over a period of 1 hour in 23 dogs with stenosed circumflex arteries. The first exponential phase of the myocardial clearance (found to be biexponential over 1 hour) was significantly different in the normal zones (half-time = 4.5 min) compared to the stenosed territories (10.2 min, $p < .05$). However, the half-times of the second exponential phase were not significantly different (160.7 min for normal zones and 140.4 min for the stenosed zones). These data demonstrated that there is a differential clearance and redistribution of Tc-99m-teboroxime in a canine model of resting hypoperfusion and this can be used to differentiate between normal and hypoperfused myocardium. The same group of authors [59] studied the regional Tc-99m-teboroxime clearance kinetics in a canine model using dipyridamole to determine if clearance kinetics could be useful in differentiating the severity of coronary artery flow restriction. A significant difference in fractional myocardial clearance between the normal zones (0.69) versus mild-to-moderate stenosis (0.61, $p < .05$) and severe flow-restricted zones (0.57, $p < .05$) was observed over a 1-hour period. After 7 minutes, the myocardial Tc-99m-teboroxime clearance was significantly different between normal and mild-to-moderate stenosis zones, whereas after 15 minutes the clearance was significantly different between mild-to-moderate and severe stenosis zones. A significant correlation was also found between blood flow and early myocardial Tc-99m-teboroxime clearance across all zones.

Biodistribution and Dosimetry

Human biodistribution data have been obtained in nine normal volunteers during a Phase I clinical trial [48]. After intravenous administration at rest, Tc-99m-teboroxime diffuses rapidly across the phospholipid cell membrane due to its neutral and highly lipophilic characteristics. Blood and lung activity clears within 1 to 2 minutes after the injection. Blood clearance is rapid with only 9.5% of the dose remaining in the circulation 15 minutes after the injection. The liver, which is the major route of elimination, shows a low activity initially but the hepatic uptake increases over time with peak activity starting about 5 minutes after injection. The hepatic half-time differs from that of Tc-99m-

sestamibi: it is approximately 1 to 1.5 hours, suggesting that the mechanisms of uptake and excretion may also differ. During the first 4 hours after the injection of Tc-99m-teboroxime, an average of 8% of the injected dose is excreted in urine, and from 4 to 24 hours 13% is found in the urine. Total urinary excretion averages 22% of the injected dose, while total fecal excretion averages 26% of the injected dose. Myocardial uptake of Tc-99m-teboroxime is rapid, with excellent myocardial visualization at 1–2 minutes after injection. The myocardial clearance, however, is also very rapid and biexponential with half-times of 2 minutes (68%) and 78 minutes (32%).

Absorbed radiation doses from a Tc-99m-teboroxime intravenous injection have been estimated from human biodistribution data obtained in a Phase I clinical trial involving nine normal volunteers [48]. The estimated absorbed radiation doses are given in Table 4.2. These numbers were calculated for an intravenous injection of Tc-99m-teboroxime at rest and are based on the following assumptions: 6-hour gallbladder emptying interval, 2-hour urinary bladder voiding interval, two-thirds of the activity leaving the liver goes directly into the small intestine and the remaining one-third is stored in the gallbladder prior to excretion, and all the activity in the liver is excreted in the feces. The results show that the upper large intestine and the gallbladder are the target organs. Obviously, a significant change in liver and gastrointestinal function can lead to a major change in dose estimations.

Technical Aspects

Preparation

Preparation of Tc-99m-teboroxime from the kit supplied by the manufacturer is relatively simple. Under aseptic and radiation safety regular conditions, a recommended maximum dose of 100 mCi (3.7 GBq) of sterile, additive-free, nonpyrogenic sodium pertechnetate Tc-99m in approximately 1 ml of solution is added into the 5 ml vial in a lead shield. The contents of the vial are swirled for a few seconds. Then the vial containing Tc-99m-teboroxime is placed upright in a boiling water bath or in a heating block for 15 minutes (100°C). After this time period, the vial is removed from the water bath, placed in a lead shield, and another period of approximately 10–15 minutes is needed to allow the vial to cool before administration to the patient. The reconstituted vial should be stored at room temperature and Tc-99m-teboroxime doses should be aseptically withdrawn within 6 hours of preparation.

The total preparation time for Tc-99m-teboroxime

usually takes at least 30 minutes, including the time required to heat the water to boiling or to heat the heating block and the time for the agent to be heated. Fast labeling method and quality control procedure have been described, similar to the procedure previously reported for Tc-99m-sestamibi preparation. Wilson et al. [60] described a microwave oven method for fast labeling (20 seconds) of Tc-99m-teboroxime. Several technical precautions need to be considered when using a microwave oven for preparing Tc-99m-teboroxime, similar to those for preparing Tc-99m-sestamibi.

Quality control

The method for evaluating the radiochemical purity of Tc-99m-teboroxime involves a two-strip paper chromatography; one to evaluate the percentage of reduced hydrolyzed Tc-99m and the second one to evaluate the percentage of soluble Tc-99m contaminants. Like the recommended labeling preparation procedure, the recommended quality control is time-consuming (10–13 min) and needs to be significantly reduced in order to use Tc-99m-teboroxime for emergency purposes or to improve laboratory efficiency. Wilson et al. [60] described a one-strip paper chromatographic procedure offering a faster (2–3 min instead of 10–13 min) and more convenient method for determining radiochemical purity of Tc-99m-teboroxime.

Tc-99m-TETROFOSMIN

Tc-99m-tetrofosmin, a new diphosphine complex of Tc-99m, was the third Tc-99m labeled myocardial perfusion imaging agent to be approved and made commercially available, following Tc-99m-teboroxime and Tc-99m-sestamibi. Tc-99m-tetrofosmin shows similar myocardial uptake, retention, and blood clearance kinetics to Tc-99m-sestamibi. However, the clearance of Tc-99m-tetrofosmin from both the liver and the lung is faster than that of Tc-99m-sestamibi. These characteristics can have an impact on the injection and imaging protocols. Furthermore, the preparation of Tc-99m-tetrofosmin does not require a heating period.

Chemistry and Constituents

Tetrofosmin is a ligand that forms a lipophilic, cationic complex with Tc-99m. Tc-99m-tetrofosmin is the generic name for 1,2,-bis [bis(2-ethoxyethyl) phosphino] ethane, also called P53 (developmental name) or Myoview (trademark name from Medi-Physics, Inc., Amersham Healthcare, Arlington Heights, Illinois). PPN1011 was also another term used to describe tetrofosmin. Tetrofosmin has a molecular weight of 382, and an empirical formula of $C_{18}H_{40}O_4P_2$. The functionalized diphosphine complex of Tc-99m has a molecular weight of 895 and a formula of $[TcO_2 (tetrofosmin)_2]^+$.

According to the product monograph, a 10 ml vial of tetrofosmin, or Myoview, supplied by Amersham Healthcare, contains a predispensed, nonpyrogenic, sterile, lyophilized mixture of the following ingredients sealed under a nitrogen atmosphere with a rubber closure: 0.23 mg of tetrofosmin or [6,9-bis(2-ethoxyethyl)-3, 12 dioxa-6,9-diphospha-tetradecane], 0.03 mg of stannous chloride dihydrate (minimum stannous tin 5.0 μg, maximum total stannous and stannic tin 15.8 μg, 1.0 mg of sodium D-gluconate, 1.8 mg of sodium hydrogen carbonate, and 0.32 mg of disodium sulphosalicylate.There is no bacteriostatic preservative. The lyophilisate is reconstituted with oxidant-free, sterile, nonpyrogenic Tc-99m-sodium pertechnetate. The pH of the reconstituted product varies from 7.5 to 9.0. There are no known contraindications to intravenous administration.

Physiologic Characteristics

Assessment of myocardial blood flow

Using an intact canine model of ischemia, Sinusas et al. [61] tested the hypothesis that Tc-99m-tetrofosmin was a reliable coronary blood flow tracer over a pathophysiologic range of flows seen in ischemia or infarction conditions. Six open-chest mongrel dogs had a complete occlusion of the left anterior descending coronary artery. Dogs were injected with 30 mCi of Tc-99m-tetrofosmin during peak pharmacologic stress performed with either adenosine or dipyridamole. Radiolabeled microspheres were also injected into the left atrium at baseline, coronary artery occlusion, and peak pharmacologic stress to measure the regional myocardial blood flow. Dynamic planar imaging and arterial sampling were performed during the radiotracer injection and up to 15 minutes after the administration. The hearts were then rapidly excised at 15 minutes for well counting of myocardial Tc-99m-tetrofosmin activity and flow. Myocardial Tc-99m-tetrofosmin activity at 15 minutes after the injection correlated linearly with radiolabeled microsphere flow during peak stress in each dog. The correlation coefficients ranged from 0.71 to 0.94 with an average of 0.84. Myocardial Tc-99m-tetrofosmin activity appeared to underestimate flow at flows exceeding 1.5–2.0 ml/min/gr. The plot of Tc-99m-tetrofosmin activity versus blood flow achieved a plateau at approximatly 2.0 ml/min/gr (see Fig. 4.2).

On the other hand, as with Tc-99m-sestamibi and Tl-201, Tc-99m-tetrofosmin activity overestimated coronary blood flow in low flow ranges, at less than 0.2 ml/min/gr. Tc-99m-tetrofosmin activity cleared rapidly from the blood with 2.8% and 0.8% of peak activity remaining in the blood at 5 and 15 minutes, respectively. During this study, the authors also assessed heart, liver, and lung clearance. The myocardial clearance between 3 and 15 minutes was similar in both ischemic and nonischemic regions. The myocardial activity cleared 18% ± 11% in the ischemic region. Lung activity remained lower than myocardial activity and the liver activity remained elevated over the initial 15 minute period following injection.

Mechanisms of myocardial uptake

Mechanisms of Tc-99m-tetrofosmin myocardial uptake have been studied by some authors using different experimental models. Dahlberg et al. [62] evaluated the effect of coronary blood flow on the uptake of Tc-99m-tetrofosmin in the isolated rabbit heart model. The maximum extraction (Emax) of 0.37 for Tc-99m-tetrofosmin suggests a capillary-tissue permeability surface (PS cap) similar to that of Tc-99m-sestamibi. In comparison, Emax value for Tl-201 is 0.73, for Tc-99m-teboroxime, 0.81, and for Tc-99m-sestamibi, 0.39. However, Tc-99m-tetrofosmin has the lowest net extraction (Enet) among the four compounds: 0.23 (Tl-201: 0.57, Tc-99m-sestamibi: 0.41, and Tc-99m-teboroxime : 0.67). This lower value of Enet for Tc-99m-tetrofosmin in rabbits suggests myocardial clearance of this compound. However, studies in humans [63] have shown a stable myocardial retention of Tc-99m-tetrofosmin, at least up to 4 hours after its intravenous injection. This difference between animal and human data is not really surprising, considering that similar interspecies variability has been previously observed for the kinetics of other Tc-99m labeled phosphine compounds, especially for Tc-99m-DMPE [64]. Unfortunately, extrapolating of data from animal or in vivo experiment results to humans may be difficult due to these species differences.

Platts et al. [65] studied the mechanism of Tc-99m-tetrofosmin uptake in isolated adult rat myocytes. They also evaluated the subcellular localization in ex vivo myocardial tissue. They found that the uptake of Tc-99m-tetrofosmin into rat myocytes was rapid, temperature dependent (an approximately fourfold decrease in uptake was observed when the incubation temperature was reduced from 37°C to 22°C), and independent of extracellular Tc-99m-tetrofosmin concentration. Metabolic inhibitors such as iodoacetic acid

and 2,4-dinitrophenol inhibited Tc-99m-tetrofosmin uptake at 30 minutes by approximately 50% depending on the dosage that was used. However, the cellular uptake was not affected by cation channel inhibitors such as ouabain, amiloride, bumetanide, and nifedipine. The lack of effect of ion channel inhibitors on Tc-99m-tetrofosmin uptake is similar to that on uptake of other cations such as Tc-99m-sestamibi. Thus Tc-99m-tetrofosmin differs from Tl-201 in that it does not appear to act as potassium analog. Based on studies performed on tissue homogenate, it seems that mitochondrial membrane potential plays a major role in the myocardial uptake and retention of Tc-99m-tetrofosmin, as seen with Tc-99m-sestamibi.

Younes et al. [66] studied the mechanism of Tc-99m-tetrofosmin uptake into isolated rat heart mitochondria. They concluded that the most probable mechanism of uptake of Tc-99m-tetrofosmin into myocytes is by potential-driven transport of the lipophilic cation. Their results did not predict the mechanism of uptake at the sarcolemmal membrane. They postulated that the myocardial uptake in vivo was related to the metabolic status of the myocytes, in particular the mitochondrial membrane and the plasma membrane potentials.

Biodistribution and Dosimetry

Human biodistribution, dosimetry, and safety of Tc-99m-tetrofosmin administration at rest and during exercise were studied in 12 male volunteers by Higley et al. [67]. Every volunteer was injected with 3.7–4.7 mCi of Tc-99m-tetrofosmin both at rest and at stress within 7–14 days. Blood, urinary, fecal, and whole-body clearances were calculated. The blood clearance was rapid for all volunteers. By 10 minutes after the injection there was less than 5% of the injected dose in the whole blood volume and less than 3.5% of the injected dose in the total plasma volume. The blood clearance was initially faster following exercise. At 2 hours after injection, the urinary clearance was 13.1% ± 2.1% in the resting study and 8.9% ± 1.7% in the exercise study (p < .001). At 48 hours postinjection, the rate of urinary clearance was almost identical for both physiological conditions: 39.0% ± 3.7% at rest and 40.0% ± 3.7% at exercise. The 48-hour cumulative fecal clearance was 34.2% ± 4.3% at rest and 25.2% ± 5.6% after exercise. The whole-body clearance at 48 hours was 67% ± 6% after exercise and 72% ± 6% at rest.

Analysis of whole-body images showed that good quality images of the heart can be obtained as early as 5 minutes after the injection of Tc-99m-tetrofosmin and this uptake persisted for several hours. Myocardial background clearance resulting from activity in the blood, liver, and lung was rapid. After exercise, there was less Tc-99m-tetrofosmin activity in certain organs, mainly liver, urinary bladder, and salivary glands, in comparison to the rest study. As with Tc-99m-sestamibi, this relative reduced liver uptake at stress can be explained by an enhanced retention in peripheral muscles as a result of the increased blood flow induced by physical exercise and by splanchnic vasoconstriction during exercise.

After a stress injection, the myocardial uptake of Tc-99m-tetrofosmin, although relatively stable over time, slightly decreases from 1.3% of the injected dose at 5 minutes to 1.0% at 2 hours after the injection. From 5 minutes to 120 minutes postinjection, liver uptake decreases from 3.2% to 0.5%, lung uptake decreases from 1.2% to 0.2%, while gallbladder activity increases from 0.5% to 3.2%, and the gastrointestinal tract activity increases from 2.0% to 8.7%. From 5 minutes to 60 minutes after Tc-99m-tetrofosmin injection, the heart-to-lung ratio increases from 4.0 ± 1.1 to 5.9 ± 1.3 and the heart-to-liver ratio increases from 0.8 ± 0.3 to 3.1 ± 3.0. After a rest injection, the myocardial activity of Tc-99m-tetrofosmin remains relatively constant over time with an uptake of 1.2% of the injected dose at 5 minutes and 1.0% at 2 hours after the injection. From 5 minutes to 120 minutes postinjection, liver uptake decreases from 7.5% to 0.9%, lung uptake decreases from 1.7% to 0.3%, while gallbladder activity increases from 0.8% to 5.3%, and the gastrointestinal tract activity increases from 2.9% to 13.8%. From 5 minutes to 60 minutes after Tc-99m-tetrofosmin injection, the heart-to-lung ratio increases from 3.1 ± 1.8 to 7.3 ± 4.4 and the heart-to-liver ratio increases from 0.4 ± 0.1 to 1.2 ± 0.8. Sridhara et al. [68] compared Tc-99m-tetrofosmin and Tl-201 myocardial imaging in patients with documented coronary artery disease. Planar imaging was performed at six different time points: 5, 30, 60, 90, 120, and 240 minutes. They showed that there was no significant Tc-99m-tetrofosmin myocardial redistribution with a slow myocardial washout of approximately 4%–5% per hour after exercise and 0.4%–0.6% per hour after a rest injection.

Absorbed radiation doses from a Tc-99m-tetrofosmin intravenous injection have been estimated from human biodistribution data obtained in a Phase II clinical trial involving 12 normal male volunteers. The estimated absorbed radiation doses at rest and at stress are given in Table 4.2. These numbers were calculated assuming a 3.5-hour bladder voiding period. The results show that, both at rest and at stress, the gallbladder wall is the target organ, followed by the other excre-

tory organs such as upper large intestine, lower large intestine, bladder wall, and small intestine. Overall, the radiation dose to most organs is significantly reduced during exercise in comparison to rest study.

Technical Aspects

Preparation

The 10 ml glass vial containing the lyophilized mixture for preparation of tetrofosmin is sealed under an inert nitrogen atmosphere with a rubber closure and should be stored at 2°C to 8°C. The preparation of Tc-99m-tetrofosmin from the kit supplied by the manufacturer is a simple procedure, since it does not require any type of heating. Under standard aseptic and radiation safety conditions, the vial is reconstituted with 4–8 ml of a sterile, additive-free, nonpyrogenic sodium pertechnetate Tc-99m solution. The radioactive concentration of the diluted Tc-99m generator eluate should not exceed 1.1 GBq/ml when added to the vial. The Tc-99m-tetrofosmin vial, placed in a lead shield, is then shaken gently to ensure complete dissolution of the lyophilized powder and the vial is allowed to stand at room temperature (15°C–25°C) for approximately 15 minutes. So far, different strategies to decrease the preparation time (although faster than Tc-99m-sestamibi or Tc-99m-teboroxime) have not been successful. The reconstituted injectate must be used within 8 hours and stored at 2°C–25°C.

Quality control

As with other Tc-99m labeled radiotracers, radiochemical purity determination should be carried out before use. The method for evaluating the radiochemical purity of Tc-99m-tetrofosmin involves single-strip paper chromatography [69]. Free Tc-99m-pertechnetate runs to the top of the strip, Tc-99m-tetrofosmin complex runs to the middle portion, and reduced hydrolyzed Tc-99m and other hydrophilic complexes will remain at the origin of the strip. Tc-99m-tetrofosmin radiochemical purity should be more than 90% before use. The manufacturer-recommended chromatography system for Tc-99m-tetrofosmin radiochemical purity assessment generally requires almost 30 minutes for completion. This time period added to the preparation time may represent a relative drawback for Tc-99m-tetrofosmin in clinical practice. Geyer et al. [70] investigated the possibility of using an alternative technique to obtain a more rapid assessment of radiochemical purity of Tc-99m-tetrofosmin preparations without altering the overall accuracy of the procedure. They used a miniaturized chromatographic system, which resulted in a significant reduction in the time required to perform the procedure. The average time required to develop the standard strip was 28 minutes, while the time needed for the miniaturized strip was approximately 4 minutes. This represents a more than six-fold reduction in developing time, related to the use of miniaturized paper strips.

Tc-99m-N-NOET

Tc-99m labeled bis (N-ethoxy, N-ethyl dithiocarbamato) nitrido technetium (II) or Tc-99m-N-NOET is another new Tc-99m labeled myocardial perfusion imaging agent that is currently undergoing Phases II and III clinical evaluation [71]. Since this is the newest of the Tc-99m labeled agents that can be used for myocardial perfusion imaging, published data are more limited than those already available for Tc-99m-sestamibi, Tc-99m-teboroxime, Tc-99m-tetrofosmin, and even Tc-99m-furifosmin. However, the biological characteristics of Tc-99-N-NOET are very interesting and different from those of the other myocardial perfusion radiopharmaceuticals.

Like Tc-99m-teboroxime (and contrary to the other Tc-99m labeled agents) Tc-99m-N-NOET is a neutral Tc-99m complex. However, in contrast to Tc-99m-teboroxime, Tc-99m-N-NOET is the first reported neutral Tc-99m complex showing long retention times in normal myocardial tissue. Furthermore, unlike Tc-99m-sestamibi, Tc-99m-tetrofosmin, and Tc-99m-furifosmin, Tc-99m-N-NOET shows a significant myocardial redistribution over time. Therefore, Tc-99m-N-NOET is the first Tc-99m labeled myocardial perfusion imaging agent that demonstrates similar characteristics to those of Tl-201.

Chemistry and Preparation

Tc-99m-N-NOET, or bis (N-ethoxy, N-ethyl dithiocarbamato) nitrido technetium (II), is a member of a class of neutral myocardial imaging agents named Tc-99m-nitrido dithiocarbamates (C5H10NOS2NaH2O), which are characterized by the presence of a triple-bond core [Tc $\equiv$ N] 2+ [72,73]. It is a neutral and highly lipophilic compound with a octanol/ water partition coefficient of approximately 3100 [74].

Tc-99m-N-NOET has not yet been approved for clinical use in humans. However, the kit for the preparation of Tc-99m-N-NOET supplied by Cis-Us Inc. (Bedford, Massachusetts) can be available in a lyophilized formulation. Each kit consists of two vials: vial A contains a lyophilized product and vial B contains a solution. The components of vial A are succinic acid dihydrazide (nitrido donator agent), stannous chloride dihydrate (reducing agent), 1,2-diaminopropane N,N,N′,N′tetraacetic acid (tin-chelating agent), sodium dihydrogen phosphate, monohydrate and disodium hydrogen phosphate, dihydrate (buffer components). The components of vial B are monohydrate of sodium N-ethoxy, N-ethyl dithiocarbamate or NOET (complexing agent), 2,6-dimethyl-B-cyclodextrin or DIMEB (solubilizing agent), and water for injection (solvent).

Tc-99m-N-NOET injection is prepared using a two-step procedure. Sterile, pyrogen-free sodium pertechnetate (1 to 3 ml) is added to vial A. The content is mixed by inverting vial A. A 15-minute period is allowed for reaction at room temperature. The content of vial B is then added to vial A. Another 5-minute period is allowed for reaction also at room temperature. Reconstituted solution can be stored at room temperature for up to 6 hours.

Quality Control

As with the other Tc-99m-labeled myocardial perfusion imaging agents, labeling efficiency of Tc-99m-N-NOET is obtained with thin-layer chromatography. The quality control procedure is performed with a silica gel thin layer chromatography (TLC) plate and ethyl acetate as a solvent. The labeled product has an Rf of approximately 0.9. Pertechnetate that has not reacted and radioactive impurities will remain at the origin.

Physiologic Characteristics

Myocardial uptake versus blood flow

Comparison between myocardial distribution of Tc-99m-N-NOET and regional myocardial blood flow was performed by Ghezzi et al. [75] in dogs after permanent and temporary partial coronary occlusion of the left anterior descending artery and dipyridamole infusion in 15 mongrel dogs. Comparative blood clearances of Tc-99m-N-NOET and Tc-99m-sestamibi and first-pass extraction fraction have also been evaluated. Like other Tc-99m labeled myocardial perfusion imaging agents, Tc-99m-N-NOET tended to overestimate coronary blood flow in the low-flow range and to underestimate flow in the high-flow range at 15 minutes after its injection, under basal conditions and with dipyridamole. The ischemic-to-nonischemic zone activity ratio was always higher with Tc-99m-N-NOET than that determined with blood flow data. The first-pass extraction fraction of Tc-99m-N-NOET was 75% $\pm$

4% under basal conditions and 85% ± 2% under hyperemic conditions. This high extraction fraction is similar to that of Tc-99m-teboroxime (although slightly less). The lipophilic properties and consequently the large permeability/surface area product explain the high extraction fraction of both radiopharmaceuticals.

Despite the persistent significant linear correlation between Tc-99m-N-NOET activity and regional myocardial blood flow during 90 minutes after the injection when partial coronary occlusion was maintained, there was an increase in myocardial Tc-99m-N-NOET activity relative to the blood flow as measured by microspheres in the 0%–20% flow range and a decrease in the 80%–100% flow range. These data suggest a continuous and slow myocardial redistribution of Tc-99m-N-NOET 15–90 minutes after the injection. Some data from this study also indirectly showed that there was an early myocardial redistribution of Tc-99m-N-NOET within the first 15 minutes following its administration. The blood clearance of Tc-99m-N-NOET and Tc-99m-sestamibi has also been evaluated by Ghezzi et al. [75] using the same experimental model. The blood activity at 30, 90, and 240 minutes after the injection of Tc-99m-N-NOET was 20%, 19%, and 14%, respectively, of that measured at 2 minutes after the injection. In contrast, Tc-99m-sestamibi blood activity decreased much faster with 10% and 4.5% (of the level measured at 2 minutes) at 30 minutes and 90 minutes postinjection, respectively. The blood clearance of Tc-99m-N-NOET was biexponential with an initial half-life of 4.7 minutes and a late half-life of 674 minutes, while the initial blood half-life of Tc-99m-sestamibi was 1.7 minutes and the late half-life was 55 minutes. No metabolite of Tc-99m-N-NOET has been detected in the blood at 2 or 60 minutes postinjection. With this animal model, in vivo imaging showed that the myocardial uptake of Tc-99m-N-NOET at 60 minutes postinjection had decreased by 43% of that measured at 5 minutes. The lung uptake was initially high but decreased faster than cardiac uptake with a heart-to-lung ratio of 1.04 at 5 minutes and 1.84 at 60 minutes postinjection. The liver uptake remained constant over time (Fig. 4.3). Glover et al. [76] studied the myocardial uptake of Tc-99m-N-NOET in nine dogs with either critical or mild left anterior descending coronary artery stenoses during adenosine infusion. Five minutes after the injection, the in vitro Tc-99m-N-NOET uptake was higher than Tl-201 over a wide range of flow. Although myocardial uptake of both agents underestimated the level of flow disparity, Tc-99m-N-NOET uptake more closely matched coronary blood flow than did Tl-201. The authors concluded that Tc-99m-N-NOET is the first Tc-99m labeled myocardial perfusion imaging agent with cardiac retention higher than that

of Tl-201 at 5 minutes postinjection. The same group of authors [77] assessed the first-pass myocardial extraction fraction of Tc-99m-N-NOET in an animal model. The mean Tc-99m-N-NOET extraction fraction was 87 ± 1% (range: 81%–90%) at normal coronary flow rate and 82 ± 1% with adenosine infusion. This extraction fraction is similar to the one reported for Tl-201 using a similar experimental model (82%–87%).

Subcellular distribution of Tc-99m-N-NOET

The subcellular distribution of Tc-99m-N-NOET was determined by Uccelli et al. [78] in Sprague-Dawley rat hearts, using standard differential centrifugation techniques. Subcellular distribution of Tc-99m-sestamibi was also assessed using the same procedures as those performed for Tc-99m-N-NOET. These authors showed that Tc-99m-N-NOET can diffuse and localize in the hydrophobic components of myocardial cells with no evidence of specific association of activity with the mitochondrial and cytosolic components.

Structural membrane integrity was found to be important in the myocardial retention of Tc-99m-N-NOET. After induction of severe cell membrane and organelle disruption, there was no release of Tc-99m-N-NOET activity in the cytosol, while approximately 70% of Tc-99m-sestamibi activity was released into the cytosolic fraction as a result of the disruption of mitochondria, as previously reported. These observations strongly support the hypothesis that Tc-99m-N-NOET, a neutral and lipophilic radiotracer, remains tightly bound to the hydrophobic components of the cell and that the cell membranes are the most probable subcellular localization site of Tc-99m-N-NOET. These results are also in agreement with those reported by Maublant et al. [79] in cell cultures from newborn rat myocytes where relatively high washin rates and long half-times for washout have been found. The concept that Tc-99m-N-NOET is localized predominantly in or on cell membranes was also validated in a study performed by Johnson et al. [80]. Using a perfused rat heart model with Triton X-100 (causing membrane disruption), the clearance of Tc-99m-N-NOET was increased markedly in conditions of membrane disruption.

Myocardial kinetics

The myocardial extraction of Tc-99m-N-NOET has been determined by Dahlberg et al. [81] in isolated rabbit hearts, using multiple indicator-dilution methods over a wide range of coronary blood flows. The maximum extraction (Emax) was 0.48 ± 0.10, the net extraction at 5 minutes (Enet) was 0.24 ± 0.08, and the capillary permeability-surface area product (PS cap)

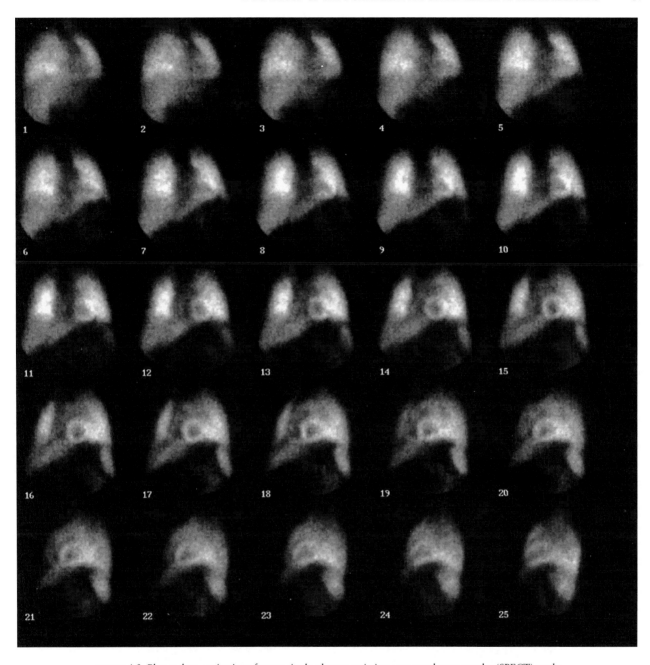

FIGURE 4.3 Planar data projections from a single-photon emission computed tomography (SPECT) study performed 20 minutes following the injection of 20 mCi of Tc-99m-N-NOET at peak stress. There is some degree of initial increased lung uptake, which decreases over time. The degree of lung uptake is unpredictable, does not seem to be related to the extent of coronary artery disease, and in the majority of patients does not interfere with the image interpretation. The liver uptake, contrary to that of Tc-99m-sestamibi or Tc-99m-tetrofosmin, remains relatively fixed for a few hours following Tc-99m-NOET administration, both at rest and at stress.

was 1.02 ± 0.32. These values were 0.75 ± 0.06, 0.57 ± 0.10 and 2.30 ± 1.02, respectively, for Tl-201. These results show that after a moderate initial extraction, there is a significant myocardial clearance of Tc-99m-N-NOET. A study from the same group of investigators [82] also showed that initial Tc-99m-N-NOET extraction and retention were moderately reduced by severe ischemic injury but unaffected after brief ischemia, demonstrating that the cardiac transport of Tc-99m-N-NOET is less sensitive than Tl-201 to ischemic injury. Uptake and release kinetics of Tc-99m-N-NOET were examined in cultures of beating myocardial cells of newborn rats [83]. The myocardial uptake appeared to be independent of extracellular Tc-99m-N-NOET concentration. Metabolic inhibition (induced by Rotenone or iodoacetic acid) and amiloride, ouabain, and bumetanide had no effect on the 1-minute or 30-minute Tc-99m-N-NOET uptake. However, verapamil and diltiazem significantly reduced the uptake of Tc-99m-N-NOET. Furthermore, BayK 8644, a calcium channel activator, increased the uptake, suggesting that Tc-99m-N-NOET uptake might be, at least partially, mediated through an interaction with calcium channels.

Myocardial redistribution and viability

In vitro experiments and studies performed in animals and in humans have demonstrated myocardial redistribution of Tc-99m-N-NOET with a similar behavior to

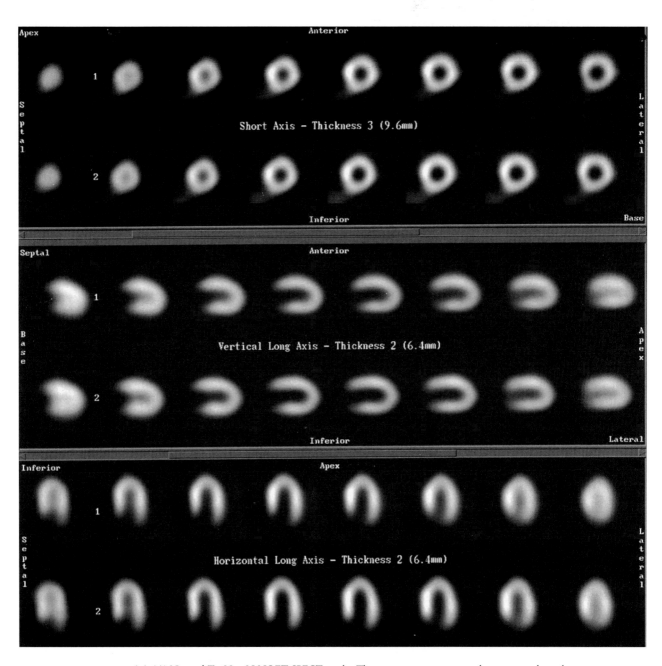

FIGURE 4.4 (A) Normal Tc-99m-N-NOET SPECT study. The upper row represents the stress study and the lower row corresponds to the rest study.

that of Tl-201. Ghezzi et al. [84] studied the myocardial distribution of Tc-99m-N-NOET and Tl-201 under conditions of low-flow ischemia (30 minute duration) in open-chest dogs with partial occlusion of the left anterior descending artery. Myocardial uptake of Tc-99m-N-NOET and Tl-201 were determined by in vitro counting and correlated with radiolabeled mi-

crospheres data. Their results clearly demonstrated that Tc-99m-N-NOET myocardial redistribution was comparable to that of Tl-201 (Fig. 4.4). Vanzetto et al. [85] also compared Tl-201 and Tc-99m-N-NOET myocardial uptake in open-chest dogs with partial occlusion of the left anterior descending coronary artery with a 50% flow reduction. In their model of sustained low

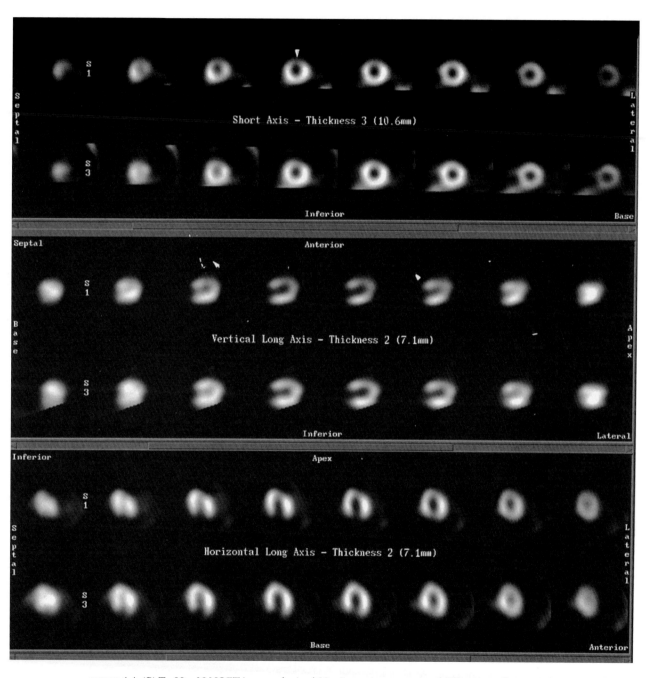

FIGURE 4.4 (B) Tc-99m-N-NOET images obtained 20 minutes (upper row) and 120 minutes (lower row) after the injection of the radiotracer at stress. There is an ischemic antero-apical wall defect (arrow) that is almost completely reversible on the "delayed" images obtained 2 hours later (without reinjection of Tc-99m-N-NOET). This patient had a left anterior descending artery stenosis.

coronary blood flow with severe regional left ventricular dysfunction, the myocardial uptake and kinetics of Tc-99m-N-NOET were comparable to those of Tl-201. They showed a trend toward resolution of the Tc-99m-N-NOET perfusion defect over time consistent with a rest redistribution. The count ratio of left anterior descending to left circumflex artery improved from 66% ± 4% at 15 minutes postinjection to 72% ± 2% at 120 minutes. The same group of authors [86] compared myocardial uptake of Tc-99m-N-NOET and Tl-201 in a canine model of acutely infarcted reperfused myocardium. Dogs were injected after 3 hours of total occlusion of the left anterior descending artery and 1 hour of reperfusion. The infarct-to-normal wall activity ratio was 0.32 ± 0.07 for Tl-201 (reflecting the extent of necrosis) and 0.74 ± 0.12 for Tc-99m-N-NOET ($p < 0.01$, reflecting reperfusion flow). The authors concluded that in the setting of acutely infarcted reperfused myocardium, Tc-99m-N-NOET uptake was a good marker of reperfused flow, whereas Tl-201 uptake appeared to be a better marker of viability.

Johnson et al. [87] investigated the effects of moderate-to-severe stenosis on Tc-99m-N-NOET kinetics at rest using an animal model (dogs) with a 90% reduction in the left circumflex flow. This study showed that resting ischemia caused by a stenosis can be detected by planar Tc-99m-N-NOET imaging. Furthermore, quantification of both ex vivo and in vivo scintigraphic data confirmed the presence of significant Tc-99m-N-NOET myocardial redistribution, which was nearly complete within 90–120 minutes. The apparent rest-redistribution of Tc-99m-N-NOET was mainly explained by differential clearance of the radiotracer where the clearance from the normally perfused myocardial region is more rapid than clearance from the ischemic zone. Although a smaller component of delayed uptake in the underperfused myocardial regions was not totally excluded in their study, it is likely that Tc-99m-N-NOET does not exhibit a true redistribution (as Tl-201 does) but rather a differential clearance. However, the final scintigraphic result will remain the same, that is, correction of the myocardial perfusion defect on delayed study. Although there is a myocardial redistribution of Tc-99m-N-NOET over time, the clinical relationship of redistribution to myocardial viability assessment is still unknown. The apparent discordance between extremely high myocardial retention of Tc-99m-N-NOET reported in isolated myocytes and perfused hearts [79,80,88] and data from canine and human studies showing washout [77,83, 89–91] seems to be related to interactions with blood elements. Although species-specific differences may explain the discordance, Johnson et al. [92] showed that

Tc-99m-N-NOET has significant affinities for binding to both albumin and red blood cells. They demonstrated a bidirectional transfer of Tc-99m-N-NOET between red blood cells and the myocardium. This finding can partially explain the phenomenon of Tc-99m-N-NOET myocardial redistribution.

Biodistribution and Dosimetry

Biodistribution of Tc-99m-N-NOET in humans was initially studied by Giganti et al. [91] in three patients with coronary artery disease and more recently by Fagret et al. [93] in 10 normal healthy volunteers (4 males, 6 females). Although there are some discrepancies between the two studies that can be explained by the small number of observations, the different types of patient populations, or the methodology, these two preliminary studies showed that the myocardial uptake of Tc-99m-N-NOET is rapid, high, and stable in time, and it is rapidly cleared from the circulating blood. Although the myocardial uptake of Tc-99m-N-NOET is higher than the uptake of other Tc-99m labeled myocardial perfusion imaging agents, the lung uptake is also higher with approximately 20% of the injected dose in the lungs 5 minutes after the injection at rest with a lung half-life of 50 minutes at rest and 77 minutes at stress. Giganti et al. [91] also reported an initial lung uptake of Tc-99m-N-NOET of 24% at 30 minutes after the injection with a lung half-life of 11 minutes. This increased lung uptake is thought to be related to the presence of cyclodextrin in the kit preparation. Cyclodextrin, as previously mentioned, is used to avoid significant adsorption of Tc-99m-N-NOET on the vial, plastic syringes, and catheters due to the lipophilic character and the neutral charge of Tc-99m-N-NOET. Ongoing studies are performed to find an alternative dispersant to decrease the lung uptake.

Besides the lung uptake of 24% of the injected dose at 30 minutes, Giganti et al. [91] also reported that the liver uptake was 21% of injected dose at 30 minutes, 27% at 2 hours, and 20% at 4 hours. The myocardial uptake of 5.2% of the injected dose at 30 minutes and 4.8 % at 4 hours was slightly higher than the one previously reported.

Only preliminary data on radiodosimetric estimation of Tc-99m-N-NOET in normal humans are currently available and published in an abstract form [93]. Two separate groups of investigators have reported their radiation dose estimates in one group of 10 normal volunteers (4 males, 6 females) with a mean age of 36 ± 11 years [93] and in a group of 3 fasted patients with coronary artery disease [94]. Table 4.2 summarizes the results of the two sets of data. Radiation dose estimates vary most significantly for liver and ovaries. Further data will be needed to complete these estimates and to compare radiodosimetry of Tc-99m-N-NOET to that of the other Tc-99m labeled myocardial perfusion imaging agents.

CONCLUSIONS

Many radionuclide myocardial perfusion imaging agents are now commercially available and others should be soon. Although many of their characteristics differ, they all share the same utilization, that is, the diagnostic and evaluation of patients with coronary artery disease. We still are learning how to obtain the best diagnostic results from Tl-201 and Tc-99m-sestamibi myocardial perfusion scintigraphy. It is likely that with the newest agents and constantly evolving technology in data acquisition and analysis, our knowledge will improve and all these agents will be able to fulfill a more specific role in clinical practice.

REFERENCES

1. Sapirstein LA. Regional blood flow by fractional distribution of indicators. Am J Physiol 1958;193:161.
2. Zimmer L, McCall D, D'Addabbo L, et al. Kinetics and characteristics of thallium exchange in cultured cells. Circulation 1979;59:138.
3. Beller GA, Watson DD. Physiological basis of myocardial perfusion imaging with the technetium99m agents. Semin Nucl Med 1991;12:173.
4. Dahlberg ST, Leppo JA. Myocardial kinetics of radiolabeled perfusion agents: basis for perfusion imaging. J Nucl Cardiol 1994; 1:189.
5. Leppo JA, Meerdink DJ. Comparison of the myocardial uptake of a technetium-labeled isonitrile analogue and thallium. Circ Res 1989;65:632.
6. Weich HF, Strauss HW, Pitt B. The extraction of Tl-201 by the myocardium. Circulation 1977;56:188.
7. Krahwinkel W, Herzog H, Feinendegen LE. Pharmacokinetics of thallium-201 in normal individuals after routine myocardial scintigraphy. J Nucl Med 1988;29:1582.
8. Deutsch E, Bushong W, Glavan KA, et al. Heart imaging with cationic complexes of technetium. Science 1981;214:85.
9. Dudczak R, Angelberger P, Homan R, et al. Evaluation of Tc-99m-dichloro bis (1,2-dimethylphosphino)ethane (Tc-99m-DMPE) for myocardial scintigraphy in man. Eur J Nucl Med 1983;8:513.
10. Gerson MC, Deutsch EA, Libson KF, et al. Myocardial scintigraphy with Tc-99m-Tris-DMPE in man. Eur J Nucl Med 1984; 9:403.
11. Jones AG, Davison A, Abram S, et al. Biological studies of a new class of technetium complexes: the hexakis (alkylisonitrile) technetium (I) cations. Int J Nucl Med Biol 1984;11:225.
12. Holman BL, Jones AG, Lister-James J, et al. A new Tc-99m labelled imaging agent, hexakis (T-butyl-isonitrile)-technetium (I) (Tc-99m-TBI): initial experience in the human. J Nucl Med 1984; 25:1350.
13. Sia STB, Holman BL, McKusick K, et al. The utilization of Tc99m TBI as a myocardial perfusion agent in exercise studies. Comparison with Tl201 thallous chloride and examination of its biodistribution in humans. Eur J Nucl Med 1986;12:333.
14. Sia STB, Holman BL, Campbell S, et al. The utilization of technetium-99m CPI as a myocardial perfusion imaging agent in exercise studies. Clin Nucl Med 1987;12:681.
15. Wackers FJ, Berman DS, Maddahi J, et al. Technetium-99m hexakis-2-methoxyisobutyl isonitrile: human biodistribution, dosimetry, safety and preliminary comparison to thallium-201 for myocardial perfusion imaging. J Nucl Med 1989;30:310.
16. Piwnica-Worms D, Kronauge JF, Chiu ML. Uptake and retention of hexakis (2-methoxyisobutyl-isonitrile) technetium (I) in cultured chick myocardial cells. Mitochondrial and plasma membrane potential dependence. Circulation 1990;82:1826.
17. Beanlands RSB, Dawood F, Wen WH, et al. Are the kinetics of technetium-99m methoxyisobutyl isonitrile affected by cell metabolism and viability? Circulation 1990;82:1802.
18. Okada RD, Glover D, Gaffney T, et al. Myocardial kinetics of technetium-99m-hexakis-2-methoxy-2-methylpropyl-isonitrile. Circulation 1988;77:491.
19. Glover DK, Okada RD. Myocardial kinetics of Tc-MIBI in canine myocardium after dipyridamole. Circulation 1990;81:628.
20. Mousa SA, Cooney JM, Williams SJ. Relationship between regional myocardial blood flow and the distribution of Tc-99m-sestamibi in the presence of total coronary artery occlusion. Am Heart J 1990;119:842.
21. Canby RC, Silber S, Pohost GM. Relations of the myocardial imaging agents Tc-99m mibi and Tl-201 to myocardial blood flow in a canine model of myocardial ischemic insult. Circulation 1990;81:289.
22. Leppo JA, Meerdink DJ. Comparison of the myocardial uptake of a technetium-labeled isonitrile analogue and thallium. Circ Res 1989;65:632.
23. Li QS, Solot G, Frank TL, et al. Myocardial redistribution of technetium-99m-methoxyisobutyl isonitrile (sestamibi). J Nucl Med 1990;31:1069.
24. Sinusas AJ, Beller GA, Smith WH, et al. Quantitative planar imaging with technetium-99m methoxy isobutyl isonitrile: comparison of uptake patterns with thallium-201. J Nucl Med 1989; 30:1456.
25. Sinusas AJ, Bergin JD, Edwards NC, et al. Redistribution of Tc-99m-sestamibi and 201Tl in the presence of a severe coronary artery stenosis. Circulation 1994;89:2332.
26. Verani MS, Jeroudi MO, Mahmarian JJ, et al. Quantification of myocardial infarction during coronary occlusion and myocardial salvage after reperfusion using cardiac imaging with technetium-99m hexakis 2-methoxyisobutyl isonitrile. J Am Coll Cardiol 1988;12:1573.
27. Rubow S, Klopper J, Wasserman H, et al. The excretion of radiopharmaceuticals in human breast milk: additional data and dosimetry. Eur J Nucl Med 1994;21:144.
28. Gagnon A, Taillefer R, Bavaria G, et al. Fast labeling of technetium-99m-sestamibi with microwave oven heating. J Nucl Med Technol 1991;19:90.
29. Hung JC, Wilson ME, Brown ML, et al. Rapid preparation and quality control method for technetium-99m-2-methoxy isobutyl isonitrile (technetium-99m-sestamibi). J Nucl Med 1991;32: 2162.
30. Porter WC, Karvelis KC. Microwave versus recon-o-stat for preparation of technetium-99m sestamibi: a comparison of hand exposure, radiochemical purity and image quality. J Nucl Med Technol 1995;23:279.

31. Hung JC, Wilson ME, Brown ML, et al. Comparison of four alternative radiochemical purity testing methods for Tc-99m-sestamibi. Nucl Med Commun 1995;16:99.

32. Patel M, Sadek S, Jahan S, et al. A miniaturized rapid paper chromatographic procedure for quality control of technetium-99m sestamibi. Eur J Nucl Med 1995;22:1416.

33. Reilly RM, So M, Polihronis J, et al. Rapid quality control of Tc-99m-sestamibi. Nucl Med Commun 1992;13:664.

34. Beller GA, Watson DD. Physiological basis of myocardial perfusion imaging with the technetium agents. Semin Nucl Med 1991;21:173.

35. Berman DS, Kiat H, Van Train KF, et al. Comparison of SPECT using technetium-99m agents and thallium-201 and PET for the assessment of myocardial perfusion and viability. Am J Cardiol 1990;66:72E.

36. Johnson LL, Seldin DW. Clinical experience with technetium-99m teboroxime, a neutral, lipophilic myocardial perfusion imaging agent. Am J Cardiol 1990;66:63E.

37. Johnson LL. Clinical experience with technetium-99m teboroxime. Semin Nucl Med 1991;21:182.

38. Johnson LL. Myocardial perfusion imaging with technetium-99m-teboroxime. J Nucl Med 1994; 35: 689.

39. Leppo JA, DePuey EG, Johnson LL. A review of cardiac imaging with sestamibi and teboroxime. J Nucl Med 1991;32:2012.

40. Narra RK, Nunn AD, Kuczynski BL, et al. A neutral technetium-99m complex for myocardial imaging. J Nucl Med 1989;30:130.

41. Nunn AD. Radiopharmaceuticals for imaging myocardial perfusion. Semin Nucl Med 1990;20:111.

42. Taillefer R. New agents labelled with technetium 99m for myocardial perfusion imaging. Can Assoc Radiol J 1992;43:258.

43. Taillefer R. Technetium-99m teboroxime. In: *New Radiotracers in Cardiac Imaging: Principles and Applications,* edited by R. Taillefer, N. Tamaki. Stamford: Appleton Lange, 1999, pp. 49–74.

44. Di Rocco RJ, Rumsey WL, Kuczynski BL, et al. Measurement of myocardial blood flow using a co-injection technique for technetium-99m-teboroxime, technetium-96-sestamibi and thallium-201. J Nucl Med 1992;33:1152.

45. Leppo JA, Meerdink DJ. Comparative myocardial extraction of two technetium-labeled BATO derivatives (SQ30217, SQ32014) and thallium. J Nucl Med 1990;31:67.

46. Meerdink DJ, Leppo JA. Experimental studies of the physiologic properties of technetium-99m agents: myocardial transport of perfusion imaging agents. Am J Cardiol 1990;66:9E.

47. Marshall RC, Leidholdt EM, Zhang DY, et al. The effect of flow on technetium-99m-teboroxime (SQ30217) and thallium-201 extraction and retention in rabbit heart. J Nucl Med 1991;32:1979.

48. Narra RK, Feld T, Nunn AD. Absorbed radiation dose to humans from technetium-99m-teboroxime. J Nucl Med 1992;33:88.

49. Beanlands R, Muzik O, Nguyen N, et al. The relationship between myocardial retention of technetium-99m teboroxime and myocardial blood flow. J Am Coll Cardiol 1992;20;712.

50. Stewart RE, Schwaiger M, Hutchins GD, et al. Myocardial clearance kinetics of technetium-99m-SQ30217: a marker of regional myocardial blood flow. J Nucl Med 1990;31:1183.

51. Pieri P, Yasuda T, Fischman AJ, et al. Myocardial accumulation and clearance of technetium 99m teboroxime at 100%, 75%, 50% and zero coronary blood flow in dogs. Eur J Nucl Med 1991;18:725.

52. Maublant JC, Moins N, Gachon P, et al. Uptake of technetium-99m-teboroxime in cultured myocardial cells: comparison with thallium-201 and technetium-99m-sestamibi. J Nucl Med 1993; 34:255.

53. Weinstein H, Reinhardt CP, Leppo JA. Teboroxime, sestamibi and thallium-201 as markers of myocardial hypoperfusion: comparison by quantitative dual-isotope autoradiography in rabbits. J Nucl Med 1993;34:1510.

54. Stewart RE, Heyl B, O'Rourke RA, et al. Demonstration of differential post-stenotic myocardial technetium-99m-teboroxime clearance kinetics after experimental ischemia and hyperemic stress. J Nucl Med 1991;32:2000.

55. Hendel RC, McSherry B, Karimeddini M, et al. Diagnostic value of a new myocardial perfusion agent, teboroxime (SQ 30,217), utilizing a rapid planar imaging protocol: preliminary results. J Am Coll Cardiol 1990;16:855.

56. Weinstein H, Dahlberg ST, McSherry B, et al. Rapid redistribution of teboroxime. Am J Cardiol 1993;71:848.

57. Yamagami H, Ishida Y, Morozumi T, et al. Detection of coronary artery disease by dynamic planar and single photon emission tomographic imaging with technetium-99m teboroxime. Eur J Nucl Med 1994;21:27.

58. Johnson G, Glover DK, Hebert CB, et al. Early myocardial clearance kinetics of technetium-99m-teboroxime differentiate normal and flow-restricted canine myocardium at rest. J Nucl Med 1993;34:630.

59. Johnson G, Glover DK, Hebert CB, et al. Myocardial clearance kinetics of technetium-99m-teboroxime following dipyridamole: differentiation of stenosis severity in canine myocardium. J Nucl Med 1995;36:111.

60. Wilson ME, Hung JC. Microwave preparation of and one-strip paper chromatography for technetium Tc 99m teboroxime. Am J Hosp Pharmacol 1993;50:2376.

61. Sinusas AJ, Shi QX, Saltzberg MT, et al. Technetium-99m-tetrofosmin to assess myocardial blood flow: experimental validation in an intact canine model of ischemia. J Nucl Med 1994;35:664.

62. Dahlberg ST, Leppo JA. Myocardial kinetics of radiolabeled perfusion agents: basis for perfusion imaging. J Nucl Cardiol 1994; 1:189.

63. Sridhara BS, Braat S, Rigo P, et al. Comparison of myocardial perfusion imaging with technetium-99m tetrofosmin versus thallium-201 in coronary artery disease. Am J Cardiol 1993;72: 1015.

64. Deutsch E, Ketring AR, Libson K, et al. The Noah's ark experiment: species dependent biodistributions of cationic Tc-99m complexes. Nucl Med Biol 1989;16:191.

65. Platts EA, North TL, Pickett RD, et al. Mechanism of uptake of technetium-tetrofosmin. I: Uptake into isolated adult rat ventricular myocytes and subcellular localization. J Nucl Cardiol 1995;2:317.

66. Younes A, Songadele JA, Maublant J, et al. Mechanism of uptake of technetium-tetrofosmin. II: Uptake into isolated adult rat heart mitochondria. J Nucl Cardiol 1995;2:327.

67. Higley B, Smith FW, Smith T, et al. Technetium-99m-1,2-bis[bis(2-Ethoxyethyl) Phosphino]ethane: human biodistribution, dosimetry and safety of a new myocardial perfusion imaging agent. J Nucl Med 1993;34:30.

68. Sridhara B, Sochor H, Rigo P, et al. Myocardial single-photon emission computed tomographic imaging with technetium-99m tetrofosmin: stress-rest imaging with same-day and separate-day rest imaging. J Nucl Cardiol 1994;1:138.

69. Jones S, Hendel RC. Technetium-99m tetrofosmin: a new myocardial perfusion agent. J Nucl Med Technol 1993;21:191.

70. Geyer MC, Zimmer AM, Spies WG, et al. Rapid quality control of technetium-99m-tetrofosmin: comparison of miniaturized and standard chromatography systems. J Nucl Med Technol 1995;23:186.

71. Taillefer R. Technetium-99m-N-NOET. In: *New Radiotracers in Cardiac Imaging: Principles and Applications,* edited by R. Taillefer, N. Tamaki. Stamford: Appleton Lange, 1999, pp. 113.

72. Pasqualini R, Comazzi V, Bellande E, et al. A new efficient method for the preparation of Tc-99m-radiopharmaceuticals containing the Tc = N multiple bond. Appl Radiat Isot 1992;43:1329.

73. Pasqualini R, Duatti A, Bellande E, et al. Bis (dithiocarbamato) nitrido technetium-99m radiopharmaceuticals: a class of neutral myocardial imaging agents. J Nucl Med 1994;35:334.

74. Bellande E, Hoffschir D, Comazzi V, et al. Interaction of the myocardial imaging agent TcN-NOET with cyclodextrins: influence of the stability of the inclusion complex on the biological properties. J Nucl Med 1994;35:261p (abstract).

75. Ghezzi C, Fagret D, Arvieux CC, et al. Myocardial kinetics of TcN-NOET: a neutral lipophilic complex tracer of regional myocardial blood flow. J Nucl Med 1995;36:1069.

76. Glover DK, Ruiz M, Calnon DA, et al. Favorable first-pass myocardial extraction fraction for technetium-99m-N-NOET: implications for pharmacologic stress imaging. J Nucl Med 1997;38:65p (abstract).

77. Glover DK, Vanzetto G, Calnon DA, et al. Kinetics of bis (N-ethoxy, N-ethyl dithiocarbamato) nitrido 99m-Tc (NOET) in a canine model of transient coronary artery occlusion: comparison with Tl-201. Circulation 1996;94:I-302 (abstract).

78. Uccelli L, Giganti M, Duatti A, et al. Subcellular distribution of technetium-99m-N-NOET in rat myocardium. J Nucl Med 1995;36:2075.

79. Maublant J, Zhang Z, Ollier M, et al. Uptake and release of bis(N-ethoxy, N-ethyl dithiocarbamato) nitrido Tc-99m(V) in cultured myocardial cells: comparison with Tl-201, MIBI, and teboroxime. Eur J Nucl Med 1992;19:597 (abstract).

80. Johnson G, Allton IL, Nguyen KN, et al. Clearance of technetium 99m N-NOET in normal, ischemic-reperfused, and membrane-disrupted myocardium. J Nucl Cardiol 1996;3:42.

81. Dahlberg ST, Gilmore MP, Flood M, et al. Extraction of technetium-99m-N-NOET in the isolated rabbit heart. Circulation 1994;90:I-368 (abstract).

82. Guillaud C, Comazzi V, Joubert F, et al. Metabolite analysis of the neutral technetium-99m nitrido dithiocarbamate complex TcN-NOET after injection in rats. J Nucl Med 1996;37:188–189p (abstract).

83. Ghezzi C, Fagret D, Mouton O, et al. In vitro uptake kinetics of bis(N-ethoxy, N-ethyl dithiocarbamato) nitrido technetium-99m (V), a myocardial perfusion imaging agent: a study in cultured cardiac cells. Circulation 1996; 90:I-301 (abstract).

84. Ghezzi C, Fagret D, Brichon PY, et al. Redistribution of bis(N-ethoxy, N-ethyl dithiocarbamato) nitrido technetium-99m-(V), a new myocardial perfusion imaging agent: comparison with Tl-201 redistribution. Circulation 1996;94:I-302 (abstract).

85. Vanzetto G, Calnon DA, Ruiz M, et al. Tc-99m-N-NOET uptake in dogs with a severe coronary artery stenosis: comparison to thallium-201 and regional blood flow. Circulation 1996; 94:I-301 (abstract).

86. Vanzetto G, Calnon DA, Ruiz M, et al. Myocardial uptake of 99Tc-NOET in dogs with reperfused acute myocardial infarction: comparison to Tl-201. J Nucl Cardiol 1997;4:S21 (abstract).

87. Johnson G, Nguyen KN, Liu Z, et al. Planar imaging of Tc-99m labeled (bis(N-ethoxy, N-ethyl dithiocarbamato) nitrido technetium (V)) can detect resting ischemia. J Nucl Cardiol 1997; 4:217.

88. Pasqualini R, Comazzi V, Bellande E, et al. A new efficient method for the preparation of Tc-99m-radiopharmaceuticals containing the Tc = N multiple bond. Appl Radiat Isot 1992; 43:1329.

89. Fagret D, Marie PY, Brunotte F, et al. Myocardial perfusion imaging with technetium-99m-Tc NOET: comparison with thallium-201 and coronary angiography. J Nucl Med 1995;36:936.

90. Glover DK, Ruiz M, Vanzetto G, et al. Myocardial uptake of Tc-99m-NOET during adenosine hyperemia in dogs with mild to moderate coronary stenoses. J Nucl Cardiol 1997;4:S65 (abstract).

91. Giganti M, Cittanti C, Colamussi P, et al. Biodistribution in man of bis [(N-Ethyl, N-Ethoxy) Dithiocarbamate] nitrido technetium (V), a promising new tracer for myocardial perfusion imaging. J Nucl Med 1994;35:155p (abstract).

92. Johnson G, Nguyen KN, Pasqualini R, et al. Interaction of technetium-99m-N-NOET with blood elements: potential mechanism of myocardial redistribution. J Nucl Med 1997;38:138.

93. Fagret D, Vanzetto G, Mathieu JP, et al. Biodistribution and dosimetry of Tc-99m-N-NOET in normal human. J Nucl Med 1996;37:229p (abstract).

94. Giganti M, Uccelli L, Cittanti C, et al. Dosimetric estimations in man of bis [(N-ehtyl, N-ethoxy) dithiocarbamate] nitrido technetium (V). J Nucl Cardiol 1997;4:S46 (abstract).

5 | Acquisition, processing, and quantification of nuclear cardiac images

DENNY D. WATSON

Most nuclear cardiac imaging today is performed using gated single-photon emission computed tomography (SPECT) technique. Data acquisition and basic software to perform reconstruction and reorientation are provided on all commercial systems and are reasonably standardized. The choices of acquisition protocols, reconstruction, and reorientation parameters are many, but they have been extensively reviewed by expert panels and recommendations are available [1,2], and can also be found on the Internet (http://www.asnc.org/policy/). These guidelines are reviewed in Chapter 25 of this book. This chapter does not repeat the recommendations but reviews some considerations, choices, and trade-offs that must be made by nuclear clinicians in adopting specific protocols for image acquisition and processing.

Many well-executed quantitative processing systems are now becoming available, and this chapter contains an overview of the characteristics of these systems. These systems add a number of additional capabilities that extend and augment the basic set of SPECT images. The first of these additional capabilities is measurement. Interpretation of images does not require measurement of image parameters. Measurements, however, provide an objective way to characterize and communicate results of the study. Measurements can also be used to compile a normal database and compare the image of an individual to the normal database. Defect severity and prognostic significance are better evaluated using measurements rather than subjective judgments. Serial studies to evaluate disease progression or response to therapy are facilitated by quantitative measurements. With gated images, regional and global ventricular function can be specified by numerical values of thickening fractions and left ventricular ejection fraction. Ventricular volume or volume index is also better expressed as a numerical value.

An important new feature of quantitative SPECT imaging systems is related to image transmission, storage, and both on-site and off-site retrieval of digitally encoded images for review and clinical evaluation. Several systems are now evolving to use nonproprietary platforms and generic image standards for reading stations and for servers to facilitate storing the image database. These systems can have economical distributed reading stations for image viewing and interpretation and for report viewing and report generation. Issues related to the growth and implementation of these systems are included in the section of this chapter on Networking.

PLANAR IMAGING

Although SPECT is now the standard approach for myocardial perfusion imaging, planar imaging can be a salvation for patients who are unsuitable for SPECT imaging because of body habitus, or for patients who cannot remain in one position long enough for a complete SPECT rotation. Gated planar images using Tc-99m perfusion agents are feasible and useful. Gated planar images are the basis for radionuclide angiography, which is covered in Chapter 17 of this book. Finally, planar projection images obtained in multiple projections provide the input data for SPECT reconstruction. As such, good planar technique is essential to good SPECT imaging.

The spatial resolution of planar images is the limiting resolution for SPECT reconstruction. As such, planar images will always have at least slightly higher resolution. Perfusion defects must be detectable in planar images in order to be detectable by SPECT reconstruction, since multiple planar images are the only source of information from which SPECT images are derived. However, because planar images include background activity and are projection images, defect contrast will be lower compared to SPECT imaging. It is therefore essential for adequate planar images to maintain the highest possible spatial resolution and good statistical definition, in order to visualize perfusion defects, which may be presented in a more subtle way compared to SPECT. A substantial increase in defect contrast can also be obtained using background subtraction. It is also important to have enough angular projections to insure adequate defect visualization. Small focal defects will tend to become obscured by overlying and underlying activity in some angular projections and be more clearly visualized in other angular projections. It could be argued that the main advantage SPECT offers over planar imaging is that it forces us to image the heart from at least 30 different angular projections. Another advantage of SPECT imaging is that it provides a mathematical way of correlating all the projections into a single three-dimensional composite. Interpreters of planar images must view the various projections and be able to mentally visualize the tracer distribution in space. Those who can do this can become quite accurate at reading planar images. However, perhaps because of the increased dependence on spatial visualization and correlation, the learning curve for planar image interpretation tends to be longer than for SPECT.

Typical standards for planar projections are 0°, 45°, and 70° left oblique. It is good to have a "best septal" angle and that is not always at 45°. We would recommend adding a best septal angle if the heart is observed to be rotated upon initial viewing of the standard projections. For those who are successful in locating the angular orientation of the heart from persistence scope images, it is feasible to start with the best septal angle and move 45° either way from that angle. It is also useful [3] to obtain a right-decubitus left lateral view. This allows a true left lateral view without arm obstruction and often allows a view of the anterior wall of the heart without obstruction by the left breast.

Gated planar images show what appears to be the ventricular cavity moving through the cardiac cycle. Wall motion can be judged from that. However, the appearance of a cavity is the result of more activity from projections that pass obliquely through myocardium near the edge and less activity from projections that pass perpendicularly through the myocardium near the center of the heart in the projected view. There is not a simple direct relationship between the actual endocardial edge and the apparent edge, which is created by an isocount contour somewhere in the transition between the center and edge of the ventricle. Because of the indirect relationship between the apparent and true endocardial border, it is probably best to treat gated planar myocardial perfusion images as qualitative and not attempt to extract precise measures of regional or global wall motion.

The basis of quantitative perfusion imaging was initially developed using planar imaging with thallium-201 (Tl-201) [4–7]. Good results for detection of coronary artery disease [3,8–10] and for prognosis [11–14] have been obtained using quantitative planar imaging techniques. Improvements realized at the time of introduction of quantitative planar imaging were probably not primarily related to the addition of quantitative measurements to the images. Imaging techniques in general were probably improved by the quantitative discipline and there was a greater accumulation of experience. Possibly one of the most powerful advantages added by planar quantification was the subtraction of background from the projection images. This produced images without interfering background and with defect contrast much closer to that of SPECT reconstructed images. From this viewpoint, quantitative planar imaging could be described as a half-way house between simple projection images and those with full three-dimensional reconstruction using SPECT methods.

SPECT IMAGING

Acquisition

Thorough discussion and recommendations for acquisition and imaging protocols are contained in "Imaging Guidelines for Nuclear Cardiology Procedures" [1,2]. The following comments are intended to clarify decisions that are made in setting up an image acquisition.

Imaging time

The total time of image acquisition is usually 15–20 minutes for SPECT rotations. Shorter imaging times give lower quality images due to increased statistical noise. For longer imaging times, patient motion starts to become the limiting factor in image quality. Experience has taught us that for total imaging times of much more than 20 minutes, patient motion will negate any gains in accumulated counts. Note, also, that one must quadruple the imaging time to decrease Poisson statistical noise by a factor of two. So, for example, going from a 20-minute acquisition to a 40-minute acquisition will reduce the image noise by a factor of 1.4, and this rather modest gain may be negated by increased patient movement.

Matrix size

The standard matrix is 64 × 64. If this covers a space of 30 cm then the matrix pixel size is 5 mm. This is adequate given that the overall instrument resolution is no more than 15 mm. However, using a large field camera without zoom can result in pixels that are spaced as wide as a centimeter. That would result in very suboptimal image resolution. Zoom should be used so that the pixel spacing is not more than 5 mm.

Angular resolution

A rule of thumb is to record as many angles as matrix elements. Sixty or 64 stops in 360° should be adequate for acquisition in a 64 square matrix.

Beat rejection

Most commercial systems reject the beat *following* the heart beat with R-R length outside the set window. This is less expensive in both hardware and software than to reject the beat *with* aberrant R-R interval. However, it rarely accomplishes anything other than the loss of good data (while keeping the suspect beats). In general this type of beat rejection should be turned off or set so wide that all beats are accepted. It is possible to use a buffer or list mode recording so that heartbeats can be recorded individually and then retrospectively chosen for inclusion or exclusion from the average. This type of beat rejection can be useful, but the user must confirm positively that the system is capable of retrospective beat rejection.

Positioning

The ability to reproduce positioning in stress and rest images is critical. Variations in arm position are a frequent cause of shifting breast shadow artifacts. Supine position should be standard. Prone position can sometimes reduce subdiaphragmatic attenuation artifact but should probably be used in conjunction with supine images. Prone imaging is subject to anterior artifacts, usually resulting from skin folds over the edge of the narrow imaging table.

Protocols

Tc-99m imaging agents present the problem of choosing between three imaging protocols: 2-day, same-day stress–rest, or same-day rest–stress. The 2-day protocol gives optimal images and allows the comparison of two equal high-dose images. The same-day protocols accommodate situations where it is undesirable to have a 2-day study. If the rest injection is performed first, it is done with low dose. The subsequent high-dose stress image makes the stress image optimal in terms of im-

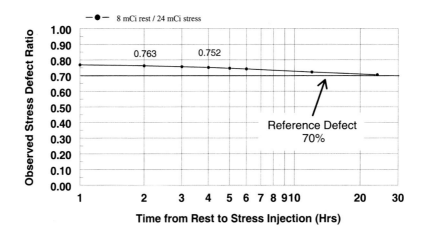

FIGURE 5.1 Defect-to-normal ratio that would be observed on a same-day protocol with 8 mCi injected at rest and 24 mCi injected at peak stress. This is for an assumed mild and completely reversible defect that would have a stress defect ratio of 0.7 using a 2-day protocol. The dilution factor from the same-day rest injection would result in an observed ratio of 0.76 with a 2-hour interval between injections. A 4-hour interval between injections would result in a ratio of 0.75. The improvement in defect resolution comparing 2 hours to 4 hours is insignificant.

age quality, which is desirable. Since there is some residual tracer left over from the previous rest injection, the magnitude of stress-induced perfusion defect will be diluted, so that transient stress-induced defects will lose some contrast compared to a 2-day protocol. Conventionally, we wait 2 hours or more for the rest injection to decay, and increase the dose of the second injection to about three times that of the prior injection. The amount of this defect dilution and the effect of waiting for the prior injection to decay can be easily calculated. Figure 5.1 shows the effect on a mild stress-induced perfusion defect that would have had a defect ratio of 70% compared to the region of maximum uptake if rest and stress injections were separated by at least 24 hours. This calculation shows that for a rest injection of 8 mCi and a stress injection of 24 mCi, the observed defect ratio would be about 0.77 with a 1-hour interval, 0.76 with a 2-hour interval, and 0.75 with a 4-hour interval between injections. This shows that the dilution is primarily related to the ratio of stress dose to rest dose. The waiting time between the two doses in terms of 1 hour versus 2 hours versus 4 hours has (surprisingly) an almost negligible effect. In fact, waiting too long for the first dose to decay will only result in buildup of activity in the large bowel, which can be a major imaging problem. The stress-first protocol can be gainfully used for patients without prior infarction and especially for those with relatively low pretest likelihood of coronary artery disease. We pre-

fer a somewhat higher initial dose (around 15 mCi) in this case to obtain adequate stress images. If the stress images are normal, rest imaging is not required. If the stress image is equivocal or abnormal, rest injection of around 30 mCi is given. This protocol will show stress-induced defects at full contrast but the contamination of stress injection in the rest images will reduce that amount of observed reversibility. This contamination can also be calculated and is shown in Figure 5.2. For illustration, we assume a severe defect with a poststress ratio of 50% of maximum tracer uptake and assume that this defect would have been completely reversible. In this case, we will observe on the same-day study that the defect has reversed from a poststress value of 50% to a post-rest-injection value of about 85%. The reduction in observed reversibility is not severe. Again, it is of surprisingly little value to wait for 1 or 2 more hours for the initial dose to decay. This protocol will easily demonstrate significant but not complete reversibility. However, having chosen patients without prior myocardial infarction, it is clinically unnecessary to distinguish partial from complete reversibility, and this protocol can frequently be useful.

Dual isotope

The dual-isotope protocol usually is performed with Tl-201 given at rest and followed by a stress Tc-99m injection. The advantage of this is greater patient

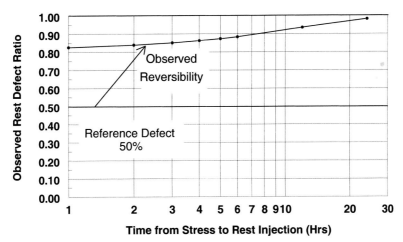

FIGURE 5.2 Calculated effect of using a 15 mCi stress injection prior to a 25 mCi rest injection. It is assumed that there is a severe stress-induced defect with defect-to-normal ratio of 0.5, and completely reversible at rest. On the stress-first study, the defect is correctly observed as 0.5. A following rest injection shows the defect to be about 0.85. An interval of 7.5 hours between injections would result in a poststress defect ratio of 0.9. The effect of waiting 2 to 4 hours between injections is almost negligible.

throughput. The disadvantage of the dual-isotope protocol is that images from Tl-201 must be compared to images from Tc-99m to determine if defects are reversible. Differences in defect resolution and photon scatter will somewhat degrade the ability to identify subtle reversibility. The ability to simultaneously image two radiotracers, one injected at stress and the other injected at rest, would be a major advance. This would not only greatly speed the procedure but would also result in exact spatial registration comparing rest and stress images. Success in doing this has been limited primarily by the fact that photon scatter causes the image obtained in an off-peak-energy window to be spatially distorted compared to the image obtained in an on-peak window. This greatly complicates any attempt to correct the lower energy image for contamination from the higher energy tracer.

Processing

Image processing parameters are also described in the "Guidelines for Nuclear Cardiology Procedures" [1,2]. The orientation for short-axis, horizontal long-axis, and vertical long-axis views is now well standardized. It is most important to maintain the ability to always review raw projection images. These are used to evaluate the potential for motion artifact, for attenuation artifact, and for the identification of many other abnormalities that can be seen in projection images but will be excluded in the reoriented SPECT views. All images should be scaled so that the most intense region of uptake in the myocardium sets the level of maximum intensity. If the image scale is set by a region of more intense uptake outside the myocardium, the perception of myocardial tracer uptake may be unacceptably distorted. The mechanisms to exclude extracardiac activity from resetting the image scale are nonstandardized and often not well developed in commercial software packages. The person processing the study may need to be skillful in order to avoid image scaling problems with Tc-99m tracers. Once this is accomplished, it is probably best to adopt a standard fixed gray scale or color scale. A standardized scale facilitates a more rapid and reliable learning curve for interpreters. Multicolor scales have no particular utility for myocardial perfusion images and abrupt color changes at color band thresholds tend to distort the perception of defect magnitude and image subtlety. Color scales, such as the hot body scale, which show uniform and intuitively perceptible gradation are suitable for myocardial perfusion imaging. Standard test patterns such as the Society of Motion Picture and Television Engineers (SMPTE) [15] pattern should be available and the monitor should be adjusted to display the more subtle features of the test pattern.

Quantification of Perfusion Images

In the mid-1980s, rotational tomography was beginning to replace planar imaging, and methods for quantification of the larger set of tomographic images were being developed [16–18]. The approach developed by Garcia at Cedars-Sinai [17,19,20] was widely distributed and later commercialized. This approach evolved into a collaborative effort with Emory University and Cedars-Sinai called CEqual (for Cedars Emory Quantitative Analysis) [21,22]. This package was developed to include same-day and 2-day protocols using Tc-99m myocardial perfusion tracers. The Emory Toolbox was subsequently developed at Emory University and includes an updated version of CEqual along with other packages to analyze function (Emory Gated SPECT), three-dimensional display (PerSPECTive), and expert system analysis (PERFEX) [23–25].

A method emphasizing fully automatic processing of gated SPECT images to obtain left ventricular ejection fraction and to analyze regional wall motion was developed by Germano at Cedars-Sinai [26,27]. This method also provides left ventricular volume measurements [28,29]. These investigators have incorporated ellipsoidal volume fitting techniques into a new comprehensive package for quantitative SPECT analysis [30,31].

A method developed at the University of Michigan, 3D-MSPECT, provides quantification of gated SPECT and attenuation corrected SPECT images [32,33]. This program emphasizes three-dimensional displays and includes analysis of attenuation corrected SPECT images associated with methods developed at the University of Michigan.

A program used at the University of Virginia (VQuant) is expected to become commercially available. This program provides quantification of perfusion, regional wall motion, and global left ventricular function using an entirely counts-based method based on the partial volume effect [34,35].

Yale University has introduced a package called Wackers-Liu CQ (http://www.eclipsesys.com). This is a comprehensive package providing quantification of perfusion and ventricular function from gated SPECT images [36].

The programs mentioned above, along with others, share many features in common. There are, however, some fundamental differences in approach taken by the developers of the software and there are strengths and weaknesses in each different approach. This discussion is an overview of the main features in common and the main features that differentiate the various approaches to SPECT quantification.

The task of quantification of perfusion images involves two processes. The first is to devise a method of measuring regional tracer uptake in the myocardial images. The second task is to devise a way of displaying the result. The similarities and differences in comparing different quantification schemes can be reduced to two questions: (1) How is the program making measurements of regional tracer activity? (2) How are the measurements being displayed to the interpreter?

Measurement of myocardial tracer activity

Two schools of thought have evolved in measuring myocardial tracer uptake. The oldest and most common method is to determine the maximum tracer activity along a ray that traverses the myocardium. This measurement was found to be reliable for quantification of planar images and has been carried over to SPECT images.

The method of searching for the maximum tracer activity along a path from endocardial to epicardial border has been robust and reproducible but it has been argued that myocardial ischemia and infarction are frequently subendocardial, and that the point of maximum uptake would indicate epicardial activity, and thus be insensitive to subendocardial defects. Computing a transmural average of tracer uptake would alleviate this potential problem and also make use of more pixel measurements, and that would provide an advantage of less statistical noise in the measurement. The disadvantage of computing a transmural average is that the measurement requires the location of the endocardial and epicardial walls. These points are often very poorly determined and the variation in locating wall positions causes measurement variation that can easily offset the increased count statistics of transmural averaging.

Both methods, in reality, provide an average of tracer uptake throughout the sampled myocardial wall. This is so because the resolution of SPECT is less than the thickness of the average myocardial wall. Consequently, the peak of uptake among pixels that lie across a myocardial wall is really the result of averaging across the wall thickness; simply because the imaging system has insufficient resolution to detect which part of the myocardial wall the activity came from. Moreover, the search for "peak" counts, in practice, uses spatial averaging to avoid sampling statistical outliers. Thus, both methods of myocardial sampling are, in reality, reflecting a transmural average and are not different in any fundamental way. There is insufficient spatial resolu-

tion in SPECT imaging to obtain samples that reflect endocardial or epicardial activity. The old method of finding the ray maximum is still probably the more robust, in that it does not require edge detection.

Ideally, the rays traversing the myocardium should be perpendicular to the myocardial wall. For SPECT, this requires some manipulation of coordinates. Probably the best and most frequently used was proposed by Garcia. This uses cylindrical coordinates for the body of the ventricle with radial rays perpendicular to the long axis, and a spherical cap at the apex with rays extending outward from the origin to remain approximately perpendicular to the apex. The spherical cap alleviates problems of sampling over the apex that occur with a full cylindrical coordinate system. Sampling can be done entirely in a spherical or elliptical system. The most recent work from Germano uses an ellipsoidal form fit to the myocardial count distribution and uses transmural averages based on the boundaries of the ellipsoidal form. Methods that use peak sampling are less sensitive to the precise direction of the ray as it crosses the myocardium.

Display and Modeling

The computer can quickly determine tracer activity along hundreds of rays. Displaying this information to a human so that it can be rapidly and accurately assimilated is a challenge. Nevertheless, it is a most important part of the quantitative process [37,38]. Garcia created a long-standing standard with the polar map display. There are many discussions of polar maps and most readers will be familiar with the technique. Polar maps are well illustrated by Van Train et al. [39]. Briefly, tracer activity at the apex is indicated in the center and then activity on successive short-axis slices is displayed around a flat annular ring with the radius of the ring increasing as the slices progress toward the base of the ventricle. The key advantage to this is that it displays all of the sampled activity on a single compact two-dimensional image. One disadvantage is that the polar map has a mapping distortion similar to a polar projection map of the earth. It is therefore difficult to visually estimate the fraction of myocardium involved in a defect.

Polar maps are not the only way to form a compact summary display of SPECT images. Yale-CQ and VQuant are packages that offer alternatives. The summed short-axis and vertical long-axis sections conventionally used to divide the ventricle into segments for visual and quantitative assessment can simply be displayed as conventional cross-sectional images. An example from VQuant is shown in Color Figure 5.3A (normal patient) and *5.3B* (abnormal patient) [see separate color insert]. This shows the summed cross sections used in the quantification of percentage tracer uptake in each segment. This results in three images (or six including both rest and stress) rather than the single (or dual stress–rest) polar map images, but has the advantage of showing anatomically correct images that can be readily appreciated and visually interpreted.

For the purpose of storing numbers representing regional myocardial tracer uptake in a database, it is useful to segment the ventricle in some fashion and record the average tracer activity in segments that can be related to standardized locations in the myocardium. It has become standard to use hexagonal sectors for radial sampling, as depicted in the graphics of Color Figure 5.3A and B. The ventricle is further divided in sections along the long axis. Usually either three sections (base, midventricle, apical) or four sections (base, proximal, distal, apical). The radial sampling in the apical section can remain with six radial sectors but is usually reduced to four (anterior, septal, inferior, lateral) or two (anterior-apical, inferior-apical) (Color Fig. 5.3). This scheme results in anywhere from 14 to 24 segments.

More segments are not necessarily better. The apical region can be adequately covered by two or four sectors. When using four sections along the long axis, the base section tends to become a narrow annulus surrounding the mitral and aortic valve planes. Measurements of tracer uptake in this region are often variable and rarely of clinical significance. It is our preference not to include these in the data set, since they tend to be "throw-away" numbers. Dropping to three long-axis sections with the "base" section extended well into the meaty part of the ventricle results in a smaller data set with all numbers in the data set being of more equal clinical importance. The restriction to six radial sectors may be a greater sampling limitation than that imposed along the long axis, but six sectors have become a de facto standard and there is a good argument to be made for adopting the smallest (and most simple) data set that will provide adequate sampling.

The Normal Database

The normal database should be the average of all subjects contained in the general database who have normal hearts. In practice, we use a sample of patients to establish a normal database. It is questionable that one normal database can be optimal or even adequate in every lab. The criteria for selecting subjects for the normal database are also a subject for discussion. We prefer to use clinically referred patients with low pretest and posttest likelihood of coronary artery disease. This sets the normal database to represent more the average weight, size, and age of patients being examined. More pristine "normals" can be found among young asymptomatic volunteers, but this data set may be unrealistic when applied to the clinically referred population. We are no longer attached to the idea of selecting normals entirely by coronary angiography. Only patients who are referred for coronary angiography with good clinical cause are available today. While some of these

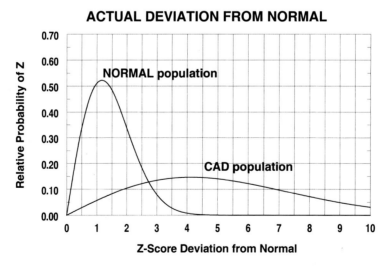

FIGURE 5.4 These curves indicate the frequency of occurrence of a perfusion defect of magnitude shown on the horizontal axis expressed in units of standard deviations from the normal database average. The two curves are for a population of patients with low likelihood of coronary artery disease (CAD) and a second population of patients with known CAD.

will turn out to have angiographlically normal coronary arteries, this is a highly selected population and may be less representative of a population with truly normal coronary arteries and normal myocardium.

Deviations from the normal database can be indicated by contrasting regions in the polar map, or as shown in Figure 5.3B, nonblank entries in the corresponding segment of the, in this example, 14 segment model. A numerical entry in a segment indicates that stress uptake was outside normal limits in this segment. The number entered in the segment represents the difference between rest defect and stress defect, and the asterisk means that the difference is statistically significant, thus indicating defect reversibility.

Sensitivity and Specificity

Comparison of a specific patient to a normal database is a feature of all quantitative programs. On the surface, we could just flag the values representing myocardial uptake in a patient as positive if they were more than two standard deviations below the normal limits. A problem with this is that we are comparing many measurements and the statistics of multiple measurements are different than those of a single measurement. The chance of finding a single specified segment more than two standard deviations below the normal average by virtue of measurement error is 2.3% (one-sided p-value for 2σ deviation). However, when multiple segments are sampled, the probability of finding any one of the sampled segments outside of two standard deviations increases. For an n segment model, and if the probability of each segment being falsely positive is $P(f+)$, then the overall specificity (probability of finding no abnormal segments in a normal subject) is $\{1 - P(f+)\}^n$. With a 14-segment model, the chance of finding at least one segment more than two standard deviations below the normal average (the false positive rate) is 28%. With a 20-segment model the predicted false positive rate would be 37%.

Normal limits can be adjusted to thresholds of more than two standard deviations, and logic requiring multiple conditions can be employed to reduce the false positive rate in comparing the images of a normal individual to the normal database. However, reducing the false positive rate will always be accompanied by a corresponding reduction in sensitivity. This can be appreciated from Figure 5.4, which shows a graph of the maximum defect deviation from normal in z-score (units of standard deviations). The graph shows a peaked curve of the normal patient population and a broad distribution of patients with coronary artery disease of varying severity. A threshold to bifurcate studies into normal and abnormal can be positioned at any point along the horizontal axis, and that will determine a possible discrete sensitivity/specificity combination. The set of all possible sensitivity/specificity pairs is conventionally plotted to form an ROC curve (Fig. 5.5). The computer can then be set to operate anywhere on the ROC curve. The makers of quantitative software are thus faced with an inevitable trade-off between sensitivity and specificity in setting the threshold for the computer to flag a study as abnormal.

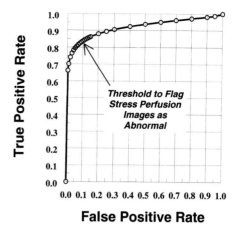

FIGURE 5.5 ROC curve representing the frequency distributions from Figure 5.4. Each choice of threshold to bifurcate studies into "normal" and "abnormal" results in a discrete point on the ROC curve pointing to the sensitivity (vertical axis) and false positive rate (horizontal axis). The computer can be set to provide any sensitivity/specificity pair along the curve.

Interpretation of myocardial perfusion images involves complex factors of pattern recognition, beyond recognition of simple normal limits. The finding of coronary artery disease (CAD) in a patient without previously known disease, is really the estimation of probability of CAD, which should include pretest probability as well as test result. Consequently, expert interpreters should be able to outperform computer interpretations. We should therefore allow and encourage interpreters to overrule the computer analysis. Most interpreters are more reluctant to downgrade a study to "normal" when the computer has flagged it as "abnormal," and less reluctant to upgrade a scan to "abnormal" when the computer finds it within normal limits. For this reason, it is the prejudice of the author to set the computer thresholds to maintain a relatively low (below 10%) false positive rate and to rely on interpreters to look for typical but subtle defects that probably represent significant CAD, but do not cross the computer threshold as being "abnormal." Alternatively, some will find that software has greater commercial appeal if it can be advertised as having very high sensitivity for detection of

CAD. The computer threshold can easily be set to provide any level of sensitivity, but only at the expense of a higher false positive rate. The marketplace tends to encourage us to set thresholds with greater sensitivity and consequently with higher false positive rates. The user needs to be aware of this, and ideally have control of where the computer threshold is set on its characteristic ROC curve.

In performing the comparison of an individual study to a normal database, the computer program can use "expert logic." Rules can be programmed that will account for at least some of the learning experience of experts [40–42]. In practice, most computer programs do employ some expert rules, which will make the computer program more agreeable to the interpreter's experience and logic. Programmers can go beyond this concept to the use of artificial intelligence [43]. It is possible to program the computer to learn from its database of experience if we feed back to it the knowledge of when it was correct in its interpretation. This is a fascinating area of investigation and development. The complexity should not be underestimated. While it is possible today to build a computer and computer program that can equal an expert at chess, it requires extravagant computer systems—and the rules of chess are certainly more explicit and probably more compact than the rules of image interpretation.

It is quite possible to incorporate conditional probability computation into quantitative analysis packages [44–46]. A built-in probability computation could serve as a handy and desirable reference to calculate the prob-

ability of coronary artery disease in a specific patient population, factoring in the current test results. One could also estimate the probability of hard events, which seems palatable if the probability is viewed as a guide to show the outcome of a population similar to the individual patient being tested. Probability calculations should be adjunctive rather than incorporated as part of a quantitative interpretation. Such predictions are useful in risk stratification and planning of treatment options. The desirability of quoting them as specific and accurate predictions of the fate of an individual patient being tested is questionable.

It is the author's opinion that image quantification should not be a substitute for image interpretation. Quantification can provide an objective indication that a study is outside or within the limits established from normal subjects. It can provide objective measures of defect extent and severity for risk stratification. Well-trained interpreters will use this as well as the other quantitative parameters along with all the other clinical information that is available to make the most informed and most nearly accurate interpretation.

Attenuation Correction

Attenuation correction is considered essential to positron emission tomography (PET) imaging. It is becoming a practical option in SPECT imaging today and has the potential to become an equally essential component [47–51]. If attenuation correction can be applied correctly, image interpretation will benefit fun-

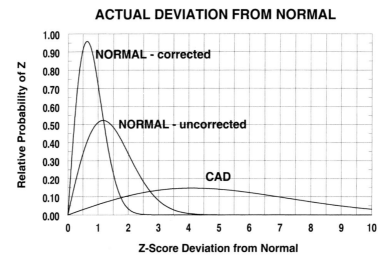

ACTUAL DEVIATION FROM NORMAL

FIGURE 5.6 Defect distribution of normal and abnormal populations before and after attenuation correction. Attenuation reduces the scatter in the normal population by removing variables of body habitus. The CAD distribution is changed only slightly by attenuation correction. The result is to reduce the overlap between the normal and CAD populations.

damentally. To better understand this, consider the distributions in Figure 5.4. These curves show the distribution of measurements of myocardial perfusion in a normal population and in a population with coronary artery disease. The coronary artery disease population has a broad distribution owing primarily to the broad range of perfusion abnormalities associated with CAD. The normal population has a more narrow distribution, but still with substantial spread owing to variations in the amount of attenuation and scatter related to the orientation of the heart, position of surrounding organs, and overall body habitus. Some of this variability has been removed by normalizing or by comparing each myocardial segment with the normal database. This, however, can only account for the average amount of attenuation and there remains substantial residual variability because the individual may differ substantially from the normal average. True attenuation correction can remove the individual variability, and this will significantly reduce the spread in the distribution of the normal population, as illustrated in Figure 5.6. As a result, the limits of normal can be reduced significantly without incurring excessive false positives. The distribution of defects in CAD patients is not substantially changed by attenuation correction. Basically, a real perfusion defect will remain a real defect both before and after attenuation correction, with attenuation correction making some a bit larger and some a bit smaller in magnitude. Thus, theoretically, the sensitivity for detection of perfusion abnormalities can be significantly increased without the expense of more false positives. The technical way of stating this is that the area under the ROC curve will become greater. Of course, images without attenuation artifact would be much easier for interpreters to learn to read as well.

QUANTIFICATION OF VENTRICULAR FUNCTION

Most SPECT studies now incorporate ECG gating and functional assessment, and there is a chapter in this book devoted to the details of gated SPECT. Most of the programs mentioned earlier for quantification of myocardial perfusion also perform quantification of function [34–36,52–54]. Accordingly, the following sections are limited to the relationships and overview of the various quantitative methods. The first quantitative parameter to be extracted from gated SPECT studies is the left ventricular ejection fraction (LVEF). It appears that LVEF can be determined from gated SPECT studies with reasonable accuracy and reproducibility [55–57]. As with the quantification of perfusion, there are three approaches to the quantification of global function. The first approach is to search for the endocardial edge at end-systole and at end-diastole and compute end-systolic and end-diastolic volumes. This is potentially an accurate method and should be good for regional function as well as global function. However, depending on the amount of image noise and the presence of perfusion defects, the techniques for finding endocardial borders must be highly sophisticated to avoid tracking errors. The second method is to fit a shape-constrained volume to the count distribution—typically an ellipsoid of revolution. This will result in approximations of the actual wall position where it is not adequately determined by sufficiently dense tracer uptake. Because of the shape constraints, this method is characteristically more robust for determination of global function, but would be expected to be more approximate for determination of regional function. A third method is to estimate LVEF from thickening fractions, which have been determined from peak counts measured at end-diastole and end-systole. This avoids edge detection entirely and tends to be more robust as a result. This method is ideal for regional function but can have potential problems underestimating LVEF in thick-walled ventricles where either the thickening fractions are actually reduced as a result of severe hypertrophy, or are being underestimated because the ventricle is too thick for the partial volume effect to work. The myocardial wall thickness limitation is not exceeded, however, in most patients [58].

Normal Values for Global LVEF

Quality control for the computation of LVEF by gated SPECT is not standardized or well developed at present. It may be difficult after the study is acquired to check for gate synchronization, arrhythmia, or even edge tracking error. Most errors will cause LVEF to be underestimated and most methods have an intrinsic tendency to yield LVEF values that are lower than those obtained by traditional methods. Nevertheless, physicians make decisions based on LVEF values obtained by traditional methods. We do not subscribe to the idea that gated SPECT can establish different standards for normal and abnormal values of LVEF. If we use the term "left ventricular ejection fraction," we should not expect clinicians to realize, for example, that 45% is within normal limits if it was obtained in my lab using gated SPECT, but not if it was measured by cardiac MRI or in the cardiac catheterization lab or by radionuclide ventriculography. We should develop methods so that the measured values of LVEF are clinically interchangeable.

To assure that values for LVEF are consistent, it seems wise for each nuclear cardiology lab to check the average values of LVEF obtained for normal patients using gated SPECT, along with standard deviations and rate of sporadic failures in the computation of LVEF. This should be relatively simple, since most patients referred for evaluation of myocardial perfusion and with normal perfusion scans will have normal ventricular function. Clinical screening can identify and remove most patients with hypertensive or idiopathic cardiomyopathy from the cohort of patients with normal perfusion, and the remaining group should be a fairly pure sample of subjects with normal ventricular function.

Regional Function

Gated SPECT imaging yields some form of cine display of regional wall motion. Wall motion can be judged either by the perception of edges or by the observation that regional myocardial thickening translates into brightening via the partial volume effect. Using the partial volume effect, we are sensing true myocardial thickening as compared to endocardial excursion. We favor this method for two reasons. First, regional endocardial excursion can be a capricious measure of regional myocardial function because it is the net result of myocardial translation, rotation, and regional thickening. Regional partial volume brightening can occur only if the myocardium actually thickens. It will not reflect myocardial translation. Second, using the counts-based method of partial volume to evaluate thickening obviates the need to judge or detect the endocardial edge. Typical resolution for SPECT imaging after reorientation and filtration is 1.5–2.0 cm. The endocardial border is ragged at best and moves only a few millimeters between diastole and systole. Tracking the endocardial border using SPECT images is a more complex and challenging operation. A disadvantage of using partial volume to estimate regional and global function is that it does not provide actual ventricular volumes. Measurement of ventricular volumes will require edge detection. Future programs may very well adopt a hybrid approach.

Regional Thickening Fractions

It is a natural extension of quantitative SPECT imaging to measure regional myocardial thickening fractions. Absolute normal values for humans are not well established. It seems likely that cardiac MRI will provide the gold-standard for thickening fractions, but there are significant problems with the definition of thickening fractions measured with MRI. The resolution of MRI is so great that we are confronted with a heavily trabeculated wall that varies in thickness from millimeter to millimeter. This can cause wild variations in the thickening fraction measurement depending on exactly what part of the myocardial wall was sampled, the gross motion of the heart, and the method of averaging multiple samples.

It is within easy grasp to obtain regional thickening fractions from the normal database and characterize regional function compared to normal. Color Figure 5.7A (see separate color insert) shows a normal image at end-diastole and at end-systole. All images are intensity scaled on the same scale. The partial volume effect results in a striking change in image brightness resulting from regional myocardial thickening. In this manner, regional wall thickening can be visualized directly from static images. The graphics below the images in Color Figure 5.7A indicate regional thickening fractions based on regional systolic and diastolic count changes. These numbers are compared to a normal database. Color Figure 5.7B shows the function study for the perfusion study shown in Color Figure 5.3B. Regions of poor contraction can be identified as having little or no change in intensity between diastole and systole, and the asterisks on the thickening fractions indicate thickening fractions that are outside the limits determined from the normal database. Global function is also indicated, and by this technique is derived from regional thickening fractions. Regional function adds considerably to myocardial perfusion imaging. For example, normal thickening in the region of a fixed defect is used to indicate attenuation artifacts. Abnormal thickening in a region without a concordant perfusion defect can indicate stunned or hibernating myocardium. Reduced thickening fractions with normal global LVEF may indicate early stages of hypertrophic myopathy. Finally, globally reduced thickening fractions in cases of severe diffuse multivessel disease may indicate hibernation with globally exhausted coronary reserve capacity. In such cases, vasodilators will fail to indicate inducible ischemia and the potential for functional recovery with revascularization.

Volume Measurements

Measurements of end-diastolic and end-systolic volumes add a significant dimension to quantitative processing of gated SPECT studies, and it is clear that absolute volume can be estimated with adequate precision using gated SPECT [59,60]. It would seem prudent, however, to use these measurements with caution. The determination of absolute volume requires absolute spatial calibration of the imaging system. The task of calibration can be demanding, and errors in linear dimension measurements will tend to magnify (be cubed) in the computation of volume.

Clinical interpretation of volume measurements should require normalization of the volumes by body surface area, since normal volumes vary according to the size of the patient. It may be clinically useful to compare ventricular volumes serially in a patient being treated or being followed for the progression of disease. This would not require accuracy of volume index measurements, but would require rigorous control of the spatial calibration of the imaging system to insure that serial volume changes were not the result of instrumental variation or changes in calibration.

It has been suggested that volume measurements would be useful to detect "transient cavity dilatation." The author considers this to be a misconception. Most "transient cavity dilatation" is not an actual change in the physical size of the left ventricle. It is the result of extended subendocardial regions of severely reduced tracer uptake owing to severely reduced subendocardial blood flow with stress. This makes the ventricular "cavity," as judged by region of absent tracer, appear to be larger compared to the rest images when the tracer is present in the subendocardial region. If the "volume" being measured by radiotracer is based on the edge of the radiotracer distribution, then it will reflect the "transient cavity dilatation." However, if this is so, the measured volume will not be the same as the actual ventricular volume. The difference between actual physical ventricular volume and volume determined by the edge of the tracer distribution can be significant. So these two measures of "volume" should not be confused.

One of the current mysteries of gated SPECT imaging is probably the result of not making a distinction between the physical volume of the ventricle and the apparent volume traced by an isocount contour. Methods that measure the edge of the tracer will indicate a higher ventricular volume in the presence of a substantial stress-induced perfusion defect. Consequently the computed LVEF will tend to be lower when there are regions of severely reduced myocardial tracer uptake. This will result in the indication of lower poststress LVEF compared to rest LVEF in patients with stress-induced perfusion defects, and this phenomenon may be erroneously attributed to poststress myocardial stunning. Methods of measuring LVEF that are not dependent on locating tracer edges will not show the effect and will indicate a lower occurrence of true protracted poststress stunning.

Nuclear cardiologists should distinguish between "ventricular dilatation" that is related to the edge of the tracer from that which is related to the true volume of the ventricle. The reason is that the former is caused by garden-variety stress-induced blood flow abnormalities and the latter reflects a prolonged stress-induced contractile failure and/or elevated filling pressures with abnormal stretching of muscle fibers. Certainly the physiology, and possibly the prognostic implications of each, may be significantly different. The frequency of occurrence is vastly different. Perhaps those of us who create programs to measure ventricular volumes could be more sensitive to this issue.

RELIABILITY OF QUANTITATIVE IMAGING METHODS

"Robust" is a favorite term, almost a cliché, used extensively to describe quantitative methods. It is a characteristic of overriding importance to the clinician who needs to have a sense of the reliability of a test result. It is a term usually defined by intuition more than science. It is often true that methods seeking a high degree of accuracy give a result that may be highly accurate but can also sporadically be in error. In such cases the substitution of a less accurate approximation that will dependably be approximately correct may be better. The latter method would be described as more robust. Figure 5.8 depicts the frequency of error in measurements performed by a highly accurate but not very robust method compared to a robust alternative, which is less accurate. The robust method can be thought of as yielding a range of values, in the hands of average users, mostly in a range of ±10% around the true value. The more accurate method will yield most results in a range of less than 5% from the true value, but can sporadically be off by 50% or 100%.

Different methods of performing a measurement differ greatly in this respect. The inventor of the method is often faced with choices that provide reliable approximations at the expense of more sophisticated and theoretically more accurate methods that provide greater accuracy but with greater potential for large error. The measurement of LVEF is an example. A robust method may be able to reliably distinguish if the LVEF is in the range of 20% or 40% or 60%. This method may not be able to distinguish an LVEF of 58% from one of 65%. A more accurate method may be able to do that, but with the disadvantage that it also can falsely indicate 40% when the true LVEF is 60%. The problem with the latter method is that it has the potential to produce incorrect clinical classifications of normal, mild, moderate, severe. If the frequency of sporadically incorrect classifications is significant, clinicians cannot be confident in using the measurement for clinical decision making.

While validation studies address these issues, a test may perform more erratically in the hands of an end-user than in the hands of the investigators performing

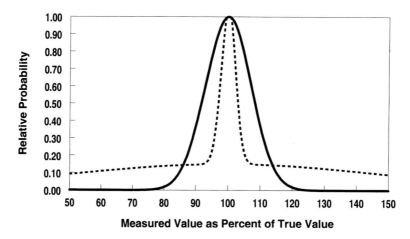

FIGURE 5.8 Distribution of values from multiple repeated measures made by a method that is robust but less accurate, shown by the solid line, and a method that is highly accurate but less robust, shown by the dashed line. The probability for very large deviations from the true value is higher for the less robust method, making it less suitable for clinically important measurements.

the validation study. Investigators, even when strictly blinded, are usually cognizant of acquisition or processing errors that will cause major error in computed values, and these will likely be corrected at the time of data acquisition and processing. Multicenter trials will provide a better estimation of real-world test performance, but each user must ultimately establish the level of confidence to be vested in a new technique as it is developed for use in the individual clinical setting.

Simplicity can be a close correlate of reliability. The field of nuclear medicine lends itself to an endless parade of colorful, animated, and multidimensional displays of data obtained using methods with myriad user-defined options. The marketing value of such display is clear, since it provides something that will be attractive to almost any potential customer. It is easy to argue passionately for rich displays that take full advantage of the intrinsic three-dimensional nature of SPECT imaging. However, in the arena of clinical interpretation, basic standardized presentations representing cross-sectional anatomy have been the reliable standard for X-ray, computed tomography (CT), and magnetic resonance imaging (MRI), and this will likely be true as well for SPECT.

Software development is enormously expensive. Because of the limited market, nuclear cardiology vendors will not be able to invest as much in software development as could be borne by larger markets. As a result, nuclear cardiology is congenitally obliged to live with relatively immature software. In the past few years, a growing number of programs from within medical centers have been commercialized to provide software packages in nuclear cardiology. These medical centers are often working in conjunction with traditional vendors and combine to provide a rich source of software, which has been developed and tested in the field, providing more options and better performance and provoking developments such as low-cost standardized networking solutions. Users, and in some ways even vendors, should benefit from these commercial developments. While we applaud these developments, it may be useful to remind potential users that the investigators who are producing and validating the new software now more frequently have a commercial interest in sales of the software packages. Users will ultimately have to judge for themselves the validity, idiosyncrasies, and usefulness of the software packages.

Networking

Nuclear cardiology computer systems have traditionally been proprietary and lacking in data transmission standards that would allow data to be exchanged between systems or stored in separate image and report archive and retrieval systems. Nuclear cardiology, to remain competitive, needs efficient methods of on-site image storage and retrieval and off-site image review. Independently developed quantification packages are now tending to prefer generic standards for image files, and most are using standard personal computer–level computers so that multiple image review stations can be inexpensively added on a network. The image files generated in nuclear cardiology are relatively small compared to most radiology images, and many years of prior studies can be stored and rapidly retrieved using affordable technology. It appears that systems developed and commercialized at university hospitals may become the catalyst for implementation and deployment of standards that will make data exchange, image storage and retrieval, and off-site networked stations an economic reality.

The adaptation of digital information technology to medical practice has been restrained by the slow development of standards for medical communications and medical imaging. The adoption of standards is prerequisite to the deployment of this technology. The explosive growth of the Internet was made possible by the adoption of transmission standards (TCP/IP) and document standards (HTML) that were implemented in the early part of 1990. Prior to that time, communications from computer to computer were chaotic and cumbersome. The adoption of data transmission standards essentially allowed many different kinds of computers to speak a common language by which they could communicate. Once the standards had been adopted, the subsequent development of Internet communications was staggering in its scope and speed. In fact, all mass communications such as radio and television have been preceded by the development and acceptance of standards, which are necessary to allow mass development of radios, TV sets, transmitters, recorders, etc. Indeed, the industrial revolution is based on standards. Consider the importance of screw thread specifications or bearing sizes, and the thousands of details that must be standardized prior to the economical production of trains, automobiles, or electric toasters.

We would argue that all of the technological possibilities we can imagine for digital data are available to medicine, but none will be economically successful until appropriate standards are adopted. Accordingly, let us review some of the current standards that are in progress.

Health level 7

Health Level 7 (HL7) was founded in 1987 to develop standards for the electronic interchange of clinical, financial, and administrative information among healthcare-oriented computer systems. HL7 was designated by the American National Standards Institute (ANSI) as an ANSI accredited standards developer in June of 1994.

The HL7 standard is supported by most system vendors and the majority of large U.S. hospitals today. It is also used in Australia, Austria, Germany, Holland, Israel, Japan, New Zealand, and the United Kingdom. HL7 seems destined to become the overriding standard for medical electronic communications. It can serve for hospital information systems, clinical laboratory systems, enterprise systems, and pharmacy systems. However, at the present time, there is no standard within

HL7 for medical images. Since we are concerned with the communication of medical images, we can forgo any further discussion of HL7.

DICOM

DICOM stands for Digital Imaging and Communications in Medicine. DICOM is now a collaboration between the American College of Radiology (ACR) and the National Electrical Manufacturers Association (NEMA). DICOM is a standard, which addresses the issue of vendor-independent data formats and data transfers for digital medical images. DICOM versions 1 and 2 were published respectively in 1985 and 1988. In both versions, data transfer was defined for point-to-point connections without consideration of networked environments. ACR and NEMA have recently completed the third version, named DICOM v3.0, which includes support for network communications.

DICOM is an extensive standard with 13 parts. The specification alone fills several hundred pages, and support documentation would amount to thousands of pages. The standard is evolving and not all the parts are complete. Radiology picture archiving and communication systems (PACs) and teleradiology systems have successfully used DICOM as an image communication standard. Many nuclear cardiology systems issue extensive DICOM compliance statements but generally cannot exchange data between different vendor systems or with radiology systems such as CT or MRI. DICOM is not a "plug and play" standard. The standard is so complex and broad ranging that it is possible for a system to be extensively "DICOM compliant" and still not have the basic capability of exchanging data or images between two systems. Nevertheless, DICOM is rapidly becoming a de facto standard for nuclear cardiology as well as for radiology.

Interfile

Interfile is a nuclear medicine file format adopted by the European community and supported by the Society of Nuclear Medicine as the nuclear medicine image file format of choice. This is a very specific format for nuclear medicine images and data. It can be easily implemented to exchange data files between two different machines. The exporting machine can simply translate its internal proprietary format into Interfile. The importing machine can then accept the Interfile transfer and translate the data back into its internal proprietary format. Because of its relative simplicity and ease of use, Interfile has been widely successful in facilitating the exchange of data between gamma imaging systems used in nuclear cardiology. All nuclear imaging vendors have access to Interfile translation capabilities.

Interfile is currently in version 3.3. A significant weakness is that there is at present only a proposal not an adopted standard for gated SPECT data. Presumably, version 4.x would contain specifications for gated SPECT data. Every major vendor of SPECT imaging equipment now uses a different method of storing gated SPECT data.

Internet Standards

Today, images are massively exchanged on the Internet. As indicated earlier, this is made possible by the adoption of a number of image and transmission standards. These standards will not encompass all the needs of the medical sector, but they are available, efficient, and economical ways to store and transmit images electronically. Because these formats are ubiquitous, there are programs for encoding and decoding readily available for every computer platform and operating system. It should be economically compelling to replace the closed proprietary image formats commonly used in nuclear medicine with these open standards, especially as new systems develop for image archive, retrieval, and review on low-cost portable clinical reading stations. A brief description of a few relevant image formats follows:

GIF

The GIF format was developed by CompuServe for transmitting graphics on its network. There are still some questions about licensing issues, but the format is used so extensively that it has become a de facto standard. This format can represent color images using a 256 level palette. This is a compressed format, which is highly efficient for nuclear cardiology images. It is important to note that the compression is lossless. The original data are recovered exactly upon decompression, so there is no issue here of losing image quality or information content.

TIFF

TIFF is usually less efficient than GIF, but it can represent virtually any kind of image with gray scale or color resolutions of over 65 million levels. TIFF also utilizes a lossless compression scheme.

JPEG

The JPEG format was developed to represent photographs. These files are compressed using a lossy tech-

nique and cannot be used in applications where the received data must be an exact duplicate of the transmitted data. Image files can be compressed more or less with image quality being traded for file size.

MPEG

MPEG is an efficient coding for video streams. This standard is about to be used for digital video broadcasting.

There are many other file format standards, but the ones discussed above may be the most useful for medical images. The use of lossy compression is feasible and economically attractive, especially for nuclear cardiology images. Wavelett compression is a relatively new method that should be noted. For medical images, it is superior to JPEG in that higher compression ratios can be achieved without loss of clinically significant information. It is not, however, as ubiquitous with respect to off-the-shelf coding and decoding software.

We have considered the acquisition, processing, and quantification of nuclear cardiac images. We no longer consider the production of an image the end product of our craft. The images must be electronically managed so as to be readily available for physicians to review and be archived to allow retrieval of old studies for comparison. Physicians should have access to relevant clinical data and be able to report and transmit findings in a nearly real-time mode.

The goal of efficient image and text management is particularly achievable in nuclear cardiology. The image and text data sets are of manageable size and the technology is intrinsically digital. Nuclear cardiology can aspire to be a leader in making digital data efficiently available to referring physicians. Efficient utilization of digital information technology would help significantly in keeping nuclear imaging relevant, cost-effective, and genuinely clinically useful.

REFERENCES

1. Imaging guidelines for nuclear cardiology procedures. J Nucl Cardiol 1996;G34.
2. Updated imaging guidelines for nuclear cardiology procedures, Part 1. J Nucl Cardiol 2001;8:G5.
3. Wackers FJ, Fetterman RC, Mattera JA, et al. Quantitative planar thallium-201 stress scintigraphy: a critical evaluation of the method. Semin Nucl Med 1985;15:46.
4. Mead RC, Bamrah VS, Horgan JD, et al. Quantitative methods in the evaluation of thallium-201 myocardial perfusion images. J Nucl Med 1978;19:1175.
5. Burow RD, Pond M, Schafer AW, et al. Circumferential profiles: a new method for computer analysis of thallium-201 myocardial perfusion images. J Nucl Med 1979;20:771.
6. Garcia EV, Maddahi J, Berman DS, et al. Space-time quantitation of thallium-201 myocardial scintigraphy. J Nucl Med 1981;22:309.

7. Watson DD, Campbell NP, Read EK, et al. Spatial and temporal quantitation of plane thallium myocardial images. J Nucl Med 1981;22:577.

8. Berger BC, Watson DD, Taylor GJ, et al. Quantitative thallium-201 exercise scintigraphy for detection of coronary artery disease. J Nucl Med 1981;22:585.

9. Kaul S, Boucher CA, Newell JB, et al. Determination of the quantitative thallium imaging variables that optimize detection of coronary artery disease. J Am Coll Cardiol 1986;7:527.

10. Maddahi J, Garcia EV, Berman DS, et al. Improved noninvasive assessment of coronary artery disease by quantitative analysis of regional stress myocardial distribution and washout of thallium-201. Circulation 1981;64:924.

11. Brown KA, Boucher CA, Okada RD, et al. Prognostic value of exercise thallium-201 imaging in patients presenting for evaluation of chest pain. J Am Coll Cardiol 1983;1:994.

12. Brown KA. Prognostic value of thallium-201 myocardial perfusion imaging. A diagnostic tool comes of age. Circulation 1991; 83:363.

13. Gibson RS, Beller GA, Gheorghiade M, et al. The prevalence and clinical significance of residual myocardial ischemia 2 weeks after uncomplicated non-Q-wave myocardial infarction; a prospective natural history study. Circulation 1986;73:1186.

14. Gibson RS, Watson DD, Carabello BA, et al. Clinical implications of increased lung uptake of thallium-201 during exercise scintigraphy 2 weeks after myocardial infarction. Am J Cardiol 1982;49:1586.

15. Society of Motion Picture and Television Engineers. URL: http://www.smpte.org.

16. Caldwell J, Williams D, Harp G, et al. Quantitation of size of relative myocardial perfusion defect by single-photon emission computed tomography: Circulation 1984;70:1048.

17. Garcia EV, Van Train K, Maddahi J, et al. Quantification of rotational thallium-201 myocardial tomography: J Nucl Med 1985;26:17.

18. DePasquale E, Nody A, DePuey G, et al. Quantitative rotational thallium-201 tomography for identifying and localizing coronary artery disease. Circulation 1988;77:316.

19. Maddahi J, Van Train KF, Prigent F, et al. Quantitative single photon emission computerized thallium-201 tomography for the evaluation of coronary artery disease: optimization and prospective validation of a new technique. J Am Coll Cardiol 1989;14:1689.

20. Van Train KF, Maddahi J, Berman DS, et al. Quantitative analysis of tomographic stress thallium-201 myocardial scintigrams: a multicnenter trial: J Nucl Med 1990;31:1168.

21. Garcia E, Cooke CD, Van Train KF, et al. Technical aspects of myocardial SPECT imaging with technetium-99m sestamibi: Am J Cardiol 1990;66:23E.

22. Berman DS, Kiat H, Van Train KF, et al. Technetium 99m sestamibi in the assessment of chronic coronary artery disease. Semin Nucl Med 1991;21:190.

23. Garcia EV, Cooke CD, Krawczynska EG, et al. Expert system interpretation of technetium-99m sestamibi myocardial perfusion tomograms: enhancement and validation. Circulation 1991; 92:1.

24. Garcia EV, Krawczynska EG, Folks RD, et al. Expert system interpretation of myocardial tomograms: validation using 288 prospective patients. J Nucl Med 1996;37:48P.

25. Garcia EV, Cooke CD, Volks RD, et al. Expert system (PERFEX) interpretation of myocardial perfusion tomograms: validation using 655 prospective patients. J Nucl Med 1991;40:126P.

26. Germano G, Kiat H, Kavanagh PB, et al. Automatic quantification of ejection fraction from gated myocardial perfusion SPECT. J Nucl Med 1995;36:2138.

27. Germano G, Erel J, Lewin H, et al. Automatic quantitation of regional myocardial wall motion and thickening from gated technetium-99m sestamibi myocardial perfusion single-photon emission computed tomography. J Am Coll Cardiol 1997;30:1360.

28. Van Kriekinge SD, Berman DS, Germano G. Automatic quantification of left ventricular ejection fraction from gated blood pool SPECT. J Nucl Cardiol 1999;6:498.

29. Iskandrian AE, Germano G, VanDecker W, et al. Validation of left ventricular volume measurements by gated SPECT 99mTc-labeled sestamibi imaging. J Nucl Cardiol 1998;5:574.

30. Germano G, Kavanagh PB, Waechter P, et al. A new algorithm for quantitation of myocardial perfusion SPECT I: technical principles and reproducibility. J Nucl Med 2000;41:712.

31. Sharir T, Germano G, Waechter PB, et al. A new algorithm for quantitation of myocardial perfusion SPECT II: validation and diagnostic yield. J Nucl Med 2000;41:720.

32. Kritzman JN, Ficaro EP, Liu YH, et al. Evaluation of 3D-MSPECT for quantification of Tc-99m sestamibi defect size. J Nucl Med 1999;5:181P(abst).

33. Ficaro EP, Kritzman JN, Corbett JR. Development and clinical validation of normal Tc-99m sestamibi database: comparison of 3D-MSPECT to CEqual. J Nucl Med 1995; 5:125P(abst).

34. Smith WH, Kastner RJ, Calnon DA, et al. Quantitative gated SPECT imaging: a counts-based method for display and measurement of regional and global ventricular systolic function. J Nucl Cardiol 1997;4:451.

35. Calnon DA, Kastner RJ, Smith WH, et al. Validation of a counts-based method for quantitating left ventricular systolic function using gated tomographic technetium-99m sestamibi perfusion images: comparison to equilibrium radionuclide angiography. J Nucl Cardiol 1997;4:464.

36. Liu YH, Sinusas AJ, DeMan P, et al. Quantification of SPECT myocardial perfusion images: methodology and validation of the Yale-CQ method. J Nucl Cardiol 1999;6:190.

37. Tuft ER. The Visual Display of Quantitative Information. Cheshire, CT: Graphics Press, 1983.

38. Tuft ER. Envisioning Information. Cheshire, CT: Graphics Press, 1990.

39. Van Train KF, Garcia EV, Cooke CD, et al. Quantitative analysis of SPECT myocardial perfusion. In: Cardiac SPECT Imaging, 2nd Edition. edited by Depuey, Garcia, Berman. Lippincott Williams & Wilkins, 2001.

40. Garcia EV, Cooke CD, Krawczynska EG, et al. Expert system interpretation of technetium-99m sestamibi myocardial perfusion tomograms: enhancement and validation. Circulation 1995; 92:1.

41. Garcia EV, Krawczynska EF, Folks RD, et al. Expert system interpretation of myocardial tomograms: validation using 288 prospective patients. J Nucl Med 1996;37:48P.

42. Garcia EV, Cooke CD, Folks RD, et al. Expert system (PERFEX) interpretation of myocardial perfusion tomograms: validation using 655 prospective patients. J Nucl Med 1999;40:126P.

43. Ezquerra NF, Garcia EV. Artificial intelligence in nuclear medicine imaging. Am J Cardiol Imaging 1989;3:130.

44. Rembold CM, Watson DD. Posttest probability calculation by weights. Ann Intern Med 1988;108:115.

45. Diamond GA, Forrester JS. Analysis of probability as an aid in the clinical diagnosis of coronary artery disease. N Engl J Med 1979;300:1350.

46. Diamond GA, Staniloff HM, Forrester JS, et al. Computer-assisted diagnosis in the noninvasive evaluation of patients with

suspected coronary artery disease. J Am Coll Cardiol 1983; 1(2 Pt 1):444.

47. Gullberg GT. Innovative design concepts for transmission CT in attenuation corrected SPECT imaging. J Nucl Med 1998;39:1344.

48. King MA, Xia W, deVries DH, et al. A Monte Carlo investigation of artifacts caused by liver uptake in single-photon emission computed tomography perfusion imaging with technetium 99m-labeled agents. J Nucl Cardiol 1996;3:18.

49. King MA, Tsui BM, Pan TS, et al. Attenuation compensation for cardiac single-photon emission computed tomographic imaging: Part 2. Attenuation compensation algorithms. J Nucl Cardiol 1996;3:55.

50. Ficaro EP, Fessler JA, Shreve PD, et al. Simultaneous transmission/emission myocardial perfusion tomography. Circulation 1996;93:463.

51. Galt JR, Cullom J, Garcia EV. Attenuation and scatter compensation in myocardial perfusion SPECT. Semin Nucl Med 1999;29:204.

52. Faber TL, Cooke CD, Folks RD, et al. Left ventricular function and perfusion from gated SPECT perfusion images: an integrated method. J Nucl Med 1999;40:650.

53. Shen MY, Liu YH, Sinusas AJ, et al. Quantification of regional myocardial wall thickening on electrocardiogram-gated SPECT imaging. J Nucl Cardiol 1999;6:583.

56. Germano G. Automatic analysis of ventricular function by nuclear imaging. Curr Opin Cardiol 1998;13:425.

57. Rozanske A, Nichols K, Yao SS, et al. Development and application of normal limits for left ventricular ejection fraction and volume measurements from 99mTc-sestamibi myocardial perfusion gated SPECT. J Nucl Med 2000;41:1445.

56. Bax JJ, Lamb H, Dibbets P, et al. Comparison of gated single-photon emission computed tomography with magnetic resonance imaging for evaluation of left ventricular function in ischemic cardiomyopathy. Am J Cardiol 2000;86:1299.

57. Nichols K, Lefkowitz D, Faber T, et al. Echocardiographic validation of gated SPECT ventricular function measurements. J Nucl Med 2000;41:1308.

58. Nichols K, DePuey EG, Friedman MI, et al. Do patient data ever exceed the partial volume limit in gated SPECT studies? J Nucl Cardiol 1998;5:484.

59. Iskandrian AE, Germano G, VanDecker W, et al. Validation of left ventricular volume measurements by gated SPECT 99mTc-labeled sestamibi imaging. J Nucl Cardiol 1998;5:574.

60. Vallejo E, Dione DP, Bruni WL, et al. Reproducibillity and accuracy of gated SPECT for determination of left ventricular volumes and ejection fraction: experimental validation using MRI. J Nucl Med 2000;41:874.

6 | Image artifacts

E. GORDON DEPUEY

Artifacts and normal variants are a significant source of false positive interpretations of myocardial perfusion single-photon emission computed tomography (SPECT) [1]. By anticipating and recognizing such findings, the astute technologist and interpreting physician can increase test specificity in the diagnosis of coronary artery disease and avoid unnecessary catheterization of normal patients.

ARTIFACTS ASSOCIATED WITH INSTRUMENTATION ERROR

Flood Field Nonuniformity

Flood field nonuniformity may be secondary to defective photomultiplier tubes, damaged collimators, faulty camera electronics, or defects in the sodium iodide crystal. To detect such abnormalities, intrinsic flood fields (3 million counts) should be obtained each day, and extrinsic flood fields with the collimator on (30 million counts) should be obtained weekly. Flood field nonuniformity can be detected either visually or quantitatively by inspection/analysis of these planar flood field images.

When a SPECT acquisition is acquired using a camera with one or more sources of nonuniformity described above, each flood field defect will be propagated into a circular arc (Fig. 6.1). Thereby "ring artifacts," consisting of alternating "hot" and "cold" rings will be created. If these "rings" pass through the myocardium in a perfusion SPECT study, irregularities in myocardial count density will be created. In extreme cases, apparent perfusion defects will result. If the heart is not positioned in the exact same location in the flood field in both stress and rest images, which is usually the case, such a defect will appear to be reversible, that is, ischemic.

Errors in Center of Rotation

The center of rotation allows SPECT data to be back-projected onto a central point in the volumetric matrix.

Exact centering of data reconstruction is critical to accurately reproduce anatomic structure and count density distribution. A correct center of rotation for each scintillation camera head should be verified weekly. Errors in the center of rotation will result in misregistration of tomographic data, image blurring, and artifactual SPECT myocardial perfusion defects (Fig. 6.2). Since data from various portions of the heart are back-projected onto different locations in the volumetric matrix, the myocardial image may appear to be misaligned or skewed (Fig. 6.3).

Camera Head Tilt

Similar to the problem with center of rotation error, with a variable-angle multiheaded detector system, if one camera head is tilted, the two (or three) detector heads do not record exactly the same image. Backprojection and reconstruction of these different images into a single cardiac image may also produce regional myocardial perfusion artifacts.

Detector-to-Patient Distance

Minimizing detector-to-patient distance is a very important technical consideration to assure optimal image quality and test sensitivity in detection of perfusion abnormalities. The technologist should strive to minimize detector-to-patient distance, using any one of circular, elliptical, or body-contoured orbits. Increased detector-to-patient distance results in suboptimal defect contrast and spatial resolution. Therefore, with increased detector-to-patient distance true perfusion abnormalities are less well defined, and test sensitivity for the detection of coronary artery disease may decrease. In obese patients, in women with large breasts, and in patients who are unable to elevate their left arm above their head, it is frequently not possible to minimize detector-to-patient distance. Under those circumstances, the interpreting physician should be aware of this technical limitation and the possible impact on test sensitivity.

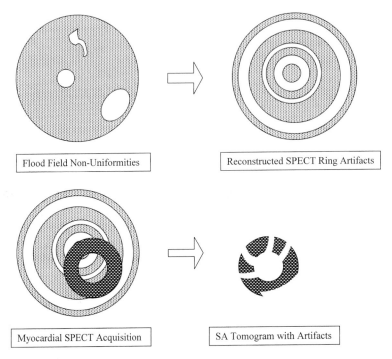

FIGURE 6.1 Flood field nonuniformity resulting in ring artifacts and artifactual myocardial perfusion defects.

PATIENT-RELATED ARTIFACTS

Patient Motion

Patient motion is one of the most common sources of SPECT myocardial perfusion artifacts [2–5]. During SPECT acquisition patients may move in the vertical (axial), lateral, or rotational direction. Unquestionably, the best means to detect patient motion is to inspect the planar projection images of the SPECT acquisition in endless loop cinematic format at the computer console. Inspection of sinograms or a summed image of the planar projections is a poor substitute.

Whether patient movement is abrupt or gradual, myocardial perfusion SPECT image artifacts may be created. The cause of the SPECT reconstruction artifacts is similar to that due to an erroneous center of rotation. However, with patient motion the heart itself is at a different location during different portions of the SPECT acquisition. With filtered back-projection, data are back-projected onto different points of the volumetric matrix, and thereby a misregistration error occurs (see Fig. 6.3). Characteristically with patient motion reconstructed perfusion SPECT images demonstrate opposed defects in contralateral walls. Frequently there are "tails" of diminishing tracer concentration "streaming" from the edges of the defect (see Fig. 6.3). The overall visual effect has been termed the "hurricane sign."

Multiheaded detector systems have been beneficial to decrease SPECT image acquisition time, improve patient

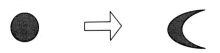

FIGURE 6.2 Error in filtered back-projection resulting in a blurred or "skewed" SPECT reconstruction of a point source. Such an error can be due to an incorrect center of rotation.

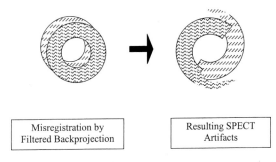

FIGURE 6.3 Schematic representation of camera center of rotation error resulting in artifactual myocardial perfusion defects.

tolerance, and thereby decrease the possibility of patient motion. However, the deleterious effects of patient motion, if it occurs, may be compounded using multiheaded detector systems. If motion occurs, it is "seen" by *each* detector, so artifacts may be compounded.

An attentive technologist can be of great help in minimizing patient motion. SPECT acquisition should be fully explained to patients. Patients should be encouraged not to talk, yawn, sigh, or fall asleep (and snore). The lumbar curvature of the back should be supported, the knees should be slightly elevated and supported to minimize back strain, and the left arm and shoulder should be supported and restrained. Commercially available arm holders are of great help in supporting the arm and shoulder and thereby minimizing patient motion. Although SPECT acquisitions can be performed with both arms at the side [6], in order to minimize detector-to-patient distance and avoid the soft tissue and bone attenuation caused by the arms, elevation of at least the left arm above the head is preferable.

If patient motion does occur, several measures can be taken to salvage the study. If Tc-99m labeled tracers are used, image acquisition can be repeated without tracer redistribution. Without repeating the acquisition, individual planar projection images of the SPECT acquisition can be manually shifted caudally or cephalad to compensate/correct for patient motion. There are also now several computer software programs available that automatically detect and correct for vertical (and sometimes lateral) patient motion [7–11]. However, if such automated programs are employed, the technologist and interpreting physician must inspect the corrected planar projection images (in rotating cinematic format) to assure that patient motion has been completely compensated for.

Soft Tissue Attenuation

The deleterious effects of soft tissue attenuation in myocardial perfusion SPECT may be generalized or localized. Generalized soft tissue attenuation, encountered in obese patients and in individuals with a large chest circumference, results in decreased count density and poor image quality (also see Filtering, below). Of particular concern in such patients are artifacts secondary to depth-dependent attenuation. In a 180° orbit (45° right anterior oblique to 45° left posterior oblique) the part of the left ventricle that is most distant from the camera detector is the base of the posterolateral wall. Consequently, it is the most attenuated portion of the heart. Therefore, in obese patients depth-dependent attenuation may result in artifactual abnormalities in the basal half of the posterolateral wall (Fig. 6.4).

More frequently encountered are fixed, localized soft tissue attenuation artifacts secondary to the left hemidiaphragm, a protuberent abdomen, the left breast, and lateral chest wall fat. Such fixed artifacts mimic myocardial scarring. To anticipate such soft tissue attenuation artifacts, it is helpful to visually evaluate the patient prior to imaging. The technologist, nurse, or physician may note pertinent body habitus characteristics (height, weight, chest circumference, bra cup size, etc.), which the interpreting physician can use to *anticipate* soft tissue attenuation artifacts. A second very useful step to anticipate localized soft tissue attenuation artifacts is to inspect the SPECT planar projection images in endless loop cinematic format at the computer console (Figs. 6.5 and 6.6). The outline and position of a large, dense breast is easily ascertained; the location of the left hemidiaphragm can generally be approximated by visualization of a photopenic defect due to air or fluid in the fundus of the stomach; and presence of excessive lateral chest wall fat can be inferred by decreased visualization of myocardial activity in the left lateral/left posterior oblique views.

Attenuation by the left breast may create artifactual fixed perfusion defects in the anterior, lateral, and even the inferior wall of the left ventricle, depending upon the location of the breast [12] (Fig. 6.7C; see Color Figs. 6.7A and B and 6.8A and B in separate color insert). The severity of the artifacts is most often dependent upon the thickness of the breast (bra cup size). For this reason, it is preferable to image women with the bra off in order to minimize the thickness of the breast.

A particularly problematical artifact is one associated with "shifting" breast attenuation. The position of the breast may differ in the stress and rest acquisitions. Such differences will result in attenuation artifacts that affect different portions of the left ventricle in the stress and rest images and thereby mimic stress-induced ischemia and/or "reverse distribution" (Fig. 6.9A; see Color Fig. 6.9B and C in separate color insert). The breasts may shift in position if a patient wears different clothing for the stress and rest image acquisitions. For instance, if the bra is worn in the stress acquisition, the breast will be positioned anteriorly, whereas if it is not worn for the rest acquisition, the breast will be more dependent and laterally positioned. Taping up the breasts may have the advantage of positioning them superior to the heart, although sometimes the breast will still "eclipse" the anterior wall of the left ventricle. Binding the breasts flattens them, although the position of the breasts under the binding may be variable and may create a "shifting" artifact.

Localized attenuation by the left hemidiaphragm generally creates a fixed inferior or inferolateral defect (Fig. 6.10C; see Color Fig. 6.10A and B in separate color insert). Unlike the breast, the position of the left

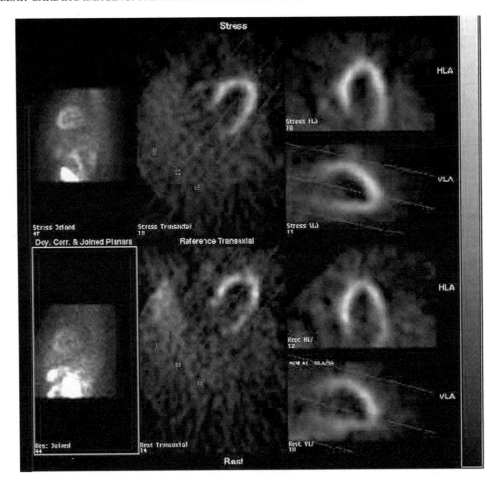

FIGURE 6.4 Depth-dependent attenuation in an obese patient resulting in an artifactual decrease in tracer concentration in basal half of the posterolateral wall.

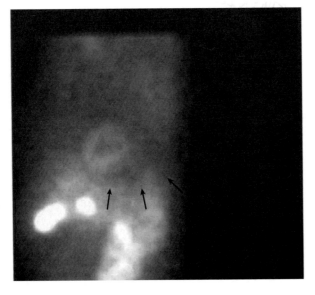

FIGURE 6.5 Planar projection image (left lateral view) demonstrating a breast "shadow" (arrows) overlying the entire left ventricle.

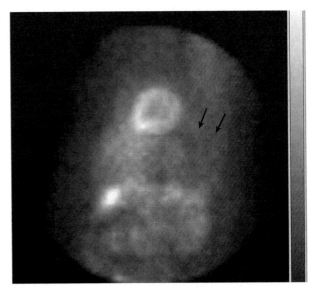

FIGURE 6.6 Planar projection image (left lateral view) in which the level of the left hemidiaphragm is defined by a photopenic defect in the fundus of the stomach (arrows).

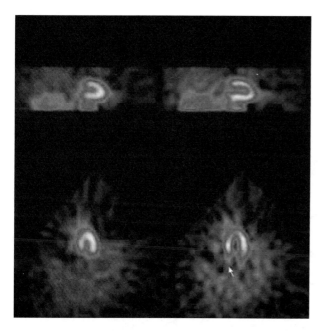

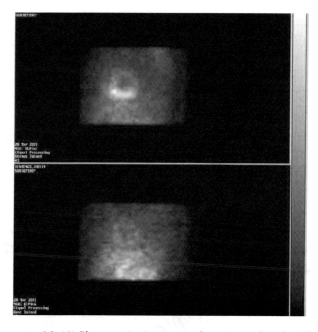

FIGURE 6.7 (C) Gated perfusion tomograms demonstrate normal anterior wall motion and thickening, favoring the presence of an attenuation artifact rather than scar.

FIGURE 6.9 (A) Planar projection images demonstrate that the left breast is positioned differently in stress (top) and rest (bottom) SPECT acquisitions.

hemidiaphragm is relatively stable. Therefore, "shifting" diaphragmatic attenuation artifacts, mimicking ischemia, are relatively rare.

Prone imaging has been demonstrated to minimize diaphragmatic attenuation artifacts [13–14]. When a patient lies prone, the heart shifts upward to a slight degree, and the diaphragm is pushed down. By increasing the distance between the inferior wall of the left ventricle and diaphragm, the diaphragmatic attenuation effect is minimized. However, a separate prone SPECT image acquisition following stress and rest acquisition is time-consuming and logistically difficult: processed images must be inspected prior to the patient's departure from the laboratory, and a decision to perform additional prone imaging must be made. Some laboratories perform prone imaging routinely. However, since the position of the heart within the thorax relative to the scintillation camera detector may differ with the patient in the prone versus the supine position, apparent regional tracer distribution may likewise differ. Frequently, septal and apical count density may be relatively increased, rendering the lateral wall relatively count-poor (Fig. 6.11).

A recently described alternative to prone imaging is upright imaging with the patient sitting in a chair and the scintillation detector(s) perpendicular to the floor, rotating around the patient's chest [15]. In the sitting position the level of the diaphragm is more caudal than

in the upright position, potentially decreasing the effect of diaphragmatic attenuation.

A unique diaphragmatic attenuation artifact (actually, more correctly, a motion artifact) peculiar to stress/delayed Tl-201 SPECT is "diaphragmatic creep" [16]. After a patient has performed dynamic exercise, respirations are deep, and at end-inspiration, the posi-

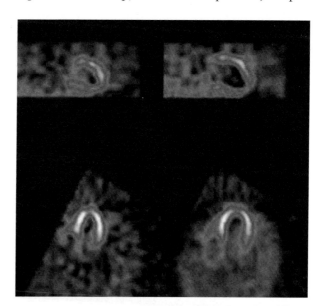

FIGURE 6.10 (C) Gated perfusion tomograms demonstrate normal inferior wall motion and thickening, favoring an attenuation artifact rather than a scar.

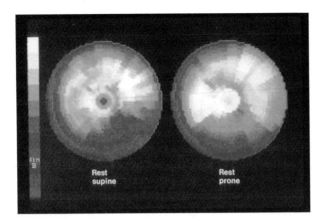

FIGURE 6.11 Stress and rest polar plots obtained in a male patient imaged supine (left) and prone (right). In the supine study diaphragmatic attenuation results in a decrease in inferior count density. This artifact is less evident in the prone study. However, there is a relative increase in apical and septal count density with the patient prone.

tion of the diaphragm is low. Therefore, when a patient lies supine for SPECT image acquisition immediately postexercise, the position of the heart is relatively caudal. However, as SPECT acquisition proceeds, respirations become less deep, and the heart gradually shifts ("creeps") upward. This "creep" of the heart results in a motion artifact. Since the motion of the heart is vertical, the artifactual defect is most apparent in the inferior wall of the left ventricle and, to a lesser degree, the contralateral anterior wall. To avoid the diaphragmatic creep artifact, immediate postexercise Tl-201 image acquisition should be delayed for approximately 15 minutes until the patient's respiratory rate has returned to baseline.

A soft tissue attenuation artifact that is less often recognized is attenuation of lateral wall count density by overlying lateral chest wall fat. In obese patients the thickness of lateral chest wall fat may be just as great as that of the breast. Such an artifact may be anticipated by interpreting physicians by a priori knowledge of the patient's body habitus and by inspection of planar projection images displayed in endless loop cinematic format on the computer console, as described earlier.

The physiologic explanation for "reverse redistribution" is described in Chapter 4. However, soft tissue attenuation may be a frequent artifactual cause of reverse distribution. In low count density images, frequently encountered in obese patients, the standard filter used for processing (see below) accentuates photon-deficient regions, whether real or artifactual [17]. Thereby, in such low count density studies attenuation artifacts may be exaggerated. Consequently, in stress/delayed Tl-201 images where delayed image count density is approximately 50% of the stress images, or

in low-dose rest–high-dose stress Tc-99m-sestamibi or tetrofosmin images, attenuation artifacts may be accentuated in the delayed or resting studies, respectively (see Color Fig. 6.12 in separate color insert). Under these circumstances, attenuation artifacts may appear more marked in resting images than in stress images, simulating a pattern of reverse distribution.

Attenuation correction, now commercially available on many scintillation camera systems, is of benefit in minimizing or eliminating artifacts secondary to soft tissue attenuation (see Chapter 7). However, the interpreting physician must be cautious of unique artifacts produced by current attenuation correction algorithms, including truncation, defects secondary to inadequate transmission source count density and uniformity, exaggeration of "apical thinning," and scatter of subdiaphragmatic activity into the inferior wall of the left ventricle.

Gated perfusion SPECT is an alternate, tried-and-true method to minimize false positive studies resulting from fixed soft tissue attenuation artifacts and to increase test specificity [18,19]. Fixed defects resulting from soft tissue attenuation will move and thicken normally, whereas myocardial scars (at least transmural scars) usually demonstrate decreased wall motion (endocardial wall excursion) and wall thickening (an increase in count density during systole) (see Figs. 6.7C and 6.10C). By incorporating gated SPECT to differentiate infarct from artifact, investigators have reported an increase in test specificity of approximately 10% [19].

IMAGE PROCESSING ARTIFACTS

Filtering

Commercially available computers have incorporated empirically determined optimal filters for commonly performed SPECT myocardial perfusion imaging protocols. Such selection of filters has generally been determined based upon SPECT images of adequate count density in patients of average body habitus. Therefore, if a laboratory uses a standard protocol, it is generally advisable to adhere to the manufacturer's filtering guidelines. Technologists and interpreting physicians should be aware of the consequences of altering filter parameters. Moreover, they should be cognizant of the effect of applying "standard" filters to images of unusually low or high count density. For example, decreasing the critical frequency will render a tomogram very smooth with loss of detail and contrast resolution, and associated decreased sensitivity in detecting perfusion abnormalities. On the other hand, increasing the critical frequency will accentuate high-frequency data and exaggerate noise, giving the tomogram an "impixelated"

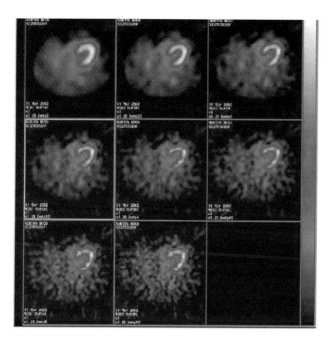

FIGURE 6.13 A midventricular transaxial tomographic slice from a resting Tc-99m-sestamibi scan in a patient with myocardial infarction is processed with a Butterworth filter and critical frequencies ranging from 0.20 to 0.72. As the critical frequency decreases, the image becomes blurred, losing contrast resolution and anatomic detail. As the critical frequency increases, the image becomes "impixelated," and true perfusion defects are exaggerated. The critical frequency recommended by the manufacturer for this particular imaging protocol is 0.52 (upper right hand image).

appearance (Fig. 6.13). Likewise, lowering the critical frequency will decrease the apparent extent and severity of the true perfusion abnormality, whereas increasing the critical frequency may appear to accentuate the defect. As described previously, the result is similar if the critical frequency is held constant and the count density of an image decreases. True perfusion abnormalities as well as localized attenuation artifacts may appear more marked and extensive. It may seem tempting to adjust a filter to match the count density of an image (so-called adaptive filtering). However, unless a laboratory is exceptionally knowledgeable regarding the effects of filters, it is probably advisable not to adjust prescribed filters but instead to anticipate filtering effects in particular patients, such as those who are obese or in whom localized attenuation artifacts may be present.

Adjacent Bowel Activity

Subdiaphragmatic tracer concentration adjacent to the inferior wall of the left ventricle may create significant image artifacts. Tl-201 localizes in the liver. The Tc-99m labeled compounds sestamibi and tetrofosmin initially localize in the liver but are then excreted via

the hepatobiliary tract and enter the duodenum. From there, tracer moves distally in the small bowel, which may be positioned in the left upper quadrant of the abdomen, and it may reflux into the fundus of the stomach, which lies immediately adjacent to the inferior wall of the left ventricle. Such subdiaphragmatic activity may create artifacts due to scatter, filtering, or tomographic image processing.

Scatter

Photons emanating from subdiaphragmatic tracer concentration may undergo Compton scattering and may be misregistered as activity in the inferior wall of the left ventricle. By this means scattered subdiaphragmatic activity may artifactually increase inferior wall count density. This phenomenon may obscure true inferior wall perfusion defects. Alternately, in normal patients the inferior wall may become relatively "hot." By subsequent image normalization an artifactual defect may be created in the contralateral anterior wall (see Color Fig. 6.14 in separate color insert). Such scatter artifacts are more common with Tl-201 than Tc-99m because of the larger Compton scatter angle, and when an all-purpose parallel-hole collimator is used instead of a high-resolution collimator.

Inclusion of subdiaphragmatic activity in the polar plot radius-of-search

To construct a polar map, the center of the left ventricle is identified. Then the maximal count density within radians extending from the ventricular center is determined. The limit of search of these radians is determined by a limiting region of interest placed around the left ventricle, conforming as closely as possible to its epicardial border. However, if this limiting region of interest encompasses extracardiac activity, particularly intense subdiaphragmatic activity or activity scattered into the inferior wall (see above), an artifactually "hot" region will be superimposed upon the polar plot (Fig. 6.15). Through the standard process of normalization, this "hot" region may appear relatively normal, and artifactual defects may be created in remote regions of the left ventricle.

Ramp-filter artifact

With filtered back-projection, the ramp-filter is employed to eliminate the "star artifact" associated with reconstruction of a finite number of projection images. This filtering process essentially minimizes count density adjacent to an intense object, thereby better defining its borders and increasing its contrast and spatial resolution. However, when the ramp-filter is applied to

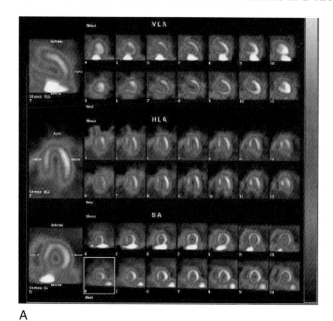

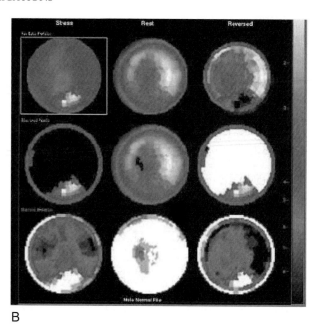

A

B

FIGURE 6.15 (A) Tomographic slices demonstrate intense, localized subdiaphragmatic tracer concentration. (B) By inclusion of this activity in the polar plot radius of search, count density of the inferior wall in the polar plots is artifactually increased. Normalization of images to the region of greatest count density (the inferior wall) results in an artifactual decrease in count density in the contralateral anterior wall as well as other regions remote from the inferior wall. Since this phenomenon is much more marked in the stress images in this patient, artifactual marked ischemia is created.

intense, localized tracer concentration adjacent to the heart, present in the liver, stomach, or small bowel, it may result in an artifactual decrease in count density in the inferior wall of the left ventricle (see Color Fig. 6.16 in separate color insert). Therefore, subdiaphragmatic activity adjacent to the inferior wall may artifactually *increase* inferior wall count density due to scatter, or *decrease* count density secondary to the ramp-filter.

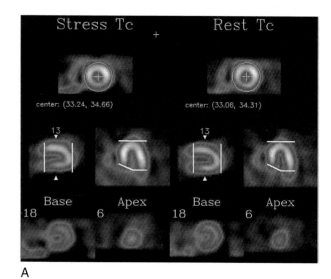

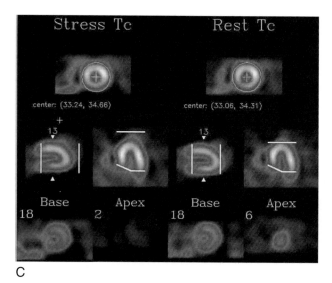

A

C

FIGURE 6.17 (A) With apical and basal slice limits correctly positioned, (B) polar plots in a normal individual demonstrate normal tracer distribution. (C) When the stress apical limit is positioned too far distally, an artifactual apical defect is created in (D) the reconstructed stress polar plot. In this case example, only the stress apical limit is positioned incorrectly, mimicking stress-induced ischemia. (See Color Fig. 6–17 for [B] and [D].)

Selection of the Apex and Base for Polar Map Reconstruction

Accurate and reproducible selection of the apex and base of the left ventricular myocardium is necessary in stress and rest images. Positioning the limits for slice selection too far basally will result in an apparent basal myocardial perfusion defect, and positioning the limits distal to the apex will result in an apparent apical defect (Fig. 6.17A,C; see B and D in separate color insert). In contrast, positioning slice limits too tightly, so that they do not encompass the entire heart, may result in underestimation of the size and extent of a defect.

Axis Selection

If the long axis of the left ventricle is defined incorrectly on either the transaxial or midventricular vertical long-axis slices, the geometry of the heart in subsequently reconstructed orthogonal tomographic slices can be distorted (Fig. 6.18). Consequently, the apparent regional count density can be altered in polar maps, resulting in apparent perfusion defects. In polar map reconstruction, such errors most often occur in basal myocardial regions at the periphery of the polar plot, due to foreshortening of one of the myocardial walls. Also, the apex, which often demonstrates physiologic thinning and decreased count density, is displaced from the exact center of the polar plot. The displaced relatively count-poor apex may also result in an artifact.

Misregistration of true myocardial perfusion defects in short-axis slices and polar maps may result in assignment of the defect to an incorrect vascular territory. Moreover, if the axes are selected differently for the stress and rest tomograms, perfusion defects will appear to be localized to different regions of the myocardium, thus mimicking ischemia or "reverse distribution" (see Fig. 6.18).

Quantitatative Analysis

Quantitative analysis aids the novice observer in recognizing subtle perfusion abnormalities. Moreover, it can increase interobserver agreement in detecting perfusion defects and characterizing their extent and severity. However, normal files, against which patient data are compared, are derived from patients with a low likelihood of coronary artery disease and an average body habitus. When body habitus deviates from gender-match normal limits, quantitative analysis may result in artifacts. For example, in a woman with very large, dense breasts, an anterior artifact will be observed with quantitative analysis. In contrast, a woman

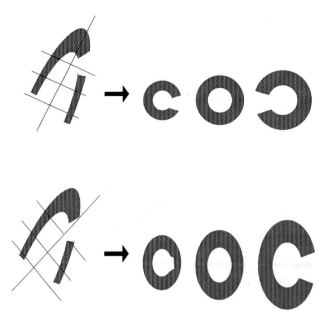

FIGURE 6.18 The long axis of the left ventricle is selected inconsistently in stress and rest transaxial tomographic images (left) of patient with myocardial infarction. In the reconstructed stress (top) and rest (bottom) tomographic slices, the location of the perfusion abnormality differs, mimicking septal ischemia and basal posterolateral reverse distribution. Also note that in the resting tomograms the left ventricular cavity appears elliptical rather than circular, because slices are created oblique to the true long axis of the ventricle.

who has undergone a left mastectomy has a thoracic body habitus more similar to a man's than a woman's. Therefore, if the perfusion scan in such a woman is compared to the female normal file, an inferior perfusion defect will be recognized by quantitative analysis because inferior attenuation, such as that normally observed in men, is characterized as abnormal in a woman (Fig. 6.19). Therefore, in women who have had left mastectomy, the normal male file should be used for quantitative analysis.

INTERPRETATION ERRORS SECONDARY TO IMPROPER IMAGE DISPLAY

Stress and rest perfusion tomograms should each be individually normalized to maximal myocardial count density so that stress and rest perfusion defects can be compared and assessed for reversibility. If images are incorrectly normalized to noncardiac activity, particularly subdiaphragmatic tracer concentration, accurate comparison of stress and rest images is not possible (Fig. 6.20).

Software on some computers provides the option of either heart-normalized or slice-normalized perfusion

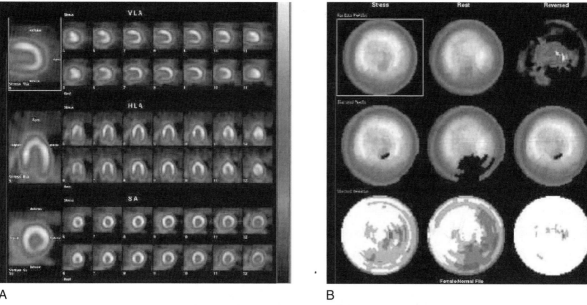

A   B

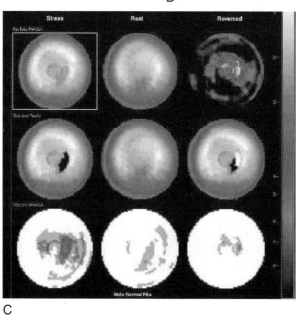

C

FIGURE 6.19 (A) Tomograms of a normal perfusion scan in a woman with prior left mastectomy demonstrate a mild decrease in inferior tracer concentration secondary to diaphragmatic attenuation. (B) In polar plots, when patient data are compared to the normal female file, an artifactual inferior perfusion defect (more marked in low-dose resting images) is created. However, when compared to (C) the normal male file, quantitative analysis is normal.

tomograms. With the former, the entire three-dimensional image data set (either stress or resting) is normalized to the hottest area of the entire myocardium. In contrast, with slice-normalization, each individual slice is normalized to its own hottest area. The potential drawback of slice-normalization is that if there is an abnormal, pathological circumferential decrease in count density in a particular slice, the abnormality may be overlooked.

ARTIFACTS RELATED TO NONCORONARY DISEASE

Left Bundle Branch Block

In exercise myocardial perfusion studies, reversible septal perfusion defects may occur in patients with left bundle branch block (LBBB) [21–22]. In dog experiments that increased heart rates associated with right ventricular pacing, investigators demonstrated that LBBB results in a relative decrease in blood flow to the

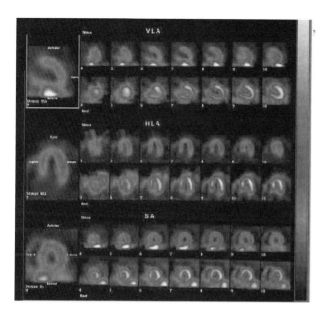

FIGURE 6.20 Stress tomographic slices are incorrectly normalized to intense subdiaphragmatic activity, whereas resting slices are appropriately normalized to maximal myocardial tracer concentration.

septum [23]. It has been postulated that the decrease in septal blood flow is due to asynchronous relaxation of the septum, which is out of phase with diastolic filling of the remainder of the ventricle, during which coronary perfusion is maximal. At higher heart rates the degree of septal asynchrony relative to the electrocardiogram (ECG) R-R interval is greater than at rest, making septal perfusion defects appear reversible (Color Fig. 6.21). It has been reported that the severity of reversible perfusion defects is most marked in LBBB patients who achieve very high heart rates (greater than 170 beats per minute) [21].

Perfusion defects associated with LBBB frequently spare the apex in patients without coronary artery disease [24]. Thus, if an apical defect is present in a patient with LBBB, disease of the left anterior descending coronary artery should be suspected. Perfusion abnormalities in the territories of the right and circumflex arteries nevertheless are associated with a high sensitivity for the presence of coronary artery disease despite the presence of LBBB [25]. To anticipate reversible septal perfusion artifacts, it is imperative that the interpreting physician inspect the ECG tracing or report for the presence of LBBB.

It has been reported that septal artifacts associated with LBBB can be minimized by substituting pharmacologic stress with intravenous dipyridamole or adenosine for exercise [26,27]. Since these agents have only a slight positive chronotropic effect, increasing the heart rate by only 10 beats per minute in most patients, there is little increase in septal asynchrony relative to the R-R interval. Thus, septal perfusion is kept rela-

tively constant, and septal artifacts are avoided. However, it should be cautioned that patients undergoing pharmacologic stress with either dipyridamole or adenosine occasionally have high resting heart rates due to underlying medical conditions, and that in other individuals there may be an unexplained marked increase in heart rate associated with pharmacologic stress. Therefore, septal artifacts may nonetheless be expected to occur if such patients also have LBBB.

Left Ventricular Hypertrophy

Concentric hypertrophy

Hypertensive patients are frequently referred for myocardial perfusion SPECT because hypertension is a significant risk factor for epicardial coronary artery disease. Diffuse myocardial hypertrophy often results from systemic hypertension. Such hypertrophy results in a generalized increase in uptake of myocardial perfusion radiopharmaceuticals. Additionally, a relative increase in septal wall count density is common in hypertensive patients [28]. This relative increase in septal count density may be due either to some degree of selective septal hypertrophy or to alterations in regional blood flow or metabolism in hypertensive patients. In patients with long-standing hypertension, a significant decrease in the lateral-to-septal wall count density ratio as compared to that in normotensive controls has been reported. Thus, in tomographic slices, raw polar maps, and quantitative plots, there may be a relative decrease in count density in the lateral wall in the territory of the circumflex coronary artery (Fig. 6.22). This defect is usually "fixed" in stress and rest images, mimicking myocardial infarction. However, occasionally, the septum may appear slightly less intense in resting images, rendering the defect partly reversible and raising a clinical suspicion of ischemia.

Interpreting physicians should anticipate this lateral wall artifact in patients with hypertension or other causes of left ventricular hypertrophy, such as valvular heart disease. Inspection of the ECG for evidence of left ventricular hypertrophy is a valuable part of patient assessment prior to scan interpretation. In gated SPECT studies in hypertensive patients without coronary artery disease, areas of relatively decreased count density, usually involving the lateral wall, will move and thicken vigorously (see Fig. 6.22).

Another cause of SPECT artifacts in hypertensive patients and others with left ventricular hypertrophy are "hot spots" in the anterolateral and posterolateral walls, which may be due to hypertrophy of the anterior and posterior papillary muscles, respectively. In the case of a prominent posterior papillary muscle, the image will be normalized to the "hot spot" in the poste-

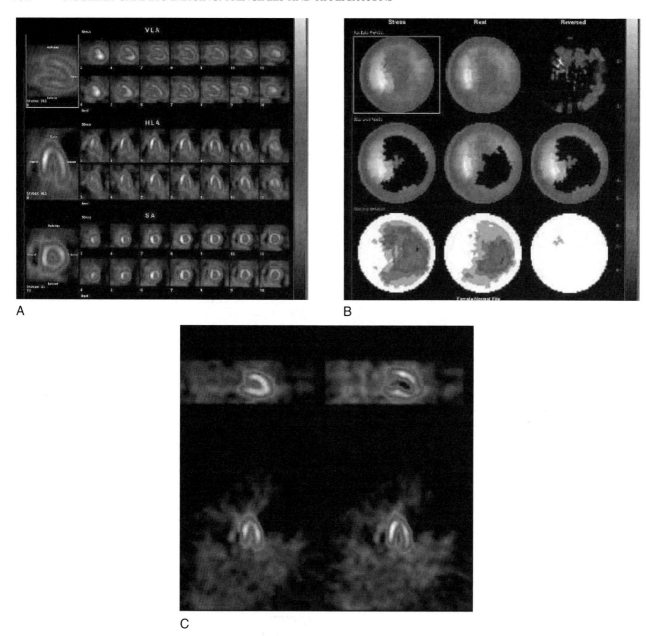

FIGURE 6.22 In this patient with longstanding hypertension and left ventricular hypertrophy, (A) tomographic slices and (B) polar plots demonstrate a relative increase in count density in the septum. Through the process of normalization, an artifactual lateral wall defect is created. (C) Gated perfusion tomograms demonstrate normal lateral wall motion and thickening, favoring presence of a normalization artifact rather than scar.

rior wall, creating a relative decrease in count density throughout the remainder of the myocardium.

Localized apical hypertrophy

Localized apical hypertrophy, a variant of hypertrophic cardiomyopathy, may also result in similar artifacts in quantitative analysis due to normalization of the tomograms and polar plots to a localized increase in count density in the apex. Consequently, there is a relative decrease in count density circumferentially in the mid and basal portions of the left ventricular myocardium, simulating perfusion abnormalities in the basal regions of the myocardium (Fig. 6.23).

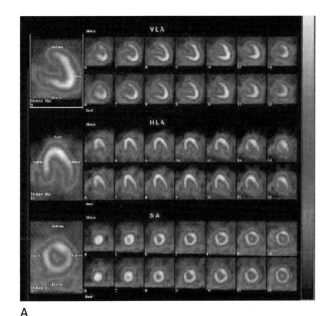

A

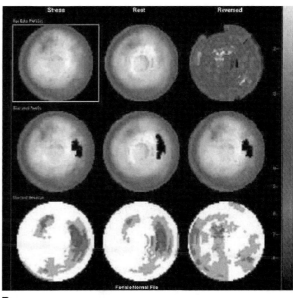

B

FIGURE 6.23 In this patient with localized apical hypertrophy, confirmed by echocardiography, (A) to-mographic slices and (B) polar plots demonstrate increased thickness and increased count density of the apex. Images are normalized to the "hot" apex, creating artifactual defects circumferentially in the basal portions of the left ventricle.

Long Membranous/Short Muscular Septum

It is well known that septum is shorter than the lateral wall in most patients because the base of the septum is comprised of membranous tissue rather than muscle. In SPECT myocardial perfusion images, this consistently results in an apparent perfusion defect at the very base of the septum. Experienced interpreting physicians readily recognize this defect and overlook it. Moreover, this basal septal defect is judged to be within normal limits by quantitative analysis. However, the length of the membranous septum, and consequently the length of the muscular septum, vary considerably among individuals. In some patients the membranous septum is unusually long, exaggerating the basal septal defect. Therefore, interpreting physicians should always view horizontal long-axis images to compare the length of the septum to that of the lateral wall to determine the length of the membranous septum and incorporate this knowledge in interpreting the orthogonal short-axis slices (see Color Fig. 6.24 in separate color insert).

Physiological Apical "Thinning"

The appearance of the apex may also be variable among patients. Such variability may be secondary to actual anatomic differences or may result from differences in spatial resolution at the apex (high-resolution) as compared to that of more basal portions of the left ventri-cle (relatively low resolution). This so-called apical thinning may produce a relative decrease in apical count density in both stress and rest tomographic images. As described earlier, gating can help to differentiate apical "thinning" from localized myocardial infarction, since regions of "thinning" will move and thicken normally, whereas localized scars should demonstrate dysynergy and decreased thickening (see Color Fig. 6.25A and B in separate color insert; Fig. 6.25C).

The 11 O'Clock Defect

Linear, transmural, apparent perfusion defects can frequently be observed at approximately 11 o'clock and 7 o'clock, particularly in short-axis tomograms. These defects are generally fixed in stress and rest images, although their appearance may vary slightly owing to differences in count density and associated contrast resolution in the two data sets. Upon close inspection (viewing images using a linear gray scale with no background subtraction is very helpful), these linear defects are localized to, or adjacent to, the anterior and inferior insertion points of the free wall of the right ventricle (Fig. 6.26). The cause of this normal variant is not known, although it may be due in part to attenuation by the right ventricle and the right ventricular blood. It is not always possible to differentiate this finding from a small area of scar; however, experienced readers generally become accustomed to this normal variant.

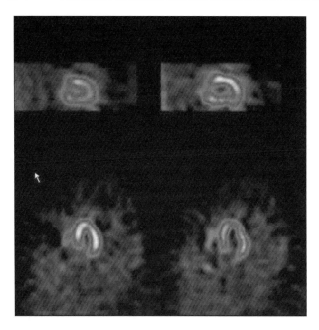

FIGURE 6.25 (C) Gated perfusion tomograms demonstrate normal apical wall motion and thickening.

GATING ARTIFACTS

If arrhythmia is present, or if the heart rate changes during SPECT acquisition, inordinately short or long cardiac cycles will be rejected during an 8- or 16-frame

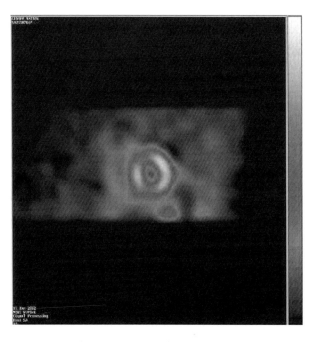

FIGURE 6.26 A short-axis tomographic slice demonstrates apparent "linear" defects at 11 o'clock and 7 o'clock (arrows), adjacent to insertion point of the free wall of the right ventricle.

gated acquisition. If the degree of irregular beat rejection varies during the SPECT acquisition, the number of cardiac cycles acquired for each projection image may differ, assuming that each projection image is acquired for the same length of time (the standard protocol for gated perfusion SPECT). Therefore, projection images will vary in count density. When viewed in endless loop cinematic format, the projection images will appear to "flash." Acquisition of a variable number of counts in the projection images may potentially result in errors in filtered back-projection and consequently perfusion artifacts. However, investigators have reported that clinically significant perfusion artifacts are encountered only with severe arrhythmias, such as associated with atrial fibrillation and trigemeny [29,30].

REFERENCES

1. DePuey EG, Garcia EV. Optimal specificity of thallium-201 SPECT through recognition of imaging artifacts. J Nucl Med 1989;30:441.
2. Friedman J, Berman DS, Van Train K, et al. Patient motion in thallium-201 myocardial SPECT imaging. An easily identified frequent source of artifactual defect. Clin Nucl Med 1988;13: 321.
3. Cooper JA, Neumann PH, McCandless BK. Effect of patient motion on tomographic myocardial perfusion imaging. J Nucl Med 1992;13:1566.
4. Botvinick EH, Yu Yz, O'Connell WJ, et al. A quantitative assessment of patient motion and its effect on myocardial perfusion SPECT images. J Nucl Med 1993;34:303.
5. Prigent FM, Hyun M, Berman DS, et al. Effect of motion on thallium-201 SPECT studies: a simulation and clinical study. J Nucl Med 1993;34:1845.
6. Toma DM, White MP, Mann A, et al. Influence of arm positioning on rest/stress technetium-99m labeled sestamibi tomographic myocardial perfusion imaging. J Nucl Cardiol 1999;6: 163.
7. Eisner RL, Churchwell A, Noever T, et al. Quantitative analysis of the tomographic thallium-201 myocardial bullseye display: critical role of correcting for patient motion. J Nucl Med 1988; 29:91.
8. Geckle WJ, Frank TL, Links JM, et al. Correction for patient and organ movement in SPECT: application to exercise thallium-201 cardiac imaging. J Nucl Med 1986;27:899.
9. Eisner RL, Noever T, Nowak D, et al. Use of cross-correlation function to detect patient motion during SPECT imaging. J Nucl Med 1987;28:97.
10. Cooper JA, Neumann PH, McCandless BK. Detection of patient motion during tomographic myocardial perfusion imaging. J Nucl Med 1993;34:1341.
11. Germano G, Chua T, Kavanagh PB, et al. Detection and correction of patient motion in dynamic and static myocardial SPECT using a multi-detector camera. J Nucl Med 1993;34: 1349.
12. Manglos SH, Thomas FD, Gagne GM, et al. Phantom study of breast tissue attenuation in myocardial imaging. J Nucl Med 1993;34:992.
13. Machac J, George T. Effect of 360 SPECT prone imaging on Tl-201 myocardial perfusion studies. J Nucl Med 1979;20:183.

14. Kiat H, Van Train KF, Friedman JD, et al. Quantitative stress-redistribution thallium-201 SPECT using prone imaging: methodologic development and validation. J Nucl Med 1992;33:1509.

15. Johnson LL, Tauxe EL, Smith KR. Comparison of supine and upright SPECT myocardial perfusion imaging. J Am Coll Cardiol 1995; 25: 363A (abstract).

16. Friedman J, Van Train K, Maddahi J, et al. "Upward creep" of the heart: a frequent source of false-positive reversible defects during thallium-201 stress-redistribution SPECT. J Nucl Med 1989;30:1718.

17. Araujo W, DePuey EG, Kamran M, et al. Artifactual reverse distribution pattern in myocardial perfusion SPECT with Tc-99m sestamibi. J Nucl Cardiol, 2000;7:633.

18. DePuey EG, Rozanski A. Using gated technetium-99m sestamibi SPECT to characterize fixed myocardial defects as infarct or artifact. J Nucl Med 1995;36:952.

19. Smanio PE, Watson DD, Segalla DL, et al. Value of gating of technetium-99m sestamibi single-photon emission computed tomographic imaging. J Am Coll Cardiol 1997;29:69.

20. Taillefer R, DePuey EG, Udelson JE, et al. Comparative diagnostic accuracy of thallium-201 and Tc-99m sestamibi (perfusion and ECG-gated SPECT) in detecting coronary artery disease in women. J Am Coll Cardiol 1997;29:69.

21. DePuey EG, Krawczynska EG, Robbins WL. Thallium-201 SPECT in coronary artery disease patients with left bundle branch block. J Nucl Med 1988;29:1479.

22. Burns RJ, Galligan L, Wright LM, et al. Improved specificity of myocardial thallium-201 single-photon emission computed tomography in patients with left bundle branch block by dipyridamole. Am J Cardiol 1991;68:504.

23. Hirzel HO, Senn M, Nuesch K, et al. Thallium-201 scintigraphy in complete left bundle branch block. Am J Cardiol 1984; 53:764.

24. Matzer LA, Kiat H, Friedman JD, et al. A new approach to the assessment of tomographic thallium-201 scintigraphy in patients with left bundle branch block. J Am Coll Cardiol 1991;17:1309.

25. Civelek AC, Gozukara I, Durski K, et al. Detection of left anterior descending coronary artery disease in patients with left bundle branch block. Am J Cardiol 1992;70:1565.

26. Rockett JF, Chadwick W, Moinuddin M, et al. Intravenous dipyridamole thallium-201 SPECT imaging in patients with left bundle branch block. Clin Nucl Med 1990;6:401.

27. Larcos G, Brown ML, Gibbons RJ. Role of dipyridamole thallium-201 imaging in left bundle branch block. Am J Cardiol 1991; 68:1097.

28. DePuey EG, Guertler-Krawczynska E, Perkins JV, et al. Alterations in myocardial thallium-201 distribution in patients with chronic systemic hypertension undergoing single-photon emission computed tomography. Am J Cardiol 1988;62:234.

29. Nichols K, Dorbala S, DePuey EG, et al. Influence of gated SPECT myocardial perfusion and function quantification. J Nucl Med 1999; 40: 924.

30. Nichols K, Yao SS, Kamran M, et al. Clinical impact of arrhythmias on gated SPECT cardiac myocardial perfusion and function assesssment. J Nucl Cardiol, 2001;37:458.

7 | Myocardial perfusion single-photon emission computed tomography attenuation correction

JAMES A. CASE, S. JAMES CULLOM, AND TIMOTHY M. BATEMAN

Myocardial perfusion imaging with single-photon emission computed tomography (SPECT) is a widely utilized modality for the diagnosis of coronary artery disease and assessment of ventricular function. The clinical potential of this modality, however, has yet to be fully realized, owing to physical limitations including photon attenuation, scatter, and limited system resolution that can produce image artifacts. Attenuation artifacts are generally regarded as the most clinically important, because they can cause unpredictable variation from expected perfusion patterns thereby affecting test accuracy and interpretative confidence. Recent advances in SPECT equipment design and associated research have resulted in the commercialization of a new generation of systems utilizing transmission imaging for patient-specific attenuation correction. These methods have the goal of removing attenuation as a factor to interpretation and obviating the reliance on inefficient adjunctive techniques currently used to identify attenuation artifacts. This approach is motivated by the recognition of cardiac perfusion positron emission tomography (PET) imaging as a gold-standard where transmission-based attenuation correction is used routinely. Although studies with early attenuation correction systems yielded mixed results, recent studies are demonstrating improving specificity, sensitivity, and simplified quantitative methods. Furthermore, this evolving technology provides the groundwork for new imaging protocols promising to improve the clinical efficiency and enhance the appeal of myocardial perfusion SPECT.

ATTENUATION ARTIFACTS: CLINICAL IMPLICATIONS

Attenuation artifacts have their origin in the physics of photon interaction within the patient and the limited mathematical framework of conventional reconstruction algorithms. Attenuation affects perfusion SPECT images in two important ways: gender-specific expected normal perfusion patterns and unpredictable artifacts arising from exaggerated soft tissue attenuation. The former is an important characteristic of SPECT perfusion images providing a baseline for interpretation and quantitation. These patterns result from "typical" distributions of attenuating soft tissue in the general population [1–3]. Artifacts occur when the attenuating anatomy deviates significantly from the expected population patterns. Diaphragmatic attenuation in males and breast attenuation in females are commonly identified attenuation artifacts. In males, photon attenuation by the left hemidiaphragm disproportionately suppresses counts from that region in the SPECT projections leading to potential perfusion artifacts in the inferior wall and right coronary artery (RCA) territory [1]. The diaphragm can appear as a count-poor "bulge" extending from the abdominal region over the inferior wall of the heart and may move independently across this region in a cine display of the projection images (Fig. 7.1). By inspecting the rotating planar projections, the interpreter can qualitatively assess the potential magnitude of diaphragmatic attenuation and adjust the clinical interpretation accordingly. In females, significant breast attenuation often affects the anterior, septal, and lateral walls of the left ventricle by disproportionately suppressing counts and is a significant source of artifact often overlying the left anterior descending (LAD) and left circumflex (LCX) artery territories (Fig. 7.2). Attenuation patterns are complicated in practice by interpatient variability and intrastudy differences that can result from changes in breast and diaphragm positioning during stress and rest imaging. Breast attenuation can often be visualized in the rotating planar projections as a

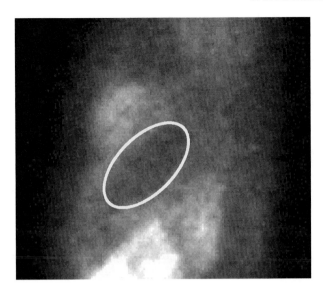

FIGURE 7.1 Example of a high and dense diaphragm in a lateral planar view. Note how the diaphragm obscures the inferior wall of the heart.

count-poor region passing over the anterior wall of the heart in the cine display. Attenuation also causes three-dimensional distortion of the reconstructed images [4]. Reconstructed vertical long-axis images can have an "arrowhead" appearance in severe cases. This distortion limits perfusion assessment by increasing uncertainty in standard landmarks and causing errors in perfusion values. It is important to note, however, that although the literature focuses on breast and diaphragmatic attenuation, all regions of the myocardium may be affected by attenuation.

DePuey et al. extended ideas developed early to identify attenuation artifacts in planar imaging to SPECT by outlining key gender-dependent body habitus factors and their correlation with potential artifacts for

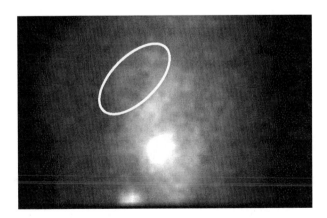

FIGURE 7.2 Example of a large, dense breast attenuation artifact.

Tl-201 [1] and later for Tc-99m SPECT [2]. Hendel et al. highlighted the importance of reviewing the rotating planar projections of the SPECT study and the abundance of clinical and quality control factors available to the interpreter [3]. The ASNC/ACC guidelines for clinical interpretation of myocardial perfusion SPECT studies make specific recommendations for the utilization of rotating planar projection images as part of a comprehensive interpretation of SPECT myocardial perfusion scans [5].

Quantitation of myocardial perfusion SPECT scans has a supportive role in differentiating attenuation artifacts from true perfusion defects. Eisner et al. and others quantified the gender-dependent myocardial perfusion patterns in normal populations [6–8]. Subsequent work developed normal databases and associated abnormality criteria based on expert interpretation and coronary angiography. This allows the interpreter to compare a given study to expected distributions and provides a measure of objectivity in assessing the likelihood of disease or attribute count deficit to excessive attenuation.

Electrocardiogram (ECG)-gating of myocardial perfusion SPECT studies has been shown to be valuable in discriminating fixed perfusion defects from attenuation artifacts in patients without prior myocardial infarction [9,10]. In segments where there is concern about the presence of fixed defects, adequate thickening and contraction can be attributed to attenuation. However, ECG-gating is not helpful in assessing patterns where attenuation may be superimposed on true perfusion defects due to ischemia.

Other adjunctive methods have been utilized to identify attenuation artifacts including the use of external breast markers and breast positioning protocols to identify and standardize breast position, recording breast (bra) size, breast density, patient body habitus, and the use of prone and left-decubitus planar imaging for diaphragmatic attenuation assessment [1–3,11,12]. Although the value of these methods has been demonstrated, they lack standardization and significantly hamper laboratory efficiency and operation.

PHYSICS OF ATTENUATION

Attenuation results from the interaction of photons (referred to as X-rays or gamma rays depending on their origin) with orbital electrons in the patient. Attenuation produces an inconsistency in the projection information and subsequent artifacts in the tomographic images. Interactions occur in two predominant ways relevant to clinical nuclear imaging:

Compton scattering and the photoelectric effect [13]. The likelihood of each interaction depends on the photon energy and the intrinsic properties of the tissue. At low energies (< 60 keV), photons are more likely to cause excitation and ionizing of the atoms in the body, known as the photoelectric effect. These photons have a significant amount of their energy transferred to the atom and can be completely destroyed or a small fraction of the incident radiation is reradiated. As photon energy increases (> 60 keV) the electrons act more like a collection of inelastic objects causing the photons to scatter and transfer a significant portion of their energy to the electrons and create a second photon of lower energy [14]. In Compton scattering, the incident photon is not destroyed, but rather it is deflected to a new trajectory at a lower energy level. These redirected photons may be detected within the energy window of the pulse height analyzer can reduce image contrast and introduce quantitative errors [14].

Photon attenuation is exponential and described by the following relation

$$I = I_0 \exp(-\mu D)$$

where I_0 is the initial count flux arising from an activity source, D is the depth of the source in the medium, and μ is the linear attenuation coefficient [13] (Fig. 7.3). μ is an intrinsic property of the medium and contains components describing Compton scattering and the photoelectric effects. I_0 is dependent on the medium and incident photon energy (Table 7.1). Tl-201 has relatively low energy emissions with Hg X-ray peaks at 69–83 keV, and gamma emissions at 135 and 167 keV compared with Tc-99m with a single gamma emission at 140 keV. Because of the energy differences, attenuation is significantly greater for Tl-201 than for Tc-99m.

TABLE 7.1 *Attenuation Coefficients for Common Radionuclides and Tissue Types*

	Tc-99m (140 keV)	Tl-201 (72 keV)
Bone (spine)	0.284 cm^{-1}	0.365 cm^{-1}
Soft tissue	0.151 cm^{-1}	0.187 cm^{-1}
Lung (typical)	0.045 cm^{-1}	0.056 cm^{-1}

PRINCIPLES OF TRANSMISSION TOMOGRAPHY

Early investigations demonstrated that patient-specific attenuation measures were required to adequately compensate for attenuation in myocardial perfusion SPECT. The commercial response has been modified SPECT hardware to acquire transmission scans similar to conventional computed tomography (CT) [15]. CT uses an X-ray tube and array of detectors to acquire projection images comprising integral attenuation values along lines through the patient (Fig. 7.4). These images are of very high signal-to-noise ratio and spatial resolution. CT image values are proportional to the linear attenuation coefficients in the body. Following this approach, SPECT attenuation correction systems use external radionuclide sources for transmission imaging and the collimated NaI detector as the detector array, although one commercial implementation utilizes a conventional X-ray source and detectors as described below. Most systems use Gd-153 (100 keV, 273 day half-life) as the external source but others are utilized commercially. Gd-153 is well suited for transmission tomography because of its relatively long half-life and emits radiation between the Tl-201 peak at 72 keV and the Tc-99m peak at 140 keV. The combination of emission and transmission energies must provide limited cross talk that can be minimized with hardware or corrected using computational techniques particularly for simultaneous emission transmission acquisition. Failure to adequately correct for the cross talk from Tc-99m

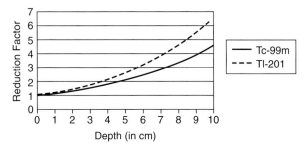

FIGURE 7.3 The attenuation factor increases as an exponential of depth in the patient. This effect is more pronounced with Tl-201 photons.

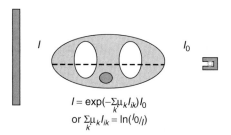

$$I = \exp\left(-\sum_k \mu_k l_{ik}\right) I_0$$
$$\text{or } \sum_k \mu_k l_{ik} = \ln(I_0/I)$$

FIGURE 7.4 Attenuation is often measured using an external source and a detector located opposite the source. This is the same geometry that is used in a conventional computed tomography scanner.

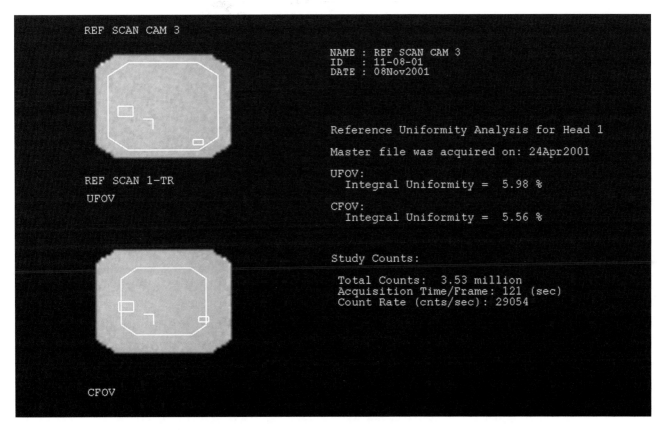

FIGURE 7.5 Example of the reference scan from the VantagePro. This scan demonstrates the uniformity analysis that is performed on the scan. The reference scan is compared to a "master reference scan" the measure if the uniformity is stable.

into Gd-153 in simultaneous acquisitions leaves artifacts in the attenuation map that significantly limit attenuation correction [16,17].

Each transmission projection is normalized to a "blank" or "reference" scan for absolute integral attenuation calculation and tomographic reconstruction (Fig. 7.5). This scan is a high-count planar transmission image acquired in the absence of attenuating medium in the field of view for each detector. Furthermore, the reference scan provides a baseline response of the detectors to the X-ray source that can be used for quality control purposes [18,19]. Since the emission and transmission images are usually acquired with sources of different energies, therefore the attenuation coefficients must be scaled to the appropriate energy dependence before attenuation correction [20]. The normalized projection data are then used to reconstruct an "attenuation map" on each transverse plane that is used for attenuation correction. Figure 7.6 shows an example of transverse attenuation maps obtained from a Gd-153 dual scanning line source system.

RECONSTRUCTION METHODS

Filtered back-projection, the algorithm commonly used for reconstruction in commercial SPECT systems, assumes that all of the radiation emitted along the line of sight to the detector is recorded. This algorithm does not model any deviation from the assumption of consistency of the projections, including photon attenuation. In order to utilize the attenuation information, iterative reconstruction methods have been developed [21]. They were proposed early in the study of SPECT reconstruction for both emission and transmission imaging but could not be implemented due to substantial computational demands. Iterative algorithms use a stepwise approach for removing attenuation artifacts from the reconstructed images. At each iteration, the accuracy of the emission image estimate is improved over previous iterations until a specified criterion is satisfied. In practice, noise and limited computational resources lead to truncation of the iterative sequence [22].

Early methods to correct myocardial perfusion

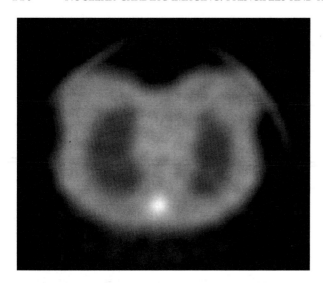

FIGURE 7.6 Example of a high count transmission scan acquired using the Vantage simultaneous transmission-emission system. This system employs two external, moving line sources of Gd-153 for measuring patient-specific attenuation.

SPECT images for attenuation applied algorithms developed initially for noncardiac imaging where the attenuation coefficient distribution could be described by a single value for all positions in the body. The method of Chang [23], successful for this application, was extended to an iterative algorithm and applied in early studies to cardiac imaging. Malko et al. showed that a uniform sheet source could be used for transmission imaging and subsequent correction of Tl-201 SPECT studies [24]. Hutton et al. later extended the idea using an iterative form of the Chang algorithm [25]. Galt et al. built upon these ideas by extending the iterative Chang method using a first order iteration with scatter correction using a secondary scatter window [26]. Although these methods demonstrated early success for attenuation correction methods, they were not easily implemented clinically. However, with current transmission scanning capabilities, a modified form of the Chang approach is utilized for one commercially available attenuation correction system [27].

The most common iterative reconstruction algorithm studied for cardiac perfusion SPECT attenuation correction is the maximum likelihood–expectation maximization (MLEM) algorithm [21,28] (Fig. 7.7). This algorithm estimates the three-dimensional distribution that most likely produced the projection data given an image formation model. It also determines an optimum correction factor from each iteration to the next. This algorithm is the basis for most commercial implementations, although other iterative algorithms have been proposed [29]. An accelerated iterative algorithm sim-

ilar to MLEM known as the ordered-subset expectation maximization (OSEM) is used on some commercial systems for attenuation correction [21]. This algorithm has been shown to reduce reconstruction time by as much as a factor of 10. However, large-scale validation of this promising algorithm on clinical studies has not yet been adequately demonstrated.

Some of the earliest techniques proposed from the scientific community were for iterative reconstruction of the transmission data. Despite early recommendations, the first generation of attenuation correction products failed to emphasize the importance of using sophisticated transmission reconstruction algorithms that appropriately model image noise and other error sources that may propagate into the corrected images [30]. It is now known that the quality of the transmission map has a critical impact on the quality of the attenuation corrected emission studies.

Artifacts in transmission reconstructions also occur and can result from either large regions of pixels being too high or too low (bias) or large variation between individual pixels (variance). At low count density, attenuation coefficients can vary up to 50% or more from one pixel to the next. This can lead to excess noise being introduced into the corrected images. However, bias is the more detrimental source of error. Typically, if a

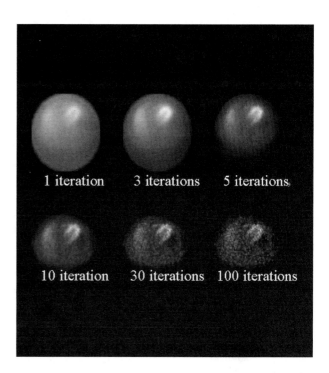

FIGURE 7.7 In the absence of noise, iterative reconstruction progressively improves the image quality at each iteration. In reality, the images reach an optimum appearance, and then for successive iterations the reconstruction is dominated by the noise.

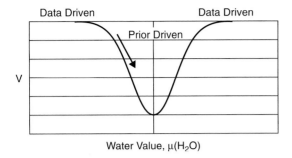

FIGURE 7.8 The Bayesian method drives those pixels that are near the water value to the water value (the prior), and those pixels that are far from the water value are driven by the data.

large number of pixels in the transmission projection have zero values, a region of artifactually reduced attenuation coefficients can emerge in the transmission reconstructions. This is most commonly present in the densely attenuating abdominal region and can have a negative impact of attenuation correction of the inferior wall [31,32]. This is why it is important to assure that the sources are appropriately serviced to prevent excessive physical decay.

A balanced approach for reducing the bias and variance of attenuation map reconstruction is to use a Bayesian iterative reconstruction technique. One such algorithm developed by our group in collaboration with Emory University exploits the property that much of the attenuation coefficients in the thorax and abdomen are similar to the value for water [32]. The algorithm "encourages" pixels that are near the water value to move closer to the water value at each iteration by mathematical constraint (Fig. 7.8). Those "far" from the water value are independently determined by the data. This algorithm was recently included in a multicenter evaluation for attenuation correction of Tc-99m-sestamibi where it was observed that in all patients studied, none had an inferior scan using this algorithm and 19% of patients had superior image quality compared with an existing back-projection-based attenuation map reconstruction method [33]. These results and other recent studies support the need for high-quality, accurate attenuation maps for successful attenuation correction.

Photo-Peak Scatter and Nonstationary Spatial Resolution

Attenuation correction is not "everything correction" [34]. As more is learned about attenuation corrected images, it is becoming clear that other physical limitations continue to challenge physicians and physicists and are likely required as part of the "total" correction. Photon scatter, partial volume effects, and depth-dependent spa-

tial resolution are factors that are important to the complete solution to correcting for physical limitations of SPECT. Spatial resolution in SPECT is limited (finite) and nonstationary (varies with source-detector distance) and the implications for orbital-dependent artifacts are well described for conventional SPECT and attenuation correction [35]. Compton scattered photons detected in the photo-peak form a greater proportion of the emission image with Tl-201 than for Tc-99m agents [14]. At least two techniques have now been commercialized for attenuation correction that include compensation for Compton scatter and the depth-dependent spatial resolution of SPECT [27,36]. Both methods use a restoration filtering technique that models the system response of the collimated detector as a preprocessing step prior to correction with the attenuation map.

Compton scattering of photons prior to detection is an important factor in conventional imaging, however, the significance is changed with attenuation correction. Scatter is present in the emission and transmission images, although collimation of the source and detector, together with energy and spatial window discrimination, provide good estimates to the narrow beam (scatter-free) estimate. Scatter correction is important for more accurate measures of myocardial uptake values and to assist in minimizing artifacts that can result from subdiaphragmatic activity in proximity to the heart with attenuation correction. Extracardiac activity adjacent to the myocardium can cause "overcorrection" of the inferior wall causing artifactual decrease in anterior wall intensity [31]. This is because attenuation in regions below the diaphragm may be several times greater than in the thorax and thereby correction may exacerbate the effect of scatter by enhancing the "blurring" of counts from these regions into the inferior or posterior wall of the myocardium. The clinical literature on attenuation correction consistently reports some small but significant complication to image interpretation from extracardiac scatter. Several methods have recently been investigated to correct for scatter. These methods use scatter information collected in a separate window for subtraction of a fraction of this from the photo-peak image [37], intrinsically model scatter in the reconstruction algorithm [38], and use of filtering methods that compensate for spatial and contrast resolution [36,39].

SPECT-BASED TRANSMISSION IMAGING SYSTEMS: TECHNICAL AND PRACTICAL DESCRIPTION

All manufacturers now provide transmission-based SPECT systems for attenuation correction. However, they differ in their hardware configuration and related software methods. Recent development has been directed toward the simultaneous acquisition of transmission and emission imaging for clinical time efficiency, although some systems utilize sequential (emission study followed or preceded by the transmission study) or interleaved sequential (alternating emission and transmission at each projection angle). Misregistration of emission and transmission image data has been shown to be a potential source of error in attenuation corrected images, which may be more likely with sequential scanning [40].

Figure 7.9 illustrates basic configurations for transmission-based imaging with SPECT. Figure 7.9A shows a fixed line source placed at the focal line of a symmetric fan beam collimator while the other two detectors are used for emission acquisition [41]. This approach provides very high system sensitivity for transmission imaging due to the geometry of the collimator-source positioning and requires a relatively small transmission source activity (usually about 60 mCi). Emission sensitivity is very efficient due to convergent collimation, although enhanced truncation of the patient's body in the field of view is an important aspect of this approach compared with other configurations. This effect is limiting, as sufficiency criteria for attenuation map reconstruction are violated that may result in artifacts in the attenuation map for some systems. These artifacts have been implicated as a limitation to diagnostic accuracy in simulation studies where "severe"

truncation was present. Reconstruction methods that use models of body boundaries or other a priori information to support the missing anatomical information have been shown to minimize the effects of truncation, permitting improved diagnostic accuracy and quantitation with attenuation correction [42,43].

A noncommercialized modification of this triple-detector approach replaces the convergent collimators for emission acquisition with parallel collimation and uses Am-241 (59 keV) as the transmission source [43,44]. This system has the advantage of a large field of view from the parallel geometry and it has been used to demonstrate the clinical value of attenuation correction for myocardial perfusion SPECT, but has not been commercialized.

A modification of this triple-detector approach was developed using a line source of activity positioned "off-center" at the focal line of an asymmetric fan beam collimator [45] (Fig. 7.9B). This approach solves the truncation problem by using the complementary opposing view to collect truncated data and therefore requires 360° of data acquisition. Another geometric solution to minimize the truncation problem utilizes a point source that scans parallel to the system axis and out of the field of view of the detectors [46]. Detector collimation of the transmission source is not utilized in this approach as the high-energy Ba-133 source (330 keV) emitted along the focal line penetrates the collimator in the asymmetric fan beam geometry.

The most widely implemented and studied configu-

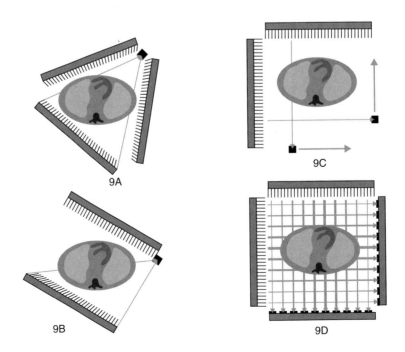

FIGURE 7.9 Common geometries used for attenuation correction in SPECT.

ration for transmission imaging in myocardial perfusion SPECT is the scanning line source approach implemented on dual 90° detector systems [47] (Fig. 7.9C). This approach achieves transmission and emission separation by collimating the source and using a narrow (5 cm) electronic window that moves simultaneously and opposite the external source, permitting photons about the transmission energy window to be counted. This system permits maximal separation of emission and transmission energies but as a result has low sensitivity due to the collimation and limited projection area on the detector. Mechanically, this arrangement is complex, potentially requiring careful monitoring for sufficient performance.

Another approach to transmission imaging that utilizes an array of line sources that span the field of view has been implemented on 90° dual-detector systems for transmission acquisition with cardiac perfusion SPECT [48] (Fig. 7.9D). Each rod has uniform activity concentration but those located toward the periphery of the field of view have lower activity. This provides improved count rates for central regions of the patient where attenuation is greatest and minimizes dead time effects from photons incident on the detector in regions not attenuated by the patient. The sources are "rotated" periodically to preserve the effective life of the sources and to optimize penetration of the densest part of the patient.

By far the most accurate (and currently most expensive) method of obtaining an attenuation map uses a traditional X-ray tube as the radiation source [49]. This technique, developed for general nuclear imaging, would provide virtually noise-free transmission data sets that could be used for attenuation correction. Though this technique has appeal, the transmission images cannot be acquired simultaneously with the emission data, because the transmission source and detector are physically separated from the emission detectors. However, this separation may be acceptable, because PET studies where attenuation correction is an integral part of all studies utilize this approach with a very high accuracy rate for myocardial perfusion imaging [50]. It is unclear whether this highly accurate transmission study is necessary for attenuation correction. Other advanced designs proposed for transmission imaging beyond those described here can be found in Bailey [51].

ATTENUATION CORRECTION QUALITY CONTROL

Quality assurance is an essential component of all imaging modalities but has not been adequately developed for SPECT attenuation correction. The American Society of Nuclear Cardiology (ASNC) and Society of Nuclear Medicine (SNM) have recently acknowledged quality control and technical performance as critical for attenuation correction systems by outlining key elements in the recent guidelines for perfusion SPECT [4].

Quantitative software tools to address this need have been developed recently for monitoring of transmission hardware performance, attenuation map, and reference scan quality as part of a comprehensive quality assurance program. Galt et al. developed automated algorithms that could be used to successfully detect the common technical errors in attenuation correction acquisition with dual scanning Gd-153 line sources on a dual detector system [52]. Associated work led to the development of a prescanning technique for transmission imaging that yielded an estimate of the required imaging time for adequate count density in the attenuation map [53]. This is important when there are patients with exceptional density or size and if the transmission sources are weakened from physical decay. Early clinical investigations of attenuation correction methods as well as recent reports do not contain quality control discussion as part of their clinical protocol [54]. Therefore, early clinical results may have been influenced by technical limitations not adequately appreciated by investigators and must be an integral part of future clinical utilization.

Reference Scan

The reference scan is similar to the flood field uniformity scan for emission imaging as a valuable tool for attenuation correction quality control. Reference scan uniformity is a measure of the combined performance of the transmission hardware, source strength, and acquisition software. It is typically acquired at the beginning of the day as part of a quality control protocol or after system maintenance. Total counts in the reference scan images for each detector should also be monitored regularly and compared to a baseline standard as a measure of transmission source decay and overall hardware performance. Sudden changes in total counts or reference scans' appearance may indicate malfunction or the need for source replacement or removal of source attenuators. The latter are placed in front of the sources to remove lower energy photons that do not contribute to the transmission energy window and to prevent count rates from exceeding detector limitations. They can be "removed" in the field to replenish the source strength after sufficient decay has occurred. Manufacturers sometimes provide specific guidelines for quality performance of transmission scanning equipment. Criteria for this important measurement are not an industry standard.

CLINICAL STATUS OF ATTENUATION CORRECTION

The potential clinical ramifications of a fully implemented attenuation correction approach are substantial: enhanced visual and quantitative analyses through improved count density distribution that approaches homogeneity in the presence of normal perfusion; higher sensitivity for detection of disease including mild-moderate, single-vessel, and multivessel disease with relative balanced flow reduction; higher specificity due to reduced artifacts from attenuation; and improved delineation of myocardial viability in terms of accuracy of assessment of tracer uptake in dysfunctional areas (Figs. 7.10 and 7.11). Unfortunately, truly clinical studies on the value of currently implemented attenuation correction methods are few and most of the studies to date are validation studies. It is likely that with recent improvements designed to overcome first generation hardware/software systems for attenuation

correction that these long-awaited investigations will soon appear in the literature.

What has been established is that the various approaches improve the relative uniformity of tracer uptake in low-likelihood subjects for a range of systems, protocols, and transmission sources. Ficaro et al. first described the impact of a transmission-based attenuation correction method on the homogeneity of perfusion in 10 normal volunteers with adenosine Tl-201 stress-reinjection using simultaneous emission-transmission 360° imaging on a triple-detector system with Am-241 as the transmission source [43]. Using a nine-segment polar map model, lateral-to-posterior and basal-to-apical wall ratios showed statistically significant improvement in homogeneity (relative value equal to 1.0) with attenuation correction compared with uncorrected images. In a later study, as part of an investigation of the diagnostic accuracy of an attenuation correction technique in stress Tc-99m-sestamibi stud-

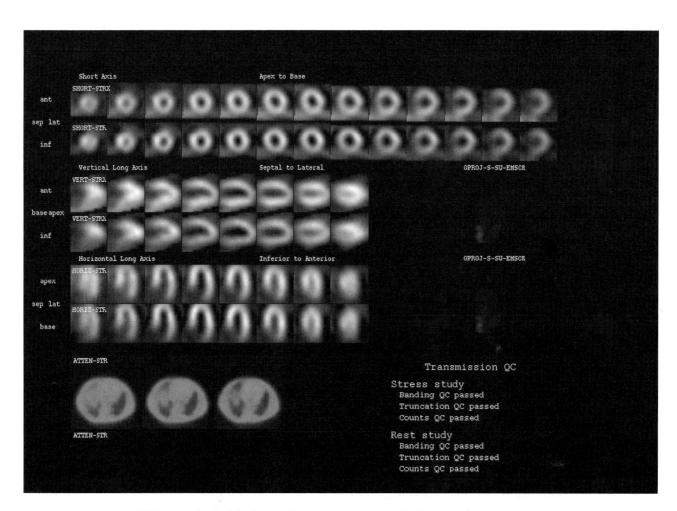

FIGURE 7.10 Example of subdiaphragmatic attenuation in a male that is corrected using attenuation correction.

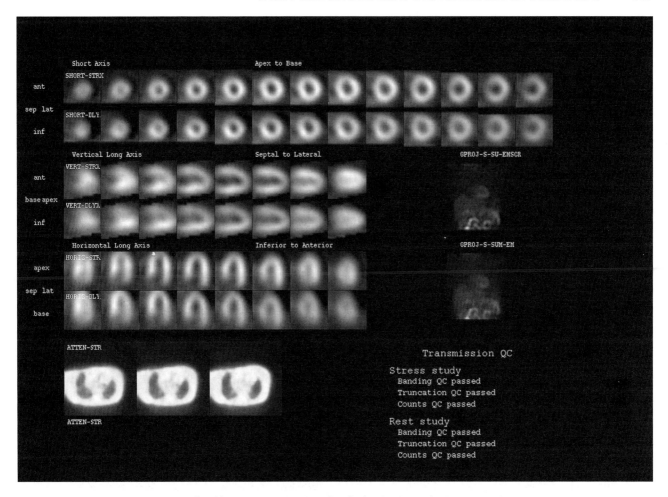

FIGURE 7.11 Example of breast attenuation in a female that is corrected using attenuation correction.

ies, the same group studied 59 patients with < 5% probability of coronary artery disease also using a triple-detector system with Am-241 as the transmission source [44]. Improved perfusion homogeneity was also demonstrated for males and females compared with uncorrected images. Statistically, this study demonstrated no significant difference for each of the segments between male and female attenuation corrected databases, and therefore a gender-composite polar map for quantitative analysis was formed. Visual and quantitative normalcy rates were significantly improved from 0.88 and 0.76 to 0.98 and 0.95, respectively.

Prvulovich et al. performed a similar analysis using pharmacologic stress on Tl-201 studies with < 5% likelihood of coronary artery disease [55]. This study used scanning Gd-153 transmission line sources and MLEM-based reconstruction for attenuation correction and filtered back projection (FBP)-based method for attenuation map reconstruction. Using a 17-segment polar map model, improved tracer homogeneity in both male and female populations as measured by septal-to-lateral wall ratios and anterior-basal wall activity was demonstrated to be significantly improved compared with the noncorrected images. Statistical equivalence between male and female normal databases was also found. Choraqui et al. showed similar results in 42 patients (29 men) with < 5% likelihood of coronary artery disease using a 31-segment model and treadmill exercise Tl-201 SPECT with scanning line source Gd-153 [56]. Matsunari et al. investigated normal perfusion distributions in rest Tl-201–stress Tc-99m-sestamibi acquired using a similar system to that of Ficaro et al. [57]. In this study, segmental analysis demonstrated significant differences in attenuation corrected stress and rest images. This finding highlighted differences that can exist with attenuation corrected studies and that method-specific considerations are required including attenuation corrected normal databases.

Studies on the diagnostic accuracy of attenuation correction techniques are more varied in their findings compared with those on low-likelihood populations. Ficaro et al. investigated the diagnostic accuracy of attenuation correction compared with uncorrected studies in 60 patients with angiographically documented coronary artery disease (CAD) using a stress Tc-99m-sestamibi–rest Tl-201 protocol [44]. For detection of CAD, sensitivity/specificity values improved from 0.78/0.46 (without correction) to 0.84/0.82 with correction, respectively, for visual analysis and 0.84/0.46 (no correction) to 0.88/0.82 with quantitation analysis using the gender-composite normal database described earlier. Receiver Operator Characteristic analysis demonstrated significantly improved discrimination for right coronary disease. Left circumflex artery discrimination was not improved significantly. Left anterior descending analysis was not performed. Significant improvement in attenuation correction to localize diseased vessels in single-vessel and multivessel disease was also demonstrated. Kluge et al. evaluated attenuation correction with 90° dual-detector and Gd-153 scanning line sources comparing attenuation corrected and uncorrected studies in two groups of males and Tc-99m-tetrofosmin stress imaging (exercise and pharmacologic) [58]. The first group consisted of 25 males with CAD of the right coronary artery and/or left circumflex arteries, all without "significant" narrowing of the left anterior descending artery (LAD). Of these, 16 had single-vessel disease (8 with left circumflex and 8 with right coronary artery lesions) and 9 had two-vessel disease. The second group (also 25 males) had < 10% likelihood for the presence of CAD. Studies were quantified using a normal database developed from 25 males with < 10% likelihood of CAD. Sensitivity improved from 65% to 88% for right coronary lesions and from 71% to 94% for left circumflex. Specificity improved from 88% and 75% to 100% for right and left circumflex disease.

Gallowitsch et al. also investigated the effect of attenuation correction on diagnostic accuracy and examined the impact on the extent and severity of perfusion abnormalities in 107 patients (69 males, 38 females) undergoing stress-rest-redistribution imaging with exercise (bicycle) or pharmacologic (dipyridamole) stress and scanning line source Gd-153 transmission imaging [59]. The patients were assigned to two groups: those with chest pain and no known disease (n = 49) and those with known CAD (n = 58). Polar map analysis was performed using a 31-segment model. Overall sensitivity, based on visual analysis, was improved with attenuation correction from 89% to 94% in the first group and 74% to 94% in the second group. Specificity was improved from 69% to 84% in the first group and 91% to 100% in the second. The

authors reported defect extent and severity were significantly influenced by attenuation correction as fewer abnormal and less severe abnormal segments were demonstrated with attenuation correction.

Hendel et al. presented results from the first prospective multicenter trial evaluating attenuation correction using dual scanning Gd-153 line sources with stress Tc-99m-sestamibi imaging obtained from dual-isotope and 1-day Tc-99m-sestamibi studies [60]. This technique of attenuation correction employed photo-peak scatter and variable spatial resolution compensation. In this study, 96 patients were studied with angiographically demonstrated CAD and 88 with low likelihood (< 5%) were studied. Detection of > 50% stenosis was similar with and without correction (76% vs 75%, p = NS). Normalcy rate, however, was significantly improved with correction using visual analysis (86% vs 96%) and quantitative analysis (86% vs 97%). There was, however, a reduction in the detection of extensive CAD.

Links et al. investigated a method that incorporated a correction technique for patient motion in conjunction with corrections for scatter, attenuation, and spatial resolution in a multicenter trial from four institutions [61]. They studied 51 patients with coronary artery disease and 61 with low likelihood (< 5%) of disease or normal angiograms. Multiple combinations of Tl-201 and Tc-99m agents were used for emission and Gd-153 or Tc-99m was used for transmission imaging with dual scanning line sources in a simultaneous or sequential interleaved acquisition protocol. Sensitivity and specificity for motion corrected only studies were 84%/69%, 64%/71%, and 32%/94% for left anterior descending, right and left circumflex, respectively, and 71%/81% overall. This was compared with 88%/92%, 77%/93%, 50%/97% for the three territories and 74%/95% overall with motion and attenuation correction. Sensitivity was not significantly changed for single- and triple-vessel disease (79%/79% and 93%/93%), respectively. Specificity was significantly improved for left anterior descending (71%/93%) and right coronary arteries (81%/95%).

Clinical studies using investigational correction components continue to report mixed results in varying populations. Harel et al. recently reported application of attenuation, scatter, and resolution recovery techniques for Tl-201 in 82 patients (42 low likelihood, 42 with known CAD) [62]. Overall, specificity and normalcy were significantly improved but sensitivity was lower owing to false positive evaluation for viability in patients with inferior infarction, attributable to overcorrection in the inferior wall. Although studies delineating the limitations of methods are reported, often on noncommercialized systems and methods, the general weight of evidence suggests that attenuation correction methods are demonstrating improved accuracy through significant improvements in specificity with a trend toward improved sensitivity [63]. This status is reflected in a position paper published by the Society of Nuclear Medicine and Journal of Nuclear Cardiology on attenuation correction for cardiac perfusion SPECT stating that this rapidly evolving technology should be considered as an important clinical adjunct to SPECT [64].

Limitations and Characteristics of Attenuation Corrected SPECT Images

As might be expected, correction for attenuation changes the balance of SPECT performance, generating new and unique image features and technical limitations. Artifacts can arise from enhanced subdiaphragmatic uptake by attenuation correction and is a common limitation cited in clinical studies with attenuation correction. Attenuation correction, without scatter correction, unmasks the presence of scatter artifacts [65,66]. During display, images may be normalized to the "hot" (overcorrected) region, causing the image to incorrectly appear suppressed in relative uptake. This may be more pronounced with pharmacologic stress protocols compared with exercise studies where subdiaphragmatic activity is more frequently observed. Therefore, efforts to minimize gut activity may be more critical with attenuation correction studies than conventional studies. Ficaro et al. reported that with 119 Tc-99m-sestamibi stress images, liver activity was problematic in 6 uncorrected studies and 12 corrected studies [44]. Kluge et al. reported that in 50 stress studies of this investigation, enhanced liver activity was observed in 2 uncorrected and 3 attenuation corrected studies [58]. Gallowitsch et al. [59] reported that enhanced gut activity affected the posterior wall in attenuation corrected studies obtained with dipyridamole compared with those studies with bicycle exercise. Most of the clinical studies suggest that scatter correction and nonstationary resolution compensation seem to be indicated to further optimize the performance clinically.

Truncation artifacts are errors in the attenuation map that occur when portions of the body move out of the field of view of the transmission projections for some of the angles [67]. They are recognizable as bright arcs of activity on the edge of the patient body outline with FBP reconstruction and a complex distortion of the attenuation map with iterative reconstruction methods. Information describing the effects of truncation on corrected image quality is limited largely technical on phantom and simulation studies. The technologist and physician should of truncation in order to minimize its occurrence. This should include reviewing the transmission images and quality of the attenuation map as part of a quality assurance protocol for attenuation correction.

The effects of patient and respiratory motion on attenuation correction are not well understood clinically, although studies demonstrate that they can increase variability in perfusion SPECT by changing degree of attenuation correction over the cardiac cycle [68]. Therefore, it may be possible to develop methods that model this inconsistency to further optimize the accuracy of attenuation correction.

Another common observation in attenuation corrected images is so-called apical-thinning that results from actual anatomical thinning of the myocardial wall in the region of the apex and partial volume effects related to finite resolution of the SPECT system [34]. Most publications on attenuation correction cite apical thinning in their analysis or describe it in discussions of the findings and may necessitate re-examination of expected distributions in this distal region.

ADVANCED APPLICATIONS

In addition to improving the diagnostic accuracy and confidence of conventional perfusion SPECT studies, attenuation correction may provide an important component to promising investigational single-acquisition imaging protocols. Stress-only imaging has been proposed for certain populations and is based on the observation that only limited information is provided by the resting scans particularly with ECG-gating [69]. Patients with normal stress scans may not require rest imaging. Attenuation correction could provide improved discrimination of true defects from attenuation artifacts thereby lessening the need for additional resting images [70].

Attenuation correction also has potential implications for patients being assessed for potential coronary events in the emergency department. Several authors have reported success in using acute imaging to differentiate between acute coronary syndromes and non-coronary chest pain [71]. However, they have realized the need to improve the specificity of acute imaging to obtain the full benefits of using nuclear cardiology to triage chest pain patients. Attenuation correction has been identified as a potential technique for improving the specificity of acute myocardial perfusion imaging. Although this has been hypothesized, it has not been broadly demonstrated clinically. This result could minimize the number of patients requiring additional testing or extended stay and thereby reduce associated cost of treatment.

SUMMARY

The enthusiasm about clinical application of attenuation correction techniques for cardiac perfusion SPECT continues to grow, especially as current developments responding to early shortcomings of transmission-based methods mature and more clinical studies emerge. A significant body of evidence now exists that transmission-based attenuation correction is a valuable new tool for the diagnosis and assessment of coronary artery disease. However, for attenuation correction methods to realize their full clinical potential, such important attributes as quality control and standards for interpretation will be required. Important, but not yet studied, is the impact that attenuation correction techniques could have on the management of cardiac patients as compared with the emphasis on diagnostic accuracy commonly reported in the literature. Attenuation correction provides an important component to the implementation of new algorithms for single-acquisition studies such as acute applications, stress-only, and attenuation corrected dual-simultaneous acquisition protocols. If successful, these developments will undoubtedly have a profound influence on the way in which nuclear cardiology studies are performed and will strengthen the clinical appeal of SPECT.

ACKNOWLEDGMENT

The authors would like to thank James R. Galt, Ph.D., of Emory University School of Medicine, Atlanta, Georgia, for supplying some of the Figures used in this manuscript.

REFERENCES

1. DePuey EG, Garcia EV. Optimal specificity of thallium-201 SPECT through recognition of imaging artifacts. J Nucl Med 1989;30:441.
2. DePuey EG. How to detect and avoid myocardial perfusion SPECT artifacts. J Nucl Med 1994;35:699.
3. Hendel RC, Gibbons RJ, Bateman TM. Use of rotating (cine) planar projection images in the interpretation of a tomographic myocardial perfusion study. J Nucl Cardiol 1999;6:234.
4. Knesaurek K, King MA, Glick SJ, et al. Investigation of causes of geometric distortion in 180° and 360° angular sampling in SPECT. J Nucl Med 1989;30:1666.
5. Updated Imaging Guidelines for Nuclear Cardiology Procedures. Part 1. DePuey EG editor. J Nucl Cardiol 2001;8:G1.
6. Eisner RL, Tamas MJ, Cloninger K, et al. Normal SPECT thallium-201 bull's eye display: gender differences. J Nucl Med 1988; 29:1901.
7. DePasquale EE, Nody AC, DePuey EG, et al. Quantitative rotational thallium-201 tomography for identifying and localizing coronary artery disease. Circulation 1988;77:316.
8. Garcia EV, Cooke CD, Van Train KF, et al. Technical aspects of myocardial SPECT imaging with technetium-99m sestamibi. Am J Cardiol 1990;13:23E.
9. DePuey EG, Rozanski AR. Using gated technetium-99m-sestamibi SPECT to characterize fixed defects as infarct or artifact. J Nucl Med 1995;36:952.
10. Smanio PE, Watson DD, Segalla DL, et al. Value of gating of technetium-99m sestamibi single-photon emission computed tomographic imaging. J Am Coll Cardiol 1997;30:1687.
11. Esquerre JP, Coca FJ, Martinez SJ, et al. Prone decubitus: a solution to inferior wall attenuation in thallium-201 myocardial tomography. J Nucl Med 1989;30:398.
12. Kiat H, Van Train KF, Friedman JD, et al. Quantitative stress-redistribution thallium-201 SPECT using prone imaging: methodologic development and validation. J Nucl Med 1992;33:1509.
13. Sorenson SA, Phelps ME. *Physics in Nuclear Medicine*, 2nd Edition. Philadelphia: W.B. Saunders, 1987, Chapter 9.
14. Gagnon D, Pouliot N, Laperriere L. Statistical and physical content of low-energy photons in holospectral imaging. IEEE Trans Med Imaging 1991;10:284.
15. Bushberg JT, Seibert JA, Leidholdt EM, et al. *The Essential Physics of Medical Imaging*. Baltimore: Williams & Wilkins, 1994.
16. Cullom SJ, L Liu, White ML. Compensation of attenuation map errors from Tc-99m-sestamibi downscatter with simultatneous Gd-153 transmission scanning. J Nucl Med 1996;37:215P.
17. Almquist H, Arheden H, Arvidsson AH, et al. Clinical implication of down scatter in attenuation corrected myocardial SPECT. J Nucl Cardiol 1999;6;406.
18. Miles J, Cullom SJ, Case JA. An introduction to attenuation correction. J Nucl Cardiol 1999;6:449.
19. Ficaro EP, Harris AJ. A quality control protocol for transmission-emission tomographic systems. J Nucl Med 1997;38:214P.
20. Ficaro EP, Rogers WL, Schwaiger M. Comparison of Am-241 and Tc-99m as transmission sources for the attenuation correction of Tl-201 SPECT imaging of the heart. J Nucl Med 1994;35; 652.
21. Lange K, Bahn M, Little R. A theoretical study of some maximum likelihood algorithms for emission and transmission tomography. IEEE Trans Med Imaging 1987;6:106.
22. Snyder DL, Miller MI, Thomas LJ Jr, et al. Noise and edge artifacts in maximum-likelihood reconstructions for emission tomography. IEEE Trans Med Imaging 1987;MI-6:228.
23. Chang LT. A method for attenuation correction in radionuclide computed tomography. IEEE Trans Nucl Sci 1978;1:638.
24. Malko JA, Van Heertum RL, Gullberg GT, et al. SPECT liver imaging using an iterative attenuation correction algorithm and an external flood source. J Nucl Med 1986;27:701.
25. Bailey DL, Hutton BF, Walker PJ. Improved SPECT using simultaneous emission and transmission tomography. J Nucl Med 1987;28:844.
26. Galt JR, Cullom SJ, Garcia EV. SPECT quantification: a simplified method of attenuation correction for cardiac imaging. J Nucl Med 1993;33:2232.
27. Rigo P, Van Boxem P, Foulon J, et al. Quantitative evaluation of a comprehensive motion, resolution, and attenuation correction program: initial experience. J Nucl Cardiol 1998;5:458.
28. Tsui BMW, Gullberg GT, Edgerton ER, et al. Correction of

nonuniform attenuation in cardiac SPECT imaging. J Nucl Med 1989;30:497.

29. Ficaro EP, Fessler JA. Statistical algorithms for reconstructing cardiac attenuation maps from simultaneous transmission-emission SPECT systems. J Nucl Med 1997;38:214P.

30. Tung CH, Gullberg GT. A simulation of emission and transmission noise propagation in cardiac SPECT imaging with nonuniform attenuation correction. Med Phys 1994;21:1565.

31. Heller EN, DeMan P, Liu YH, et al. Extracardiac activity complicates quantitative cardiac SPECT imaging using a simultaneous transmission-emission approach. J Nucl Med 1997;38:1882.

32. Case JA, Cullom SJ, Galt JR, et al. Impact of transmission scan reconstruction using an iterative algorithm (BITGA) versus FBP: clinical appearance of attenuation-corrected myocardial perfusion SPECT images. J Nucl Med 2001;42:51P.

33. Galt JR, Arram SM, Case JA, et al. Multicenter evaluation of automated quality control of transmission scans for attenuation correction in myocardial perfusion SPECT. J Am Coll Cardiol 2001;37:425A.

34. Hutton BF. Cardiac single-photon emission tomography: is attenuation correction enough? Eur J Nucl Med 1997;24:713.

35. Maniawski PJ, Morgan HT, Whackers FJTh, et al. Orbit-related variation in spatial resolution as a source of artifactual defects in thallium-201 SPECT. J Nucl Med 1991;32:871.

36. Liu L, Cullom SJ, White ML. A modified wiener filter method for nonstationary resolution recovery with scatter and iterative attenuation correction for cardiac SPECT. J Nucl Med 1996;37:210P.

37. Jaszczak RJ, Greer KL, Floyd CE, et al. Improved SPECT quantification using compensation for scattered photons. J Nucl Med 1984;25:893.

38. Bowsher JE, Floyd CE Jr. Treatment of Compton scattering in maximum-likelihood, expectation-maximization reconstructions of SPECT images. J Nucl Med 1991;32:1291.

39. Links JM, Becker LC, Rigo P, et al. Combined corrections for attenuation, depth-dependent blur, and motion in cardiac SPECT: a multicenter trial. J Nucl Cardiol 2000;7:414.

40. Stone CD, McCormick JW, Gilland DR, et al. Effect of registration errors between transmission and emission scans on a SPECT system using sequential scanning. J Nucl Med 1998;39:365.

41. Tung CH, Gullberg GT, Zeng GL, et al. Non-uniform attenuation correction using simultaneous transmission and emission converging tomography. IEEE Trans Nucl Sci 1992;39:1134.

42. Case JA, Pan TS, O'Brian-Penney B, et al. Reduction of truncation artifacts in fan beam transmission imaging using a spatially varying gamma prior. IEEE Trans Nucl Sci 1995;42:1310.

43. Ficaro EP, Fessler JA, Ackermann RJ, et al. Simultaneous transmission-emission thallium-201 cardiac SPECT: effect of attenuation correction on myocardial tracer distribution. J Nucl Med 1995;36:921.

44. Ficaro EP, Fessler JA, Shreve PD, et al. Simultaneous transmission/emission myocardial perfusion tomography. Diagnostic accuracy of attenuation-corrected 99mTc-sestamibi single-photon emission computed tomography. Circulation 1996;93:463.

45. Chang W, Loncaric S, Huang, et al. Asymmetrical-fan transmission CT on SPECT to derive μ-maps for attenuation correction. J Nucl Med 1994;35:92P.

46. Beekman FJ, Kamphuis C, Hutton BF, et al. Half-fanbeam collimators combined with scanning point sources for simultaneous emission-transmission imaging. J Nucl Med 1998;39:1996.

47. Tan P, Bailey DL, Meikle SR, et al. A scanning line source for simultaneous emission and transmission measurements in SPECT. J Nucl Med 1993;34:1752.

48. Celler A, Sitek A, Stoub E, et al. Multiple line source array for SPECT transmission scans: simulation, phantom and patient studies. J Nucl Med 1998;39:2183.

49. Lang TF, Hasegawa BH, Liew SC, et al. Description of a prototype emission-transmission computed tomography imaging system. J Nucl Med 1992;33:1881.

50. Bachrach SL, Buvat I. Attenuation correction in cardiac positron emission tomography and single-photon emission computed tomography. J Nucl Cardiol 1995;2:246.

51. Bailey DL. Transmission scanning in emission tomography. Eur J Nucl Med 1998;25:774. Review.

52. Galt JR, Blais M, Cullom SJ, et al. Quality control of transmission scans for attenuation correction in cardiac SPECT. J Nucl Med 1999;40:286P.

53. Shao L, Ye J, Durbin MK. Use of a prestudy information density scan to improve transmission map acquisition for attenuation correction. J Nucl Med 2000;5:177P.

54. Cullom SJ, Case JA, Bateman TM. Invited Commentary: Attenuation correction for myocardial perfusion SPECT. J Nucl Med 2000;41:860.

55. Prvulovich EM, Lonn AHR, Bomanji JB, et al. Effect of attenuation correction on myocardial thallium-201 distribution in patients with a low-likelihood of coronary artery disease. Eur J Nucl Med 1997;266.

56. Chouraqui P, Livschitz S, Sharir T, et al. Evaluation of an attenuation correction method for thallium-201 myocardial perfusion tomographic imaging of patients with low-likelihood of coronary artery disease. J Nucl Cardiol 1998;5:369.

57. Matsunari I, Boning G, Ziegler SI, et al. Attenuation corrected thallium-201/stress technetuim 99m sestamibi myocardial SPECT in normals. J Nucl Cardiol 1998;5:48.

58. Kluge R, Sattler B, Seese A, et al. Attenuation correction by simultaneous emission-transmission myocardial single-photon emission tomography using a technetium-99m-labelled radiotracer: impact on diagnostic accuracy. Eur J Nucl Med 1997;24:1107.

59. Gallowitsch HJ, Syokora J, Mikosch P, et al. Attenuation corrected thallium-201 single-photon emission tomography using a gadolinium-153 moving line source: clinical value and the impact of attenuation correction on the extent and severity of perfusion abnormalities. Eur J Nucl Med 1998;25:220.

60. Hendel RC, Berman DS, Cullom SJ, et al. A multicenter trial to evaluate the efficacy of correction for photon attenuation and scatter in SPECT myocardial perfusion imaging. Circulation 2002;99(21), 2742.

61. Links JM, Becker LC, Rigo P, et al. Combined corrections for attenuation, depth-dependent blur, and motion in cardiac SPECT: a multicenter trial. J Nucl Cardiol 2000;7:414.

62. Harel F, Genin R, Daou D, et al. Clinical impact of combination of scatter, attenuation correction, and depth-dependent resolution recovery for Tl-201 studies. J Nucl Med 2001;42:1451.

63. Corbett JR, Ficaro EP. Clinical review of attenuation-corrected cardiac SPECT. J Nucl Cardiol 1999;6:54.

64. Hendel RC, Corbett JR, Cullom SJ, et al. The value and practice of attenuation correction for myocardial perfusion SPECT imaging: a joint position paper from the American Society of Nuclear Cardiology and the Society of Nuclear Medicine (to be published simultaneously J Nucl Med and J Nucl Cardiol 2001).

65. King MA, Tsui BMW, Pan TS. Attenuation compensation for cardiac single-photon emission computed tomographic imaging: Part 1. Impact of attenuation and methods of estimating attenuation maps. J Nucl Cardiol 1995;2:513.

66. King MA, Tsui BMW, Pan TS, et al. Attenuation compensation

for cardiac single-photon emission computed tomographic imaging: Part 2. Attenuation compensation algorithms. J Nucl Cardiol 1995;3:55.

67. Maniawski PJ, Morgan HT, Gullbert GT, et al. Performance evaluation of a transmission reconstruction algorithm with simultaneous transmission-emission SPECT system in a presence of data truncation. Proceedings of the IEEE Nuclear Science Symposium and Medical Imaging Conference 1994;4:1578.

68. Cho K, Shin-ichiro K, Okada S, et al. Development of a respiratory gated myocardial SPECT system. J Nucl Cardiol 1999;6:20.

69. Chua T, Kiat H, Germano G, et al. Gated technetium-99m sestamibi for simultaneous assessment of stress myocardial perfusion, post-exercise regional ventricular function and myocardial viability. Correlation with echocardiography and rest thallium-201 scintigraphy. J Am Coll Cardiol 1995;23:1107.

70. Bateman TM, Heller GV, Hayes S, et al. Diagnostic accuracy of stress-only attenuation-corrected SPECT myocardial perfusion scintigraphy: results of a multicenter interpretation.

71. Tatum JL. Cost effective nuclear scanning in a comprehensive and systematic approach to the evaluation of chest pain in the emergency department. Md Med J 1997;Suppl:25.

8 | Gated single-photon emission computed tomography

GUIDO GERMANO AND DANIEL S. BERMAN

Gated myocardial perfusion single-photon emission computed tomography (SPECT) provides an accurate and reproducible method for measuring left ventricular ejection fraction and absolute left ventricular volumes. It also provides a means of assessing regional wall motion abnormality, either at rest or poststress. These capabilities of gated SPECT complement the strength of myocardial perfusion SPECT in coronary artery disease (CAD) diagnosis as well as risk stratification. This chapter briefly addresses several issues related to the acquisition of a gated perfusion SPECT study, presents a comprehensive review of gated SPECT quantification, and discusses the clinical value of assessing left ventricular function from gated SPECT. In addition, the emerging modality of gated blood SPECT and its relationship to gated perfusion SPECT are discussed.

GATED PERFUSION SPECT ACQUISITION

As explained in Chapter 5, a gated SPECT acquisition is similar to a standard SPECT acquisition, except that, in the former, a number (8 to 16) of projection images is acquired at each projection angle, with each image (also called interval or frame) corresponding to a specific portion of the cardiac cycle (Fig. 8.1). All projection images for a given interval are reconstructed into a SPECT image volume using standard filtered backprojection or iterative reconstruction, and the SPECT volumes relative to the various acquisition intervals can be displayed in four-dimensional format (x, y, z, and time) allowing for the assessment of dynamic cardiac function. In addition, summing all individual intervals' projections at each angle before reconstruction is essentially equivalent to having acquired a static perfusion SPECT study, and results in what is generally referred to as the "ungated" or summed gated SPECT image volume. Thus, a gated SPECT acquisition results

in a standard SPECT data set ("summed" gated SPECT), from which perfusion is assessed, and a larger gated SPECT data set, from which function is evaluated. The strong appeal of gating is a direct consequence of the ease and modest expense with which perfusion assessment is "upgraded" to perfusion/function assessment.

It is the authors' belief that, as long as adequate count statistics are achieved, there is no limitation as to the specific perfusion agent that can be imaged with the gated SPECT technique. Gated Tc-99m-sestamibi and Tc-99m-tetrofosmin SPECT imaging are routinely performed at a steadily increasing number of institutions, and accounted for over two-thirds of all SPECT studies in the United States in 1999, as shown in Figure 8.2. Gated Tl-201 SPECT imaging, originally considered not feasible, is now performed at a number of clinical sites, especially using multidetector cameras, with quantitative results not substantially different from gated Tc-99m-based SPECT [1,2] (see Tables 8.4 and 8.5). No matter what radiopharmaceutical is used, the quality of the gated SPECT study will be closely and directly related to the number of counts in its individual frames. Count statistics are influenced by numerous factors, including injected dose, acquisition time, patient size, camera configuration and sensitivity, collimation, number of frames, and count acceptance criteria.

Ideally, the length of acquisition (expressed in seconds per projection) for a gated Tc-99m-based SPECT study needs not exceed that traditionally employed for a nongated SPECT study. For gated Tl-201 SPECT, extending the acquisition time may be necessary, especially for gated redistribution acquisitions. While many other factors are involved, Table 8.1 gives the values currently used at Cedars-Sinai for gated SPECT acquisitions using a variety of cameras, low-energy–high-resolution (LEHR) collimation, 3° projection spacing, and 8-frame gating. It is clear that, although in principle any type of acquisition can be gated, practical con-

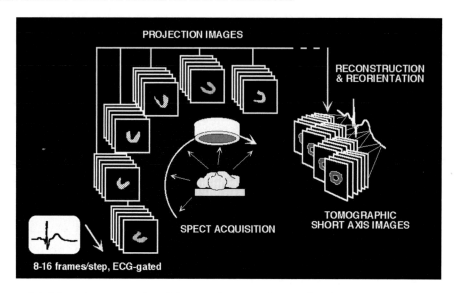

FIGURE 8.1 Schematic representation of electrocardiogram (ECG)-gated perfusion SPECT acquisition and processing. (Reproduced with permission from Germano G, Berman D. Acquisition and processing for gated perfusion SPECT: technical aspects. In: G Germano and D Berman, eds. Clinical gated cardiac SPECT. Futura Publishing Company, Armonk, NY; 1999:93–113.) [133]

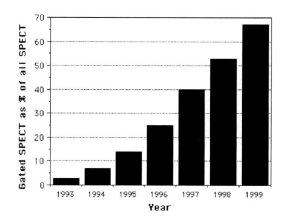

FIGURE 8.2 Growth in the percentage of all perfusion SPECT studies acquired using the ECG-gated technique. (Modified and reproduced with permission from Germano G, Berman D. Acquisition and processing for gated perfusion SPECT: technical aspects. In: G Germano and D Berman, eds. Clinical gated cardiac SPECT. Futura Publishing Company, Armonk, NY; 1999:93–113.) [133]

TABLE 8.1 *Injected Dose and Total Gated Perfusion SPECT Study Duration for Different Camera/Detector Configurations and Commonly Used Radiopharmaceuticals*

| Isotope | Dose (mCi) | No. Projs. | Sec/ Proj. | TOTAL STUDY DURATION (MIN) | | |
				1-det., 2-det @ 180°	2-det. @ 90°	3-det. @ 120°
Tc-99m-based	25–40	60	25	25	12.5	16.7
Tl-201	3–4.5	60	35	35	17.5	23.3
Tl-201 (redistribution)	3–4.5	60	45	45	22.5	30

(Reproduced with permission from Germano G, Berman D. Acquisition and processing for gated perfusion SPECT: technical aspects. In: G Germano and D Berman, eds. Clinical gated cardiac SPECT. Futura Publishing Company, Armonk, NY; 1999:93–113) [133].

Proj, projection; det, detector.

siderations on patient tolerance and avoidance of motion limit some acquisitions to multidetector cameras. Also, our approach leaves the acquisition time constant across patients for a given radioisotope and protocol, while the injected dose and the parameter of the pre-reconstruction filter are varied, as indicated in Tables 8.1 and 8.2. Other centers acquire a planar ungated image at the beginning of the study, calculate the total counts within the image or (by using a region of interest) in the myocardium, and adjust the acquisition time accordingly. Of course, both approaches aim at ensuring that adequate counts are collected.

Setting the Cardiac Beat Length Acceptance Window

The usual variation of the cardiac beat length during gated acquisitions has led to the building of tolerances in the count collection process. The beat length acceptance window aims at eliminating data from beats that are "too short" or "too long," while still accepting a sensible range of beat lengths. As Figure 8.3 shows, a beat length acceptance window of 20% allows accumulation of data from cardiac beats having a duration within ±10% of the expected duration. An acceptance window of 100%, somewhat counterintuitively, allows accumulation of data from beats of duration within ±50% of the expected. This is *not* equivalent to accepting 100% of the beats, which is instead consistent with having a window of infinite width.

In order to understand why a wide window would be desirable at all, it bears reminding that the perfusion SPECT data are derived by summing the various intervals of the gated study (Fig. 8.4). If too many counts

TABLE 8.2 *Butterworth Filter Parameter Employed at the Authors Institution Using the 0-0.05 Cutoff Range, Epital Size of 0.53-0.64 cu, and the Isotype Doses and Aquisition Tissues Described in Table 8.1*

| | Tc-99m-Based Agents | | Tl-201 | |
	Nongated	Gated	Nongated	Gated
Order	2.5		5	
Cutoff	0.33	0.3	0.25	0.2

(Reproduced with permission from Germano G, Berman D. Acquisition and processing for gated perfusion SPECT: technical aspects. In: G Germano and D Berman, eds. Clinical gated cardiac SPECT. Futura Publishing Company, Armonk, NY; 1999:93–113) [133].

are rejected due to arrhythmias or gating problems, not only would the gated information be unreliable but artifacts might appear in the summed SPECT data. This is not an issue if all rejected counts are automatically accumulated in an extra frame (a 9th frame in 8-frame gated SPECT imaging), and added back during generation of the "summed" perfusion SPECT study. While only a minority of camera manufacturers currently provide the "extra frame" feature, the consensus of the academic and clinical community is that this capability is necessary, and its diffusion is expected to increase in the future. In summary, our advice is to use as wide an acceptance window as possible if no extra frame is available to "save" rejected counts, or a 20%–30% acceptance window if that feature is available. If a 20%–30% beat acceptance window is used in conjunction with the "extra frame" feature, things are easier in that (*1*) the gated intervals surely do not contain data from arrhythmic beats, and (*2*) the extra frame (if accessible by itself) provides a convenient additional tool to assess

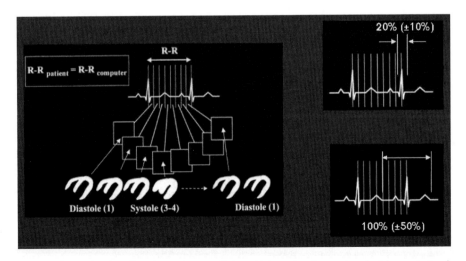

FIGURE 8.3 The cardiac beat length acceptance window. (Adapted and reproduced with permission from Cullom SJ, et al. Electrocardiographically gated myocardial perfusion SPECT: technical principles and quality control considerations. Journal of Nuclear Cardiology 1998;5(4):418–25.) [3]

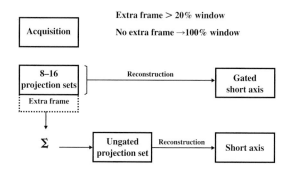

FIGURE 8.4 Setting the cardiac beat length acceptance window.

how many counts were rejected, both globally and on a projection-by-projection basis. In this situation, the gated SPECT data set is essentially reliable if it contains enough counts. If, on the other hand, a wide open acceptance window is used because no extra frame is available, the following options exist: (1) the technologist can monitor the electrocardiogram (ECG) during acquisition, and note the occurrence of abnormalities in the cardiac rhythm—some laboratories recommend the exclusion of gated data acquired from patients with more than one premature ventricular contraction (PVC) per six cardiac beats [3]; (2) software can be developed or obtained that aims at detecting gating errors from

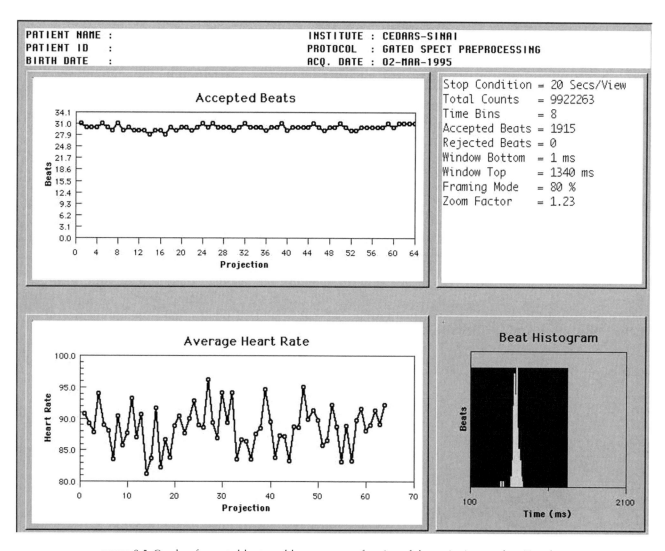

FIGURE 8.5 Graphs of accepted beats and heart rate as a function of the projection number. Together with the cardiac beat length histogram, these tools are useful to assess the reliability of the gated data sets. (Reproduced with permission from Germano G, Berman D. Acquisition and processing for gated perfusion SPECT: technical aspects. In: G Germano and D Berman, eds. Clinical gated cardiac SPECT. Futura Publishing Company, Armonk, NY; 1999:93–113.) [133]

postacquisition analysis of the relative counts and count patterns in the various gated frames [4]; (3) when provided by the camera manufacturer, graphs of accepted counts or heart rate as a function of the projection angle (as well as beat length histograms) can provide immediate evidence of gating abnormalities (Fig. 8.5). The lack of standardized, automatic quality control tools for the determination of the reliability of gated SPECT data is a well-recognized problem [5] that is likely to be targeted by camera manufacturers soon.

QUANTIFICATION OF MYOCARDIAL FUNCTION

Global and regional parameters of function quantified from gated perfusion SPECT images include left ventricular ejection fraction (LVEF), end-diastolic and end-systolic volumes, and left ventricular (LV) myocardial wall motion and thickening. Diastolic function assessment is generally not performed with gated SPECT, as it would require too large a number of gating intervals [6]. Also, right ventricular (RV) quantification is generally not performed with gated SPECT, because (1) the RV myocardium is thinner and takes up less activity compared to the LV, hence it is not always visible; and (2) the geometric shape of the RV is less straightforward to model than that of the LV. Several algorithms have been developed for the quantification of gated SPECT, as shown in Table 8.3. They are based on different principles and mathematical operators, re-

flect different degrees of automation and validation, and are becoming increasingly available on commercial gamma cameras and computer systems. The few studies analyzing cross-algorithm agreement have shown strong linear correlation between measurements of the same parameters by different algorithms [7–10]. However, it has also been suggested that systematic differences between the measurements may exist, preventing the direct merging of differently analyzed data in the context of multicenter trials [11,12].

Left Ventricular Ejection Fraction

Unlike gated planar blood pool approaches, quantitative measurements of LVEF using gated perfusion SPECT are usually volume-based rather than count-based. The goal of most quantitative algorithms is that of estimating the location of the LV endocardium in the two- or three-dimensional space (Fig. 8.6), so that the LV cavity volume can be measured as the territory bound by the endocardium and its valve plane. Having done this for every interval in the cardiac cycle, the time-volume curve allows to identify the end-diastolic (EDV) and end-systolic (ESV) LV cavity volumes (Fig. 8.7), from which the ejection fraction is calculated as

$$\% \text{ LVEF} = (\text{EDV-ESV})/\text{EDV} * 100$$

All English language validation studies of gated perfusion SPECT LVEF published to date are presented

TABLE 8.3 *A Review of Published Quantitative Algorithms for Gated Perfusion SPECT*

	Cedars-Sinai	St. Luke's	Stanford U.	(Various)	(Various)	U. of Chicago
Operation	Automatic	Semi-automatic	Semi-automatic	Semi-automatic	Semi-automatic, automatic	Semi-automatic
Dimensionality	3-D	2-D (biplanar)	3-D	3-D	2-D, 3-D	2-D (summed biplanar)
Method	Gaussian fit [13]	Threshold [42,134]	Moment [48,135]	Gradient [59]	Partial volume [54,136–140]	Image inversion [56]
Validation of LVEF	First-pass, MUGA, 3-D MUGA, 2-D echo, 3-D echo, contrast ventriculography, MRI, EBCT, thermodilution	First-pass, MUGA, 2-D echo, contrast ventriculography, MRI	First-pass, MUGA, 2-D echo	Contrast ventriculography	First-pass, MUGA, 2-D echo, MRI	First-pass, contrast ventriculography
Volumes	MUGA, 3-D MUGA, 2-D echo, 3-D echo, contrast ventriculography, MRI, thermodilution	2-D echo, contrast ventriculography	First-pass, MUGA, contrast ventriculography	Contrast ventriculography, MRI	First-pass, 2-D echo, MRI	

LVEF, left ventricular ejection fraction; MUGA, gated planar blood pool; echo, echocardiography; MRI, magnetic resonance imaging; EBCT, electron beam computed tomography.

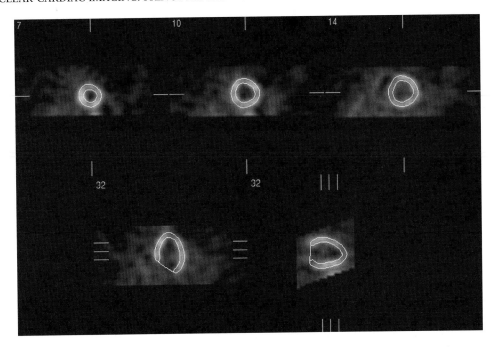

FIGURE 8.6 Reconstructed and reoriented short axis (top row, left to right = apex to base), midventricular horizontal (bottom left), and vertical (bottom right) long-axis images for a gated perfusion SPECT study, at end-diastole, with automatically computed endocardial and epicardial contours overlaid.

in Table 8.4, along with details about the studies [7,12–56]. It is apparent that the agreement between gated SPECT and gold-standard measurements of LVEF is generally very good-to-excellent. Indeed, it has been pointed out that two-dimensional gold-standards may be intrinsically less accurate than gated SPECT algorithms operating in the three-dimensional space, because of geometric assumptions required by the former [13].

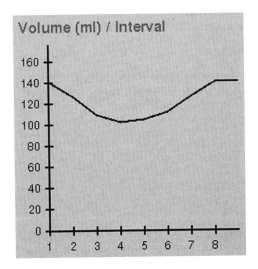

FIGURE 8.7 Time-volume curve for an 8-interval gated perfusion SPECT study.

Volumes

It might be assumed that validating quantitative measurements of LVEF from gated perfusion SPECT images implicitly validates the absolute end-diastolic and end-systolic volume measurements from which the LVEF is derived. This assumption, however, is not necessarily correct. Errors in the determination of end-diastolic and end-systolic volumes would be expected to occur in the same general direction, and therefore would at least partially cancel out when the volumes are ratioed [13]. In essence, one can more accurately measure ratios of volumes, such as LVEF or the transient ischemic dilation (TID) ratio [57], than the absolute volumes themselves. This notwithstanding, a growing body of published evidence appears to suggest that quantitative measurements of absolute LV cavity volumes from gated perfusion SPECT images agree well with established standards, as summarized in Table 8.5 [9,12, 21–26,28,30,33–37,39–41,44,47,49,50,52,54,55,58,59].

Reproducibility and Limitations of Global Function Measurements

The accuracy of LVEF and volumes measurements from gated SPECT images has been validated with respect to a variety of radiopharmaceuticals (Tc-99m-sestamibi, Tc-99m-tetrofosmin, Tl-201) against a large number of

TABLE 8.4 *Validation of Quantitative Measurements of LVEF from Gated Myocardial Perfusion SPECT*

"Gold-Standard"	No. Reports	No. Patients	Spearman's r (LVEF)	Isotope	References
MUGA	15	585	0.7–0.94	99mTc-sestamibi, 99mTc-tetrofosmin, 201-Tl	[7,18–21,29,30,42,48–50,53]
First-pass	12	533	0.82–0.92	99mTc-sestamibi, 201-Tl, I-123 BMIPP	[13–17,42,43,47,54,56]
2-D echo	11	643	0.72–0.90	99mTc-sestamibi, 99mTc-tetrofosmin, 201-Tl	[12,23–28,31,51]
MRI	11	238	0.71–0.94	99mTc-sestamibi, 99mTc-tetrofosmin, 201-Tl	[34–37,39,45,54,55,141]
Contrast ventriculography	8	357	0.26–0.97	99mTc-sestamibi, 99mTc-tetrofosmin, 201-Tl	[22,31,32,44,50,52,56, 142]
3-D echo	1	18	0.80	201-Tl	[33]
3-D MUCA	1	10	0.97	99mTc-tetrofosmin	[22]
Thermodilution	1	21	0.84	99mTc-sestamibi	[40]
EBCT	1	10	0.94	99mTc-sestamibi	[38]
Total	61	2415	0.86		

BMIPP, beta-methyl-iodophenyl-pentedecanoic acid.

gold-standards (MUGA, first-pass, MRI, contrast ventriculography, 2-D echocardiography, 3-D echocardiography, 3-D MUGA, thermodilution, and electron beam computed tomography) [7,13–15,18–20,23–25, 28,31–38,40–49,51–54,56,58]. The reproducibility of these measurements is by definition perfect if the algorithm used to derive them is completely automatic [13], but is generally very good even if some degree of manual operation is required [21,30,42,43,46–48,53,56]. The repeatability (agreement of the quantitative measurements from separate gated SPECT studies of the same patient) is also excellent [26,60–64], making

gated SPECT an ideal technique for serial assessment of patients undergoing medical or surgical therapy.

There are some limitations to quantification of global function from gated SPECT. For example, it has been shown that the relatively low resolution of nuclear cardiology images can lead to the apparent underestimation of the LV cavity size in patients with small ventricles, the end result being an underestimation of cavity volumes (particularly the ES volume), with consequent overestimation of the LVEF [65]. This phenomenon can be alleviated by magnifying the LV either in acquisition (by employing a larger acquisition zoom) and/or

TABLE 8.5 *Validation of Quantitative Measurements of Volumes from Gated Myocardial Perfusion SPECT*

"Gold-Standard"	No. Reports	No. Patients	Spearman's r (EDV)	Spearman's r (ESV)	Isotope	References
2-D echo	11	564	0.70–0.92	0.71–0.94	99mTc-sestamibi, 201-Tl	[9,12,23–26,28]
MRI	9	185	0.81–0.97	0.90–0.99	99mTc-sestamibi, 99mTc-tetrofosmin, 201-Tl	[34–37,39,54,55]
MUGA	4	123	0.7–0.88	0.7–0.95	99mTc-sestamibi, 99mTc-tetrofosmin, 201-Tl	[21,30,49]
Contrast ventriculography	3	117	0.86–0.89	0.90–0.95	99mTc-sestamibi, 201-Tl	[44,50,52]
3-D echo	2	26	0.94–0.99	0.97–0.99	99mTc-sestamibi, 201-Tl	[33,58]
First-pass	2	99	0.85–0.93	0.91–0.92	99mTc-sestamibi	[47,54]
Thermodilution	2	45	0.86–0.89	0.94	99mTc-sestamibi	[40,41]
Total	33	1159	0.87	0.90		

in reconstruction (by employing zoomed centered or zoomed off-axis reconstruction) [66–69], or by applying numerical modeling and compensation of blurring [70,71]. Conversely, gated SPECT imaging is usually performed with 8-frame gating, which leads to mild underestimation of the LVEF (due to the smoothing of the time-volume curve) compared to 16-frame gating. However, the degree of underestimation has been shown to be small (3–4 LVEF percentage points) and remarkably uniform over a wide range of ejection fractions [13,29,72–74]. Finally, it is remarkable that several published reports exist that deny the presence of major discrepancies between true and quantitatively measured LVEF in patients with large perfusion defects and/or low LVEF [7,34,44,45,51,74–77]. While most quantitative algorithms tend to cut off aneurysms by assuming a regular or smooth LV shape in areas with severely reduced or absent perfusion, the consequent error in measured LVEF is generally mild.

Regional Function Measurements

Quantification and validation of regional myocardial function measurements from gated perfusion SPECT are more challenging, compared to global function. To begin with, there is no agreement as to whether one should concentrate on myocardial wall motion or thickening: the former has traditionally been evaluated by nuclear cardiologists in conjunction with blood pool studies (and is found by many as being easier to score), while the latter is uniquely suited to turn the relatively low resolution of gated tomographic cardiac perfusion images into an advantage. Many think the two measurements are essentially equivalent, because, in order to thicken, the myocardium must necessarily move (and vice versa). This is mostly true, but there are exceptions. For instance, small infarcted portions of the myocardium can be "tethered" by surrounding healthy cardiac muscle, thus appearing as having normal motion but absent thickening. On the other hand, it is well known that typically postcardiac surgery patients have septal dyskinesis in the presence of normal septal thickening [78,79]. The authors believe that it is important to evaluate both regional motion and thickening, whether the assessment is done visually or quantitatively.

Special technical difficulties associated with the measurement of regional function from gated perfusion SPECT are related to the rotation and translation of the heart, as well as to the choice of an appropriate reference system. The very nature of cardiac motion causes areas of the myocardium to move between image slices from diastole to systole, thus requiring accurate evaluation of regional function to be performed in three-dimensional space. Even three-dimensional quantitative algorithms like those described in this chapter, how-

ever, do not account for the rotation of the heart during systole [80]. Methods for the correction of myocardial rotation have been proposed for other modalities [81], but we consider similar developments for nuclear cardiology to be problematic, because of the insufficient resolution of the gated SPECT image set. Incidentally, it has been demonstrated that correction for myocardial rotation has very little effect in the assessment of the basal two-thirds of the left ventricle [82,83], and its clinical relevance in assessing the distal one-third of the left ventricle is uncertain [83]. The authors believe that the adoption of the three-dimensional, coordinateless "centerline" approach utilized by our and other algorithms previously described [84–86] avoids the inaccuracies deriving from the use of a fixed or floating reference system [83], albeit without specifically addressing cardiac rotation and translation.

Overall, reports of validation of quantitative measurements of regional function from gated perfusion SPECT images are few and heterogeneous, differing greatly as to number of myocardial segments assessed and gold-standard and validation criteria [46,59,86–88]. Validations of semiquantitative assessments are also not numerous [36,37,45,88–90]. Of interest, semiquantitative categorization of myocardial wall motion and thickening can now be performed automatically and has been validated against analogous semiquantitative visual assessment [91]. Ideally, one would first want to ensure that the quantitative measurements of regional wall motion and thickening from gated perfusion SPECT are accurate, as quantitatively confirmed by a three-dimensional anatomic technique with excellent resolution. Then, these accurate numerical determinations should be translated into an assessment of function abnormality, which would include the development of normal limits [92–96] and criteria for abnormality [91].

CORONARY ARTERY DISEASE DIAGNOSIS AND GATED PERFUSION SPECT

With respect to the diagnosis of coronary artery disease, the principal contribution of gating to myocardial perfusion SPECT is to increase specificity by allowing the more effective detection of attenuation artifacts. In general, if apparent nonreversible defects that may be artifactual demonstrate normal contraction by gated SPECT, they are considered attenuation artifacts. Taillefer and associates [97] evaluated the specificity of thallium-201 (Tl-201) SPECT and technetium (Tc-99m)-sestamibi SPECT with gating for detection of 50% or 70% coronary artery stenoses in women. With either definition of significant stenosis, the addition of gated SPECT significantly improved the specificity of myocardial perfusion imaging in this population. This improvement in specificity was associated with a slight but not significant fall in sensitivity. Smanio et al. from the University of Virginia also demonstrated the added value of gated SPECT in diagnosis. These investigators interpreted myocardial perfusion SPECT studies using perfusion data alone and then by combining the gated study and the perfusion information. The investigators found a significant reduction in equivocal interpretation categories in the final interpretation, when consideration of the gated data was utilized in addition to perfusion information [98]. The limitation of this application is that regions with subendocardial infarction and recanalized infarct-related arteries may contract normally or near normally and demonstrate only nonreversible defects. Clinical correlations are particularly useful in arriving at the correct diagnosis in this setting.

Another application of gated myocardial perfusion SPECT in diagnosis is the use of the technique to identify patients with dilated, poorly contracting left ventricles in whom the diagnosis of an occult nonischemic cardiomyopathy can be made. Since more accurate detection of severe coronary disease has importance in risk stratification, this improved identification of the patient with severe coronary artery disease is likely to be beneficial. In a preliminary evaluation, Hachamovitch et al., evaluating data from Cedars-Sinai Medical Center, documented that the measurement of the poststress ejection fraction provides incremental prognostic value for the prediction of heart events over the prognostically important perfusion measurement of the summed stress score [99].

RISK STRATIFICATION AND GATED PERFUSION SPECT

With respect to risk stratification, there are several ways in which the assessment of ventricular function complements the assessment of myocardial perfusion. Johnson et al. [60] demonstrated that patients with coronary artery disease commonly had a significantly lower left ventricular ejection fraction on poststress gated SPECT imaging than at rest. This finding is most likely secondary to postexercise stunning, and is likely to be a marker of severe coronary artery disease. Sharir et al. from our group have presented preliminary data documenting that poststress wall motion abnormalities in areas with normal perfusion are a sensitive and specific marker for the presence of severe coronary artery disease (> 90% stenosis) [100]. We found that the assessment of regional function from gated SPECT provides added information to perfusion defect assessment in the detection of severe coronary artery disease. Since the extent of severe coro-

nary artery disease is likely to have prognostic information, this assessment of poststress wall motion abnormality may be of value in risk assessment. Similarly, Mazzanti et al. [57] demonstrated that the finding of transient ischemic dilation of the left ventricle, automatically measured using the gated SPECT software on the nongated data, provides an accurate marker of severe and extensive coronary artery disease (proximal LAD or multiple vessels with ≥ 90% stenosis), which also is complementary to the information provided by myocardial perfusion SPECT.

The potent information contained in the ejection fraction assessed from gated SPECT is likely to enhance the prognostic content of myocardial perfusion SPECT. Since gated SPECT has become routine only recently, there are few reports of its incremental value over perfusion in assessing prognosis. Evidence that gated SPECT is likely to add to prognostic assessment is provided by prior ejection fraction data. Left ventricular ejection fraction has been shown to risk-stratify suspected disease patients according to their risk of subsequent cardiac death. In a series of reports from the Duke databank using rest and exercise first-pass radionuclide angiography, suspected disease patients could be risk-stratified using a diagnostic threshold of 50% ejection fraction [101–106].

In a preliminary communication, Hachamovitch et al. demonstrated that after risk adjustment for pretest likelihood of coronary artery disease and results of perfusion SPECT, LVEF provides significant incremental value in prediction of cardiac death or nonfatal myocardial infarction in patients with known or suspected chronic coronary artery disease [99]. In the first manuscript on this subject, Sharir et al., studying 1680 patients, demonstrated that poststress LVEF, as measured by gated SPECT, provides significant information over the extent and severity of perfusion defect as measured by the summed stress score [107]. Furthermore, these authors demonstrated that LV end-systolic volume provides added information over poststress LVEF in prediction of cardiac death. The relatively low cardiac death rate in patients with abnormal perfusion and normal left ventricular function in this study is probably explained by a referral bias in which patients with greatest ischemia by summed stress score (SSS) were preferentially sent for early revascularization and thus censored from assessment of the prognostic value of the test. In a subsequent preliminary report of 2600 patients, Sharir et al. have shown that while poststress EF provides incremental information over prescan and perfusion variables in prediction of cardiac death, the perfusion variables are stronger predictors of nonfatal myocardial infarction. Once prescan and perfusion variables were known, poststress EF did not provide incremental information with respect to the risk of non-fatal myocardial infarction [108].

In the future, complex algorithms will need to be developed that incorporate all of the information from gated SPECT for purposes of guiding patient management. In this regard, it is likely that poststress EF (related predominately to the size of myocardial infarction) and summed difference score (an expression of the amount of stress-induced ischemia) will provide the greatest complementary information. As an initial approach, Sharir et al. [108] have reported the combination of the ejection fraction and reversible ischemia in the prediction of cardiac events. If poststress ejection fraction is less than 30%, cardiac death or nonfatal myocardial infarction rates appear to be high regardless of the amount of ischemia as assessed by the summed difference score. In patients with poststress LVEF of 30% to 50%, mild amounts of ischemia were associated with relatively high cardiac event rates. In patients with ejection fractions of greater than 50%, only patients with moderately extensive ischemia were at high risk of cardiac events. Still to be defined is a simple way to facilitate integration of poststress end-systolic volume with the information regarding ejection fraction and reversible ischemia.

Finally, supporting the above-noted work by Johnson indicating the common occurrence of postexercise stunning, O'Keefe and associates have demonstrated that there may be additional information derived by measuring both rest and poststress ejection fractions [109]. These investigators demonstrated that a poststress drop in ejection fraction on gated SPECT Tl-201 scintigraphy (fall $\geq$ 8 LVEF points) occurred in approximately 25% of patients and was associated with other findings consistent with severe and extensive coronary artery disease, including a multivessel ischemic pattern, transient ischemia dilation of the left ventricle, and a higher mortality rate than those patients in whom there was no fall in left ventricular ejection fraction. Dakik et al. have demonstrated incremental prognostic value of ventricular ejection fraction when combined with exercise and Tl-201 SPECT after myocardial infarction, and Mahmarian et al. from the same group have demonstrated incremental information of ejection fraction over adenosine Tl-201 SPECT for assessment of prognosis following acute myocardial infarction [110]. With gated SPECT, these measurements can be made during one examination.

GATED BLOOD POOL SPECT

Gating of nuclear cardiology studies had originally been applied to planar blood pool imaging using Tc-99m-albumin [111] and Tc-99m labeled red blood cells [112],

and was successfully extended to blood pool SPECT following the gain in popularity of perfusion SPECT over perfusion planar imaging [113–115]. The main potential advantage of the SPECT approach is that the separation of left ventricle (LV) and right ventricle (RV) conceptually allows gated blood pool SPECT to measure right ventricular function parameters. Moreover, the absence of overlap of different cardiac chambers with gated blood pool SPECT translates in the elimination of the need for background subtraction, a requirement of gated blood pool planar imaging. Finally, due to the larger dimension of the left ventricular blood pool compared to the myocardial thickness, partial volume effects [116] would be expected to be less of a problem, and measurements of volume (especially end-diastolic) could be potentially more accurate with gated blood pool SPECT than with gated perfusion SPECT.

Most of the technical issues examined in this chapter with respect to gated perfusion SPECT imaging also apply to gated blood pool SPECT imaging. In particular, a gated blood pool SPECT acquisition is usually accomplished with 8-frame or 16-frame temporal resolution. Acquisition follows an injection of Tc-99m labeled red blood cells in dosages similar to those described in Table 8.1 for gated Tc-99m-based perfusion imaging. Acquisition is generally performed with the patient in the resting state, although acquisitions after nitroglycerin [117] or during low-dose dobutamine, to assess myocardial contractile reserve, are clearly feasible. It should be noted that, although the injected dose and the specific patient's attenuation characteristics may be the same in perfusion and blood pool imaging, the number of cardiac counts collected per millicurie of injected radioactivity is higher for the latter, because a lesser amount of activity is taken up by the myocardium in perfusion studies than is present in the blood pool with blood pool radiopharmaceuticals. In contrast with gated perfusion SPECT, in blood pool imaging no perfusion information is acquired, and therefore it is advisable to always set the cardiac beat length acceptance window to 20%–30% in order to minimize the effects of arrhythmia. With the use of 10%–20% acceptance windows and 16-frame studies, assessment of diastolic function could be both feasible and accurate.

The three-dimensional nature of the gated blood pool SPECT data lends itself naturally to space-based rather than count-based analysis. Several quantitative algorithms have been recently introduced that aim at identifying the endocardial surfaces of the LV and (in a minority of cases) of the RV throughout the cardiac cycle (Fig. 8.8), so as to determine ventricular volumes and ejection fractions in a manner similar to gated perfusion SPECT. While reported validations of these algorithms' measurements are generally satisfactory

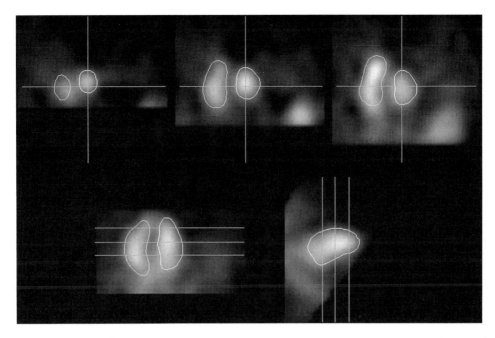

FIGURE 8.8 Short- and long-axis slices with automatically determined and overlayed contours for the LV and RV endocardium. (Reproduced with permission from Germano G, Berman D. Acquisition and processing for gated perfusion SPECT: technical aspects. In: G Germano and D Berman, eds. Clinical gated cardiac SPECT. Futura Publishing Company, Armonk, NY; 1999:93–113.) [133]

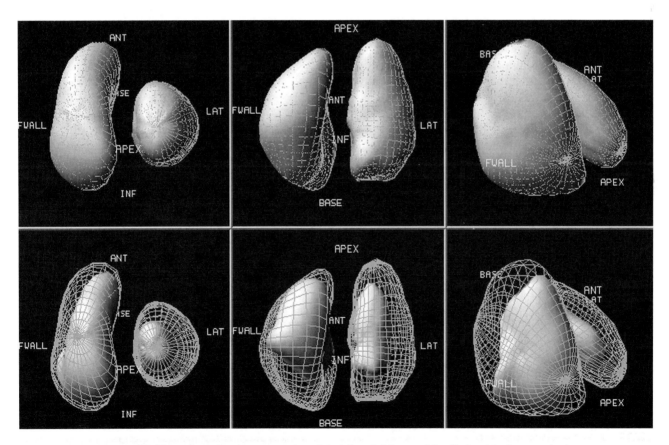

FIGURE 8.9 Three-dimensional representation of the left and right ventricles displayed in three standard orientations at end-diastole (top row) and end-systole (bottom row). (Reproduced with permission from Germano G, Berman D. Acquisition and processing for gated perfusion SPECT: technical aspects. In: G Germano and D Berman, eds. Clinical gated cardiac SPECT. Futura Publishing Company, Armonk, NY; 1999:93–113.) [133]

131

[59,118–132], the gold-standards used are almost invariably planar, and right ventricular parameters are rarely validated. Still, the increase in computer speed, the greater diffusion of multidetector cameras, and the general acceptance of state-of-the-art three-dimensional analysis and display techniques (Fig. 8.9) have already considerably strengthened the case for gated blood pool SPECT imaging.

Because of the ease of SPECT acquisition and processing, and given the growing widespread use of gated SPECT in myocardial perfusion scintigraphy, we believe that gated blood pool SPECT will become the most commonly utilized nuclear cardiology method for blood pool scintigraphy. The clinical circumstances in which this procedure is likely to become effective are the same as those in which resting blood pool scintigraphy is currently applied. Chief among these is the assessment of adriamycin cardiotoxicity. Blood pool scintigraphy is also commonly employed in serial assessment of patients with aortic insufficiency, congestive heart failure, and patients who have undergone cardiac transplantation.

REFERENCES

1. Germano G, Erel J, Kiat H, et al. Quantitative LVEF and qualitative regional function from gated thallium-201 perfusion SPECT. J Nucl Med 1997;38:749.

2. Maunoury C, Chen CC, Chua KB, et al. Quantification of left ventricular function with thallium-201 and technetium-99m-sestamibi myocardial gated SPECT. J Nucl Med 1997;38:958.

3. Cullom SJ, Case JA, Bateman TM. Electrocardiographically gated myocardial perfusion SPECT: technical principles and quality control considerations. J Nucl Cardiol 1998;5:418.

4. Nichols K, DePuey E, Dorbala S, et al. Prevalence of gating errors in myocardial perfusion SPECT data. J Nucl Med 1998 (abstract);39:45P.

5. Nichols K, DePuey E, Yoon J, et al. Relative influence of gating errors on myocardial perfusion and function computed by QGS software. J Nucl Med 1999 (abstract);40:157P.

6. Germano G, Van Train K, Kiat H, et al. Digital techniques for the acquisition, processing, and analysis of nuclear cardiology images. In: *Diagnostic Nuclear Medicine*, edited by MP Sandler. Baltimore: Williams & Wilkins, 1995, pp. 347.

7. Everaert H, Bossuyt A, Franken PR. Left ventricular ejection fraction and volumes from gated single photon emission tomographic myocardial perfusion images: comparison between two algorithms working in three-dimensional space. J Nucl Cardiol 1997;4:472.

8. Vera P, Koning R, Cribier A, et al. Comparison of two three-dimensional gated SPECT methods with thallium in patients with large myocardial infarction. J Nucl Cardiol 2000;7:312.

9. Nichols K, Lefkovitz D, Faber T, et al. Ventricular volumes compared among three gated SPECT methods and echocardiography. J Am Coll Cardiol 1999 (abstract);33(2(Suppl.A)):409A.

10. Sias T, Calnon D, Beller G, et al. Comparison of two algorithms for calculation of left ventricular ejection fraction using gated single photon emission tomography (SPECT) myocardial perfusion images. J Am Coll Cardiol 1999 (abstract);33(2(Suppl.A)):436A.

11. Nichols K, Folks R, Cooke D, et al. Comparisons between "ECTb" and "QGS" software to compute left ventricular function from myocardial perfusion gated SPECT data. J Nucl Cardiol 2000 (abstract);7:S20.

12. Nichols K, Lefkowitz D, Faber T, et al. Echocardiographic validation of gated SPECT ventricular function measurements. J Nucl Med 2000;41:1308.

13. Germano G, Kiat H, Kavanagh PB, et al. Automatic quantification of ejection fraction from gated myocardial perfusion SPECT. J Nucl Med 1995;36:2138.

14. He Z, Mahmarian J, Preslar J, et al. Correlations of left ventricular ejection fractions determined by gated SPECT with thallium and sestamibi and by first-pass radionuclide angiography. J Nucl Med 1997 (abstract);38:27P.

15. Inubushi M, Tadamura E, Kudoh T, et al. Simultaneous assessment of myocardial fatty acid utilization and LV function using I-123 BMIPP gated SPECT (GSPECT). J Nucl Cardiol 1999 (abstract);6(1(Part 2)):S66.

16. Inubushi M, Tadamura E, Kudoh T, et al. Simultaneous assessment of myocardial free fatty acid utilization and left ventricular function using 123I-BMIPP-gated SPECT. Journal of Nuclear Medicine 1999;40:1840.

17. He ZX, Cwajg E, Preslar JS, et al. Accuracy of left ventricular ejection fraction determined by gated myocardial perfusion SPECT with Tl-201 and Tc-99m sestamibi: comparison with first-pass radionuclide angiography. J Nucl Cardiol 1999;6:412.

18. Moriel M, Germano G, Kiat H, et al. Automatic measurement of left ventricular ejection fraction by gated SPECT Tc-99m sestamibi: a comparison with radionuclide ventriculography. Circulation 1993 (abstract);88:I-486.

19. Bateman T, Case J, Saunders M, et al. Gated SPECT LVEF measurements using a dual-detector camera and a weight-adjusted dosage of thallium-201. J Am Coll Cardiol 1997 (abstract);29(2(Suppl.A)):263A.

20. Carpentier P, Benticha H, Gautier P, et al. Thallium 201 gated SPECT for simultaneous assessment of myocardial perfusion, left ventricular ejection fraction and qualitative regional function. J Nucl Cardiol 1999 (abstract);6(1(Part 2)):S39.

21. Yoshioka J, Hasegawa S, Yamaguchi H, et al. Left ventricular volumes and ejection fraction calculated from quantitative electrocardiographic-gated Tc-99m-tetrofosmin myocardial SPECT. J Nucl Med 1999;40:1693.

22. Paul A, Hasegawa S, Yoshioka J, et al. Left ventricular volume and ejection fraction from quantitative gated SPECT: comparison with gated pool SPECT and contrast ventriculography. J Nucl Med 1999 (abstract);40:178P.

23. Zanger D, Bhatnagar A, Hausner E, et al. Automated calculation of ejection fraction from gated Tc-99m sestamibi images—comparison to quantitative echocardiography. J Nucl Cardiol 1997 (abstract);4(1, Part 2):S78.

24. Bateman T, Magalski A, Barnhart C, et al. Global left ventricular function assessment using gated SPECT-201: comparison with echocardiography. J Am Coll Cardiol 1998 (abstract);31(2(Suppl.A)):441A.

25. Cwajg E, Cwajg J, He Z, et al. Comparison between gated-SPECT and echocardiography for the analysis of global and regional left ventricular function and volumes. J Am Coll Cardiol 1998 (abstract);31(2(Suppl.A)):440A.

26. Cwajg E, Cwajg J, He ZX, et al. Gated myocardial perfusion tomography for the assessment of left ventricular function and volumes: comparison with echocardiography. Journal of Nuclear Medicine 1999;40:1857.

27. Bacher-Stier C, Müller S, Pachinger O, et al. Thallium-201 gated single-photon emission tomography for the assessment of left ventricular ejection fraction and regional wall motion abnormalities in comparison with two-dimensional echocardiography. Eur J Nucl Med 1999;26:1533.

28. Mathew D, Zabrodina Y, Mannting F. Volumetric and functional analysis of left ventricle by gated SPECT: a comparison with echocardiographic measurements. J Am Coll Cardiol 1998 (abstract);31(2(Suppl.A)):44A.

29. Manrique A, Koning R, Cribier A, et al. Effect of temporal sampling on evaluation of left ventricular ejection fraction by means of thallium-201 gated SPET: comparison of 16- and 8-interval gating, with reference to equilibrium radionuclide angiography. Eur J Nucl Med 2000;27:694.

30. Chua T, Yin L, Thiang T, et al. Accuracy of the automated assessment of left ventricular function with gated perfusion SPECT in the presence of perfusion defects and left ventricular dysfunction: correlation with equilibrium radionuclide ventriculography and echocardiography. J Nucl Cardiol 2000;7:301.

31. Di Leo C, Bestetti A, Tagliabue L, et al. Tc-99m-tetrofosmin gated-SPECT LVEF: correlation with echocardiography and contrastographic ventriculography. J Nucl Cardiol 1997 (abstract);4(1, Part 2):S56.

32. Atsma D, Croon C, Dibbets-Schneider P, et al. Good correlation between left ventricular ejection fraction and wall motion score assessed by gated SPECT as compared to left ventricular angiography. J Am Coll Cardiol 1999 (abstract);33(2(Suppl.A)):409A.

33. Akinboboye O, El-Khoury Coffin L, Sciacca R, et al. Accuracy of gated SPECT thallium left ventricular volumes and ejection fractions: comparison with three-dimensional echocardiography. J Am Coll Cardiol 1998 (abstract);31(2(Suppl.A)):85A.

34. He Z, Vick G, Vaduganathan P, et al. Comparison of left ventricular volumes and ejection fraction measured by gated SPECT and by cine magnetic resonance imaging. J Am Coll Cardiol 1998 (abstract);31(2(Suppl.A)):44A.

35. Atsma D, Kayser H, Croon C, et al. Good correlation between left ventricular ejection fraction, endsystolic and enddiastolic volume measured by gated SPECT as compared to magnetic resonance imaging. J Am Coll Cardiol 1999 (abstract);33(2(Suppl.A)):436A.

36. Vaduganathan P, He ZX, Vick GW 3rd, et al. Evaluation of left ventricular wall motion, volumes, and ejection fraction by gated myocardial tomography with technetium 99m-labeled tetrofosmin: a comparison with cine magnetic resonance imaging. J Nucl Cardiol 1999;6:3.

37. Tadamura E, Kudoh T, Motooka M, et al. Assessment of regional and global left ventricular function by reinjection T1-201 and rest Tc-99m sestamibi ECG-gated SPECT: comparison with three-dimensional magnetic resonance imaging. J Am Coll Cardiol 1999;33:991.

38. Toba M, Ishida Y, Fukuchi K, et al. Application of ECG-gated Tc-99m sestamibi cardiac imaging to patients with arrhythmogenic right ventricular dysplasia (ARVD). J Nucl Cardiol 1999 (abstract);6(1(Part 2)):S41.

39. Tadamura E, Kudoh T, Motooka M, et al. Use of technetium-99m sestamibi ECG-gated single-photon emission tomography for the evaluation of left ventricular function following coronary artery bypass graft: comparison with three-dimensional magnetic resonance imaging. Eur J Nucl Med 1999;26:705.

40. Germano G, VanDecker W, Mintz R, et al. Validation of left ventricular volumes automatically measured with gated myocardial perfusion SPECT. J Am Coll Cardiol 1998 (abstract);31(2(Suppl.A)):43A.

41. Iskandrian AE, Germano G, VanDecker W, et al. Validation of left ventricular volume measurements by gated SPECT Tc-99m-labeled sestamibi imaging. J Nucl Cardiol 1998;5:574.

42. Nichols K, DePuey EG, Rozanski A. Automation of gated tomographic left ventricular ejection fraction. J Nucl Cardiol 1996;3(6 Pt 1):475.

43. Nichols K, DePuey EG, Rozanski A, et al. Image enhancement of severely hypoperfused myocardia for computation of tomographic ejection fraction. J Nucl Med 1997;38:1411.

44. Nichols K, Tamis J, DePuey EG, et al. Relationship of gated SPECT ventricular function parameters to angiographic measurements. J Nucl Cardiol 1998;5:295.

45. Stollfuss JC, Haas F, Matsunari I, et al. Regional myocardial wall thickening and global ejection fraction in patients with low angiographic left ventricular ejection fraction assessed by visual and quantitative resting ECG-gated Tc-99m-tetrofosmin single-photon emission tomography and magnetic resonance imaging. Eur J Nucl Med 1998;25:522.

46. Yang KT, Chen HD. Evaluation of global and regional left ventricular function using technetium-99m sestamibi ECG-gated single-photon emission tomography. Eur J Nucl Med 1998;25:515.

47. Schwartz R, Thompson C, Mixon L, et al. Gated SPECT analysis with 3-D wall parametrization method: accurate and reproducible evaluation of left ventricular volumes and ejection fraction. Circulation 1995 (abstract);92:I-449.

48. Everaert H, Franken PR, Flamen P, et al. Left ventricular ejection fraction from gated SPECT myocardial perfusion studies: a method based on the radial distribution of count rate density across the myocardial wall. Eur J Nucl Med 1996;23:1628.

49. Daou D, Helal B, Colin P, et al. Are LV ejection fraction (EF), end diastolic (EDV) and end systolic volumes (ESV) measured with rest Tl-201 gated SPECT accurate? J Nucl Cardiol 1999 (abstract);6(1(Part 2)):S31.

50. Vera P, Manrique A, Pontvianne V, et al. Thallium-gated SPECT in patients with major myocardial infarction: effect of filtering and zooming in comparison with equilibrium radionuclide imaging and left ventriculography. J Nucl Med 1999;40:513.

51. Schwartz R, Eckdahl J, Thompson C. 3-D wall parametrization method for quantitative LVEF of gated SPECT sestamibi with LV dysfunction and severe perfusion defects. J Nucl Cardiol 1995 (abstract);2:S114.

52. Adiseshan P, Corbett J. Quantification of left ventricular function from gated tomographic perfusion imaging: development and testing of a new algorithm. Circulation 1994 (abstract);90:I-365.

53. Calnon DA, Kastner RJ, Smith WH, et al. Validation of a new counts-based gated single photon emission computed tomography method for quantifying left ventricular systolic function: comparison with equilibrium radionuclide angiography. J Nucl Cardiol 1997;4:464.

54. Faber TL, Cooke CD, Folks RD, et al. Left ventricular function and perfusion from gated SPECT perfusion images: an integrated method. J Nucl Med 1999;40:650.

55. Vansant J, Pettigrew R, Faber T, et al. Comparison and accuracy of two gated-SPECT techniques for assessing left ventricular function defined by cardiac MRI. J Nucl Med 1999 (abstract);40:166P.

56. Williams KA, Taillon LA. Left ventricular function in patients with coronary artery disease assessed by gated tomographic myocardial perfusion images. Comparison with assessment by contrast ventriculography and first-pass radionuclide angiography. J Am Coll Cardiol 1996;27:173.

57. Mazzanti M, Germano G, Kiat H, et al. Identification of severe and extensive coronary artery disease by automatic measurement of transient ischemic dilation of the left ventricle in dual-isotope myocardial perfusion SPECT. J Am Coll Cardiol 1996;27:1612.

58. Cittanti C, Mele D, Colamussi P, et al. Determination of left ventricular volume and ejection fraction by g-SPECT myocardial perfusion scintigraphy. A comparison with quantitative 3-D echocardiography. J Nucl Cardiol 1999 (abstract);6(1(Part 2)):S34.

59. Faber TL, Stokely EM, Peshock RM, et al. A model-based four-dimensional left ventricular surface detector. IEEE Trans Med Imaging 1991;10:321.

60. Johnson LL, Verdesca SA, Aude WY, et al. Postischemic stunning can affect left ventricular ejection fraction and regional wall motion on post-stress gated sestamibi tomograms [see comments]. J Am Coll Cardiol 1997;30:1641.

61. Berman D, Germano G, Lewin H, et al. Comparison of post-stress ejection fraction and relative left ventricular volumes by automatic analysis of gated myocardial perfusion single-photon emission computed tomography acquired in the supine and prone positions. J Nucl Cardiol 1998;5:40.

62. Germano G, Kavanagh PB, Kavanagh JT, et al. Repeatability of automatic left ventricular cavity volume measurements from myocardial perfusion SPECT. J Nucl Cardiol 1998;5:477.

63. Hyun I, Kwan J, Park K, et al. Reproducibility of gated perfusion SPECT for the assessment of myocardial function: comparison with 201Tl and Tc-99m-MIBI. J Nucl Med 2000 (abstract);41:125P.

64. Everaert H, Vanhove C, Franken PR. Gated SPECT myocardial perfusion acquisition within 5 minutes using focussing collimators and a three-head gamma camera. Eur J Nucl Med 1998;25:587.

65. Case J, Cullom S, Bateman T, et al. Overestimation of LVEF by gated MIBI myocardial perfusion SPECT in patients with small hearts. J Am Coll Cardiol 1998 (abstract);31(2(Suppl.A)):43A.

66. Schwartz R, Mixon L, Germano G, et al. Gated SPECT reconstruction with zoom and depth dependent filter improves accuracy of volume and LVEF in small hearts. J Nucl Cardiol 1999 (abstract);6(1, Part 2):S17.

67. Ezuddin S, Sfakianakis G, Pay L, et al. Comparative study to determine the effect of different zoom factors on the calculation of LVEF from gated myocardial perfusion SPECT with Tl-201 and Tc-99m-sestamibi in patients with small hearts. J Nucl Med 1999 (abstract);40:169P.

68. Nakajima K, Taki J, Higuchi T, et al. Factors affecting volume measurement of small heart by gated SPECT. J Nucl Med 2000 (abstract);41:99P.

69. Nakajima K, Taki J, Higuchi T, et al. Gated SPECT quantification of small hearts: mathematical simulation and clinical application. Eur J Nucl Med 2000;27:1372.

70. Case J, Bateman T, Cullom S, et al. Improved accuracy of SPECT LVEF using numerical modeling of ventricular image blurring for patients with small hearts. J Am Coll Cardiol 1999 (abstract);33(2(Suppl.A)):436A.

71. Faber T, Cooke C, Folks R, et al. Correction of artifactually high EF from gated perfusion SPECT in small ventricles. J Nucl Cardiol 2000 (abstract);7:S20.

72. Imai K, Azuma Y, Nakajima S, et al. Frames a cardiac cycle in quantitative gated SPECT (QGS) for clinical use: 8 versus 16. J Nucl Cardiol 1999 (abstract);6(1(Part 2)):S17.

73. Cohade C, Taillefer R, Gagnon A, et al. Effect of the number of frames per cardiac cycle and the amount of injected dose of radionuclide on the determination of left ventricular ejection fraction (LVEF) with gated SPECT myocardial perfusion imaging (GS). J Nucl Med 2000 (abstract);41:154P.

74. Manrique A, Vera P, Hitzel A, et al. 16-interval gating improves thallium-201 gated SPECT LVEF measurement in patients with large myocardial infarction. J Am Coll Cardiol 1999 (abstract);33(2(Suppl.A)):436A.

75. Al-Khori F, McNelis P, Van Decker W. Reliability of gated SPECT in assessing left ventricular ejection fraction in ventricles with scarred myocardium. J Nucl Cardiol 1999 (abstract); 6(1(Part 2)):S26.

76. Giubbini R, Terzi A, Rossini P, et al. Gated myocardial perfusion single photon emission tomography (GSPECT) in the evaluation of left ventricular ejection fraction in CAD patients with previous myocardial infarction. J Nucl Cardiol 1999 (abstract);6(1(Part 2)):S58.

77. Bax J, Lamb H, Dibbets P, et al. Comparison between LV volumes and LVEF assessed by MRI and gated SPECT in patients with severe ischemic LV dysfunction. J Nucl Med 1999 (abstract); 40:45P.

78. De Nardo D, Caretta Q, Mercanti C, et al. Effects of uncomplicated coronary artery bypass graft surgery on global and regional left ventricular function at rest. Study by equilibrium radionuclide angiocardiography. Cardiology 1989;76:285.

79. Canclini S, Rossini P, Terzi A, et al. Gated SPECT (GSPECT) evaluation of septal wall motion after cardiac surgery. J Nucl Med 2000 (abstract);41:125P.

80. Nichols K, Cooke C, Faber T, et al. Detection of cardiac torque from gated myocardial perfusion tomograms. J Nucl Med 2000 (abstract);41:45P.

81. Perman WH, Creswell LL, Wyers SG, et al. Hybrid DANTE and phase-contrast imaging technique for measurement of three-dimensional myocardial wall motion. J Magn Reson Imaging 1995;5(1):101.

82. Mirro MJ, Rogers EW, Weyman AE, et al. Angular displacement of the papillary muscles during the cardiac cycle. Circulation 1979;60:327.

83. Katz A, Force T, Folland E, et al. Echocardiographic assessment of ventricular systolic function. In: *Marcus Cardiac Imaging: A Companion to Braunwald's Heart Disease*, edited by ML Marcus and E Braunwald. Philadelphia: W.B. Saunders, 1996, pp. 297.

84. Sheehan FH, Dodge HT, Mathey D, et al. Application of the centerline method: analysis of change in regional left ventricular wall motion in serial studies. Computers in Cardiology. Ninth Meeting of Computers in Cardiology 1983;97.

85. Faber TL, Akers MS, Peshock RM, et al. Three-dimensional motion and perfusion quantification in gated single-photon emission computed tomograms. J Nucl Med 1991;32:2311.

86. Germano G, Erel J, Lewin H, et al. Automatic quantitation of regional myocardial wall motion and thickening from gated technetium-99m sestamibi myocardial perfusion single-photon emission computed tomography. J Am Coll Cardiol 1997;30:1360.

87. Fukuchi K, Uehara T, Morozumi T, et al. Quantification of systolic count increase in technetium-99m-MIBI gated myocardial SPECT. J Nucl Med 1997;38:1067.

88. Nichols K, DePuey EG, Krasnow N, et al. Reliability of enhanced gated SPECT in assessing wall motion of severely hypoperfused myocardium: echocardiographic validation. J Nucl Cardiol 1998;5:387.

89. Chua T, Kiat H, Germano G, et al. Gated technetium-99m sestamibi for simultaneous assessment of stress myocardial perfusion, postexercise regional ventricular function and myo-

cardial viability. Correlation with echocardiography and rest thallium-201 scintigraphy. J Am Coll Cardiol 1994;23:1107.

90. Gunning MG, Anagnostopoulos C, Davies G, et al. Gated technetium-99m-tetrofosmin SPECT and cine MRI to assess left ventricular contraction. J Nucl Med 1997;38:438.

91. Sharir T, Lewin H, Germano G, et al. Automatic quantitation of wall motion and thickening by gated SPECT: validation and application in identifying severe coronary artery disease. J Am Coll Cardiol 1999 (abstract);33(2(Suppl.A)):418A.

92. Cooke C, Garcia E, Folks R, et al. Myocardial thickening and phase analysis from Tc-99m sestamibi multiple gated SPECT: development of normal limits. J Nucl Med 1992 (abstract);33:926.

93. Shirakawa S, Hattori N, Tamaki N, et al. [Assessment of left ventricular wall thickening with gated Tc-99m-MIBI SPECT—value of normal file]. Kaku Igaku 1995;32:643.

94. Itoh Y, Adachi I, Kohya T, et al. Heterogeneity in myocardial perfusion, wall motion and wall thickening with Tc-99m-sestamibi quantitative gated SPECT in normal subjects. J Nucl Med 1999 (abstract);40:165P.

95. Fujino M, Masuyama K, Kanayama S, et al. Early and delayed technetium-99m labeled sestamibi myocardial ECG-gated SPECT by QGS program in normal volunteers. J Nucl Med 1999 (abstract);40:180P.

96. Everaert H, Vanhove C, Franken PR. Effects of low-dose dobutamine on left ventricular function in normal subjects as assessed by gated single-photon emission tomography myocardial perfusion studies. Eur J Nucl Med 1999;26:1298.

97. Taillefer R, DePuey EG, Udelson JE, et al. Comparative diagnostic accuracy of Tl-201 and Tc-99m sestamibi SPECT imaging (perfusion and ECG-gated SPECT) in detecting coronary artery disease in women. J Am Coll Cardiol 1997;29:69.

98. Smanio PE, Watson DD, Segalla DL, et al. Value of gating of technetium-99m sestamibi single-photon emission computed tomographic imaging. J Am Coll Cardiol 1997;30:1687.

99. Hachamovitch R, Berman D, Lewin H, et al. Incremental prognostic value of gated SPECT ejection fraction in patients undergoing dual-isotope exercise or adenosine stress SPECT. J Am Coll Cardiol 1998 (abstract);31(2(Suppl.A)):441A.

100. Sharir T, Bacher-Stier C, Dhar S, et al. Post exercise regional wall motion abnormalities detected by Tc-99m sestamibi gated SPECT: a marker of severe coronary artery disease. J Nucl Med 1998 (abstract);39:87P.

101. Johnson SH, Bigelow C, Lee KL, et al. Prediction of death and myocardial infarction by radionuclide angiocardiography in patients with suspected coronary artery disease. American Journal of Cardiology 1991;67:919.

102. Lee KL, Pryor DB, Pieper KS, et al. Prognostic value of radionuclide angiography in medically treated patients with coronary artery disease. A comparison with clinical and catheterization variables. Circulation 1990;82:1705.

103. Upton MT, Palmeri ST, Jones RH, et al. Assessment of left ventricular function by resting and exercise radionuclide angiocardiography following acute myocardial infarction. Am Heart J 1982;104:1232.

104. Pryor DB, Harrell FE Jr, Lee KL, et al. Prognostic indicators from radionuclide angiography in medically treated patients with coronary artery disease. Am J Cardiol 1984;53:18.

105. Jones RH, Johnson SH, Bigelow C, et al. Exercise radionuclide angiocardiography predicts cardiac death in patients with coronary artery disease. Circulation 1991;84(3 Suppl):I52.

106. Morris KG, Palmeri ST, Califf RM, et al. Value of radionuclide angiography for predicting specific cardiac events after acute myocardial infarction. Am J Cardiol 1985;55:318.

107. Sharir T, Germano G, Kavanagh PB, et al. Incremental prognostic value of post-stress left ventricular ejection fraction and volume by gated myocardial perfusion single photon emission computed tomography. Circulation 1999;100:1035.

108. Sharir T, Germano G, Lewin H, et al. Prognostic value of myocardial perfusion and function by gated SPECT in the prediction of non-fatal myocardial infarction and cardiac death. Circulation 1999 (abstract);100:I-383.

109. O'Keefe J, Case J, Moutray K, et al. Post-stress drop in ejection fraction on ECG-gated SPECT thallium-201 scintigraphy predicts poor prognosis. J Am Coll Cardiol 1999 (abstract); 33(2(Suppl.A)):469A.

110. Mahmarian JJ, Mahmarian AC, Marks GF, et al. Role of adenosine thallium-201 tomography for defining long-term risk in patients after acute myocardial infarction. J Am Coll Cardiol 1995;25:1333.

111. Strauss HW, Zaret BL, Hurley PJ, et al. A scintiphotographic method for measuring left ventricular ejection fraction in man without cardiac catheterization. Am J Cardiol 1971;28:575.

112. Berman DS, Salel AF, DeNardo GL, et al. Clinical assessment of left ventricular regional contraction patterns and ejection fraction by high-resolution gated scintigraphy. J Nucl Med 1975;16:865.

113. Moore ML, Murphy PH, Burdine JA. ECG-gated emission computed tomography of the cardiac blood pool. Radiology 1980;134:233.

114. Tamaki N, Mukai T, Ishii Y, et al. Multiaxial tomography of heart chambers by gated blood-pool emission computed tomography using a rotating gamma camera. Radiology 1983; 147:547.

115. Maublant J, Bailly P, Mestas D, et al. Feasibility of gated single-photon emission transaxial tomography of the cardiac blood pool. Radiology 1983;146:837.

116. Hoffman EJ, Huang SC, Phelps ME. Quantitation in positron emission computed tomography: 1. Effect of object size. J Comput Assist Tomogr 1979;3:299.

117. Salel AF, Berman DS, DeNardo GL, et al. Radionuclide assessment of nitroglycerin influence on abnormal left ventricular segmental contraction in patients with coronary heart disease. Circulation 1976;53:975.

118. Bunker SR, Hartshorne MF, Schmidt WP, et al. Left ventricular volume determination from single-photon emission computed tomography. Am J Roentgenol 1985;144:295.

119. Barat JL, Brendel AJ, Colle JP, et al. Quantitative analysis of left-ventricular function using gated single photon emission tomography. J Nucl Med 1984;25:1167.

120. Underwood SR, Walton S, Ell PJ, et al. Gated blood-pool emission tomography: a new technique for the investigation of cardiac structure and function. Eur J Nucl Med 1985;10:332.

121. Stadius ML, Williams DL, Harp G, et al. Left ventricular volume determination using single-photon emission computed tomography. Am J Cardiol 1985;55:1185.

122. Corbett JR, Jansen DE, Lewis SE, et al. Tomographic gated blood pool radionuclide ventriculography: analysis of wall motion and left ventricular volumes in patients with coronary artery disease. J Am Coll Cardiol 1985;6:349.

123. Gill JB, Moore RH, Tamaki N, et al. Multigated blood-pool tomography: new method for the assessment of left ventricular function. J Nucl Med 1986;27:1916.

124. Chin BB, Bloomgarden DC, Xia W, et al. Right and left ventricular volume and ejection fraction by tomographic gated blood-pool scintigraphy. J Nucl Med 1997;38:942.

125. Vanhove C, Everaert H, Bossuyt A, et al. Automatic determination of LV ejection fraction and volumes by gated blood pool SPECT. J Nucl Med 2000 (abstract);41:187P.

126. Van Kriekinge SD, Berman DS, Germano G. Automatic quantification of left ventricular ejection fraction from gated blood pool SPECT. J Nucl Cardiol 1999;6:498.

127. Van Kriekinge S, Berman D, Germano G. Automatic quantification of left and right ventricular ejection fractions from gated blood pool SPECT. Circulation 1999 (abstract);100:I-26.

128. Schwartz R, Le Guludec D, Holder L, et al. Blood pool gated SPECT: validation of left ventricular volumes and ejection fraction with planar radionuclide angiography. J Nucl Cardiol 2000 (abstract);7:S2.

129. Groch M, Belzberg A, DePuey E, et al. Evaluation of ventricular performance using gated blood pool SPECT: a multicenter study. J Nucl Med 2000 (abstract);41:5P.

130. Groch M, Marshall R, Erwin W, et al. Left ventricular ejection fraction computed from gated SPECT blood pool imaging correlates with conventional planar imaging. J Nucl Med 2000 (abstract);41:98P.

131. Keng F, Tan H, Chua T. Gated SPECT blood pool imaging: a comparison with equilibrium blood pool imaging. J Nucl Cardiol 2000 (abstract);7:S3.

132. Bartlett ML, Srinivasan G, Barker WC, et al. Left ventricular ejection fraction: comparison of results from planar and SPECT gated blood-pool studies. J Nucl Med 1996;37:1795.

133. Germano G, Berman D. Acquisition and processing for gated perfusion SPECT: technical aspects. In: *Clinical Gated Cardiac SPECT,* edited by G Germano and D Berman. Armonk, NY: Futura Publishing Company, 1999, pp. 93–113.

134. DePuey EG, Nichols K, Dobrinsky C. Left ventricular ejection fraction assessed from gated technetium-99m-sestamibi SPECT. J Nucl Med 1993;34:1871.

135. Goris ML, Thompson C, Malone LJ, et al. Modelling the integration of myocardial regional perfusion and function. Nucl Med Commun 1994;15:9.

136. Marcassa C, Marzullo P, Parodi O, et al. A new method for noninvasive quantitation of segmental myocardial wall thickening using technetium-99m 2-methoxy-isobutyl-isonitrile scintigraphy—results in normal subjects. J Nucl Med 1990;31:173.

137. Smith WH, Kastner RJ, Calnon DA, et al. Quantitative gated single photon emission computed tomography imaging: a counts-based method for display and measurement of regional and global ventricular systolic function. J Nucl Cardiol 1997;4:451.

138. Cooke CD, Garcia EV, Cullom SJ, et al. Determining the accuracy of calculating systolic wall thickening using a fast Fourier transform approximation: a simulation study based on canine and patient data. J Nucl Med 1994;35:1185.

139. Mochizuki T, Murase K, Fujiwara Y, et al. Assessment of systolic thickening with thallium-201 ECG-gated single-photon emission computed tomography: a parameter for local left ventricular function. J Nucl Med 1991;32:1496.

140. Buvat I, Bartlett ML, Kitsiou AN, et al. A "hybrid" method for measuring myocardial wall thickening from gated PET/SPECT images. J Nucl Med 1997;38:324.

141. Stollfuss JC, Haas F, Matsunari I, et al. Tc-99m-tetrofosmin SPECT for prediction of functional recovery defined by MRI in patients with severe left ventricular dysfunction: additional value of gated SPECT. J Nucl Med 1999;40:1824.

142. Ficaro E, Quaife R, Kritzman J, et al. Accuracy and reproducibility of 3D-MSPECT for estimating left ventricular ejection fraction in patients with severe perfusion abnormalities. Circulation 1999 (abstract);100:I-26.

9 | Exercise treadmill testing and exercise myocardial perfusion imaging

AMI E. ISKANDRIAN

Part 1

Exercise Treadmill Testing

OXYGEN CONSUMPTIONS AND METS

At rest, approximately 25% of the arterial oxygen content is extracted by tissues, or roughly 250 ml/min. The 250 ml of oxygen in a 70 kg subject represents approximately 3.5 ml/kg per minute. This value has come to be known as the MET (metabolic equivalent), which is the oxygen consumption per kilogram per minute in the basal state.

Nearly 75 ml of carbon dioxide is produced for each 100 ml of oxygen used. The ratio of carbon dioxide production to oxygen consumption is known as the *respiratory gas exchange ratio (R)* and this ratio, therefore, is 0.75. During exercise, oxygen consumption increases steadily; the VO_2 max may be as high as 60 ml/kg per minute or higher, that is, roughly 4 l/min—a nearly twentyfold increase over baseline value! The VO_2 max is age-dependent and gender-dependent, being higher in men than women at any age and decreasing in both sexes with aging. The VO_2 max declines roughly by 5% per decade of life, but tends to increase by 20% with training.

The minute ventilation may increase eight times or more during exercise, and ventilatory reserve is not a limitation to sustained aerobic work in normal subjects. The functional aerobic impairment (FAI) is an index that represents the difference between the observed VO_2 max and predicted VO_2 max (based on age, gender, and intensity of the stress); in healthy individuals, it is $0 \pm 14\%$.

If oxygen delivery during exercise is not sufficient to maintain aerobic metabolism, lactate production (from anaerobic metabolism) begins. The lactate is converted to carbon dioxide, which therefore adds to carbon dioxide production; the carbon dioxide to oxygen ratio therefore increases above 0.75. To maintain the carbon dioxide level and the blood pH in normal range, ventilation increases. The anaerobic threshold can be determined by several methods, such as lactate production, disproportionate rise in VCO_2 relative to VO_2, respiratory gas exchange ratio, minute ventilation, and ventilatory equivalent for oxygen.

Increased oxygen delivery to muscles during exercise is achieved via increased cardiac output, increased oxygen extraction, and redistribution of the cardiac output from inactive vascular beds (such as the skin, subcutaneous tissue, splanchnic tissue, and nonexercising muscles) to exercising muscle groups. Although the muscle blood flow is only 20% of the rest cardiac output, it may be as high as 80% during strenuous exercise. A decrease in the muscle blood flow is an important reason for the decrease in exercise tolerance in patients with congestive heart failure. The peak VO_2 is reduced even in asymptomatic patients with left ventricular (LV) dysfunction [1].

HEMODYNAMIC RESPONSES TO EXERCISE

During dynamic exercise, the heart rate, cardiac output, and systolic blood pressure increase. The mean peak systolic blood pressure (BP) in normal subjects is 180 ± 10 mm Hg (mean $\pm$ 1 SD). During exhaustive exercise, there may be a slight (approximately 10 mm Hg) decrease in BP, the so-called drift phase. It is thought that vasodilatation in the cutaneous vasculature is responsible for this decline; the dilatation is mediated by the heat-regulating center to rid the body of excessive heat accumulated during the exercise. The diastolic BP often changes little (≤ 10 mm Hg) in either direction. The systolic BP often returns to normal within 6 minutes. The systemic vascular resistance decreases in the exercising muscle beds but increases in other muscle beds because of reflex vasoconstriction. In some subjects, an exaggerated hypertensive response is seen with systolic BP > 200 mm Hg. The exaggerated pressure response may be due to higher than normal cardiac output for a given level of vascular resistance. The cardiac output at peak exercise is similar in those with and without exaggerated BP response, but the change (from rest to exercise) in vascular resistance is different [2].

Systolic BP during daily activity or during exercise is a better predictor of LV hypertrophy than the resting BP. We found a significantly better correlation between the exercise systolic BP and LV mass than between the resting BP and LV mass [1]. Lauer and associates, based on the Framingham experience, suggested that there are important confounding problems that affect the relationship between LV mass and exercise systolic BP. If these factors are not considered, then patients with exaggerated BP response have 10% higher LV mass than patients with normal BP response. If these confounding factors are taken into consideration, then only a 5% difference is noted in the LV mass [3].

Cardiac output increases almost linearly with exercise intensity and is also linearly related to oxygen consumption. At each level of exercise, however, the increase in oxygen consumption is greater than the corresponding increase in cardiac output (because of increased oxygen extraction). The peak cardiac output is roughly threefold to fivefold higher than baseline during treadmill exercise; most of the increase is the result of an increase in heart rate, but a slight increase in stroke volume also occurs. The increase in stroke volume is caused by increased inotropism (a decrease in end-systolic volume), and the Frank-Starling mechanism with LV dilatation. It is interesting to note that despite a decrease in the RR cycle and diastolic filling period (because of tachycardia) during exercise, a slight increase in end-diastolic volume and stroke volume still occur. This may be the result of improvement in diastolic function.

The increase in myocardial oxygen demand during exercise causes a twofold to threefold increase in coronary blood flow. The coronary blood flow attained during exercise is *not* the maximum attainable coronary blood flow. In fact, coronary vasodilation with papaverine, adenosine, nitric oxide, or dipyridamole may result in fourfold to fivefold increases in coronary blood flow or even higher [1].

EFFECTS OF AGING AND TRAINING

With aging, there are decreases in peak exercise heart rate, stroke volume, cardiac output, and VO$_2$ max; the relative magnitude is similar in men and women. The VO$_2$ max declines by approximately 0.9 ml/min per kilogram per year of life, and the decline is more accentuated in sedentary than active individuals. Training (20–30 minutes of brisk walking three to five times per week) results in improvement in exercise capacity, a decrease in heart rate and BP for any given workload, a decrease in sympathetic discharge activity and systemic vascular resistance, and an increase in oxygen extraction. In addition, there is increased sense of well-being, increased muscle tone and efficiency, and probably also a decrease in osteoporosis in the elderly. Physical training attenuates the decreases in heart rate and arteriovenous oxygen difference with aging. The age and training effects cannot be fully explained by differences in body composition. Alterations in beta-adrenergic receptors may explain the age-related decrease in cardiac output, which is a primary age-related process and is not related to inactivity [1].

TYPES OF EXERCISE TESTS

Exercise may be dynamic (isotonic), isometric, or combined. Dynamic muscular exercise consists of rhythmic contractions of alternating extensor and flexor muscles [3,4]. This is the common type of exercise and includes treadmill testing, bicycle exercise, and other more familiar forms of exercise such as walking, jogging, swimming, and rowing. In contrast, isometric exercise consists of a sustained muscular contraction of extensor or flexor muscle groups, or both, against a fixed resistance. The most familiar type of isometric exercise is the handgrip test. The combination of dynamic and isometric exercises occurs in daily activity such as carrying a weight while walking. Exercise may be performed with the patient in the supine, semierect, or upright position. Upright exercise is most commonly performed on a treadmill or a bicycle ergometer. The first examples of supervised exercise tests were the Master one-step and two-steps tests.

The exercise may either be symptom limited, or submaximal. In symptom-limited exercise testing, the exercise is terminated based on development of symptoms or signs. In contrast, a submaximal exercise test is terminated when an arbitrary end point is reached. The end point is determined before testing begins and may involve a predetermined target heart rate or exercise workload. Submaximal exercise is usually performed in patients who have experienced recent acute myocardial infarction, and occasionally may be combined with pharmacologic stress testing. Many of the parameters used to judge maximal exercise, such as VO_2 max and the maximum heart rate have considerable variability; for example, the 95% confidence limit for heart rate based on age is roughly 50 beats per minute. Exercise testing may be categorized as single-level (constant workload) or multilevel, in which exercise workload is progressively increased until a maximum or an end point is reached. The exercise work pattern may be continuous or intermittent; the alternating exercise–rest protocol is now rarely used [1].

EXERCISE PROTOCOLS

There are several treadmill exercise protocols, although none may be suited for all patients and the choice of exercise protocol must be individualized. For instance, patients unable to walk fast may prefer a protocol that increases the treadmill inclination but not its speed. Of the various treadmill protocols available (Bruce, Ellestad, Kattus, McHenry, Naughton, Sheffield, Reeves, and Balke), the Bruce protocol (or its modification) is the one most commonly employed. This protocol is multistaged, providing progressive increments in workload by increasing the speed and inclination of the treadmill. At each stage, the patient walks on the treadmill at a certain speed and at an incline varying from 0° to 20° or more. The incline of the treadmill is expressed in grade percentage and not in degrees. The grade percentage is calculated by dividing the height of the treadmill by its length multiplied by 100. Each stage lasts 3 minutes.

Exercise testing on a bicycle ergometer can be performed in the upright, supine, or semierect position. The ergometer is braked either manually or electrically. The choice of the protocol can be individualized to a patient's symptoms, body habitus, and physical fitness. Initial workload may start at 150–300 kilopound-meters per minute (25 to 50 W) and is increased by 25 to 50 W every 2 to 3 minutes depending on conditioning. The use of 3-minute stages is particularly popular in laboratories using blood pool imaging because data acquisition during exercise requires at least 2 minutes during each stage [4].

Protocols with rapid increments of workload (such as the Bruce) may falsely lower estimates of exercise capacity (exercise capacity is defined as observed MET divided by predicted MET times 100) and are less reliable for studying the effect of drug therapy. It is unclear, however, if they also lower the sensitivity for detecting coronary artery disease (CAD) compared to a protocol like the Balke, which has slow increments; the treadmill speed is kept at a constant speed between 2 to 3.3 mph, and workload is increased by equal increments of 2.5% to 5% every 2 to 3 minutes.

An individualized ramp protocol employs a steady increase in workload rather than the interrupted and sudden changes as in conventional protocols. The aim of this protocol is to complete the exercise in 10 minutes. In patients with heart failure, the relation between measured and observed VO_2 is better with the ramp than with other protocols (especially those with marked changes in workloads at each stage, such as the Bruce protocol).

GENERAL CONSIDERATIONS FOR EXERCISE TESTING

Guidelines are available for establishing laboratories to conduct exercise testing in both adult and pediatric patients. The physical environment should be conducive to exercise testing. The room should be well ventilated, the temperature between 68°F and 75°F, and the humidity comfortable (< 60%). The exercise test must be supervised by an individual who has knowledge of exercise testing and who can assume responsibility for the safety and performance of the test. The rhythm should be constantly monitored (a 12-lead ECG is often obtained at the end of each exercise stage) during exercise and the BP should be measured regularly. To obtain high-quality electrocardiographic recordings, proper electrodes should be used and skin preparation should be adequate (cleansing the site with alcohol followed by removal of the superficial epidermal layer by light abrasion). Emergency equipment and drugs must be available, and the staff should be well trained in cardiopulmonary resuscitation. The patient should be instructed to wear loose-fitting clothes and to refrain from eating or smoking for at least 3 hours prior to testing. The risks and benefits of exercise testing and

TABLE 9.1 *Common Indications of Exercise Testing*

1. Diagnosis of coronary artery disease
2. Risk assessment
3. Assessment of functional capacity
4. Symptom reproducibility
5. Evaluation of results of therapy
6. Detection of cardiac arrhythmias
7. Disability evaluation

alternative diagnostic techniques should be explained to the patient [4].

Indications and Contraindications

According to ACC/AHA guidelines, the indications for exercise testing are listed in Tables 9.1–9.3 [4].

TABLE 9.2 *More Specific Indications for Exercise Testing**

1. Exercise testing in diagnosis of CAD: see Table 9.3
2. Exercise testing in prognosis of CAD
   Class I: Initial evaluation; change in clinical status since last evaluation
   Class IIa: None
   Class IIb: WPW; pacemakers; > 1 mm ST depression; LBBB; diagnosis is already established; periodic testing in otherwise stable course
   Class III: Severe comorbidity
3. Exercise testing in postacute MI
   Class I: Before discharge for evaluation of risk, activity, or medical therapy; early after discharge if above was not done; late after discharge if above was submaximal
   Class II: Before discharge to detect ischemia in borderline lesions by angiography; WPW; LVH; digoxin therapy; > 1 mm ST depression; pacemaker; periodic monitoring of patient in rehabilitation
   Class III: Severe comorbidity
4. Asymptomatic patients with no known CAD
   Class I: None
   Class IIa: None
   Class IIb: Multiple risk factors; men > 40, women > 50; before vigorous exercise program; special occupations; high risk for CAD due to other reasons such as chronic renal failure
   Class III: Routine
5. Exercise testing in valvular disease
   Class I: None
   Class IIa: None
   Class IIb: Evaluation of exercise capacity
   Class III: Diagnosis of CAD
6. Exercise testing before and after revascularization
   Class I: Detect ischemia before; recurrent ischemia after
   Class IIa: Activity counseling/rehabilitation after
   Class IIb: Detect restenosis in high-risk patients early after PTCA
   Class III: Localizing ischemia for determining site of PTCA; routine periodic monitoring after
7. Exercise testing in rhythm disorders
   Class I: Identify appropriate setting in rate-adaptive pacemakers
   Class IIa: Known or suspected exercise-induced arrhythmias; evaluate results of medical, surgical, or ablative therapy
   Class IIb: Isolated VPC without evidence of CAD
   Class III: Isolated VPC in young patients

CAD, coronary artery disease; WPW, Wolf-Parkinson-White syndrome; LBBB, left bundle branch block; MI, myocardial infarct; LVH, left ventricular hypertrophy; PTCA, percutaneous transluminal coronary angioplasty; VPC, ventricular premature contractions.
   *Class I: Evidence/agreement. . . . "useful and effective"
   Class II: Conflicting evidence/agreement
        IIa: In favor
        IIb: Less well established
   Class III: Evidence/agreement . . . "not useful or effective and may even be harmful"

TABLE 9.3 *Recommendation for Diagnosis of Obstructive CAD with Exercise ECG Testing without an Imaging Modality*

Class I: Patients with an intermediate pretest probability of CAD based on age, gender, and symptoms, including those with complete right bundle branch block or < 1 mm of ST depression at rest (exceptions are listed in Classes II and III) (level of evidence B).

Class IIa: Patients with suspected vasospastic angina (level of evidence C).

Class IIb: Patients with a high pretest probability of CAD by age, gender, and symptoms (level of evidence B); patients with a low pretest probability of CAD by age, gender, and symptoms (level of evidence: B); patients taking digoxin whose ECG has < 1 mm of baseline ST-segment depression (level of evidence B); patients with ECG criteria for LV hypertrophy and < 1 mm of baseline ST-segment depression (level of evidence B).

Class III: Patients with the following baseline ECG abnormalities: Preexcitation Wolff-Parkinson-White syndrome (level of evidence B); electronically paced ventricular rhythm, (level of evidence B); paced ventricular rhythm (level of evidence B); complete left bundle branch block (level of evidence B); patients with an established diagnosis of CAD due to prior MI or coronary angiography; however, testing can assess functional capacity and prognosis, as discussed in Section III (level of evidence B).

Level of evidence A, high; B, intermediate; C, low.

Complications

Complications secondary to exercise testing are uncommon. Bradyarrhythmias such as atrioventricular block, junctional rhythm, ventricular escape rhythm, or asystole may occasionally occur. Serious cardiac complications such as myocardial infarction, shock, congestive heart failure, and sudden death from ventricular tachycardia or fibrillation are very rare. In a meta analysis of more than 71,000 tests over 16 years, the rate of serious complications was 0.8 in 10,000 tests. Most complications occur in patients with unstable angina pectoris, left main CAD, severe LV dysfunction, critical aortic stenosis, or in those with serious arrhythmias.

Safety of exercise testing (usually submaximal) shortly after acute infarction was examined in 151,000 tests, 76% of which were performed within 2 weeks of infarction. The death rate was 0.03%, major nonfatal complications occurred in 0.09%, and other complications were observed in 1.4%. Overall, major complications were more common after maximal than submaximal testing [4].

NORMAL RESPONSES

In healthy individuals, several changes occur in the ECG during exercise. For example, the Q-wave magnitude increases, especially in the inferior leads; the P vector becomes more vertical (the P-wave duration does not change); and the PR segment shortens. The repolarization of the atrium (Ta wave) may cause J-point or ST-segment depression, which is one of the mechanisms of a false positive response. Subjects with a resting J-point elevation may develop an isoelectric J junction during exercise. There is a decrease in the R-wave amplitude, especially in the lateral leads. Also, the S wave becomes deeper. There is a gradual decrease in the amplitude of the T wave, but at peak exercise, the T-wave amplitude increases and a further increase may be observed 1 minute into recovery. There is a decrease in the QT interval corrected for heart rate (0.4 times the square root of the RR interval). The QT interval is highly dependent on the heart rate, varies with age and sex, and is influenced by medications and serum concentrations of potassium, calcium, and hydrogen ions. The QT interval may also be difficult to measure, especially at fast heart rates, with superimposition of the T and P waves. Factors that contribute to changes in various electrocardiographic wave forms during exercise are controversial. They include different positions of the recording electrodes relative to the heart at rest and during exercise, alterations in the action potentials of the atrial and ventricular activation patterns, and changes in cardiac and pulmonary blood volume [4].

ST-SEGMENT CHANGES

Exercise-induced ischemia can result in ST-segment depression or elevation during exercise or recovery. ST-segment depression or elevation is measured 60–80 msec from the J point relative to the isoelectric PR segment. J-point depression alone is normal, as discussed earlier. ST depression may be horizontal (flat), downsloping, or upsloping.

Based on the ST-segment changes during exercise or recovery, exercise ECGs are interpreted as positive, negative, or nondiagnostic (inconclusive). A positive ECG indicates the presence of ≥ 1 mm of ST-segment depression (or elevation) of the horizontal or downsloping variety, or ≥ 1.5 mm of the upsloping variety seen in at least three consecutive beats. The lower the workload and the double product at onset of ST-segment depression, the more likely that CAD is present and that the disease involves multiple vessels. In some patients, the ST shift occurs in the recovery period only or becomes more prominent in the recovery period. The precise reasons for why this happens are not clear. Possible mechanisms include: increased wall stress (due to LV distension as heart rate slows down but venous return continues to be high); coronary spasm superimposed on stenosis (due to withdrawal of sympathetic tone); or a

decrease in coronary driving pressure (aortic diastolic pressure minus LV filling pressure). In our experience, these patients tend not to have extensive CAD [1].

A negative exercise ECG implies the absence of ischemic ST-segment abnormalities in a patient attaining at least 85% of the maximum predicted heart rate. (The maximum predicted heart rate = 220 − patient age).

A nondiagnostic exercise ECG is considered to be present when any of the following occurs:

1. There are baseline electrocardiographic abnormalities that preclude interpretation of the ST-segment changes, such as LV hypertrophy, left bundle branch block, Wolff-Parkinson-White syndrome, or a pacemaker rhythm. In patients with right bundle branch block, the left (V4 to V6) but not the right (V1 to V3) precordial leads can be used to detect ischemic changes. Digitalis therapy may produce false positive ST response even when ST shift is not detected in the resting ECG.

2. The presence of ST-segment depression at rest.

3. Failure to achieve at least 85% of the maximum predicted heart rate in the absence of ST-segment depression or elevation during exercise or recovery.

Nondiagnostic exercise ECGs are seen in 30%–40% of patients referred for exercise testing for the diagnosis of CAD [4].

EXERCISE-INDUCED ST-SEGMENT ELEVATION

ST-segment elevation during exercise occurs most often in leads with Q waves as a result of a previous myocardial infarction; it is thought to reflect regional asynergy and thus it is not considered evidence of ischemia. Approximately 50% of patients with previous anterior Q-wave infarction and 15% of patients with previous inferior Q-wave myocardial infarction exhibit this finding during exercise. Patients with prior infarction and ST-segment elevation during exercise often have larger infarcts and lower ejection fraction (EF) than those without ST-segment elevation. ST elevation may result in reciprocal ST-segment depression simulating ischemia in the opposite leads. ST-segment elevation without Q waves frequently indicates the presence of severe and transmural ischemia resulting from proximal coronary stenosis, exercise-induced spasm, or both. The site of ST-segment elevation predicts the site of coronary artery stenosis, unlike ST-segment depression during exercise, which does not [5–8]. These patients often have large reversible perfusion defects. Ventricular arrhythmias appear to be more frequent in patients with ST-segment elevation than with ST-segment depression [4].

OTHER ABNORMALITIES

Pseudonormalization of inverted T waves or normalization of ST-segment depression has been noted in some patients with CAD during exercise or during episodes of spontaneous angina [9]. However, these findings are nonspecific and cannot be considered reliable markers of ischemia. Occasionally, patients with CAD have been noted to have U-wave inversion during exercise. Inversion of the U wave has also been noted in patients with LV hypertrophy and valvular heart disease.

Atrial repolarization (Ta) is opposite in direction to the P wave, may have a magnitude of 100 to 200 μV, and may extend into the ST segment and T waves. If exaggerated during exercise, Ta can cause ST-segment depression that may mimic ischemia. The repolarization of the atrium is expected more often, however, to produce its maximum effect on the J point, resulting in an upsloping ST segment, but if the P waves and the Ta waves exceed 400 msec, which occurs occasionally, it may cause horizontal ST-segment depression. These changes are more pronounced in the inferior leads, suggesting a lower reliability of ST-segment changes in these leads as markers of CAD [4].

ST-SEGMENT DEPRESSION DURING PHARMACOLOGIC TESTING

ST-segment depression occurs less frequently during adenosine, dipyridamole, or dobutamine infusion than during exercise testing. The prevalence and significance of these findings are discussed in Chapter 10.

ARRHYTHMIAS DURING EXERCISE

Arrhythmias, both atrial and ventricular, may occur in some patients during exercise. The precise mechanism is not well understood, although changes in heart rate, enhanced sympathetic activity, increased catecholamine secretion, and development of myocardial ischemia may be important. Ventricular tachycardia may occur in normal subjects though it is more common in the setting of CAD [10–15].

Atrioventricular block is very rare during exercise and is probably secondary to ischemia of the AV node or the conduction system.

The effect of coronary revascularization on exercise-induced ventricular arrhythmias is debatable; if the arrhythmias are ischemia-mediated, then coronary revascularization may abolish them. More often than not,

however, the arrhythmias are the result of scarring and LV dysfunction and therefore do not respond to revascularization. The prognostic relevance of exercise-induced arrhythmias in medically treated patients with CAD is not clear, with some (but not all) studies suggesting a relationship between them and subsequent events [9–13,14].

In a recent study, frequent exercise-induced ventricular premature beats (defined as couplets or at least 10% of depolarizations during any 30-second period of recording) increased the risk of cardiac death by a factor of 2.5 in asymptomatic men during a 20-year follow-up. The presence of such arrhythmia before or after the exercise did not carry an increased risk. There was no association between ventricular arrhythmia and ischemia (~5% overlap) and each increased risk independently by the same magnitude [16].

HYPOTENSION DURING EXERCISE

Hypotension during exercise is defined as a decrease of $\geq$ 20 mm Hg in systolic BP compared to an earlier measurement. A change in systolic blood BP from rest to peak exercise of < 20 mm Hg is defined as a blunted response. Hypotension during exercise has been noted in patients with stable CAD, hypertrophic cardiomyopathy, aortic stenosis, severe dilated cardiomyopathy, and after acute myocardial infarction. Cardiac medications such as beta-blockers, ACE inhibitors, nitrates, and other hypotensive medications may cause or contribute to hypotension in some patients. In patients with CAD, a hypotensive response is a marker of extensive disease and poor outcome. The hypotensive response is corrected after coronary revascularization.

Approximately 8% of CAD patients may develop hypotension during exercise. Hypotension during supine exercise is also a marker of severe CAD but is less frequent than that observed during upright exercise [17–20]. We observed, by multivariate discriminant analysis, that the number of diseased vessels, EF, and ischemic burden by perfusion imaging are independent predictors of hypotensive response during exercise [18].

Since not all patients with left main or three-vessel CAD develop hypotension during exercise, other factors may be important. We compared a group of patients who had a hypotensive response to an age-matched and sex-matched control group, who also had CAD but who had a normal BP response to exercise [18]. The two groups had comparable extent of CAD and comparable extent of perfusion abnormality (Fig. 9.1). It is therefore possible that ischemia may not be the only mechanism for hypotension during ex-

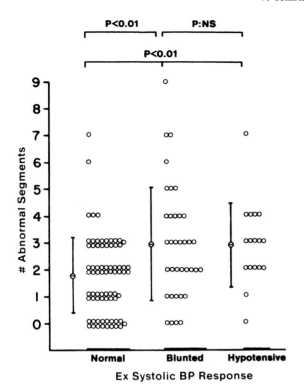

FIGURE 9.1 The exercise perfusion defect size in patients with coronary artery disease (CAD) who had hypotensive pressure response, blunted response, or normal pressure response. Even large ischemia may be associated with normal pressure response, suggesting other factors may be important in producing hypotension during exercise in some patients. Ex, exercise. (Reproduced from Hakki et al. [18].)

ercise in CAD patients. Activation of the Bezold-Jarisch reflex may be another mechanism. Neurally mediated hypotension is a documented mechanism of syncope and involves reflex activation of mechanoreceptors in the myocardium that triggers vagally induced slowing of the heart rate, a decrease in systemic vascular resistance, or both. This response has been implicated as the mechanism of hypotension in normal subjects and patients with aortic stenosis or hypertrophic cardiomyopathy. Vigorous LV contraction (especially in the presence of reduced end-diastolic volume) has been thought to be the mechanism that initiates this reflex activation. These mechanoreceptors are more predominant in the inferior and posterior segments of the myocardium. Of interest, the patients in our study with hypotensive response had inferior and posterior ischemia by perfusion imaging during exercise. Lele and coworkers measured the peripheral vascular resistance and concluded that hypotension during exercise in patients with CAD may be due to inappropriate vasodilation rather than a decrease in cardiac output [20].

SENSITIVITY, SPECIFICITY, PREDICTIVE VALUE, AND RELATIVE RISK

Sensitivity is defined as TP/(TP + FN) × 100, where TP (true positive) is a patient with CAD and a positive response and FN (false negative) is a patient with CAD and a negative response. *Specificity* is defined as TN/(FP + TN) × 100, where TN (true negative) is a patient with no CAD and a negative response, and FP (false positive) is a patient with no CAD but a positive response. Positive predictive value is TP/(TP + FP) × 100; negative predictive value is TN/(TN + FN) × 100; predictive accuracy is defined as (TP + TN)/(TP + FN + FP + FN) × 100. The overall test accuracy is defined as TP + TN/total number of patients tested × 100.

BAYESIAN ANALYSIS IN THE INTERPRETATION OF TEST RESULTS

Bayes's theorem states that although the reliability of a less-than-perfect diagnostic test is defined by the test's sensitivity and specificity, a test cannot be adequately interpreted without reference to the prevalence of the disease in the population under study [4].

Bayes's theorem expresses the posttest likelihood of disease as a function of the sensitivity and the specificity of the test and the prevalence of disease in the population being tested (Fig. 9.2). The posttest probability of a negative test is

(1 − Sensitivity) × (Prevalence)/(1 − Sensitivity)
    × (Prevalence) + Specificity (1 − Prevalence) × 100

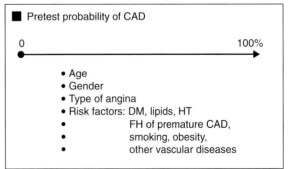

FIGURE 9.2 Estimation of pretest probability of CAD based on clinical evaluation and risk factors. DM, diabetes mellitus; HT, hypertension; FH, family history. (Adapted from Gibbons et al. [4].)

The posttest probability of a positive test is

(Sensitivity) × (Prevalence)/(Sensitivity) × (Prevalence)
    + (1 − Specificity) × (1 − Prevalence) × 100.

Other biases may affect test results, such as pretest and posttest biases. The pretest bias refers to patient selection before testing. For example, the sensitivity will be higher if patients with more extensive and severe disease are selected compared to patients with moderate stenosis in a single vessel. Also the specificity will be higher if young, healthy subjects are studied compared to elderly patients with multiple coronary risk factors but no "significant" angiographic stenosis. Posttest bias refers to selective use of coronary angiography in patients with positive results. This will increase sensitivity and lower the specificity, since patients are referred to angiography because of abnormal tests.

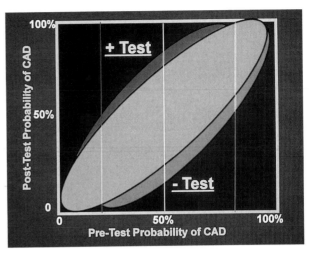

FIGURE 9.3 The posttest probability of disease is relative to test result (positive or negative) and pretest likelihood of CAD. The graph lines will vary depending on sensitivity and specificity of the test used.

Prediction of CAD by Bayesian Analysis

Diamond and Forrester reported the prevalence of CAD in 4952 patients from the angiographic literature. From this information, the pretest probability of CAD can be determined based on age, sex, and symptoms (Table 9.4). The pretest probability can then be used to address the implication of test results. For example, if the sensitivity of exercise electrocardiography is 60% and its specificity is 80%, a negative test will yield a posttest probability of 33% for having CAD, while a positive test will yield a posttest probability of 75% for having CAD in a patient who started out with a 50% pretest prevalence of disease (Fig. 9.3).

The matter simply is that in any diagnostic test that is not perfect, that is, with a sensitivity and specificity < 100%, test results are affected by the pretest likelihood of disease. One can also conclude that an abnormal ST-segment response may not provide a definitive answer as to the presence or absence of CAD, but may rather provide a probability statement that is dependent on the pretest likelihood of disease. Furthermore, this probability can be used as a continuous spectrum, depending not only on the presence or absence of ST-segment depression but also on the magnitude of ST changes and on the presence of other hemodynamic changes, such as the response of BP, exercise level, and duration of ST-segment abnormalities.

RESULTS OF EXERCISE TESTING

In the ACC/AHA guidelines on exercise testing, the average sensitivity was 68% (range = 23%–100%) and the average specificity was 77% (range = 17%–100%) (Table 9.5). The results from more recent data suggest that the sensitivity is lower (50%–60%), especially in women (Fig. 9.4).

The causes of false positive and false negative exercise

TABLE 9.4 *Pretest Probability of Coronary Artery Disease by Age, Gender, and Symptoms*

Age (y)	Gender	Typical/Definite Angina Pectoris*	Atypical/Probable Angina Pectoris*	Nonanginal Chest Pain*	Asymptomatic*
30–39	Men	Intermediate	Intermediate	Low	Very low
	Women	Intermediate	Very low	Very low	Very low
40–49	Men	High	Intermediate	Intermediate	Low
	Women	Intermediate	Low	Very low	Very low
50–59	Men	High	Intermediate	Intermediate	Low
	Women	Intermediate	Intermediate	Low	Very low
60–69	Men	High	Intermediate	Intermediate	Low
	Women	High	Intermediate	Intermediate	Low

*High indicates > 90%; intermediate 10%–90%; low < 10%; and very low < 5%.
Source: From the ACC/AHA Guidelines [4], with permission.

TABLE 9.5 *Sensitivity and Specificity of Exercise ECG*

	Sensitivity (%)	Specificity (%)
All patients	68	77
No prior MI	67	72
Rest-ST depression	69	70
Digoxin therapy	68	74
LVH	68	69

MI, myocardial infarction; LVH, left ventricular hypertrophy.
Source: From Gibbons et al. [4].

ECGs are not well known [4,21–31], although false negative exercise ECGs are more common in patients with single-vessel disease than in those with less extensive disease. However, false negative results may also be seen in patients with multivessel disease and in patients with objective evidence of ischemia by other tests, such as reversible perfusion defects. We found that patients with CAD and ST-segment depression have larger perfusion abnormality than patients with false negative results. (Fig. 9.5). In general, mild CAD, submaximal exercise, and anti-ischemic cardiac medications may lower the sensitivity. We reported that ST-segment depression is unusual (~10%) in CAD patients with small R-wave amplitude (< 11 mm) [1]. Finally, if the criteria of positive results are made less rigid, the sensitivity may improve, but obviously the specificity will also decrease.

The causes of false positive results are not always clear, though some may be indicative of true ischemia due to microvascular disease, in the absence of large vessel CAD. Patients with left ventricular hypertrophy, digitalis therapy, electrolyte imbalance, WPW, and abnormal baseline electrocardiograms are more likely to

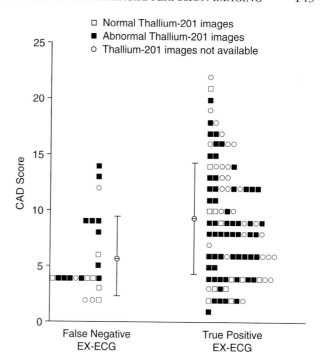

FIGURE 9.5 Comparison of perfusion defect size in CAD patients with true positive versus false negative exercise EKG responses. The patients with true positive responses had larger ischemic burden [1].

have false positive results. One study suggested that incorporation of right precordial leads increased the test sensitivity from 52% to 89% without loss of specificity [32] (Fig. 9.6). These findings could not be confirmed by other investigators [33].

Duke Treadmill Exercise Score

The Duke treadmill exercise score is *derived* as follows: = Exercise Time (minutes) − 5 (ST shift in

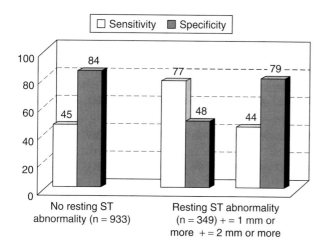

FIGURE 9.4 Results of exercise ECG in patients with and without ST abnormalities at rest. The sensitivity is low regardless of presence or absence of ST depression. (Adapted from Fearon et al. [23].)

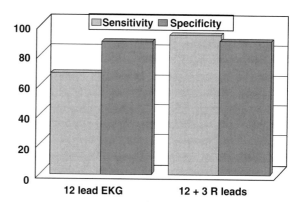

FIGURE 9.6 Sensitivity and specificity of exercise ECG with and without right precordial leads. Sensitivity improves with inclusion of right precordial leads. (Adapted from Michaelides et al. [32].)

mm) − 4 (angina severity) (where 0 denotes angina; 1 mild angina; and 2 limiting angina). The score has been used to detect severe and extensive CAD. In the low-risk group (score > 4), Shaw et al. showed that 60% of patients had no severe stenosis and 16% had one-vessel disease. By comparison, 74% of the high-risk group (score < −10) had three-vessel or left main disease. The 5-year mortality was 3%, 10%, and 35% in the low, intermediate, and high-risk groups [34–41].

ST/Heart Rate Relationship

There are several types of heart rate adjustments of ST depression: The ST-segment/heart rate index, maximal ST-segment/heart rate slope, rate recovery loop, and time recovery loop. The heart rate adjustment of ST depression was reported to be superior to ST-segment depression in detecting CAD and identifying patients who are at high risk. In addition, it was useful in identifying patients with CAD but equivocal for negative ST-segment response. For example, in 150 patients, the sensitivity of the ST-segment/heart rate slope was 95% in men and 82% in women, the slope had 95% sensitivity in men and 93% in women, and the rate recovery was reported to be 90% sensitive in men and 87% in women. These results were better than the sensitivity of 67% in men and 60% in women for ST-segment depression [42–45].

When both the ST-segment/heart rate index and the rate recovery loops were abnormal, the relative risk of cardiac events was 3.6 times higher than when both were negative. When only one of the two indexes was abnormal, the relative risk was 1.9. Other investigators have not found similar results. Lachterman and associates, using the ST-segment/heart rate index, observed a sensitivity of 54% and a specificity of 73%. The corresponding sensitivity of ST-segment analysis at the same specificity was 58% [44]. Bobbio and colleagues in a multicenter European study involving 2270 patients of whom 401 had left main artery or three-vessel disease, reported that the sensitivity of the ST-segment/heart rate index was 78%, and that the sensitivity of the ST-segment analysis alone was 75% at the specificity of 64% [43].

Sex-Related Differences

Several studies show that exercise testing is less accurate in diagnosing CAD in women than in men [28–30,38]. Morise and associates reported a sensitivity of 47% in women versus 56% in men, and a specificity of 73% in women versus 81% in men [30]. When results were analyzed in relation to posttest bias "un-

biased results," the sensitivity in women was only 33% and in men 40%, though the specificity increased to 83% in women and 96% in men [30]. Even in patients with similar prevalence of disease, the positive predictive value of ST-segment depression is significantly higher in men than women (77% versus 47%, $p <$ .05). Prevalence rates of CAD in women with typical angina pectoris and with atypical chest pains are reported to be 72% and 6%, respectively. These rates are lower than in men, which are 93% and 54%, respectively [1]. The difficulty in interpreting the results of these studies is to determine whether the higher rate of false positive ST-segment changes during exercise in women is a true difference or a Bayesian effect. We examined the gender differences in exercise responses in 1035 men and 594 women who underwent symptom-limited treadmill exercise testing with single-photon emission computed tomography (SPECT) perfusion imaging. Men had more frequent ST-segment depression than women (20% versus 16%; $p <$ .05). Men and women were divided into tertiles based on pretest probability of CAD. More men than women in each group had ST-segment depression. Further, with SPECT imaging, reversible defects were also more frequent in men than women in each of the three groups (17% vs 8%, 30% vs 17%, and 56% vs 30%, $p <$ .001 for all differences), respectively. In patients who had coronary angiography, there were no differences between men and women in severity and extent of disease. Women had lower exercise duration (6.4 vs 8.7 minutes, $p <$ .001), lower exercise heart rate ($p <$ .001), and smaller body weight (156 vs 183 lb, $p <$ .001). These results suggest that there are other differences beyond disease prevalence that may affect the exercise responses in women [1].

Other studies have examined the ability of additional criteria for the diagnosis of CAD in women such as R-wave response to exercise, ST-segment/heart rate slope, and QRS score. The results have not been consistently better. Stepwise, logistic analysis is often used to incorporate multiple independent variables available from exercise treadmill testing. A model derived from workload, peak heart rate, and ST-segment depression had a sensitivity (70% vs 59%) and specificity (89% vs 72%) which were higher than ST-segment depression alone. Another model based on ST-segment depression, angina during exercise, and workload had a sensitivity of 44% and a specificity of 90% in women compared to a sensitivity of 59% and a specificity of 77% for ST-segment depression alone. Alexander et al. reported that the Duke treadmill score was useful in diagnostic and prognostic assessment of women as well as men [28].

PROGNOSTIC IMPLICATIONS

The information derived from exercise testing can also be used in risk assessment [46–54]. The markers of poor outcome are listed in Table 9.6. The probability of subsequent angina pectoris or myocardial infarction is likely to be higher in patients with positive tests. Recent data suggest that chronotropic incompetence, delayed heart rate recovery after termination of exercise, and delayed BP recovery are also prognostically important (Fig. 9.7). An exaggerated hypertensive response is not associated with increased mortality [17].

In the Seattle Heart Watch Study of 2365 healthy men (reported by Bruce and colleagues) [47], the predictors of subsequent CAD were chest pain during exercise, duration of exercise below 6 minutes, failure to achieve >90% of maximal predicted heart rate for age, and the presence of ischemic ST-segment depression. The 10 years' experience of the Seattle Heart Watch Study was later reported by Bruce and coworkers, who found that of 3611 men and 547 women who were initially free of clinical heart disease, subsequent cardiac events occurred in 4.9% of patients at a mean follow-up of 6.1 years. The incidence of cardiac events was 2.9% among asymptomatic healthy persons, 5.5% among patients with atypical or nonanginal chest pains, and 10% among hypertensive patients. The presence of any conventional risk factor, in conjunction with two or more selective maximal exercise test predictors, significantly increased the cumulative 6-year incidence rate. Survival, however, correlates better with exercise tolerance than with the degree of ST-segment depression, peak exercise heart rate, or peak blood pressure during exercise. Weiner and associates observed in the Coronary Artery Surgery Study (CASS) study that surgical benefit was greater in patients with ST-segment depression than in patients with poor exercise tolerance. Of the 398 patients with three-vessel disease and the above criteria, the 7-year survival was 58% with medical therapy and 81% with surgical therapy. On

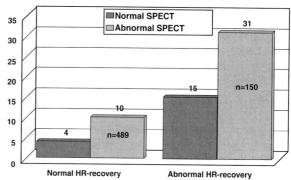

FIGURE 9.7 Estimates of the relative risk of death within six years according to heart-rate recovery one minute after cessation of exercise in relation to pressure of normal or abnormal SPECT images. (Adapted from Cole et al. [45].)

the other hand, no benefit was seen in 1545 patients who were able to exercise into stage 3 or more of the Bruce protocol with no ST-segment changes. In this cohort of patients, ST-segment elevation was more frequent in patients with prior infarction, LV enlargement, and dysfunction. These patients, in general, had poor prognosis [53].

The Duke exercise score has been used to predict the prognosis (Table 9.7). Patients in the high-risk group had a higher cardiac event rate than patients with intermediate or low-risk scores. We examined the coronary arteriographic and perfusion correlates of the Duke score in 834 patients. Based on the score, 369 patients were in the low-risk group, 384 in the moderate-risk group, and 81 in the high-risk group. The extent of CAD was 2.1 ± 1 diseased vessels in the high-risk group, 1.7 ± 1 in the moderate-risk group, and 1.4 ± 1.1 in the low-risk group ($p < .01$). The extent of the perfusion abnormality was greater in the high-risk group. Although the mean CAD score and ischemic burden differed in the various risk groups, considerable overlap was noted [36].

In a recent study based on a multicenter registry, patients with an intermediate score but who had normal exercise perfusion images were found to have an event

TABLE 9.6 *Exercise Testing: Poor Predictors of Outcome*

1. Impaired chronotropic response
2. Abnormal HR recovery (≤ 12 bpm decrease from peak to 1 min)
3. Delayed recovery of SBP (3 min/1 min ratio > 1.0)
4. HR adjusted ST depression
5. Hypotensive response
6. High-risk Duke treadmill score
7. Low workload or exercise time
8. Strongly positive ST response at submaximal exercise

HR, heart rate; SBP, systolic blood pressure.

TABLE 9.7 *Survival According to Risk Groups Based on Duke Treadmill Score*

Risk Group (Score)	% of Total Patients	4-Year Survival	% Annual Mortality
Low (> 4)	62	0.99	0.25
Moderate (−10 to +4)	34	0.95	1.25
High (< −10)	4	0.79	5.0

Source: From Mark et al. [34].

rate of < 1%/year. Other studies used ST/heart rate index and the rate recovery loop to predict events in patients with CAD. Although marked abnormalities predicted future events, most events nevertheless occurred in patients with negative test results, and only 23% of the patients with events were identified by the ST-segment/heart rate index, 15% by the rate recovery loop, and 20% by the ST-segment criteria. Most patients with positive results did not suffer events in the subsequent 4 years.

These data suggest that no single variable consistently predicts prognosis. Independent predictors of cardiac events in patients with stable CAD include the presence of congestive heart failure; Q-wave myocardial infarction; exercise workload; ventricular premature beats; low maximum heart rate; 2 mm or more ST-segment depression; less than 3 stages on the Bruce protocol; angina severity; history of prior infarction; angina during exercise; low maximum BP response; rest ST-segment depression; ST-segment elevation during exercise; heart rate during recovery; and BP during recovery.

EXERCISE TESTING AFTER MYOCARDIAL INFARCTION

Exercise testing is an important element of risk stratification after acute myocardial infarction. It may be done before or after hospital discharge [4]. In addition to its use in risk assessment, it is also useful for exercise prescription in patients enrolled in cardiac rehabilitation programs, and it provides encouragement and assurance to the patients, and their spouses, to return to a normal lifestyle. At the present time, most predischarge exercise tests are done submaximally. The test is terminated at roughly 70% of the maximum predicted heart rate in the absence of other, more serious indications to discontinue the test, such as hypotension, arrhythmias, angina pectoris, or ST-segment shifts.

After discharge (4 to 6 weeks), the exercise is symptom limited. There are pros and cons for using either of these two tests (submaximal and maximal) or a combination of both. The predischarge submaximal study may not identify all patients with potential ischemia, but since most events occur within the first 3 months (especially the first month after infarction), it may, nevertheless, identify those at the highest risk. Postdischarge, symptom-limited exercise may detect more ischemic responses, but events may have occurred between discharge and the time of the exercise study. What is more important is that after infarction, patients who are not candidates for exercise testing are exactly the ones who are at the highest risk for future events.

The role of pharmacologic stress testing is discussed in Chapter 10.

Mortality is often greater in the patients who are unable to perform exercise testing because of cardiac limitation. In those who can exercise, the presence of ST-segment elevation of ≥ 1 mm, inadequate blood pressure response, ventricular premature beats, and inability to exercise beyond stage 1 of the modified Bruce protocol identifies them as high-risk patients in the first year after infarction. If none of these variables is present, the risk is low. Patients who have one or two of the four markers are in the intermediate-risk group [4].

In a meta analysis of published exercise testing studies, the following markers were found to indicate poor prognosis: abnormal blood pressure response to exercise, ventricular premature beats or ventricular tachycardia, a low exercise tolerance, angina pectoris during exercise, and ST-segment depression [4]. Again not a single variable was consistently a predictor of events after acute infarction. These studies also showed a higher event rate after discharge in patients with non-Q-wave infarction than in patients with Q-wave infarction.

SUMMARY

(1) The sensitivity of exercise ECG is suboptimal. (2) The site of ST depression does not localize the site of coronary stenosis. (3) With rare exceptions, the severity of ST depression does not predict severity of CAD. (4) The Duke score is an improvement but most patients fall in the intermediate group. (5) The value of right precordial leads and heart rate adjusted ST depression requires further studies and cannot be recommended for routine use. (6) Other exercise variables such as heart rate response, exercise time, BP response, and symptoms are useful in patient management. The latter point may account for the continued popularity of the test despite its suboptimal performance.

REFERENCES

1. Iskandarian AS. *Nuclear Cardiac Imaging: Principles and Applications* edited by AS Iskandarian. Philadelphia: FA Davis Co., 1986.
2. Iskandarian AS, Heo J. Exaggerated systolic blood pressure response to exercise: a normal variant or a hyperdynamic phase of essential hypertension? Int J Cardiol 1988;18:207.
3. Lauer MS, Levy D, Anderson KM, et al. Is there a relationship between exercise systolic blood pressure response and left ventricular mass? The Framingham Heart Study. Ann Intern Med 1992;116:203.
4. Gibbons RJ, Balady GJ, Beasley JW, et al. ACC/AHA Guidelines for exercise testing: executive summary: a report of the American College of Cardiology/American Heart Association

Task Force on Practice Guidelines (Committee on Exercise Testing). Circulation 1997;96:345.

5. Abouantoun S, Ahnve S, Savvides M, et al. Can areas of myocardial ischemia be localized by the exercise electrocardiogram? A correlative study with thallium-201 scintigraphy. Am Heart J 1984;108:933.

6. Kang X, Berman DS, Lewin HC, et al. Comparative localization of myocardial ischemia by exercise electrocardiography and myocardial perfusion SPECT. J Nucl Cardiol 2000;7:140.

7. Tavel ME, Shaar C. Relation between the electrocardiographic stress test and degree and location of myocardial ischemia. Am J Cardiol 1999;84:119.

8. Weiner DA, Ryan TJ, McCabe CH, et al. ST-segment elevation with exercise: a marker for poor ventricular function and poor prognosis. Coronary Artery Surgery Study (CASS) confirmation of Seattle Heart Watch results. Circulation 1988;77:897.

9. Lee JH, Crump R, Ellestad MH. Significance of precordial T-wave increase during treadmill stress testing. Am J Cardiol 1995;76:1297.

10. Busby MJ, Shefrin EA, Fleq JL. Prevalence and long-term significance of exercise-induced frequent or repetitive ventricular ectopic beats in apparently healthy volunteers. J Am Coll Cardiol 1989;14:1659.

11. Califf RM, McKinnis RA, McNeer JF, et al. Prognostic value of ventricular arrhythmias associated with treadmill exercise testing in patients studied with cardiac catheterization for suspected ischemic heart disease. J Am Coll Cardiol 1983;2:1060.

12. Lehrman KL, Tilkian AG, Hutgren HN. Effect of coronary arterial bypass surgery on exercise-induced ventricular arrhythmias. J Cardiol 1979;44:1056.

13. Schweikert RA, Pashkow FH, Snader CE, et al. Association of exercise-induced ventricular ectopic activity with thallium myocardial perfusion and angiographic coronary artery disease in stable, low-risk populations. Am J Cardiol 1999;83:530.

14. Weiner DA, Ryan TJ, McCabe CH, et al. The role of exercise testing in identifying patients with improved survival after coronary artery bypass surgery. J Am Coll Cardiol 1986;8:741.

15. Bhadha K, Marchlinski F, Iskandrian AS. Ventricular tachycardia in patients without structural heart disease. Am Heart J 1993;126:1194.

16. Jouven X, Zureik M, Desnos M, et al. Long-term outcome in asymptomatic men with exercise-induced premature ventricular depolarizations. N Engl J Med 2000;343:826.

17. Campbell L, Marwick TH, Pashkow FJ, et al. Usefulness of an exaggerated systolic blood pressure response to exercise in predicting myocardial perfusion defects in known or suspected coronary artery disease. Am J Cardiol 1999;84:1304.

18. Hakki A-H, Munley BM, Hadjimiltiades S, et al. Determinants of abnormal blood pressure response to exercise in coronary artery disease. Am J Cardiol 1986;57:71.

19. Go BM, Sheffield D, Krittayaphong R, et al. Association of systolic blood pressure at time of myocardial ischemia with angina pectoris during exercise testing. Am J Cardiol 1997;79:954.

20. Lele SS, Scalia G, Thompson H, et al. Mechanism of exercise hypotension in patients with ischemic heart disease. Role of neuro-cardiogenically mediated vasodilation. Circulation 1994; 90:2701.

21. Do D, West JA, Morise A, et al. An agreement approach to predict severe angiographic coronary artery disease with clinical and exercise test data. Am Heart J 1997;134:672.

22. Elhendy A, van Domburg RT, Bax JJ, et al. The significance of stress-induced ST segment depression in patients with inferior Q wave myocardial infarction. J Am Coll Cardiol 1999;33:1909.

23. Fearon WF, Lee DP, Froelicher VF. The effect of resting ST segment depression on the diagnostic characteristics of the exercise treadmill test. J Am Coll Cardiol 2000,35:1206.

24. Gerber AM, Solomon NA. Cost-effectiveness of alternative test strategies for the diagnosis of coronary artery disease. Ann Intern Med 1999;130:719.

25. Kong B, Heo J, Iskandrian AS. The duration of ST-segment depression as an indicator of the pathophysiology of myocardial ischemia. Am Heart J 1989;118:195.

26. Lachterman B, Lehmann KG, Abrahamson D, et al. "Recovery only" ST segment depression and the predictive accuracy of the exercise test. Ann Intern Med 1990;112:11.

27. Simoons ML, Hugenholtz PG. Gradual changes of ECG waveform during and after exercise in normal subjects. Circulation 1975;52:570.

28. Alexander KP, Shaw LJ, Shaw LK, et al. Value of exercise treadmill testing in women. J Am Coll Cardiol 1998;32:1657.

29. Lauer MS, Pashkow FJ, Snader CE, et al. Sex and diagnostic evaluation of possible coronary artery disease after exercise treadmill testing at one academic teaching center. Am Heart J 1997;134:807.

30. Morise AP, Diamond GA. Comparison of the sensitivity and specificity of exercise electrocardiography in biased and unbiased populations of men and women. Am Heart J 1995;135:741.

31. Colby J, Hakki A-H, Iskandrian As, et al. Hemodynamic angiographic and scintigraphic correlates of positive exercise electrocardiograms: Emphasis on strongly positive exercise of coronary disease. Circulation 1979;59:286.

32. Michaelides AP, Psomadaki ZD, Dilaveris PE, et al. Improved detection of coronary artery disease by exercise electrocardiography with the use of right precordial leads. N Engl J Med 1999;340:340.

33. Bokkari S, Blood DK, Bergmann SR. Failure of right precordial electrocardiography during stress testing to identify coronary artery disease. J Nucl Cardiol 2001,8:325.

34. Mark DM, Shaw L, Harrell FF Jr, et al. Prognostic value of a treadmill exercise score in outpatients with suspected coronary artery disease. N Engl J Med 1991;325:849.

35. Pilote L, Pashkow F, Thomas JD, et al. Clinical yield and cost of exercise treadmill testing to screen for coronary artery disease in asymptomatic adults. Am J Cardiol 1998;81:219.

36. Iskandrian AS, Ghods M, Helfeld H, et al. The treadmill exercise score revisited: coronary arteriographic and thallium perfusion correlates. Am Heart J 1992;124:1581.

37. Shaw LJ, Hachamovitch R, Iskandrian AE. Treadmill test scores: attributes and limitations. J Nucl Cardiol 1997;4:74.

38. Allen WH, Aronow WS, Goodman P, et al. Five-year follow-up of maximal treadmill stress test in asymptomatic men and women. Circulation 1980;62:522.

39. Ho KT, Miller TD, Holmes DR, et al. Long-term prognostic value of Duke treadmill score and exercise thallium-201 imaging performed one to three years after percutaneous transluminal coronary angioplasty. Am J Cardiol 1999;84:1323.

40. Kwok JM, Miller TD, Christian TF, et al. Prognostic value of a treadmill exercise score in symptomatic patients with nonspecific ST-T abnormalities on resting ECG. JAMA 1999;282:1047.

41. Shaw LJ, Peterson ED, Shaw LK, et al. Use of a prognostic treadmill score in identifying diagnostic coronary disease subgroups. Circulation 1998;98:1622.

42. Kligfield P, Ameisen O, Okin PM. Heart rate adjustment of ST segment depression for improved detection of coronary artery disease. Circulation 1989;79:245.

43. Bobbio M, Detrano R, Schmid JJ, et al. Exercise-induced ST depression and ST/heart rate index to predict triple-vessel or left main coronary disease: a multicenter analysis. J Am Coll Cardiol 1992;19:11

44. Lachterman B, Lehmann KG, Detrano R, et al. Comparison of ST segment/heart rate index to standard ST criteria for analysis of exercise and electrocardiograms. Circulation 1990;82:44.

45. Cole CR, Blackstone EH, Pashkow FJ, et al. Heart-rate recovery immediately after exercise as a predictor of mortality. N Engl J Med 1999;341:1351.

46. Gibbons, RJ, Hodge DO, Berman DS, et al. Long-term outcome of patients with intermediate-risk exercise electrocardiograms who do not have myocardial perfusion defects on radionuclide imaging. Circulation 1999;100:2140.

47. Bruce RA, Hossack KF, DeRouen TA, et al. Enhanced risk assessment for primary coronary heart disease events by maximal exercise testing: 10 years experience of Seattle Heart Watch. J Am Coll Cardiol 1983;2:565.

48. Lauer MS, Okin PM, Larson MG, et al. Impaired heart rate response to graded exercise. Prognostic implications of chronotropic incompetence in the Framingham Heart Study. Circulation 1996;93:1520.

49. Lauer MS, Francis GS, Okin PM, et al. Impaired chronotropic response to exercise stress testing as a predictor of mortality. JAMA 1999;281:524.

50. McHam SA, Marwick TH, Pashkow FJ, et al. Delayed systolic blood pressure recovery after graded exercise: an independent correlate of angiographic coronary disease. J Am Coll Cardiol 1999;34:754.

51. Roger VL, Jacobsen SJ, Pellikka PA, et al. Prognostic value of treadmill exercise testing: a population-based study in Olmsted County, Minnesota. Circulation 1998;98:2836.

52. Sox HC, Littenberg B, Garber AM. The role of exercise testing in screening for coronary artery disease. Ann Intern Med 1989;110:456.

53. Weiner DA. Screening for latent coronary artery disease by exercise testing. Circulation 1991;83:1104.

54. Weiner DA, McCabe CH, Ryan TJL. Identification of patients with left main and three-vessel coronary disease with clinical and exercise test variables. Am J Cardiol 1980;46:21.

Part 2

Exercise Myocardial Perfusion Imaging

The number of myocardial perfusion studies has shown a steady ~10% per year growth rate and there is no end in sight. The latest Medicare data show that stress perfusion imaging is used far more frequently than treadmill exercise testing (without imaging), stress echocardiography, and coronary angiography [1] (Table 9.8). This growth rate was predictable and unavoidable once the diagnostic and prognostic values of perfusion imaging were fully established and divulged to the medical community. Exercise myocardial perfusion imaging remains the most popular form of stress nuclear testing accounting for 60%–70% of all stress tests. Most are done with single-photon emission computed tomography (SPECT).

PRINCIPLES AND METHODS

As discussed earlier, peak exercise in normal subjects produces an increase in myocardial oxygen demand, and roughly a threefold increase in myocardial blood flow (MBF). In the presence of coronary stenosis, the MBF is often normal at rest but fails to increase proportionally in response to the increase in demand. The peak MBF is inversely proportional to the degree of stenosis [2] (Fig. 9.8). The variation in regional MBF during stress is the mechanism that is responsible for the production of perfusion defects irrespective of the presence or absence of ischemia. The regional variation in MBF will result in regional variation in tracer concentration. Obviously the relation between MBF and tracer concentration is not linear for several reasons: the reduction in extraction fraction at high flow rates, tracer clearance, attenuation, scatter, partial volume, and depth resolution effects, to mention a few [3].

TABLE 9.8 *Medicare Volume of Cardiac Procedures*

Treadmill exercise tests	689,851
Stress echocardiography	303,047
Stress SPECT	1,158,389
Coronary angiography	664,936

SPECT, single-photon emission computed tomography.
Source: Gibbons et al. [1].

The method of exercise perfusion imaging is simple; the tracer is injected via an indwelling intravenous line and flushed with saline at peak exercise and the patient is asked to continue exercising for 1–2 additional minutes at the same or reduced workload to allow tracer uptake at peak hyperemia. Imaging is subsequently done within 10 minutes with thallium, 30–60 minutes with sestamibi or tetrofosmin, and within 2 minutes with teboroxime.

INDICATIONS

Several ACC/AHA and ASNC guidelines have addressed this topic [1]. The major indications are listed in Table 9.9. Only the diagnostic use is discussed in this chapter. The ACC/AHA guidelines favor treadmill exercise testing alone as "first line" test and reserve imaging for patients in whom the ECG response is not likely to be helpful. These recommendations do not reflect the reality of clinical practice (see Table 9.8). In our institution, a large tertiary referral center, SPECT

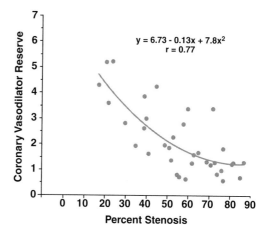

FIGURE 9.8 Relationship between degree of coronary artery stenosis by angiography and myocardial blood flow measured by positron emission tomography (PET). An inverse relation is noted but considerable scatter, especially in moderate stenosis. (Reproduced from Uren et al. [2], with permission.)

151

TABLE 9.9 *Major Indications for Exercise SPECT*

1. Diagnosis of CAD in patients with symptoms
2. Diagnosis of CAD in high-risk asymptomatic patients
3. Determining the physiologic significance of equivocal coronary angiogram
4. Assessment of risk
5. Stable symptoms
6. Acute coronary syndromes
7. Before major noncardiac surgery
8. Assessment of patients after coronary revascularization
9. Assessment of patients with heart failure
10. Assessment of patients with serious arrhythmia or survivors of sudden cardiac death
11. Assessment of effect of therapeutic interventions

TABLE 9.11 *Comparison between SPECT and Treadmill Exercise Testing*

Variable	SPECT	Treadmill
Availability	++	++++
Cost	++++	+
Familiarity	++	++++
Accuracy	+++	+
Localization	++++	+
Extent of disease	++++	+
Viable myocardium	++++	+
LV function	++++	+
Follow-up testing	++++	+
Risk assessment	++++	+

(++++ is better or more than +)

is done ~20 times more frequently than treadmill testing alone. The advantages of SPECT over treadmill testing alone are listed in Tables 9.10 and 9.11.

PERFUSION PATTERNS

How is the site of perfusion abnormality related to coronary anatomy? The left anterior descending artery (LAD) provides blood supply to the anterior wall and anterior two-thirds of the septum; the right coronary artery (RCA) to the inferior wall, part of the posterior wall, and the posterior third of the septum; and the left circumflex artery (LCX) to the lateral wall (Fig. 9.9; see Color Figs. 9.10–9.12 in separate color insert). The LV apex may be nourished by any of the three vessels and hence an apical defect is not helpful in localizing the site of coronary stenosis. Variations of the above themes are common. For example, the RCA may supply the basal part of the lateral wall, the LAD may supply the anterolateral wall, and the LCX may supply the basal parts of the inferior wall [3].

Several studies show that there is considerable variability in the size of the perfusion abnormality in relation to coronary stenosis [4–9]. These observations are consistent regardless of the methods used, which include stress testing, injection of tracer at the time of

TABLE 9.10 *Advantages of SPECT Compared to Treadmill Testing Alone*

1. SPECT has higher sensitivity and diagnostic accuracy
2. SPECT is capable of localizing the site of ischemia and the culprit lesion
3. SPECT can quantify the ischemic burden and the degree of scarring
4. SPECT is a much more powerful tool for risk stratification
5. SPECT provides quantitative indexes of LV size and function

LV, left ventricular.

balloon occlusion during percutaneous transluminal coronary angioplasty (PTCA), and in patients with acute infarction, in whom the tracer is injected before thrombolytic therapy or primary PTCA (during the time when the coronary artery is likely to be occluded). Examples shown in Color Figure 9.13 (in separate color insert) and Fig. 9.14 were obtained with tracer injection at the time of balloon occlusion during PTCA in two patients with LCX stenosis. Based on coronary anatomy, one would have predicted a larger defect in the patient with the dominant LCX shown in Figure 9.13 than in the patient with a marginal disease shown in Figure 9.14, but the opposite was actually observed. The results in patients with CAD undergoing exercise testing are shown in Figures 9.15 and 9.16. The data show: (*1*) the average defect size is larger in patients with isolated LAD than isolated LCX or RCA disease; (*2*) the average defect size is similar in patients with LCX and RCA disease; (*3*) the average defect size is larger in patients with proximal than with distal stenosis and in patients with severe stenosis than with mild stenosis; (*4*) the average defect size is larger in patients with multivessel than one-vessel disease; and (*5*) the perfusion abnormality was smaller in the presence of collaterals. An important observation that should not be overlooked is the considerable scatter and overlap between these values in any of the groups. Further, it was not possible to predict the size of the defect from coronary angiography or by the presence or absence of ST-segment depression or angina [8].

A possible reason for such variations in defect size (which is discussed subsequently) is the function of collateral vessels and the degree of endothelial dysfunction [9–13]. Collaterals (collateral vessels or collateral circulation) are either intercoronary (between a donor and a recipient vessel) or intracoronary (same vessel); jeopardized or nonjeopardized (no stenosis before take off), and subepicardial or subendocardial in location [3].

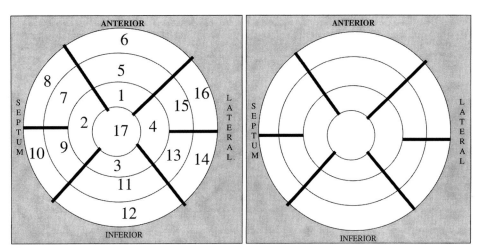

A **Single Photon Emission Computed Tomography (SPECT)**

Planes of the Heart

PERFUSION   :0- absent (<25%);   1- severe (25-49%);   2- moderate (50-60%);
                                     3- mild (60-80%);   4- normal

WALL MOTION: 0- dyskinesia;   1- akinesia;   2- severe hypokinesia;
                      3- mild-moderate hypokinesia; 4- normal

WALL THICKENING: 0- absent;   1- almost absent;   2- severely reduced;
                      3- mild-moderately reduced;   4- normal

FIGURE 9.9 Traditional SPECT projections. (A) Schematic presentation of SPECT images using 17-segment model. (B) Segments 1, 5, 6 = anterior wall (distal, mid, basal); 3, 11, 12 = inferior wall (distal, mid, basal); 2 = distal septum; 4 = distal lateral wall; 7, 8 = anteroseptal (mid, basal);9, 10 = inferoseptal (mid, basal); 13, 14 = inferolateral (mid, basal); 15, 16 = anterolateral (mid, basal); 17 = apex.

They are variable in size and those smaller than 100 microns are not visible by angiography. They are often capable of maintaining resting MBF but are unlikely to augment the MBF high enough to prevent against ischemia during stress. There is evidence also to suggest that the appearance of collaterals on angiography and their size are not reliable predictors of their physiologic role. It is possible that well-functioning collaterals may protect against development of ischemia during less strenuous activity and that regular physical exercise may promote collateral development [12].

SENSITIVITY AND SPECIFICITY

The early data were obtained with planar imaging, which is now rarely used. SPECT imaging improves sensitivity when compared with planar imaging. Most

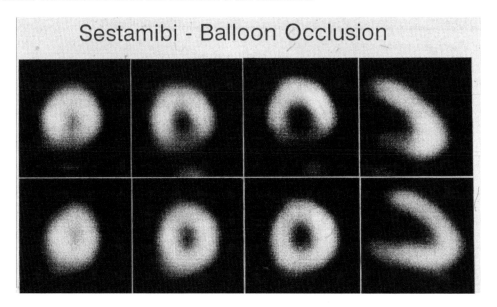

FIGURE 9.14 The same as in Figure 9.11 but in a different patient. The abnormality is smaller than that in Figure 9.13, though by angiography the vessel was larger.

early data were also obtained with thallium and without gating. Gated SPECT imaging with technetium tracers improves specificity. A case in point is the data shown in Figure 9.17, which were obtained in women, using thallium, nongated sestamibi, and gated sestamibi. The specificity increased from 67% to 84% and to 92%, respectively [14]. Artifacts due to patient motion and soft tissue attenuation may have contributed to the lower specificity by SPECT than planar imaging in the early studies.

The average results from exercise planar thallium, SPECT thallium, and SPECT sestamibi are shown in

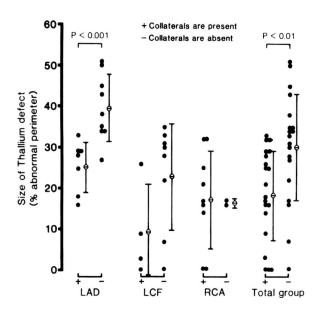

FIGURE 9.15 Variation in size of perfusion abnormality in patients with one-vessel disease. The images were obtained during exercise. (Reproduced from DePace et al. [5], with permission].)

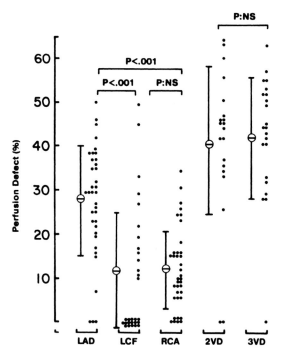

FIGURE 9.16 Variation in size of perfusion abnormality among patients with one-, two-, and three-vessel disease. Format as in Figure 9.15. Considerable variability is noted in each group. (Reproduced from Iskandrian et al. [6], with permission.)

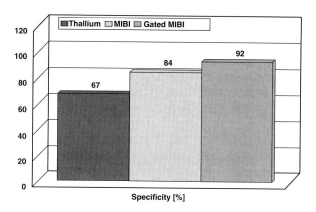

FIGURE 9.17 The specificity of SPECT in women using thallium, non-gated sestamibi, and gated sestamibi. An increase in specificity is evident. (Reproduced from Taillefer et al. [14], with permission.)

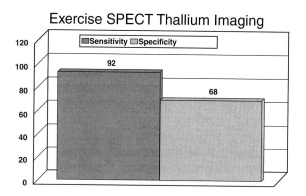

FIGURE 9.19 The average sensitivity and specificity of exercise SPECT thallium in detecting CAD.

Figures 9.18–9.20. The sensitivity by quantitative planar thallium is higher than by visual analysis (91% vs 82%) with similar specificity (89% vs 88%) [3,15,16–31]. The sensitivity by SPECT thallium is 92% and specificity is 68%. The sensitivity and specificity by SPECT sestamibi are 90% and 83%, respectively. The normalcy rates for thallium and sestamibi are 90%–100%, respectively. The results of a meta analysis of many published reports show a sensitivity of 87% and a specificity of 64% [32] (Fig. 9.21). As discussed earlier, normalcy rates are often used as surrogates for specificity because of posttest referral bias, which tends to lower specificity. The sensitivity is higher in three-vessel disease (95%) than one-vessel disease (83%) or two-vessel disease (93%). The results by and large are similar regardless of protocol used (stress–rest, rest–stress, or dual isotope) [33–40]. The

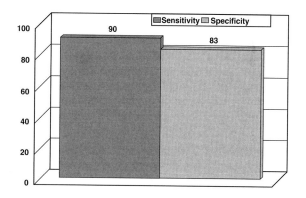

FIGURE 9.20 The average sensitivity and specificity of exercise SPECT sestamibi in detecting CAD.

Planar Thallium-201 Imaging

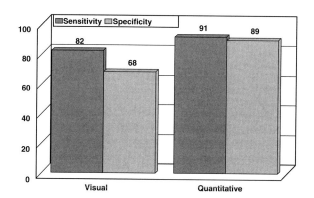

FIGURE 9.18 The average results of sensitivity and specificity by visual and quantitative planar thallium imaging.

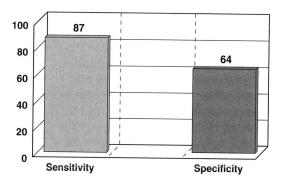

FIGURE 9.21 Meta analysis of 44 perfusion studies regardless of method or tracer [32].

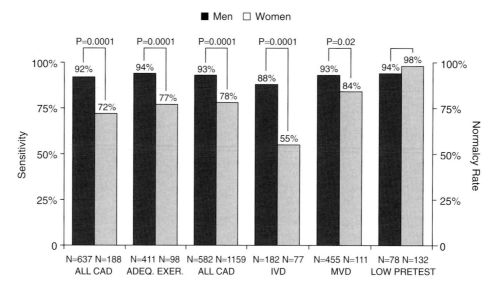

FIGURE 9.22 The results of exercise SPECT perfusion imaging in men and women according to the extent of CAD. The sensitivity is lower in women. (Reproduced from Iskandrian et al. [43], with permission.)

sensitivity is lower in women than men, especially in patients with one-vessel disease [14,17,41–45] (Fig. 9.22). This difference may be due in part to smaller heart size.

Hansen et al. reported that the area under the receiver operating characteristics (ROC) curve was 0.85 in small hearts and 0.92 in normal-sized hearts, regardless of gender [43,44]. This issue is discussed further in Chapter 13. The factors that may increase sensitivity are listed in Table 9.12 and those that may decrease sensitivity in Table 9.13. Submaximal exercise tends to lower sensitivity, underestimate the presence or extent of ischemia, and affect the ability to identify patients with multivessel disease [45–50]. The results of a study from our group regarding the importance of submaximal versus maximal exercise are shown in Figure 9.23 [47].

Gated SPECT improves specificity and decreases the number of nondiagnostic results (more on that in Chapter 8) [51,52]. In one study, which used a high-dose, 2-day sestamibi protocol, the perfusion pattern was ex-

amined on end-diastolic gated images [41]. The sensitivity (84% versus 74%) and the number of reversible defects increased with gating (173 versus 106). These observations are preliminary and evaluation of perfusion on end-diastolic images cannot be recommended at this time.

Attenuation, scatter, and depth resolution compensation have been shown to increase specificity and in one center to improve sensitivity as well (more on this in Chapter 7).

The specificity may be affected by several factors (Table 9.14). Not all false positive scans are "false," as ischemia due to microvascular disease may be present despite normal epicardial arteries. Thus, it may be important to divide the false positive scans into those of a technical nature and those due to true ischemia [53–56].

The sensitivity and specificity for detecting individual diseased vessels vary between 60% and 90% in dif-

TABLE 9.12 *Factors that May Increase Sensitivity*

1. Prior myocardial infarction
2. Multivessel disease
3. Severe stenosis
4. Proximal stenosis
5. Maximal exercise
6. High-quality images
7. Experience
8. Quantitative analysis

TABLE 9.13 *Factors that May Lower Sensitivity*

1. No prior myocardial infarction
2. Female gender
3. Small heart
4. Submaximal exercise
5. One-vessel or branch disease
6. Distal stenosis
7. Mild stenosis
8. Anti-ischemic medications
9. Poor-quality images
10. Lack of experience
11. Visual analysis

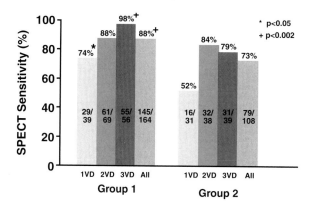

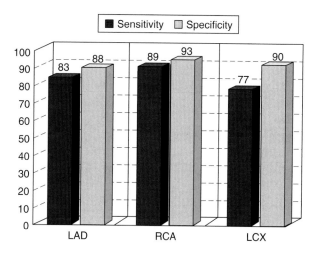

FIGURE 9.23 The results of exercise SPECT thallium in relation to the intensity of exercise. The sensitivity is lower at submaximal exercise (Group 2) than maximal exercise (Group 1). VD = vessel disease.) (Reproduced from Iskandrian et al. [47], with permission.)

FIGURE 9.24 The average results of SPECT imaging in detecting disease in individual diseased vessels. (LAD = left anterior descending artery; RCA = right coronary artery; LCX = left circumflex artery.) (Reproduced from Mahmarian et al. [25], with permission.)

ferent reports, and such variation may be explained on the basis of prior MI, severity of stenosis, site of stenosis, collaterals, level of exercise, visual versus quantitative analysis, quality of images, reader's experience, termination of exercise because of ischemia in only the vessel with the most severe stenosis, variation in coronary anatomy, and difficulty in assigning the appropriate vascular territory. For example, an abnormality in inferior and inferolateral walls is assumed to be due to RCA disease rather than RCA and LCX disease. As a rule of thumb, an abnormality that involves more than one-half of two vascular territories should be assumed to reflect disease in two vascular territories rather than an extension of the abnormality from a single territory (Fig. 9.24).

TABLE 9.14 *Factors that Lower Specificity**

1. Poor-quality images
2. Obesity
3. Artifacts
4. Misinterpretation of images
5. Misinterpretation of coronary angiograms
6. Lack of gating
7. Coronary artery spasm
8. Myocardial bridging
9. Hypertrophic cardiomyopathy
10. Left bundle branch block
11. Pacemaker rhythm
12. Spontaneous coronary artery dissection
13. Clot formation and spontaneous lysis
14. Endothelial dysfunction
15. Congenital coronary anomalies
16. Vasculitis
17. Infiltrative disorders of the myocardium

* Some of these factors cause true ischemia even though the coronary angiogram is normal. Therefore, they are not false positives.

MODERATE CORONARY STENOSIS

As shown in Figure 9.8, the peak MBF and coronary flow reserve (ratio of peak MBF/resting MBF) vary considerably in patients with moderate stenosis (40%–70% diameter stenosis). The reasons are not clear but multiple factors can be invoked (Table 9.15). Because of this variation, one should not expect to see a perfusion abnormality in all vessels with moderate stenosis. In several studies, a very good relationship between the results of SPECT and MBF has been found, which was far better than the relationship between SPECT and coronary angiography (% diameter stenosis) [54,56]. This fact again emphasizes that perfusion imaging is a physiologic measurement and one should not expect that it would correlate very well with coronary angiography. Nishioka et al. observed a good correlation between intravascular ultrasound imaging and SPECT imaging, with a sensitivity of 80% and a specificity of 90% (for the ultrasound method) [53]. In this study, the authors used SPECT as the gold-standard to compare the results of ultrasound imaging.

There are limited data to recommend the "ideal"

TABLE 9.15 *Reasons for Variability in Myocardial Blood Flow in Moderate Coronary Stenosis*

. Underestimation of severity because of focal stenosis superimposed upon diffuse disease
. Errors in measurement due to eccentricity or overlap
. Vasomotor changes during exercise
. Endothelial dysfunction downstream
. Multiple lesions in series

tracer or protocol for detecting moderate stenosis. Based on physiologic principles of MBF and tracer kinetics, one can conclude that tracers with higher first-pass extraction (teboroxime, NOET, or thallium) are better than sestamibi or tetrofosmin; vasodilator imaging is better than exercise, and a stress–rest protocol is better than rest–stress protocol. These assumptions have not been clinically tested, because patients with moderate stenosis or vessels with moderate stenosis are often lumped together with more severe stenosis and their unique features are lost in the pool data analysis. Proper identification of such vessels has more than theoretical advantages, as these moderate lesions may be more likely to fissure and rupture causing acute coronary syndromes. Moreover, they are more likely to undergo regression with appropriate therapy than the more advanced lesions.

One of our challenges in the future will be to try to distinguish between perfusion defects due to abnormal MBF on the basis of a hemodynamically significant coronary stenosis and those due to endothelial dysfunction superimposed on a borderline lesion. In the catheterization laboratory, this could be done by measuring the fractional flow reserve (FFR), which is the ratio of the distal to proximal coronary pressure measured during adenosine-induced hyperemia. Pijls et al. reported that an FFR < 0.75 is associated with evidence of ischemia by noninvasive testing. This index, therefore, is a useful marker of the functional severity of coronary stenosis [55]. Clearly, endothelial dysfunction or microvascular disease may produce myocardial ischemia due to impairment of MBF. This is due to deficiency in nitric oxide, which has been demonstrated in many groups of patients with CAD risk factors, such as diabetes, hyperlipidemia, hypertension, smoking, and family history of premature atherosclerosis. Recent data also show that such patients are also at increased risk for cardiovascular events.

LEFT MAIN/THREE-VESSEL CAD

There are two main issues in patients with left main/three-vessel CAD. First, is it possible that "diffuse ischemia" could produce normal images? While this is a possibility, it is a rare cause of false negative SPECT. As mentioned earlier, the sensitivity is higher in three-vessel than one-vessel CAD. The reason for this rarity is that the physiologic significance of stenoses is unlikely to be identical even though the percentage stenosis appears similar in different vessels. A rare exception is the patient with isolated left main stenosis with left dominant circulation. In these patients other

markers of severe ischemia may be present, such as the presence of poststress stunning; transient left ventricular dilatation; increased tracer lung uptake; ischemic ST-segment changes; hypotensive blood pressure response; and angina [57–64]. Second, how often is the presence of left main/three-vessel disease correctly identified? There is no specific pattern for left main disease on SPECT; though one would argue that the presence of LAD and LCX abnormality, especially at a low workload, could raise the suspicion of left main disease. It is unlikely that a perfusion abnormality would be detected in all three vascular territories in all or most patients with three-vessel disease for the reasons discussed earlier, but roughly two-thirds of these patients will have a perfusion abnormality in more than one vascular territory. In our study, which used a multivariable analysis model in a large group of patients, three variables were the most important predictors of left main/three-vessel disease [63]. These were the presence of a perfusion abnormality in more than one vascular territory, exercise workload, and ST-segment depression. Clearly, the presence of a single vascular abnormality at submaximal exercise cannot rule out extensive CAD. Kwok et al. found four clinical and exercise variables to be predictors of left main/three-vessel disease among patients with a single perfusion abnormality history of diabetes or hypertension, magnitude of ST-segment depression, and low exercise double product [64]. It should be noted, however, that the outcome of all patients with left main/three-vessel disease is not the same, and therefore those with limited ischemia may be at low risk for future events. One should distinguish between the ability to diagnose versus predict outcome in left main/three-vessel CAD, as the criteria are different. A large abnormality in one vascular territory predicts a poor outcome regardless of extent of CAD by angiography.

OTHER SUBGROUPS

There is no reason to suspect that left ventricular hypertrophy (LVH), either by ECG (which is insensitive) or by two-dimensional echocardiography, affects the results of exercise SPECT in detecting CAD, although LVH itself increases the risk for cardiac events. In one study, the sensitivity was 84% and the specificity 82% in 200 patients with echocardiographic evidence of LVH [30].

There are limited data on patients with diabetes, but in one study the results were similar in those with and without diabetes (sensitivity 90% and specificity 50%). It is possible, however, that diabetic patients, especially those with a long history and those with evidence of neuropathy, retinopathy, or nephropathy, are more likely to have microvascular disease or diffuse large-vessel disease that may cause false positive results. It is also possible that these patients may have exercise limitations and, therefore, may have false negative results because of submaximal stress [29].

Patients with LBBB and pacemaker rhythms may have septal reversible defects related to the conduction abnormality in the absence of LAD disease in ~40% of patients. The perfusion abnormality is the result of a reduction in diastolic flow in the LAD. These patients should be studied with vasodilator imaging, as discussed in Chapter 10. Other conduction abnormalities do not affect the results of imaging. Similarly, the stress SPECT results are not different in patients with, compared to those without, mitral valve prolapse; breast attenuation artifacts should not be confused with true defects, as mitral valve prolapse is more common in women than men [65–68].

SIZE (EXTENT) VERSUS SEVERITY OF DEFECT

Size and severity defect are not the same; a defect may be large (involves multiple segments or a large area) but of mild degree (tracer activity > 70% of normal segment), moderate degree (50%–70% activity), or severe degree (< 50% activity). Conversely, a small defect (involving a small area of the myocardium) may be mild, moderate, or severe. The severity reflects the degree of flow disparity, which in turn is a reflection of stenosis severity, while the extent reflects the area at risk, which is a reflection of the vascular distribution. In several outcome studies, these two variables are combined and called summed stress score. In our opinion, the extent is more important than severity in patient outcome.

PATIENTS WITH NORMAL BASELINE ELECTROCARDIOGRAMS

The Mayo Clinic investigators suggested that in patients with normal baseline ECGs, treadmill exercise testing alone provides comparable diagnostic and prognostic data to exercise SPECT [18]. Our results are different (Fig. 9.25) [69]. In our experience, the sensitivity of SPECT was significantly higher than that of ST-segment changes. It is possible that in patients with a low pretest probability of CAD, the two methods provide similar data. In patients with intermediate or high pretest probability of CAD, the data favor SPECT over

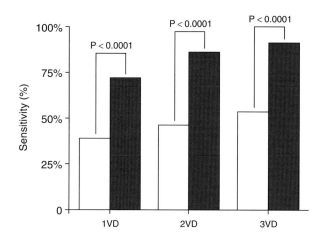

FIGURE 9.25 The results of exercise ST changes and SPECT imaging in patients with normal resting electrocardiograms. SPECT is more sensitive. (Reproduced from Nallamothu et al. [69], with permission.)

ST-segment shifts in terms of diagnosis. A recent study showed that exercise SPECT is cost-effective in patients with normal resting electrocardiograms who have intermediate or high pre-test probability of CAD [69a].

ADDITIONAL FINDINGS ON SPECT

Transient left ventricular dilatation, increased lung uptake, poststress stunning, regional and global left ventricular dysfunction, right ventricular dilatation, hypertrophy and dysfunction, and localized extracardiac masses such as lung tumors, breast tumors, and axillary nodes may be found on SPECT [38,70–73]. Transient ischemic dilatation (TID) refers to a larger left ventricular cavity on the tomographic slices of the post-exercise images, compared to rest images. The presence of TID can be assessed visually or by automated quantitative methods based on volume measurements of the summed images. In dual-isotope imaging, the upper limit of normal is 1.22; it is less (~1.1) in stress–rest sestamibi or tetrofosmin imaging [34]. TID is often associated with reversible (ischemic) defects and suggests extensive ischemia and multivessel CAD. It is also a marker of poor outcome.

Mazzanti et al. showed that the presence of TID had a sensitivity of 71% and a specificity of 95% in predicting severe and extensive CAD [60]. Occasionally TID is an isolated finding and as such does not have serious implications. The reason TID may be observed in patients without large-vessel CAD is not clear but may be due to differences in fluid balance (which affect left ventricular volume) and variations in image acquisition or reconstruction, for example, acquiring the stress and rest images on two different gamma cameras, or variation in the radius of rotation of the detectors. It is possible that microvascular disease may produce subendocardial ischemia and TID in some patients.

TID should be distinguished from persistent or fixed left ventricular dilatation, which in patients with CAD implies poor left ventricular function. Left ventricular dilatation may also be due to mitral or aortic regurgitation, dilated cardiomyopathy, or obesity. The left ventricular size increases in proportion to the body surface area, especially in men, and therefore it is important to index the left ventricular size to the body surface area. The ability to gate the SPECT images and measure ejection fraction is very helpful in obese patients in whom the dilatation could be physiological rather than pathological.

Poststress stunning, which occurs in about 15% of patients with CAD, is defined as wall motion/thickening abnormality that is present in poststress images but not in rest images. This implies a severe stenosis and severe ischemia that persist 30–60 minutes after the termination of stress (when the gated SPECT images are obtained). The poststress ejection fraction may or may not be lower than the rest ejection fraction, as the difference depends on the size of the abnormality and any compensatory hyperkinesia in the remote zones. To demonstrate stunning requires gating both the rest and stress images, which we strongly recommend.

Increased lung tracer uptake was originally described with Tl-201. Similar to TID, increased lung tracer uptake can be assessed visually or by resting automated quantitative methods based on separate regions of interest [72]. Increased lung thallium uptake signifies elevated left ventricular filling pressure, which can be caused by a large area of ischemia or severe left ventricular systolic dysfunction. In the absence of perfusion defects and LV elevated filling pressure due to left ventricular dysfunction, it may represent left ventricular hypertrophy, hypertension (such as due to aortic stenosis, hypertrophic cardiomyopathy), restrictive cardiomyopathy, or mitral stenosis. Increased lung thallium uptake is not seen in patients with chronic obstructive lung disease.

The meaning of lung uptake of sestamibi and tetrofosmin is less clear, as a mild increase is not unusual in normal subjects; a marked increase (lung/heart ratio > 60%) is, on the other hand, useful and provides data comparable to thallium [33]. In one study a lung-to-heart ratio of sestamibi images obtained during exercise > 44% yielded a sensitivity of 63% and a specificity of 81% for severe and extensive CAD [50]. Traditionally, a ratio > 0.50 is considered abnormal. TID and lung uptake, though indirect markers of tran-

sient or persistent left ventricular dysfunction in most patients, do not often occur together in the same patient. Both have been noted to add incremental value to the ability of SPECT to identify patients with more extensive CAD or those at high risk, although their independent value is much less powerful than the perfusion pattern by SPECT.

OTHER TRACERS

Tc-99m-teboroxime was approved by the Food and Drug Administration but was subsequently withdrawn from the market. It is again undergoing trials. Early experience identified two problems with teboroxime imaging: rapid myocardial clearance and high liver activity. Despite these problems, however, several studies, including a multicenter trial, showed good agreement (80–86%) between stress–rest teboroxime and stress–redistribution Tl-201 images [74,75]. There are recent innovative methods to correct the high liver activity. If successful, and combined with attenuation and scatter correction, adenosine-teboroxime imaging may emerge as a useful, rapid imaging protocol for assessment of myocardial ischemia [74,75].

Tc-99m-furifosmin has not yet received FDA approval even though a multicenter trial showed good concordance with Tl-201 and the image quality was quite acceptable [76].

Tc-99m-N-NOET is currently undergoing a large multicenter trial in the United States. This tracer has unique features of being a technetium tracer (like sestamibi and tetrofosmin) but it shows redistribution at 4 hours (like Tl-201) [77,78].

VISUAL VERSUS QUANTITATIVE ANALYSIS

We recommend using both visual and quantitative analysis because quantitative analysis (using raw and normal database polar maps) improves accuracy and reproducibility but cannot correct for artifacts or marked variations in body habitus. Quantitation also allows for a more meaningful report (see Chapter 24). The results with tetrofosmin are comparable in general to sestamibi [79–82].

SUMMARY

Exercise SPECT perfusion imaging is highly reliable in detecting CAD and extensive CAD, provided that patients achieve an adequate exercise level and appropriate imaging protocols are used. These include gating the perfusion images and using a combination of visual and quantitative methods to interpret the images. Not only is there substantial variability in the ischemic burden in relation to coronary angiography but also one needs to keep in mind the many factors that affect sensitivity and specificity of myocardial perfusion imaging.

REFERENCES

1. Gibbons RJ, Chatterjee K, Dailey J, et al. ACC/AHA Guidelines for the management of patients with chronic stable angina. J Am Coll Cardiol 1999;33:2098.
2. Uren NG, Melin JA, DeBruyne B, et al. Relation between myocardial blood flow and the severity of coronary-artery stenosis. N Engl J Med 1994;330:1782.
3. Iskandrian AE, Verani MS (eds). *Nuclear Cardiac Imaging: Principles and Applications*, 2nd Edition. Philadelphia: FA Davis Publishing Co., 1996.
4. DePace NL, Iskandrian AS, Hakki A-H, et al. One-vessel coronary artery disease: anatomic functional, and prognostic considerations. Arch Intern Med 1984;144:1233.
5. DePace NL, Iskandrian AS, Nadell R, et al. Variation in size of jeopardized myocardium in patients with isolated left anterior descending artery disease. Circulation 1983;67:988.
6. Iskandrian AS, Hakki AH, Segal BL, et al. Assessment of the myocardial perfusion pattern in patients with multivessel coronary artery disease. Am Heart J 1983;106:1089.
7. Iskandrian AS, Lichtenberg R, Segal BL, et al. Assessment of jeopardized myocardium in patients with one-vessel disease. Circulation 1982;65:242.
8. Mahmarian JJ, Pratt CM, Verani MS, et al. Altered myocardial perfusion in patients with angina pectoris or silent ischemia during exercise as assessed by quantitative thalium-201 single-photon emission computed tomography. Circulation 1990;82:1305.
9. Mahmarian JJ, Pratt CM, Boyce T, et al. The variable extent of jeopardized myocardium in patients with single vessel coronary artery disease: quantification by thallium-201 single-photon emission computed tomography. J Am Coll Cardiol 1991;17:355.
10. Gould KL. Coronary collateral function assessed by PET. In: Coronary Artery Stenosis: A Textbook of Coronary Pathophysiology, Quantitative Coronary Angiography, Perfusion Imaging and Reversal of Coronary Artery Disease, edited by KL Gould. New York: Elsevier Science Publishing Co., 1991, p. 169.
11. Hurrell DG, Nobrega TP, Christian TF, et al. Reversible perfusion defects on exercise tomographic thallium imaging in patients with and without collateral flow. Am J Cardiol 1998;82:234.
12. Niebauer J, Hambrecht R, Marburger C, et al. Impact of intensive physical exercise and low-fat diet on collateral vessel formation in stable angina pectoris and angiographically confirmed coronary artery disease. Am J Cardiol 1995;76:771.
13. Sand NPR, Rehling M, Bagger JP, et al. Functional significance of recruitable collaterals during temporary coronary occlusion evaluated by Tc-99m sestamibi SPECT. J Am Coll Cardiol 2000;35:624.
14. Taillefer R, DePuey EG, Udelson JE, et al. Comparative diagnostic accuracy of Tl-201 and Tc-99m sestamibi SPECT imaging (perfusion and ECG-gated SPECT) in detecting coronary artery disease in women. J Am Coll Cardiol. 1997;29:69.
15. Beller GA, Zaret BL. Contributions of nuclear cardiology to diagnosis and prognosis of patients with coronary artery disease. Circulation 200;101:1465.
16. Heo J, Iskandrian AS. Technetium-labeled myocardial perfusion agents. Cardiol Clin 1994;12:187.
17. Santana-Boado C, Candell-Riera J, Castell-Conesa J, et al. Diagnostic accuracy of technetium-99m-MIBI myocardial SPECT in women and men. J Nucl Med 1998;39:751.
18. Christian TF, Miller TD, Bailey KR, et al. Exercise thallium-201 tomographic imaging in patients with severe coronary artery disease and normal electrocardiograms. Ann Intern Med 1994:121:825.
19. Iskandrian AS, Heo J, Long B, et al. Use of technetium 99-m isonitrile (RP-30A) in assessing left ventricular perfusion and function at rest and during exercise in coronary artery disease and comparison with coronary arteriography and exercise thallium-201 SPECT imaging. Am J Cardiol 1989;64:270.
20. Iskandrian AS, Hakki AH. Thallium-201 myocardial scintigraphy. Am Heart J 1985;109:113.
21. Iskandrian AS, Haaz W, Segal BL. Exercise thallium-201 imaging: clinical implications of normal exercise images. Arch Intern Med 1981;141:501.
22. Kaul S, Boucher CA, Newell JB, et al. Determination of the quantitative thallium imaging variables that optimize detection of coronary artery disease. J Am Coll Cardiol 1986;7:527.
23. Kang X, Berman DS, Lewin H, et al. Comparative ability of myocardial perfusion single-photon emission computed tomography to detect coronary artery disease in patients with and without diabetes mellitus. Am Heart J 1999;137:949.
24. Maddahi J, VanTrain K, Prigent F, et al. Quantitative single photon emission computed thallium-201 tomography for detection and localization of coronary artery disease: optimization and prospective validation of a new technique. J Am Coll Cardiol 1989;14:1689.
25. Mahmarian JJ, Boyce TM, Goldberg RK, et al. Quantitative exercise thallium-201 single-photon emission computed tomography for the enhanced diagnosis of ischemic heart disease. J Am Coll Cardiol 1990;15:318.
26. Mahmarian JJ. State of the art for coronary artery disease detection: thallium-201. In: *Nuclear Cardiology: State of the Art and Future Directions*, 2nd Edition, edited by BL Zaret and GA Beller. St Louis: Mosby, 1999, pp. 237–272.
27. Morise AP, Diamond GA, Detrano R, et al. Incremental value of exercise electrocardiography and thallium-201 testing in men and women for the presence and extent of coronary artery disease. Am Heart J 1995;135:267.
28. Santoro GM, Sciagra R, Buonamici P, et al. Head-to-head comparison of exercise stress testing, pharmacologic stress echocardiography, and perfusion tomography as first-line examination for chest pain in patients without history of coronary artery disease. J Nucl Cardiol 1998;5:19.
29. Van Train KF, Maddahi J, Berman DS, et al. Quantitative analysis of tomographic stress thallium-201 myocardial scintigrams: a multicenter trial. J Nucl Med 1990;31:1168.
30. Vaduganathan P, He ZX, Mahmarian JJ, et al. Diagnostic accuracy of stress thallium-201 tomography in patients with left ventricular hypertrophy. Am J Cardiol 1998;81:1205.
31. DePuey EG, Garcia EV. Optimal specificity of thallium-201 SPECT through recognition of imaging artifacts. J Nucl Med 1989;30:441.
32. Fleischmann KE, Hunink MG, Kuntz KM, et al. Exercise echocardiography or exercise SPECT imaging? A meta-analysis of diagnostic test performance. JAMA 1998;280:913.
33. Van Train KF, Areeda J, Gercia EV, et al. Quantitative same-day rest-stress technetium-99m sestamibi SPECT: definition and

validation of stress normal limits and criteria for abnormality. J Nucl Med 1993;34:1494.

34. Berman DS, Kiat H, Friedman JD, et al. Separate acquisition rest thallium-201/stress technetium-99m sestamibi dual-isotope myocardial perfusion single-photon emission computed tomography: a clinical validation study. J Am Coll Cardiol 1993;22:1455.

35. DePasquale EE, Nody AC, DePuey EG, et al. Quantitative rotational thallium-201 tomography for identifying and localizing coronary artery disease. Circulation 1988;77:316.

36. Fox RM, Hakki AH, Iskandrian AS, et al. Relation between electrocardiographic and scintigraphic location of myocardial ischemia during exercise in one-vessel coronary artery disease. Am J Cardiol 1984;53:1529.

37. Hakki AH, DePace NL, Colby J, et al. Implications of normal exercise electrocardiograms in patients with angiographically documented coronary artery disease: correlation with left ventricular function and myocardial perfusion. Am J Med 1983;75:439.

38. Morise AP. An incremental evaluation of the diagnostic value of thallium single-photon emission computed tomographic imaging and lung/heart ratio concerning both the presence and extent of coronary artery disease. J Nucl Cardiol 1995;2:238.

39. Borges-Neto S, Shaw LJ, Kesler KL, et al. Prediction of severe coronary artery disease by combined rest and exercise radionuclide angiocardiography and tomographic perfusion imaging with technetium 99m-labeled sestamibi: a comparison with clinical and electrocardiographic data. J Nucl Cardiol 1997;4:189.

40. Levine MG, Ahlberg AW, Mann A, et al. Comparison of exercise, dipyridamole, adenosine, and dobutamine stress with the use of Tc-99m tetrofosmin tomographic imaging. J Nucl Cardiol 1999;6:389.

41. Taillefer R, DePuey EG, Udelson JE, et al. Comparison between the end-diastolic images and the summed images of gated 99mTc-sestamibi. J Nucl Cardiol 1999;6:169.

42. Friedman TD, Greene AC, Iskandrian AS, et al. Exercise thallium-201 myocardial scintigraphy in women: correlation with coronary arteriography. Am J Cardiol 1982;49:1632.

43. Iskandrian AE, Heo J, Nallamothu N. Detection of coronary artery disease in women with use of stress single-photon emission computed tomography myocardial imaging. J Nucl Cardiol 1997;4:329.

44. Hansen CL, Kramer M, Rastogi A. Lower accuracy of Tl-201 SPECT in women is not improved by size-based normal databases or Wiener filtering. J Nucl Cardiol 1999;6:177.

45. Hakki AH, Iskandrian AS, Colby J, et al. Similarity between women and men in manifestation of myocardial ischemia during exercise. Int J Cardiol 1984;5:721.

46. Iskandrian AS, Segal BL. Value of exercise thallium-201 imaging in patients with diagnostic and nondiagnostic exercise electrocardiograms. Am J Cardiol 1981;48:233.

47. Iskandrian AS, Heo J, Kong B, et al. Effect of exercise level on the ability of thallium-201 tomographic imaging in detecting coronary artery disease: analysis of 461 patients. J Am Coll Cardiol 1989;14:1477.

48. Heller GV, Ahemd I, Tilkemeier PL, et al. Comparison of chest pain, electrocardiographic changes and thallium-201 scintigraphy during varying exercise intensities in men with stable angina pectoris. Am J Cardiol 1991;68:569.

49. Esquivel L, Pollock SG, Beller GA, et al. Effect of the degree of effort on the sensitivity of the exercise thallium-201 stress test in symptomatic coronary artery disease. Am J Cardiol 1982;49:733.

50. Maddahi J, Kiat H, Friedman JD, et al. Technetium-99m-sestamibi myocardial perfusion imaging for evaluation of coronary artery disease. In: Nuclear Cardiology—State of the Art and Future Directions, edited by BL Zaret and GA Beller. St. Louis: CV Mosby, 1993, p 191.

51. Smanio PEP, Watson DD, Segalla DL, et al. Value of gating of technetium-99m sestamibi single-photon emission computed tomographic imaging. J Am Coll Cardiol 1997;30:1687.

52. Wackers FJT, Maniawski P, Sinusas AJ. Evaluation of left ventricular regional wall function by ECG-gated technetium-99m sestamibi imaging. In: Nuclear Cardiology—State of the Art and Future Directions, edited by BL Saret and GA Beller. St Louis: CV Mosby, 1993, p 216.

53. Nishioka T, Amanullah AM, Luo H, et al. Clinical validation of intravascular ultrasound imaging for assessment of coronary stenosis severity: comparison with stress myocardial perfusion imaging. J Am Coll Cardiol 1999;33:1870.

54. White CW, Wright CG, Doty DB, et al. Does visual interpretation of the coronary arteriogram predict the physiologic importance of a coronary stenosis? N Engl J Med 1984;310:819.

55. Pijls NHJ, DeBruyne B, Peels K, et al. Measurement of fractional flow reserve to assess the functional severity of coronary artery stenosis. N Engl J Med 1996;334:1703.

56. Miller DD, Donohue TJ, Younis LT, et al. Correlation of pharmacological Tc-99m sestamibi myocardial perfusion imaging with post-stenotic coronary flow reserve in patients with angiographically intermediate coronary artery stenosis. Circulation 1994;89:2150.

57. Bacher-Stier C, Sharir T, Kavanagh PB, et al. Post-exercise lung uptake of Tc-99m sestamibi determined by a new automatic technique: validation and application in detection of severe and extensive coronary artery disease and reduced left ventricular function. J Nucl Med 2000;41:1190.

58. Iskandrian AS, Chae SC, Heo J, et al. Independent and incremental prognostic value of exercise single-photon emission computed tomographic (SPECT) thallium imaging in coronary artery disease. J Am Coll Cardiol 1993;22:665.

59. Maddahi J, Abdulla A, Garcia EV, et al. Noninvasive identification of left main and triple vessel coronary artery disease: improved accuracy using quantitative analysis of regional myocardial stress redistribution and washout of thallium-201. J Am Coll Cardiol 1986;7:53.

60. Mazzanti M, Germano G, Kiat H, et al. Identification of severe and extensive coronary artery disease by automatic measurement of transient dilation of the left ventricle in dual isotope myocardial perfusion SPECT. J Am Coll Cardiol 1996;27:1612.

61. Chae SC, Heo J, Iskandrian AS, et al. Identification of extensive coronary artery disease in women by exercise single-photon emission computed tomography (SPECT) thallium imaging. J Am Coll Cardiol 1993;21:1305.

62. Christian TF, Miller TD, Bailey KR, et al. Noninvasive identification of severe coronary artery disease using exercise tomographic thallium-201 imaging. Am J Cardiol 1991;70:14.

63. Iskandrian AS, Heo J, Lemlek J, et al. Identification of high risk patients with left main and three-vessel coronary artery disease using stepwise discriminant analysis of clinical exercise and tomographic thallium data. Am Heart J 1993;125:221.

64. Kwok JM, Christian TF, Miller TD, et al. Identification of severe coronary artery disease in patients with a single abnormal coronary territory on exercise thallium-201 imaging: the importance of clinical and exercise variables. J Am Coll Cardiol 2000;35:335.

65. Ono S, Mohara R, Kambara H, et al. Regional myocardial per-

fusion and glucose metabolism in experimental left bundle branch block. Circulation 1992;85:1125.

66. DePuey EG, Guertler-Krawczynska E, et al. Thallium-201 SPECT in coronary artery disease patients with left bundle branch block. J Nucl Med 1988;29:1479.

67. Burns RJ, Galligan L, Wright LM, et al. Improved specificity of myocardial thallium-201 single-photon emission computed tomography in patients with left bundle branch block by dipyridamole. Am J Cardiol 1991;68:501.

68. O'Keefe JH, Bateman TM, Barnhart CS. Adenosine thallium-201 is superior to exercise thallium-201 for detecting coronary artery disease in patients with left bundle branch block. J Am Coll Cardiol 1993;21:1332.

69. Nallamothu N, Ghods M, Heo J, et al. Comparison of thallium-201 single photon emission computed tomography and electrocardiographic response during exercise in patients with normal rest electrocardiographic results. J Am Coll Cardiol 1995;25:830.

69a. Hachamovitch R, Berman DS, Kiat H et al: Value of stress myocardial perfusion single photon computed tomography in patients with normal resting electrocardiograms. Circulation 2002;105:823.

70. Iskandrian AE, Hartsell DU. Cardiac-gated single photon emission computed tomography (SPECT), technical considerations, pitfalls and advantages. J Women Imaging 2000;2:39.

71. Kuschner FG, Okada RD, Kirshenbaum HD, et al. Lung thallium-201 uptake after stress testing in patients with coronary artery disease. Circulation 1981;63:341.

72. Hansen CL, Sangrigoli R, Nkadi E, at al. Comparison of pulmonary uptake with transient cavity dilation after exercise thallium-201 perfusion imaging. J Am Coll Cardiol 1999;33:1323.

73. Boucher CA, Zir LM, Beller GA, et al. Increased lung uptake of thallium-201 during exercise myocardial imaging: clinical, hemodynamic and angiographic implication in patients with coronary artery disease. Am J Cardiol 1980;46:189.

74. Heo J, Iskandrian AS. Tc-99m teboroxime imaging using SPECT. In: *Cardiac SPECT Imaging*, edited by EG DePuey, DS Berman, and EV Garcia. New York: Raven Press, 1995, p. 147.

75. Iskandrian AS, Heo J, Nguyen T, et al. Tomographic myocardial perfusion imaging with teboroxime during adenosine-induced coronary hyperemia: correlation with thallium-201 imaging. J Am Coll Cardiol 1992;19:1968

76. Hendel RC. Technetium-99m furifosmin (Q12). In: *New Developments in Cardiac Nuclear Imaging*, edited by AE Iskandrian and MS Verani. Armonk: Future Publishing Co., Inc., 1998, p. 59.

77. Fagret D, Marie P-Y, Giganti M, et al. Myocardial perfusion imaging with technetium-99-Tc Noet: comparison with thallium-201 and coronary angiography. J Nucl Med 1995;36:936.

78. Vanzetto G, Galnon DA, Ruiz M, et al. Myocardial uptake and redistribution of 99mTc-N-Noet in dogs with either sustained coronary low flow or transient coronary occlusion: comparison with 201T1 and myocardial blood flow. Circulation 1997;96:2325.

79. Acampa W, Cuocolo A, Sullo P, et al. Direct comparison of technetium 99m-sestamibi and technetium 99m-tetrofosmin cardiac single photon emission computed tomography in patients with coronary artery disease. J Nucl Cardiol 1998;5:265.

80. Azzareli S, Galassi AR, Foti R, et al. Accuracy of 99mTc-tetrofosmin myocardial tomography in the evaluation of coronary artery disease. J Nucl Cardiol 1999;6:183.

81. Zaret BL, Rigo P, Wackers FJT, et al. Myocardial perfusion imaging with Tc-99m tetrofosmin. Comparison to T1-201 and coronary angiography in a phase III multicenter trial. Circulation 1995;91:313.

82. Sacchetti G, Inglese E, Bongo AS, et al. Detection of moderate and severe coronary artery stenosis with technetium-99m tetrofosmin myocardial single-photon emission tomography. Eur J Nucl Med 1997;24:1230.

10 | Pharmacologic stress testing and other alternative techniques in the diagnosis of coronary artery disease

MARIO S. VERANI

Although exercise remains the preferred stress modality, many patients with suspected or documented coronary artery disease (CAD) cannot perform exercise testing because of conditions such as arthritis, peripheral vascular disease, other severe musculoskeletal diseases, cerebrovascular disease, asthma, chronic obstructive lung disease, congestive heart failure, and other systemic diseases. In the United States, approximately one-third of all stress myocardial perfusion imaging studies use pharmacologic rather than exercise stress. Several nonexercise stressors have been combined with myocardial perfusion scintigraphy (Table 10.1). In most cases a pharmacologic stress is chosen as a substitute for exercise testing. The other types of stresses listed in Table 10.1 are used only occasionally and in selected patients. Among the pharmacologic stresses, coronary vasodilation using dipyridamole or adenosine has been the most widely used. Positive inotropic agents, such as dobutamine, have also been successfully used in large numbers of patients. This chapter discusses the physiologic basis, hemodynamic changes, safety, and diagnostic value of pharmacologic stress imaging. The prognostic value of these techniques is discussed in Chapters 11 and 13.

PHARMACOLOGIC STRESS MYOCARDIAL PERFUSION SCINTIGRAPHY

Experimental Basis of Myocardial Perfusion Scintigraphy with Pharmacologic Coronary Vasodilation

Strauss and Pitt [1] were the first investigators to propose the use of coronary vasodilation in association with Tl-201 perfusion scintigraphy to detect CAD. These investigators used an infusion of ethyl adenosine in dogs with experimental coronary stenosis of the left circumflex artery. In the baseline state, they demonstrated that the mean flow ratio between the vascular territory perfused by the stenotic left circumflex artery and the normal vascular territory perfused by the left anterior descending artery was nearly the unit (0.96) as measured by the radioactive microspheres technique. After the administration of the vasodilator ethyl adenosine, there was a marked decrease in the ratio of stenotic-to-normal vessel flow, which fell to 0.43. In these experiments, when Tl-201 was injected during coronary vasodilation, the Tl-201 uptake ratio between the stenotic-to-normal artery was 0.56. In the few animals in which myocardial perfusion scintigraphy was performed, a perfusion defect was detected in the territory of the stenotic artery.

Shortly after Strauss and Pitt's report, Albro and colleagues [2] and Gould and associates [3–7] published a series of landmark reports that solidly established the experimental foundation of pharmacologic perfusion imaging. These investigators administered dipyridamole intravenously to instrumented dogs with partial coronary stenosis at a dose of 0.56 mg/kg of weight. Tl-201 was then injected intravenously, and imaging demonstrated perfusion defects in the territory of the stenosed artery. Myocardial perfusion images obtained after removal of the coronary stenosis showed a normal, homogeneous Tl-201 distribution. These authors also demonstrated a higher myocardial uptake of Tl-201 after dipyridamole infusion than in the basal state.

Gould's experiments established that the mechanism of perfusion defects induced by dipyridamole in the presence of a partial coronary stenosis was heterogeneous myocardial perfusion resulting from a marked increase of coronary blood flow in the vascular territory perfused by the normal coronary arteries and a

TABLE 10.1 *Nonexercise Stress Cardiac Imaging*

Pharmacologic stress
   Coronary vasodilation (adenosine, dipyridamole, adenosine
      triphosphate)
   Inotropic/chronotropic augmentation (dobutamine, arbutamine,
      dopamine, epinephrine, isoproterenol)
   Coronary vasoconstriction (spasm) (ergonovine,
      hyperventilation, acetylcholine, tobacco)
Atrial pacing
   Transvenous
   Transesophageal
Mental stress
   Speech, arithmetic, Color-Stroop test
Cold pressor test

much smaller increase (or no increase) in the territory perfused by the stenotic artery. This is illustrated in Figure 10.1. The flow increase in the normal artery after dipyridamole ranged from three- to fivefold, whereas the increase in the stenosed artery ranged from 0 to twice the baseline values. The smaller flow increase during coronary vasodilation in a partially stenotic artery is explained by the distal arteriolar dilation that follows the establishment of a severe stenosis. Such an arteriolar vasodilation reduces the coronary resistance and thereby maintains the myocardial blood flow within the normal limits in the resting state, although this requires using part or all of the coronary flow reserve. The arterioles located distally to a stenosis are thus already dilated in the basal state (in order to maintain the flow); consequently, these arterioles will only be able to dilate by a small additional fraction after administration of a potent coronary vasodilator, and the flow will increase only slightly. In contrast, in a normal coronary artery (without stenosis) the arterioles will dilate maximally and allow a three- to fivefold increase in flow. Gould and Lipscomb [3] had previously demonstrated that the coronary flow reserve begins to fall when the coronary artery luminal diameter is re-

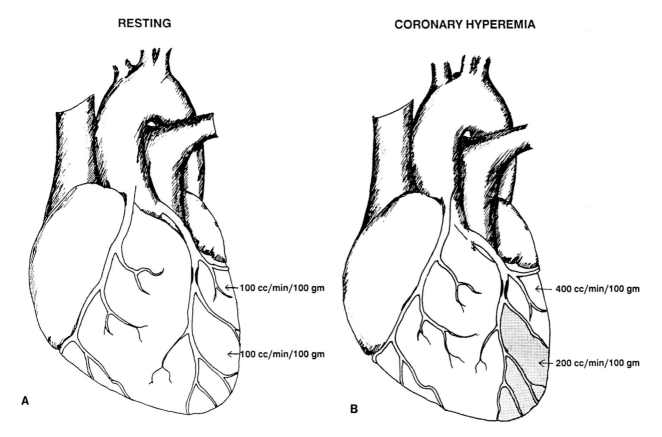

RESTING

CORONARY HYPEREMIA

← 100 cc/min/100 gm

← 100 cc/min/100 gm

← 400 cc/min/100 gm

← 200 cc/min/100 gm

A

B

FIGURE 10.1 *(A)* Myocardial perfusion at rest. The myocardial zone distal to the coronary lesion (arrow) has a flow rate equal to that of the normal zones. *(B)* Myocardial perfusion under the influence of coronary hyperemia. While the normal zones' flow increased four times above the resting flow, the flow in the zone perfused by the stenetre artery only increased by twofold. The latter zone will present with a relatively decreased thallium-201 uptake, that is, perfusion defect (illustrated by the strippled area). (From Boyce TM, et al. Adenosine cardiac imaging. J Nucl Med Tech 1991;19:203.)

duced by 45% to 50% of the normal diameter, or approximately 75% of the cross-sectional luminal area. The resting coronary blood flow, however, is maintained within normal limits, at least until the coronary stenosis surpasses 80% or 90%.

Several years after Gould's pioneering investigations, Leppo and coworkers [8] tested for the first time the use of adenosine in combination with Tl-201 perfusion imaging in the scintigraphic identification of experimental coronary stenosis. These investigators produced partial coronary stenosis in dogs and administered adenosine, which produced a fourfold increase in coronary blood flow in the normal coronary artery, but no increase in the stenosed artery. Perfusion defects corresponding to the stenosed artery were readily identified by planar Tl-201 scintigraphy obtained immediately after adenosine administration and filled in after 2 hours.

In summary, all of these landmark experiments clearly established heterogeneity of myocardial blood flow as the mechanism of perfusion defects during pharmacologic coronary vasodilation, consisting of a large increase through the normal arteries and a smaller increase or no increase through the stenosed arteries.

Relationship between Myocardial Tracer Uptake and Myocardial Blood during Pharmacologic Coronary Vasodilation

The large increase in myocardial blood flow through the normal coronary arteries, in contrast with the lack of increase through stenosed arteries, would, theoretically, create an ideal scenario to allow identification of coronary stenosis noninvasively. As discussed in Chapter 2, the myocardial Tl-201 uptake holds a linear correlation with the microsphere-determined myocardial blood flow. However, the excellent linear correlation between Tl-201 uptake and myocardial flow holds only for normal, increased, or slightly decreased coronary blood flows [1,9]. If the Tl-201 uptake were to increase in proportion to the increase in coronary blood flow, an ideal situation would be created to enable detection of perfusion defects, in that if the uptake increased linearly with flow, it would increase from three- to fivefold in the normal regions, with little or no increase in the myocardium perfused by the stenosed artery. Thus, a high contrast would exist between the normal and abnormal regions, which would allow the detection of perfusion defects. Inspection of the tracer uptake equation below would lend further support to this hypothesis. In this equation, the myocardial tracer uptake (U_m) is determined by the relation:

$$U_m = \frac{\text{coronary blood flow}}{\text{cardiac output}}$$
$$\times \text{ tracer dose} \times \text{ tracer extraction}$$

According to this equation, a large increase in coronary blood flow with little change in cardiac output (which is the usual response after a potent coronary vasodilator) would tend to increase the myocardial tracer uptake, provided the injected dose and the extraction fraction remained constant. However, the extraction fraction of most tracers, including Tl-201, Tc-99m-sestamibi or tetrofosmin, and Rb-81, falls substantially when the coronary flow increases markedly. When the coronary flow surpasses approximately 2.5 times the baseline values, the extraction of Tl-201 decreases and causes a "roll-off" in the uptake–flow relationship (Fig. 10.2) [10]. The mechanism underlying this fall in extraction with increasing coronary blood flow is not totally clear, but it may be related to the excessive blood flow velocity in the presence of normal or only slightly augmented myocardial oxygen demands during coronary vasodilation. The practical effect of this fall in extraction with increase in coronary flow is that it imposes a physiologic constraint on the ability of the test to detect mild-to-moderate coronary stenosis (30% to 60% narrowings). In such mild-to-moderate stenosis, a very high increase in tracer uptake in the normal vascular territories would be required to create enough difference in tracer uptake between the normal and abnormal vascular territories, since in those arteries with a mild-to-moderate stenosis the increase in coronary flow may still be in the order of two- or threefold.

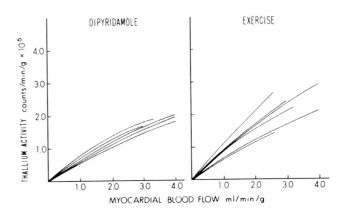

FIGURE 10.2 Dipyridamole versus microspheres flow. (From Mays et al. [10], reproduced from the Journal of Clinical Investigation, 1984, vol 73, p 1359, by copyright permission of The Society of Clinical Investigation.)

The fall in tracer extraction fraction with high coronary flows explains why pharmacologic coronary vasodilation has not yet been shown to be superior to exercise stress testing, despite the fact that pharmacologic vasodilation is a much more potent stimulus to create myocardial blood flow heterogeneity than exercise stress, which typically increases the coronary flow through normal arteries by only two- to threefold. In fact, reinspection of the tracer uptake equation above would suggest that coronary vasodilation would lead to a much higher myocardial tracer uptake, since during pharmacologic stress the ratio between coronary blood flow and cardiac output increases markedly, whereas during exercise this ratio remains approximately constant. In practice, the advantage of pharmacologic stress over exercise, namely, a higher coronary blood flow/cardiac output ratio, is counterbalanced by a lower extraction fraction during pharmacologic vasodilation.

During exercise, the linear relationship between Tl-201 uptake and myocardial blood flow is fairly well maintained, even at high levels of flow [11]. Thus, the trade-off between coronary blood flow/cardiac output ratio and extraction fraction may explain why pharmacologic perfusion scintigraphy is in practice comparable to exercise perfusion imaging.

Thallium-201 Redistribution and Washout after Pharmacologic Vasodilation

The intrinsic clearance of Tl-201 after an intracoronary injection of dipyridamole is faster than after Tl-201 administration at rest or during exercise. This may depend on the persistent increase in coronary blood flow produced by dipyridamole, which may enhance the washout of Tl-201. After intravenous dipyridamole administration, however, the Tl-201 blood levels remain higher than those during exercise, and this slightly opposes the washout, with the result that the measured Tl-201 washout is slightly lower after dipyridamole injection (40% at 4 hours) than during exercise (50% at 4 hours). The washout from normally perfused vascular territories is faster than in the hypoperfused regions, and therefore defects that are initially present after dipyridamole fill in over a period of a few hours, much like the phenomenon of redistribution after exercise perfusion imaging.

Technetium-99m-Sestamibi and Tetrofosmin during Pharmacologic Vasodilation

The roll-off phenomenon explained earlier for Tl-201 is more severe when tracers such as Tc-99m-sestamibi

2, 6-BIS-(DIETHANOL-AMINO)-4,8-DIPIPERIDINO-(5,4-D) PYRIMIDINE

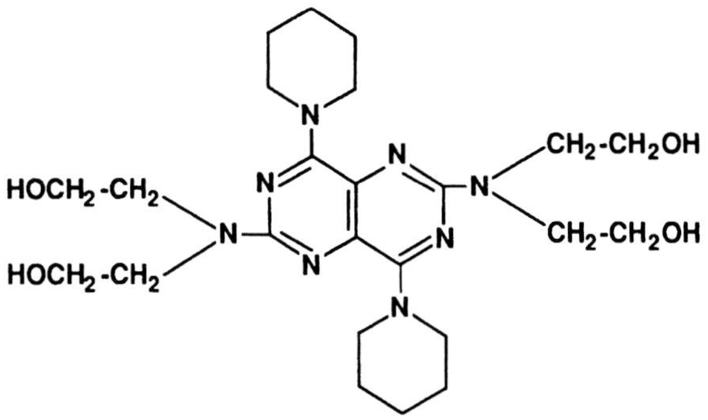

FIGURE 10.3 Dipyridamole: chemical structure and formula. (From Verani [85], with permission.)

and tetrofosmin, which have a lower first-pass extraction than Tl-201, are used in combination with pharmacologic vasodilation. This has been clearly demonstrated in animal experiments performed by Glover et al. [12,13] (Figs. 10.3 and 10.4) and raises questions whether these Tc-99m labeled compounds can be used as tracers during pharmacologic vasodilation. One would predict that it may be particularly difficult to detect mild-to-moderate lesions with Tc-99m tracers during pharmacologic vasodilation.

The newest Tc-99m labeled myocardial perfusion agent is Tc-99m-N-NOET which is still not approved by the FDA in the United States. Experimental studies show that this agent, which has a higher extraction than either sestamibi or tetrofosmin, does exhibit a better flow–uptake relationship during coronary vasodilation with adenosine. In fact, the flow–uptake curve for NOET is quite similar to that of Tl-201 and substantially better than those of sestamibi or tetrofosmin. When

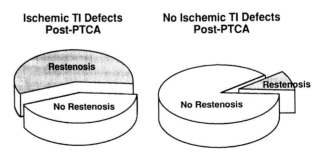

FIGURE 10.4 Of 14 patients with transient perfusion defects after coronary angioplasty, 10 (71%) developed recurrent angina and restenosis after a mean follow-up of 21 months *(left)*. Of the 26 patients without reversible thallium defects after angioplasty, only 3 (11.5%) developed documented restenosis *(right)*. The difference was significant at the $p = .007$ level. (From Verani [85], with permission.)

Tc-99m-N-NOET was combined with dobutamine, the flow–uptake characteristics were also better than for the combination of sestamibi and dobutamine [14].

The clinical experience of pharmacologic vasodilation in combination with these tracers is discussed later in this chapter.

Coronary Steal during Pharmacologic Vasodilation

Coronary steal is the phenomenon that occurs when the coronary flow distal to a stenosis is reduced by shifting some of the flow to a different coronary territory. This phenomenon has been well described in the experimental animal laboratory. Two types of steal have been described: an *intercoronary steal*, which occurs when the coronary bed distal to a high-grade stenosis or a total occlusion is perfused by collateral vessels originating from a different coronary artery. During maximal vasodilatation, the coronary resistance would decrease more in the normal, collateral-supplying artery than in the collateral-perfused area, leading to an increase in flow in the normal area and a decrease in the stenosed area [15,16]. In their work using experimental coronary stenosis, Becker et al. [15] created a coronary steal phenomenon after dipyridamole administration by ligating the left anterior descending artery while concomitantly producing a mild proximal stenosis in the collateral-supplying artery.

The second type of steal is a *subendocardial-to-subepicardial steal*, denoting a shift of blood from the endocardium to the epicardium in the vascular territory perfused by a stenotic artery. Gewirtz and associates [17] documented this type of steal in closed-chest swine with experimental coronary stenosis, following infusion of adenosine. This type of steal occurs when the subepicardial arterioles retain some residual vasodilatory reserve while the subendocardial reserve has already been exhausted in order to maintain the baseline flow within normal limits. As emphasized by Beller and colleagues [18,19], the endocardial-to-epicardial steal phenomenon is exacerbated when systemic hypotension is concomitantly induced by the vasodilator drug. During coronary steal, if the flow reduction is severe and, especially, if the myocardial oxygen demands are simultaneously increased, myocardial ischemia and lactate production may occur [20,21].

In addition to coronary steal, other factors may contribute to myocardial ischemia during coronary pharmacologic vasodilation. These factors include decrease in coronary perfusion pressure secondary to systemic hypotension, an increase in myocardial oxygen demands from reflex tachycardia, and possibly stenosis collapse because of decreased intraluminal pressure resulting from the increased blood velocity distal to the stenosis.

Whatever its mechanism, if true myocardial ischemia occurs during pharmacologic vasodilation in the presence of a coronary stenosis, it may lead to a decrease in left ventricular wall thickening and wall motion abnormalities. Local electrophysiologic changes of ischemia have been described during dipyridamole administration [22]. Fung and associates [23] observed a decrease in left ventricular contraction in a minority of their experimental animals. Because of the low occurrence of true myocardial ischemia during dipyridamole administration, these investigators suggested that perfusion imaging, which relies on heterogeneity of myocardial blood flow, may be superior to techniques that rely on the demonstration of wall motion abnormalities, such as dipyridamole or adenosine echocardiography. Poststress stunning, manifested as reduced wall motion and wall thickening, may also be seen during pharmacologic vasodilation stress [24].

Myocardial Perfusion Imaging during Pharmacologic Coronary Vasodilation

Extensive experience has been accumulated in the United States and elsewhere with both dipyridamole and adenosine in combination with myocardial perfusion imaging. As of this writing, adenosine and dipyridamole remain the only vasodilator agents approved by the Food and Drug Administration in the United States for use with myocardial perfusion imaging. Adenosine is also approved for treatment of supraventricular tachyarrhythmias. In Japan, adenosine triphosphate (ATP) has been used successfully to induce pharmacologic vasodilation.

Dipyridamole Myocardial Perfusion Imaging

Pharmacology of dipyridamole

Dipyridamole is a pyrimidine base with a molecular weight of 504.62 (see Fig. 10.3). It is believed that most, if not all, of the vasodilator effect of dipyridamole is secondary to an elevation of the interstitial and blood levels of adenosine. At high doses, dipyridamole is also a phosphodiesterase inhibitor, but it is not clear whether this contributes to the vasodilator effect in the doses currently used in humans. Dipyridamole blocks the facilitated transport of adenosine into the cells, thereby raising the extracellular levels of adenosine, which in turn causes coronary vasodilation by interacting with the adenosine A_2 receptors in the cell membrane. This interaction, which is mediated by G proteins, leads to a complex series of events, including an increase in adenylate cyclase, stimulation of potassium channels, and a decrease in intracellular calcium uptake, culminating with coronary vasodilatation [25,26].

After an intravenous injection of dipyridamole, the drug is completely distributed within 15 minutes and eliminated with a variable biological half-life that ranges from 88 to 136 minutes [27]. When dipyridamole is given orally in high doses (300 to 400 mg), it reaches a peak blood level at 30 to 90 minutes after administration. The mean blood levels achieved with these oral doses may be similar to those obtained by an intravenous injection, but with the oral administration there is a much greater variability in blood levels because of variable bioavailability [28].

In addition to its coronary vasodilatory effects, dipyridamole has well-known antiplatelet actions. Several mechanisms may be implicated in these antiplatelet actions, including inhibition of phosphodiesterase, increase in adenosine triphosphate (ATP) levels, potentiation of the antiplatelet effects of aspirin, and finally, an increase in the extracellular levels of adenosine, which has antiplatelet effects.

Clinical experience

Dipyridamole is usually given intravenously at a dose of 0.57 mg/kg over 4 minutes. This was the dose originally proposed by Gould and associates [2,7] and remains the dose with which the greatest experience has been accumulated. Some investigators have used higher doses (0.85 mg/kg for 4 minutes), especially in combination with two-dimensional echocardiography. Although this higher dose appears safe, the experience with it during perfusion imaging is limited, since it is not recommended in the drug's package insert.

Dipyridamole is available in 2 ml vials containing 10 mg of dipyridamole. Prior to administration it is diluted into 20 to 50 ml of normal saline or 5% dextrose solution in water. The infusion of dipyridamole is often performed with the aid of an infusion pump, but it may be given through a slow intravenous push over 4 minutes. The perfusion tracer is typically injected intravenously 3 to 4 minutes after the completion of the dipyridamole infusion. Imaging is initiated within 5 to 10 minutes when Tl-201 is used as the tracer, within 1 to 2 hours when Tc-99m-sestamibi or tetrofosmin are used, and within 2 minutes when Tc-99m-teboroxime is the chosen tracer.

Hemodynamic changes.
The hemodynamic effects of dipyridamole are fairly modest and have been summarized by Leppo [29]. Intravenous administration of the standard 0.56 mg/kg dose of dipyridamole results in a slight increase in heart rate (ranging from 12% to 38%) and a decrease in mean systemic arterial blood pressure (ranging from 6% to 10%). There is often a slight increase (ranging from 9% to 27%) in the rate-pressure product (double product), depending on the reciprocal changes in heart rate and blood pressure. There is also a significant yet modest increase (average 34%) in cardiac output over the baseline values, and a slight increase (average 21%) in pulmonary arterial wedge pressure above the baseline values.

Dipyridamole produces a marked increase of coronary blood flow through the normal arteries and a smaller increase or no increase through stenosed arteries. Earlier measurements of coronary blood flow in humans using a coronary sinus thermodilution technique by Brown and colleagues [30] showed a mean increase in coronary blood flow of 2.4-fold above the baseline values. They obtained a further increase in coronary blood flow by having patients perform isometric exercise (handgrip exercise at 25% of maximal tension for 4 or 5 minutes) after dipyridamole administration, to a maximum of 3.3-fold above the resting values. This study provided a basis for the strategy of combining dipyridamole with handgrip exercise, a strategy that is now rarely used. More recently, an intracoronary Doppler flow catheter has been used to assess the coronary blood flow velocity after dipyridamole administration. Rossen and coworkers [31,32] demonstrated a 3.7-fold increase in coronary blood flow velocity in normal coronary arteries. The time-to-peak flow augmentation after dipyridamole was 287 seconds after an intravenous injection. Although the Doppler flow catheter technique does not measure flow per se, the coronary flow velocity is linearly related to absolute coronary blood flow [33]. Studies using this more modern technique have shown only a minimal, statistically insignificant further increase in coronary blood flow with the addition of handgrip exercise after dipyridamole administration. In these studies, dipyridamole alone increased the flow by a factor of 3.8-fold, whereas the combination of dipyridamole and handgrip exercise increased the flow by a factor of fourfold above the baseline flow [32].

The standard dose of dipyridamole is capable of inducing maximal or near maximal coronary vasodilation in many patients. However, Rossen et al. observed a submaximal coronary vasodilation in 5 of 12 patients receiving a standard intravenous dose of dipyridamole [32].

Several investigators [34–37] have also combined dipyridamole administration with submaximal bicycle or treadmill exercise. Even maximal exercise has been used occasionally in combination with dipyridamole [38]. These investigators claim the following advantages of combining dipyridamole and exercise: First, exercise further increases the myocardial oxygen demands and hence may trigger myocardial ischemia. Second, exercise leads to a lower splanchnic uptake of radioactive tracers, with a resulting improvement in image quality. Third, the combination of dipyridamole with exercise has been reported to result in fewer side effects than dipyridamole alone [34].

A recent study using positron emission tomography found a decrease instead of an increase in coronary blood flow when exercise was added to dipyridamole [39].

Occasionally, dipyridamole and dobutamine have been combined [40]. As expected, the addition of dobutamine to dipyridamole results in a much greater increase in heart rate, systolic blood pressure, and the rate-pressure product than with dipyridamole alone. More patients may also have ischemic electrocardiographic changes during the combined test than with dipyridamole alone. Chest pain and premature atrial and ventricular beats may also be more common with the combined test. Although more abnormal results have been reported with this combined test than with dipyridamole alone, the net increase in stress defect score was relatively small. No data on sensitivity or specificity of this combined test are currently available. More studies on this and other combinations of stresses would be of interest.

Electrocardiographic changes. Ischemic ST-segment depression occurs in 6% to 34% of patients receiving intravenous dipyridamole and is significantly associated with higher patient age, presence of CAD, and reversible defects. Villaneuva and associates [41] reported that patients with ST-segment depression during dipyridamole administration were significantly more likely to have Tl-201 redistribution than those without ST-segment depression (64% vs 38%, *p* < .02). A multivariate analysis showed the number of myocardial segments demonstrating Tl-201 redistribution to be the most powerful predictor of ischemic ST-segment depression, followed by higher patient age and higher heart rate at the time of tracer injection. Chambers and colleagues [42] found the presence of coronary collateral vessels and the rate-pressure product after dipyridamole administration to be the most important predictors of ST-segment depression. Although it is not very sensitive, ST-segment depression that occurs during dipyridamole administration is highly specific for the presence of CAD.

Increased Lung Thallium Uptake and Transient Left Ventricular Cavity Dilatation

Increased lung Tl-201 uptake during exercise is a marker of exercise-induced left ventricular dysfunction, and as such it is an indirect evidence of multivessel CAD. More important, increased lung Tl-201 uptake during exercise is a marker of poor prognosis. Increased Tl-201 lung uptake has also been noted after dipyri-

damole administration, where it occurs in 22% [41] to 38% [43] of patients with CAD. Increased lung Tl-201 uptake after dipyridamole may be associated with other markers of myocardial ischemia, such as myocardial Tl-201 redistribution and transient left ventricular cavity dilatation.

Transient left ventricular cavity dilatation during exercise is a marker of severe multivessel CAD. A similar phenomenon has been noticed in 24% of patients with CAD undergoing imaging during dipyridamole administration and is associated with the presence of three-vessel CAD, collateral vessels, and more extensive reversible defects [44].

Increased Lung Sestamibi Uptake and Transient Cavity Dilatation after Dipyridamole

Because sestamibi images are typically acquired 1 hour or more after dipyridamole administration, one would expect this indirect evidence of ischemia to have dissipated by the time of imaging. However, transient left ventricular cavity dilatation has been described with dipyridamole sestamibi imaging [45]. Increased lung MIBI uptake has also been described after dipyridamole [46].

Side effects

Side effects occur in approximately 50% of patients undergoing dipyridamole scintigraphy (Table 10.2), but there is a wide variation in the frequency of side effects in different reports [29]. The most common side effects are chest pain (18% to 42%), flushing (15% to 38%),

TABLE 10.2 *Adverse Events Reported by Patients Who Underwent Intravenous Dipyridamole Thallium Imaging*

Adverse Event	No. Patients (%)
Chest pain	770 (19.7)
Headache	476 (12.2)
Dizziness	460 (11.8)
ST-T changes on electrocardiogram	292 (7.5)
Ventricular extrasystoles	204 (5.2)
Nausea	180 (4.6)
Hypotension	179 (4.6)
Flushing	132 (3.4)
Tachycardia	127 (3.2)
Pain (nonspecified)	102 (2.6)
Dyspnea	100 (2.6)
Blood pressure lability	61 (1.6)
Hypertension	59 (1.5)
Paresthesia	49 (1.3)
Fatigue	45 (1.2)
Dyspepsia	38 (1.0)

Source: From Ranhosky et al. [47], with permission.

nausea (8% to 12%), dizziness (5% to 21%), and headaches (5% to 22%). The chest pain may be similar in quality and location to the patient's anginal symptoms. In many patients, however, chest pain induced by dipyridamole has a nonanginal quality. Because chest pain occurs often in patients without angiographically significant CAD, as well as in those with significant disease, this symptom is not considered a good marker of CAD during pharmacologic stress. Cardiac arrhythmias, including atrioventricular AV block, are rare during dipyridamole administration (0.3%).

Serious side effects may rarely occur after dipyridamole administration. In the series of 3900 patients from the dipyridamole registry reported by Ranhosky and coworkers [47], four patients sustained a myocardial infarction, which was fatal in two patients. Occasionally, severe bronchospasm can be precipitated by dipyridamole, especially in patients with asthma or severe chronic obstructive pulmonary disease who require intensive use of bronchodilators or corticosteroid agents. Severe bronchospasm occurred in 0.2% of patients in the dipyridamole registry [47]. Rarely, bronchospasm may lead to rapid onset of respiratory failure culminating in respiratory arrest. This, as well as most other side effects of dipyridamole, can usually be rapidly reversed by the slow intravenous administration of theophylline (100 to 300 mg), which is a competitive blocker of the adenosine receptors. To enhance the safety of the test, in some laboratories theophylline is routinely given several minutes after the tracer injection. In patients in whom the chest pain persists despite theophylline administration, sublingual nitroglycerin may be of value.

The safety of high-dose dipyridamole infusion (0.84 mg/kg) has been reported by Picano and associates [48], in combination with two-dimensional echocardiography in a multicenter study of more than 10,000 patients. Side effects were rare in this study and occurred in only 1.2% of patients. Most of these serious side effects consisted of cardiac ischemic events, including three cases of myocardial infarction and one death. It should be emphasized that during echocardiography with high-dose dipyridamole administration, the patients are routinely monitored by echocardiography after the initial standard dipyridamole dose of 0.56 mg/kg. Only patients in whom wall motion deterioration does not occur after the standard dose should receive a supplemental dose of 0.28 mg/kg of dipyridamole. Obviously, one is less certain about the safety of a high-dose dipyridamole scan, since the wall motion is not routinely monitored during drug administration.

The safety of dipyridamole testing was further demonstrated in a very large population of 73,806 pa-tients included in the Multicenter Dipyridamole Safety Study [49] from 59 centers in 19 countries. The great majority of these patients received the standard dose of 0.56 mg/kg, but 6551 received a dose of 0.74 mg/kg and 2515 patients a dose of 0.84 mg/kg. In this series, there were a total of 7 cardiac deaths (rate of 0.95/10,000 patients), 13 known fatal myocardial infarctions (1.76/10,000), 6 sustained ventricular arrhythmias (0.1/10,000), 9 transient cerebral ischemic attacks (1.22/10,000), and 9 episodes of severe bronchospasm (1.22/10,000). Although these data demonstrate a good safety record, the study was retrospective and patients were not actively questioned during the study. Furthermore, as acknowledged by the authors, reporting of severe reactions was dependent on physicians' recollection. Nonetheless, this large study demonstrates the relative safety of dipyridamole testing when performed with the necessary precautions.

Lette and coworkers [50] further investigated the safety of dipyridamole testing in a cohort of 400 patients with known cerebrovascular disease who were undergoing dipyridamole imaging. Only one episode of transient cerebral ischemic attack occurred after dipyridamole infusion. Thus, dipyridamole imaging appears safe in patients with previous evidence of cerebrovascular disease. This is not surprising, in view of the well-known increase in regional cerebral blood flow produced by dipyridamole, which appears to be mediated by increased levels of adenosine.

Thus, dipyridamole perfusion scintigraphy has a very good safety record. Considering that patients receiving pharmacologic stress tend to be older and sicker than those undergoing exercise, its safety record is quite remarkable. However, serious side effects, even life-threatening ones, may rarely occur and for this reason it is extremely important to monitor and observe the patients during and after dipyridamole administration. As mentioned, theophylline is nearly always an efficacious antidote, but occasionally it must be given repeated times because the half-life of dipyridamole is longer than that of theophylline.

Diagnostic value of dipyridamole perfusion scintigraphy

The diagnostic value of dipyridamole perfusion scintigraphy has been summarized in several excellent reviews [6,29,51–57]. Most of the reported experience with dipyridamole imaging has been with the tracer Tl-201 and planar imaging. A more limited experience has been reported with Tc-99m sestamibi as the perfusion tracer and with single-photon emission computed tomography (SPECT).

TABLE 10.3 *Sensitivity and Specificity of Intravenous Dipyridamole Perfusion Scintigraphy*

Study	Definition of CAD(%)	% with MI	Method	Overall	Sensitivity MI	Sensitivity No MI	Specificity
Albro et al. [2] n = 62	≥ 50	NA	Planar	34/51 (67%)	NA	NA	10/11 (91%)
Francisco et al. [58] n = 86	≥ 70	29	Planar	41/51 (80%)	24/25 (96%)	17/26 (65%)	16/24 (67%)
			SPECT (V)	39/51 (76%)	23/25 (92%)	16/26 (62%)	16/24 (67%)
			SPECT (Q)	47/51 (92%)	23/25 (100%)	21/26 (81%)	23/24 (96%)
Huikuri et al. [59] n = 93	≥ 70	27	SPECT	78/81 (96%)	NA	NA	9/12 (75%)
Kong et al. [60] n = 114	≥ 50	7	Planar	86/94 (91%)	NA	NA	12/2 (60%)
Lam et al. [61] n = 141	≥ 70	15	Planar	93/110 (85%)	NA	NA	22/31 (71%)
Leppo et al. [62] n = 56	≥ 50	29	Planar	37/40 (93%)	16/16 (100%)	21/24 (88%)	16/20 (80%)
Mendelson et al. [63] n = 79	≥ 70	70	Planar	51/76 (67%)	41/55 (75%)	11/22 (50%)	NA
			SPECT	68/76 (89%)	51/55 (93%)	18/22 (82%)	
Okada et al. [43] n = 30	≥ 50	30	Planar	21/23 (91%)	12/13 (92%)	9/10 (90%)	7/7 (100%)
Taillefer et al. [64] n = 50	≥ 70	NA	Planar	32/39 (82%)	NA	NA	10/11 (91%)
Total Planar				395/484 (82%)	93/109 (85%)	58/82 (71%)	93/124 (75%)
Total SPECT				185/208 (89%)	74/80 (93%)	34/48 (71%)	25/32 (78%)

CAD, coronary artery disease; MI, myocardial infarction; NA, not available; SPECT, single-photon emission computed tomography; V, visual; Q, quantitative.
Source: From Mahmarian and Verani [65], with permission.

Table 10.3 reviews the reported experience with intravenous dipyridamole scintigraphy. Overall, Tl-201 scintigraphy has an average sensitivity of 82% by planar scintigraphy and 89% by SPECT, with specificities of 75% and 78%, respectively. As is true with exercise scintigraphy, different values reported in the literature for sensitivity and specificity undoubtedly depend on patient selection, including presence of previous myocardial infarction, frequency of multivessel disease, and variable stenosis severity. It is also remarkable that most studies with dipyridamole Tl-201scintigraphy have used a visual rather than a quantitative analysis.

More limited experience is available with oral dipyridamole scintigraphy. This is now only of historic value in the United States, since intravenous dipyridamole is now widely available. Nonetheless, oral dipyridamole testing can be performed safely, albeit with some increase in gastrointestinal side effects, with good sensitivity and specificity. Overall, a sensitivity of 88% and specificity of 82% can be calculated from the available reports. Using a quantitative SPECT analysis, Borges-Neto and associates [66] found an overall sensitivity of 92% and specificity of 88%.

Several studies have compared the sensitivity and specificity of dipyridamole Tl-201 scintigraphy with exercise Tl-201 scintigraphy [29,67,68] in patients who underwent both tests at different times. These studies showed similar sensitivity and specificity for exercise or dipyridamole scintigraphy.

Diagnosis of CAD in Patients with Left Bundle Branch Block

The exercise ECG is notoriously inaccurate for CAD detection in patients with an underlying left bundle branch block. Thus, myocardial perfusion scintigraphy is often used as a noninvasive diagnostic alternative in these patients. Unfortunately, myocardial perfusion defects commonly occur during exercise in these patients, with or without CAD. These defects often involve the interventricular septum, but may at times involve the anterior wall and apex and are often reversible (i.e., they show redistribution on delayed or rest imaging), but on occasion can be fixed [69–75]. The mechanism of exercise-induced perfusion defects in patients with left bundle branch block is controversial. Several studies [71,76–80] have now suggested that during pharmacologic perfusion imaging with dipyridamole or adenosine, patients with a left bundle branch block have a much lower prevalence of reversible septal defects. Thus, pharmacologic coronary vasodilation appears to be a preferred modality of testing for patients with left bundle branch block. However, one needs to keep in mind that perfusion defects may still occur in some of these patients in the absence of CAD. Moreover, the true prevalence of perfusion defects in patients with a left bundle branch block may be lower than suggested by the existing reports, because of a posttest referral bias (patients without defects rarely undergo coronary angiography). To date, little is known about the use of pharmacologic vasodilator stress in patients with other types of conduction abnormalities, such as ventricular pre-excitation.

Tc-99m-sestamibi imaging

Because sestamibi has a lower extraction fraction than Tl-201, it has been speculated that it might not be ideally combined with vasodilator stress, since a further fall in extraction at very high flows could potentially compromise the ability of the test to identify the presence of CAD. However, several reports indicate that the combination of sestamibi and dipyridamole works rather well [55,81–84]. In fact, Parodi and coworkers [82] reported the results of a multicenter study in 101 patients receiving either standard low-dose or high-dose ($n = 62$ patients) dipyridamole sestamibi imaging. Sestamibi scintigraphy had a sensitivity of 81%, specificity of 90%, and predictive accuracy of 93%.

Adenosine Myocardial Perfusion Imaging

Pharmacology of adenosine

Adenosine is a ubiquitous substance that is produced in small amounts as part of the normal cellular metabolism and in large amounts during tissue ischemia or hypoxia. Adenosine is a small heterocyclic compound (molecular weight = 267.25), containing a purine base and the sugar ribose (Fig. 10.5) [85].

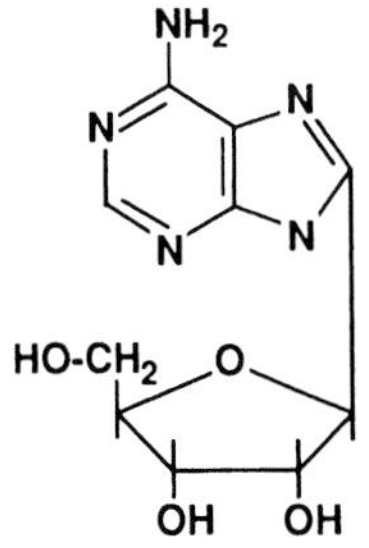

6-AMINO-9-β-D-RIBOFURANOSYL-9H-PURINE

FIGURE 10.5 Adenosine's chemical structure and formula. (From Verani [85], with permission.)

TABLE 10.4 *Physiologic Properties of Adenosine*

- Vagal inhibition (low doses): increase in heart rate
- Inhibition of the sinus node and atrioventricular conduction (high doses): bradycardia, atrioventricular block
- Antiadrenergic effect
- Potent vasodilation in all arteriolar beds, except in preglomerular arterioles of kidneys (vasoconstriction)
- Decrease in reperfusion injury

Source: From Verani [26], with permission.

Adenosine is available for use in combination with myocardial perfusion scintigraphy as 30 ml vials that contain 90 mg of adenosine and 20 ml vials that contain 60 mg of adenosine.

Table 10.4 summarizes the physiologic actions of adenosine in the cardiovascular system [26]. Adenosine is an important mediator of the coronary blood flow during ischemia and hypoxia, although its role in normal coronary autoregulation is controversial. That adenosine is a potent coronary vasodilator has been known since the classic report by Drury and Szent-Gyorgyi [86] in 1929. Although the coronary vasodilation produced by adenosine has been extensively used in the animal laboratory, only recently has it been used in human investigation. The powerful inhibitory effect of adenosine on the AV node explains why adenosine is initially used for the treatment of supraventricular tachycardia. The drug is highly effective and is, in fact, considered the drug of choice for this arrhythmia. Adenosine (Adenoscan) has been approved by the Food and Drug Administration for perfusion imaging in humans since 1995. Another clinical application, pioneered by Swedish investigators [87], is the use of adenosine to induce controlled, systemic hypotension during intracranial vascular operations.

When adenosine is infused intravenously, it has an ultrashort half-life (< 2 seconds). Endogenous adenosine is produced intracellularly through two pathways, the ATP and the S-adenosyl methionine (SAM) pathways [26,85]. For adenosine to function, it must cross the cell membrane and interact with the adenosine receptors in the outer cell wall. Interaction with the A_2 receptors that abound in the coronary arteries triggers several reactions, including an increased production of adenylate cyclase and cyclic adenosine monophosphate, and decreased intracellular calcium uptake, ultimately leading to coronary vasodilation [25,26]. Adenosine A_1 receptors abound in the proximal regions of the AV node. Their stimulation leads to a slowing of AV conduction [25]. Theophylline and caffeine are nonselective competitive blockers of the adenosine receptors and thus block the effects of adenosine.

Clinical experience

Siffring and colleagues [88] used adenosine infusion in combination with Tl-201 scintigraphy in normal volunteers. Verani and coworkers [89] first reported the use of adenosine Tl-201 imaging for the noninvasive diagnosis of CAD. In their initial series of 89 patients, adenosine was administered intravenously by pump infusion, starting with a dose of 50 μg/kg per minute, which was titrated upward to a maximal dose of 140 μg/kg per minute. After 1 minute at the highest dose, Tl-201 was injected intravenously and the adenosine infusion was maintained for 2 more minutes and then discontinued. Routine early and 4-hour delayed SPECT images were obtained (see Color Fig. 10.6 in separate color insert). This infusion technique proved to be remarkably safe and was subsequently simplified to a continuous infusion of 140 μg/kg per minute for 6 minutes, with the tracer injection made halfway into the infusion. However, for patients with a potentially higher risk of developing complications (e.g., patients with recent myocardial infarction, complicated coronary angioplasty, known three-vessel disease or left main coronary stenosis, past history of asthma or severe chronic obstructive pulmonary disease, borderline hypotension, or recent cerebrovascular accident), a stepwise infusion of adenosine is still a good option.

Because of the remarkable short half-life of adenosine, the time-to-peak effect occurs within the first minute of the infusion, and thus even shorter infusion times may be acceptable. A 4-minute infusion of adenosine at 140 μg/kg/minute has been found to perform just as well as the standard 6-minute infusion [90]. Even a 3-minute infusion may be as effective as a 6-minute infusion.

An important caveat: it is essential to refrain from injecting and flushing the radionuclide dose in the same intravenous line where adenosine is being infused, to avoid a rapid bolus of adenosine, which may cause advanced AV block, hypotension, and intensification of the expected side effects. To this end, the tracer is best administered into a different vein from that where adenosine is being infused. It is possible, however, to inject the tracer in the same intravenous line as the adenosine infusion (using dual port intravenous lines), provided the tracer is not flushed in [91].

Hemodynamic changes.

Intravenous adenosine produces significant, although modest, decreases in systolic and diastolic blood pressure and an increase in heart rate. The rate-pressure product also increases significantly, although mildly [89]. Significant increases in cardiac output (average of 56%) and in pulmonary arterial wedge pressure were reported by Ogilby and associates [92] in normal subjects as well as in patients with CAD. In the latter patients, substantial increases in pulmonary arterial wedge pressure (average increase of 13 mm Hg) were observed, without any concomitant changes in ventricular volumes or ejection fraction. This observation suggested a reduction in ventricular compliance during adenosine infusion, possibly explained by an engorgement of the ventricular walls by the massive increase in coronary blood flow. Another possibility would be that these patients effectively develop myocardial ischemia, and the changes in ventricular compliance may be secondary to ischemia. Ogilby and colleagues [92] also documented little change in the coronary epicardial artery diameter during adenosine infusion. Importantly, these authors were not able to document any stenosis collapse during adenosine infusion.

Changes in coronary blood flow.

Wilson and associates [93] have documented an average 4.4-fold increase in coronary flow velocity measured by a Doppler flow catheter, at the dose of 140 μg/kg per minute of adenosine intravenously. This coronary flow reserve was similar to the maximal reserve, elicited by an intracoronary injection of papaverine (Fig. 10.7) [93]. The potency of adenosine is such that even a low dose of 70 μg/kg per minute produces maximal vasodilation in 84% of normal subjects, whereas maximal or near maximal hyperemia occurred in 92% of patients at a dose of 140 μg/kg per minute.

Rossen and colleagues [31] compared the coronary vasodilatory effect of adenosine (140 μg/kg per minute) and dipyridamole (0.56 mg/kg over 4 minutes) in 15 patients being evaluated for chest pain who were shown

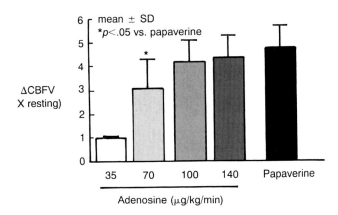

FIGURE 10.7 Change in coronary blood flow velocity (ΔCBFV) during intravenous adenosine infusion and after intracoronary papaverine. (Reproduced from Wilson et al. [93]. Copyright 1990 by American Heart Association.)

to have normal coronary arteries. Adenosine produced a greater fall in mean arterial blood pressure than dipyridamole, with similar increase in heart rate. The ratio of peak-to-rest coronary blood flow velocity was higher with papaverine (average ratio 3.9) than with adenosine (average ratio 3.4) or dipyridamole (average ratio 3.1). The maximal coronary blood flow velocity was reached more rapidly after the start of adenosine infusion (average 55 seconds) than after the start of dipyridamole injection (average 287 seconds). A larger decrease in coronary resistance occurred with papaverine or adenosine than with dipyridamole.

Chan and coworkers [94] quantified myocardial blood flow by positron emission tomography using nitrogen 13–labeled ammonia in 20 normal volunteers (average age 34.5 years, range 18 to 84). Myocardial blood flow at rest averaged 1.1 ± 0.2 ml/min per gram and increased to 4.4 ± 0.9 ml/min per gram after adenosine infusion (140 μg/kg per minute intravenously) and to 4.3 ± 1.3 ml/min per gram after dipyridamole administration (0.56 mg/kg over 4 minutes). Hyperemic-to-baseline flow ratio averaged 4.3 for adenosine and 4.0 for dipyridamole. These investigators concluded that the two drugs were equally effective in producing myocardial hyperemia.

Side effects. In the large series reported by Abreu and associates [95] adenosine perfusion imaging was well tolerated, despite a high frequency of side effects, which occurred in 79% of the patients. These untoward effects were very transient and typically subsided within 1 or 2 minutes after stopping the adenosine infusion and rarely required administration of aminophylline. A similar high frequency of side effects has been reported by Nguyen and colleagues [96], Coyne and associates [97], Iskandrian and coworkers [98], Nishimura and colleagues [99], and Gupta and associates [100], although none of these investigators reported any serious untoward reactions. More recently, Cerqueira and coworkers [101] summarized the national adenosine perfusion scintigraphy registry. In this report, which included more than 9000 patients, a high frequency of side effects was noted, but for the most part they were transient, well tolerated, and not associated with any significant complications.

Table 10.5 summarizes the most common side effects that occurred during adenosine infusion in the multicenter registry [101]. As can be seen, chest pain occurred quite frequently, but was not specific for CAD, since normal volunteers may also develop chest pain during adenosine infusion. Sylven and colleagues [102] have shown a dose–effect relationship between adenosine and presence of chest pain. It has also been sug-

TABLE 10.5 *Frequency of Adverse Events (> 2%) during Adenosine Infusion* (n = 9256)

Event	No. of Events	Percent
Flushing	3377	36.5
SOB/dyspnea	3260	35.2
Chest pain	3207	34.6
GI discomfort	1352	14.6
Headache	1318	14.2
TNJ discomfort	1078	11.6
Lightheadedness	783	8.5
AV block	706	7.6
ST-T changes	531	5.7
Arrhythmia	309	3.3
UE discomfort	213	2.3

SOB, shortness of breath; GI, gastrointestinal; TNJ, throat, neck, jaw; AV, atrioventricular; UE, upper extremity

Source: From Cerqueira et al. [101]. Reprinted with permission from Am Coll Cardiol [JACC 1994, vol 23, p 384].

gested that adenosine may be the elusive chemical substance ("substance P") that causes chest pain during myocardial ischemia by a direct stimulation of the cardiac A_1 adenosine receptors [103].

Dyspnea also occurs frequently and is believed to be the result of adenosine-induced hyperventilation, acting through stimulation of the carotid chemoreceptors [104]. Occasionally, adenosine may induce bronchospasm in patients with a history of asthma or severe chronic obstructive pulmonary disease.

Ischemic ST-segment depression on the ECG occurs more frequently in patients who also develop transient perfusion defects during adenosine administration. Overall, ST-segment depression occurs in 8% to 25% of patients during adenosine infusion. The ST-segment depression is considered a good marker of coronary steal and holds a strong association with high-grade stenosis and the presence of collateral circulation (Table 10.6) [105]. Thus, although ST-segment depression is not sensitive, it is a specific marker for CAD. It may also be a powerful prognostic marker of future cardiovascular events [106].

Changes in AV conduction have been extensively studied during adenosine infusion. First-degree AV block occurred in approximately 10% of the patients and second-degree AV block in 4% in the series reported by Abreu and associates [95]. Third-degree AV block occurred in only 0.6% in the series of 858 patients studied by Lee and colleagues [107], and in 0.8% in the large multicenter registry experience [101]. Second- or third-degree AV block is usually apparent during the first 2 minutes of infusion [107], is often intermittent, and commonly disappears despite continuation of the infusion. In most patients, AV block is an incidental finding, but occasionally severe bradycardia and

TABLE 10.6 *Potential Predictors of ST-Segment Depression during Adenosine Infusion*

	Univariate Analyses		After Three Predictors in Model	
	F	p	F	p
Presence of collaterals*	28.7	.0001	6.9	.01
Systolic blood pressure at baseline*	16.7	.0001	4.7	.03
Anginal chest pain*	16.0	.0002	4.0	.05
Rate-pressure product at 3 minutes	14.3	.0004	0.7	.42
Systolic blood pressure at 3 minutes	12.2	.001	0.1	.77
Heart rate increase	7.2	.01	3.0	.09
Maximal stenosis severity	6.9	.01	0.1	.78
Rate-pressure product at baseline	6.8	.01	0.4	.51
Heart rate at 32 minutes	4.3	.04	0.9	.36
Rate-pressure product increase	4.1	.05	2.8	.10
Increased Tl-201 lung uptake	2.8	.10	1.7	.19
Diastolic blood pressure at baseline	2.7	.10	0.1	.73
Age	2.3	.13	0.4	.52
Systolic blood pressure decrease	2.0	.17	0.1	.77
Number of diseased vessels	0.3	.57	<0.1	.97

*Presence of collaterals, systolic blood pressure at baseline, and typical chest pain are in model.
Source: From Nishimura et al. [105], with permission.

syncope may occur. In the large series reported by Lee and colleagues [107], AV block necessitated premature termination of the adenosine infusion in only one patient.

Increased lung Tl-201 uptake occurred in 52% of patients in the study by Iskandrian and associates [108,109], in 30% of the patients studied by Nishimura and colleagues [110], and in 30% of patients in the series reported by O'Keefe and coworkers [79]. Increased Tl-201 lung uptake is more likely to occur in patients with multivessel CAD, more extensive areas of hypoperfused myocardium, more segments with redistribution, and larger overall perfusion defect size than in those with normal lung uptake [110]. Transient left ventricular cavity dilatation has also been observed after adenosine infusion [79,89,98,110]. O'Keefe and associates [79] observed it in 33% of their patients. The prognostic value of both an increased Tl-201 lung uptake and transient cavity dilatation during adenosine infusion remains to be determined.

Because of the frequent side effects of adenosine, which are believed to be predominantly due to stimulation of adenosine A_1 receptors, it has been suggested that the combination of a selective A_1 receptor antagonist with adenosine might increase the tolerance and perhaps broaden the indications of adenosine perfusion imaging. Glover and colleagues [21] have demonstrated in an animal model that N6-endonorboman-2yl-9-methyladenine (N-0861) might be useful to counteract some of the undesirable side effects due to stimulation of the A_1 receptors, such as AV block, bronchospasm, and possibly angina. Using a combination of N-0861 and adenosine, Glover and coworkers observed no change in the hemodynamics and coronary flow in the compromised vascular territory or in control vascular territories relative to the changes produced by adenosine alone. Thus, N-0861 pretreatment did not adversely affect adenosine A_2–mediated vasodilation and therefore did not hamper the detection of critical stenosis by Tl-201 imaging. At this writing, N-0861 has not been used as yet in combination with adenosine in human beings, but it certainly appears a promising strategy that opens a window of opportunity for new clinical trials using pharmacologic coronary vasodilation [111].

Several selective A_2 adenosine agonists have been recently synthesized and tested experimentally as to their ability to function as pharmacologic stressors [12,112]. Because most of the undesirable side effects produced by adenosine are thought to be due to activation of the adenosine A_1 receptors (which cause chest pain and AV block), A_{2B} (which cause hypotension), and A_3 (which possibly cause bronchospasm and/or hypotension), it is very likely that new, selective A_{2A} agonists will be used as pharmacologic stressors in the future, possibly without any of the undesirable side effects of adenosine. Some of these "second generation" adenosinelike compounds may be administered as an intravenous bolus, rather than by infusion.

Diagnostic accuracy of adenosine myocardial perfusion scintigraphy. Several groups have reported their experience with adenosine perfusion SPECT using Tl-201 as a tracer (Table 10.7). An average sensitivity of 88% and specificity of 85% were found.

Adenosine SPECT appears to be equally sensitive in

TABLE 10.7 *Diagnostic Value of Adenosine Thallium-201 Tomography*

Study	No. of Patients	Sensitivity (%)	Specificity (%)
Coyne et al. [97]	100	83	75
Gupta et al. [100]	144	83	82
Iskandrian et al. [98]	148	92	88
Nguyen et al. [96]	60	92	100
Nishimura et al. [99]	101	87	90
O'Keefe et al. [79]	121	98	64
Verani et al. [89]	89	83	94
Iskandrian et al. [115]	223 (F)	84	84
	327 (M)	94	85
Total	1318	88	85

F, females; M, males.
Source: Modified from Verani [85], with permission.

patients with or without substantial changes in heart rate and systolic blood pressure. In elderly patients, adenosine appears to be also quite effective and safe [113]. The sensitivity of adenosine Tl-201 SPECT may be slightly lower in women than in men, although it may still be higher than that of exercise SPECT [114,115].

Adenosine versus exercise Tl-201 scintigraphy. The efficacy of adenosine versus exercise stress as adjuncts to Tl-201 scintigraphy has been compared by several investigators [96,97,100,115A]. In these studies, all patients underwent SPECT imaging with adenosine and, on a separate day, during exercise. The interpretation agreement between these two stress modalities was high. Table 10.8 summarizes two studies that compared exercise to adenosine Tl-201 scintigraphy.

Furthermore, computer-quantified perfusion defect sizes during adenosine scintigraphy correlated well (r = .80) with defect sizes during exercise scintigraphy in the multicenter trial reported by Nishimura and coworkers [115A]. The average defect size, however, was significantly larger with adenosine than with exercise imaging. In particular, several patients with small defects detected by adenosine SPECT failed to show any defects during exercise imaging, suggesting that adenosine may be more sensitive than exercise for detection of small perfusion defects.

Pennell and associates [116] investigated the combination of exercise and adenosine infusion. They found an insignificant trend toward improved sensitivity (98% vs 93%) and a significant reduction in noncardiac side effects and cardiac dysrhythmias with the combination of these two stressors. They also reported a higher heart/background ratio and more defect reversibility with this combination. Other groups have reported similar results [117,118].

Contraindications to adenosine scintigraphy

Adenosine is contraindicated in patients with asthma or severe obstructive chronic pulmonary disease who also have bronchospasm. In these patients, adenosine may precipitate or aggravate bronchospasm. At the Mayo Clinic, investigators have reported the use of bronchodilators (given as inhalers) in patients with moderate-to-severe chronic obstructive pulmonary disease just prior to the adenosine infusion. Using this technique, they were able to perform adenosine imaging without any serious problems [119]. Patients with baseline arterial hypotension (systolic pressure < 100 mm Hg) may have their hypotension aggravated by the systemic vasodilatory effect of adenosine and, thus, ordinarily should not receive this drug. Patients with sick sinus syndrome may be at increased risk for developing severe bradycardia during adenosine infusion. Patients with second- or third-degree AV block on the baseline ECG should not receive adenosine unless they have an artificial pacemaker. Finally, patients who take oral dipyridamole preparations should not receive adenosine for at least 24 hours following the last dipyridamole dose, because, by blocking the cellular uptake of adenosine, dipyridamole may raise adenosine's interstitial and blood levels to potentially dangerous values. Patients who have used aminophylline or caffeine prior to the testing (including those who had a cup of coffee the morning of the test) should not undergo adenosine perfusion imaging for at least another 12

TABLE 10.8 *Adenosine Versus Exercise Thallium-201 Single-Photon Tomography: Diagnostic Accuracy*

	COYNE ET AL. [97] (N = 100)		GUPTA ET AL. [100] (N = 144)	
	Exercise (%)	*Adenosine (%)*	*Exercise (%)*	*Adenosine (%)*
Sensitivity	81	83	82	83
Specificity	74	75	80	87
Normalcy rate	80	80	—	—
Positive predictive accuracy	73	75	90	93
Negative predictive accuracy	81	83	67	70
Overall accuracy	77	79	81	84

hours. Because these drugs block the adenosine receptors, they may invalidate the results of adenosine perfusion scintigraphy.

In patients with severe aortic stenosis, there may be some concern about administering a potent vasodilator such as adenosine. However, Samuels et al. [120] have reported their experience with adenosine SPECT in patients with severe aortic stenosis. Adenosine SPECT allowed recognition or exclusion of CAD in such patients without any untoward effect.

Dobutamine Myocardial Perfusion Imaging

Dobutamine is a potent cardiac inotropic agent that is ordinarily used for treatment of severe congestive heart failure and low cardiac output states. Dobutamine hydrochloride is a synthetic catecholamine that chemically is the ($\pm$)-4-[-2-[[3-(p-hydroxylphenyl)-l-methyl-propyl]amino]ethyl] procathechol hydrochloride, which has a molecular weight of 337.85. It is available in 20 ml vials containing 20 mg of dobutamine hydrochloride and a small amount of sodium bisulfide.

The onset of action of dobutamine occurs within 1 or 2 minutes after starting an intravenous infusion, but the peak effect is achieved several minutes later. The plasma half-life of dobutamine is approximately 2 minutes, and the drug is metabolized through methylation of the catechol group (by the enzyme catechol-o-methyltransferase) and conjugation [85]. Hypersensitivity reactions may occasionally occur with dobutamine, such as a skin rash, eosinophilia, fever, and bronchospasm. Because the preparation contains a small amount of sodium bisulfide, it can cause allergic reactions, including anaphylactic symptoms and even life-threatening bronchospasm in susceptible persons, especially those with a history of asthma. How often these allergic reactions occur is not known, but presumably they are extremely rare.

Although dobutamine was until recently considered to act predominantly on the beta$_1$ adrenergic receptors, increasing both the rate and the force of myocardial contraction, and to have only a secondary effect on the beta$_2$ receptors (responsible for peripheral vasodilatation) and on the alpha$_1$ receptors (producing peripheral vasoconstriction but also increasing the force of cardiac contraction) [121], evidence has shown that dobutamine is a powerful stimulant of both alpha$_1$ and beta$_2$ adrenergic receptors [122]. Nevertheless, the net effect of dobutamine at doses < 20 μg/kg per minute in the peripheral circulation is small because of a balanced stimulation of the alpha$_1$ and beta$_2$ adrenergic receptors. Since dobutamine increases the stroke volume because of its positive inotropic effects, there is

a secondary reflex withdrawal of sympathetic tone, which results in a decrease in systemic resistance [123]. The hemodynamic effects of dobutamine at low-to-moderate doses (5 to 20 μg/kg per minute) consist of a substantial increase in cardiac output and stroke volume, with little change in mean arterial pressure and heart rate. At higher doses (> 20 μg/kg per minute) there is a substantial increase in heart rate. Dobutamine also decreases the systemic and pulmonary venous pressures and resistances [124].

The intravenous administration of dobutamine (10 μg/kg per minute) to open-chest dogs increased the coronary blood flow by 138% and the heart rate by 122% of the baseline values [124]. The increase in coronary blood flow is believed to be due to increased myocardial metabolic demands, and from direct coronary beta$_2$ and alpha receptor stimulation.

The effect of dobutamine (doses up to 20 μg/kg per minute) in the presence of experimental coronary stenosis is controversial. Willerson and associates [125] reported an increase in coronary blood flow in both the nonischemic and ischemic zones. Vatner and Baig [126], on the other hand, have reported an augmentation of coronary flow through the normal arteries and in moderately ischemic zones, with no change in severely ischemic zones. In this regard, the presence or absence of tachycardia during dobutamine infusion may be critical, since tachycardia accentuates ST-segment elevation and paradoxical systolic bulging, and decreases myocardial blood flow and endocardial/epicardial flow ratio to the severely ischemic zones [125,126]. In anesthetized dogs, dobutamine (20 μg/kg per minute) produced substantial tachycardia and increased myocardial ischemic injury.

In the presence of CAD, the increase in coronary blood flow produced by dobutamine is blunted. In patients with CAD, dobutamine (at a dose of 8 μg/kg per minute) led to a heterogeneous regional myocardial perfusion [127]. In the study by Pozen and colleagues [128] lactate production occurred during dobutamine infusion in 11% of patients with congestive heart failure and CAD, whereas 17% of these patients developed angina. Ultimately, it is this heterogeneous perfusion that enables detecting CAD by perfusion imaging. The perfusion defects present during dobutamine do undergo redistribution, much like those during exercise or vasodilator stresses.

More recently coronary blood flow has been studied during the very high doses of dobutamine used for stress testing (up to 40 μg/kg per minute) in humans. Krivokapich and coworkers [129] assessed the myocardial blood flow by nitrogen 13-labeled ammonia at rest and during high-dose (40 μg/kg per minute) dobutamine infusion in 21 normal subjects. These investigators observed a threefold increase in myocardial blood flow (range 2.0- to 4.8-fold). The myocardial blood flow was significantly related to the heart rate (r = .59), systolic blood pressure (r = .86) and rate-pressure product (r = .77). Thus, this study suggests that high-dose dobutamine infusion is capable of increasing the coronary blood flow to the same levels that are ordinarily experienced with exercise stress testing. Furthermore, when high-dose dobutamine (40 μg/kg/min) was combined with atropine (0.25 to 1.0 mg), the increase in coronary blood flow appeared to surpass that produced by dipyridamole (0.56 mg/kg) in normal men [129A]. Coronary steal has also been reported during high-dose dobutamine administration in patients with ischemic heart disease [129B].

Clinical experience

Dobutamine was first used as a stress agent when Mason and associates [130] combined it with Tl-201 myocardial perfusion imaging in 1984. These investigators infused dobutamine at a maximal dose of 20 μg/kg per minute in 24 patients being evaluated for chest pain, 16 of whom had CAD and 8 of whom had normal coronary arteries. Reversible Tl-201 perfusion defects by planar scintigraphy occurred in 15 of 16 coronary patients and in only 1 of 8 normal patients, yielding a sensitivity of 94% and specificity of 87%.

Pennell and colleagues [131] used dobutamine (20 μg/kg per minute) in combination with Tl-201 tomography in 50 patients who also underwent coronary arteriography. A reversible Tl-201 defect was observed in 39 of 40 patients who had CAD, for a sensitivity of 97%, whereas 8 of 10 patients with normal coronary arteries had a normal scan (specificity 80%). Dobutamine has been generally well tolerated without major complications. Transient side effects are quite frequent. In the study reported by Pennell and associates [131], 78% of the patients developed chest pain during dobutamine infusion and 38% of the patients had cardiac arrhythmias (especially premature ventricular beats).

Hays and colleagues [132] have reported a study on dobutamine Tl-201 SPECT in 144 patients. Dobutamine was administered up to 40 μg/kg per minute, beginning with a low dose of 10 μg/kg per minute and increasing at 3-minute intervals to 20, 30, and finally 40 μg/kg per minute. A dose-dependent increase in systolic blood pressure, decrease in diastolic blood pressure, and increase in heart rate were observed (Fig. 10.8) [132]. Most patients (74%) were able to tolerate a dose of 40 μg/kg per minute, but the test had to be prematurely terminated at a lower dose because of the severity of

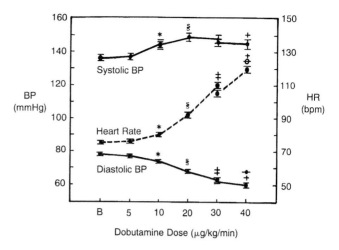

FIGURE 10.8 Hemodynamic changes during dobutamine infusion. Symbols denote significant changes from baseline. (From Hays et al. [132], with permission.)

side effects in 26% of patients. Overall, side effects occurred in 75% of all patients. Ventricular premature beats occurred in 44% of the patients, and nonsustained ventricular tachycardia in 3%. Paroxysmal atrial fibrillation with a fast ventricular response occurred in one patient. Ischemic ST-segment depression occurred with a higher frequency (50%) than that which is ordinarily seen after dipyridamole or adenosine infusion. The sensitivity and specificity for detection of CAD in this study were 86% and 90%, respectively. An example of a dobutamine Tl-201 SPECT image is shown in Color Figure 10.9 (in separate color insert).

Dakik et al. [133] have reported detailed safety data on a series of more than 1000 patients who underwent dobutamine SPECT imaging. Table 10.9 summarizes their findings.

Marwick and colleagues [134] have reported a comparative study using Tc-99m-sestamibi SPECT during adenosine or dobutamine stress, in combination with two-dimensional echocardiography. Dobutamine sestamibi had a sensitivity of 80% and specificity of 74%, compared to a sensitivity of 86% and specificity of 71% for adenosine sestamibi SPECT. In this study, dobutamine stress with two-dimensional echocardiography also had good sensitivity and specificity (85% and 82%, respectively), whereas adenosine stress with two-dimensional echocardiography had a lower sensitivity (58%), although it had the best specificity (87%).

Marwick and coworkers [135] expanded on their initial experience with dobutamine stress in combination with both scintigraphy and echocardiography. In their most recent study of 217 patients without previous infarction, dobutamine echocardiography and Tc-99m-

TABLE 10.9 *Incidence of Side Effects during Dobutamine Stress Testing and Frequency of Arrhythmias during Dobutamine Infusion*

Side Effects	No.	%	Frequency of Arrhythmias	No.	%
Chest pain	309	30.5	Nonsustained ventricular tachycardia	43	4.2
Headache	138	13.6	Premature ventricular complexes	121	12.0
Dyspnea	123	12.2	Premature atrial complexes	16	1.6
Flushing	104	10.3	Atrial fibrillation	11	1.1
Palpitation	98	9.7	Atrial flutter	1	0.1
Nausea	81	8.0			
Tremors	11	1.1			

Source: Modified from Dakik et al. [133], with permission.

sestamibi SPECT imaging were compared to coronary angiography. CAD was present in 142 patients. In these patients, the sensitivity of dobutamine sestamibi SPECT was 76% and that of dobutamine echocardiography was 72%. The specificity was 67% and 83%, respectively. Most of the patients with false positive SPECT had left ventricular hypertrophy. Interestingly enough, in this study, the sensitivity was lower (59%) by two-dimensional echocardiography in patients unable to complete the test because of side effects, whereas sestamibi scintigraphy had a higher sensitivity (71%) in these patients. Importantly, patients with a negative submaximal dobutamine stress echocardiogram (*n* = 31) were detected by sestamibi scintigraphy with a sensitivity of 80%.

Forster and associates [136] have reported a series of 105 patients who were studied with a combination of Tc-99m-sestamibi SPECT and stress echocardiography during dobutamine infusion. The response to dobutamine was concordant by the two techniques in 68% of the patients. In the 21 patients without previous infarction who underwent coronary angiography, the sensitivity and specificity of sestamibi SPECT for the diagnosis of CAD were 83% and 89%, respectively, compared with 75% and 89%, respectively, for dobutamine echocardiography.

Gunlap and colleagues [137] have also compared dobutamine Tc-99m-sestamibi SPECT with dobutamine electrocardiography and echocardiography in 27 patients who underwent coronary angiography. Sensitivity and specificity were 94% and 88% for dobutamine SPECT, 61% and 55% for dobutamine electrocardiography, and 84% and 88% for dobutamine echocardiography, respectively.

Thus, there are now several studies comparing dobutamine stress in combination with sestamibi SPECT and echocardiography. In these papers, there seems to be no clear-cut superiority of one technique over the other; the sensitivity may be somewhat higher with SPECT, but this comes at the expense of a slightly lower specificity. However, the study of Marwick and colleagues

[135] suggests that dobutamine SPECT may be more sensitive than echocardiography in patients who perform a "submaximal" dobutamine test.

Risk stratification with dobutamine Tl-201 scintigraphy prior to vascular surgery

Elliott and associates [138] investigated the use of dobutamine Tl-201 tomography in the risk stratification of 126 patients being evaluated as prospective candidates for vascular surgery. Dobutamine was infused in doses up to 20 μg/kg per minute, and atropine was given to 47 patients to further increase the heart rate. In the 84 patients with either a normal scan or only a fixed defect, cardiac event rates were 1.8% and 11%, respectively. Tl-201 redistribution occurred in 42 patients, 15 of whom were denied surgery, 18% went on with the scheduled vascular procedures, and 9 underwent coronary revascularization. Of the patients with Tl-201 redistribution who underwent vascular surgery without prior revascularization, 9 (50%) had a postoperative event.

Dobutamine Tl-201 scintigraphy after myocardial infarction

Coma-Canella and colleagues [139] reported a study including 63 patients who underwent dobutamine Tl-201 SPECT followed by dobutamine radionuclide angiography (RNA) a mean of 16 days after an acute myocardial infarction. Tl-201 redistribution was present in 45 patients. This study did not assess the prognostic value of dobutamine scintigraphy.

Contraindication to dobutamine stress testing

Because a high intravenous dose of dobutamine may increase, as well as decrease, the systemic blood pressure, patients with either severe hypertension or hypotension should not receive this test. Patients with recent dissection of the aorta, coronary arteries, or other large vessels should not receive dobutamine infusion in view of the possibility of aggravating the dissection.

Patients with uncontrolled atrial fibrillation or atrial flutter may develop very severe tachycardia because of the faster AV conduction produced by dobutamine. Patients with a history of recurrent ventricular tachycardia should also be excluded from a dobutamine test, at least until more experience is available. Finally, in patients with left ventricular outflow obstruction (aortic stenosis or hypertrophic cardiomyopathy) dobutamine will increase the pressure gradient and thus is contraindicated.

Other Pharmacologic Stress Agents

Although the present experience with pharmacologic perfusion imaging is focused nearly exclusively on dipyridamole, adenosine, and dobutamine, it is likely that other pharmacologic stressors will be tested and developed. Preliminary experience using ATP in combination with Tl-201 or tetrofosmin SPECT by investigators in Japan has been encouraging, with high sensitivity and specificity for detection of CAD in a limited number of patients [140]. ATP rapidly dissociates into adenosine, which appears to be the active moiety of the ATP molecule. Thus, ATP may be a convenient vehicle for administration of adenosine, especially where a pure form of adenosine is not available or approved for intravenous administration.

Several A_2-specific adenosine agonists are currently being tested in Phase I and II studies. Arbutamine, a new, potent, synthetic beta agonist, has been investigated in combination with Tl-201 SPECT in a multicenter trial in the United States. Preliminary results with this new agent have indicated high sensitivity (87% overall and 79% in patients without a prior infarction) and normalcy rate (90%) in a total of 112 patients with CAD and 63 subjects with low likelihood for CAD. In a group of subjects who underwent both arbutamine and exercise Tl-201 scintigraphy, high concordance was demonstrated between those two stress modalities. A high frequency of side effects has been noted with arbutamine, but no serious complications have been reported [141]. Administration of arbutamine is somewhat more complex than with dobutamine and thus the drug has not found a clinical niche, despite being approved as a pharmacologic stress by the Food and Drug Administration.

PHARMACOLOGIC STRESS IN COMBINATION WITH RADIONUCLIDE ANGIOGRAPHY

Perfusion defects may be elicited during pharmacologic stress solely on the basis of unequal distribution of coronary blood flow without necessarily requiring the presence of myocardial ischemia. In contrast, techniques that assess wall motion, such as radionuclide angiography (RNA), echocardiography, magnetic resonance imaging, or ultrafast computerized tomography imaging, require the provocation of myocardial ischemia in order to detect the presence of CAD. Hence, one would anticipate that myocardial perfusion may be more sensitive than techniques that depend on wall motion deterioration (due to ischemia) during pharmacologic coronary vasodilation.

Dipyridamole Radionuclide Angiography

Harris and associates [142] compared the sensitivity and specificity of planar Tl-201 imaging to that of blood pool RNA after intravenous dipyridamole in 38 patients, 21 with and 17 without CAD. An abnormal RNA response was defined as wall motion deterioration during dipyridamole, noted in any of the three standard views, while an abnormal Tl-201 scan required the presence of reversible defects. The sensitivity and specificity of Tl-201 imaging were 88% and 65%, respectively, compared to 13% and 100% with RNA.

Sochor and colleagues [143] studied 194 patients with both dipyridamole Tl-201 scintigraphy and coronary angiography. The overall sensitivity was 92% in the 149 patients with CAD and the specificity 81% in the 45 patients without CAD. In a subgroup of 40 patients (32 with reversible Tl-201 defects and 8 normal subjects), RNA was also performed after dipyridamole. Only 19% of patients had a fall in left ventricular ejection fraction ($\geq$ 8 units) after dipyridamole and only 31% developed wall motion abnormalities. The sensitivity for identifying the location of coronary stenosis was 70% for Tl-201 imaging and 26% for RNA (defined as deterioration of regional function).

Cates and coworkers [144] compared RNA performed after dipyridamole infusion with that during exercise in 31 patients who also underwent coronary angiography. Among these patients, 10 were normal and 21 had significant CAD ($\geq$ 50% stenosis); of the latter, 19 had severe CAD, defined as $\geq$ 70% stenosis. In normal subjects, the left ventricular ejection fraction increased during exercise (5 $\pm$ 2 units) and during dipyridamole (7.1 $\pm$ 1 units), whereas it failed to increase during either stress in patients with CAD. In the latter, regional wall motion deteriorated during exercise and during dipyridamole, although the deterioration was greater during exercise. In patients with $\geq$ 70% coronary stenosis, the sensitivity for exercise and dipyridamole was 89% and 67%, respectively, and specificity 67% and 92%, respectively. The authors concluded that dipyridamole RNA was moderately sensitive and highly specific for detecting severe CAD. These results were remarkable, particularly because 26 of the patients were receiving anti-ischemic drugs at the time of the study.

Klein and colleagues [145] performed rest and dipyridamole RNA in 113 patients with angina pectoris and 32 presumably normal subjects. Among the 113 patients, 71 had a prior myocardial infarction and 70 had coronary angiography that showed multivessel coronary disease in two-thirds of them. The left ventricular ejection fraction increased significantly in 29 normal subjects (average from 57% ± 6% to 64% ± 10%) and decreased in 98 patients (from 49% ± 11% to 43% ± 13%). Wall motion deterioration occurred in 75 patients (66%). The peak systolic pressure–end-systolic volume ratio increased in 69% of normal subjects and decreased in 72% of CAD patients.

Thus, these four published reports on dipyridamole RNA are evenly divided into those studies that found the test useful [144,145] and those that found little value in it [142,143]. However, even in the best-case scenario, deterioration of wall motion occurred in only two-thirds of the patients, and hence it is unlikely that the test would be competitive today with the higher sensitivity achieved with pharmacologic myocardial perfusion imaging.

Dobutamine Radionuclide Angiography

One might anticipate that a stress that is more likely to provoke myocardial ischemia and thereby produce wall motion deterioration is more appropriate to be used in combination with RNA than pharmacologic coronary vasodilation with dipyridamole or adenosine, which elicit heterogeneity of coronary blood flow without necessarily producing myocardial ischemia. Theoretically, then, dobutamine may be a better stress for RNA studies, provided that the increase in myocardial oxygen consumption produced by this drug outstrips the capacity of the stenotic coronary arteries to augment coronary flow. Otherwise, an increase in myocardial contractility may be the preponderant effect, and one may see an increase rather than a decrease in regional ventricular function.

Surprisingly little has been published about dobutamine RNA. Freeman and coworkers [146] in 1984 compared dobutamine RNA (maximal dose of 20 μg/kg per minute) to exercise RNA in 24 patients being evaluated for chest pain. Dobutamine RNA had a sensitivity of 89% and specificity of 100%, whereas for exercise RNA the corresponding values were 94% and 90%. In marked contrast with Freeman's excellent results with dobutamine RNA, Konishi and associates [147] found that only 2 of 21 patients with CAD had

dobutamine-induced regional wall motion abnormalities. Moreover, the left ventricular ejection fraction increased both in normal subjects and in those with CAD. This response was different from that produced by exercise, when the CAD patients failed to increase the ejection fraction.

Movahed and colleagues [148] reported 15 patients with angiographically documented CAD and global and regional left ventricular dysfunction (mean ejection fraction = 30%) who underwent dobutamine RNA (maximal dose of 20 μg/kg per minute). The ejection fraction increased (to 38%) during dobutamine infusion and all except 1 patient had an increase in ejection fraction. The ejection fraction increased by 5 units or more in 11 of 15 patients; 8 of these 11 patients had concurrent improvement in the wall motion of the asynergic area. Thus, in this cohort of patients with depressed left ventricular ejection fraction, dobutamine enhanced rather than decreased the global and regional function. Two patients in this study underwent coronary artery bypass graft surgery and one had coronary angioplasty after dobutamine RNA. After revascularization, repeat RNA showed recovery of global and regional left ventricular function to levels seen during dobutamine testing. Hence, this study should be regarded as more appropriately addressing the issue of viability rather than detection of CAD.

Coma-Canella and coworkers [139] performed both Tl-201 SPECT and RNA during dobutamine infusion (doses up to 40 μg/kg per minute) in 63 patients at a mean of 16 days after an acute myocardial infarction. Sixty patients had coronary angiography within 1 week of cardiac scintigraphy. In the entire group, left ventricular ejection fraction increased significantly from 46% ± 12% to 56% ± 14%. The regional ejection fraction of asynergic areas increased from 27% to 41% and showed no change or a decrease in 13 patients. Interestingly, the 44 patients with perinfarct redistribution (the scintigraphic equivalent of ischemia) by Tl-201 scintigraphy had a greater increase in regional function than those patients without redistribution.

Simultaneous first-pass RNA and perfusion SPECT were performed in 92 patients using Tc-99m-sestamibi. Perfusion defects occurred in 78% of patients during dobutamine SPECT. Left ventricular ejection fraction increased significantly in normal subjects and in patients with CAD. In the latter, deterioration of regional ventricular function occurred in only 32% [149].

Thus, the few studies assessing dobutamine RNA are controversial. This may be because of the bimodal response of the myocardium perfused by a stenosed coronary artery, which exhibits an early increase in function, later followed by wall motion deterioration as ischemia develops. However, it is very possible that in some patients only an increase in regional function will occur, and in these cases, the diagnosis of CAD may be missed. Comparative studies of perfusion SPECT and two-dimensional echocardiography during dobutamine infusion have been reported [150,151].

ATRIAL PACING STRESS AS AN ADJUNCT TO CARDIAC RADIONUCLIDE IMAGING

Atrial pacing as a stress modality should be reserved for patients who are not candidates for either exercise or pharmacologic stress imaging. However, the tests could also be considered in patients with a permanent dual-chamber sequential pacemaker, since the heart rate can be programmed externally.

Atrial pacing produces little, if any, change in mean and diastolic blood pressure. In normal subjects, atrial pacing to a maximally tolerated rate leads to an average two-fold increase in coronary blood flow [152]. In patients with CAD, the increase in coronary blood flow is blunted [153,154]. This blunting effect may be particularly prominent in vascular regions perfused by stenotic vessels [154]. There is no doubt that atrial pacing is a potent stimulus to the provocation of myocardial ischemia, as evidenced by the occurrence of ischemic ST-segment depression (ranging from 17% to 94%, average 57%), provocation of angina (ranging

from 44% to 100%, average 67%), and lactate production (average 57%) [154].

Atrial pacing has been used in combination with Tl-201 scintigraphy, RNA, digital subtraction ventriculography, and two-dimensional echocardiography (Table 10.10) [152,155–167]. It appears that pacing to a maximal rate of 85% to 100% of the maximal predicted heart rate is important to achieve the highest possible sensitivity for the test.

Several investigators have assessed the sensitivity and specificity of atrial pacing with Tl-201 scintigraphy in the diagnosis of CAD [158,164,167–170]. Most of these studies have included only a few highly selected patients, which may explain the wide variability of reported sensitivity (55% to 94%) and specificity (60% to 83%).

Feldman and colleagues [170] have used external ventricular pacing in combination with Tl-201 scintigraphy in a pilot study of nine patients. All eight patients with significant coronary stenoses had reversible perfusion defects by Tl-201 scintigraphy. Exercise Tl-201 scintigraphy performed on the same patients revealed transient perfusion defects in only four patients.

Stratmann and coworkers [171] assessed the prognostic value of atrial pacing in combination with Tl-201 scintigraphy in 210 patients with stable chest pain followed-up for an average of 19 months. In this study, cardiac events occurred in 38 patients and consisted of unstable angina in 20, cardiac death in 12,

TABLE 10.10 *Sensitivity and Specificity of Atrial Pacing Stress Test in Combination with Various Techniques*

Study	NO. Normal	NO. CAD	ECG Sen (%)	ECG Spec (%)	ANGINA Sen (%)	ANGINA Spec (%)	Imaging Technique	FIXED OR REVERSIBLE DEFECT Sen (%)	FIXED OR REVERSIBLE DEFECT Spec (%)	EF ≥ 5% Sen (%)	EF ≥ 5% Spec (%)	NEW WMA Sen (%)	NEW WMA Spec (%)
Chapman et al. [155]	5	16	21	100	44	—	2-DE	—	—	—	—	81	100
Dehmer et al. [156]	10	27	59	100	59	60	RVG	—	—	59	100	67	100
Hecht et al. [157]	0	12	—	—	100	—	RVG	—	—	—	—	75	—
Heller et al. [158]	6	16	94	83	56	67	Thal	94	67	—	—	—	—
Iliceto et al. [159]*	25	56	—	—	—	—	2-DE	—	—	—	—	87	88
Iliceto et al. [160]*	19	39	—	—	—	—	2-DE	—	—	—	—	85	84
Iskandrian et al. [161]	0	12	17	—	67	—	RVG	—	—	67	—	58	—
Johnson et al. [162]	17	44	—	—	—	—	DVG	—	—	—	—	67	94
Mancini et al. [152]	5	17	—	—	—	—	DVG	—	—	47	100	82	100
Markham et al. [163]	10	18	56	80	67	60	RVG	—	—	1 00	100	100	100
Stratmann et al. [164]	3	33	55	67	61	100	Thal	82	100	—	—	—	—
Tzivoni et al. [165]	7	11	64	71	—	—	RVG	—	—	91	100	82	100
Wasserman et al. [166]	12	28	—	—	71	67	DVG	—	—	—	—	82	100
Weiss et al. [167]	10	31	55	60	77	—	Thal	94	80	—	—	—	—

CAD, coronary artery disease (one or more lesions ≥ 50%); ECG, ST depression ≥ 1mm; Sen, sensitivity; Spec, specificity; EF, ejection fraction; WMA, wall motion abnormality; 2-DE, two-dimensional echocardiography; RVG, radionuclide ventriculography; Thal, thallium 201 scintigraphy; DVG, digital ventriculography.

*Transesophageal pacing studies

Source: From Strattman et al [164], with permission.

and nonfatal acute myocardial infarction in 6 patients. Reversible defects as determined by Tl-201 scintigraphy were present in 19 of the 38 patients with cardiac events, as compared with 42 of 157 patients without events ($p < .01$). Thus, as is also the case with exercise and pharmacologic scintigraphy, the demonstration of reversible defects during atrial pacing identifies patients who are more likely to develop subsequent events.

Although the experience with myocardial perfusion scintigraphy in combination with atrial pacing is limited, the results appear sufficiently encouraging to continue to apply the technique in appropriately selected patients.

Transesophageal pacing potentially could also be used to accomplish atrial pacing in combination with perfusion scintigraphy. LeFeuvre and associates [168] compared Tl-201 scintigraphy during transesophageal atrial pacing and, on a separate day, during exercise in 49 patients who also underwent coronary angiography. In the 16 patients with CAD with a previous myocardial infarction, the sensitivity was 87% for transesophageal pacing and 62% for exercise Tl-201 scintigraphy. The specificities were 71% and 78%, respectively. In patients with prior infarction ($n = 19$), reversible ischemia was elicited in 10 and 11 patients, respectively.

INDUCTION OF CORONARY VASOCONSTRICTION IN COMBINATION WITH MYOCARDIAL PERFUSION SCINTIGRAPHY

Several exogenous stimuli may induce coronary vasoconstriction. The most frequently used stimuli for this purpose have been hyperventilation, administration of ergonovine, and administration of acetylcholine. Patients susceptible to provocation of coronary vasoconstriction or coronary spasm with any of these stimuli often present with Prinzmetal's angina. Myocardial perfusion defects can be observed if Tl-201 or another tracer is injected during spontaneous Prinzmetal's angina [172] and may also be elicited by ergonovine administration prior to Tl-201 injection or by administration of intracoronary acetylcholine preceding the Tl-201 injection [173].

COLD PRESSOR STRESS AS AN ADJUNCT TO MYOCARDIAL PERFUSION SCINTIGRAPHY

The cold pressor test produces a generalized sympathetic stimulation and coronary vasoconstriction [174]. This stimulus is also apt to provoke focal coronary spasm in susceptible patients. To date, only one study has investigated the use of the cold pressor test in combination with Tl-201 perfusion scintigraphy. Ahmad and colleagues [175] studied 31 patients with CAD, 77% of whom had reversible perfusion defects during a cold pressor test. Conversely, none of the 5 patients without CAD developed a perfusion defect. In this small series, the sensitivity of the test was 40% in patients with one-vessel disease but increased to 100% in patients with three-vessel disease. Although encouraging, this study has neither been confirmed nor refuted by other investigators.

REFERENCES

1. Strauss HW, Pitt B. Noninvasive detection of subcritical coronary arterial narrowing with a coronary vasodilator and myocardial perfusion imaging. Am J Cardiol 1977;39:403.
2. Albro PC, Gould KL, Westcott RJ, et al. Noninvasive assessment of coronary stenoses by myocardial imaging during pharmacologic coronary vasodilatation. III. Clinical trial. Am J Cardiol 1978;42:751.
3. Gould KL, Lipscomb K. Effects of coronary stenosis on coronary flow reserve and resistance. Am J Cardiol 1978;34:48.
4. Gould KL. Assessment of coronary stenoses by myocardial perfusion imaging during pharmacologic coronary vasodilation: IV. Limits of stenosis by idealized, experimental, cross-sectional myocardial imaging. Am J Cardiol 1978;42:761.
5. Gould KL. Noninvasive assessment of coronary stenoses by myocardial perfusion imaging during pharmacologic coronary vasodilatation: I. Physiologic basis and experimental validation. Am J Cardiol 1978;41:267.
6. Gould KL. Pharmacologic interventions as an alternative to exercise stress. Semin Nucl Med 1987;17:121.
7. Gould KL, Westcott RJ, Albro PC, et al. Noninvasive assessment of coronary stenosis by myocardial imaging during pharmacologic coronary vasodilatation: II. Clinical methodology and feasibility. Am J Cardiol 1978;41:279.
8. Leppo J, Rosenkrantz J, Rosenthal R, et al. Quantitative thallium-201 redistribution with a fixed coronary stenosis in dogs. Circulation 1981;63:632.
9. Mueller TM, Marcus ML, Ehrhardt JC, et al. Limitations of thallium-201 myocardial perfusion scintigrams. Circulation 1976;54:640.
10. Mays AE, Cobb FR. Relationship between regional myocardial blood flow and thallium-201 redistribution in the presence of coronary artery stenosis and dipyridamole-induced vasodilation. J Clin Invest 1984;23:1359.
11. Nielsen AP, Morris KG, Murdock R, et al. Linear relationship between the distribution of thallium-201 and blood flow in ischemia and nonischemic myocardium during exercise. Circulation 1980;61:797.
12. Glover DK, Ruiz M, Yang JY, et al. Pharmacological stress thallium scintigraphy with 2-cyclohexylmethylidenehydrazinoadenosine (WRC-0470). A novel, short-acting adenosine A2A receptor agonist. Circulation 1996;94:1726.
13. Glover DK, Ruiz M, Yang JY, et al. Myocardial 99mTc-tetrofosmin uptake during denosine-induced vasodilatation with either a critical or mild coronary stenosis: comparison with 201Tl and regional myocardial blood flow. Circulation 1997;96:2332.

14. Calnon DA, Ruiz M, Vanzetto G, et al. Myocardial uptake of (99m) Tc-N-NOET and (201) Tl during dobutamine infusion. Comparison with adenosine stress. Circulation 1999;100:1653.

15. Becker, LC: Conditions for vasodilator-induced coronary steal in experimental myocardial ischemia. Circulation 1978;57:1103.

16. Patterson RE, Kirk ES. Coronary steal mechanisms in dogs with one-vessel occlusion and other arteries normal. Circulation 1983;67:1009.

17. Gewirtz H, Gross SL, Williams DO, et al. Contrasting effects of nifedipine and adenosine on regional myocardial flow redistribution and metabolism distal to a severe coronary arterial stenosis: observations in sedated, closed-chest, domestic swine. Circulation 1984;69:1048.

18. Beller GA. Pharmacologic stress myocardial perfusion imaging. Curr Probl Cardiol 1993;18:481 (Commentary).

19. Beller GA, Holzgrefe HH, Watson DD. Effects of dipyridamole-induced vasodilation on myocardial uptake and clearance kinetics of thallium-201. Circulation 1983;68:1328.

20. Feldman RL, Nichols WW, Pepine CJ, et al. Acute effect of intravenous dipyridamole on regional coronary hemodynamics and metabolism.Circulation 1981;64:333.

21. Glover DK, Ruiz M, Sansoy KV, et al. Effect of N-0861, a selective A1 receptor antagonist, on pharmacologic stress imaging with adenosine. J Nucl Med 1995;36:270.

22. John RM, Taggart PI, Sutton PM, et al. Vasodilator myocardial perfusion imaging: demonstration of local electrophysiological changes of ischemia. Br Heart J 1992;68:21.

23. Fung A, Gallagher K, Buda A. The physiologic basis of dobutamine as compared to dipyridamole stress interventions in the assessment of critical stenosis. Circulation 1987;76:943.

24. Lee DS, Yeo JS, Chung JK, et al. Transient prolonged stunning induced by dipyridamole and shown on 1- and 24-hour post-stress 99mTc-MIBI gated SPECT. J Nucl Med 2000;41:27.

25. Bellardinelli L, Lindel J, Beme RM. The cardiac effects of adenosine. Prog Cardiovasc Dis 1989;32:73.

26. Verani MS. Adenosine thallium-201 myocardial perfusion scintigraphy. Am Heart J 1991;122:269.

27. Nielsen-Kudsk F, Pedersen AK. Pharmacokinetics of dipyridamole. Acta Pharmacol Toxicol 1979;44:391.

28. Homma S, Callahan RJ,Ameer B, et al.Usefulness of oral dipyridamole suspension for stress thallium imaging without exercise in the detection of coronary artery disease. Am J Cardiol 1986;57:503.

29. Leppo JA. Dipyridamole-thallium imaging: the lazyman's stress test. J Nucl Med 1989;30:281.

30. Brown BG, Josephson MA, Petersen RB, et al. Intravenous dipyridamole combined with isometric handgrip for near maximal acute increase in coronary flow in patients with coronary artery disease. Am J Cardiol 981;48:1077.

31. Rossen JD, Quillen JE, Lopez JAG, et al. Comparison of coronary vasodilation with intravenous dipyridamole and adenosine. J Am Coll Cardiol 1991;18:485.

32. Rossen JD, Simonetti I, Marans ML, et al. Coronary dilation with standard dose dipyridamole and dipyridamole combined with hand-grip. Circulation 1989;79:566.

33. Wilson RF, Laughlin DE, Ackett PH, et al. Transluminal, subselective measurement of coronary artery blood flow velocity and vasodilator reserve in man. Circulation 1985;72:82.

34. Casale PN, Guiney TE, Strauss HW, et al. Simultaneous low level treadmill exercise and intravenous dipyridamole stress thallium imaging. Am J Cardiol 1988;62:799.

35. Verzijlbergen JF, Vermeersch PHMJ, Laarman G-J, et al. In-adequate exercise leads to suboptimal imaging. Thallium-201 myocardial perfusion imaging after dipyridamole combined with low-level exercise unmasks ischemia in symptomatic patients with non-diagnostic thallium-201 scans who exercise submaximally. J Nucl Med 1991;32:2071.

36. Walker PR, James MA, Wilde RPH, et al. Dipyridamole combined with exercise for thallium-201 myocardial imaging. Br Heart J 1986;55:321.

37. Wilde P, Walker P, Watt I, et al. Thallium myocardial imaging: recent experience using a coronary vasodilator. Clin Radiol 1982;33:43.

38. Candell-Riera J, Santana-boado c, Castell-Conesa J. Simultaneous dipyridamole/maximal subjective exercise with 99mTc-MIBI SPECT: improved diagnostic yield in coronary artery disease. J Am Coll Cardiol 1997;29:531.

39. Czernin J, Auerbach M, Sun K, et al. Effects of modified pharmacologic stress approaches on hyperemic myocardial blood flow. J Nucl Med 1995;36:575.

40. Shehata AR, Ahlberg AW, White MP, et al. Dipyridamole-dobutamine stress with Tc-99m sestamibi tomographic myocardial perfusion imaging. Am J Cardiol 1998;82:520.

41. Villaneuva FS, Kaul S, Smith WH, et al. Prevalence and correlates of increased lung/heart ratio of thallium-201 during dipyridamole stress imaging for suspected coronary artery disease. Am J Cardiol 1990;66:1324.

42. Chambers CE, Brown KA. Dipyridamole-induced ST segment depression during thallium-201 imaging in patients with coronary artery disease: angiographic and hemodynamic determinants. J Am Coll Cardiol 1988;12:37.

43. Okada RD, Dai Y, Boucher CA, et al. Significance of increased lung thallium-201 activity on serial cardiac images after dipyridamole treatment in coronary artery disease. Am J Cardiol 1984;53:470.

44. Chouraqui P, Rodrigues EA, Berman DS, et al. Significance of dipyridamole-induced transient dilation of left ventricle during thallium-201 scintigraphy in suspected coronary artery disease. Am J Cardiol 1990;66:689.

45. McClellan JR, Travin MI, HermanSD, et al. Prognostic importance of scintigraphic left ventricular cavity dilation during intravenous dipyridamole technetium-99m sestamibi myocardial tomographic imaging in predicting coronary events. Am J Cardiol 1997;79:600.

46. Hurwitz GA, Ghali SK, Husni M, et al. Pulmonary uptake of technetium-99m-sestamibi induced by dipyridamole-based stress or exercise. J Nucl Med 1998;39:339.

47. Ranhosky A, Kempthorne-Rawson J, Intravenous Dipyridamole Thallium Imaging Study Group. The safety of intravenous dipyridamole thallium myocardial perfusion imaging. Circulation 1990;81:1205.

48. Picano E, Marini C, Pirelli S, et al. Safety of intravenous high-dose dipyridamole echocardiography Am J Cardiol 1992;70:252.

49. Lette J, Tatum JL, Fraser S, et al. Safety of dipyridamole testing in 73,806 patients: the Multicenter Dipyridamole Safety Study. J Nucl Cardiol 1995;2:3.

50. Lette J, Carini G, Tatum JL et al. Safety of dipyridamole testing in patients with cerebrovascular disease. Am J Cardiol 1995;75:535.

51. Bateman TM, O'Keefe JH Jr. Pharmacological (stress) perfusion scintigraphy: methods, advantages, and applications. Am J Cardiac Imaging 1992;6:3.

52. Botvinick E, Dae WM. Dipyridamole perfusion scintigraphy. Semin Nucl Med 1991;21:242.

53. Eagle KA, Strauss W, Boucher CA. Dipyridamole myocardial perfusion imaging for coronary artery disease. Am J Cardiac Imaging 1988;2:292.

54. Iskandrian AS, Heo J, Askenase A, et al. Dipyridamole cardiac imaging. Am Heart J 1988;115:432.

55. Iskandrian AS. Dipyridamole sestamibi myocardial imaging. Am J Cardiol 1991;68:674.

56. Stratmann HG, Kennedy HL. Evaluation of coronary artery disease in the patient unable to exercise: alternatives to exercise stress testing. Am Heart J 1989;117:1344.

57. Travin MI, Wexler JP. Pharmacological stress testing. Semin Nucl Med 1999;29:298.

58. Francisco DA, Collins SM, Go RT. Tomographic thallium-201 myocardial perfusion scintigrams after maximal coronary artery vasodilation with intravenous dipyridamole: comparison of qualitative and quantitative approaches. Circulation 1982; 66:370.

59. Huikuri HV, Korhonen RU, Airaksinen J, et al. Comparison of dipyridamole-handgrip test and bicycle exercise test for thallium tomographic imaging. Am J Cardiol 1988;61:264.

60. Kong BA, Shaw L, Miller DD, et al. Comparison of accuracy for detecting coronary artery disease and side-effect profile of dipyridamole thallium-201 myocardial perfusion imaging in women versus men. Am J Cardiol 1992;70:168.

61. Lam JY, Chaitman BR, Glaenzer M, et al. Safety and diagnostic accuracy of dipyridamole-thallium imaging in the elderly. J Am Coll Cardiol 1988;11:585.

62. Leppo J, Boucher CA, Okada RD, et al. Serial thallium-201 myocardial imaging after dipyridamole infusion: diagnostic utility in detecting coronary stenoses and relationship to regional wall motion. Circulation 1982;66:649.

63. Mendelson MA, Spies SM, Spies WG, et al. Usefulness of single photon emission computed tomography of thallium-201 uptake after dipyridamole infusion for detection of coronary artery disease. Am J Cardiol 1992;69:1150.

64. Taillefer R, Lette J, Phaneuf DC, et al. Thallium-201 myocardial imaging during pharmacologic coronary vasodilation: comparison of oral and intravenous administration of dipyridamole. J Am Coll Cardiol 1986;8:76.

65. Mahmarian JJ, Verani MS. Myocardial perfusion imaging during pharmacologic stress testing. Cardiol Clin 1994;12:223.

66. Borges-Neto S, Mahmarian JJ, Jain A, et al. Quantitative thallium-201 single-photon emission computed tomography after oral dipyridamole for assessing the presence, anatomic location and severity of coronary artery disease. J Am Coll Cardiol 1988;11:962.

67. Martin W, Tweddel AC, Main G, et al. A comparison of maximal exercise and dipyridamole thallium-201 planar gated scintigraphy. Eur J Nucl Med 1992;19:258.

68. Varma SK, Watson DD, Beller GA. Quantitative comparison of thallium-201 scintigraphy after exercise and dipyridamole in coronary artery disease. Am J Cardiol 1989;64:871.

69. Matzer L, Kiat H, Friedman JD, et al. A new approach to the assessment of tomographic thallium-201 scintigraphy in patients with left bundle branch block. J Am Coll Cardiol 1991; 17:1309.

70. Braat SH, Brugada P, Barr FW, et al. Thallium-201 exercise scintigraphy and left bundle branch block. Am J Cardiol 1985; 55:224.

71. Burns RJ, Galligan L, Wright LM, et al. Improved specificity of myocardial thallium-201 single photon emission computed tomography in patients with left bundle branch block by dipyridamole. Am J Cardiol 1991;68:504.

72. DePuey EG, Guertler-Krawczynska E, Robbins WL. Thallium-201 SPECT in coronary disease patients with left bundle branch block. J Nucl Med 1988;29:1479.

73. Hirzel HO, Msenn N, Nuesch K, et al. Thallium-201 scintigraphy in complete left bundle branch block. Am J Cardiol 1984;53:764.

74. Huerta EM, Rodriguez PL, Castro BJM, et al. Thallium-201 exercise scintigraphy in patients having complete left bundle branch block with normal coronary arteries. Int J Cardiol 1987; 16:43.

75. Rockett JF, Wood WC, Moihuddin M, et al. Intravenous dipyridamole thallium-201 SPECT imaging in patients with left bundle branch block. Clin Nucl Med 1990;15:401.

76. Jukema JW, Van de Wall E-E, Van Der Vis Meesen MJ, et al. Dipyridamole thallium-201 scintigraphy for improved detection of left anterior descending coronary artery stenosis in patients with left bundle branch block. Eur Heart J 1993;14:53.

77. Larcos G, Brown ML, Gibbons RJ. Role of dipyridamole thallium-201 imaging in left bundle branch block. Am J Cardiol 1991;68:1097.

78. Morais J, Soucy JP, Sestier F, et al. Dipyridamole testing compared to exercise stress for thallium-201 imaging in patients with left bundle branch block. Can J Cardiol 1990;6:5.

79. O'Keefe JH Jr, Bateman TM, Silvestri R, et al. Safety and diagnostic accuracy of adenosine thallium-201 scintigraphy in patients unable to exercise and those with left bundle branch block. Am Heart J 1992;124:614.

80. O'Keefe JH, Bateman TM, Barnhart CS. Adenosine thallium-201 is superior to exercise thallium-201 for detecting coronary artery disease in patients with left bundle branch block. J Am Coll Cardiol 1993;21:1332.

81. Kettunen R, Huikuri HV, Keikkila J, et al. Usefulness of technetium-99m-MIBI and thallium-201 in tomographic imaging combined with high-dose dipyridamole and handgrip exercise for detecting coronary artery disease. Am J Cardiol 1991; 68:575.

82. Parodi O, Marcassa C, Casucci R, et al. Accuracy and safety of technetium-99m hexakis 2-methoxy-2-isobutyl isonitrile (Sestamibi) myocardial scintigraphy with high dose dipyridamole test in patients with effort angina pectoris: a multicenter study. J Am Coll Cardiol 1991;18:1439.

83. Primeau M, Taillefer R, Essiambre R, et al. Technetium-99m sestamibi myocardial perfusion imaging: comparison between treadmill, dipyridamole and trans-oesophageal atrial pacing "stress" test in normal subjects. Eur J Nucl Med 1991;18:247.

84. Tartagni F, Dondi M, Limonetti P, et al. Dipyridamole technetium-99m-2-methoxy isobutyl isonitrile tomoscintigraphic imaging for identifying diseased coronary vessels: comparison with thallium-201 stress-rest study. J Nucl Med 1991;32:369.

85. Verani MS. Pharmacologic stress myocardial perfusion imaging. Curr Prob Cardiol 1993;18:481.

86. Drury AN, Szent-Gyorgyi A. The physiological activity of adenine compounds with special reference to their action upon the mammalian heart. J Physiol 1929;68:213.

87. Sollevi A, Langerkranser M, Irestedt L, et al. Controlled hypotension with adenosine in cerebral aneurysm surgery. Anesthesiology 1984;61:400.

88. Siffring PA, Gupta NC, Mohiuddin SM, et al. Myocardial uptake and clearance of Tl-201 in healthy subjects: comparison of adenosine-induced hyperemia and exercise stress. Radiology 1989;173:769.

89. Verani MS, Mahmarian JJ, Hixson JB, et al. Diagnosis of coronary artery disease by controlled coronary vasodilation with adenosine and thallim-201 scintigraphy in patients unable to exercise. Circulation 1990;82:80.

90. O'Keefe JH Jr, Bateman TM, Handlin LR, et al. Four-versus 6-minute protocol for adenosine thallium-201 single photon emission computed tomography imaging. Am Heart J 1995; 129:482.

91. Korkmaz ME, Mahmarian JJ, Guidry GW, et al. Safety of single-site adenosine thallium-201 scintigraphy. Am J Cardiol 1994;73:200.

92. Ogilby JD, Iskandrian AS, Untereker WJ, et al. Effect of intravenous adenosine infusion on myocardial perfusion and function: hemodynamic, angiographic and scintigraphic study. Circulation 1992;86:887.

93. Wilson RF, Wyche K, Christensen GV, et al. Effects of adenosine on human coronary arterial circulation. Circulation 1990; 82:1595.

94. Chan SY, Brunken RC, Czernin J, et al. Comparison of maximal myocardial blood flow during adenosine infusion with that of intravenous dipyridamole in normal men. J Am Coll Cardiol 1992;20:979.

95. Abreu A., Mahmahrian JJ, Nishimura S., et al. Tolerance and safety of pharmacologic coronary vasodilation with adenosine in association with thallium-201 scintigraphy in patients with suspected coronary artery disease. J Am coll Cardiol 1991:18:730.

96. Nguyen T, Heo J, Ogilby JD, et al. Single-photon emissiomn computed tomography with thallium-201 during adenosine-induced coronary hyperemia: correlation with coronary arteriography, exercise thallium imaging and two-dimensional echocardiography. J Am Coll Cardiol 1990:;16:1375.

97. Coyne EP, Belvedere DA, Vande-Streek PR, et al. Thallium-201 scintigraphy after intravenous infusion of adenosine compared with exercise thallium testing in the diagnosis of coronary artery disease. J Am Coll Cardiol 1991;17:1289.

98. Iskandrian AS, Heo J, Nguyen T, et al. Assessment of coronary artery disease using single-photon emission tomography with thallium-201 during adenosine-induced coronary hyperemia. Am J Cardiol 1991;67:1190.

99. Nishimura S. Mahmarian JJ, Boyce TM, et al. Quantitative thallium-201 single photon emission computed tomography during maximal pharmacologic coronary vasodilation with adenosine for assessing coronary artery disease. J Am Coll Cardiol 1991;18:736.

100. Gupta NC, Esterbrooks DJ, Hilleman DE, et al. Comparison of adenosine and exercise thallium-201 single-photon emission computed tomography (SPECT) myocardial perfusion imaging. J Am Coll Cardiol 1992;19:248.

101. Cerqueira MD, Verani MS, Schwaiger M, et al. Safety profile of adenosine stress perfusion imaging: results from the Adenoscan Multicenter Trial Registry. J Am Coll Cardiol 1994; 23:384.

102. Sylven C, Jonzon B, Brandt R, et al. Dose-effect relationship of adenosine provoked angina pectoris-like pain—a study of the psychophysical power function. Eur Heart J 1988;9:87.

103. Crea F, Pupita G, Galassi AR, et al. Role of adenosine in pathogenesis of anginal pain. Circulation 1990;81:164.

104. Watt AH, Reid PG, Stephens MR, et al. Adenosine-induced respiratory stimulation depends on site of infusion. Evidence for an action on the carotid body? Br J Clin Pharmacol 1986; 22:486.

105. Nishimura S, Kimball KT, Mahmarian JJ, et al. Angiographic and hemodynamic determinants of myocardial ischemia during adenosine thallium-201 and scintigraphy in coronary artery disease. Circulation 1993;87:1211.

106. Marshall ES, Raichlen JS, Kim SM, et al. Prognostic significance of ST-segment depression during adenosine perfusion imaging. Am Heart J 1995;130:55.

107. Lee J, Heo J, Ogilby JD, et al. Atrioventricular block during adenosine thallium imaging. Am Heart J 1992;123:1569.

108. Iskandrian AS, Heo J, Nguyen T, et al. Left ventricular dilatation and pulmonary thallium uptake after single-photon emission computed tomography using thallium-201 during adenosine-induced coronary hyperemia. Am J Cardiol 1990;66:807.

109. Iskandrian AS, Verani MS, Heo J. Pharmacologic stress testing: mechanisms of action, hemodynamic responses, and results in detection of coronary artery disease. J Nucl Cardiol 1994; 1:94.

110. Nishimura S, Mahmarian JJ, Verani MS. Significance of increased lung thallium uptake during adenosine thallium-201 scintigraphy. J Nucl Med 1992;33:1600.

111. Iskandrian AS. New directions in pharmacologic stress imaging. (Editorial). J Nucl Med 1995;36:276.

112. He ZX, Cwajg E, Hwang W, et al. Myocardial blood flow and myocardial uptake of (201) Tl and 99m (Tc) sestamibi during coronary vasodilation induced by CGS-21680, a selective adenosine A (2A) receptor agonist. Circulation 2000;102:438.

113. Wang FP, Amanullah AM, Kiat H, et al. Diagnostic efficacy of stress technetium 99m-labeled sestamibi myocardial perfusion single-photon emission computed tomography in detection of coronary artery disease among patients over age 80. J Nucl Cardiol 1995;2:380.

114. Amanullah AM, Kiat H, Friedman JD, et al. Adenosine technetium-99m sestamibi myocardial perfusion SPECT in women: diagnostic efficacy in detection of coronary artery disease. J Am Coll Cardiol 1996;27:803.

115. Iskandrian AE, Heo J, Nallamothu N. Detection of coronary artery disease in women with use of stress single-photon emission computed tomography myocardial perfusion imaging. J Nucl Cardiol 1997;4:329.

115a. Nishimura S, Mahmarian JJ, Boyce TM, et al. Equivalence between adenosine and exercise thallium-201 myocardial tomography. A multicenter, prospective, crossover trial. J Am Coll Cardiol 1992;20:265.

116. Pennell DJ, Mavrogeni SI, Forbat SM, et al. Adenosine combined with dynamic exercise for myocardial perfusion imaging. J Am Coll Cardiol 1995;25:1300.

117. Cramer MJ, Verzijlbergen JF, van der Wall EE, et al. Comparison of adenosine and high-dose dipyridamole both combined with low-level exercise stress for 99Tcm-MIBI SPECT myocardial perfusion imaging. Nucl Med Comm 1996;17:97.

118. Jamil G, Ahlberg AW, Elliott MD, et al. Impact of limited treadmill exercise on adenosine Tc-99m sestamibi single-photon emission computed tomographic myocardial perfusion imaging in coronary artery disease. Am J Cardiol 1999;84:400.

119. Johnston DL, Scanlon PD, Hodge DO, et al. Pulmonary function monitoring during adenosine myocardial perfusion scintigraphy in patients with chronic obstructive pulmonary disease. Mayo Clin Proc 1999;74:339.

120. Samuels B, Kiat H, Friedman JD, et al. Adenosine pharmacologic stress myocardial perfusion tomographic imaging in patients with significant aortic stenosis: diagnostic efficacy and comparison of clinical, hemodynamic and electrocardiographic variables with 100 age-matched control subjects. J Am Coll Cardiol 1995;25:99.

121. Sonneblick EH, Frishman WH, LeJemetel TH. Dobutamine: a new synthetic cardioactive sympathetic amine. N Engl J Med 1979;300:17.

122. Ruffolo RR Jr, Spradlin TA, Pollock DG, et al. Alpha and beta-adrenergic effects of the stereoisomers of dobutamine. J Pharmacol Exp Ther 1981;219:447.

123. Liang CS, Hood WB Jr. Dobutamine infusion in conscious dogs

with and without autonomic nervous systemic inhibition: effects on systemic hemodynamics, regional blood flows and cardiac metabolism. J Pharmacol Exp Ther 1979;211:698.

124. Chatterjee K. *Effects of Dobutamine on Coronary Hemodynamics and Myocardial Energetics in Dobutamine—A Ten Year Review.* New York: NCM Publishers, 1989, p. 49.

125. Willerson JT, Hutton I, Watson JT, et al. Influence of dobutamine on regional myocardial blood flow and ventricular performance during acute and chronic myocardial ischemia in dogs. Circulation 1976;53:828.

126. Vatner SF, Baig H. Importance of heart rate in determining the effects of sympathomimetic amines on regional myocardial function and blood flow in conscious dogs with acute myocardial ischemia. Circ Res 1979;45:793.

127. Meyer SL, Curry GC, Donsky MS, et al. Influence of dobutamine on hemodynamics and coronary blood flow inpatients with and without coronary artery disease. Am J Cardiol 1976; 38:103.

128. Pozen RG, DiBianco R, Katz RJ, et al. Myocardial metabolic and hemodynamic effects of dobutamine in heart failure complicating coronary artery disease. Circulation 1981;63:1279.

129. Krivokapich J, Huang S-C, Schelbert HR. Assessment of the effects of dobutamine on myocardial blood flow and oxidative metabolism in normal human subjects using nitrogen-13 ammonia and carbon-11 acetate. Am J Cardiol 1993;71:1351.

129a. Tadamura E, Iida H, Matsumoto K, et al. Comparison of myocardial blood flow during dobutamine-atropine infusion with that after dipyridamole administration in normal men. J Am Coll Cardiol 2001;37:130.

129b. Skopicki HA, Abraham SA, Picard MH, et al. Effects of dobutamine at maximally tolerated dose on myocardial blood flow in humans with ischemic heart disease. Circulation 1997;96:3346.

130. Mason JR, Palac RT, Freeman ML, et al. Thallium scintigraphy during dobutamine infusion: nonexercise-dependent screening test for coronary disease. Am Heart J 1984;107:481.

131. Pennell DJ, Underwood SR, Swanton RH, et al. Dobutamine-thallium myocardial perfusion tomography. J Am Coll Cardiol 1991;18:1471.

132. Hays JT, Mahmarian JJ, Cochran AJ, et al. Dobutamine thallium-201 tomography for evaluating patients with suspected coronary artery disease unable to undergo exercise or vasodilatory pharmacologic testing. J Am Coll Cardiol 1993;21:1583.

133. Dakik HA, Vempathy H, Verani MS. Tolerance, hemodynamic changes, and safety of dobutamine stress perfusion imaging. J Nucl Cardiol 1996;3:410.

134. Marwick T, Willemart B, D'Hondt AM, et al. Selection of the optimal nonexercise stress for the evaluation of ischemic regional myocardial dysfunction and malperfusion: comparison of dobutamine and adenosine using echocardiography and 99mTc MIBI single photon emission computed tomography. Circulation 1993;87:345.

135. Marwick T, D'Hondt A-M, Baudhuin T, et al. Optimal use of dobutamine stress for the detection and evaluation of coronary artery disease: combination with echocardiography or scintigraphy, or both? J Am Coll Cardiol 1993;22:159.

136. Forster T, McNeill AJ, Salustri A, et al. Simultaneous dobutamine stress echocardiography and technetium-99m isonitrile single-photon emission computed tomography in patients with suspected coronary artery disease. J Am Coll Cardiol 1993;21:1591.

137. Gunalp B, Dokumaci B, Uyan C, et al. Value of dobutamine technetium-99m-sestamibi SPECT and echocardiography in the detection of coronary artery disease compared with coronary angiography. J Nucl Med 1993;34:889.

138. Elliott BM, Robinson JG, Zellner JL, et al. Dobutamine-thallium-201 imaging: assessing cardiac risks associated with vascular surgery. Circulation 1991;84 (suppl III):54.

139. Coma-Canella I, Martinez MVG, Rodrigo F, et al. The dobutamine stress test with thallium-201 single-photon emission computed tomography and radionuclide angiography: post infarction study. J Am Coll Cardiol 1993;22:399.

140. Takeishi Y, Takahashi N, Fujiwara S, et al. Myocardial tomography with technetium-99m-tetrofosmin during intravenous infusion of adenosine triphosphate. J Nucl Med 1998; 39:582.

141. Kiat H, Iskandrian AS, Villegas BJ, et al. Arbutamine stress thallium-201 single-photon emission computed tomography using a computerized closed-loop delivery system. Multicenter trial for evaluation of safety and diagnostic accuracy. The International Arbutamine Study Group. J Am Coll Cardiol 1995; 26:1159.

142. Harris D, Taylor D, Condon B, et al. Myocardial imaging with dipyridamole: comparison of the sensitivity and specificity of Tl-201 versus MUGA. Eur J Nucl Med 1982;7:1.

143. Sochor H, Pacinger O, Ogris E, et al. Radionuclide imaging after coronary vasodilation: myocardial scintigraphy with thallium-201 and radionuclide angiography after administration of dipyridamole. Eur Heart J 1984;5:500.

144. Cates CV, Kronenberg MW, Collings HW, et al. Dipyridamole radionuclide ventriculography: a test with high specificity for severe coronary artery disase. J Am Coll Cardiol 1989;13:841.

145. Klein HO, Ninio R, Eliyahu S, et al. Effects of the dipyridamole test on left ventricular function in coronary artery disease. Am J Cardiol 1992;69:482.

146. Freeman ML, Palac R, Mason J. A comparison of dobutamine infusion and supine bicycle exercise for radionuclide cardiac stress testing. Clin Nucl Med 1984;9:251.

147. Konishi T, Koyama T, Aoki T, et al. Radionuclide assessment of left ventricular function during dobutamine infusion in patients with coronary artery disease: comparison with ergometer exercise. Clin Cardiol 1990;13:183.

148. Mohaved A, Reeves WC, Rose GC, et al. Dobutamine and improvement of regional and global left ventricular function in coronary artery disease. Am J Cardiol 1990;66:375.

149. Iftikhar I, Koutelou M, Mahmarian JJ, et al. Simultaneous perfusion tomography and radionuclide angiography during dobutamine stress. J Nucl Med 1996;37:1306.

150. O'Keefe JH Jr, Barnhart CS, Bateman TM. Comparison of stress echocardiography and stress myocardial perfusion scintigraphy for diagnosing coronary artery disease and assessing its severity. Am J Cardiol 1995;75:25D.

151. Verani MS. Myocardial perfusion imaging versus two-dimensional echocardiography: comparative value in the diagnosis of coronary artery disease. J Nucl Cardiol 1994;1:399.

152. Mancini GB, Peterson KL, Gregoratos G, et al. Effects of atrial pacing on global and regional left ventricular function in coronary heart disease assessed by digital intravenous ventriculography. Am J Cardiol 1984;53:456.

153. Schmidt DH, Weiss MB, Casarella WJ, et al. Regional myocardial perfusion during atrial pacing in patients with coronary artery disease. Circulation 1976;53:807.

154. Wilson JR, Martin JL, Untereker WJ, et al. Sequential changes in regional coronary flow during pacing-induced angina pectoris: coronary flow limitations precedes angina. Am Heart J 1984;107:269.

155. Chapman PD, Doyle TP, Troup PJ, et al. Stress echocardiog-

raphy with transesophageal atrial pacing: preliminary report of a new method for detection of ischemic wall motion abnormalities. Circulation 1984;70:445.

156. Dehmer GJ, Firth BG, Nicod P, et al. Alterations in left ventricular volumes and ejection fraction during atrial pacing in patients with coronary artery disease: assessment with radionuclide ventriculography. Am Heart J 1983;106:114.

157. Hecht HS, Chew CY, Burnam M, et al. Radionuclide ejection fraction and regional wall motion during atrial pacing in stable angina pectoris: comparison with metabolic and hemodynamic parameters. Am Heart J 1981;101:726.

158. Heller GV, Aroesty JM, Parker JA, et al. The pacing stress test: thallium-201 myocardial imaging after atrial pacing. Diagnostic value in detecting coronary artery disease compared with exercise testing. J Am Coll Cardiol 1984;3:1197.

159. Iliceto S, Sorino M, D'Ambrosio G, et al. Detection of coronary artery disease by two-dimensional echocardiography and transesophageal atrial pacing J Am Coll Cardiol 1985;5:1188.

160. Iliceto S, D'Ambrosio G, Sorino M, et al. Comparison of postexercise and transesophageal atrial pacing two-dimensional echocardiography for detection of coronary artery disease. Am J Cardiol 1986;57:547.

161. Iskandrian AS, Bemis CE, Hakki AH, et al. Ventricular systolic and diastolic impairment during pacing-iduced myocardial ischemia in coronary artery disease. simultaneous hemodynamic, electrocardiographic, and radionuclide angiographic evaluation. Am Heart J 1986;112:382.

162. Johnson RA, Vasserman AG, Leiboff RH, et al. Intravenous digital left ventriculography at rest and with atrial pacing as a screening procedure for coronary artery disease. J Am Coll Cardiol 1983;2:905.

163. Markham RV, Winniford MD, Firth BG, et al. Symptomatic, electrocardiographic, metabolic, and hemodynamic alterations during pacing-induced myocardial ischemia. Am J Cardiol 1983;51:1589.

164. Stratmann HG, Mark AL, Walter KE, et al. Atrial pacing and thallium-201 scintigraphy: combined use for diagnosis of coronary artery disease. Angiology 1987;38:807.

165. Tzivoni D, Weiss AT, Solomon J, et al. Diagnosis of coronary artery disease by multigated radionuclide angiography during right atrial pacing. Chest 1981;80:562.

166. Wasserman AG, Johnson RA, Katz RJ, et al. Detection of left ventricular wall motion abnormalities for the diagnosis of coronary artery disease: a comparison of exercise radionuclide and pacing intravenous digital ventriculography. Am J Cardiol 1984;54:497.

167. Weiss AT, Tzivoni D, Sagie A, et al. Atrial pacing thallium scintigraphy in the evaluation of coronary artery disease. Isr J Med Sci 1983;19:495.

168. Le Feuvre C, Vacheron A, Metzger JP, et al. Comparison of thallium myocardial scintigraphy after exercise and transesophageal atrial pacing in the diagnosis of coronary artery disease. Eur Heart J 1992;13:794.

169. Le Helloco A, Nicol N, Leborgne O, et al. Diagnosis of coronary artery disease by thallium-201 myocardial scintigraphy during atrial pacing. Arch Mal Coeur Vaiss 1991;84:801.

170. Feldman MD, Warren SE, Gervino EV, et al. Noninvasive external cardiac pacing for thallium-201 scintigraphy. Am J Physiol Imaging 1988;3:172.

171. Stratmann HG, Mark AL, Walter KE, et al. Prognostic value of atrial pacing and thallium-201 scintigraphy in patients with stable chest pain. Am J Cardiol 1989;64;985.

172. Maseri A, Parodi O, Severi S, et al. Transient transmural reduction of myocardial blood flow demonstrated by thallium-201 scintigraphy, as a cause of variant angina. Circulation 1976;54:280.

173. Kugiyama K, Yasue H, Okumura K, et al. Simultaneous multivessel coronary artery spasm demonstrated by quantitative analysis of thallium-201 single photon emission computed tomography. Am J Cardiol 1987;60:1009.

174. Raizner AE, Chahine RA, Ishimori T, et al. Provocation of coronary artery spasm by the cold pressor test. Hemodynamic, arteriographic and quantitative angiographic observation. Circulation 1980;62:925.

175. Ahmad M, Dubiel JP, Hiabach H. Cold pressor thallium-201 myocardial scintigraphy in the diagnosis of coronary artery disease. Am J Cardiol 1982;50:1253.

11 | Risk assessment in CAD

KENNETH A. BROWN, JOHN J. MAHMARIAN, AND JEFFREY LEPPO

Part 1

Suspected CAD/Known Stable CAD

KENNETH A. BROWN

Over the past decade there has been a gradual expansion in the use of stress nuclear myocardial perfusion imaging (MPI) among patients with suspected or known coronary artery disease (CAD) from a diagnostic tool to a prognostic risk assessor. As constraints in medical resources and the demand for cost-effective care increase, the need for a noninvasive test that can identify those patients with chronic CAD who will most benefit from the expense and risk of additional invasive or interventional procedures has grown. With its now well-established prognostic value, stress nuclear MPI has become an invaluable adjunct to clinicians for making management decisions by distinguishing those patients at high risk for future cardiac events who will most benefit from further interventions from patients at low risk for cardiac events, who are very unlikely to benefit.

DETERMINANTS OF CARDIAC RISK

The two most important determinants of the risk of future cardiac death or myocardial infarction in patients with coronary heart disease are left ventricular function and extent of jeopardized viable myocardium. The former is an index of the extent of prior damage from infarction and remodeling, while the latter reflects additional myocardium at risk for future damage. Since nuclear cardiac imaging can identify the presence and extent of jeopardized viable myocardium, as well as measure ventricular function either indirectly or directly, it has unique advantages for the determination of prognosis in patients with chronic CAD.

Left Ventricular Function

Ejection fraction is the most direct and simplest measure of systolic function. Measurement of resting ejec-

tion fraction using either first-pass or equilibrium radionuclide cineangiography has been shown to be an important predictor of cardiac events, particularly cardiac death [1–26]. The Multicenter Postinfarction Research Group showed a representative strong inverse relationship between resting ejection fraction and 1-year cardiac death rate (Fig. 11.1) [7]. However, for the most part, identifying reduced left ventricular function, although helpful at defining cardiac risk, has limited remedial options: we cannot bring back to life what is already dead. That is why identification of additional jeopardized viable myocardium is so important. Not only does it identify risk of cardiac events, it allows potential modification of such risk by revascularization either with bypass surgery or coronary interventional procedures.

Jeopardized Viable Myocardium

The presence and extent of transient defects on stress nuclear MPI, reflecting jeopardized viable myocardium, are probably the most consistent predictors of important cardiac events described in the literature [27,28]. A direct relationship between cardiac risk and the presence and extent of jeopardized viable myocardium determined from stress nuclear MPI was first described by Brown and colleagues in 1983 [29]. In a series of 100 patients without known prior myocardial infarction who presented for evaluation of chest pain, the predictive value of exercise thallium-201 (Tl-201) imaging was compared to clinical, exercise electrocardiographic, and angiographic data. The best predictor of cardiac death or myocardial infarction was the extent of jeopardized viable myocardium reflected in the number of myocardial segments with transient Tl-201 defects (Fig. 11.2). Importantly, although angiographic

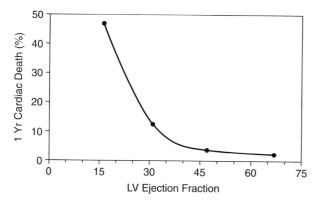

FIGURE 11.1 One-year cardiac death rate as a function of resting left ventricular ejection fraction. Risk begins to increase substantially when ejection fraction falls below 35%. (Adapted from The Multicenter Postinfarction Research Group [7].)

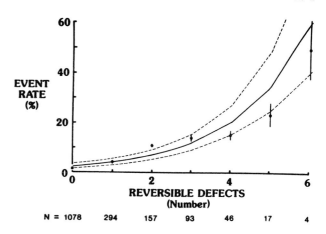

FIGURE 11.3 The relationship of cardiac events as a function of the number of reversible thallium-201 defects is exponential (r = .99, p < .001). (Reprinted from Ladenheim et al. [30].)

data had significant univariate predictive value, they added no significant prognostic value to the noninvasive marker of jeopardized viable myocardium.

These initial observations have been confirmed and extended by many subsequent studies for both stress Tl-201 and Tc-99m-based MPI [27,28]. Representative studies include a large series of over 1000 patients reported by Ladenheim and colleagues, who found that among clinical and scintigraphic variables, the number of reversible Tl-201 defects was the best predictor of future cardiac events (Fig. 11.3) [30]. Staniloff et al. showed that transient Tl-201 defects were associated with a 6- to 12-fold increased risk of cardiac death or myocardial infarction compared to normal stress MPI [31]. Similarly, Heller and colleagues found that reversible defects on stress Tc-99m-sestamibi MPI were the best predictor of cardiac death or myocardial infarction (MI) [32]. In a series of reports by Iskandrian

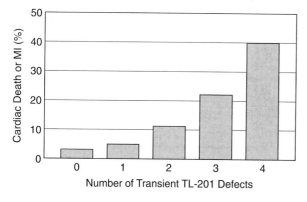

FIGURE 11.2 Risk of cardiac death or myocardial infarction (MI) as a function of the number of myocardial segments with transient thallium-201 defects. Risk increases as the extent of transient defects increases. (Adapted from Brown et al. [29].)

and colleagues, the extent of stress perfusion defects was the best predictor of cardiac events compared to clinical and exercise electrocardiographic data [33–35]. Interestingly, such stress image perfusion defects reflect a combination of infarction (fixed component) and jeopardized viable myocardium (transient component). In fact, one might expect jeopardized myocardium to carry a worse outcome in the setting of prior infarction, although this concept has not been fully evaluated.

There are other, less direct indexes of jeopardized viable myocardium that have also been demonstrated to have important prognostic value. Increased lung uptake on exercise Tl-201 imaging reflects exercise-induced left ventricular dysfunction, extent of angiographic disease, as well as resting left ventricular dysfunction [36–41], and has been associated with an increased risk of cardiac events [42,43]. Kaul et al. found that among clinical, electrocardiographic, and angiographic data, increased Tl-201 lung uptake was the best predictor of cardiac events [42]. Similarly, Gill and colleagues found that increased Tl-201 lung uptake was the best predictor of cardiac events in a series of patients with suspected CAD [43]. The cardiac death/myocardial infarction (MI) rate in patients with increased Tl-201 lung uptake over a 5-year follow-up was 40% compared to only 7% in patients with normal lung uptake (Fig. 11.4). Although the presence and extent of transient Tl-201 defects also was a strong predictor of cardiac events, it did not add to the prognostic value of increased Tl-201 lung uptake.

Transient ischemic dilation of the left ventricle with stress also reflects severe diffuse CAD or jeopardized myocardium and is a marker of increased cardiac risk [44–48]. Lette and colleagues found that transient left ventricular dilation during dipyridamole Tl-201 imag-

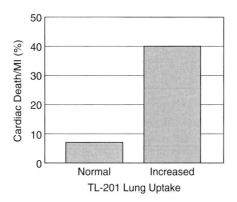

FIGURE 11.4 Cardiac death or myocardial infarction (MI) rate in patients with normal versus increased lung uptake on exercise thallium-201 imaging studies. (Adapted from Gill et al. [43].)

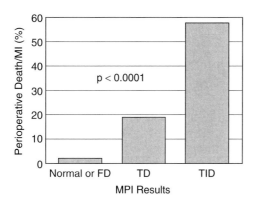

FIGURE 11.5 Perioperative cardiac death or myocardial infarction (MI) rate as a function of dipyridamole-thallium-201 myocardial perfusion imaging (MPI) results. The event rate was low in patients with normal studies or with only fixed defects (FD), intermediate in patients with transient defects (TD) and highest in patients with transient ischemic dilation of the left ventricle (TID) (p < .001). (Adapted from Lette et al. [47].)

ing was associated with a high risk of perioperative and long-term cardiac events [47]. Perioperative death or MI occurred in 58% of patients with transient ischemic dilation on dipyridamole Tl-201 imaging compared to 19% in patients with reversible defects and only 2% with normal studies or fixed defects (p < .0001) (Fig. 11.5). Furthermore among patients with transient ischemic dilation who did not undergo coronary revascularization, 50% suffered cardiac death an average of 4 months later.

Exercise Radionuclide Ventriculography

Ejection fraction response to exercise has been shown to reflect the extent of underlying CAD and inducible ischemia [49–53], and consequently has important prognostic value [54–65]. Several studies have found that a peak exercise ejection fraction < 50% is the best predictor of cardiac events [54–56] (Fig. 11.6). Furthermore, when compared to clinical and cardiac catheterization data, peak exercise ejection fraction had incremental prognostic value that was equal to cardiac catherization data (Fig. 11.7). Interestingly, although jeopardized viable myocardium might correspond best to exercise-induced *changes* in ejection fraction, studies have found that the absolute ejection fraction at peak exercise is the best predictor of cardiac events [54–62]. Borer and colleagues suggest that this is explained by the failure to account for low resting ejection fraction in many patients [63]. They point out that ejection fraction during exercise is tied to resting ejection fraction with the relationship strongest and exercise-induced changes least among patients with a low resting ejection fraction [63,64]. Thus, the prog-

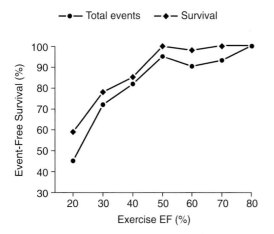

FIGURE 11.6 Cardiac event-free survival as a function of peak exercise left ventricular ejection fraction (EF). Death and all cardiac events increase substantially as peak exercise EF falls below 50%. (Adapted from Pryor et al. [54].)

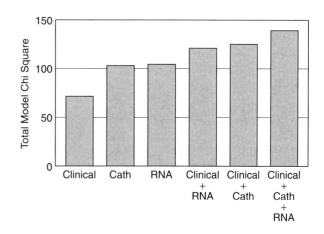

FIGURE 11.7 Incremental prognostic value of clinical, cardiac catheterization (cath), and radionuclide angiography (RNA). The prognostic value of RNA data was superior to clinical data and comparable to catheterization data. (Adapted from Lee et al. [57].)

nostic influence of resting ejection fraction on exercise ejection fraction will be greatest when the resting ejection fraction is very low, for example, < 30% [7]. In fact, when resting ejection fraction is > 30%, exercise-induced changes in ejection fraction have been shown to be highly predictive of cardiac events [65,66]. Among such patients a fall in ejection fraction of 10% from rest to exercise was associated with a 12-fold increase in cardiac events compared to patients with a fall of < 5%, and an annual mortality rate of 6% in the absence of coronary revascularization. In addition, some of the prognostic power of peak exercise ejection fraction may come from the fact that, like peak stress myocardial perfusion images, it reflects both prior myocardial damage (resting function) and additional jeopardized viable myocardium (exercise-induced fall).

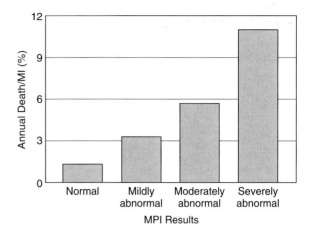

FIGURE 11.8 Annualized cardiac death/myocardial infarction (MI) rate as a function of results of adenosine thallium-201 myocardial perfusion imaging (MPI). (Adapted from Amanullah et al. [71].)

PHARMACOLOGIC STRESS

A series of studies have now established that nuclear MPI using vasodilator stress has similar prognostic value compared to exercise imaging [27,28,67–69]. Compared with angiographic and clinical data, reversible defects on dipyridamole Tl-201 MPI were found to be the only significant predictor of cardiac events in asymptomatic patients with coronary artery disease [69]. Those with only fixed defects or normal images had a low event rate. Similar to what Iskandrian and colleagues [33–35] reported for exercise MPI (see above), these investigators found that the size of the perfusion defect on stress imaging was the best predictor of hard cardiac events (cardiac death or MI) using adenosine single-photon emission computed tomography (SPECT) MPI [70]. Other investigators also found that an index of the extent and severity of stress image perfusion defects on adenosine SPECT MPI was the best predictor of hard cardiac events, distinguishing a low-risk group with an annual event rate of 0%–2% from a high-risk group with an event rate of 11% [71] (Fig. 11.8). Using dipyridamole Tl-201 imaging, Shaw et al. showed that while reversible defects predicted cardiac death or MI, the combination of reversible and fixed defects was a better predictor [72]. This study further supports the concept that jeopardized viable myocardium carries the greatest risk in the setting of prior damage.

Dobutamine stress nuclear MPI offers an alternative mode of pharmacologic stress that can be used in conjunction with nuclear MPI. It can be of particular benefit in patients who are unable to exercise and also have contraindications to vasodilator stress, such as those with severe bronchospastic disease. While a number of studies have established the diagnostic value of dobu-

tamine MPI for detecting CAD [73–78], fewer have evaluated its prognostic value. In a study that included soft end points of unstable angina and heart failure, Senior et al. reported that the number of reversible defects on dobutamine SPECT Tc-99m-sestamibi MPI and vascular territories ischemia were significant multivariate predictors of cardiac events in patients with suspected CAD [79]. In a larger study, Geleijnse and colleagues, using dobutamine stress Tc-99m-sestamibi SPECT MPI in a series of 418 patients who presented with chest pain, found that an abnormal imaging study or the presence of reversible defects were significant predictors of death or MI [80]. Compared to patients with normal studies, abnormal MPI results increased the risk of hard cardiac events by 10-fold, while the presence of reversible defects increased the hard event rate by threefold. Importantly, the risk of cardiac events was directly related to the extent and severity of reversible defects.

NORMAL MYOCARDIAL PERFUSION IMAGING

An extensive literature now firmly establishes that normal uptake on stress Tl-201 or Tc-99m-based MPI is associated with a very benign outcome, even in the setting of other markers of increased cardiac risk [27–29,31,34,42,43,69,81–97]. Brown reviewed 16 studies comprising over 3500 patients with known or suspected CAD who had normal stress nuclear MPI [27]. The annual death or MI rate was < 1% per year. Recent data suggest that the benign prognosis of a normal study is preserved over a long period of time. Steinberg and colleagues found that the normalized cardiac event rate over a 10-year follow-up in 309 patients with normal stress Tl-201 imaging was 0.1% per year for cardiac death and 0.6% per year for nonfatal MI [98].

Patients with Positive Stress EKG

Even in patients with exercise electrocardiographic evidence of ischemia (ST-segment depression), prognosis remains benign when stress nuclear MPI is normal [99–104]. Fagan and colleagues found an annual cardiac event rate of 0.7% per year in 70 patients with positive results on exercise electrocardiography but normal stress Tl-201 imaging [99]. Several studies showed that the cardiac event rate remains low with normal stress nuclear MPI even if exercise electrocardiography is markedly positive (≥ 2 mm ST-segment depression) [100,101]. Schalet et al. found no death or MI over a mean follow-up of 34 months in 154 patients with ≥ 2 mm ST-segment depression but normal Tl-201 imaging with exercise testing [100]. Similarly, no cardiac events were observed over a mean of 38 months follow-up in a smaller group of 32 patients with > 2 mm ST-segment depression but no reversible defects on exercise Tl-201 imaging [101]. These results may be explained in part by a low prevalence of underlying CAD in patients with a positive stress electrocardiogram when imaging is normal. A series of 52 patients with a strongly positive exercise electrocardiogram (but no conditions known to be associated with a false positive test) and normal nuclear MPI underwent coronary angiography [105]. Only 38% had significant angiographic disease, and when it was present, less than 10% had severe ($\geq 95\%$ stenosis) lesions. Disease was less prevalent in women than men.

Angiographic CAD

Even if angiographic CAD is known to be present, the cardiac event rate remains very low when stress nuclear MPI is normal [69,82,83,102–104,106,107]. Brown and Rowen described the outcome of 75 patients with significant angiographic (including 36 with multivessel) disease who had normal stress Tl-201 MPI [102]. Over a mean 2-year follow-up, only 1 cardiac event (death or MI) occurred, resulting in an annualized event rate of 0.7% per year. This event rate was not significantly different compared to a contemporaneous series of 101 patients with normal MPI and no CAD based on angiography or a very low probability of CAD determined from clinical and stress electrocardiography data. Brown summarized the data in this and other studies comprising 290 patients with significant angiographic disease [106]. These studies and new data [107] are presented in Table 11.1. The annual cardiac death or MI rate was 0.7% per

TABLE 11.1 *Outcome of Patients with Coronary Artery Disease and Normal Stress Myocardial Perfusion Imaging: Summary of Prior Studies*

Study	Patients (n)	Annual Cardiac Event Rate (% per year)
Brown and Rowen [102]	75	0.7
Abdel-Fattah et al. [103]	97	1.1
Doat et al. [104]	52	0.7
Wahl et al. [82]	8	0
Pamelia et al. [83]	22	3.2
Younis et al. [84]	36	0
Chatziioannou et al. [107]	86	0
Total	376	0.7

year, an event rate not different from the overall event rate described in patients with normal studies at-large.

By definition, normal MPI in patients with angiographic CAD is a false negative result. However, these studies tarnish angiography's gold-standard as the determinant of significant CAD and indicate that when it comes to prognosis, the functional significance of a coronary lesion appears to be more important than anatomic features, particularly the degree of stenosis.

IMPACT OF LEVEL OF STRESS ON PROGNOSTIC VALUE OF MPI

Perfusion defects on nuclear MPI result from stress-induced heterogeneous coronary blood flow in the setting of coronary artery disease. Low levels of stress could result in relatively less heterogeneity of blood flow and consequently smaller perfusion defects on MPI. Thus, inadequate stress can theoretically lead to underestimation of jeopardized viable myocardium and, consequently, the risk for cardiac events. However, available data suggest that the clinical impact of low stress on the prognostic value of MPI appears to be small, if present at all. Brown and Rowen examined the outcome of 261 patients with normal exercise Tl-201 imaging over a mean 2-year follow-up as a function of level of stress achieved [108]. The overall death or MI rate was 1.2% per year, comparable to prior studies. Importantly, the cardiac event rate was not significantly higher in patients with either a low peak heart rate or peak workload when MPI was normal (Table 11.2). Similarly, Murphy et al. found that the outcome of patients without ischemia on exercise Tl-201 MPI was not different in those who could not achieve Bruce stage 3 compared to those who did [109]. These observations probably reflect the fact that exercise MPI is very sensitive for the detection of CAD and that the sensitivity is not highly related to the level of stress achieved [110–112]. Esquivel and colleagues found no significant reduction in sensitivity for detecting CAD even in patients failing to reach 65% of their maximal predicted heart rate, remaining high at 89% [111]. Others have reported a modest reduction in sensitivity with inadequate stress (< 85% predicted maximal heart rate), but overall sensitivity was still fairly high at 73% [112]. Thus, current data suggest that a normal exercise MPI predicts a benign outcome even when the level of stress is traditionally considered "inadequate." However, additional studies are necessary to fully address this issue, particularly in patients who are on the extreme margins of poor exercise level achieved.

The converse issue is also of interest: does exercise MPI have the same prognostic value in patients who achieve a *high* level of stress? This is a group whose achieved level of exercise predicts a benign outcome. Do the results of MPI modulate their prognosis? Current data are mixed. Chatziioannou and colleagues found that among 388 patients undergoing exercise MPI who reached at least Bruce stage 4, imaging was a highly significant ($p < .001$) predictor of cardiac events, whereas exercise electrocardiography and the Duke Treadmill Score were not (Fig. 11.9) [107]. In addition, Snader and colleagues found that the results of exercise Tl-201 imaging had significant incremental prognostic value compared to functional capacity [113]. However, Murphy et al. found that patients who reached Bruce stage 3 had

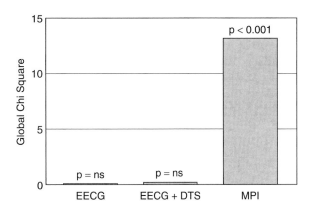

FIGURE 11.9 Independent and incremental prognostic value of exercise electrocardiography (EECG), Duke Treadmill Score (DTS), and stress myocardial perfusion imaging results (MPI). (Adapted from Chatziioannou et al. [112].)

the same low event rate whether they had Tl-201 imaging evidence of ischemia or not [109]. Additional data are necessary to clarify this issue.

IMPACT OF ANTI-ISCHEMIC MEDICATION

Previous studies have shown that anti-ischemic medication, including nitrates, beta-blockers, and calcium channel blockers can suppress ischemia seen on stress MPI [114–120]. It is also known, as previously described, that extent of ischemia detected by stress MPI is directly related to risk of cardiac events. This raises important questions: does anti-ischemic medication taken at the time of stress MPI lead to an underestimation of cardiac risk? Or do the results of MPI on anti-ischemic medications reflect a true but reduced cardiac risk? Preliminary data provide us some answers to these questions. In the study of Brown and Rowen, patients with a normal stress Tl-201 study who were taking anti-ischemic medications (including specifically beta-blockers) had the same low event rate as patients who were not (see Table 11.2) [108]. Thus, medications did not appear to be masking increased risk by "normalizing" images. Dakik and colleagues showed that reduction in perfusion defect score on adenosine Tl-201 SPECT MPI by either medical therapy or coronary angioplasty was associated with a lower cardiac event rate [121], suggesting that under the influence of anti-ischemic medication, the results of stress MPI reflect actual rather than underestimated patient risk. Presumably, this relationship will apply so long as medications are continued after imaging. A study provides some insight into what may happen if anti-ischemic medications are added *after* MPI. In a series of 352 pa-

TABLE 11.2 *Annual Cardiac Death or Myocardial Infarction Rate as a Function of Level of Exercise Achieved, Peak Heart Rate, and Anti-ischemic Medication in Patients with Normal Exercise Myocardial Perfusion Imaging Studies*

Variable	Frequency of CD/MI	Annualized Event Rate	p Value
Peak heart rate			
≥ 85% MPHR	4/178	1.2	ns (> .6)
84–60% MPHR	2/71	1.2	
< 60% MPHR	0/12	0	
Final Bruce stage			
≥ 3	3/152	1.0	ns (> .6)
≤ 2	3/109	1.4	
≤ 1	0/39	0	
Anti-ischemic medications			
Yes	3/133	1.2	ns (> .6)
No	2/128	1.2	
Beta-blocker treatment			
Yes	2/77	1.4	ns (> .6)
No	4/184	1.1	

CD, cardiac death; MI, myocardial infarction; MPHR, maximal predicted heart rate.

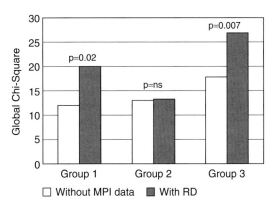

FIGURE 11.10 Incremental prognostic value of reversible defects on exercise myocardial perfusion imaging as a function of anti-ischemic medications before and after imaging. Group 1 = no change in medications. Group 2 = beta blockers added after imaging. Group 3 = anti-ischemic medications other than beta blockers added after imaging. In each group, global chi-square is shown for the predictive model without myocardial perfusion imaging (MPI) data (open bar) and for predictive model after reversible thallium-201 defects (RD) was added (solid bar). Reversible defects had significant incremental predictive value for cardiac death or myocardial infarction in Groups 1 and 3 but not in Group 2 (after beta blockers). (Adapted from Marie et al. [122].)

tients with stable coronary heart disease the prognostic value of exercise Tl-201 MPI over a 5-year follow-up was evaluated, taking into account the patients' anti-ischemic medications before and after imaging [122]. Three specific subgroups of patients were examined: Group 1, in whom medications were not changed after MPI; Group 2, in whom anti-ischemic medications including beta-blockers were added after MPI; Group 3, in whom anti-ischemic medications other than beta-blockers were added after MPI. Not surprisingly, ischemia on stress MPI (i.e., transient defects) predicted late cardiac events in Group 1 (Fig. 11.10). However, when beta-blockers were added after imaging, transient defects lost their predictive value and were associated with a lower relative risk (Group 2). This effect was not seen with other anti-ischemic medications (Group 3). These data suggest that anti-ischemic medication with beta-blockers can ameliorate the adverse prognostic implications of provokable ischemia identified on stress MPI. Presumably, if stress MPI had been repeated on beta-blockers it would have showed less ischemia, reflecting the lower risk.

FIXED TL-201 DEFECTS

The medical literature has most consistently shown that, in contrast to reversible defects, perfusion defects that are fixed on standard 2–4-hour delayed imaging generally do not predict cardiac events [27,28,67,

123–143]. A representative study is shown in Figure 11.11. In a series of 896 patients, the cardiac death rate was equally low in the 217 patients with fixed defects compared to the 310 patients with normal studies [143]. In contrast, those with reversible defects had a much higher cardiac event rate ($p < 0.001$). This may reflect the fact that, in general, fixed perfusion defects on stress Tl-201 imaging reflect scar rather than jeopardized viable myocardium.

However, it has become apparent over the last decade that some defects that appear fixed on 2–4-hour poststress imaging do not represent infarction, especially when Q waves are not present or regional wall motion is preserved [144–148]. In this setting, defects that appear fixed at 2–4 hours can be made to appear reversible with reinjection or late delayed imaging. However, the prognostic implication of fixed defects that are made reversible is unclear. Initial studies suggest that such defects do not have the same predictive value as defects that are reversible at 2–4 hours [149–152]. Brown and colleagues described the outcome of 100 patients without previous MI who had isolated fixed defects or standard stress-delayed Tl-201 imaging [149]. Because the fixed defects in this setting did not represent scar, this cohort would be likely to show reversibility with reinjection or late delayed imaging. However, over a mean follow-up of 2 years only 1 nonfatal MI occurred and no cardiac deaths, yielding a hard annual cardiac event rate of 0.5% per year, comparable to patients with a normal study. Tisselli et al. examined the predictive value of stress-rest-reinjection Tl-201 MPI in patients with remote MI and suspected ischemia [150]. The presence of fixed defects that became reversible after reinjection did not identify patients at increased risk. However, extensive defects that remained fixed after reinjection, indicating exten-

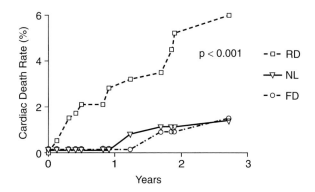

FIGURE 11.11 Cardiac death rate as a function of results of exercise thallium-201 imaging. Patients with reversible defects (RD) had significantly higher cardiac death rate than patients with normal studies (NL) or with only fixed defects (FD) ($p = .0017$). (Adapted from Bodenheimer et al. [143].)

sive infarction, was the best predictor of death or MI. Other investigators lumped reinjection-induced reversible defects with fixed defects that had moderate reduction in regional activity (consistent with preserved viability) and found that this had multivariate predictive value for death or MI (151). More recently, Zafrir et al. found that Tl-201 reinjection did not contribute independent prognostic value for hard cardiac events compared with stress-delayed redistribution imaging [152]. In summary, while reinjection Tl-201 imaging can detect viability, its prognostic significance remains unclear, but it does not appear to have the same implications as standard stress-delayed redistribution imaging. Thus, caution should be used in revising imaging protocols that eliminate the standard delayed images until more data are available.

LOCATION OF PERFUSION DEFECT AND SITE OF FUTURE MI

Although one might conclude that jeopardized viable myocardium on stress MPI identifies the actual myocardium at risk for future damage, very little data exist regarding this relationship. However, some insight is provided by two studies. Miller and colleagues examined 25 patients with acute MI who had undergone earlier stress Tc-99m-sestamibi MPI [153]. The majority of patients (17/25; 68%) had perfusion defects that corresponded to the coronary territory of the subsequent MI. The large majority of these (14/17) were reversible defects. More recently, Galvin and Brown described 34 patients with acute MI who had reversible defects on prior stress MPI [154]. The duration of time between the imaging study and the MI influenced the relationship between the site of the transient defect and the subsequent MI. When there was less than 2 years time interval, most patients (11/14; 79%) had an MI in the same coronary territory as the antecedent transient defect ($p < .0005$). However, when the time interval was 2 years or more, only 5 of 20 (25%) had corresponding MI and defect sites, suggesting that new disease may have developed in that time interval. Interestingly, there was no relationship between severity of angiographic disease and site of MI regardless of time frame between angiography and MI.

INCREMENTAL PROGNOSTIC VALUE

In the context of the current health-care environment where all procedural expenses come under increasing scrutiny, it is necessary not only to demonstrate that stress MPI has significant prognostic value, but more importantly to show that it *adds* significant prognostic value to less costly clinical and exercise electrocardiographic data. Additionally, it is important to ask what more costly invasive procedures add to the prognostic value of noninvasive cardiac imaging. Probably the first to evaluate this concept in the context of cardiac stress testing and imaging were Ladenheim and colleagues in 1987 [155]. They examined the hierarchical and incremental prognostic value of stress MPI in over 1500 patients with suspected CAD. MPI had the greatest incremental impact in predicting cardiac events in patients with abnormal resting electrocardiograms and in patients with intermediate-to-high probability of having CAD based on historical parameters. Cardiac risk was increased 5- to 10-fold by finding abnormal MPI results. Furthermore, exercise testing and MPI could be applied selectively in a strategy that stratified individual cardiac risk 10-fold (from 2% to 22%) with a reduction in cost of 64% compared to uniformly performing both tests. Pollock et al. took the analysis one step further in 1992, examining the hierarchical incremental prognostic value of exercise MPI in the context of angiographic as well as clinical and stress testing variables [156]. They found that the addition of MPI data improved the power of the predictive model by a factor of 2 compared to clinical and exercise data (Fig. 11.12). Importantly, the incremental increase in prognostic value was not different from what angiographic data added. In addition, MPI data provided significant improvement to the predictive model beyond what angiographic, clinical, and exercise data offered.

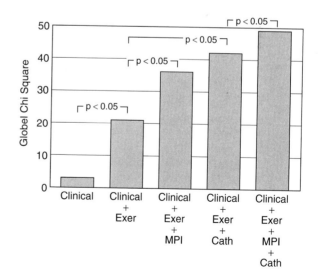

FIGURE 11.12 The hierarchical incremental prognostic value of clinical, exercise (exer), myocardial perfusion imaging (MPI), and cardiac catheterization (cath) data. The addition of MPI data to clinical and exercise data significantly increased the predictive model to a similar degree compared to catheterization data. (Adapted from Pollock et al. [156].)

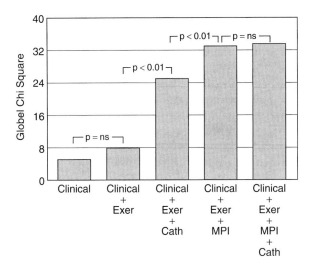

FIGURE 11.13 Incremental prognostic value of clinical, exercise (exer), myocardial perfusion imaging (MPI), and cardiac catheterization (cath) data. MPI data added significantly prognostic value to clinical, exercise, and even cardiac catheterization data. (Adapted from Iskandrian et al. [157].)

Subsequently, the principle of incremental prognostic value for MPI has been confirmed by others with both exercise and vasodilator stress and with both Tl-201 and Tc-99m-based MPI [157–164]. In a series of patients with known CAD, Iskandrian and colleagues found that MPI had the most prognostic value [157]. More importantly, MPI improved the predictive value compared to stress and clinical data by a factor of 4, and it provided significantly greater incremental prognostic value than cardiac catheterization data (Fig. 11.13). Furthermore, the catheterization data did not improve the predictive value of MPI data. Thus, not only did noninvasive MPI greatly improve the predictive value of clinical and stress data alone, it was more valuable than invasive data. Other recent studies have demonstrated that the best MPI risk-stratifying predictors take into account not just whether imaging is normal or abnormal but rather the extent of jeopardized viable myocardium defined by defect reversibility [158,159], consonant with established principles of prognostic value previously discussed. In addition, several long-term studies have confirmed that the incremental prognostic value of MPI persists for at least 6 years [159,161].

Several studies have demonstrated significant incremental prognostic value of MPI in patients with prior coronary artery bypass surgery [158,160,162,165, 166]. In a small study of 75 patients, the extent and severity of defect reversibility on stress MPI performed 3 years after bypass was the best predictor of outcome and added significantly to the prognostic value of clin-

ical and stress variables [160]. In a larger study of 255 patients undergoing stress MPI a mean of 5 years after bypass surgery, Nallamothu et al. showed that MPI results added significantly to the predictive model generated by clinical, stress, and even angiographic data [162] (Fig. 11.14). Over a 41-month follow-up, MPI results could stratify patients into high-risk (10% annual death/MI rate) and low-risk (1.7% annual death/MI rate) subgroups. Even when performed early postbypass (mean 11 months), stress MPI was highly predictive of cardiac death or MI [165]. Similarly, in a series of patients undergoing stress MPI 1 year after revascularization with bypass surgery or coronary angioplasty, reversible defects predicted hard and soft cardiac events over the next 2 years [166].

Finally, several studies have evaluated the incremental value of left ventricular function compared to perfusion and clinical data [159,163,164]. Marie and colleagues found that left ventricular (LV) function determined from both radionuclide ventriculography and MPI data had significant incremental prognostic value over clinical data [159]. Interestingly, while MPI data did not add significantly to ventricular function for predicting cardiac death, the extent of reversible defects did have significant incremental prognostic value for predicting overall cardiac events including future myocardial infarction. This suggests that risk of cardiac death may be most related to extent of prior myocardial damage (LV function), whereas risk of ischemic

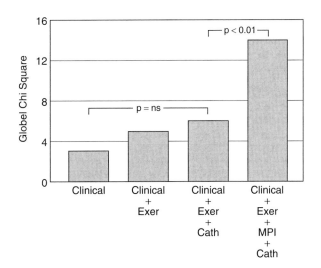

FIGURE 11.14 Incremental prognostic value of clinical, exercise (exer), myocardial perfusion imaging (MPI), and cardiac catheterization (cath) data in patients with prior coronary bypass surgery. MPI added significant incremental prognostic value to clinical, exercise, and catheterization data. Exercise and catheterization data did not have significant incremental value compared to clinical data in this study. (Adapted from Nallamothu et al. [162].)

events like acute myocardial infarction is better related to extent of jeopardized viable myocardium. In contrast, Nallamothu et al. found that ejection fraction had no significant predictive value for outcome compared to MPI data [163]. However, there were very few cardiac deaths in this cohort, probably limiting the value of LV function. More recently, Sharir and colleagues examined the incremental prognostic value of LV function and perfusion derived from gated MPI compared to clinical data [164]. In this study perfusion data surprisingly had no significant predictive value for cardiac death or MI, whereas LV function and end-systolic volume were the principal determinants of outcome and had incremental prognostic value over clinical and perfusion data. Gated MPI with Tc-99m-based agents allow determination of both perfusion and ventricular function. Since the major determinants of outcome in patients with coronary heart disease are ventricular function and jeopardized viable myocardium, it is likely that taking both factors into consideration will optimize our ability to predict risk and type of future cardiac events, but more data are necessary to clarify these issues.

CLINICAL OUTCOMES

Clearly, the body of literature at-large establishes that stress nuclear MPI predicts cardiac events and that this technique can be used to identify low-risk and high-risk subgroups. However, relevant clinical questions remain: what is the impact of nuclear MPI on patient management and outcome? Is MPI actually acting as a gatekeeper to more expensive diagnostic and interventional procedures in clinical practice? Does identification of the high-risk patient lead to a better outcome by allowing intervention with revascularization? In recent years data have become available that begin to answer these important questions.

Hachamovitch and colleagues examined the relationship of the prognostic value of stress MPI to its influence on referral rates for early cardiac catheterization and revascularization [167]. In a series of 2200 patients without documented CAD, nuclear MPI doubled the prognostic information available from clinical and exercise data. The rates of referral for angiography or revascularization were very low when MPI was normal even if clinical or stress test results suggested that CAD was present (Fig. 11.15*B, C*). As MPI results worsened, referral rates increased. Thus, clinicians were using MPI in an appropriate manner to select high-risk patients for referral to catheterization and coronary revascularization. Importantly, the referral rates for

catheterization and revascularization corresponded closely to the observed risk of hard cardiac events (Fig. 11.15*A*) based on clinical and exercise data (postexercise test probability of CAD) and MPI results. One exception appears to be patients with high-risk imaging results (severely abnormal) who had a low clinical risk.

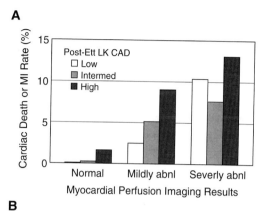

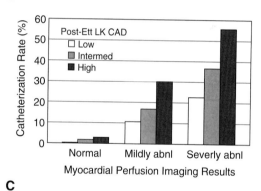

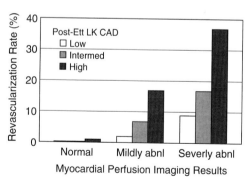

FIGURE 11.15 (*A*) Cardiac event rate as a function of postexercise treadmill test (ETT) likelihood (LK) of coronary artery disease (CAD) and myocardial perfusion imaging results. (*B*) Rate of referral to cardiac catheterization, and (*C*) coronary revascularization as a function of the same variables. Referral rates were low when imaging results were normal even if the likelihood of CAD was high, reflecting the low cardiac event rate. Utilization of catheterization and revascularization increased as the degree of imaging abnormality increased, reflecting the higher cardiac event rates. (Adapted from Hachamovitch et al. [167].)

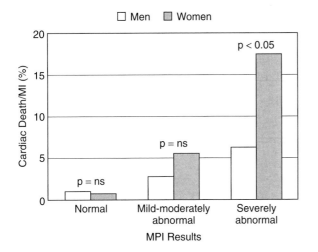

FIGURE 11.16 Cardiac death or myocardial infarction (MI) rate as a function of gender and results of stress myocardial perfusion imaging (MPI). The risk of cardiac events was directly related to the degree of imaging abnormality ($p < .0001$). With severely abnormal imaging results, the cardiac event rate was higher in women compared to men.

Although these patients had a probability of cardiac death or MI that was comparable to those with intermediate or high clinical risk, the referral rates for catheterization and revascularization were considerably lower (Fig. 11.15B, C). This appears to be a subgroup in whom clinicians are underestimating cardiac risk. Women may be another group in whom risk may be underestimated by clinicians. These investigators showed that gender-related differences in referral rates for cardiac catheterization and coronary revascularization generally reflected differences in the prevalence and degree of imaging abnormalities [168]. However, in the setting of severe abnormalities on MPI, while women and men had comparable rates of referral to revascularization (18% and 15%, respectively), the cardiac event rate was much higher in women (18% versus 6%, respectively, $p < .05$) (Fig. 11.16). Thus, the cardiac risk in women appears to have been underappreciated. The authors called for more vigilance in identifying and appropriately treating the high-risk woman with CAD.

Other investigators have also showed a direct link between MPI results and referral rates to invasive procedures. In a large series of 4162 patients undergoing stress Tl-201 imaging, only 3.5% of patients without reversible defects underwent cardiac catheterization compared with 32% who had reversible defects [169]. Among those with reversible defects, the degree of abnormality also had an impact on referral rates. Those with high-risk results (multiple coronary territories, increased lung uptake, left anterior descending territory) were referred for catheterization 60% of the time, while

only 9% without these findings were referred. Similarly, Nallamothu et al. found that only 3% of patients with normal MPI results went on to cardiac catheterization compared to 36% with abnormal results, and among those with abnormal MPI results, the referral rate was directly related to the extent of the abnormality [170]. In a questionnaire-based study, Steingart et al. showed that the results of exercise MPI influenced clinicians' perceived need to refer for cardiac catheterization, particularly in the patients with a low-to-intermediate probability of CAD, although the impact of MPI on influencing decisions regarding cardiac catheterization was greatest in patients with known CAD [171]. These studies clearly show that stress nuclear MPI is having an important measurable impact on decisions that clinicians make regarding sending their patients for invasive procedures.

Having identified the high-risk patient with MPI and having sent the patient for cardiac catheterization and revascularization, is there evidence that such an approach leads to a better clinical outcome? Initial data suggest that it does. Hachamovitch and colleagues have studied 5183 patients with suspected CAD who underwent stress MPI [172]. Annual hard cardiac event rates were directly related to MPI results. However, in patients with severely abnormal MPI results, the annual cardiac death rate in patients who underwent early coronary revascularization was quite low, only ~1% per year, and was significantly lower than patients

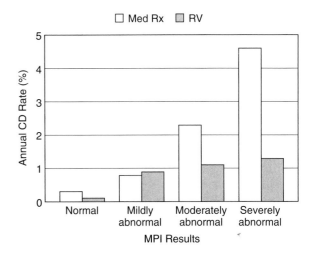

FIGURE 11.17 Annual cardiac death (CD) rate as a function of myocardial perfusion imaging (MPI) results and early postscan management. Open bars represent patients treated medically after MPI (med RX); solid bars represent patients undergoing coronary revascularization (RV) early after MPI. The cardiac death rate was lower in patients with severely abnormal (abnl) imaging results who underwent coronary revascularization compared to medical treatment ($p < .01$). (Adapted from Hachamovitch et al. [172].)

treated medically after nuclear imaging (Fig. 11.17). This suggests that coronary revascularization had an ameliorating effect on cardiac risk. Furthermore, a recent study suggests that when the revascularization rate is low in the setting of high-risk imaging results, the observed cardiac event rate increases [173]. Among 8411 patients undergoing stress nuclear MPI, Shaw et al. reported that the referral rates for coronary revascularization were similar (~25%) for patients with ischemia in single versus multiple coronary territories [173]. However, the cardiac death or MI rate was 2–4 times higher with multivessel ischemia, suggesting that revascularization in this group may be inappropriately low. More data are needed before we can make definitive conclusions regarding the impact of revascularization on prognosis in the high-risk patient identified by stress MPI.

In summary, stress nuclear MPI results appear to significantly influence clinician decisions regarding referral for cardiac catheterization and revascularization. Such influence appears to correspond directly to documented risk for cardiac events, indicating that clinicians understand the connection between MPI abnormality and risk. Patients at low risk for cardiac events with normal or near-normal MPI are rarely referred for cardiac catheterization even if clinical and exercise data suggest a high likelihood of CAD. Conversely, those with high-risk MPI results are much more likely to be referred for angiography and coronary revascularization. Early data suggest that the higher referral rate may lead to a better outcome with a lower cardiac death rate. There are some subgroups with high-risk MPI results, such as women and those with a low clinical risk, in which cardiac risk may be underestimated by clinicians, leading to a referral rate that may be inappropriately low. Nevertheless, stress nuclear MPI appears to be playing an important role in limiting health-care costs by appropriately controlling access to more expensive procedures and interventions and is likely to have a growing value in the triage of medical procedures in the future.

SUMMARY

The prognostic value of stress nuclear cardiac imaging in patients with stable CAD is now well established. These radionuclide techniques have powerful ability to distinguish high-risk from low-risk patients and add important measurable predictive value to standard clinical and exercise data. Such function-based noninvasive models have consistently provided prognostic information that equals or exceeds that provided by anatomy-based invasive data. There is growing evidence that radionu-

clide techniques are playing an important gatekeeper function in management decisions made by clinicians, allowing a rational approach to utilizing more expensive invasive, interventional, and surgical procedures.

REFERENCES

1. Rigo P, Murray M, Strauss HW, et al. Left ventricular function in acute myocardial infarction by gated scintigraphy. Circulation 1974;50:678.
2. Schelbert HR, Henning H, Ashburn W, et al. Serial measurements of left ventricular ejection fraction by radionuclide angiography early and late after myocardial infarction. Am J Cardiol 1976;38:407.
3. Schulze RA, Strauss HW, Pitt B. Sudden death in the year following myocardial infarction: relation to ventricular premature contractions in the late hospital phase and left ventricular ejection fraction. Am J Med 1977;62:192.
4. Reduto LA, Berger HJ, Cohen LS, et al. Sequential radionuclide assessment of left and right ventricular performance after acute transmural myocardial infarction. Ann Intern Med 1978;89:441.
5. Borer JS, Rosing DR, Miller RH, et al. Natural history of left ventricular function during 1 year after acute myocardial infarction: comparison with clinical, electrocardiographic and biochemical determination. Am J Cardiol 1980;46:1.
6. Corbett JR, Dehmer GJ, Lewis SE, et al. The prognostic value of submaximal exercise testing with radionuclide ventriculography before hospital discharge in patients with recent myocardial infarction. Circulation 1981;64:535.
7. Multicenter Postinfarction Research Group. Risk stratification and survival after myocardial infarction. N Engl J Med 1983;309:331.
8. Nicod P, Corbett JR, Firth BG, et al. Prognostic value of resting and submaximal exercise radionuclide ventriculogram after acute myocardial infarction in high-risk patients with single and multivessel disease. Am J Cardiol 1983;52:30.
9. Dewhurst NG, Muir AL. Comparative prognostic value of radionuclide ventriculography at rest and during exercise in 100 patients after first myocardial infarction. Br Heart J 1983;49:111.
10. Morris KG, Palmeri ST, Califf RM, et al. Value of radionuclide angiography for predicting specific cardiac events after acute myocardial infarction. Am J Cardiol 1985;55:318.
11. Ong L, Green S, Reiser P, et al. Early prediction of mortality in patients with acute myocardial infarction: a prospective study of clinical and radionuclide risk factors. Am J Cardiol 1986;57:33.
12. Starling MR, Crawford MH, Henry RL, et al. Prognostic value of electrocardiographic exercise testing and noninvasive assessment of left ventricular ejection fraction soon after acute myocardial infarction. Am J Cardiol 1986;57:532.
13. Stadius ML, Davis K, Maynard C, et al. Risk stratification for 1 year survival based on characteristics identified in the early hours of acute myocardial infarction: the western Washington intracoronary streptokinase trial. Circulation 1986;74:703.
14. Ahnve S, Gilpin E, Henning H, et al. Limitations and advantages of the ejection fraction for defining high risk after acute myocardial infarction. Am J Cardiol 58:872, 1986.
15. White HD, Norris RM, Brown MA, et al. Left ventricular end-systolic volume as the major determinant of survival after recovery from myocardial infarction. Circulation 1987;76:44.

16. Kuchar DL, Thorburn CW, Sammel NL. Prediction of serious arrhythmic events after myocardial infarction: signal averaged electrocardiogram, Holter monitoring and radionuclide ventriculography. J Am Coll Cardiol 1987;9:531.

17. Hakki AH, Nestico PF, Heo J, et al. Relative prognostic value of rest thallium 201 imaging radionuclide ventriculography and 24-hour ambulatory electrocardiographic monitoring after acute myocardial infarction. J Am Coll Cardiol 1987;10:25.

18. Gomes JA, Winters SL, Steward D, et al. A new noninvasive index to predict sustained ventricular tachycardia and sudden death in the first year after myocardial infarction: based on signal-averaged electrocardiogram radionuclide ejection fraction and Holter monitoring. J Am Coll Cardiol 1987;10:3498.

19. Abraham RD, Harris PJ, Roubin GS, et al. Usefulness of ejection fraction response to exercise one month after acute myocardial infarction in predicting coronary anatomy and prognosis. Am J Cardiol 1987;60:225.

20. Kuchar DL, Freund J, Yeates M, et al. Enhanced prediction of major cardiac events after myocardial infarction using exercise radionuclide ventriculography. Aust NZ J Med 1987;17:228.

21. Gabsboll N, Hoilund-Carlsen PF, Madsen EB, et al. Right and left ventricular ejection fractions: relation to one-year prognosis in acute myocardial infarction. Eur Heart J 1987;8:1201.

22. Zaret BL, Wackers FJ, Terrin M, et al. Does left ventricular ejection fraction following thrombolytic therapy have the same prognostic impact described in the prethrombolytic era? Results of the TIMI II Trial (abstr). J Am Coll Cardiol 1991;17:214A.

23. Mazzotta G, Camerini A, Scopinaro G, et al. Predicting cardiac mortality after uncomplicated myocardial infarction by exercise radionuclide ventriculography and exercise-induced ST-segment elevation. Eur Heart J 1992;13:330.

24. Harris PJ, Harrell FE, Lee KI, et al. Survival in medically treated coronary artery disease. Circulation 1979;60:1259.

25. Mock MB, Ringqvist I, Fisher LD, et al. Survival of medically treated patients in the coronary artery surgery study (CASS) registry. Circulation 1982;66:562.

26. Bonow RO, Epstein SE. Indications for coronary artery bypass surgery: implications of the multicenter randomized trials. Circulation 1985;72 (suppl):V.

27. Brown KA. Prognostic value of Tl-201 myocardial perfusion imaging. A diagnostic tool comes of age, Circulation 1991;83:363.

28. Brown KA. Prognostic value of myocardial perfusion imaging: state of the art and new developments, J Nucl Cardiol 1996;3:516.

29. Brown KA, Boucher CA, Okada RD, et al. Prognostic value of exercise Tl-201 imaging in patients presenting for evaluation of chest pain, J Am Coll Cardiol 1983;1:994.

30. Ladenheim ML, Pollock BH, Rozanski A, et al. Extent and severity of myocardial hypoperfusion as predictors of prognosis in patients with suspected coronary artery disease, J Am Coll Cardiol 1986;7:464.

31. Staniloff HM, Forrester JS, Berman DS, et al. Prediction of death, myocardial infarction, and worsening chest pain using thallium scintigraphy and exercise electrocardiography. J Nucl Med 1986;27:1842.

32. Heller GV, Herman SD, Travin MI, et al. Independent prognostic value of intravenous dipyridamole with technetium-99m sestamibi tomographic imaging in predicting cardiac events and cardiac-related hospital admissions. J Am Coll Cardiol 1995;26:1202.

33. Iskandrian AS, Hakki AH, Kane-Marsch S. Prognostic implications of exercise thallium 201 scintigraphy in patients with suspected or known coronary artery disease. Am Heart J 1985;110:135.

34. Iskandrian AS, Hakki AH, Kane-Marsch S. Exercise thallium 201 scintigraphy in men and nondiagnostic exercise electrocardiograms: prognostic implications. Arch Intern Med 1986;146:2189.

35. Felsher J, Meissner MD, Hakki AH, et al. Exercise thallium imaging in patients with diabetes mellitus: prognostic implications. Arch Intern Med 1987;147:313.

36. Boucher CA, Zir LM, Beller GA, et al. Increased lung uptake of thallium 201 during exercise myocardial imaging: clinical, hemodynamic and angiographic implications in patients with coronary artery disease. Am J Cardiol. 1980;46:189.

37. Bingham JB, McKusick KA, Strauss HW, et al. Influence of coronary artery disease on pulmonary uptake of thallium 201. Am J Cardiol 46:821, 1980.

38. Kushner FG, Okada RD, Kirshenbaum HD, et al. Lung thallium 201 uptake after stress testing in patients with coronary artery disease. Circulation 1981;63:341.

39. Gibson RS, Watson DD, Carabello BA, et al. Clinical implications of increased lung uptake of thallium 201 during exercise scintigraphy 2 weeks after myocardial infarction. Am J Cardiol 1982;49:1586.

40. Brown KA, Boucher CA, Okada RD, et al. Quantification of pulmonary thallium 201 activity after upright exercise in normal persons: importance of peak heart rate and propranolol usage in defining normal values. Am J Cardiol 1984;53:1678.

41. Liu P, Kiess M, Okada RD, et al. Increased thallium lung uptake after exercise in isolated left anterior descending coronary artery disease. Am J Cardiol 1985;55:1469.

42. Kaul S, Finkelstein DM, Homma S, et al. Superiority of quantitative exercise thallium 201 variables in determining long-term prognosis in ambulatory patients with chest pain: a comparison with cardiac catheterization. J Am Coll Cardiol 1988;12:25.

43. Gill JB, Ruddy TD, Newell JB, et al. Prognostic importance of thallium uptake by the lungs during exercise coronary artery disease. N Engl J Med 1987;317:1485.

44. Stolzenberg J. Dilatation of left ventricular cavity on stress thallium scan as an indicator of ischemic disease. Clin Nucl Med 1980;5:289.

45. Lette J, Lapointe J, Waters D, et al. Transient left ventricular cavity dilatation during dipyridamole-thallium imaging as an indicator of severe coronary artery disease. Am J Cardiol 1990;66:1163.

46. Krawczynska EG, Weintraub WS, Garcia EV, et al. Left ventricular dilatation and multivessel coronary artery disease on thallium 201 SPECT are important prognostic indicators in patients with large defects in the left anterior descending distribution. Am J Cardiol 1994;74:1233.

47. Lette J, Lapointe J, Waters D, et al. Transient left ventricular cavitary dilation during dipyridamole-thallium imaging as an indicator of severe coronary artery disease. Am J Cardiol 1990;66:1163.

48. Weiss AT, Berman DS, Lew AS, et al. Transient ischemic dilation of the left ventricle on stress thallium 201 scintigraphy: a marker of severe and extensive coronary artery disease. J Am Coll Cardiol 1987;9:752.

49. Gibbons RJ. Rest and exercise radionuclide angiography for diagnosis in chronic ischemic heart disease. Circulation 1991;84:193.

50. Beller GA, Gibson RS. Sensitivity, specificity and prognostic significance of noninvasive testing for occult or known coronary disease. Prog Cardiovasc Dis 1987;29:241.

51. Borer JS, Bacharach SL, Green MV. Radionuclide cineangiography in the evaluation of patients with heart disease: the perspective of the decade. Cardiovasc Rev Rep 1991;12:14,31,70.

52. Dymond DS. Radionuclide assessment of ventricular function in patients with coronary artery disease: clinical perspective. Br Med Bull 1989;45:881.

53. Iskandrian AS, Hakki AH. Radionuclide evaluation of exercise left ventricular performance in patients with coronary artery disease. Am Heart J 110:851, 1985.

54. Pryor DB, Harrell FE Jr, Lee KL, et al. Prognostic indicators from radionuclide angiography in medically treated patients with coronary artery disease. Am J Cardiol 1984;53:18.

55. Iskandrian AS, Hakki AH, Goel IP, et al. The use of rest and exercise radionuclide ventriculography in risk stratification in patients with suspected coronary artery disease. Am Heart J 1985;110:864.

56. Iskandrian AS, Hakki AH, Schwartz JS, et al. Prognostic implications of rest and exercise radionuclide ventriculography in patients with suspected or proven coronary heart disease. Int J Cardiol 1984;6:707.

57. Lee KL, Pryor DB, Pieper KS, et al. Prognostic value of radionuclide angiography in medically treated patients with coronary artery disease: a comparison with clinical and catheterization variables. Circulation 1990;82:1705.

58. Jones RH, Johnson SH, Bigelow C, et al. Exercise radionuclide angiocardiography predicts cardiac death in patients with coronary artery disease. Circulation 84:152, 1991.

59. Clements IP, Brown Martin M, LeWinter MD, et al. Influence of left ventricular diastolic filling on symptoms and survival in patients with decreased left ventricular systolic function. Am J Cardiol 1991;67:1245.

60. Johnson SH, Bigelow C, Lee KL, et al. Prediction of death and myocardial infarction by radionuclide angiocardiography in patients with suspected coronary artery disease. Am J Cardiol 1991;67:919.

61. Mazzotta G, Bonow RO, Pace L, et al. Relation between exertional ischemia and prognosis in mildly symptomatic patients with single or double vessel coronary artery disease and left ventricular dysfunction at rest. J Am Coll Cardiol 1989;13:567.

62. Wallis JB, Holmes JR, Borer JS. Prognosis in patients with coronary artery disease and low ejection fraction at rest: impact of exercise ejection fraction. Am J Cardiol Imaging 1990; 4:1.

63. Borer JS, Supino P, Wencker D, et al. Assessment of coronary artery disease by radionuclide cineangiography: history, current applications, and new directions, In: Cardiology Clinics, Nuclear Cardiology: State of the Art edited by MH Crawford. Philadelphia: WB Saunders, 1994, pp. 333–357.

64. Braegelmann F, Herrold EM, Wallis J, et al. Ejection fraction change with exercise: variation dependent on ejection fraction at rest (abstr). Clin Res 1992;40:272A.

65. Borer JS, Wallis J, Hochreiter C, et al. Prognostic value of left ventricular dysfunction at rest and during exercise in patients with coronary artery disease. Adv Cardiol 1986;34:179.

66. Borer JS, Wallis J, Holmes J, et al. Prognostication in patients with coronary artery disease: preliminary results of radionuclide cineangiographic studies. Bull NY Acad Med 1983;59: 847.

67. Hendel RC, Layden JJ, Leppo JA. Prognostic value of dipyridamole thallium scintigraphy for evaluation of ischemic heart disease, J Am Coll Cardiol 1990;15:10.

68. Shaw L, Chaitman BR, Hilton TC, et al. Prognostic value of dipyridamole Tl-201 imaging in elderly patients, J Am Coll Cardiol 1992;19:1390.

69. Younis LT, Byers S, Shaw L, et al. Prognostic importance of silent myocardial ischemia detected by intravenous dipyridamole thallium myocardial imaging in asymptomatic patients with coronary artery disease. J Am Coll Cardiol 1989;14:1635.

70. Kamal A, Fattah A, Pancholy S, et al. Prognostic value of adenosine single-photon emission computed tomographic thallium imaging in medically treated patients with angiographic evidence of coronary artery disease. Am Soc Nucl Cardiol 1994;1:254.

71. Amanullah A, Berman D, Erel J, et al. Incremental prognostic value of adenosine myocardial perfusion single-photon emission computed tomography in women with suspected coronary artery disease. Am J Cardiol 1998;82:725.

72. Shaw L, Chaitman B, Hilton T, et al. Prognostic value of dipyridamole Tl-201 imaging in elderly patients. J Am Coll Cardiol 1992;19:1390.

73. Forster T, McNeill AJ, Salustri A, et al. Simultaneous dobutamine stress echocardiography and 99m-technetium isonitrile single photon emission computed tomography in patients with suspected coronary artery disease. J Am Coll Cardiol 1993;21: 1591.

74. Gunalp B, Dokumaci B, Uyan C, et al. Value of dobutamine technetium-99m-sestamibi SPECT and echocardiography in the detection of coronary artery disease compared with coronary angiography. J Nucl Med 1993;34:889.

75. Marwick T, D'Hondt A, Baudhuin T, et al. Optimal use of dobutamine stress for the detection and evaluation of coronary artery disease: combination with echocardiography or scintigraphy, or both? J Am Coll Cardiol 1993;22:159.

76. Herman SD, Labresh KA, Santos-Ocampo CD, et al. Comparison of dobutamine and exercise using technetium-99m sestamibi imaging for the evaluation of coronary artery disease. Am J Cardiol 1994;73:164.

77. Senior R, Sridhara BS, Anagnostou E, et al. Synergistic value of simultaneous stress dobutamine sestamibi single-photon emission computerized tomography and echocardiography in the detection of coronary artery disease. Am Heart J 1994;128:713.

78. Voth E, Baer FM, Theissen P, et al. Dobutamine 99m-Tc-MIBI single-photon emission tomography: non-exercise-dependent detection of hemodynamically significant coronary artery stenoses, Eur J Nucl Med 1994;21:537.

79. Senior R, Raval U, Lahiri A. Prognostic value of stress dobutamine technetium-99m sestamibi single-photon emission computed tomography (SPECT) in patients with suspected coronary artery disease. Am J Cardiol 1996;78:1092.

80. Geleijnse M, Elhendy A, van Domburg R, et al. Prognostic value of dobutamine-atropine stress technetium-99m sestamibi perfusion scintigraphy in patients with chest pain. J Am Coll Cardiol 1996;28:447.

81. Fleg JL, Gerstenblith G, Zonderman AB, et al. Prevalence and prognostic significance of exercise-induced silent myocardial ischemia detected by thallium scintigraphy and electrocardiography in asymptomatic volunteers. Circulation 1990;81:428.

82. Wahl JM, Hakki A-H, Iskandrian AS. Prognostic implications of normal exercise Tl-201 images. Arch Intern Med 1985;145: 263.

83. Pamelia FX, Gibson RS, Watson DD, et al. Prognosis with chest pain and normal Tl-201 exercise scintigrams. Am J Cardiol 1985;55:920.

84. Wackers FJTh, Russo DJ, Russo D, et al. Prognostic significance of normal quantitative planar Tl-201 stress scintigraphy in patients with chest pain. J Am Coll Cardiol 1985:6:27.

85. Heo J, Thompson WO, Iskandrian AS. Prognostic implications of normal exercise thallium images. Am J Noninvasive Cardiol 1987;1:209.

86. Bairey CN, Rozanski A, Maddahi J, et al. Exercise-Tl-201 scintigraphy and prognosis in typical angina pectoris and negative exercise electrocardiography. Am J Cardiol 1989;64:282.

87. Koss JH, Kobren SM, Grunwald AM, et al. Role of exercise Tl-201 myocardial perfusion scintigraphy in predicting prognosis in suspected coronary artery disease. Am J Cardiol 1987; 59:531.

88. Hendel RC, Layden JJ, Leppo JA. Prognostic value of dipyridamole-thallium scintigraphy for evaluation of ischemic heart disease. J Am Coll Cardiol 1990;15:109.

89. Younis LT, Byers S, Shaw L, et al. Prognostic value of intravenous dipyridamole-thallium scintigraphy after acute myocardial ischemic events. Am J Cardiol 1989;64:161.

90. Stratman HG, Mark AL, Walter KE, et al. Prognostic value of atrial pacing and Tl-201 scintigraphy in patients with stable chest pain. Am J Cardiol 1989;64:985.

91. Geleijnse M, Elhendy A, van Domburg R, et al. Prognostic significance of normal dobutamine-atropine stress sestamibi scintigraphy in women with chest pain. Am J Cardiol 1996;77: 1057.

92. Nigam A, Humen D. Prognostic value of myocardial perfusion imaging with exercise and/or dipyridamole hyperemia in patients with preexisting left bundle branch block. J Nucl Med 1998; 39:579.

93. Gil V, Almeida M, Ventosa A, et al. Prognosis in patients with left bundle branch block and normal dipyridamole Tl-201 scintigraphy. J Nucl Cardiol 1998;5:414.

94. Gibbons R, Hodge D, Berman D, et al. Long-term outcome of patients with intermediate-risk exercise electrocardiograms who do not have myocardial perfusion defects on radionuclide imaging. Circulation 1999;100:2140.

95. Alkeylani A, Miller D, Shaw L, et al. Influence of race on the prediction of cardiac events with stress technetium-99m sestamibi tomographic imaging in patients with stable angina pectoris. Am J Cardiol 1998;81:293.

96. Brown KA, Altland E, Rowen M. Prognostic value of normal technetium-99m-sestamibi cardiac imaging. J Nucl Med 1994; 35:554.

97. Iskander S, Iskandrian A. Risk assessment using single-photon emission computed tomographic technetium-99m sestamibi imaging. J Am Coll Cardiol 1998; 32:57.

98. Steinberg EH, Koss JH, Lee M, et al. Prognostic significance from 10-year follow-up of a qualitatively normal planar exercise thallium test in suspected coronary artery disease. Am J Cardiol 1993;71:1270.

99. Fagan LF Jr, Shaw L, Kong BA, et al. Prognostic value of exercise thallium scintigraphy in patients with good exercise tolerance and a normal or abnormal exercise electrocardiogram and suspected or confirmed coronary artery disease. Am J Cardiol 1992;69:607.

100. Schalet BD, Kegel JG, Heo J, et al. Prognostic implications of normal exercise SPECT thallium images in patients with strongly positive exercise electrocardiograms. Am J Cardiol 1993;72:1201.

101. Krishnan R, Lu J, Dae M, et al. Does myocardial perfusion scintigraphy demonstrate clinical usefulness in patients with markedly positive exercise tests? An assessment of the method in a high-risk subset. Am Heart J 1994;127(4 pt 1):804.

102. Brown KA, Rowen M. Prognostic value of a normal exercise myocardial perfusion imaging study in patients with angiographically significant coronary artery disease, Am J Cardiol 1993;71:865.

103. Abdel-Fattah A, Kamal AM, Pancholy S, et al. Prognostic implications of normal exercise tomographic thallium images in patients with angiographic evidence of significant coronary artery disease. Am J Cardiol 1994;74:769.

104. Doat M, Podio V, Pavin D, et al. Long term prognostic significance of normal or abnormal exercise T1-201 myocardial scintigraphy in patients with or without significant coronary stenosis. J Am Coll Cardiol 1994;158A (abstract).

105. He Z, Dakik H, Vaduganathan P, et al. Clinical and angiographic significance of a normal Tl-201 tomographic study in patients with a strongly positive exercise electrocardiogram. Am J Cardiol 1996;78:638.

106. Brown, KA. Prognosis in stable coronary artery disease. In: Nuclear Cardiology: State of the Art and Future Directions, 2nd Edition. edited by BL Zaret and GA Beller. Philadelphia: Mosby, 1999.

107. Chatziioannou S, Moore W, Ford P, et al. Prognostic value of myocardial perfusion imaging in patients with high exercise tolerance. Circulation 1999;99:867.

108. Brown K, Rowen M. Impact of antianginal medications, peak heart rate and stress level on the prognostic value of a normal exercise myocardial perfusion imaging study. J Nucl Med 1993; 34:1467.

109. Murphy J, Krone R, Multicenter Study of Myocardial Ischemia Group (MSMI). Importance of exercise capacity in the interpretation of a myocardial ischemic response to exercise testing. Am J Cardiol 1998;82:1525.

110. Pohost GM, Alpert NS, Ingwall JS, et al. Thallium redistribution: mechanisms and clinical utility. Semin Nucl Med 1980; 20:70.

111. Esquivel L, Pollock SG, Beller GA, et al. Effect of the degree of effort on the sensitivity of the exercise Tl-201 stress test in symptomatic coronary artery disease. Am J Cardiol 1989;63: 160.

112. Iskandrian AS, Heo J, Kong B, et al. Effect of exercise level on the ability of Tl-201 tomographic imaging in detecting coronary artery disease: analysis of 461 patients. J Am Coll Cardiol 1989;14:1477.

113. Snader C, Marwick T, Pashkow F, et al. Importance of estimated functional capacity as a predictor of all-cause mortality among patients referred for exercise thallium single-photon emission computed tomography: report of 3,400 patients from a single center. J Am Coll Cardiol 1997;30:641.

114. Rainwater J, Steele P, Kirch D, et al. Effect of propranolol on myocardial perfusion images and exercise ejection fraction in men with coronary artery disease. Circulation 1982;65:77.

115. Steele P, Sklar J, Kirch D, et al. Tl-201 myocardial imaging during maximal and submaximal exercise: comparison of submaximal exercise with propranolol. Am Heart J 1983;106: 1353.

116. Hockings B, Saltissi S, Croft DN, et al. Effect of beta adrenergic blockade on Tl-201 myocardial perfusion imaging. Br Heart J 1983;49:83.

117. Stegaru B, Loose R, Keller H, et al. Effects of long-term treatment with 120 mg of sustained-release isosorbide dinitrate and 60 mg of sustained-release nifedipine on myocardial perfusion. Am J Cardiol 1988;61:74E.

118. Göller V, Clausen M, Henze E, et al. Reduction of exercise-induced myocardial perfusion defects by isosorbide-5-nitrate: assessment using quantitative Tc-99m-MIBI-SPECT. Coron Artery Dis 1995;6:245.

119. Madias JE, Lee VW, Song SS. Acute effects of oral isosorbide dinitrate on exercise Tl-201 myocardial imaging in patients with stable angina pectoris. A randomized double-blind placebo-controlled clinical trial. Am J Noninvasive Cardiol 1992;6:215.

120. Mahmarian J, Fenimore N, Marks G, et al. Transdermal nitroglycerine patch therapy reduces the extent of exercise-induced myocardial ischemia: results of a double-blind, placebo-controlled trial using quantitative thallium-2-1 tomography. J Am Coll Cardiol 1994;24:25.

121. Dakik H, Kleiman N, Farmer J, et al. Intensive medical therapy versus coronary angioplasty for suppression of myocardial ischemia in survivors of acute myocardial infarction. Circulation 1998;98:2017.

122. Marie P, Danchin N, Branly F, et al. Effects of medical therapy on outcome assessment using exercise Tl-201 single photon emission computed tomography imaging. J Am Coll Cardiol 1999;34:113.

123. Bosch X, March R, Magrina J, et al. Prediction of in-hospital cardiac events using dipyridamole perfusion scintigraphy after myocardial infarction. Circulation 1989;80 (suppl II):II-307 (abstract).

124. Boucher CA, Brewster DC, Darling RC, et al. Determination of cardiac risk by dipyridamole-thallium imaging before peripheral vascular surgery. N Engl J Med 1985; 312:389.

125. Brown KA, O'Meara J, Chambers CE, et al. Ability of dipyridamole-Tl-201 imaging one to four hours after myocardial infarction to predict in-hospital and later recurrent myocardial ischemic events. Am J Cardiol 1990;65:160.

126. Brown KA, Weiss RM, Clements JP, et al. Usefulness of residual ischemic myocardium within prior infarct zone for identifying patients at high risk late after acute myocardial infarction. Am J Cardiol 1987;60:15.

127. Eagle KA, Coley CM, Newell JB, et al. Combining clinical and thallium data optimizes preoperative assessment of cardiac risk before major vascular surgery, Ann Intern Med 1989;110:859.

128. Eagle KA, Singer DE, Brewster DC, et al. Dipyridamole-thallium scanning in patients undergoing vascular surgery. Optimizing preoperative evaluation of cardiac risk. JAMA 1987; 257:2185.

129. Gibson RS, Beller GA, Gheorghiade M, et al. The prevalence and clinical significance of residual myocardial ischemia 2 weeks after uncomplicated non-Q-wave myocardial infarction: a prospective natural history study, Circulation 1986;73:1186.

130. Gill JB, Ruddy TD, Newell JB, et al. Prognostic importance of thallium uptake by the lungs during exercise in coronary artery disease, N Engl J Med 1987;317:1486.

131. Gimple LW, Hutter AM Jr, Guiney TE, et al. Prognostic utility of predischarge dipyridamole-thallium imaging compared to predischarge submaximal exercise electrocardiography and maximal exercise imaging after uncomplicated acute myocardial infarction. Am J Cardiol 1989;64:1243.

132. Kaul S, Lilly DR, Gasho JA, et al. Prognostic utility of the exercise thallium-201 test in ambulatory patients with chest pain: comparison with cardiac catheterization. Circulation 1988;77:745.

133. Lane SE, Lewis SM, Pippin JJ, et al. Predictive value of quantitative dipyridamole-thallium scintigraphy in assessing cardiovascular risk after vascular surgery in diabetes mellitus. Am J Cardiol 1989;64:1275.

134. Leppo J, Plaja J, Gionet M, et al. Noninvasive evaluation of cardiac risk before elective vascular surgery. J Am Coll Cardiol 1987;9:269.

135. Leppo JA, O'Brien J, Rothendler JA, et al. Dipyridamole-thallium-201 scintigraphy in the prediction of future cardiac events after acute myocardial infarction, N Engl J Med 1984;310:1014.

136. Lette J, Waters D, Lapointe J, et al. Usefulness of the severity and extent of reversible perfusion defects during thallium-dipyridamole imaging for cardiac risk assessment before noncardiac surgery. Am J Cardiol 1989;64:276.

137. Lette J, Waters D, Lassonde J, et al. Postoperative myocardial infarction and cardiac death. Predictive value of dipyridamole-thallium imaging and five clinical scoring systems based on multifactorial analysis. Ann Surg 1990;211:84.

138. Pirelli S, Inglese E, Suppa M, et al. Dipyridamole-thallium-201 scintigraphy in the early post-infarction period, (Safety and accuracy in predicting the extent of coronary disease and future recurrence of angina in patients suffering from their first myocardial infarction). Eur Heart J 1988;9:1324.

139. Sachs RN, Tellier P, Larmignat P, et al. Assessment by dipyridamole-thallium-201 myocardial scintigraphy of coronary risk before peripheral vascular surgery. Surgery 1988;103:584.

140. Stratmann HG, Mark AL, Walter KE, et al. Prognostic value of atrial pacing and thallium-201 scintigraphy in patients with stable chest pain. Am J Cardiol 1989;64:985.

141. Wilson WW, Gibson RS, Nygaard TW, et al. Acute myocardial infarction associated with single vessel coronary artery disease: an analysis of clinical outcome and the prognostic importance of vessel patency and residual ischemic myocardium. J Am Coll Cardiol 1988;11:223.

142. Younis LT, Byers S, Shaw L, et al. Prognostic value of intravenous dipyridamole thallium scintigraphy after an acute myocardial ischemic event. Am J Cardiol 1989;64:161.

143. Bodenheimer MM, Wackers FJTh, Schwartz RG, et al. Prognostic significance of a fixed thallium defect one to six months after onset of acute myocardial infarction or unstable angina. Multicenter Myocardial Ischemia Research Group. Am J Cardiol 1994;74:1196.

144. Botvinick EH. Late reversibility: a viability issue, J Am Coll Cardiol 1990;15:341.

145. Brunken R, Schwaiger M, Grover-McKay M, et al. Positron emission tomography detects tissue metabolic activity in myocardial segments with persistent thallium perfusion defects. J Am Coll Cardiol 1987;10:557.

146. Dilsizian V, Rocco TP, Freedman NMT, et al. Enhanced detection of ischemic but viable myocardium by the reinjection of thallium after stress-redistribution imaging. N Engl J Med 1990;323:141.

147. Liu P, Kiess MC, Okada RD. The persistent defect on exercise thallium imaging and its fate after myocardial revascularization: does it represent scar or ischemia? Am Heart J 1985;110:996.

148. Yang LD, Berman DS, Kiat H, et al. The frequency of late reversibility in SPECT thallium-201 stress-redistribution studies. J Am Coll Cardiol 1990;15:334.

149. Brown KA, Rowen M, Altland E. Prognosis of patients with an isolated fixed thallium-201 defect and no prior myocardial infarction. Am J Cardiol 1993;72:1199.

150. Tisselli A, Pierliugi P, Moscatelli G, et al. Prognostic value of persistent thallium-201 defects that become reversible after reinjection in patients with chronic myocardial infarction. J Nucl Cardiol 1997; 4:195.

151. Petretta M, Cuocolo A, Bonaduce D, et al. Incremental prognostic value of thallium reinjection after stress-redistribution imaging in patients with previous myocardial infarction and left ventricular dysfunction. J Nucl Med 1997;38:195.

152. Zafrir Nili, Leppo J, Reinhardt C, et al. Thallium reinjection versus standard stress/delay redistribution imaging for prediction of cardiac events. J Am Coll Cardiol 1998;31:1280.

153. Miller GL, Herman SD, Heller GV, et al. Relation between perfusion defects on stress technetium-99m sestamibi SPECT scintigraphy and the location of a subsequent acute myocardial infarction. Am J Cardiol 1996;78:26.

154. Galvin GM, Brown KA. The site of acute myocardial infarction is related to the coronary territory of transient defects on prior myocardial perfusion imaging. J Nucl Cardiol 1996;3: 382.

155. Ladenheim ML, Kotler TS, Pollock BH, et al. Incremental prognostic power of clinical history, exercise electrocardiography and myocardial perfusion scintigraphy in suspected coronary artery disease. Am J Cardiol 1987;59:270.

156. Pollock SG, Abbott RD, Boucher CA, et al. Independent and incremental prognostic value of tests performed in hierarchical order to evaluate patients with suspected coronary artery disease. Validation of models based on these tests, Circulation 1992;85:237.

157. Iskandrian AS, Chae SC, Heo J, et al. Independent and incremental prognostic value of exercise single-photon emission computed tomographic (SPECT) thallium imaging in coronary artery disease. J Am Coll Cardiol 1993;22:665.

158. Palmas W, Bingham S, Diamond GA, et al. Incremental prognostic value of exercise thallium-201 myocardial single-photon emission computed tomography late after coronary artery bypass surgery. J Am Coll Cardiol 1995;25:403.

159. Marie PY, Danchin N, Durand JF, et al. Long-term prediction of major ischemic events by exercise thallium-201 single-photon emission computed tomography. Incremental prognostic value compared with clinical, exercise testing, catheterization and radionuclide angiographic data. J Am Coll Cardiol 1995; 26:879.

160. Desideri A, Candelpergher G, Zanco P, et al. Exercise technetium 99m sestamibi single-photon emission computed tomography late after coronary artery bypass surgery: long-term follow-up. Clin Cardiol 1997;20:779.

161. Vanzetto G, Ormezzano O, Fagret D, et al. Long-term additive prognostic value of thallium-201 myocardial perfusion imaging over clinical and exercise stress test in low to intermediate risk patients. Circulation 1999;100:1521.

162. Nallamothu N, Johnson J, Bagheri B, et al. Utility of stress single-photon emission computed tomography (SPECT) perfusion imaging in predicting outcome after coronary artery bypass grafting. Am J Cardiol 1997;80:1517.

163. Nallamothu N, Araujo L, Russel J, et al. Prognostic value of simultaneous perfusion and function assessment using technetium-99m sestamibi. Am J Cardiol 1996;78-562.

164. Sharir T, Germano G, Kavanagh P, et al. Incremental prognostic value of post-stress left ventricular ejection fraction and volume by gated myocardial perfusion single photon emission computed tomography. Circulation 1999;100:1035.

165. Miller T, Christian T, Hodge D, et al. Prognostic value of exercise thallium-201 imaging performed within 2 years of coronary artery bypass graft surgery. J Am Coll Cardiol 1998;31:848.

166. Alazraki N, Krawczynska E, Kosinski A, et al. Prognostic value of thallium-201 single-photon emission computed tomography for patients with multivessel coronary artery disease after revascularization (The Emory angioplasty versus surgery trial [East]). Am J Cardiol 1999;84:1369.

167. Hachamovitch R, Berman DS, Kiat H, et al. Exercise myocardial perfusion SPECT in patients with known coronary artery disease: incremental prognostic value and use in risk stratification. Circulation 1996;93:905.

168. Hachamovitch R, Berman DS, Kiat H, et al. Gender-related differences in clinical management after exercise nuclear testing. J Am Coll Cardiol 1995;26:1457.

169. Bateman TM, O'Keefe JH Jr, Dong VM, et al. Coronary angiographic rates after stress single-photon emission computed tomographic scintigraphy, J Nucl Cardiol 1995;2:217.

170. Nallamothu N, Pancholy SB, Lee KR, et al. Impact on exercise single-photon emission computed tomographic thallium imaging on patient management and outcome. J Nucl Cardiol 195;2:334.

171. Steingart RM, Wassertheil-Smoller S, Tobin JN, et al. Nuclear exercise testing and the management of coronary artery disease. J Nucl Med 199;32:753.

172. Hachamovitch R, Berman D, Shaw L, et al. Incremental prognostic value of myocardial perfusion single photon emission computed tomography for the prediction of cardiac death. Differential stratification for risk of cardiac death and myocardial infarction. Circulation 1998; 97:535.

173. Shaw L, Hachamovitch R, Heller G, et al. Noninvasive strategies for the estimation of cardiac risk in stable chest pain patients. Am J Cardiol 2000;86:1.

Part 2

Risk Assessment in Acute Coronary Syndromes

JOHN J. MAHMARIAN

Acute coronary syndromes represent a wide spectrum of disorders ranging from nonischemic chest pain to acute myocardial infarction (AMI). Over 5 million emergency room visits occur each year in the United States alone for evaluation of chest pain and other related symptoms [1]. Annual hospital admissions exceed 1.5 million for unstable angina and non-ST-segment elevation AMI [2]. Each year an additional 400,000 patients suffer acute ST-segment elevation AMI.

The initial treatment of these conditions has evolved tremendously over the last decade, with the development of thrombolytic agents to achieve early coronary artery patency during ST-segment elevation AMI and the more recent use of primary coronary angioplasty for patients admitted to hospitals with this capability. Advances in the treatment of unstable angina and non-ST-segment elevation AMI include the incorporation of platelet glycoprotein IIb/IIIa inhibitors to standard treatment with heparin and aspirin. The use of angiotensin converting enzyme (ACE) inhibitors, lipid-lowering therapy, beta-blockers, nitrates, and calcium channel blockers in selected patients has enhanced clinical stability and improved survival. Nuclear cardiac imaging continues to play a pivotal role in assessing risk and guiding therapeutics in stabilized patients with acute coronary syndromes.

CLINICAL PREDICTORS OF RISK IN ACUTE CORONARY SYNDROMES

Unstable Angina and Non-ST Elevation Acute Myocardial Infarction

Several clinical classifications provide a framework for risk assessment in patients presenting with acute chest pain not associated with ST-segment elevation [3,4]. The Braunwald risk classification assesses (1) angina severity within specific clinical settings; (2) whether electrocardiographic (ECG) changes are present; (3) the intensity of medical therapy required to achieve clinical stability; and (4) troponin results as an indicator of AMI (Table 11.3) [3]. This classification method has

been prospectively validated, demonstrating a high incidence of in-hospital recurrent chest pain among patients who have acute angina at rest (64%) (Class III) as compared to those with accelerating exertional angina (28%) (Class I) or subacute angina at rest (45%) (Class II) [5]. Although 6-month survival and infarct-free survival are not significantly different between severity classes, patients with recurrent chest pain post infarction (Class C) have a higher event rate (11% and 20%), than those with primary unstable angina (Class B) (3% and 11%) ($p = 0.01$), respectively [5]. Another classification based on clinical and ECG criteria also predicts risk for in-hospital events in patients admitted with unstable angina [4]. In the study by Rizik et al., event rates among 1387 patients increased with worsening clinical class (Fig. 11.18) [4]. Patients who develop hemodynamic instability or congestive heart failure are also at significantly higher risk for early death or nonfatal infarction.

Beyond clinical variables, the presence and extent of AMI both predict outcome in patients presenting with acute coronary syndromes [6,7]. Results from the Global Use of Strategies to Open Occluded Arteries in Acute Coronary Syndromes (GUSTO IIa) [6] and Thrombolysis in Myocardial Infarction (TIMI) IIIB trials [7] indicate a strong relationship between troponin T and I levels and early mortality (Fig. 11.19A and B). Short-term risk can therefore be determined based on these clinical considerations as well as on biochemical markers (Table 11.4) [8].

ST-Segment Elevation AMI

Clinical models have been developed to assist in risk stratification among patients with acute ST-segment elevation AMI. Two recent trials in 55,135 patients receiving thrombolytic therapy reported a 30-day mortality rate of 6.9% [9,10]. Data from the GUSTO I in 41,021 patients indicate that patient age is the most significant risk factor influencing 30-day mortality, followed by markers of myocardial dysfunction (i.e., lower systolic blood pressure, higher Killip class, elevated heart rate, and presence of anterior infarction)

TABLE 11.3 *Classification of Unstable Angina*

	CLINICAL CIRCUMSTANCES		
	A	B	C
Severity	*Develops in Presence of Extracardiac Condition that Intensifies Myocardial Ischemia (Secondary UA)*	*Develops in Absence of Extracardiac Condition (Primary UA)*	*Develops within 2 Weeks of Acute Myocardial Infarction (Postinfarction UA)*
I New onset of severe angina or accelerated angina; no rest pain	IA	IB	IC
II Angina at rest within past month but not within preceding 48 hr (angina at rest, subacute)	IIA	IIB	IIC
III Angina at rest within 48 hr (angina at rest, acute)	IIIA	IIIB-T$_{negative}$ IIIB-T$_{positive}$	IIIC

UA, unstable angina; T, troponin.

Source: From Hamm CW, Braunwald E. A classification of unstable angina revised. Circulation 2000;102:118–122, with permission.

[9]. These five variables contained 90% of the prognostic information derived from all baseline clinical information (Fig. 11.20). Patients aged < 60 years had a 2.4% 30-day mortality as compared to a 20.5% mortality in those aged > 75. Mortality increased dramatically with increasing Killip class from I (5.1%) to IV (57.8%).

A similar and simpler "bedside" prognostic tool was derived from the 14,114 patients enrolled in the Intravenous nPA for Treatment of Infarcting Myocardium Early II (INTIME II) trial [10]. This TIMI risk score also identified patient age ≥ 75 as the most important predictor of early (30-day) mortality, followed by increasing Killip class, heart rate ≥ 100 beats/minute, anterior

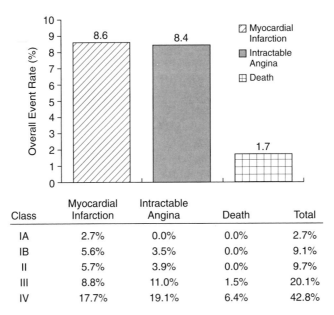

Class	Myocardial Infarction	Intractable Angina	Death	Total
IA	2.7%	0.0%	0.0%	2.7%
IB	5.6%	3.5%	0.0%	9.1%
II	5.7%	3.9%	0.0%	9.7%
III	8.8%	11.0%	1.5%	20.1%
IV	17.7%	19.1%	6.4%	42.8%

FIGURE 11.18 Bar graph demonstrates overall rate of myocardial infarction, intractable angina, and death for 1387 patients. Table shows further categorization of all major cardiac events within the classification scheme. IA, accelerating angina without new electrocardiographic changes; IB, accelerating angina with new electrocardiographic changes; II, exertional angina of new onset; III, new onset rest angina; IV, patients with protracted chest pain (> 20 minutes per episode) with electrocardiographic evidence of ischemia. (From Rizik DG, Healy S, Margulis A, et al. A new clinical classification for hospital prognosis of unstable angina pectoris. Am J Cardiol 1995;75;993, with permission.)

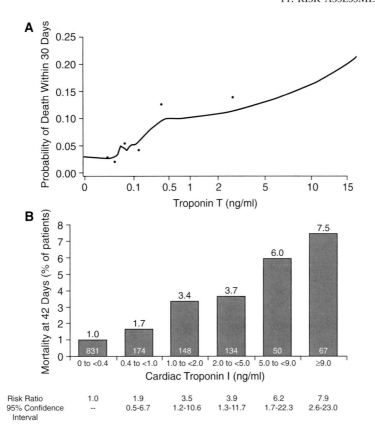

FIGURE 11.19 (A) Probability of death within 30 days according to the troponin T level at hospital admission. Smoothed nonparametric estimates are shown. The troponin T levels are plotted on a cube-root scale. The density of the data is indicated at the top, with each mark representing one patient. The dots represent simple estimates of mortality derived from ranges of the troponin T level that contained at least 70 patients. (From Ohman EM, Armstrong PW, Christenson RH, et al. for the GUSTO-IIa Investigators. Cardiac troponin T levels for risk stratification in acute myocardial ischemia. N Engl J Med 1996;335:1333, with permission.) (B) Mortality rates at 42 days according to the level of cardiac troponin I measured at enrollment. Mortality rates at 42 days (without adjustment for baseline characteristics) are shown for ranges of cardiac troponin I levels measured at baseline. The numbers at the top of each bar are the percentages. $p < 0.001$ for the increase in the mortality rate (and the risk ratio for mortality) with increasing levels of cardiac troponin I at enrollment. (From Antman EM, Tanasijevic MJ, Thompson B, et al. Cardiac-specific troponin I levels to predict the risk of mortality in patients with acute coronary syndromes. N Engl J Med 1996;335:1342, with permission.)

AMI, and systolic hypotension (< 100 mm Hg) [10]. Ten clinical variables accounted for 97% of all prognostic risk (Fig. 11.21). The TIMI score predicted both 30-day and 1-year mortality (Fig. 11.22). These trials indicate that beyond patient age, hemodynamic instability strongly affects survival. The causes of hemodynamic instability are multifactorial and include persistent or recurrent ischemic chest pain, reinfarction, myocardial rupture, ventricular septal defect, left ventricular failure, right ventricular infarction, valvular abnormalities, bradyarrhythmias and other conduction disturbances, and ventricular tachyarrhythmias. Current ACC/AHA guidelines recommend coronary angiography in such patients who are clinically unstable [11].

RISK ASSESSMENT AFTER ACUTE MYOCARDIAL INFARCTION

In clinically stable survivors of AMI, the most important predictors of subsequent patient outcome are infarct size [12,13], left ventricular ejection fraction (LVEF) [12,14–16], LV volumes [17,18], and the presence and extent of residual myocardial ischemia [19–22]. All of these variables can be determined by scintigraphic approaches.

Infarct Size

Rest myocardial perfusion scintigraphy is an attractive method for assessing infarct size, since the uptake of

TABLE 11.4 *Short-Term Risk of Death or Nonfatal MI in Patients with Unstable Angina**

Feature	High Risk At least 1 of the following features must be present	Intermediate Risk No high-risk feature but must have 1 of the following	Low Risk No high- or intermediate-risk feature but may have any of the following features
History	Accelerating tempo of ischemic symptoms in preceding 48 hr	Prior MI, peripheral or cerebrovascular disease, or CABG, prior aspirin use	
Character of pain	Prolonged ongoing (> 20 min) rest pain	Prolonged (> 20 min) rest angina, now resolved, with moderate or high likelihood of CAD Rest angina (< 20 min) or relieved with rest or sublingual NTG	New-onset CCS Class III or IV angina in the past 2 weeks without prolonged (> 20 min) rest pain but with moderate or high likelihood of CAD
Clinical findings	Pulmonary edema, most likely due to ischemia New or worsening MR murmur S_3 or new/worsening rales Hypotension, bradycardia, tachycardia Age > 75 years	Age > 70 years	
ECG	Angina at rest with transient ST-segment changes > 0.05 mV Bundle-branch block, new or presumed new Sustained ventricular tachycardia	T-wave inversion > 0.2 mV Pathological Q waves	Normal or unchanged ECG during an episode of chest discomfort
Cardiac markers	Markedly elevated (e.g., TnT or TnI > 0.1 ng/ml)	Slighty elevated (e.g., TnT > 0.01 but < 0.1 ng/ml)	Normal

MI, myocardial infarction; CABG, coronary artery bypass grafting; CAD, coronary artery disease; NTG, nitroglycerin; CCS, Canadian Cardiovascular Society; MR, mitral regurgitation; ECG, electrocardiogram; Tn, troponin.

*Estimation of the short-term risks of death and nonfatal cardiac ischemic events is a complex multivariable problem that cannot be fully specified in a table such as this; therefore, this table is meant to offer general guidance and illustration rather than rigid algorithms.

Source: From Braunwald E, Antman EM, Beasley JW, et al. ACC/AHA guidelines for the management of patients with unstable angina and non-ST segment elevation myocardial infarction: a report of the American College of Cardiology/American Heart Association Task Force on Practice Guidelines. (Committee on the Management of Patients with Unstable Angina). J Am Coll Cardiol 2000;36:970-1062, with permission.

thallium (Tl)-201 and more recently developed technetium (Tc)-99m-based radiopharmaceuticals is solely dependent on coronary blood flow and myocardial viability [23–25]. In animal models of permanent coronary occlusion, initial Tl-201 activity within the infarct zone correlates very well with coronary blood flow as measured by radiolabeled microspheres [26]. However, the relative gradient in Tl-201 activity between normal and infarcted myocardium decreases over time as this isotope washes out from normal regions (Fig. 11.23). Due to the kinetics of Tl-201, the relative count activity within the infarct zone might appear to improve over time, simulating an artifactual reduction in scintigraphic infarct size.

An alternative radiopharmaceutical for assessing infarct size is Tc-99m-sestamibi, since this isotope minimally redistributes once it is taken up by the myocardium [25,27–29]. Imaging can be performed even several hours after the initial rest injection. Recent animal investigations with sestamibi demonstrate close correlations between its initial uptake and occluded flows by microspheres, and the gradient in count activity between normally perfused and infarcted zones remains relatively constant over time [27,29]. In animal models of coronary occlusion, several investigators have demonstrated a close correlation between scintigraphic and pathologic infarct size (Fig. 11.24), which is not influenced by the early reactive hyperemia observed following rapid reperfusion [27,29,30]. These series of experiments indicate that sestamibi imaging during AMI can estimate infarct size following coronary reperfusion independent of temporal restraints.

Two studies have addressed the importance of infarct size on subsequent survival. In the Western Washington Study, 307 survivors of AMI had rest Tl-201 single-photon emission computed tomograpy (SPECT) imaging a mean of 8.1 ± 6.4 weeks after enrollment [12]. Patients with a quantified LV infarct size ≥ 20% had a significantly higher mortality rate than those with smaller infarcts (Fig. 11.25). Miller et al. prospectively followed 274 patients who received thrombolytic therapy for AMI and had rest Tc-99m-sestamibi imaging a

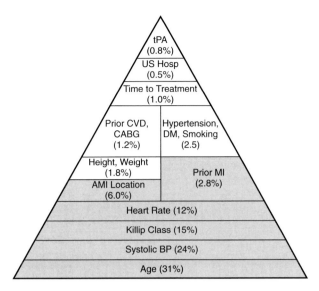

FIGURE 11.20 This pyramid depicts the importance of clinical characteristics on 30-day mortality after AMI as calculated from a regression analysis in the GUSTO I trial. Numbers in parentheses indicate the proportion of 30-day mortality risk associated with each particular characteristic; shaded blocks indicate variables that constitute 90% of mortality seen in post AMI patients with ST elevation receiving thrombolytic therapy. AMI, acute myocardial infarction; BP, blood pressure; CABG, coronary artery bypass graft; CVD, cardiovascular disease; DM, diabetes mellitus; tPA, tissue-type plasminogen activator; US Hosp, patients treated in a US hospital. (From Ryan TJ, Antman EM, Brooks NH, et al. ACC/AHA guidelines for the management of patients with acute myocardial infarction: 1999 update: a report of the American College of Cardiology/American Heart Association Task Force on Practice Guidelines [Committee on Management of Acute Myocardial Infarction]. Available at http://www.acc.org.)

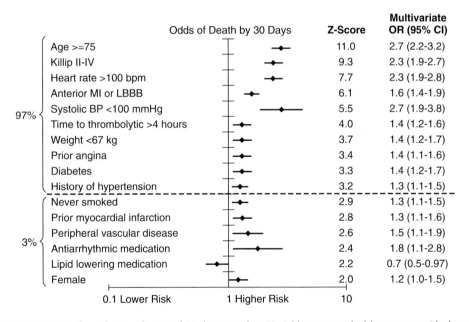

FIGURE 11.21 Independent predictors of 30-day mortality. Variables were ranked by z score, with those above dashed line selected for TIMI risk score for STEMI. Proportion of prognostic information captured by variables enclosed by braces is shown to the left. STEMI, ST elevation myocardial infarction. (From Morrow DA, Antman EM, Charlesworth A, et al. TIMI risk score for ST-elevation myocardial infarction: a convenient, bedside, clinical score for risk assessment at presentation. An Intravenous nPA for Treatment of Infarcting Myocardium Early II trial substudy. Circulation 2000;102:2031, with permission.)

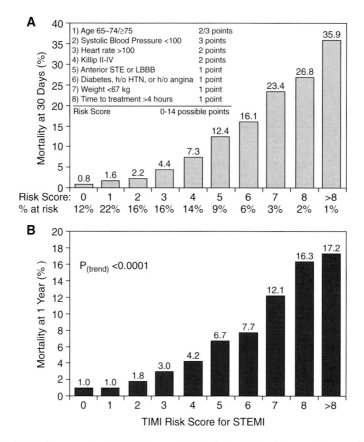

FIGURE 11.22 TIMI risk score for STEMI for predicting 30-day (*A*) and 1-year (*B*) mortality. STEMI, ST elevation myocardial infarction; h/o, history of. (From Morrow DA, Antman EM, Charlesworth A, et al. TIMI risk score for ST-elevation myocardial infarction: a convenient, bedside, clinical score for risk assessment at presentation. An Intravenous nPA for Treatment of Infarcting Myocardium Early II trial substudy. Circulation 2000;102:2031, with permission.)

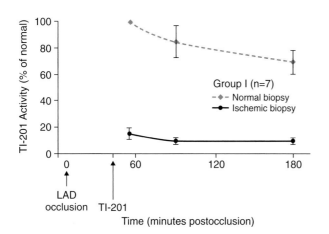

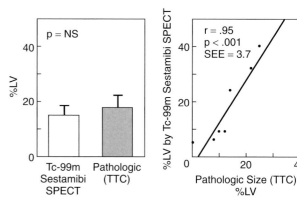

FIGURE 11.23 Myocardial thallium (Tl)-201 time-activity curves in dogs after 3 hours of sustained coronary artery occlusion. Note the constancy of low counts in the area of the infarct zone (ischemic biopsy) versus the decrease in counts from the normal myocardium over time. (From Granato JE, Watson DD, Flanagan TL, et al. Myocardial thallium-201 kinetics during coronary occlusion and reperfusion: Influence of method of reflow and timing of thallium-201 administration. Circulation 1986;73:150, with permission.)

FIGURE 11.24 Comparison of tomographic (SPECT) and pathologic infarct sizes in 13 dogs with permanent coronary occlusion. LV, left ventricle, Tc, technetium, TTC, triphenyltetrazolium chloride. (From Verani MS, Jeroudi MO, Mahmarian JJ, et al. Quantification of myocardial infarction during coronary occlusion and myocardial salvage after reperfusion using cardiac imaging with technetium-99m hexakis 2-methoxyisobutyl isonitrile. J Am Coll Cardiol 1988;12:1573, with permission.)

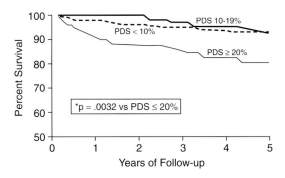

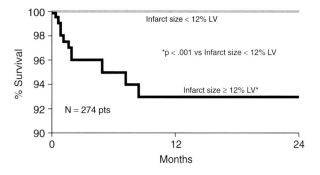

FIGURE 11.25 Kaplan-Meier survival curves based on cutoffs of total resting left ventricular perfusion defect size (PDS) as assessed by thallium-201 tomography. Patients with a ≥ 20% PDS had a significantly higher mortality rate than those with smaller infarct sizes. (From Cerqueira MD, Maynard C, Ritchie JL, et al. Long-term survival in 618 patients from the Western Washington streptokinase in myocardial infarction trials. J Am Coll Cardiol 1992;20:1452, with permission.)

mean of 7 ± 8 days after hospital admission [13]. The median LV infarct size for the entire cohort was 12% (range 0% to 68%) with a mortality rate at 2 years of 3%. Patients with a ≥ 12% LV infarct size had significantly higher mortality rates as compared to those with a smaller infarction (7% vs 0%, respectively) (Fig. 11.26). Thus, infarct size as assessed by either Tl-201 or Tc-99m-sestamibi SPECT predicts mortality. This result is not unexpected, since infarct size and LVEF are inversely related [31].

Left Ventricular Ejection Fraction

The LVEF remains the best long-term predictor of mortality in survivors of AMI [12,14–16]. Numerous studies have demonstrated excellent survival in patients with preserved LV function but a marked increase in mortality as the LVEF decreases below 40%. One of the largest patient series exploring the relationship between survival and LVEF was reported by the Multicenter Post Infarction Research Group (MPRG) [14]. The 1-year mortality among 799 patients was 9%, but 60% of all deaths occurred in the 33% of patients with an LVEF < 40%. This exponential rise in mortality was most apparent in the 3% of patients with an LVEF < 20% where the mortality rate dramatically increased to 47% (Fig. 11.27).

The important prognostic information obtained from LVEF in early studies is now reported in patients receiving thrombolytic therapy or primary angioplasty during AMI [12,15,32–34]. The resultant LVEF and subsequent mortality rate are clearly dependent on the degree to which early coronary artery patency is

achieved. In the GUSTO I trial, LVEF and 30-day survival were both significantly higher in patients who achieved TIMI Grade 3 flow (61 ± 14%, 95.6%) versus TIMI 0/I (55 ± 14%, 91.1%), or TIMI 2 (56 ± 14%, 92.6%) flows, respectively [35]. In the Survival and Ventricular Enlargement (SAVE) study, gated radionuclide angiography (RNA) was performed within the first 2 weeks of AMI and patients with an LVEF < 40% were randomized to receive either placebo or captopril therapy [36]. One-third of all patients had thrombolytic therapy during AMI. The mean LVEF in patients randomized to placebo was 31% and the associated 1-year mortality approximately 12%—similar to the 15% mortality reported by the MPRG in patients with an LVEF < 40% [14]. Likewise, in the Western Washington Streptokinase Trials, LVEF measured 8.7 ± 6 weeks after enrollment was the best univariate and multivariate predictor of survival [12]. In the 20% of patients with an LVEF < 35%, the 1-year mortality was 15%, which increased to 22% by 3 years—virtually identical to the 22% placebo mortality reported in SAVE (Fig. 11.28).

Similar results are reported by Simoons et al. in 422 patients randomized to intracoronary streptokinase versus placebo where the LVEF was measured 10 to 40 days after AMI [15]. In patients with LVEF ≥ 40%, the 3-year mortality rate remained low (4.3%). Conversely, in patients with an LVEF < 40%, the 1- and 3-year mortality rates increased with worsening LVEF, but irrespective of initial therapy (Fig. 11.29). Dakik et al. reported that the relative risk of a cardiac event doubled for every 10% decrease in LVEF [32].

Results from the TIMI II [33] and Grupo Italiano per lo Studio della Streptochinase Nell'Infarcto Miocardico (GISSI) 2 [34] trials indicate that survival at any given

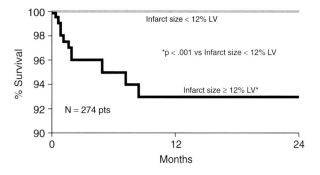

FIGURE 11.26 Kaplan-Meier survival curves based on infarct size as assessed by Tc-99m-sestamibi tomography. LV, left ventricle. (From Miller TD, Christian TF, Hopfenspirger MR, Hodge DO, Gersh BJ, Gibbons RJ. Infarct size after acute myocardial infarction measured by quantitative tomography Tc-99m sestamibi imaging predicts subsequent mortality. Circulation 1995;92:334, with permission.)

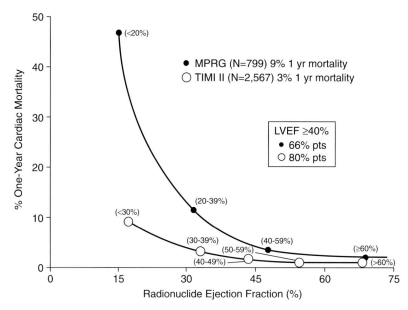

FIGURE 11.27 Impact of left ventricular ejection fraction (LVEF) on mortality after myocardial infarction. Comparison of Multicenter Postinfarction Research Group (MPRG) with Thrombolysis in Myocardial Infarction (TIMI) trial. (Adapted from The Multicenter Postinfarction Research Group: Risk stratification and survival after myocardial infarction. N Engl J Med 1983;309:331; and Zaret BL, Wackers FJT, Terrin ML, et al. for the TIMI Study Group. Value of radionuclide rest and exercise left ventricular ejection fraction in assessing survival of patients after thrombolytic therapy for acute myocardial inarction: Results of Thrombolysis in Myocardial Infarction (TIMI) Phase II Study. J Am Coll Cardiol 1995;26:73, with permission.)

LVEF is better in patients who receive thrombolytic therapy as compared to historic controls in the prethrombolytic era [14] (see Fig. 11.27). This may be due to a host of factors ranging from patient selection to refinements in risk stratification and improvements in therapeutics. Thrombolytic therapy itself may improve survival by maintaining arterial patency and thereby preventing long-term remodeling effects. One

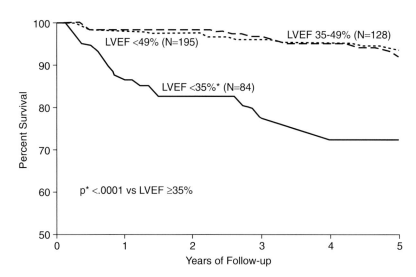

FIGURE 11.28 Kaplan-Meier survival curves based on cutoffs of left ventricular ejection fraction (LVEF) assessed by gated radionuclide angiography. Patients with an LVEF < 35% had a significantly higher mortality rate than those with better preserved LV function. (From Cerqueira MD, Maynard C, Ritchie JL, et al. Long-term survival in 618 patients from the Western Washington streptokinase in myocardial infarction trials. J Am Coll Cardiol 1992;20:1452, with permission.)

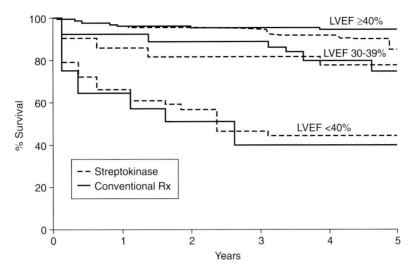

FIGURE 11.29 Survival of patients based on various LVEF cutoffs and initial therapy during acute infarction. No difference in survival was observed between patients treated with streptokinase (solid lines) or conventional therapy (dashed lines) within a given range of LVEF. (From Simoons ML, Vos J, Tijssen JG, et al. Long-term benefit of early thrombolytic therapy in patients with acute myocardial infarction: 5 year follow-up of a trial conducted by the Interuniversity Cardiology Institute of the Netherlands. J Am Coll Cardiol 1989;14:1609, with permission.)

additional factor is that regional stunning in viable myocardium frequently occurs, and can persist for weeks, in patients who achieve early coronary reperfusion during AMI [31,37]. Patients with minimal LV dysfunction (i.e., LVEF > 40%) are expected to have a low subsequent mortality rate. The TIMI II [33] and GISSI 2 [34] data also show a similar and comparably low mortality rate in patients with normal LV function (LVEF > 50%) (1.2%) as that reported by the MPRG [14] (see Fig. 11.27). However, if the LVEF is reduced due to extensive myocardial stunning which later resolves, cardiac risk could be spuriously overestimated. This may partially explain the lower 1-year mortality rate in patients with LV dysfunction in the TIMI II and GISSI 2 studies as compared to the MPRG. Measuring LVEF 1–2 months after infarction, rather than within the first 2 weeks, would reduce the likelihood of stunning and offer a more reliable estimate of risk. Despite these caveats, current data indicate that the final LVEF remains an important predictor of long-term survival irrespective of initial therapy during AMI.

Left Ventricular Volumes

Left ventricular enlargement adversely affects survival in patients with AMI and particularly when myocardial dysfunction is also present. White et al. showed that survival decreased with progressive LV dilation and decrease in LVEF [17]. However, LV dilation influenced survival only in patients with LVEF < 50%

(Fig. 11.30). Likewise, the SAVE investigators demonstrated in 512 patients with LVEF < 40% that 1-year survivors had a significantly smaller increase in LV dimensions as compared to patients who died [18].

LV dilation may develop even within the initial 24 hours of AMI, presumably as a compensatory mechanism for maintaining stroke volume [38]. This is particularly true in patients with anterior infarction, who generally have the greatest degree of initial LV dysfunction and are therefore most likely to develop early infarct zone expansion [38,39]. Over the ensuing months, structural and geometric changes occur that entail scar formation and thinning of the infarct zone as well as hypertrophy and dilatation of noninfarcted regions [40–42]. The initial loss of myocardium, if large enough, leads to progressive LV dilation, increasing wall stress, further LV dysfunction, and ultimately end-stage heart failure. In a recent trial of 291 survivors of AMI who had sequential gated RNA at baseline and again at 6 months, both LV end-diastolic and end-systolic volume indexes increased over time, but this occurred almost exclusively in patients with an initial LVEF ≤ 40% [43] (Fig. 11.31).

Various therapeutics limit LV dilation and thereby improve survival in patients with depressed LV function. In the SAVE study, patients randomized to captopril therapy had a significantly smaller LV end-diastolic volume and end-systolic volume at 1 year compared to those who received placebo [18]. Patients who responded favorably to captopril with limitation in LV

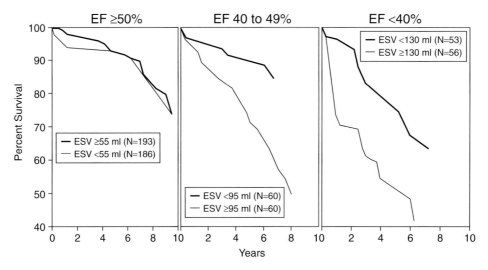

FIGURE 11.30 Interaction of end-systolic volume (ESV) and left ventricular ejection fraction (LVEF) on survival in patients with acute myocardial infarction. In patients with an abnormal LVEF ($<$ 50%), LV dilation resulted in a significantly higher mortality rate. (From White HD, Norris RM, Brown MA, Brandt PWT, Whitlock RML, Wild CJ. Left ventricular end-systolic volume as the major determinant of survival after recovery from myocardial infarction. Circulation 1987;76:44, with permission.)

dilation also had improved survival. Similar effects on LV remodeling are reported with enalapril in patients with chronic LV dysfunction [44]. Nitrates also limit LV dilation when administered early after AMI [45,46]. In a recent placebo-controlled trial, both end-diastolic and end-systolic volume indexes were significantly reduced with transdermal nitroglycerin patches (Fig. 11.32), but the nitrate effect was limited to patients with an initial LVEF $\leq$ 40% [43] (Fig. 11.33). Nitrates were most effective in preventing LV dilation in patients not taking ACE inhibitors, but a beneficial effect was also observed in those taking concomitant therapy.

These results imply that nitrates may prevent LV dilation beyond that achieved with ACE inhibitors alone. Whether nitrates, like ACE inhibitors, improve survival as a result of their salutary effects on LV remodeling remains to be determined.

Myocardial Ischemia

The presence and extent of myocardial ischemia are strong predictors of both fatal and nonfatal cardiac events, and beyond clinical variables alone [19–22]. Myocardial ischemia can be detected by various tech-

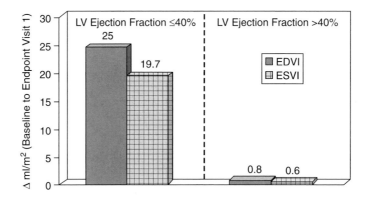

FIGURE 11.31 Changes in placebo left ventricular (LV) end-diastolic volume index (EDVI) and end-systolic volume index (ESVI) from baseline to end point visit 1 (6 month analysis) based on initial left ventricular ejection fraction (LVEF). (Adapted from Mahmarian JJ, Moye LA, Chinoy DA, et al. Transdermal nitroglycerin patch therapy improves left ventricular function and prevents remodeling after acute myocardial infarction: Results of a multicenter prospective randomized double-blind placebo controlled trial. Circulation 1998;97:2017, with permission.)

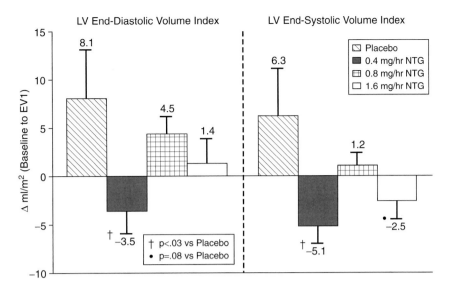

FIGURE 11.32 Changes in left ventricular (LV) end-diastolic volume index (EDVI) and end-systolic volume index (ESVI) (ml/m^2) from baseline to end point visit (EV) 1 in the four randomized treatment groups. Only the 0.4 mg/hr nitroglycerin (NTG) patch dose significantly reduced cardiac volumes. Data are presented as mean ± SEM. (Adapted from Mahmarian JJ, Moye LA, Chinoy DA, et al. Transdermal nitroglycerin patch therapy improves left ventricular function and prevents remodeling after acute myocardial infarction: Results of a multicenter prospective randomized double-blind placebo controlled trial. Circulation 1998;97:2017, with permission.)

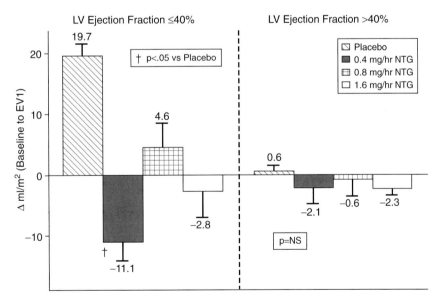

FIGURE 11.33 Changes in left ventricular (LV) end-systolic volume index (ESVI) from baseline to end point visit 1 based on initial LV ejection fraction (EF). No significant changes in LV ESVI were noted in patients with an LVEF > 40%. However, in patients with an LVEF ≤ 40%, LV ESVI dramatically increased in patients assigned to placebo but was significantly reduced in those randomized to 0.4 mg/hr nitroglycerin (NTG) patch therapy. Data are presented as mean ± SEM. (Adapted from Mahmarian JJ, Moye LA, Chinoy DA, et al. Transdermal nitroglycerin patch therapy improves left ventricular function and prevents remodeling after acute myocardial infarction: Results of a multicenter prospective randomized double-blind placebo controlled trial. Circulation 1998;97:2017, with permission.)

niques, including ambulatory ECG monitoring [47], submaximal exercise treadmill testing [48], stress echocardiography [49,50], exercise RNA [51,52], and stress myocardial perfusion scintigraphy [19–22].

AMBULATORY ELECTROCARDIOGRAPHY

Ambulatory ECG monitoring during the initial hospitalization can identify high-risk patients who have underlying myocardial ischemia [47,53–55]. Approximately 25% of patients will have ischemic ST-segment depression detected by this method. Gill et al. reported a high 11.6% 1-year mortality in the 23% of patients who had ambulatory ECG ischemia early after AMI [47]. In those without ECG ischemia, the mortality rate was significantly lower at 3.9% ($p < .01$). The composite end point of death, recurrent infarction, and rehospitalization for unstable angina occurred in 44% of those with ischemia, as compared to only 19% without ($p < .001$). The presence of ambulatory ECG ischemia provided significant prognostic information beyond that available from standard clinical information. Langer et al. reported a similar prevalence of ambulatory ECG ischemia in patients who did (37%) or did not (26%) receive thrombolytic therapy for AMI [55]. Death and recurrent AMI were also more frequent in patients with, versus those without, ECG ischemia (27% vs 6%, $p < .03$), respectively. At present, routine ECG monitoring in patients postinfarction is not recommended [11].

EXERCISE STRESS TESTING

Exercise stress testing has been extensively studied for separating high- from low-risk patients after AMI [48,56–64]. Predictors of high risk include failure to achieve a workload of at least four metabolic equivalents (METS); and exercise-induced angina, ischemic ($\geq$ 1 mm) ST-segment depression, hypotension, and ventricular arrhythmias. Inability to perform a predischarge exercise test is, in itself, a poor prognostic finding [34,65]. In the TIMI II trial, the mortality rate at 1 year was 7.7% in those who did not perform an exercise test as compared to 1.8% in those who did ($p < .001$) [65]. Likewise, in the GISSI 2 trial, the mortality rate at 6 months increased from 1.3% to 9.8% based on whether patients could perform an exercise test [34].

Electrocardiographic ischemia during submaximal exercise predicts subsequent cardiac death [48]. In an early study from the Montreal Heart Institute, the 1-year mortality rate among all patients was 9.5%, but death occurred almost exclusively in the 30% of patients with ECG ischemia. Patients without ischemia had only a 2.1% mortality compared to a 27% mortality in those with ST-segment depression [48].

Low-level exercise ECG testing may predict mortality in seemingly low-risk groups post AMI, but it is of limited value in predicting other morbid events for several reasons. The stress ECG has at best modest sensitivity for detecting significant coronary artery disease (CAD) [57,66], which may be further reduced in patients who perform only submaximal exercise [67]. It is also difficult to interpret in patients who already have an underlying rest abnormality. Furthermore, recent trials indicate a lower rate of positivity with treadmill testing than in the previous years. In the prethrombolytic era, approximately 31% of patients with uncomplicated AMI exhibited ECG ischemia on predischarge exercise testing [19,20,68,69]. However, this has decreased to approximately 15% among patients evaluated in the thrombolytic era [32,65,70–73]. All of these factors limit the ability of the treadmill test to accurately predict which stable patients after AMI are at increased risk for subsequent events (Fig. 11.34).

GATED RADIONUCLIDE ANGIOGRAPHY

Gated RNA allows assessment of LVEF at rest and during dynamic exercise. The rest LVEF identifies patients at high risk for death [12,14–16,32–34], and the presence of exercise-induced ischemia adds further prognostic information beyond the rest function alone [51,52,74–79] (Table 11.5). The peak LVEF during exercise and the change in LVEF from rest to exercise can be used to risk-stratify stable patients after AMI. Morris et al. studied 106 patients, of whom 24 died and an additional 38 had recurrent AMI, readmission for unstable angina, or refractory angina necessitating coronary revascularization [79]. The rest and exercise LVEF both predicted survival but did not predict any other clinical event. The change in LVEF from rest to exercise predicted subsequent refractory angina and need for coronary revascularization. Abraham et al. reported a 58% event rate at 2 years in patients with an exercise LVEF < 50% as compared to a 17% event rate among those with normal LV function [74]. Furthermore, a > 5% increase in the LVEF during exercise identified a very low risk group for subsequent cardiac events, particularly if the rest function was > 40%.

Whether a < 5% increase in exercise LVEF predicts high risk depends largely on the population studied and the types of subsequent events considered (see Table 11.5). Hung et al. studied 115 patients with rest/exercise RNA 3 weeks post AMI [76]. Twenty-two patients either died ($n = 3$) or had recurrent infarction ($n = 5$), readmission for unstable angina ($n = 4$), congestive

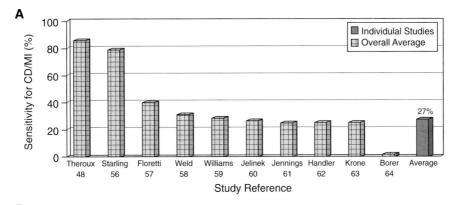

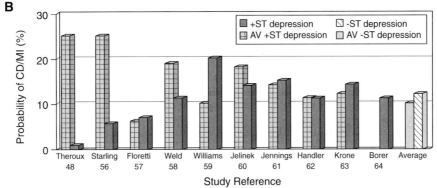

FIGURE 11.34 Sensitivity (*A*) and predictive value (*B*) of predischarge exercise electrocardiography after acute myocardial infarction (MI) for detection of patients who had subsequent cardiac death (CD) or recurrent MI. The overall sensitivity (27%) and predictive value of the exercise electrocardiogram were low for identifying patients at risk for events. DEP, depression. (From Brown KA. Prognostic value of myocardial perfusion imaging: State of the art and new developments. J Nucl Cardiol 1996;3:516, with permission.)

heart failure (*n* = 1), or bypass surgery (*n* = 9). Six of the latter 9 patients had refractory angina. The change in LVEF during exercise was a significant predictor of both hard (i.e., death, recurrent infarction) and all cardiac events. In the study by Corbett et al., 97% of patients who failed to increase their LVEF during exercise returned with a cardiac event by 6 months; however, most of these events were ischemic (i.e.,

angina or recurrent infarction) [52]. Conversely, in the series by Nicod et al. where the majority of events were death or recurrent infarction (65%), the exercise LVEF was less discriminating (positive predictive accuracy = 46%) [77]. Despite these differences, knowing the extent of rest and inducible LV dysfunction can help stratify risk and identify patients who might best be further evaluated with coronary angiography.

TABLE 11.5 *Gated Exercise Radionuclide Angiography for Risk Assessment after Acute Myocardial Infarction*

Study	N	Follow-up (mos)	Events	Predictor	Positive Predictive Accuracy (%)	Negative Predictive Accuracy (%)	Overall Accuracy (%)
Candell-Riera et al. [51]	115	12	D/RMI/A/CHF/REV	EX LVEF < 40%	—	—	82
Corbett et al. [52]	61	9.6	D/RMI/A/UA/CHF	Δ LVEF < 5%	97	92	95
Corbett et al. [75]	117	8.3	D/RMI/A/UA/CHF	Δ LVEF < 5%	95	91	93
Nicod et al. [77]	42	8	D/RMI/UA	Δ LVEF < 5%	46	86	52
Roig et al. [78]	93	16	D/RMI/UA	Δ LVEF < 5%	26	94	62
Hung et al. [76]	115	11.6	D/RMI/UA/CHF/REV	Δ LVEF < 5%	63	84	83

mos, months; D, death; RMI, recurrent myocardial infarction; A, exertional angina; CHF, congestive heart failure; REV, revascularization; EX, exercise; LVEF, left ventricular ejection fraction; UA, unstable angina.

Source: Adapted from Mahmarian JJ. Prediction of myocardium at risk. Clinical significance during acute infarction and in evaluating subsequent prognosis. In Kleiman NS (ed.), Acute Myocardial Infarction, Cardiol Clin 1994;13:355–378, with permission.

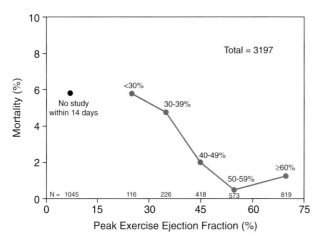

FIGURE 11.35 Relation of all-cause mortality to peak exercise ejection fraction. (From Zaret BL, Wackers FJT, Terrin ML, et al. for the TIMI Study Group. Value of radionuclide rest and exercise left ventricular ejection fraction in assessing survival of patients after thrombolytic therapy for acute myocardial inarction: Results of Thrombolysis in Myocardial Infarction (TIMI) Phase II Study. J Am Coll Cardiol 1995;26:73, with permission.)

Patients who receive thrombolytic therapy commonly have exercise-induced ischemic LV dysfunction. In the TIMI II trial, 59% of 2143 patients who had rest and exercise RNA prior to hospital discharge had an ischemic response defined as either a < 5% increase (48%) or a > 5% decrease (11%) in exercise LVEF [33]. The 1-year mortality rate in the total TIMI cohort of 3197 patients was 3%, which decreased to 2.2% in the 2567 who underwent gated RNA and 1.7% in those who had both rest and exercise RNA. The rest (see Fig. 11.27) and peak exercise (Fig. 11.35) LVEF predicted survival as did the change in LVEF with exercise. However, by multivariate analysis, the exercise variables did not improve predictive accuracy over the rest LVEF alone. These results may be biased, since the 1045 patients who could not undergo exercise RNA had a significantly higher mortality rate (5.8%) as compared to those who exercised (1.7%) (Fig. 11.35). Furthermore, the exercise LVEF variables may better predict nonfatal ischemic cardiac events, which were not evaluated in this trial. Although important from a historical perspective, exercise gated RNA has been largely supplanted by gated SPECT perfusion imaging for risk stratification.

EXERCISE MYOCARDIAL PERFUSION SCINTIGRAPHY

Exercise myocardial perfusion scintigraphy can accurately define risk in stable survivors of AMI (Table 11.6) [19,20,69,73,80]. Patients without scintigraphic ischemia have a very low cardiac event rate (< 5%), whereas 40% to 50% of patients with ischemia will de-

TABLE 11.6 *Comparison of Exercise vs Pharmacologic Coronary Vasodilators for Risk Assessment after Acute Myocardial Infarction*

Study	N	Follow-up (mos)	Events	Predictor	Positive Predictive Accuracy (%)	Negative Predictive Accuracy (%)
Exercise						
Wilson et al. [69]	97	39	D/MI/UA	IZRD	42	77
Brown et al. [80]	59	37	D/MI/UA	IZRD	28	100
Gibson et al. [19]	140	15	D/MI/UA	RD	59 (86)*	
Gibson et al. [20]	241	27	D/MI	IZRD	31	97
Travin et al. [73]	87	15	D/MI/UA	RD	20	96
Overall	624				37	93
Dipyridamole						
Gimple et al. [68]	36	6	D/MI/UA	NIZRD	26 (42)*	88
Younis et al. [81]	68	12	D/MI	RD	22	94
Leppo et al. [82]	51	19	D/MI	RD	33	94
Brown et al. [83]	50	12	D/MI/UA	RD	45	100
Overall	205				30	94
Adenosine						
Mahmarian et al. [21]	92	15	D/MI/UA/CHF	RD (5% LV)	50	97

MI, myocardial infarction; IZ, infarct zone; RD, redistribution; NIZ, noninfarct zone; LV, left ventricle.

*Positive predictive accuracy for ischemia in multiple vascular territories.

Source: Adapted from Mahmarian JJ. Prediction of myocardium at risk: Clinical significance during acute infarction and in evaluating subsequent prognosis. In Kleiman NS (ed.), Acute Myocardial Infarction, Cardiol Clin 1994;13:355–378, with permission.

velop subsequent cardiac events. Early reports demonstrated increased lung uptake of Tl-201, and ischemia in multiple vascular territories as additional high-risk predictors [20]. With the advent of quantitative SPECT analysis, the size of the stress-induced perfusion defect, in relation to the presence and quantified extent of scintigraphic ischemia, have added a new dimension to risk stratification [21]. Furthermore, with gated SPECT the important prognostic variables of LVEF and LV volumes can be directly derived from the perfusion images.

Gibson et al. reported some of the most compelling initial data with exercise scintigraphy. In this study, 140 seemingly low-risk patients were evaluated with submaximal exercise Tl-201 scintigraphy and coronary angiography [20]. Over 15 ± 12 months of follow-up, 36% of patients either died ($n = 7$), had recurrent AMI ($n = 9$), or had readmission for unstable angina ($n = 34$). The presence of scintigraphic ischemia, particularly when involving multiple vascular territories, was the most powerful prognosticator. The scintigraphic variables were superior to the treadmill exercise variables in determining high- and low-risk individuals. Although 49% of patients with exercise-induced ST-segment depression had a subsequent cardiac event, so did 26% of those with a low-risk exercise test (Fig. 11.36). However, in patients with either a normal myocardial perfusion study or a nonreversible perfusion defect the total event rate was only 6%. Conversely, 59% of patients with evidence of Tl-201 redistribution and 86% of those with redistribution in multiple vascular beds had a subsequent cardiac event (Fig. 11.36).

These data were the first to imply that patients with the largest ischemic burden were also at highest risk.

More recently, Travin et al. demonstrated the value of exercise Tc-99m-sestamibi SPECT in stratifying risk after AMI [73]. Submaximal exercise SPECT was performed in 134 stable patients within 14 days (mean 7.5 ± 2 days) of AMI. Ischemic ECG changes were observed in only 23% of patients, whereas 70% had scintigraphic ischemia. Thirty-three patients who had early coronary revascularization were excluded from analysis and most (79%) of these patients had ischemia by SPECT. Cardiac events occurred in 13 patients over 15 ± 10 months of follow-up. Patients without scintigraphic ischemia had a very low 7% event rate. In patients with ischemia, both the presence and extent of this variable predicted outcome. Overall, 19% of patients with ischemia had a subsequent cardiac event, but this increased from 12% in those with one or two ischemic defects to 38% in patients with three or more ischemic defects. By Cox regression analysis of clinical, exercise treadmill, and scintigraphic variables, only the number of ischemic defects on SPECT predicted outcome.

PHARMACOLOGIC STRESS PERFUSION SCINTIGRAPHY

Dipyridamole and adenosine SPECT are effective alternative methods for assessing risk in patients after AMI and have some distinct advantages over exercise

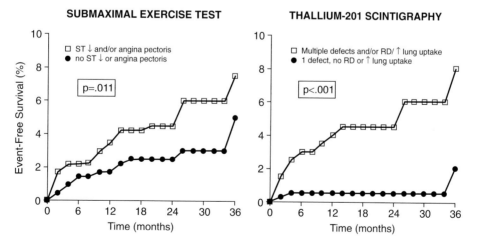

FIGURE 11.36 Kaplan-Meier event-free survival curves in 140 stable patients with acute myocardial infarction based on the presence of ischemia as assessed by the submaximal exercise test and thallium-201 scintigraphy. The thallium-201 scintigraphic results best predicted risk for subsequent cardiac events. RD, redistribution. (Adapted from Gibson RS, Watson DD, Craddock GB, et al. Prediction of cardiac events after uncomplicated myocardial infarction: A prospective study comparing predischarge exercise thallium-201 scintigraphy and coronary angiography. Circulation 1983;68:321, with permission.)

perfusion imaging [21,68,81–83]. Pharmacologic vasodilators maximize heterogeneity in coronary blood flow and can thereby more accurately identify the extent of LV hypoperfusion and residual ischemia [84,85]. Furthermore, these tests can be safely performed even within 1–2 days after AMI, allowing rapid triage of high-risk patients for coronary angiography and low-risk patients for early hospital discharge [86–88]. The scintigraphic risk variables identified with exercise stress have been confirmed in studies using dipyridamole and adenosine (see Table 11.6).

Dipyridamole SPECT

In the initial series by Leppo et al., dipyridamole Tl-201 scintigraphy was performed in 51 patients 1–2 weeks after uncomplicated AMI [82]. The presence of Tl-201 redistribution was the only significant predictor of cardiac death or recurrent AMI. Brown et al. performed dipyridamole imaging in 50 stable patients very early (mean 62 ± 121 hours) after hospitalization [83]. None of these patients had a complication from the test. When clinical, scintigraphic, and angiographic variables were compared, the only significant predictor of in-hospital cardiac events was the presence of infarct-zone Tl-201 redistribution. Events occurred in 45% of patients with, but in none of the 30 without redistribution. Importantly, those without scintigraphic ischemia remained event-free over a year's follow-up

period; whereas 3 additional patients with Tl-201 redistribution had a cardiac event. Other investigators have likewise confirmed the prognostic importance of Tl-201 redistribution on dipyridamole imaging post infarction [89,90].

Brown et al. reported the results of a large multicenter trial evaluating dipyridamole SPECT for predicting early and late cardiac events [22]. Stable patients post infarction underwent 3:1 randomization to either early (2–4 days) dipyridamole Tc-99m-sestamibi SPECT followed by exercise SPECT (at 6–12 days) (n = 284) versus submaximal exercise SPECT alone (n = 309). Twenty-nine patients who had in-hospital cardiac events and 24 who had early coronary revascularization were excluded from long-term follow-up. Following hospital discharge, death or recurrent AMI occurred in 37 patients assigned to dipyridamole testing and in 31 who had submaximal exercise SPECT. Semiquantitative visual analysis of the perfusion images was reported as a summed stress score (SSS) and summed difference score (SDS) to assess the size of the stress-induced perfusion defect and the extent of scintigraphic ischemia, respectively. By multivariate analysis of clinical, dipyridamole stress ECG, and scintigraphic variables, only the SSS, SDS, and peak creatine kinase were independent predictors of in-hospital events. Multivariate predictors of postdischarge cardiac death or recurrent AMI were the dipyridamole SPECT derived SSS and SDS, and anterior infarction location. The extent

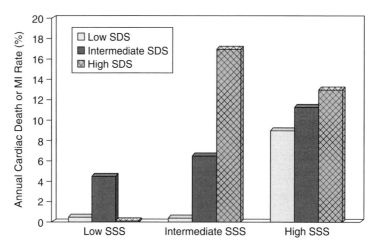

FIGURE 11.37 Annual cardiac death or myocardial infarction (MI) rate as a function of summed difference score (SDS) for a given summed stress score (SSS). For each SSS subgroup, cardiac event risk increased as SDS increased. The effect of SDS was greatest in the intermediate SSS group. (Adapted from Brown, KA, Heller GV, Landin RS, et al. Early dipyridamole 99mTc-sestamibi single photon emission computed tomographic imaging 2 to 4 days after acute myocardial infarction predicts in-hospital and postdischarge cardiac events: comparison with submaximal exercise imaging. Circulation 1999;100: 2060, with permission.)

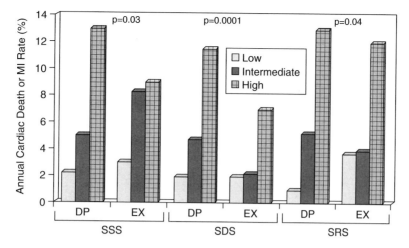

FIGURE 11.38 Annual cardiac death or recurrent myocardial infarction (MI) rate as a function of summed stress score (SSS), summed difference score (SDS), and summed rest score (SRS) for dipyridamole (DP) and submaximal exercise (EX) Tc-99m-sestamibi tomographic imaging. Event rate increased as scores increased. The ability to predict cardiac events was better for dipyridamole studies than for exercise studies for each summed score (p value depicted). All event rates are derived from risk-adjusted Cox survival scores. (Adapted from Brown, KA, Heller GV, Landin RS, et al. Early dipyridamole 99mTc-sestamibi single photon emission computed tomographic imaging 2 to 4 days after acute myocardial infarction predicts in-hospital and postdischarge cardiac events: comparison with submaximal exercise imaging. Circulation 1999;100:2060, with permission.)

of scintigraphic ischemia (i.e., SDS) further improved risk stratification—particularly in patients with intermediate sized perfusion defects (Fig. 11.37). Risk stratification was significantly better with dipyridamole than with submaximal exercise SPECT (Fig. 11.38). ECG ischemia during submaximal exercise testing did not predict subsequent death or recurrent AMI. This study emphasizes that pharmacologic stress testing post infarction is safe and effective at predicting high- and low-risk groups based on the extent of stress-induced hypoperfusion and scintigraphic ischemia. This is the first study to demonstrate improved risk stratification with dipyridamole stress as compared to submaximal treadmill exercise in the same patients.

Adenosine SPECT

Adenosine is a potent direct coronary artery vasodilator that predictably induces maximal hyperemia [84,85] and thereby produces a similar perfusion defect extent as observed with maximal exercise stress in patients who have CAD [91,92]. Based on these considerations, its high safety profile [88], and exceedingly short half-life [84], this agent is well suited for evaluating patients after AMI for residual myocardial ischemia.

Mahmarian et al. evaluated the role of adenosine Tl-201 SPECT for detecting residual ischemia and predicting in-hospital cardiac events in 120 stable survivors of AMI who were imaged early (5 ± 3 days) after infarction [87]. The overall sensitivity for detecting significant (> 50%) CAD was 87%. Sixty-three percent of patients with double-vessel and 91% of patients with triple-vessel CAD were accurately predicted to have multivessel involvement. Scintigraphic ischemia was common within the infarct zone (59%), but also in noninfarct zone (63%) territories in patients with multivessel CAD. Neither angiographic patency of the infarct and noninfarct related arteries (Table 11.7) nor the presence of collaterals (Table 11.8) predicted the presence of scintigraphic ischemia.

In-hospital cardiac events occurred in 41 patients. The adenosine-induced LV perfusion defect size (PDS) was significantly larger in patients with (45 ± 15%) as compared to those without (22 ± 15%) in-hospital complications (Table 11.9). No patient with a < 10% LV PDS had an in-hospital cardiac event as compared to 51% of those with a ≥ 10% PDS. A positive predictive value of 43% and a negative predictive value of 91% were observed when the ischemic PDS was dichotomized at 12%. These data emphasize that (1) SPECT can readily identify patients with multivessel CAD; (2) the angiographic information alone is a poor predictor of myocardial viability and may be misleading when trying to decide the appropriateness of coronary revascularization; and (3) the scintigraphic total and ischemic PDS identify patients at high and low risk for in-hospital events.

TABLE 11.7 *Redistribution Patterns in Infarct and Noninfarct Zones: Relation to Vessel Patency*

	PARENT ARTERY (N = 86)			OCCLUDED ARTERY (N = 54)		
Zone	Complete R	Partial R	No R	Complete R	Partial R	No R
Infarct zone	8 (13%)	27 (45%)	25 (42%)	5 (13%)	19 (47%)	16 (40%)
Noninfarct zone	13 (50%)*	12 (46%)	1 (4%)†	6 (43%)†	6 (43%)	2 (14%)
Infarct/Noninfarct zones	21 (24%)	39 (45%)	26 (31%)	11 (21%)	25 (46%)	18 (33%)

R, redistribution.

*$p = .0005$ vs infarct zone.

†$p = .02$ vs infarct zone.

Source: From Mahmarian JJ, Pratt CM, Nishimura S, et al: Quantitative adenosine Tl-201 single-photon emission computed tomography for the early assessment of patients surviving acute myocardial infarction. Circulation 1993;87:1197–1210, with permission.

In a subsequent trial [21], 92 stable patients underwent adenosine Tl-201 SPECT a mean of 5 ± 3 days after AMI. Cardiac events occurred in 30 (33%) patients over 15.7 ± 4.9 months of follow-up (8 deaths, 12 recurrent infarctions, 7 admissions for unstable angina, and 3 for congestive heart failure). Clinical predictors of risk were patient age, gender, prior history of AMI, and prior coronary revascularization. Scintigraphic predictors of all events were the quantified LV PDS ($p < .0001$), LVEF ($p < .0001$), and absolute extent of scintigraphic ischemia ($p < .000001$) (Fig. 11.39). This was also true when events were restricted to hard cardiac events of death and recurrent MI.

Multivariate analysis incorporating clinical, angiographic, and scintigraphic variables identified several models for predicting risk. The most powerful model was based on the absolute extent of scintigraphic ischemia and LVEF. For every 10% increment in these variables, risk increased by 82% or decreased by 24%, respectively. Only female gender added to the model at a p value of .03. At any given LVEF, risk increased dramatically according to the extent of LV ischemia (Fig. 11.40A). A second model based solely on scintigraphic perfusion variables showed increased risk with increasing total LV PDS and infarct zone ischemia (Fig. 11.40B). Chi square analysis using a baseline model of clinical variables demonstrated improved risk stratification when LVEF

and total and ischemic PDS were added in an incremental fashion. The addition of coronary angiographic findings did not improve the clinical model (Fig. 11.41).

To further validate these retrospective results, the same group of investigators prospectively risk-stratified 133 stable patients after AMI according to their initial PDS and the extent of scintigraphic ischemia (Fig. 11.42) [93]. Patients with a small (< 20%) adenosine-induced LV PDS were classified as low risk (Group 1), those with a large ($\geq$ 20%) but nonischemic (< 10%) PDS, as intermediate risk (Group 2), and patients with a large ($\geq$ 20%) and ischemic ($\geq$ 10%) LV PDS, as high risk (Group 3). Group 3 patients were further divided based on whether they were (3A) or were not (3B) good revascularization candidates. Patients in Group 3A were randomized to receive either intensive anti-ischemic medical therapy or coronary revascularization.

Patients classified as low risk (Group 1) had a relatively low overall cardiac event rate (17%) with no deaths and few reinfarctions (7%) over 11 ± 5 months; whereas patients classified as intermediate risk (Group 2) had an overall higher event rate (29%). Patients in Group 3B had a significantly higher event rate than those with scintigraphic scar (Group 2) (78% vs 29%, $p < .001$, respectively), despite a comparable LVEF of 36%. This was also true when events were limited to death and nonfatal reinfarction (see Fig. 11.42). Of

TABLE 11.8 *Prevalence of Redistribution Associated with Occluded Infarct and Noninfarct Arteries: Relation to Coronary Collaterals*

COLLATERALS (N = 43)			NO COLLATERALS (N = 11)		
IRA	NIRA	Total	IRA	NIRA	Total
22/31 (71%)*	11/12 (92%)	33/43 (77%)†	2/9 (22%)	1/2 (50%)	3/11 (27%)

IRA, infarct-related artery; NIRA, non-infarct-related artery.

*$p = .009$ vs no collaterals

†$p = .002$ vs no collaterals.

Source: From Mahmarian JJ, Pratt CM, Nishimura S, et al: Quantitative adenosine Tl-201 single-photon emission computed tomography for the early assessment of patients surviving acute myocardial infarction. Circulation 1993;87:1197–1210, with permission.

TABLE 11.9 *Adenosine SPECT Perfusion Defect Size: Cardiac Events*

	No Complications (n = 52)	Chest Pain (n = 14)	CHF/Death/VT (n = 25/1/2)	Total Complications (n = 41)
PDS (total)	22 ± 15%	33 ± 19%*	51 ± 14%‡	45 ± 18%‡
PDS (ischemia)	10 ± 10%	21 ± 16%†	18 ± 14%§	19 ± 14%P
PDS (scar)	12 ± 10%	12 ± 8%	33 ± 10%‡	26 ± 16%‡

CHF, congestive heart failure; VT, ventricular tachycardia; PDS, perfusion defect size.
*p = .047 vs no complications.
†p = .0001 vs no complications.
‡p = .01 vs no complications.
§p = .001 vs no complications.
Pp = .004 vs no complications.
Source: From Mahmarian JJ, Pratt CM, Nishimura S, et al. Quantitative adenosine Tl-201 single-photon emission computed tomography for the early assessment of patients surviving acute myocardial infarction. Circulation 1993;87:1197–1210, with permission.

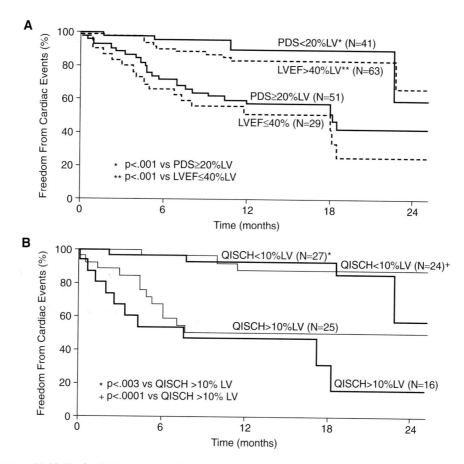

FIGURE 11.39 Kaplan-Meier curves depicting freedom from cardiac events on the basis of (*A*) left ventricular (LV) perfusion defect size (PDS) and ejection fraction (EF); and (*B*) quantified extent of left ventricular ischemia (QISCH). The total PDS and global LVEF were inversely related and provided similar prognostic information. QISCH was the best univariate predictor of risk and did so irrespective of initial therapy during acute infarction. Thick lines in (*B*) = early reperfusion therapy, thin lines = no early reperfusion therapy. (From Mahmarian JJ, Mahmarian AC, Marks GF, Pratt CM, Verani MS. Role of adenosine thallium-201 tomography for defining long-term risk in patients after acute myocardial infarction. J Am Coll Cardiol 1994;25:1333, with permission.)

225

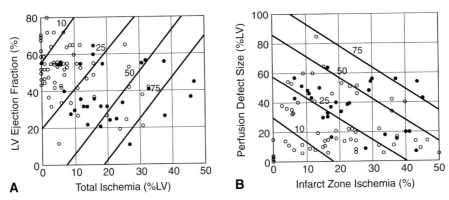

FIGURE 11.40 Cox regression models displaying 1-year risk for a cardiac event according to left ventricular (LV) ejection fraction and total LV ischemia (*A*) or scintigraphic variables (*B*). Diagonal lines = representative isobars of percentage risk. Patient risk for any cardiac event increases as total LV ischemia increases and LV ejection fraction decreases (*A*); or as total perfusion defect size and percentage infarct zone ischemia increase (*B*). For any given LV ejection fraction (*A*) or perfusion defect size (*B*), risk varies widely depending on the amount of ischemia. LV ejection fraction and scintigraphic results for each of the 92 patients who did (solid circles) or did not (open circles) have a subsequent cardiac event over the entire follow-up period are plotted against their calculated risk at 1 year (*A,B*). (From Mahmarian JJ, Mahmarian AC, Marks GF, Pratt CM, Verani MS. Role of adenosine thallium-201 tomography for defining long-term risk in patients after acute myocardial infarction. J Am Coll Cardiol 1994;25:1333, with permission.)

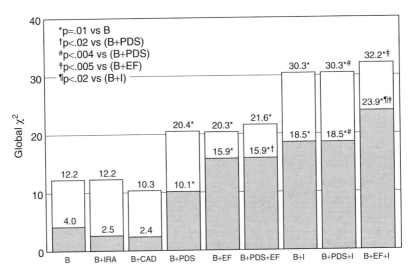

FIGURE 11.41 Incremental prognostic power of scintigraphic variables and left ventricular ejection fraction (LVEF) compared with that of a baseline clinical model (B) for predicting all events (cross-hatched and open bars) or death and reinfarction (cross-hatched bar). The LVEF and perfusion defect size (PDS), and particularly the extent of scintigraphic ischemia (I), predicted risk significantly better than the baseline clinical model (B). Furthermore, extent of ischemia improved the predictive power of the combined baseline clinical model and PDS (B+PDS) or baseline model and LVEF (B+LVEF) for all events and for death and reinfarction. LVEF added to the combined baseline model and PDS (B+PDS) or the baseline model and extent of ischemia (B+I) for predicting death and reinfarction. CAD, extent coronary artery disease; IRA, infarct artery patency; χ^2, chi-square analysis. (From Mahmarian JJ, Mahmarian AC, Marks GF, Pratt CM, Verani MS. Role of adenosine thallium-201 tomography for defining long-term risk in patients after acute myocardial infarction. J Am Coll Cardiol 1994;25:1333, with permission.)

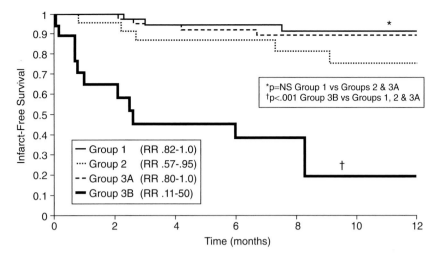

FIGURE 11.42 Infarct-free survival based on the total left ventricular (LV) perfusion defect size (PDS) and the extent of scintigraphic ischemia. Group 1 = LV PDS < 20% (low risk); Group 2 = LV PDS ≥ 20%, ischemia < 10% (intermediate risk); Group 3A = LV PDS ≥ 20%, ischemia ≥ 10% (high risk, randomized); Group 3B = LV PDS ≥ 20%, ischemia ≥ 10% (high risk, nonrandomized).

note, the high-risk but intensely treated patients in Group 3A had as low a subsequent cardiac event rate as those with an initially small PDS (Group 1). These data imply that stable patients after AMI who have a small or nonischemic PDS can generally be managed conservatively, with aggressive anti-ischemic therapy reserved for those with large reversible defects who are known to be at high risk for subsequent cardiac events.

RISK STRATIFICATION IN THE THROMBOLYTIC ERA

The important prognostic information obtained with scintigraphy in the prethrombolytic era has recently been challenged in patients postthrombolysis. This stems from (1) the lower event rate in patients who receive acute reperfusion therapy versus conventional management; (2) the unproven accuracy of noninvasive techniques for detecting residual ischemia in patients given thrombolytic therapy; and (3) the perceived lower predictive accuracy of scintigraphic variables for identifying high-risk patients.

Patients currently presenting with AMI have a lower cardiac mortality rate than their predecessors for several reasons: (1) patients who are eligible to receive thrombolytic therapy are generally younger, have a lower incidence of prior MI, and have less extensive CAD, all of which profile a patient population at lower risk for subsequent cardiac death; and (2) thrombolytic therapy and primary angioplasty reduce infarct size [94,95], preserve LV function [35,96], and thereby lower post infarction mortality [35]. In the TIMI II trial, over 50% of all deaths occurred within the first 3 weeks with only an additional 4.5% mortality by 2 years [97]. This low late mortality rate has also been confirmed by the GUSTO I investigators [98]. Thus, most cardiac events after hospital discharge reported in current studies [97,98] and in those from the prethrombolytic era [19,20,68,69,80–83] are attributable to recurrent AMI and particularly readmission for unstable angina rather than death (Table 11.10). In the latter studies this is due to the proper initial exclusion of clinically high-risk patients from scintigraphic evaluation.

Another issue is that the prevalence of ischemia in

TABLE 11.10 *Prethrombolytic vs Thrombolytic Era Cardiac Events after Hospital Discharge*

	PRETHROMBOLYTIC*		TIMI-II† [72]		GUSTO-I† [98]	
Event	*Absolute*	*(%)*	*Absolute*	*(%)*	*Absolute*	*(%)*
Death	5.7%	14	2.6%	15	2.9%	11
Recurrent myocardial infarction	8.5%	22	2.4%	14	3.5%	13
Recurrent ischemia	25%	64	12%	71	20%	76

*Eight trials in Table 11.6 [references 19,20,68,69,80–83], mean 2-year follow-up.
†1-year follow-up.

TABLE 11.11 *Incidence of Scintigraphic Ischemia Post Infarction*

Study	Stressor	− Thrombolytic Therapy	+ Thrombolytic Therapy
Brown (n = 50) [83]	Dipyridamole	10/25 (40%)	10/25 (40%)
Tilkemeier (n = 171) [70]	Submaximal exercise	70/107 (65%)	26/64 (42%)
Mahmarian (n = 146) [21]	Adenosine	43/74 (58%)	30/72 (42%)
Haber (n = 67) [71]	Submaximal exercise	—	32/67 (48%)
Dakik (n = 71) [32]	Submaximal exercise	—	27/71 (38%)
Travin (n = 134) [73]	Submaximal exercise	61/80 (76%)	36/54 (67%)
Total		184/286 (64%)	161/353 (46%)

patients receiving thrombolytic therapy is significantly lower than that previously reported. This is apparently true for exercise-induced ECG ischemia, which has decreased from a prevalence of approximately 31% to 15% [19,20,32,65,69–73]. The prevalence of scintigraphic ischemia has also decreased but to a much lesser degree than observed with treadmill testing, with approximately 46% of patients still demonstrating ischemia on perfusion scintigraphy [21,32,70,71,73,83] (Table 11.11). In the study by Grines et al. comparing primary angioplasty to thrombolytic therapy in AMI, 38% of patients receiving tissue plasminogen activator (tPA) had exercise-induced scintigraphic ischemia in the infarct zone and 24% in the noninfarct zone [96]. Of note, 24% of patients who had primary angioplasty of the infarct-related artery also had residual ischemia.

Two initial patient series demonstrated little benefit of scintigraphy for predicting subsequent cardiac events in patients receiving thrombolytic therapy [99,100]. However, both studies had design limitations that may have led to these conclusions. In the study by Krone et al. [99], 936 patients with unstable angina or AMI were evaluated of whom 31% received thrombolytic therapy. Sixty-seven percent of patients had coronary angiography and 39% had angioplasty prior to scintigraphy. Patients who underwent bypass surgery or had resting ST-T wave changes on the baseline ECG were excluded. Since scintigraphy was performed relatively late after AMI (2.7 months), many patients already had events prior to noninvasive testing. In the study by Miller et al. [100], 73% of patients had coronary angiography, with subsequent coronary angioplasty prior to (35%) or early after (17%) scintigraphy. In both of these studies most of the anticipated high-risk patients were effectively excluded or treated prior to noninvasive testing, thereby limiting the ability of scintigraphic results to predict outcome.

More recent studies have clarified the role of both exercise and pharmacologic stress myocardial perfusion imaging in predicting outcome in patients receiving thrombolytic therapy. Tilkemeier et al compared sub-

maximal planar Tl-201 scintigraphy in 171 patients who did or did not have interventions (i.e., primary angioplasty or thrombolytic therapy) during AMI [70]. The positive predictive value of exercise-induced scintigraphic ischemia was similar in both groups (36% vs 33%, respectively). Furthermore, the presence of scintigraphic ischemia identified 80% (4 out of 5) of intervened patients who died or had recurrent infarction. Within the limitations of this study (i.e., submaximal exercise, planar imaging, no quantification of ischemia), Tl-201 perfusion imaging did equally well in predicting events in intervened and nonintervened patients. Travin et al. followed 87 patients after submaximal exercise SPECT of whom 34 received thrombolytic therapy [73]. The number of ischemic segments predicted subsequent cardiac events equally well irrespective of initial therapy.

Dakik et al. performed quantitative SPECT analysis on 71 patients who received thrombolytic therapy during AMI and had exercise Tl-201 SPECT and coronary angiography prior to hospital discharge [32]. Twenty-five (37%) patients either died (n = 2), had recurrent MI (n = 5), or were rehospitalized due to unstable angina (n = 11) or heart failure (n = 7). The exercise-induced total (p = .002) and ischemic (p < .0005) SPECT PDS, as well as the LVEF (p < .0005) were all strong univariate predictors of subsequent cardiac events over 26 ± 18 months of follow-up (Fig. 11.43). This is despite the fact that 45% of patients had coronary revascularization prior to SPECT imaging. None of the treadmill exercise variables predicted subsequent outcome. By multivariate analysis, the best predictors of risk were the LVEF (RR 1.85 for a 10% decrease) and quantified ischemic PDS (RR 1.38 for a 5% increase). The LVEF and scintigraphic variables significantly contributed to predicting risk beyond the clinical variables alone, with no additional information gained from the angiographic results (Fig. 11.44).

These results with submaximal exercise testing have been confirmed in patients studied with pharmacologic vasodilators. Brown et al. [22] reported better separa-

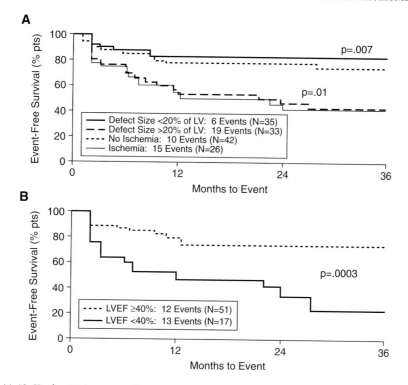

FIGURE 11.43 Kaplan-Meier curves showing event-free survival as a function of left ventricular (LV) perfusion defect size and presence of myocardial ischemia (A); and LV ejection fraction (LVEF) (B). Events were defined as cardiac death, myocardial reinfarction, unstable angina, or congestive heart failure. (Adapted from Dakik HA, Mahmarian JJ, Kimball KT, Koutelou MG, Medrano R, Verani MS. Prognostic value of exercise thallium-201 tomography in patients treated with thrombolytic therapy during acute myocardial infarction. Circulation 1996;94:2735, with permission.)

tion of high and low risk with dipyridamole sestamibi SPECT in patients receiving thrombolytic therapy (*p* = .02). Mahmarian et al. likewise showed that adenosine Tl-201 SPECT imaging could predict events comparably well in patients who did or did not receive thrombolytic therapy during AMI based on the quantified ischemic PDS [21] (see Fig. 11.39*B*).

The prognostic value of SPECT is evident even in seemingly very low risk patients [101]. One study enrolled 203 patients (of whom 62% received thrombolytic therapy) who had both low-risk submaximal exercise test and coronary angiographic results prior to dipyridamole SPECT. Most patients either had no significant CAD (23%) or only single-vessel involvement (52%). Over a mean follow-up of 15 ± 3 months, cardiac events occurred in 69 patients (34%) with 1 cardiac death, 7 recurrent infarctions, 26 admissions for unstable angina, and 35 subsequent revascularization procedures. Multivariate predictors of all events were the angiographic extent of CAD and presence of scintigraphic ischemia (Fig. 11.45). The scintigraphic data provided greater prognostic value than the angio-

graphic results (Fig. 11.46). These data all indicate that the resultant extent of residual scintigraphic ischemia, rather than the initial thrombolytic strategy per se, best predicts future cardiac risk.

Since patients postthrombolysis who lack ischemia by noninvasive testing have an excellent prognosis, it seems unlikely that coronary revascularization in this population would further improve outcome. Ellis et al. studied 87 patients with residual high-grade stenosis of the infarct-related artery following thrombolytic therapy but who had no objective ischemia by subsequent noninvasive testing (48% by Tl-201 scintigraphy) [102]. These patients were randomized to receive either medical therapy or coronary angioplasty. The 1-year mortality rate for the total group was 0% with only 5 recurrent infarctions—4 in the angioplasty group. The infarct-free 1-year survival was 98% in the medically treated patients versus 91% in the percutaneous transluminal coronary angioplasty (PTCA) group. Absence of ischemia in these patients conferred an excellent prognosis post infarction which was not improved with coronary revascularization.

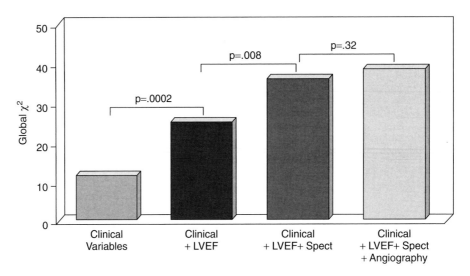

FIGURE 11.44 Incremental prognostic value of left ventricular ejection fraction (LVEF) and thallium-201 single-photon emission computed tomography (SPECT) variables. The bars depict the χ^2 statistics for clinical variables; clinical variables and LVEF; clinical, LVEF, and SPECT variables; and clinical, LVEF, SPECT, and angiographic variables. (From Dakik HA, Mahmarian JJ, Kimball KT, Koutelou MG, Medrano R, Verani MS. Prognostic value of exercise thallium-201 tomography in patients treated with thrombolytic therapy during acute myocardial infarction. Circulation 1996;94:2735, with permission.)

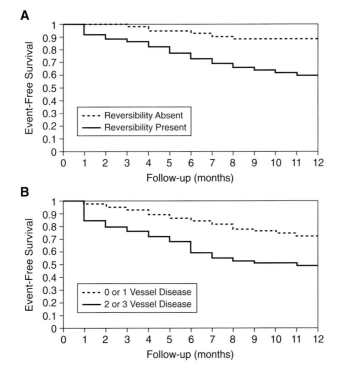

FIGURE 11.45 Event-free survival based on presence or absence of scintigraphic reversibility (A); and number of coronary arteries with ≥ 70% stenosis (B). (From Chiamvimonvat V, Goodman SG, Langer A, Barr A, Freeman MR. Prognostic value of dipyridamole SPECT imaging in low-risk patients after myocardial infarction. J Nucl Cardiol 2001;8:136, with permission.)

RISK STRATIFICATION IN UNSTABLE ANGINA

Unstable angina represents a large, heterogeneous group of patients who are hospitalized each year due to chest pain symptoms thought to be of ischemic origin. The identification of patients with true ischemia remains imprecise. Even in clinical trials of unstable angina where stringent enrollment criteria were utilized, the percentage of patients with normal coronary arteries has ranged from 10% to 20% [103–106]. One proposed strategy for identifying patients with ischemic chest pain is to perform rest scintigraphic imaging in the emergency department. This technique should be reserved for patients who have acute chest pain and nondiagnostic electrocardiograms. Patients with dynamic ST-segment changes (i.e., either ST-segment elevation or depression), a history of prior MI, or pathologic Q waves on the 12-lead ECG are not candidates for this type of evaluation. In this scenario, patients receive a rest injection of radiopharmaceutical during or in close temporal proximity to their chest pain symptoms.

Patients with chest pain who have a normal rest myocardial perfusion study can be safely discharged home from the emergency department [107–109]. In a recent study of over 1000 patients utilizing rest Tc-99m-sestamibi imaging, those with normal studies had no subsequent death or myocardial infarction and only a 3% revascularization rate over the ensuing year [107].

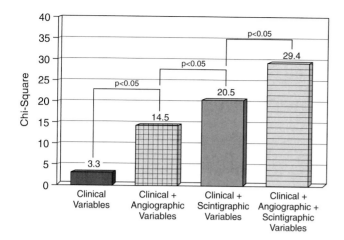

FIGURE 11.46 Incremental prognostic power (depicted by global χ^2 on y-axis) of angiographic and scintigraphic variables over clinical model in predicting all cardiac events after myocardial infarction. (From Chiamvimonvat V, Goodman SG, Langer A, Barr A, Freeman MR. Prognostic value of dipyridamole SPECT imaging in low-risk patients after myocardial infarction. J Nucl Cardiol 2001;8:136, with permission.)

However, the event rate was significantly higher in the 100 patients with abnormal or equivocal studies who were subsequently admitted for further evaluation. In this group, 11 patients had AMI, 9 had cardiac death, and 32 had revascularization procedures for a total event rate of 42%. Overall the pooled negative predictive value for a normal rest sestamibi study is 100% for AMI and 97% for all cardiac events [107–109].

In patients hospitalized with a high likelihood of myocardial ischemia, all underlying precipitating medical conditions need to be meticulously excluded. The pathophysiology of unstable angina in patients without increased cardiac demand revolves around plaque instability with intermittent coronary vasospasm due to endothelial dysfunction [110], arterial inflammation [111], or plaque rupture with varying degrees of vessel thrombosis [112]. Maximizing medical therapy can

stabilize the vast majority of patients admitted with unstable angina [113]. Patients generally respond to aspirin, heparin, and anti-ischemic drug therapy consisting of nitrates, beta-blockers, and calcium antagonists. Platelet IIb-IIIa antagonists have also been shown to reduce morbidity in patients who receive standard medical therapy [114,115]. The small percentage of patients who do not clinically stabilize are at very high risk for in-hospital cardiac events [113].

The role of nuclear stress imaging in risk stratification of medically stabilized patients with unstable angina is similar to that observed in stable patients recovering from AMI. The premise of such an evaluation is to identify which seemingly stable patients are at high risk for subsequent cardiac events and who might benefit from an invasive evaluation or intensive anti-ischemic medical therapy. Likewise, the identification of low-risk patients would streamline patient care and allow for early hospital discharge.

Trials evaluating stress myocardial perfusion imaging in patients with unstable angina are shown in Tables 11.12 and 11.13 [81,116–120]. These trials have used varying combinations of stressors and radiopharmaceuticals. Overall event rates typically after 1 year of follow-up approach 45% (from death, nonfatal MI, and unstable angina) and 13% from death and nonfatal MI. These event rates are remarkably similar to those reported in large randomized clinical trials of patients with acute coronary syndromes [104,121]. As demonstrated in stable patients surviving AMI, those with a normal perfusion scan result are at very low risk for subsequent death or MI (2%), whereas patients with either an abnormal study or one demonstrating ischemia have a significantly higher event rate (20% and 25%, respectively). When readmission for unstable angina is included, 58% of patients with an abnormal study and 73% of those with scintigraphic ischemia had a subsequent cardiac event. The negative predictive accuracy remained high at 88% (for a normal study) and 79% (for no evidence of ischemia).

TABLE 11.12 *Unstable Angina: Stress Myocardial Perfusion Scintigraphy for Predicting All Events*

Study	Stressor	N	Follow-up (mos)	Event Rate	SCAN Abnormal PPA	SCAN Normal NPA	SCAN + Ischemia PPA	SCAN − Ischemia NPA
Strattman [120]	DIP Tc-99m	128	16 ± 11	68 (53%)	62/99 (66%)	26/29 (90%)	53/71 (75%)	42/57 (74%)
Younis [81]	DIP Tl-201	68	12	40 (59%)	39/54 (72%)	13/14 (93%)	31/37 (84%)	22/31 (71%)
Strattman [119]	Ex Tc-99m	126	12 ± 7	35 (28%)	29/74 (39%)	46/52 (88%)	24/40 (60%)	75/86 (87%)
Brown [116]	Ex Tl-201	52	39 ± 11	24 (46%)	20/37 (54%)	12/15 (80%)	16/23 (70%)	22/29 (76%)
Total		374		167 (45%)	153/264 (58%)	97/110 (88%)	124/171 (73%)	161/203 (79%)

PPA, positive predictive accuracy; NPA, negative predictive accuracy; DIP, dipyridamole; Tc, technetium; Tl, thallium-201; Ex, exercise.

TABLE 11.13 *Unstable Angina: Stress Myocardial Perfusion Scintigraphy for Predicting Death/Myocardial Infarction*

Study	Stressor	N	Follow-Up (mos)	Event Rate	Predictor	SCAN ABNORMAL/NORMAL		SCAN	
								+ ISCHEMIA	−ISCHEMIA
						PPA	NPA	PPA	NPA
Brown [116]	Ex Tl-201	52	39 ± 11	7 (13%)	RD	7/37 (19%)	15/15 (100%)	6/23 (26%)	28/29 (96%)
Madsen [117]	Ex Tl-201	158	14	10 (6%)	RD	8/61 (13%)	95/97 (98%)	6/29 (21%)	125/129 (97%)
Strattman [119]	Ex Tc-99m	126	12 ± 7	11 (9%)	RD	10/74 (14%)	51/52 (98%)	10/40 (25%)	85/86 (99%)
Younis* [81]	DIP Tl-201	68	12	10 (15%)	RD	10/54 (19%)	14/14 (100%)	4/21 (19%)	41/47 (87%)
Miller† [118]	DIP Tc-99m	137	10 ± 5	20 (15%)	RD fixed defect	20/110 (18%)	27/27 (100%)	13/66 (20%)	64/71 (90%)
Strattman [120]	DIP Tc-99m	128	16 ± 11	32 (25%)	RD fixed defect	30/99 (30%)	27/29 (93%)	17/47 (36%)	66/81 (82%)
Total		669		90 (13%)		85/435 (20%)	229/234 (98%)	56/226 (25%)	409/443 (92%)

RD, redistribution.

*65% with unstable angina.

†77% with unstable angina.

The studies by Brown [116] and Madsen [117] using exercise Tl-201 scintigraphy prior to hospital discharge demonstrated similar results with death or AMI in 26% and 21% of patients who had scintigraphic ischemia, respectively. Virtually no patient with a normal study returned with a subsequent cardiac event. By multivariate analysis, Tl-201 redistribution was the only predictor of cardiac death or AMI when compared to clinical and angiographic variables [116]. The only predictors of all events were the number of segments showing Tl-201 redistribution and a prior history of MI. These data emphasize that the extent of ischemia is an important predictor of events beyond its mere presence.

Dipyridamole Tl-201 scintigraphy yields comparable results to exercise stress. In the series by Younis et al., of whom 65% had unstable angina, no patient with a normal study died or had MI, whereas 19% with an abnormal scan or one demonstrating ischemia had a hard cardiac event [81]. By multivariate analysis of clinical, angiographic, and scintigraphic variables, only a reversible perfusion defect ($p < .001$) and CAD extent ($p < .009$) predicted a subsequent cardiac event.

Technetium-99m-sestamibi has been studied with both exercise [119] and dipyridamole [120] SPECT in medically stabilized patients admitted with unstable angina who were considered at intermediate risk for cardiac events based on clinical criteria (see Table 11.4). In the series by Stratmann et al., 128 patients were followed 16 ± 11 months after dipyridamole Tc-99m SPECT [120]. The 68 patients with subsequent

cardiac events either died ($n = 26$), had nonfatal AMI ($n = 6$), or returned with unstable angina ($n = 36$). Patients with a normal study had a very low total event rate (10%) as compared to those with abnormal results (66%) (Table 11.12) (Fig. 11.47). Univariate clinical predictors of events were a history of congestive heart failure, prior MI, and diabetes mellitus (all $p < .05$). By multivariate analysis, only an abnormal scan result (relative risk 4.3, 1.5 to 12.0, $p < .05$); and a reversible (relative risk 1.8, 1.1 to 2.9, $p < .05$) or fixed (relative risk 2.9, 1.6 to 5.4, $p < .05$) perfusion defect were predictors of all events. Multivariate predictors of death/AMI were the presence of fixed (relative risk 3.4, 1.3 to 8.8) and reversible (relative risk 2.4, 1.1 to 5.2) perfusion defects and a history of congestive heart failure (relative risk 4.0, 1.9 to 8.3, all $p < .05$).

Stratmann et al. also studied 126 patients with exercise Tc-99m-sestamibi SPECT [119]. Thirty-five cardiac events occurred over 12 ± 7 months of follow-up. In this series, as compared to the previous one [120], subsequent events were more commonly due to unstable angina (69% vs 53%) than death (14% vs 38%). Patients who had a normal study had a very low death or AMI event rate (2%) as compared to 14% of those with an abnormal study and 25% with a reversible perfusion defect (Table 11.13). Likewise, 39% of patients with an abnormal study had a subsequent event but this increased to 60% of those with evidence of scintigraphic ischemia (Table 11.12) (Fig. 11.48). A fixed perfusion defect was not associated with increased cardiac risk, probably due to the lower mortality rate in

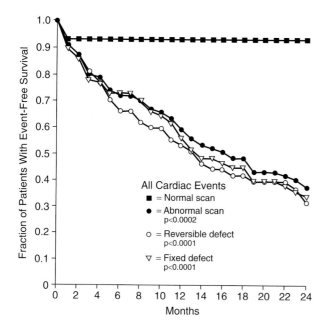

FIGURE 11.47 Two-year survival curves for occurrence of any cardiac event in patients with normal and abnormal scans. Event-free survival was significantly less in patients with abnormal scans (all $p < .0002$). (From Stratmann HG, Tamesis BR, Younis LT, Wittry MD, Amato M, Miller DD: Prognostic value of predischarge dipyridamole technetium 99m sestamibi myocardial tomography in medically treated patients with unstable angina. Am Heart J 1995; 130:734, with permission.)

this trial. By multivariate analysis, the only scintigraphic variable with independent predictive value was the presence of a reversible defect for any cardiac event (relative risk 3.8, 1.6 to 8.6) or death and nonfatal myocardial infarction (relative risk 19.2, 2.2 to 167).

All of these studies demonstrate the great potential for using noninvasive perfusion imaging, particularly with pharmacologic vasodilator stress, to identify low- and high-risk patient subsets among those admitted with the heterogeneous diagnosis of unstable angina.

TRACKING CARDIAC RISK WITH SEQUENTIAL PERFUSION IMAGING

Myocardial perfusion scintigraphy is a reproducible and accurate method to assess quantitative changes in stress-induced perfusion defects following anti-ischemic medical and revascularization therapies [122] (see Color Fig. 11.49 in separate color insert). An important remaining question is whether a reduction in quantified PDS in patients at high scintigraphic risk is simply cosmetic or actually infers a reduction in risk for subsequent cardiac events. Dakik et al. performed a prospective, randomized pilot study that compared intensive medical therapy with coronary angioplasty for suppressing myocardial is-

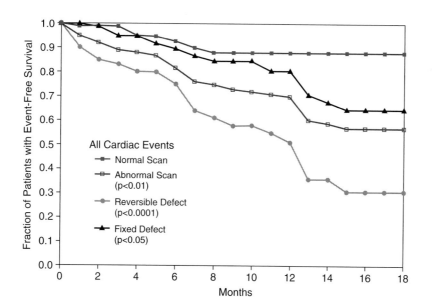

FIGURE 11.48 Eighteen-month survival curves for occurrence of any cardiac event in patients with normal and abnormal scans. Compared with patients with normal scans, event-free survival was significantly less in patients with any type of abnormal scan ($p < .01$), and with the specific presence of a reversible ($p < .0001$) or fixed ($p < .05$) perfusion defect. (From Stratmann HG, Younis LT, Wittry MD, et al. Exercise technetium-99m myocardial tomography for the risk stratification of men with medically treated unstable angina pectoris. Am J Cardiol 1995;76:236, with permission.)

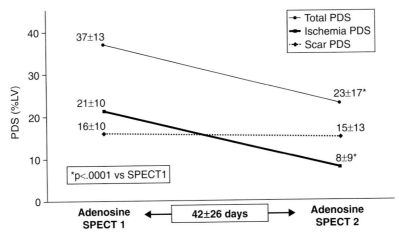

FIGURE 11.50 Mean quantified total, ischemia, and scar perfusion defect size(s) (PDS) at baseline (SPECT 1) and following anti-ischemic medical or revascularization therapies (SPECT 2). (From Dakik HA, Kleiman NS, Farmer JA, et al. Intensive medical therapy versus coronary angioplasty for suppression of myocardial ischemia in survivors of acute myocardial infarction. A prospective, randomized pilot study. Circulation 1998;98:2017, with permission.)

chemia in 44 stable patients after AMI who had large ($\geq$ 20%) and ischemic ($\geq$ 10%) LV perfusion defects [123]. SPECT was repeated at 42 $\pm$ 26 days after therapy was optimized. The adenosine-induced LV PDS was significantly reduced from 37 $\pm$ 13% (at baseline) to 23 $\pm$ 17% (posttherapy) ($p < .0001$), which was almost entirely attributable to a reduction in ischemic PDS (Fig. 11.50). The total PDS was comparably reduced with medical therapy (from 38 $\pm$ 13% to 26 $\pm$ 16%, $p < .0001$) and coronary angioplasty (from 35 $\pm$ 12% to 20 $\pm$ 16%, $p < .0001$). The overall reduction in ischemic PDS was also similar in both groups. Event-free

survival was superior in the 25 patients (13 revascularized, 12 medically treated) who had a significant ($\geq$ 9%) reduction in PDS (96%) as compared to those who did not (65%, $p = .007$) (Fig. 11.51). A 40% 1-year event rate was anticipated based on the initial SPECT results. Thus, patients who did not reduce their PDS with anti-ischemic therapy continued to have events at an expected rate. A representative patient is shown in Color Figure 11.52 (see separate color insert). These preliminary data indicate that myocardial perfusion scintigraphy can be used to assess not only initial risk but also to track subsequent risk by evaluating the efficacy of various

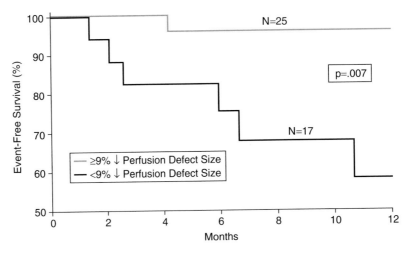

FIGURE 11.51 Kaplan-Meier curves depicting event-free survival based on changes in perfusion defect size after anti-ischemic therapy. (From Dakik HA, Kleiman NS, Farmer JA, et al. Intensive medical therapy versus coronary angioplasty for suppression of myocardial ischemia in survivors of acute myocardial infarction. A prospective, randomized pilot study. Circulation 1998;98:2017, with permission.)

therapies on myocardial ischemia. A large multicenter postinfarction trial currently underway (INSPIRE) will further explore the effects of various treatment strategies on scintigraphic ischemia and subsequent patient outcome [124].

ROUTINE INVASIVE VERSUS A CONSERVATIVE APPROACH IN ACUTE CORONARY SYNDROMES

Coronary angiography is an acceptable approach for evaluating patients with acute coronary syndromes who are at high clinical risk and would appear to benefit from urgent revascularization [8,11]. The 15% to 20% of patients with ongoing or recurrent ischemic chest pain despite medical therapy, and those with congestive heart failure or hemodynamic instability represent such a high-risk group. However, controversy continues as to whether stabilized patients with acute coronary syndromes benefit more from routine coronary angiography versus noninvasive testing followed by selective angiography only in patients found to be at high scintigraphic risk.

The rationale behind a routine invasive approach is that patients with high-risk coronary anatomy can be readily identified early after hospital admission and that appropriate coronary revascularization can be performed in an expeditious fashion. Implicit to this approach is that revascularization will improve survival and reduce morbidity from CAD, and do so more effectively than intensive medical therapy. This should lead to a more cost-effective strategy by limiting the initial hospital stay and preventing subsequent admissions due to recurrences of clinical instability.

The rationale behind a noninvasive conservative approach is that most patients with acute coronary syndromes do not have subsequent cardiac events, and that various medical therapies can prevent anginal symptoms and improve event-free survival. Although exercise treadmill testing is insensitive for detecting patients with residual myocardial ischemia who are at risk for morbid events, stress myocardial perfusion scintigraphy readily identifies patients with residual myocardial ischemia (see Tables 11.6 and 11.12) and accurately identifies those with multivessel CAD [87]. Based on the scintigraphic PDS, the extent of myocardial ischemia, and the LVEF by gated SPECT, risk can be readily determined and appropriate patients can be selected for invasive procedures.

Patients without scintigraphic ischemia and preserved LV function have a very low cardiac event rate, which is not improved with coronary revascularization—thereby precluding the need for angiography

[102]. Furthermore, with the introduction of pharmacologic vasodilators in lieu of exercise stress, perfusion imaging can be performed safely within 1–2 days of admission thereby allowing rapid risk stratification and triage of patients to early coronary angiography, if need be, or hospital discharge [21,22,86,88].

The widespread acceptance of an invasive strategy as the community standard for evaluating patients with acute coronary syndromes has occurred despite the lack of definitive clinical trials supporting this strategy over a conservative approach. In fact, results of randomized trials comparing an early invasive approach to a conservative approach have generally determined no advantage to routine angiography for either improving LV function (a strong determinant of survival) or patient outcome.

In the TIMI IIB study, 3339 patients with acute ST-segment elevation received thrombolytic therapy and were then randomized to either early coronary angiography or a conservative strategy where coronary angiography was performed only in patients who had spontaneous ischemia or inducible ischemia on treadmill testing [125]. Although twice as many patients had either angioplasty or coronary artery bypass surgery by 1 year in the invasive (72%) versus the conservative limb (35%), 1- [72] and 3-year [97] infarct-free survival were virtually identical in both groups (Fig. 11.53).

Similar results were reported in the Should We Intervene Following Thrombolysis (SWIFT) study where 800 patients with AMI received anistreplase and were then randomized to either a conservative or invasive strategy [126]. Coronary revascularization was performed in 57% of patients randomized to the invasive strategy, which increased to 61% by 1 year. In the conservative strategy, 5% of patients had coronary revascularization at hospital discharge and only 15% by 1 year. As in TIMI IIB, the conservative therapy group did as well as those assigned to an invasive strategy, with a 1-year infarct-free survival of 83.4% versus 80.9% (p = NS), respectively.

The Veterans Affairs Non Q-Wave Infarction Strategies in Hospital (VANQWISH) trial was the first study to select myocardial perfusion scintigraphy as the noninvasive testing modality in 920 patients randomized to either an invasive or conservative strategy following non-Q wave AMI [105]. During the trial, significantly higher rates of coronary angiography (94% vs 48%) and revascularization (44% vs 33%) were observed in the invasive versus conservative limbs despite a comparable 1-year infarct-free survival (76% vs 81%) (Fig. 11.54).

In the Medicine versus Angiography in Thrombolytic Exclusion (MATE) trial, 201 patients with acute chest pain who were ineligible for thrombolysis were ran-

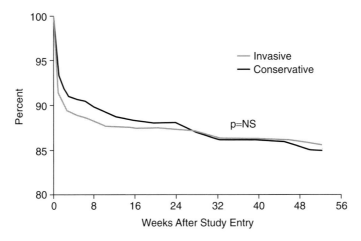

FIGURE 11.53 Kaplan-Meier infarct-free 1-year survival curves in patients randomized to the invasive and conservative strategies of TIMI II. (From Williams DO, Braunwald E, Knatterud G, et al. One-year results of the Thrombolysis in Myocardial Infarction Investigation (TIMI) Phase II trial. Circulation 1992;85:533, with permission.)

domized [127]. In the invasive strategy, 58% of patients were revascularized as compared to 37% in the conservative medical therapy limb (*p* = .004). Of note, 27 of 54 patients who underwent coronary angiography in the conservative group did so due to physician preference, and not because of clinical instability. After 21 months of follow-up, no significant differences in death (11% vs 10%) or infarct-free survival (14% vs 12%) were observed between the two groups. TIMI IIIB randomized patients with unstable angina or

non-Q-wave infarction [103]. Although angiography rates at 1 year were higher in the conservative limb of this trial (73%) than in TIMI IIB (45%), coronary revascularization was still significantly greater in those assigned to the invasive versus the conservative strategy (69% vs 40%). Once again survival (94.8% vs 93.7%) and infarct-free survival (88.9% vs 86%) were similar in both groups [121].

These large randomized trials are further supported by subgroup analyses from the SAVE [128] and

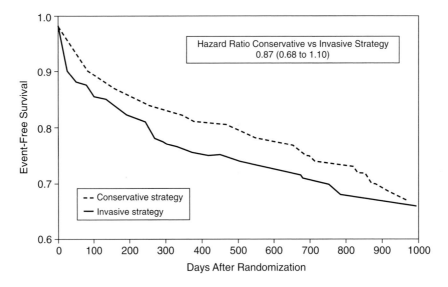

FIGURE 11.54 Kaplan-Meier infarct-free survival curves in patients randomized to the invasive and conservative strategies of VANQWISH. (From Boden WE, O'Rourke RA, Crawford MH, et al. Outcomes in patients with acute non-Q-wave myocardial infarction randomly assigned to an invasive as compared with a conservative management strategy. Veterans Affairs Non-Q-Wave Infarction Strategies in Hospital (VANQWISH) Trial Investigators. N Engl J Med 1998;338:1785, with permission.)

GUSTO I trials [129], which showed comparable infarct-free survival among patients treated in the United States and Canada despite a two- to threefold higher rate of coronary revascularization in the former country. In SAVE, only effort-related angina was less frequent in the United States than Canada (27% vs 33%) [128]. Data from the Organization to Assess Strategies for Ischemic Syndromes (OASIS) registry also show no difference in 6-month outcome among patients admitted to hospitals in countries where coronary angiography and revascularization are more frequently performed [130]. A sobering report from the GUSTO I investigators indicated that the high rate of coronary angiography in this trial (71%) was primarily driven by younger patient age and the availability of catheterization facilities [131].

Two recent trials have demonstrated a benefit with routine coronary angiography over a conservative strategy in patients with acute chest pain symptoms [104,106]. The Fragmin and Fast Revascularisation During Instability in Coronary Artery Disease (FRISC) II trial was a randomized multicenter study enrolling 2457 patients [104]. Most patients (96%) randomized to the invasive strategy had coronary angiography within 7 days of admission and 78% had either coronary artery bypass surgery (35%) or coronary angioplasty (43%) with placement of stents in most of these latter patients (61%). Conversely, coronary angiography was performed in only 47% of patients assigned to the conservative limb, with 36% undergoing coronary revascularization. Infarct-free survival was significantly better at 6 months (90.6% vs 87.9%, $p = .031$) and at 1 year (89.6% vs 85.9%, $p = .005$) in patients assigned to the invasive versus the conservative strategy, respectively (Fig. 11.55).

The FRISC II study design was biased in favor of the invasive strategy by comparing state-of-the-art interventional techniques versus substandard noninvasive testing and anti-ischemic therapy in the conservative limb. Treadmill exercise testing was chosen as the method to identify high-risk individuals. Not only is this technique poor at detecting ischemia [57,66] but the criteria used for patient crossover were inordinately strict and do not follow the ACC/AHA guidelines [11]. Crossover to angiography required (1) ≥ 3 mm exercise-induced ST-segment depression; (2) exercise-limiting chest pain or a

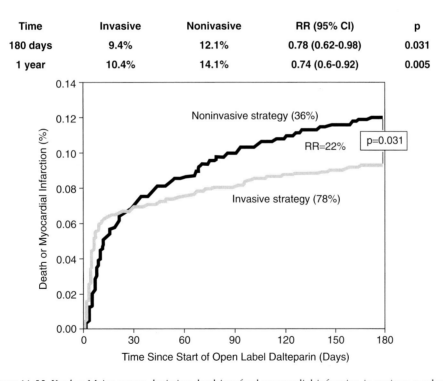

Time	Invasive	Noninvasive	RR (95% CI)	p
180 days	9.4%	12.1%	0.78 (0.62-0.98)	0.031
1 year	10.4%	14.1%	0.74 (0.6-0.92)	0.005

FIGURE 11.55 Kaplan-Meier curves depicting death/nonfatal myocardial infarction in patients randomized to the invasive or noninvasive strategies of FRISC-II. ( ) = percentage of patients with coronary revascularization at hospital discharge. (Adapted from FRagmin and Fast Revascularisation during InStability in Coronary artery disease (FRISC II) Investigators. Invasive compared with non-invasive treatment in unstable coronary-artery disease: FRISC II prospective randomised multicentre study. Lancet 1999;354:708, with permission.)

decrease in blood pressure at a low workload; or (3) exercise-induced ST-segment elevation. No prospective therapeutic regimen was proposed as to the number or doses of anti-ischemic medications to be given to patients randomized to the conservative limb. Further, there is no mention as to the anti-ischemic therapy administered to patients with < 3 mm ST-segment depression who, by protocol design, did not undergo coronary angiography. It is now well recognized that higher doses of combination anti-ischemic medical therapy are needed to effectively treat myocardial ischemia as compared to angina alone [132,133].

In the Treat Angina with Aggrastat and Determine Cost of Therapy with an Invasive or Conservative Strategy (TACTICS) trial, 2200 patients with unstable angina and non-Q-wave AMI were randomized to an invasive strategy of coronary angiography with the intent to revascularize versus a conservative approach where angiography was only performed for clinical instability or an abnormal stress test result [106]. An exercise treadmill test was performed prior to hospital discharge and 83% included nuclear perfusion imaging or echocardiography. Stress test criteria for crossover to angiography were (1) the development of angina with accompanying 1 mm ST-segment depression; (2) isolated 2 mm ST-segment depression without angina; (3) exercise-induced hypotension; (4) one "large" or two "smaller" regions of ischemia on nuclear testing; or (5) a new stress-induced regional wall motion abnormality on echocardiography.

In the invasive strategy, 97% of patients had coronary angiography prior to hospital discharge and 61% had either coronary angioplasty with stenting (41%) or bypass surgery (20%). In the conservative limb, 51% had coronary angiography and 37% had either angioplasty (24%) or bypass surgery (13%) during the initial hospitalization. At 6 months, the primary end point of death, nonfatal AMI, and readmission for unstable angina was significantly lower in the invasive (15.9%) versus the conservative strategy (19.4%) group (p = .025) as was the end point of death/nonfatal myocardial infarction (4.7% vs 7%, respectively, p = .02). Of note, the prognostic advantage of the invasive strategy was observed only during the first 30 days, after which cardiac events occurred at a similar rate in both groups (Table 11.14).

As with FRISC II, the TACTICS study was biased in favor of the invasive strategy. Noninvasive testing was performed in the conservative group without standardization of the results to determine the presence or absence of significant ischemia. The allocation, timing, and intensity of medical therapy were not prospectively defined. This may possibly explain why cardiac event rates were only lower in the first 30 days when medical therapy was variably titrated. Treadmill testing does not allow for very early (within 2–3 days) patient assessment as can be achieved with pharmacologic stress testing. Indeed, 44% of patients in the conservative limb who crossed over to coronary angiography during the initial hospitalization did so due to a recurrent cardiac event before treadmill testing could be performed. Despite these issues, the difference in the primary end point at 6 months was only 3 patients per 100 in favor of the invasive strategy. It is also to be noted that 40% of the patients in the invasive strategy did not undergo coronary revascularization, indicating the overuse of this procedure when performed routinely in patients with acute coronary syndromes. Furthermore, subgroup analysis demonstrated that patients in the invasive limb who were treated medically actually had a lower event rate by hospital discharge (5.6% vs 8.5%) and at 6 months (10.8% vs 21%) than those who had undergone revascularization procedures, respectively.

A trial currently underway will assess state-of-the-art interventional and noninvasive techniques for assessing risk and guiding therapeutics in patients with AMI.

TABLE 11.14 *TACTICS—Cardiac Event Rates at 30 Days and 6 Months*

	30 DAYS		30 DAYS–6 MONTHS	
Cardiac Event	Invasive Strategy (n = 1114)	Conservative Strategy (n = 1106)	Invasive Strategy (n = 1114)	Conservative Strategy (n = 1106)
Primary end point*	82 (7.4%)	116 (10.5%)†	95 (8.5%)	99 (8.9%)
Death or nonfatal MI	52 (4.7%)	77 (7.0%)‡	29 (2.6%)	28 (2.5%)
Death	25 (2.2%)	18 (1.6%)	12 (1.0%)	21 (1.9%)
Rehospitalization for ACS	38 (3.4%)	61 (5.5%)‡	85 (7.6%)	91 (8.2%)

*Death, nonfatal myocardial infarction (MI), readmission for acute coronary syndrome (ACS).
†p = .009
‡p = .02
Source: Adapted from Cannon CP, Weintraub WS, Demopoulos LA, et al for the TACTICS - Thrombolysis in Myocardial Infarction 18 Investigators: Comparison of early invasive and conservative strategies in patients with unstable coronary syndromes treated with the glycoprotein IIb/IIIa inhibitor tirofiban. N Engl J Med 2001;344:1879, with permission.

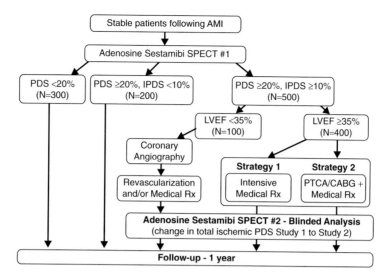

FIGURE 11.56 The adenosINe Sestamibi Post-InfaRction Evaluation (INSPIRE) trial study design. AMI, acute myocardial infarction; CABG, coronary artery bypass graft; IPDS, ischemic perfusion defect size; PDS, perfusion defect size; PTCA, percutaneous transluminal coronary angioplasty; SPECT, single-photon emission computed tomography.

The Adenosine Sestamibi Post-Infarction Evaluation (INSPIRE) trial is a prospective, multicenter, randomized study that will evaluate the role of nuclear cardiology in defining initial risk and subsequent patient outcome following anti-ischemic therapies (Fig. 11.56). This trial will enroll 1000 clinically stable patients with Q-wave and non-Q-wave AMI who will then undergo adenosine Tc-99m-sestamibi gated SPECT within the first several days of AMI. Therapeutic decision making will be based on the quantified size of the total LV PDS, the extent of residual ischemia, and LVEF. A core laboratory is currently set up to interpret all nuclear studies online so that sites can be notified of patient SPECT results the day of imaging. Patients with a small quantified PDS (< 20%) will be considered low risk and will be medically managed. Patients with a large (≥ 20%) and ischemic (≥ 10%) LV PDS will be considered at high risk for subsequent cardiac events. High-risk patients with an LVEF < 35% will undergo coronary angiography with the intent to revascularize whereas those with LVEF ≥ 35% will be randomized to either intensive medical therapy or coronary revascularization. Crossover to coronary angiography will be driven only by clinical indications. As in other trials, INSPIRE will use state-of-the-art interventional approaches. However, unlike other studies, the medical therapy regimen in this trial is intensive and prospectively defined. In the group with ischemia, SPECT will be repeated at 6 to 8 weeks to assess the effects of therapy on PDS and determine whether a reduction in scintigraphic ischemia predicts a low subsequent cardiac event rate. All patients will have

at least a 1 year follow-up. The results of INSPIRE should be ready in early 2003.

In conclusion, controversy continues as to the best approach for initially assessing risk in patients with acute coronary syndromes. Whether the use of glycoprotein IIb/IIIa inhibitors and coronary artery stenting were the reason for improved patient outcome in the invasive strategy of TACTICS, as compared to TIMI IIB and IIIB, or whether this was the inevitable result due to study design issues remains to be determined.

REFERENCES

1. Braunwald E, Mark DB, Jones RH, et al. Unstable angina: diagnosis and management. Rockville, MD: Agency for Health Care Policy and Research and the National Heart, Lung, and Blood Institute, US Public Health Service, US Department of Health and Human Services 1994;1: AHCPR Publication No 94-0602.
2. Detailed diagnoses, and procedures, National Hospital Discharge Survey. National Center for Health Statistics. Vital Health Stat 1998;1996:13:138.
3. Hamm CW, Braunwald E. A classification of unstable angina revised. Circulation 2000;102:118.
4. Rizik DG, Healy S, Margulis A, et al. A new clinical classification for hospital prognosis of unstable angina pectoris. Am J Cardiol 1995;75:993.
5. vanMiltenburg-vanZijl AJM, Simoons ML, Veerhoek RJ, et al. Incidence and follow-up of Braunwald subgroups in unstable angina pectoris. J Am Coll Cardiol 1995;25:1286.
6. Ohman EM, Armstrong PW, Christenson RH, et al. for the GUSTO-IIa Investigators. Cardiac troponin T levels for risk stratification in acute myocardial ischemia. N Engl J Med 1996; 335:1333.

7. Antman EM, Tanasijevic MJ, Thompson B, et al. Cardiac-specific troponin I levels to predict the risk of mortality in patients with acute coronary syndromes. N Engl J Med 1996;335:1342.

8. Braunwald E, Antman EM, Beasley JW, et al. ACC/AHA guidelines for the management of patients with unstable angina and non-ST segment elevation myocardial infarction: a report of the American College of Cardiology/American Heart Association Task Force on Practice Guidelines. (Committee on the Management of Patients with Unstable Angina). J Am Coll Cardiol 2000;36:970.

9. Lee KL, Woodlief LH, Topol EJ, for the GUSTO-I Investigators. Predictors of 30-day mortality in the era of reperfusion for acute myocardial infarction. Results from an international trial of 41,021 patients. Circulation 1995;91:1659.

10. Morrow DA, Antman EM, Charlesworth A, et al. TIMI risk score for ST-elevation myocardial infarction: a convenient, bedside, clinical score for risk assessment at presentation. An Intravenous nPA for Treatment of Infarcting Myocardium Early II trial substudy. Circulation 2000;102:2031.

11. Ryan TJ, Antman EM, Brooks NH, et al. ACC/AHA guidelines for the management of patients with acute myocardial infarction: 1999 update: a report of the American College of Cardiology/American Heart Association Task Force on Practice Guidelines (Committee on Management of Acute Myocardial Infarction). Available at http://www.acc.org.

12. Cerqueira MD, Maynard C, Ritchie JL, et al. Long-term survival in 618 patients from the Western Washington streptokinase in myocardial infarction trials. J Am Coll Cardiol 1992;20:1452.

13. Miller TD, Christian TF, Hopfenspirger MR, et al. Infarct size after acute myocardial infarction measured by quantitative tomography Tc-99m sestamibi imaging predicts subsequent mortality. Circulation 1995;92:334.

14. The Multicenter Postinfarction Research Group. Risk stratification and survival after myocardial infarction. N Engl J Med 1983;309:331.

15. Simoons ML, Vos J, Tijssen JG, et al. Long-term benefit of early thrombolytic therapy in patients with acute myocardial infarction: 5 year follow-up of a trial conducted by the Interuniversity Cardiology Institute of the Netherlands. J Am Coll Cardiol 1989;14:1609.

16. Sanz G, Castaner A, Betriu A, et al. Determinants of prognosis in survivors of myocardial infarction. A prospective clinical angiographic study. N Engl J Med 1987;306:1065.

17. White HD, Norris RM, Brown MA, et al. Left ventricular end-systolic volume as the major determinant of survival after recovery from myocardial infarction. Circulation 1987;76:44.

18. St. John Sutton M, Pfeffer MA, Plappert T, et al. for the SAVE investigators. Quantitative two-dimensional echocardiographic measurements are major predictors of adverse cardiovascular events after acute myocardial infarction. The protective effects of captopril. Circulation 1994;89:68.

19. Gibson RS, Beller GA, Gheorghiade M, et al. The prevalence and clinical significance of residual myocardial ischemia 2 weeks after uncomplicated non-Q wave infarction: a prospective natural history study. Circulation 1986;73:1186.

20. Gibson RS, Watson DD, Craddock GB, et al. Prediction of cardiac events after uncomplicated myocardial infarction: a prospective study comparing predischarge exercise thallium-201 scintigraphy and coronary angiography. Circulation 1983;68:321.

21. Mahmarian JJ, Mahmarian AC, Marks GF, et al. Role of adenosine thallium-201 tomography for defining long-term risk in patients after acute myocardial infarction. J Am Coll Cardiol 1994;25:1333.

22. Brown, KA, Heller GV, Landin RS, et al. Early dipyridamole 99mTc-sestamibi single photon emission computed tomographic imaging 2 to 4 days after acute myocardial infarction predicts in-hospital and postdischarge cardiac events: comparison with submaximal exercise imaging. Circulation 1999;100:2060.

23. Leppo JA, Meerdink DA. Comparison of the myocardial uptake of a technetium-labeled isonitrile analogue and thallium. Circ Res 1989;65:632.

24. Nishiyama H, Adolph RJ, Gabel M, et al. Effect of coronary blood flow on thallium-201 uptake and washout. Circulation 1982;65:534.

25. Okada RD, Glover D, Gaffney T, et al. Myocardial kinetics of technetium-99m-hexakis-2-methoxy-2-methylpropyl-isonitrile. Circulation 1988;77:491.

26. Granato JE, Watson DD, Flanagan TL, et al. Myocardial thallium-201 kinetics during coronary occlusion and reperfusion: influence of method of reflow and timing of thallium-201 administration. Circulation 1986;73:150.

27. DeCoster PM, Wijns W, Cauwe F, et al. Area-at-risk determination by technetium-99m-hexakis-2-methoxyisobutyl isonitrile in experimental reperfused myocardial infarction. Circulation 1990;82:2152.

28. Liu P, Houle S, Mills L, et al. Kinetics of Tc-99m MIBI in clearance in ischemia-reperfusion: comparison with Tl-201 (abstr). Circulation 1987;76(suppl IV):IV-216.

29. Sinusas AJ, Trautman KA, Bergin JD, et al. Quantification of area at risk during coronary occlusion and degree of myocardial salvage after reperfusion with technetium-99m methoxyisobutyl isonitrile. Circulation 1990;82:1424.

30. Verani MS, Jeroudi MO, Mahmarian JJ, et al. Quantification of myocardial infarction during coronary occlusion and myocardial salvage after reperfusion using cardiac imaging with technetium-99m hexakis 2-methoxyisobutyl isonitrile. J Am Coll Cardiol 1988;12:1573.

31. Christian TF, Behrenbeck T, Pellikka PA, et al. Mismatch of left ventricular function and infarct size demonstrated by technetium-99m isonitrile imaging after reperfusion therapy for acute myocardial infarction: identification of myocardial stunning and hyperkinesia. J Am Coll Cardiol 1990;16:1632.

32. Dakik HA, Mahmarian JJ, Kimball KT, et al. Prognostic value of exercise thallium-201 tomography in patients treated with thrombolytic therapy during acute myocardial infarction. Circulation 1996;94:2735.

33. Zaret BL, Wackers FJT, Terrin ML, et al. for the TIMI Study Group. Value of radionuclide rest and exercise left ventricular ejection fraction in assessing survival of patients after thrombolytic therapy for acute myocardial inarction: results of Thrombolysis in Myocardial Infarction (TIMI) Phase II Study. J Am Coll Cardiol 1995;26:73.

34. Volpi A, DeVita C, Franzosi MG, et al., the Ad hoc Working Group of the Gruppo Italiano per lo Studio della Sopravivenza nell'Infarto Miocardico (GISSI)-2 Data Base. Determinants of 6-month mortality in survivors of myocardial infarction after thrombolysis: results of the GISSI-2 Data Base. Circulation 1993;88:416.

35. The GUSTO Angiographic Investigators. The effects of tissue plasminogen activator, streptokinase, or both on coronary-artery patency, ventricular function, and survival after acute myocardial infarction. N Engl J Med 1993;329;1615.

36. Pfeffer MA, Braunwald E, Moye LA, et al. Effect of captopril on mortality and morbidity in patients with left ventricular dysfunction after myocardial infarction. Results of the Survival and Ventricular Enlargement Trial. N Engl J Med 1992;327:669.

37. Santoro GM, Bisi G, Sciagra R, et al. Single photon emission computed tomography with technetium-99m hexakis 2-methoxyisobutyl isonitrile in acute myocardial infarction before and after thrombolytic treatment: assessment of salvaged myocardium and prediction of late functional recovery. J Am Coll Cardiol 1990;15:301.

38. Seals AA, Pratt CM, Mahmarian JJ, et al. Relation of left ventricular dilation during acute myocardial infarction to systolic performance, diastolic dysfunction, infarct size and location. Am J Cardiol 1988;61:224.

39. Pfeffer MA, Lamas GA, Vaughan DE, et al. Effect of captopril on progressive left ventricular dilation after anterior myocardial infarction. N Engl J Med 1988;319:80.

40. Pfeffer MA, Braunwald E. Ventricular remodeling after myocardial infarction. Experimental observations and clinical implications. Circulation 1990;81:1161.

41. Erlebacher JA, Weiss JL, Weisfeldt ML, et al. Early dilation of the infarcted segment in acute transmural myocardial infarction: role of infarct expansion in acute left ventricular enlargement. J Am Coll Cardiol 1984;4:201.

42. Erlebacher JA, Weiss JL, Eaton LW, et al. Late effects of acute infarct dilation on heart size: a two-dimensional echocardiographic study. Am J Cardiol 1982;49:1120.

43. Mahmarian JJ, Moye LA, Chinoy DA, et al. Transdermal nitroglycerin patch therapy improves left ventricular function and prevents remodeling after acute myocardial infarction: results of a multicenter prospective randomized double-blind placebo controlled trial. Circulation 1998;97:2017.

44. Konstam MA, Rousseau MF, Kronenberg MW, et al. for the SOLVD Investigators: Effects of the angiotensin converting enzyme inhibitor enalapril on the long-term progression of left ventricular dysfunction in patients with heart failure. Circulation 1992;86:431.

45. Jugdutt BI, Warnica JW. Intravenous nitroglycerin therapy to limit myocardial infarct size, expansion and complications. Effect of timing, dosage and infarct location. Circulation 1988;78:906.

46. Jugdutt BI, Khan MI. Effect of prolonged nitrate therapy on left ventricular remodeling after canine acute myocardial infarction. Circulation 1994;89:2297.

47. Gill JB, Cairns JA, Roberts RS, et al. Prognostic importance of myocaridal ischemia detected by ambulatory monitoring early after acute myocardial infarction N Engl J Med 1996;334:65.

48. Theroux P, Waters DD, Halphen C, et al. Prognostic value of exercise testing soon after myocardial infarction. N Engl J Med 1979;301:341.

49. Applegate RJ, Dell'Italia LJ, Crawford MH. Usefulness of two-dimensional echocardiography during low-level exercise testing early after uncomplicated acute myocardial infarction. Am J Cardiol 1987;60:10.

50. Picano E, Landi P, Bolognese L, et al. Prognostic value of dipyridamole echocardiography early after uncomplicated myocardial infarction: a large-scale, multicenter trial. Am J Med 1993;95:608.

51. Candell-Riera J, Permanyer-Miralda G, Castell J, et al. Uncomplicated first myocardial infarction: strategy for comprehensive prognostic studies. J Am Coll Cardiol 1991;18:1207.

52. Corbett JR, Nicod P, Lewis SE, et al. Prognostic value of submaximal exercise radionuclide ventriculography after myocardial infarction. Am J Cardiol 1983;52:82A.

53. Gottlieb SO, Gottlieb SH, Achuff SC, et al. Silent ischemia on Holter monitoring predicts mortality in high-risk postinfarction patients. JAMA 1988;259:1030.

54. Hakki AH, Nestico PF, Heo J, et al. Relative prognostic value of rest thallium-201 imaging, radionuclide ventriculography and 24 hour ambulatory electrocardiographic monitoring after acute myocardial infarction. J Am Coll Cardiol 1987;10:25.

55. Langer A, Minkowitz J, Dorian P, et al. Pathophysiology and prognostic significance of Holter-detected ST segment depression after myocardial infarction. J Am Coll Cardiol 1992;20:1313.

56. Starling MR, Crawford MH, Kennedy GT, et al. Exercise testing early after myocardial infarction: predictive value of subsequent unstable angina and death. Am J Cardiol 1980;46:909.

57. Fioretti P, Brower RW, Simoons ML, et al. Prediction of mortality during the first year after acute myocardial infarction from clinical variables and stress test at hospital discharge. Am J Cardiol 1984;55:1313.

58. Weld FM, Chu K-L, Bigger JT, et al. Risk stratification with low-level exercise testing 2 weeks after acute myocardial infarction. Circulation 1981;64:306.

59. Williams WL, Nair RC, Higginson LA, et al. Comparison of clinical and treadmill variables for the prediction of outcome after myocardial infarction. J Am Coll Cardiol 1984;4:477.

60. Jelinek VM, McDonald IG, Ryan WF, et al. Assessment of cardiac risk 10 days after uncomplicated myocardial infarction. Br Med J 1982;284:227.

61. Jennings K, Reid DS, Hawkins T, et al. Role of exercise testing early after myocardial infarction in identifying candidates for coronary surgery. Br Med J 1984;288:185.

62. Handler CE. Submaximal predischarge exercise testing after myocardial infarction: prognostic value and limitations. Eur Heart J 1985;6:510.

63. Krone RJ, Gillespie JA, Weld FM, et al. Low-level exercise testing after myocardial infarction: usefulness in enhancing clinical risk stratification. Circulation 1985;71:80.

64. Borer JS, Rosing DR, Miller RH, et al. Natural history of left ventricular function during 1 year after acute myocardial infarction: comparison with clinical, electrocardiographic and biochemical determinations. Am J Cardiol 1980;46:10.

65. Chaitman BR, McMahon RP, Terrin M, et al. Impact of treatment strategy on predischarge exercise test in the Thrombolysis in Myocardial Infarction (TIMI) II Trial. Am J Cardiol 1993;71:131.

66. Gianrossie R, Detrano R, Mulvihill D, et al. Exercise induced ST depression in the diagnosis of coronary artery disease: a meta-analysis. Circulation 1989;80:87.

67. Heller GV, Ahmed I, Tilkemeier PL, et al. Influence of exercise intensity on the presence, distribution, and size of thallium-201 defects. Am Heart J 1992;123:909.

68. Gimple LW, Hutter AM, Guiney TE, et al. Prognostic utility of predischarge dipyridamole-thallium imaging after uncomplicated acute myocardial infarction. Am J Cardiol 1989;64:1243.

69. Wilson WW, Gibson RS, Nygaard TW, et al. Acute myocardial infarction associated with single vessel coronary artery disease. An analysis of clinical outcome and the prognostic importance of vessel patency and residual ischemic myocardium. J Am Coll Cardiol 1988;11:223.

70. Tilkemeier PL, Guiney TE, LaRaia PJ, et al. Prognostic value of predischarge low-level exercise thallium testing after thrombolytic treatment of acute myocardial infarction. Am J Cardiol 1990;66:1203.

71. Haber HL, Beller GA, Watson DD, et al. Exercise thallium-201 scintigraphy after thrombolytic therapy with or without angioplasty for acute myocardial infarction. Am J Cardiol 1993;71:1257.

72. Williams DO, Braunwald E, Knatterud G, et al. One-year results of the Thrombolysis in Myocardial Infarction Investigation (TIMI) Phase II trial. Circulation 1992;85:533.

73. Travin MI, Dessouki A, Cameron T, et al. Use of exercise technetium-99m sestamibi SPECT imaging to detect residual ischemia and for risk stratification after acute myocardial infarction. Am J Cardiol 1995;75:665.

74. Abraham RD, Harris PJ, Roubin GS, et al. Usefulness of ejection fraction response to exercise one month after acute myocardial infarction in predicting coronary anatomy and prognosis. Am J Cardiol 1987;60:225.

75. Corbett JR, Dehmer GJ, Lewis SE, et al. The prognostic value of submaximal exercise testing with radionuclide ventriculography before hospital discharge in patients with recent myocardial infarction. Circulation 1981;64:535.

76. Hung J, Goris ML, Nash E, et al. Comparative value of maximal treadmill testing, exercise thallium myocardial perfusion scintigraphy and exercise radionuclide ventriculography for distinguishing high- and low-risk patients soon after acute myocardial infarction. Am J Cardiol 1984;53:1221.

77. Nicod P, Corbett JR, Firth BG, et al. Prognostic value of resting and submaximal exercise radionuclide ventriculography after acute myocardial infarction in high-risk patients with single and multivessel disease. Am J Cardiol 1983;52:30.

78. Roig E, Magrina J, Armengol X, et al. Prognostic value of exercise radionuclide angiography in low-risk acute myocardial infarction survivors. Eur Heart J 1993;14:213.

79. Morris KG, Palmeri ST, Califf RM, et al. Value of radionuclide anigography for predicting specific cardiac events after acute myocardial infarction. Am J Cardiol 1985;55:318.

80. Brown KA, Weiss RM, Clements JP, et al. Usefulness of residual ischemic myocardium within prior infarct zone for identifying patients at high risk late after acute myocardial infarction. Am J Cardiol 1987;60:15.

81. Younis LT, Byers S, Shaw L, et al. Prognostic value of intravenous dipyridamole-thallium scintigraphy after acute myocardial ischemic events. Am J Cardiol 1989;64:161.

82. Leppo JA, O'Brien J, Rothendler JA, et al. Dipyridamole-thallium-201 scintigraphy in the prediction of future cardiac events after acute myocardial infarction. N Engl J Med 1984;310:1014.

83. Brown KA, O'Meara J, Chambers CE, et al. Ability of dipyridamole-thallium-201 imaging 1 to 4 days after acute myocardial infarction to predict in-hospital and late recurrent myocardial ischemic events. Am J Cardiol 1980;65:160.

84. Wilson RF, Wyche K, Christensen BV, et al. Effects of adenosine on human coronary arterial circulation. Circulation 1990;82:1595.

85. Rossen JD, Quillen JE, Lopez AG, et al. Comparison of coronary vasodilation with intravenous dipyridamole and adenosine. J Am Coll Cardiol 1991;18:485.

86. Heller GV, Brown KA, Landin RJ, et al., and the Early Post MI IV Dipyridamole Study (EPIDS): Safety of early intravenous dipyridamole technetium 99m sestamibi SPECT myocardial perfusion imaging after uncomplicated first myocardial infarction. Am Heart J 1997;134:105.

87. Mahmarian JJ, Pratt CM, Nishimura S, et al. Quantitative adenosine Tl-201 single-photon emission computed tomography for the early assessment of patients surviving acute myocardial infarction. Circulation 1993;87:1197.

88. Abreu A, Mahmarian JJ, Nishimura S, et al. Tolerance and safety of pharmacologic coronary vasodilation with adenosine in association with thallium-201 scintigraphy in patients with suspected coronary artery disease. J Am Coll Cardiol 1991;18:730.

89. Bosch X, Magrina J, March R, et al. Prediction of in-hospital cardiac events using dipyridamole-thallium scintigraphy performed very early after acute myocardial infarction. Clin Cardiol 1996;19:189.

90. Pirelli S, Inglese E, Suppa M, et al. Dipyridamole-thallium-201 in the early post-infarction period: safety and accuracy in predicting the extent of coronary disease and future recurrence of angina in patients suffering from their first myocardial infarction. Eur Heart J 1988;9:1324.

91. Mahmarian JJ. State of the art for coronary artery disease detection: Thallium-201. In: Nuclear Cardiology: State of the Art and Future Directions, 2nd Edition. edited by GA Beller and BL Zaret. St. Louis: Mosby, 1999, pp. 237.

92. Nishimura S, Mahmarian JJ, Boyce TM, et al. Equivalence between adenosine and exercise thallium-201 myocardial tomography: a multicenter, prospective, crossover trial. J Am Coll Cardiol 1992;20:265.

93. Dakik HA, Farmer JA, He Z-X, et al. Quantitative adenosine thallium-201 single photon tomography accurately predicts risk following acute myocardial infarction: the results of a prospective trial (abstr). J Am Coll Cardiol 1997;29 (Suppl A):228A.

94. Gibbons RJ, Holmes DR, Reeder GS, et al. Immediate angioplasty compared with the administration of a thrombolytic agent followed by conservative treatment for myocardial infarction. N Engl J Med 1993;328:685.

95. Gibbons RJ, Verani MS, Behrenbeck T, et al. Feasibility of tomographic 99mTc-hexakis-2-methoxy-2-methylpropyl-isonitrile imaging for the assessment of myocardial area at risk and the effect of treatment in acute myocardial infarction. Circulation 1989;80:1277.

96. Grines CL, Browne KF, Marco J, et al. A comparison of immediate angioplasty with thrombolytic therapy for acute myocardial infarction. N Engl J Med 1993;328:673.

97. Terrin ML, Williams DO, Kleiman NS, et al. Two- and three-year results of the Thrombolysis in Myocardial Infarction (TIMI) Phase II clinical trial. J Am Coll Cardiol 1993;22:1763.

98. Califf RM, White HD, VandeWerf F, et al. for the GUSTO-I Investigators. One-year results from the Global Utilization of Streptokinase and TPA for Occluded Coronary Arteries (GUSTO-I) Trial. Circulation 1996;94:1233.

99. Krone RJ, Gregory JJ, Freedland KE, et al. Limited usefulness of exercise testing and thallium scintigraphy in evaluation of ambulatory patients several months after recovery from an acute coronary event: implications for management of stable coronary heart disease. Multicenter Myocardial Ischemia Research Group. J Am Coll Cardiol 1994;24:1274.

100. Miller TD, Gersh BJ, Christian TF, et al. Limited prognostic value of thallium-201 exercise treadmill testing early after myocardial infarction in patients treated with thrombolysis. Am Heart J 1995;130:259.

101. Chiamvimonvat V, Goodman SG, Langer A, et al. Prognostic value of dipyridamole SPECT imaging in low-risk patients after myocardial infarction. J Nucl Cardiol 2001;8:136.

102. Ellis SG, Mooney MR, George BS, et al. Randomized trial of late elective angioplasty versus conservative management for patients with residual stenoses after thrombolytic treatment of myocardial infarction. Treatment of Post Thrombolytic Stenoses (TOPS) Study Group. Circulation 1992;86:1400.

103. The TIMI IIIB Investigators. Effects of tissue plasminogen activator and a comparison of early invasive and conservative strategies in unstable angina and non-Q-wave myocardial infarction. Results of the TIMI IIIB Trial. Circulation 1994;89:1545.

104. FRagmin and Fast Revascularisation during InStability in Coronary artery disease (FRISC II) Investigators. Invasive compared with non-invasive treatment in unstable coronary-artery disease: FRISC II prospective randomised multicentre study. Lancet 1999;354:708.

105. Boden WE, O'Rourke RA, Crawford MH, et al. Outcomes in patients with acute non-Q-wave myocardial infarction randomly assigned to an invasive as compared with a conservative management strategy. Veterans Affairs Non-Q-Wave Infarction Strategies in Hospital (VANQWISH) Trial Investigators. N Engl J Med 1998;338:1785.

106. Cannon CP, Weintraub WS, Demopoulos LA, et al. for the TACTICS - Thrombolysis in Myocardial Infarction 18 Investigators. Comparison of early invasive and conservative strategies in patients with unstable coronary syndromes treated with the glycoprotein IIb/IIIa inhibitor tirofiban. N Engl J Med 2001; 344:1879.

107. Tatum JL, Jesse RL, Kontos MC, et al. A comprehensive strategy for the evaluation and triage of the chest pain patient. Ann Emerg Med 1997;29:116.

108. Hilton TC, Thompson RC, Williams HJ, et al. Technetium-99m sestamibi myocardial perfusion imaging in the emergency room evaluation of chest pain. J Am Coll Cardiol 1994;23:1016.

109. Varetto T, Cantalupi D, Altieri A, et al. Emergency room technetium-99m sestamibi imaging to rule out acute myocardial ischemic events in patients with nondiagnostic electrocardiograms. J Am Coll Cardiol 1993;22:1804.

110. Bogaty P, Hackett D, Davies G, et al. Vasoreactivity of the culprit lesion in unstable angina. Circulation 1994;90:5.

111. vanderWal AC, Becker AE, vanderLoos CM, et al. Site of intimal rupture or erosion of thrombosed coronary atherosclerotic plaques is characterized by an inflammatory process irrespective of the dominant plaque morphology. Circulation 1994;89:36.

112. deFeyter PJ, Ozaki Y, Baptista J, et al. Ischemia-related lesion characteristics in patients with stable or unstable angina. A study with intracoronary angioscopy and ultrasound. Circulation 1995;92:1408.

113. Grambow DW, Topol EJ. Effect of maximal medical therapy on refractoriness of unstable angina pectoris. Am J Cardiol 1992;70:577.

114. Platelet Receptor Inhibition in Ischemic Syndrome Management in Patients Limited by Unstable Signs and Symptoms (PRISM-PLUS) Study Investigators. Inhibition of the platelet glycoprotein IIb/IIIa receptor with tirofiban in unstable angina and non-Q-wave myocardial infarction. (Erratum appears in N Engl J Med 1998;339:415.) N Engl J Med 1998;338;1488.

115. The PURSUIT Trial Investigators. Inhibition of platelet glycoprotein IIb/IIIa with eptifibatide in patients with acute coronary syndromes. The PURSUIT Trial Investigators. Platelet Glycoprotein IIb/IIIa in Unstable Angina: receptor suppression using integrilin therapy. N Engl J Med 1998;339:436.

116. Brown KA. Prognostic value of thallium-201 myocardial perfusion imaging in patients with unstable angina who respond to medical treatment. J Am Coll Cardiol 1991;17:1053.

117. Madsen JK, Stubgaard M, Utne HE, et al. Prognosis and thallium-201 scintigraphy in patients admitted with chest pain without confirmed acute myocardial infarction. Br Heart J 1988;59:184.

118. Miller DD, Stratmann HG, Shaw L, et al. Dipyridamole technetium 99m sestamibi myocardial tomography as an independent predictor of cardiac event-free survival after acute ischemic events. J Nucl Cardiol 1994;1:172.

119. Stratmann HG, Younis LT, Wittry MD, et al. Exercise technetium-99m myocardial tomography for the risk stratificaiton of men with medically treated unstable angina pectoris. Am J Cardiol 1995;76:236.

120. Stratmann HG, Tamesis BR, Younis LT, et al. Prognostic value

121. of predischarge dipyridamole technetium 99m sestamibi myocardial tomography in medically treated patients with unstable angina. Am Heart J 1995;130:734.

121. Anderson HV, Cannon CP, Stone PH, et al. for the TIMI IIIB Investigators. One-year results of the Thrombolysis in Myocardial Infarction (TIMI) IIIB clinical trial. A randomized comparison of tissue-type plasminogen activator versus placebo and early invasive versus early conservative strategies in unstable angina and non-Q wave myocardial infarction. J Am Coll Cardiol 1995;26:1643.

122. Mahmarian JJ, Moye LA, Verani MS, et al. High reproducibility of myocardial perfusion defects in patients undergoing serial exercise thallium-201 tomography. Am J Cardiol 1994;75:1116.

123. Dakik HA, Kleiman NS, Farmer JA, et al. Intensive medical therapy versus coronary angioplasty for suppression of myocardial ischemia in survivors of acute myocardial infarction. A prospective, randomized pilot study. Circulation 1998;98: 2017.

124. Iskander SS, Pratt, CM, Filipchuk NG, et al. for the INSPIRE investigators. Therapies for suppression of post-infarction myocardial ischemia. Preliminary results from the Adenosine Sestamibi Post-infarction Evaluation (INSPIRE) Trial (abstr). Circulation 2001. Volume 104, Suppl. II, II-455.

125. TIMI Study Group. Comparison of invasive and conservative strategies after treatment with intravenous tissue plasminogen activator in acute myocardial infarction: results of the Thrombolysis in Myocardial Infarction (TIMI) Phase II Trial. N Engl J Med 1989;320:618.

126. SWIFT (Should We Intervene Following Thrombolysis?) Trial Study Group. SWIFT trial of delayed elective intervention v conservative treatment after thrombolysis with anistreplase in acute myocardial infarction. BMJ 1991;302:555.

127. McCullough PA, O'Neill WW, Graham M, et al. A prospective randomized trial of triage angiography in acute coronary syndromes ineligible for thrombolytic therapy. Results of the Medicine Versus Angiography in Thrombolytic Exclusion (MATE) Trial. J Am Coll Cardiol 1998;32:596.

128. Rouleau JL, Moyé LA, Pfeffer MA, et al. for the SAVE Investigators. A comparison of management patterns after acute myocardial infarction in Canada and the United States. N Engl J Med 1993;328:779.

129. Mark DB, Naylor CD, Hlatky MA, et al. Use of medical resources and quality of life after acute myocardial infarction in Canada and the United States. N Engl J Med 1994;331:1130.

130. Piegas LS, Flather M, Pogue J, et al. for the OASIS Registry Investigators. The Organization to Assess Strategies for Ischemic Syndromes (OASIS) Registry in patients with unstable angina. Am J Cardiol 1999;84:7M.

131. Pilote L, Miller DP, Califf RM, et al. Determinants of the use of coronary angiography and revascularization after thrombolysis for acute myocardial infarction. N Engl J Med 1996; 335:1198.

132. Knatterud GL, Bourassa MG, Pepine CJ, et al. for the ACIP Investigators. Effects of treatment strategies to suppress ischemia in patients with coronary artery disease: 12-week results of the Asymptomatic Cardiac Ischemia Pilot (ACIP) study. J Am Coll Cardiol 1994;24:11.

133. Pratt CM, McMahon RP, Goldstein S, et al. for the ACIP Investigators. Comparison of subgroups assigned to medical regimens used to suppress cardiac ischemia (the Asymptomatic Cardiac Ischemia Pilot [ACIP] study). Am J Cardiol 1996;77: 1302.

Part 3

Risk Assessment before Noncardiac Surgery

JEFFREY LEPPO

The evaluation of preoperative cardiac risk inpatients undergoing noncardiac surgery has been a challenging and important topic over the past 25 years. The medical parameters and clinical factors first reported by Goldman et al. [25] have evolved into a more systematic approach and recently into American College of Cardiology/ American Heart Association guidelines [14]. Although prospective or randomized clinical trials are lacking for this clinical area, there are many retrospective reports and a few meta analyses that demonstrate the ability of nuclear cardiology testing in this field.

This chapter reviews the current preoperative guidelines as they deal with nuclear cardiology studies and the utility of such evaluation for both short-term (preoperative) and long-term follow-up. The focus is on coronary artery disease (CAD) as the main feature of preoperative cardiac assessment. In patients with CAD, the evaluations of ischemia and left ventricular (LV) function have been shown to have significant prognostic utility for cardiac events such as myocardial infraction (MI) or cardiac death [9]. Therefore, we focus on the detection of ischemia-induced perfusion defects and LV function, as determined by ejection fraction, LV cavity size, or other appropriate scintigraphic markers.

CLINICAL EVALUATION OF PREOPERATIVE CARDIAC RISK

Reports have shown that cardiac risk for noncardiac surgery can be determined by a careful history and physical examination, which often are summarized as clinical indexes [13,17,25]. Typical clinical parameters that have been shown to have useful prognostic importance in predicting perioperative events include a history of angina, congestive heart failure (CHF), myocardial infarction, and diabetes. If the symptomatic level of angina or failure is moderate to severe and the myocardial infarction is recent (less than 3 months), then most guidelines would suggest that the cardiac problem requires attention and resolution before the patient undergoes elective surgery. In contrast, the absence of these clinical parameters in an otherwise low-

risk surgical patient is often associated with a low cardiac event rate after elective surgery. As in most type of risk assessments, it is also important to consider the specific patient population that you are evaluating. In general, those patients having minor procedures and no cardiac symptoms or history have fewer events than those patients having vascular surgery or major procedures with a history of CAD.

SPECIFIC CLINICAL RISK ASSESSMENT

Although the clinical question that is often posed to the medical or cardiac consultant is whether or not to "clear" the patient for noncardiac surgery, the ACC/AHA guidelines [14] suggest an overall conservative approach to the use of expensive tests and interventions. There are specific algorithms that describe a clinical pathway for the medical consultant to use, but these should be viewed in the setting of a team approach involving the primary care physician, surgeon, anesthesiologist, and patient.

There is little that can be done for patients who must undergo emergency surgery other than attempting to manage acute medical problems in the perioperative period. However, after surgical recovery it may be helpful in long-term follow-up to complete an appropriate evaluation in those patients with significant or major cardiac problems. For instance, a patient with unstable angina or a nontransmural MI during emergency abdominal surgery should undergo routine diagnostic studies to assess cardiac function and residual ischemia before discharge.

The real challenge is in symptomatic or mildly symptomatic patients who are being evaluated for elective surgical procedures. It is best to begin by obtaining a detailed medical history, physical examination, and electrocardiogram (ECG). Particular attention should be paid to obtaining information about angina, MI, CHF, symptomatic arrhythmia, diabetes, peripheral vascular disease, and prior history of coronary angiography or revascularization procedures. Even in the presence of a known history of CAD, it is recommended to proceed with elective surgery if the patient has had

244

successful coronary revascularization within the previous 5 years [16] and is without recurrent signs or symptoms. It is also reasonable to proceed to surgery if the patient has had a recent coronary angiogram or stress test that reveals favorable results or a stable (low-risk) clinical situation. However, the presence of major cardiac symptoms, as noted above, should alert the consulting physician to reconsider a decision to allow the patient to undergo any elective procedure.

VASCULAR SURGERY

Although it is important to detect CAD and assess its severity in most routine preoperative evaluations [25], it is clearly a very prominent feature of elective vascular surgery. This is the result of the high prevalence (~60%) of CAD in many large series of vascular surgery patients [24] and has been well documented in a series of 1000 patients who routinely underwent coronary angiography before vascular surgery [32]. The incidence of nonfatal myocardial infarction (MI) or cardiac death in this population has been summarized in Table 11.15. It is clear that cardiac death was a relatively high risk in the earlier published literature but, in the early 1990s, the death rate fell to less than 2%. During the same time period, the rate of nonfatal MIs generally decreased but the incidence is still twofold to threefold higher than cardiac death. Although it appears that overall patient care (involving preselection

TABLE 11.16 *25 Year Trends in AAA Resections*

Year	(n)	70 years	AAA size (cm)	Oper Death (%)
1971–75	43	35%	7.7	7%
1976–80	84	41%	7.4	10%
1981–85	139	44%	6.5	5%
1986–90	149	55%	6.1	3%
1991–95	159	59%	6.0	5%
Total	574	50%	6.4	5.4%

AAA, abdominal aortic aneurysm; Oper, operative.
Source: Killen et al. [39].

and more intense perioperative management) has resulted in a lower death rate, prediction and prevention of infarctions is much more difficult. It would seem reasonable at this point to conclude that aggressive interventions to further lower the death rate will be difficult and will probably fail to be cost-effective because of the low incidence. However, the observation that nonfatal MI in the postoperative period is a powerful predictor of late cardiac events [36] suggests the need to combine preoperative screening plans with longer-term coronary management. This point is further supported by the data in Table 11.16. In this 25-year study at a single site, the operative death rate fell from 7%–10% over the first 10 years to 3%–5% over the last 10 years of the study. It is interesting to note that over this study period aortic rupture decreased from 14% to 9% and the prevalence of prior coronary bypass surgery (CABG) increased from 9% to 36%. Preoperative testing and appropriate revascularization were given credit for the reduction in mortality, despite the presence of older patients with more comorbidity.

Shaw et al. reviewed the utility of preoperative noninvasive testing in a large meta analysis [65]. These authors review studies from 1985 to 1994 in which either dipyridamole thallium ($n = 1994$) or dobutamine echocardiography ($n = 455$) was used as a pharmacologic stressor. Reversible perfusion defects were noted in 26% of patients, and nonfatal MI or cardiovascular death occurred in 9% of these postoperative cases. In contrast, 430 (22%) patients had normal perfusion scans and an event rate of 1.4%. Similar prognostic utility was noted in the dobutamine echocardiography studies. New wall motion abnormalities during dobutamine-induced stress were noted in 39% of the patients, and 11% of these cases had a major cardiac event. In the 270 (61%) patients without new regional wall motion abnormalities, the event rate was 0.4%. The authors of this meta analysis concluded that (*1*) reversible perfusion defects have significant positive predictive accuracy but the overall accuracy depends on the prevalence of CAD and clinical risk factors; (*2*) dobutamine-induced wall motion abnormalities predict

TABLE 11.15 *Perioperative Cardiac Events in Noncardiac Surgery*

Study	No. Patients	INCIDENCE	
		NFMI (%)	CV Death (%)
Young 1977 [74] 1958–68	75	12.5	8.0
1968–76	143	12.5	8.0
Hertzer 1980 [30] Aortic	343	n/a	6.1
Peripheral	273	n/a	3.3
Cutler 1987 [12]	116	7.8	0
Raby 1989 [59]	176	2.3	0.6
Eagle 1989 [15]	200	4.5	3.0
Younis 1990 [76]	111	3.6	3.6
Hendel 1992 [28]	327	6.7	2.1
Taylor 1991 [67]	491	3.5	0.8
Kresowik 1993 [41]	170	2.4	0.6
McFalls 1993 [56]	116	17.0	1.7
Baron 1994 [2]	457	4.8	2.2
Bry 1994 [8]	237	5.9	1.3
Seeger 1994 [63]	172 (no test	1.1	0.6
	146 (test)	3.4	0.7
Fleisher 1995 [20]	109	3.7	0.9

No, number; NFMI, nonfatal myocardial infarction; CV, cardiovascular.

adverse outcomes but the relatively small population size yields wider confidence limits; (3) the use of semi-quantitative image analysis for perfusion imaging should improve its prognostic utility; and (4) fixed defects predict long-term cardiac events with an accuracy equal to reversible defects for perioperative events.

In summary, this background review confirms that cardiac events are a significant risk during elective surgery. In certain high-risk surgery populations (vascular), CAD is quite common. It is also clear that the most common perioperative cardiac event is a nonfatal MI, which implies that the extent of ischemic burden would be a useful predictor of these types of outcomes. Therefore the addition of noninvasive testing in this population should be able to definitively quantify the degree of ischemia to enhance the clinical information. If LV function can also be evaluated, it will prove helpful in the long-term evaluation of cardiac risk as well.

WHEN TO OBTAIN PREOPERATIVE TESTING

The preoperative guidelines [14] are fairly straightforward about recommendations for patients about to undergo emergency surgery, the presence of prior cardiac revascularization, or the occurrence of major cardiac predictors. However, the majority of patients will fall into the large group of patients who have either intermediate or minor clinical predictors of increased perioperative cardiovascular risk. Table 11.17 presents a shortcut approach to a large number of patients in whom the decision to recommend testing prior to surgery can be difficult. Basically, if two of the three listed factors are true, then the guidelines suggest the use of noninvasive cardiac testing as part of the preoperative evaluation. In any patients with an intermediate clinical predictor, the presence of either a low functional capacity or high surgical risk should lead the consulting physician to perform noninvasive testing.

In the absence of intermediate clinical predictors, noninvasive testing should be performed when both the surgical risk is high and the functional capacity is low.

TABLE 11.17 *Shortcut to Noninvasive Testing in Preoperative Patients if Any Two Factors Are Present*

1. Intermediate clinical predictors are present (Canadian class 1 or 2 angina, prior MI based on history or athologic Q waves, compensated or prior CHF, or diabetes).
2. Poor functional capacity (< 4 METS) [21,35].
3. High surgical risk procedure (emergency major operations; aortic repair or peripheral vascular; prolonged surgical procedures with large fluid shifts and or blood loss).

METS, metabolic equivalents.

The guidelines define minor clinical predictors as advanced age, abnormal ECG, rhythm other than sinus, history of stroke, or uncontrolled systemic hypertension. These factors do not by themselves suggest the need for further testing, but when combined with low functional capacity and high-risk surgery, there is a recommendation for preoperative testing.

A summary of pharmacologic (dipyridamole or adenosine) myocardial perfusion imaging in more than 3000 patients is shown in Table 11.18. In the upper section, all studies involved vascular surgery and the incidence of thallium redistribution was 42%. The overall positive predictive accuracy is 12%, but its value has clearly decreased over the past decade (from the mid-1980s). In this vascular surgery population, the prevalence of CAD is 60% to 70%, and 38% (930/2417) of these patients have a normal stress perfusion scan. It is important to note that the average negative predictive accuracy is 99%, which implies that a normal stress perfusion study has powerful prognostic utility.

The importance of negative predictive accuracy is emphasized by the observation that two of these publications concluded that perfusion imaging was not accurate in detecting risk. In studies by Mangano et al. [51] and Baron et al. [2], event sensitivity and negative predictive accuracy were relatively low, which suggest that the application of myocardial perfusion imaging is not universally appropriate. In laboratories where the sensitivity for CAD is low and the cardiac event rate in patients with normal scans exceeds 2%, the prognostic utility for perfusion imaging will not be this good. There may also be a bias in patient selection for noninvasive testing, as well as whether the studies were prospective or retrospective. In addition, there are probably differences in imaging techniques and expertise.

In the lower section of Table 11.18, the population has been expanded to include patients who did not have vascular surgery. Most patients in this section were studied because there was an increased risk of CAD, and the overall event rate (7%) was the same as in the vascular surgery group. It is interesting to note that the incidence of thallium redistribution was somewhat lower but the positive predictive value was similar to that noted in the nonvascular surgery group

CLINICAL APPLICATION OF THE PREOPERATIVE GUIDELINES

Although there are no randomized studies that have initially tested the guidelines, there are some studies that demonstrate the clinical consequences of utilizing these guidelines in a practical way. Lee et al. [45] eval-

TABLE 11.18 *Pharmacologic Perfusion Imaging for Preoperative Assessment of Cardiac Risk*

Study	Thallium Redist (%)	Periop Events MI/Dead (%)	Ischemia + Pred(%)	Normal Scan − Pred (%)
Vascular surgery only				
Boucher 1985 [6]	33	6	19	100
Cutler 1987 [12]	47	10	20	100
Fletcher 1988 [22]	22	4	37	100
Sachs 1988 [61]	31	4	14	100
Eagle 1989 [15]	41	8	16	98
Younis 1990 [76]	36	7	15	100
Mangano 1991 [52]	37	5	5	95
Lette 1992 [48]	45	8	17	99
Hendel 1992 [28]	51	9	14	99
Kresowik 1993 [41]	39	3	4	98
Baron 1994 [2]	35	5	4	96
Bry 1994 [8]	46	7	11	100
Koutelou 1995 [40]	44	3	6	100
Marshall 1995 [53]	47	10	16	97
Total (weighted avg) 2417 Total pts	42	7	12	99
Other surgery				
Coley 1992 [10]	36	4	11	99
Shaw 1992 [64]	47	10	21	100
Brown 1993 [7]	33	5	13	99
Younis 1994 [75]	31	9	18	98
Stratman 1996 [66]	29	4	6	99
Van Damme 1997 [68]	34	2	n/a	n/a
Total (weighted avg) 923 Total patients	33	6	13	99

Redist, redistribution; Periop, perioperative; MI, myocardial infarction; +Pred, positive predictive accuracy; −Pred, negative predictive accuracy.

uated a total of 4315 patients undergoing elective noncardiac surgery. They reported a simple clinical index of six factors that could predict perioperative cardiac events: specifically, the presence of high-risk surgery, a history of CAD, CHF, or cerebrovascular disease as well as treatment with insulin, or a creatinemia of greater than 2.0 mg. In a validation population trial, the authors noted that when none or only one of these six factors was present (74% of all patients), the postoperative cardiac event rate was less than 1%. In contrast the event rate in patients with any two factors was 7% (18% of all patients), and in those patients with three or more factors (8% of all patients), the event rate was 11%.

In another study, Vanzetto et al. [69] conducted a prospective clinical trial of patients undergoing abdominal aortic surgery and identified a subgroup of high-risk CAD. This classification of high risk was based on the presence of two or more of the following predictors: age over 70 years; history of MI, angina, CHF, diabetes, hypertension with LV hypertrophy; or a resting ECG that shows Q waves or ST-segment ischemia. Of 457 patients, 32% (147) were classified as high risk and subsequently 134 (of the 147) patients underwent surgery after dipyridamole (SPECT) thal-

lium scans. The remaining 310 patients underwent elective aortic surgery without any further testing based on the presence of no more than a single high-risk parameter. On the basis of these clinical criteria alone, 9% of the high-risk patients had cardiac events. In contrast, there was a 4% event rate in patients with one risk factor and a rate of approximately 2% in patients without any CAD risk predictors. In this study the classification of high risk is equivalent to intermediate clinical predictors in the ACC/AHA preoperative guidelines [14]. The combination of aortic vascular surgery with these clinical risk factors should result in preoperative testing, and the observed event rate of 23% in patients with thallium redistribution confirms the prognostic utility of scintigraphy in this subgroup. It is also important to add that Vanzetto et al. [69] performed a multivariate analysis that showed that the number of ischemic segments was the single best predictor of perioperative events.

It is equally important to note that a normal perfusion scan in this clinical high-risk group is associated with a low event rate, which is equivalent to that observed in patients without any clinical risk predictors. Therefore the presence of a normal stress perfusion scan in high-risk vascular surgery patients appears to identify an otherwise undetected low-risk subgroup that is equivalent to a group with no clinical risk factors. In comparison with the observations of Lee et al. [45], this report emphasizes the higher inherent cardiac risk when the evaluations involve only vascular surgery patients.

In another preoperative cardiac risk study, Bartels et al. [3] evaluated a strategy that emulated the ACC/AHA recommendations. Clinical risk classifications were assigned to 201 patients who were to undergo major vascular surgery. Approximately 10% of the patients were defined as high risk based on the presence of an MI within the prior 6 months, decompensated CHF, Canadian class 3–4 angina, significant arrhythmias, or severe valvular disease. This is consistent with major clinical CAD risk predictors in the guidelines [14]. In 40% of the patients, an intermediate cardiac risk was assigned based on the presence of a remote MI, compensated CHF, Canadian class 1–2 angina, diabetes (insulin-dependent), or elevated serum creatine level. In the remaining half of the patients, none of these factors were present and they were defined as low risk. All the low-risk patients and the intermediate-risk patients (52%) with a functional capacity of > 5 metabolic equivalents based on a questionnaire (Duke Activity Status Index) [35] proceeded directly to major aortic surgery without further testing. The remaining intermediate-risk patients (48%) who had a functional capacity of < 5 metabolic equivalents on the questionnaire underwent noninvasive testing (40%) or intensified medical care (60%) before surgery. In the high-risk group, approximately one-half underwent noninvasive testing and the other half received intensified medical treatment. Subsequently 5 (6%) intermediate-risk and 2 (9%) high-risk patients underwent preoperative coronary angiography, resulting in one coronary bypass procedure and two cancellations of further elective surgery.

Cardiac events occurred in 5% of the high-risk group and in 9% of the intermediate-risk group patients. The low-risk group had an event rate of 2%. In addition, intensified medical treatment or additional testing and intervention in the high-risk patients can also be appropriately guided by test results. Furthermore, this report confirms the value of testing to evaluate intermediate-risk patients. Overall, this study does support the clinical algorithm suggested by the published guidelines, but there were some protocol alterations that resulted in poor outcomes. Further studies are needed to determine whether preoperative patients at higher risk can be appropriately treated and have a lower event rate during their perioperative period.

These two imaging articles [3,69] support the use of selective testing of vascular surgery patients according to a clinical algorithm that is similar to the ACC/AHA

guidelines. These data [3,69] also suggest that increased risk is associated with larger segmental perfusion abnormalities. However, some other articles [5,58] have stressed that the use of beta-blockers alone is sufficient to adequately manage most preoperative patients. In these reports [5,58], the results of the DECREASE trial show that intermediate-risk (based on the extent of dobutamine-induced segmental wall motion abnormalities) vascular surgery patients have a significantly lower event rate if treated with bisoprolol prior to surgery. These articles are limited by a retrospective methodology and high prevalence of prior MIs as well as a relatively high postoperative cardiac death rate. In addition, other reports by Wallace et al. [70] and Mangano et al. [50], using prospective, random, and blinded methodology, show that beta-blockers do not decrease perioperative cardiac events. At present, it would still seem reasonable to follow the current ACC/AHA guidelines for perioperative risk assessment, and as we see below, there is additional utility for preoperative testing in long-term follow-up of these patients.

SPECIAL SUBGROUPS AND GENDER CONSIDERATIONS

The question of routine screening for all patients undergoing renal or liver transplants is more an issue of long-term follow-up and cardiac prognosis. There is little immediate risk to performing the transplant surgery, but it is clear that cardiac morbidity and mortality can have a significant impact during the postoperative follow-up period. This seems to be especially true for patients with diabetes [71] and can result in routine noninvasive or coronary angiogram testing in many patients before transplantation. Heston et al. [34] has shown that an "expert system" using clinical risk predictors and thallium stress testing can achieve an overall accuracy of 89% in predicting 4-year cardiac mortality among 189 renal transplant candidates. This observation is supported by prior publications [37,44] and suggests that no further cardiac evaluation is needed if there are no clinical risk predictors such as a history of CHF, angina, insulin-dependent diabetes, age over 50 years, or an abnormal ECG (excluding LV hypertrophy).

In patients being evaluated for cardiac problems prior to liver transplantation, there has been little published experience. There is a long-term cardiac risk, but a recent study from Kryzhanovski and Beller [42] suggests that this risk is too low to warrant routine stress myocardial perfusion imaging or radionuclide angiogram in all patients. There were no cardiac events in 63 liver transplant procedures and only one patient had a high-risk scan. Therefore cardiac evaluations should be used in this patient subgroup only when there is clear evidence for CAD or significant (intermediate) clinical risk predictors are present.

The effect of gender differences was reviewed by Hendel et al. [26]. It is clear from this study of 567 vascular surgery patients that overall cardiac events in both the perioperative and the long-term follow-up period were similar for men and women. However, significant differences in various clinical factors for the prediction of cardiac events were noted. Multivariate analysis of clinical and scintigraphic factors for perioperative MI or cardiac death showed that Q waves, a history of CHF, thallium redistribution, and ST-segment depression during parenteral dipyridamole administration were the best predictors in men. In contrast, only thallium redistribution was a significant predictor in women, and the presence of angina (not significant in men) was also of value.

These observations on gender differences suggest that overall clinical risk assessment might be improved by application of different specific predictors for each subpopulation. For instance, ST depression is a very powerful predictor of perioperative events in male patients but lacks such an impact in a female population. In contrast, perfusion imaging has a significant prognostic ability for both male and female patients and may well explain why this factor is the best overall predictor in the entire population. This report by Hendel et al. [26] also evaluated long-term (4–5 year) follow-up in this population and again noted gender differences in clinical but not scintigraphic predictors of cardiac events. Overall, this study suggests that scintigraphic findings are effective in both male and female populations but clinical factors need to be specific to gender differences. In addition, scintigraphic findings that correlate with ischemia (transient defects) are more powerful predictors of perioperative events, whereas late events are best predicted by the extent of injured myocardium or scar (fixed defects). This is discussed in greater detail in the following section on long-term follow-up of elective surgery patient consultations.

PREOPERATIVE EVALUATIONS AND CORONARY ANGIOGRAPHY

The presence of a positive test should not be used simply as a justification to proceed with cardiac catheterization and revascularization. There are no controlled studies or randomized data to properly evaluate the utility of coronary angiography. In addition, the precise role of coronary bypass surgery or angioplasty in patients undergoing coronary angiography is not yet determined and consequently is unclear. However, there are some recommendations that have been made in the ACC/AHA guidelines [14] In patients with known or suspected CAD, there are class I (strongly supported) indications for coronary angiography when there is (1) evidence for high risk or adverse outcomes based on noninvasive test results; (2) angina that is unresponsive to medical therapy; (3) unstable angina in situations where there is intermediate- or high-risk noncardiac surgery; and (4) nondiagnostic noninvasive test results in those patients with high clinical risk who are undergoing high-risk surgery.

There are class II (moderately supported) indications for coronary angiography when there are (1) multiple intermediate clinical risk parameters and planned vascular surgery even though noninvasive testing should be the first consideration; (2) moderate-to-large ischemic areas on noninvasive testing but without high-risk findings or reduced LVEF; (3) nondiagnostic noninvasive test results in intermediate clinical risk patients who are undergoing high-risk noncardiac surgery; (4) urgent noncardiac surgery in patients recovering from an acute MI; (5) patients having a perioperative MI; and (6) patients who are medically stable with class II or IV angina who are having low-risk or minor surgery.

These guidelines also suggest that there is no indication (class III) for coronary angiography in patients (1) with low-risk noncardiac surgery who have a known history of CAD and demonstrate no high-risk noninvasive test results; (2) with no symptoms after coronary revascularization with excellent exercise capacity (greater than or equal to 7 METs); (3) with mild stable angina who have good left ventricular function and demonstrate no high-risk noninvasive test results; (4) with concomitant medical illness that precludes coronary revascularization or those who refuse to consider such therapy; and (5) who are candidates for liver, lung, or renal transplant who are less than 40 years old as part of an evaluation for transplant, unless noninvasive testing reveals high risk for adverse outcomes.

LATE FOLLOW-UP AFTER NONCARDIAC SURGERY

Background

Once a preoperative consultation for cardiac risk is completed, it is important to consider how any of the clinical or testing data collected for surgical evaluation can be of further use. In fact, it may be even more important to evaluate the long-term risk assessment in

TABLE 11.19 *Cardiac Event Rate in Long-Term Postoperative Follow-Up*

Study	Avg FU Years	No. Patients	NFMI (%)	CV Death (%)
Hertzer 1980 [29]	6–7	286	n/a	22.0
Hertzer 1981 [30]	7–8	256	n/a	22.0
Roger 1989 [60]	8	75 no CAD	12.0	12.0
		47 CAD	28.0	38.0
Hertzer 1987 [33]	4.6	228	n/a	6.1
Younis 1990 [76]	1.5	127	—12%—	
Lette 1992 [49]	1.3	355	5.4	6.8
Mangano 1992 [50]	2	444	2.5	5.4
Seeger 1994 [63]	2.8	171 (no test)	n/a	1.2
		144 (test)	n/a	3.6
Hendel 1995 [26]	4.2	556	5.0	7.7
Fleisher 1995 [20]	1.4	108	6.5	3.7
Poldermans 1997 [58]	1.6	316	3.5	3.5

Avg FU, average follow-up; No. Pts, number patients in each study; NFMI, nonfatal myocardial infractions; CV death, cardiac death; CAD, coronary artery disease.

contrast to the short-term preoperative consultation. This is especially pertinent to the vascular surgery population, since many longitudinal studies have been published and the future risk of cardiac mortality and morbidity is well recognized.

Table 11.19 summarizes late cardiac events that occurred in a population dominated by vascular surgery procedures. It appears that cardiac mortality during long-term follow-up has been decreasing over the past decade, which was also noted previously for postoperative events (see Table 11.15). The impact of better patient selection and perioperative care for those who undergo vascular surgery has been a likely factor in reducing mortality in these large patient studies. However, despite the trend for reduced event rates over time, it is still observed that subgroups with known CAD have a worse prognosis.

In a review of the vascular surgery literature from 1975 to 1987, Hertzer [31] noted that late mortality in patients with aortic aneurysms was 44% in those with probable CAD but was only 22% in those without CAD. This review also noted a large increase in mortality among patients having infrainguinal or carotid surgery based on the presence of symptomatic CAD. L'Italien et al. [43] completed a dual-center comparison of perioperative and long-term follow-up (5 years) based in part on the type of vascular surgery (aortic, infrainguinal, or carotid) performed. These authors noted that patients undergoing infrainguinal or carotid surgery had significantly lower cumulative survival and more perioperative events compared with aortic surgery patients. However, in patients without any CAD risk factors, survival was above 95% in all three surgical groups and perioperative events occurred in less than 1%. When the surgical groups were adjusted for comorbid factors, the differences in cardiac event rates were significantly reduced. These authors concluded that cardiac and diabetic status were critical predictors for long- and short-term cardiac events. Specifically, a history of angina or CHF, diabetes, fixed dipyridamole thallium defects, and perioperative MI were identified as the best predictors of long-term events. Therefore the type of vascular surgery performed may not be as important as the extent of cardiac risk factors as determined by clinical and stress scintigraphic factors.

Clinical Challenges in Long-Term Follow-up

There is evidence that both the data that are collected and the process of evaluation and subsequent work-up or intervention (medical or surgical) have resulted in better outcomes and predictions. A review of a national Medicare population sample identified a cohort of patients ($n = 6895$) who underwent elective vascular surgery during a 17-month period in 1991 and 1992. The authors noted a relatively high mortality (14%) at 1 year of follow-up. However, in those patients undergoing preoperative stress testing with or without coronary bypass surgery, the mortality rate was lower ($< 6\%$) [19]. In another follow-up study of peripheral vascular surgery patients ($n = 343$) for a mean of 40 months, cardiac events were significantly more frequent in those who had an LVEF of $< 35\%$ or ischemia on dipyridamole-thallium imaging [62]. Other studies [46,18,54] also confirm the value of semiquantitative analysis of myocardial perfusion imaging when using these type of preoperative tests to predict future cardiac events. All these studies have the ability to combine an assessment of myocardial ischemia and left ventricular function into a more useful clinical index.

UTILIZING PREOPERATIVE TESTING FOR LONG-TERM PROGNOSIS

In the evaluation of cardiac risk for elective surgery, it is clear that clinical CAD risk factors, noninvasive cardiac imaging, and coronary angiography can all provide useful information in the appropriate patient subgroup. As noted previously, both assessment of LV function and the extent of myocardial ischemia are critical factors in the determination of risk. This is especially pertinent when intermediate or major clinical predictors are present. However, it is also clear that cardiac events are a greater problem in the long-term (3–5 years) medical management of these patients and merit attention.

Therefore we should evaluate which (if any) of the clinical and noninvasive testing parameters could possibly be used to better predict long-term follow-up. If predictive information about perioperative, as well as long-term risk can be combined, it could be more cost-effective and timely to provide all this information to the referring physician before the elective surgery decision is finalized. As previously noted, a large meta analysis [65] on preoperative testing (echocardiography and scintigraphy) has shown that indexes of ischemia (transient perfusion defects and new wall motion abnormalities) are strongly associated with perioperative cardiac risk. Both echocardiographic and scintigraphic techniques can determine whether ischemia and infarction (reduced LV function) are present. Although

myocardial perfusion imaging has previously utilized indirect measurements of LV function (increased LV size [18,47,48] and extent of fixed defects [28,65]), it is now fairly routine to obtain left ventricular ejection fraction (LVEF) calculations from gated cardiac studies using technetium-based perfusion agents [23]. As we will demonstrate, the combination of LV function and ischemia evaluation can provide important prognostic information about short- and long-term outcomes in preoperative patients.

Figures 11.57–11.60 show the prediction of long-term survival after aortic vascular surgery in different patient studies using various clinical parameters that have demonstrated significant preoperative prognostic utility. In Figure 11.57, the clinical risk index (as per Goldman et al. [25]) can be divided into low-, intermediate-, and high-risk groups and there is a significant survival difference between low- and high-risk patients. As expected, the mortality is elevated in the high-risk group but the low-risk patients have 22% mortality over 5 years. This is the same group of patients who are often sent directly to elective surgery without cardiac testing and typically have low (2%) event rates. However, the guidelines (and shortcut) recommend obtaining a functional capacity measurement in low-risk patients if there is high-risk surgery. It is possible that further risk stratification of this group might have helped to detect those low clinical risk patients who could have benefited from further cardiac testing. It is evident that intermediate-risk patients also

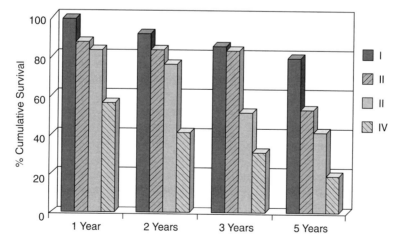

FIGURE 11.57 Summary data from White et al. [73] that shows the cumulative survival (1–5 years) after aortic surgery in patients based on their clinical risk as classified by the Goldman Index (I = lowest and IV = highest risk).

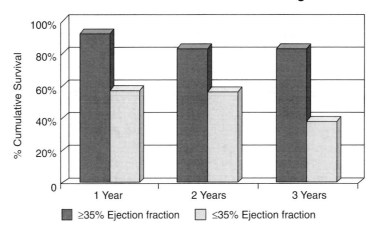

FIGURE 11.58 Summary data from Kazmers et al. [38] that shows the cumulative survival (1–3 years) after aortic surgery in patients based on a left ventricular ejection fraction of greater or less than 35%.

have a fairly high (> 50%) mortality over the 5-year follow-up period and may warrant further investigation. It is interesting to note that Hendel and Leppo [27] showed that scintigraphic findings could provide more prognostic information in the follow-up of vascular surgery patients compared with clinical indexes [15,17] alone.

This is not to suggest that all patients should be tested by cardiac stress imaging; but if the overall guidelines are followed, the resulting information can be used for more surgical patients (especially vascular surgery patients), and it is important for the medical consultant to carefully consider the long-term consequences and risk as well as the immediate ones. Our group has also looked at the short- and long-term impact of coronary angiogram referral based on positive test results [53]. Our data suggest that more invasive cardiac intervention does not result in improved short- or long-term follow-up in vascular surgery patients. Therefore it seems appropriate to continue to recommend that in-

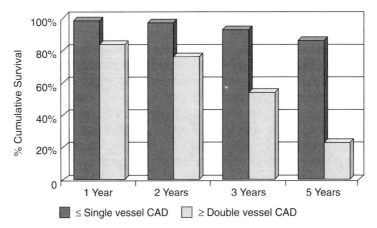

FIGURE 11.59 Summary data from Hertzer et al. [31] that shows the cumulative survival (1–5 years) after aortic surgery in patients based on the presence of multivessel CAD as compared to single-vessel or no CAD.

Prediction of Long-Term Survival
Following Aortic Reconstruction
Based on Dipyridamole Thallium Scan

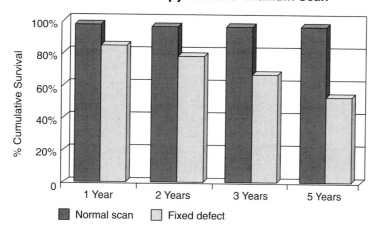

FIGURE 11.60 Summary data from Cutler et al. [11] that shows the cumulative survival (1–5 years) after aortic surgery in patients based on the presence of a normal dipyridamole-thallium scan as compared to a fixed defect on the scan.

vasive interventions after preoperative clinical or testing evaluation should be based on the ACC/AHA practice guidelines [56]. Specifically, patients with increased clinical or stress-testing risk do not need to be routinely sent for interventions just because elective surgery is contemplated.

LVEF is another powerful predictor of survival in patients with CAD. In Figure 11.58, Kazmers et al. [38] noted that at a cut point of 35%, the 3-year survival was significantly better in those with an LVEF of greater than 35%. This is not surprising, but over the same time period, mortality in those patients with preserved LVEF was approximately 6% per year. Therefore the observation of having an LVEF of > 35% does not necessarily imply an excellent event-free survival. In these types of analyses, it is important not only to detect the patients at highest risk for mortality but also to identify the subgroup with very low (< 2%/year) risk.

The long-term prognostic power of multivessel CAD has been demonstrated by Hertzer et al. [31]. In Figure 11.59, a summary of data collected after vascular surgery is shown. These investigators noted that patients with two- or three-vessel CAD had a 5-year event-free survival of only 22%. In contrast, those patients with only single-vessel CAD or normal coronary angiograms had a survival of 85%. This results in a fairly low-risk group with a 3% per year cardiac event rate, but coronary angiography is rarely a routine perioperative screening methodology.

In Figure 11.60, a long-term follow-up study by Cutler et al. [11] is presented. The authors reported a very low event rate in vascular patients who had a normal stress perfusion scan (< 1%/year). Patients in the higher-risk group were noted to have fixed perfusion defects. In a subsequent study, Emlein et al. [18] reported that the extent of LV cavity dilation was the most important factor in predicting cardiac death among patients with abnormal scans. These studies clearly show that patients with a normal scan have a very low risk of long-term follow-up events, and we have already shown (Table 11.19) that this observation

TABLE 11.20 *Proposed Prognostic Gradient of Abnormal Results from Stress (Pharmacologic or Exercise) Perfusion Imaging*

In all patients even those with suspected or proven CAD:
Very low risk
  Normal stress perfusion study
Low risk
  Stress-induced or fixed perfusion defects of small size
Intermediate risk
  Stress-induced or fixed perfusion defects of moderate size
  Stress-induced perfusion defects of small to moderate size with LVEF < 35%
High risk
  Stress-induced perfusion defects (ischemia) of greater than moderate size
Fixed perfusion defects (scar) of greater than moderate size with LVEF < 35%
Moderate size stress-induced perfusion defects in any patients with diabetes or LVEF < 35%

Source: Based in part on summary recommendations from International Nuclear Cardiology Retreat [4].

(normal scan) has a high negative predictive value in the preoperative evaluation period. Therefore pharmacologic stress myocardial perfusion imaging can be used to assess appropriate patient populations for both perioperative and long-term events by use of slightly different predictors. The extent of transient defects affects the short-term events, which typically involve nonfatal MI, whereas large cavity size and fixed defects predict long-term events, which usually involve cardiac death. Perhaps the current use of gated perfusion imaging will provide a valuable objective parameter (LVEF) for evaluating long-term cardiac risk. It is likely that a technique that can quantitate (as proposed in Table 11.20) the extent of ischemia as well as determine the LVEF should prove to be a most reliable method to evaluate short- and long-term prognosis in patients being considered for elective surgery.

REFERENCES

1. Heitzman RJ, Hibbitt KG. Effects of starvation on intermediary metabolism in the lactating cow. Biochem J 1972; 128:1311.
2. Baron J-F, Mundler O, Bertrand M, et al. Dipyridamole-thallium scintigraphy and gated radionuclide angiography to assess cardiac risk before abdominal aortic surgery. N Engl J Med 1994; 330:663.
3. Bartels C, Bechtel JFM, Hossmann V, et al. Cardiac risk stratification for high-risk vascular surgery. Circulation 1997; 95:2473.
4. Beller GA, Brown KA, Hendel RC, et al. Unresolved issues in risk stratification: chronic coronary artery disease including preoperative testing. J Nucl Cardiol 1997; 4:92.
5. Boersma E, Poldermans D, Bax JJ, et al. Predictors of cardiac events after major vascular surgery: role of clinical characteristics, dobutamine echocardiography, and beta-blocker therapy. JAMA 2001; 285:1865.
6. Boucher CA, Brewster DC, Darling C, et al. Determination of cardiac risk by dipyridamole-thallium imaging before peripheral vascular surgery. N Engl J Med 1985; 312:389.
7. Brown KA, Rowen M. Extent of jeopardized viable myocardium determined by myocardial perfusion imaging best predicts perioperative cardiac events in patients undergoing noncardiac surgery. J Am Coll Cardiol 1993; 21:325.
8. Bry JDL, Belkin M, O'Donnell TFJr, et al. An assessment of the positive predictive value and cost-effectiveness of dipyridamole myocardial scintigraphy in patients undergoing vascular surgery. J Vasc Surg 1994; 19:112.
9. Califf RM, Armstrong PW, Carver JR, et al. Task force 5: stratification of patients into high, medium and low risk subgroups for purposes of risk factor management. J Am Coll Cardiol 1996; 27:1007.
10. Coley CM, Field TS, Abraham SA, et al. Usefulness of dipyridamole-thallium scanning for preoperative evaluation of cardiac risk for nonvascular surgery. Am J Cardiol 1992; 69:1280.
11. Cutler BS, Hendel RC, Leppo JA. Dipyridamole-thallium scintigraphy predicts perioperative and long-term survival after major vascular surgery. J Vasc Surg 1992; 15:972.
12. Cutler BS, Leppo JA. Dipyridamole thallium 201 scintigraphy to detect coronary artery disease before abdominal aortic surgery. J Vasc Surg 1987; 5:91.

13. Detsky AS, Abrams HB, Forbath N, et al. Cardiac assessment for patients undergoing noncardiac surgery: a multifactorial clinical risk index. Arch Intern Med 1986; 146:2131.
14. Eagle KA, Berger PB, Calkins H, et al. ACC/AHA Guideline update for perioperative cardiovascular evaluation for noncardiac surgery-executive summary: A report of the American College of Cardiology/American Heart Association Task Force on Practice Guidelines (Committee to update the 1996 Guidelines on Perioperative Cardiovascular Evaluation for Noncardiac Surgery). JACC 2002;39:542.
15. Eagle KA, Coley CM, Newell JB, et al. Combining clinical and thallium data optimizes preoperative assessment of cardiac risk before major vascular surgery. Ann Intern Med 1989; 110:859.
16. Eagle KA, Rihal CS, Mickel MC, et al. Cardiac risk of noncardiac surgery: influence of coronary disease and type of surgery in 3368 operations. Circulation 1997; 96:1882.
17. Eagle KA, Singer DE, Brewster DC, et al. Dipyridamole-thallium scanning in patients undergoing vascular surgery: optimizing preoperative evaluation of cardiac risk. JAMA 1987; 257:2185.
18. Emlein G, Villegas B, Dahlberg S, et al. Left ventricular cavity size determined by preoperative dipyridamole thallium scintigraphy as a predictor of late cardiac events in vascular surgery patients. Am Heart J 1996; 131:907.
19. Fleisher LA, Eagle KA, Shaffer T, et al. Perioperative- and long-term mortality rates after major vascular surgery: the relationship to preoperative testing in the medicare population. Anesth Analg 1999; 89:849.
20. Fleisher LA, Rosenbaum SH, Nelson AH, et al. Preoperative dipyridamole thallium imaging and ambulatory electrocardiographic monitoring as a predictor of perioperative cardiac events and long term outcome. Anesthesiology 1995; 83:906.
21. Fletcher GF, Balady G, Froelicher VF, et al. Exercise standards: a statement for healthcare professionals from the American Heart Association. Circulation 1995; 91:580.
22. Fletcher JP, Antico VF, Gruenewald S, et al. Dipyridamole-thallium scan for screening of coronary artery disease prior to vascular surgery. J Cardiovasc Surg 1988; 29:666.
23. Garcia EV, Bacharach SL, Mahmarian JJ, et al. Imaging guidelines for nuclear cardiology procedures. Part 1. J Nucl Cardiol 1996; 3:G1.
24. Gersh BJ, Rihal CS, Rooke TW, et al. Evaluation and management of patients with both peripheral vascular and coronary artery disease. J Am Coll Cardiol 1991; 18:203.
25. Goldman L, Caldera DL, Nussbaum SR, et al. Multifactorial index of cardiac risk in noncardiac surgical procedures. N Engl J Med 1977; 297:845.
26. Hendel RC, Chen MH, L'Italien GJ, et al. Sex differences in perioperative and long-term cardiac event-free survival in vascular surgery patients: an analysis of clinical and scintigraphic variables. Circulation 1995; 91:1044.
27. Hendel RC, Leppo JA. The value of perioperative clinical indexes and dipyridamole thallium scintigraphy for the prediction of myocardial infarction and cardiac death in patients undergoing vascular surgery. J Nucl Cardiol 1995; 2:18.
28. Hendel RC, Whitfield SS, Villegas BJ, et al. Prediction of late cardiac events by dipyridamole thallium imaging in patients undergoing elective vascular surgery. Am J Cardiol 1992; 70:1243.
29. Hertzer NR. Fatal myocardial infarction following abdominal aortic aneurysm resection: three hundred forty-three patients followed 6–11 years postoperatively. Ann Surg 1980; 192:667.
30. Hertzer NR. Fatal myocardial infarction following lower extremity revascularization: two hundred seventy-three patients followed six to eleven postoperative years. Ann Surg 1981; 193:492.

31. Hertzer NR. Basic data concerning associated coronary artery disease in peripheral vascular patients. Ann Vasc Surg 1987; 1: 616.

32. Hertzer NR, Beven EG, Young JR, et al. Coronary artery disease in peripheral vascular patients: a classification of 1000 coronary angiograms and results of surgical management. Ann Surg 1984; 199:223.

33. Hertzer NR, Young JR, Beven EG, et al. Late results of coronary bypass in patients with infrarenal aortic aneurysms: the Cleveland Clinic study. Ann Surg 1987; 205:360.

34. Heston TF, Norman DJ, Barry JM, et al. Cardiac risk stratification in renal transplantation using a form of artificial intelligence. Am J Cardiol 1997; 79:415.

35. Hlatky MA, Boineau RE, Higginbotham MB, et al. A brief self-administered questionnaire to determine functional capacity (the Duke Activity Status Index). Am J Cardiol 1989; 64:651.

36. Hollenberg M, Mangano DT, Browner WS, et al. Predictors of postoperative myocardial ischemia in patients undergoing noncardiac surgery. JAMA 1992; 268:205.

37. Iqbal A, Gibbons RJ, McGoon MD, et al. Noninvasive assessment of cardiac risk in insulin-dependent diabetic patient being evaluated for pancreatic transplantation using thallium-201 myocardial perfusion scintigraphy. Transplant Proc 1991; 23:1690.

38. Kazmers A, Cerqueira MD, Zierler RE. Perioperative and late outcome in patients with left ventricular ejection fraction of 35% or less who require major vascular surgery. J Vasc Surg 1988; 8:307.

39. Killen DA, Reed WA, Gorton ME, et al. 25-year trends in resection of abdominal aortic aneurysms. Ann Vasc Sur 1998; 12:436.

40. Koutelou MG, Asimacopoulos PJ, Mahmarian JJ, et al. Preoperative risk stratification by adenosine thallium 201 single-photon emission computed tomography in patients undergoing vascular surgery. J Nucl Med 1995; 2:389.

41. Kresowik TF, Bower TR, Garner SA, et al. Dipyridamole thallium imaging in patients being considered for vascular procedures. Arch Surg 1993; 128:299.

42. Kryzhanovski VA, Beller GA. Usefulness of preoperative noninvasive radionuclide testing for detecting coronary artery disease in candidates for liver transplantation. Am J Cardiol 1997; 79:986.

43. L'Italien GJ, Cambria RP, Cutler BS, et al. Comparative early and late cardiac morbidity among patients requiring different vascular surgery procedures. J Vasc Surg 1995; 21:935.

44. Le A, Wilson R, Douek K, et al. Prospective risk stratification in renal transplant candidates for cardiac death. Am J Kidney Dis 1994; 24:65.

45. Lee TH, Marcantonio ER, Mangione CM, et al. Derivation and prospective validation of a simple index for prediction of cardiac risk of major noncardiac surgery. Circulation 1999; 100: 1043.

46. Lette J, Waters D, Bernier H, et al. Peroperative and long-term cardiac risk assessment. Ann Surg 1991; 216:192.

47. Lette J, Waters D, Cerino M, et al. Preoperative coronary artery disease risk stratification based on dipyridamole imaging and a simple three-step, three-segment model for patients undergoing noncardiac vascular surgery or major general surgery. Am J Cardiol 1992; 69:1553.

48. Lette J, Waters D, Champagne P, et al. Prognostic implications of a negative dipyridamole-thallium scan: results in 360 patients. Am J Med 1992; 92:615.

49. Mangano DT, Browner WS, Hollenberg M, et al. Long-term cardiac prognosis following noncardiac surgery. JAMA 1992; 268: 233.

50. Mangano DT, Layug EL, Wallace A, et al. Effect of atenolol on mortality and cardiovascular morbidity after noncardiac surgery. N Engl J Med 1996; 335:1713.

51. Mangano DT, London MJ, Tubau JF, et al. Study of perioperative ischemia research group: dipyridamole thallium-201 scintigraphy as a preoperative screening test: a reexamination of its predictive potential. Circulation 1991; 84:493.

52. Marshall ES, Raichlen JS, Forman S, et al. Adenosine radionuclide perfusion imaging in the preoperative evaluation of patients undergoing peripheral vascular surgery. Am J Cardiol 1995; 76: 817.

53. Massie MT, Rohrer MJ, Leppo JA, et al. Is coronary angiography necessary for vascular surgery patients who have positive results of dipyridamole thallium scans? J Vasc Surg 1997; 25: 975.

54. Matzer L, Kiat H, Friedman JD, et al. A new approach to the assessment of tomographic thallium-201 scintigraphy in patients with left bundle branch block. J Am Coll Cardiol 1991; 17:1309.

55. McFalls EO, Doliszny KM, Grund F, et al. Angina and persistent exercise thallium defects: independent risk factors in elective vascular surgery. J Am Coll Cardiol 1993; 21:1347.

56. Pepine CJ, Allen HD, Bashore TM, et al. ACC/AHA guidelines for cardiac catheterization and cardiac catheterization laboratories. J Am Coll Cardiol 1991; 18:1149.

57. Poldermans D, Arnese M, Fioretti PM, et al. Sustained prognostic value of dobutamine stress echocardiography for late cardiac events after major noncardiac vascular surgery. Circulation 1997; 95:53.

58. Polderman D, Boersma E, Bax JJ, et al. The effect of bisoprolol on perioperative mortality and myocardial infarction in high-risk patients undergoing vascular surgery. N Engl J Med 1999;341:1789.

59. Raby KE, Goldman L, Creager MA, et al. Correlation between preoperative ischemia and major cardiac events after peripheral vascular surgery. N Engl J Med 1989; 321:1296.

60. Roger VL, Ballard DJ, Hallett JW Jr, et al. Influence of coronary artery disease on morbidity and mortality after abdominal aortic aneurysmectomy: a population-based study, 1971–1987. J Am Coll Cardiol 1989; 14:1245.

61. Sachs RN, Tellier P, Larmignat P, et al. Assessment by dipyridamole-thallium-201 myocardial scintigraphy of coronary risk before peripheral vascular surgery. Surgery 1988; 103:584.

62. Schueppert MT, Kresowik TF, Corry DC, et al. Selection of patients for cardiac evaluation before peripheral vascular operations. J Vasc Surg 1996; 23:802.

63. Seeger JM, Rosenthal GR, Self SB, et al. Does routine stress-thallium cardiac scanning reduce postoperative cardiac complications? Ann Surg 1994; 219:654.

64. Shaw L, Miller DD, Kong BA, et al. Determination of perioperative cardiac risk by adenosine thallium-201 myocardial imaging. Am Heart J 1992; 124:861.

65. Shaw LJ, Eagle KA, Gersh BJ, et al. Meta-analysis of intravenous dipyridamole-thallium-201 imaging (1985 to 1994) and dobutamine echocardiography (1991 to 1994) for risk stratification before vascular surgery. J Am Coll Cardiol 1996; 27:787.

66. Stratmann HG, Younis LT, Wittry MD, et al. Dipyridamole technetium 99m sestamibi myocardial tomography for preoperative cardiac risk stratification before major or minor nonvascular surgery. Am Heart J 1996; 132:536.

67. Taylor LM Jr, Yeager RA, Moneta GL, et al. The incidence of perioperative myocardial infarction in general vascular surgery. J Vasc Surg 1991; 15:52.

68. Van Damme H, Pierard L, Gillain D, et al. Cardiac risk assessment

before vascular surgery: a prospective study comparing clinical evaluation, dobutamine stress echocardiography, and dobutamine Tc-99m sestamibi tomoscintigraphy. Cardiovasc Surg 1997;5:54.

69. Vanzetto G, Machecourt J, Blendea D, et al. Additive value of thallium single-photon emission computer tomography myocardial imaging for prediction of perioperative events in clinically selected high cardiac risk patients having abdominal aortic surgery. Am J Cardiol 1996; 77:143.

70. Wallace A, Layug B, Tateo I, et al. Prophylactic atenolol reduces postoperative myocardial ischemia. McSPI Research Group. [see comments]. Anesthesiology 1998; 88:7.

71. Weinrauch LA, D'Elia JA, Healy RW, et al. Asymptomatic coronary artery disease: angiography in diabetic patients before renal transplantation: relations of findings to postoperative survival. Ann Intern Med 1978; 88:346.

73. White GH, Advani SM, Williams RA, et al. Cardiac risk index as a predictor of long-term survival after repair of abdominal aortic aneurysm. Am J Surg 1988; 156:103.

74. Young AE, Sandberg GW, Couch NP. The reduction of mortality of abdominal aortic aneurysm resection. Am J Surg 1977; 134:585.

75. Younis L, Stratmann H, Takase B, et al. Preoperative clinical assessment and dipyridamole thallium-201 scintigraphy for prediction and prevention of cardiac events in patients having major noncardiovascular surgery and known or suspected coronary artery disease. Am J Cardiol 1994; 74:311.

76. Younis LT, Aguirre F, Byers S, et al. Perioperative and long-term prognostic value of intravenous dipyridamole thallium scintigraphy in patients with peripheral vascular disease. Am Heart J 1990; 119:1287.

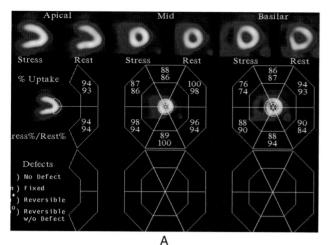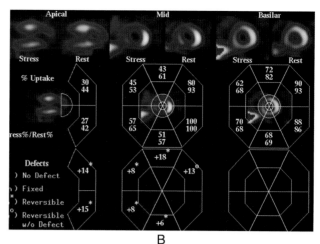

A
B

COLOR FIGURE 5.3 (A) Normal patient. Images at top show sections used for quantitative analysis of perfusion. Graphic below shows hexagonal segments in base and mid portion of left ventricle and apical segments shown on vertical long-axis view. Upper number in each segment is the percentage tracer activity of the stress images, and lower number is the activity of the rest images. Blanks in the lower graphic indicate that all values were within normal limits compared to the normal database. (B) Abnormal study. Entry of numbers in the lower graphic indicate that the stress values were outside of normal limits. The value of the number is the difference between rest and stress uptake. The asterisks mean that the difference is statistically significant, indicating reversibility. The superscript zero indicates that reversibility was significant in this segment, but that the poststress activity would not have been outside of normal limits.

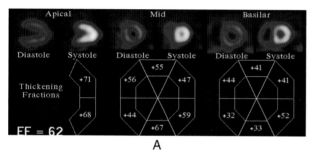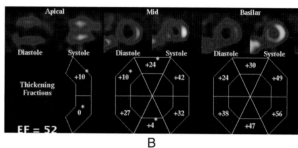

A
B

COLOR FIGURE 5.7 (A) Same sections as on the quantitative perfusion images of Color Figure 5.3(A), except the images are at end-systole and end-diastole. A constant normalization factor is used so the partial volume effect can be seen to cause apparent image brightening wherever there is myocardial thickening. Thickening fractions (actually brightening fractions) are indicated in the graphics below. Global LVEF, shown below, is derived from the regional thickening fractions. (B) Function images of the abnormal patient shown in Color Figure 5.3(B). Regional thickening fractions are compared to a normal database; values outside normal limits are indicated by an asterisk.

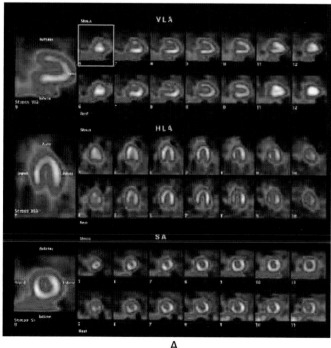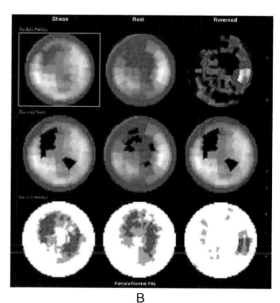

A
B

COLOR FIGURE 6.7 (A) Tomographic slices and (B) quantitative polar plots demonstrating an anterior breast attenuation artifact.

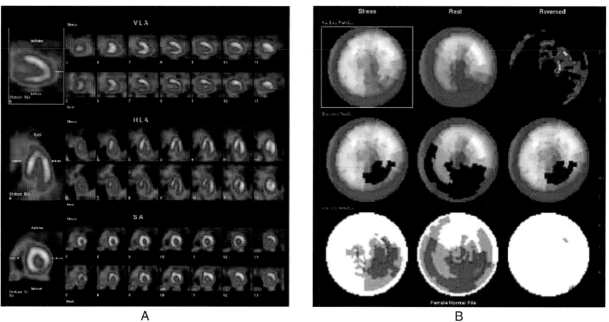

COLOR FIGURE 6.8 (A) Tomographic slices and (B) quantitative polar plots demonstrating an inferolateral breast attenuation artifact in a woman with large, very pendulous breasts. The breast attenuation artifact is more marked in the resting tomograms.

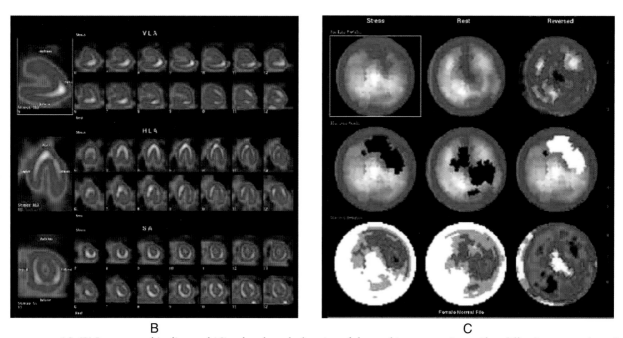

COLOR FIGURE 6.9 (B) In tomographic slices and (C) polar plots, the location of the resulting attenuation artifact differs in stress and rest images, thereby mimicking both ischemia and "reverse distribution."

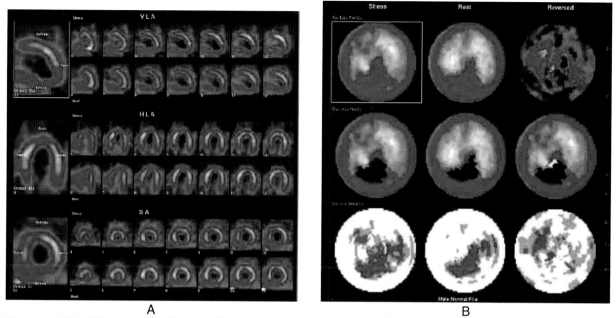

COLOR FIGURE 6.10 (A) Tomographic slices and (B) polar plots demonstrate a fixed inferior defect secondary to left hemidiaphragmatic attenuation.

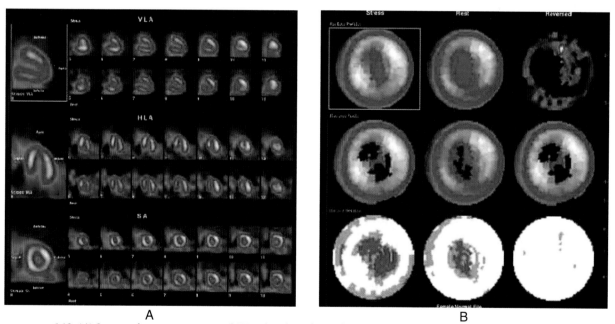

COLOR FIGURE 6.12 (A) Stress and rest tomograms and (B) polar plots obtained in an obese woman undergoing single-day low-dose rest–high-dose stress SPECT with Tc-99m sestamibi. An apical breast attenuation artifact is more apparent in the resting tomograms, simulating a pattern of "reverse distribution."

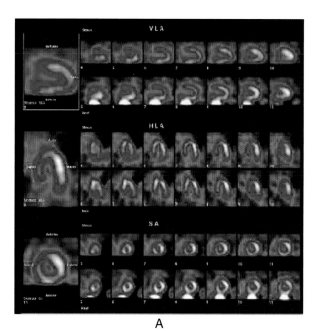
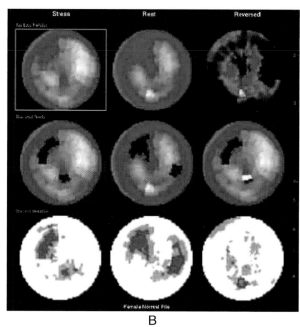

A

B

COLOR FIGURE 6.14 (*A*) In stress tomographic slices and (*B*) polar plots scatter from subdiaphragmatic tracer concentration artifactually increases left ventricular inferior wall count density. Normalization of images to the region of greatest count density (the inferior wall) results in an artifactual decrease in count density in the contralateral anterior wall. Since subdiaphragmatic activity is more intense in resting images, the stress anterior artifactual defect appears more marked at rest.

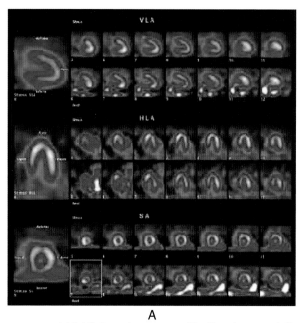
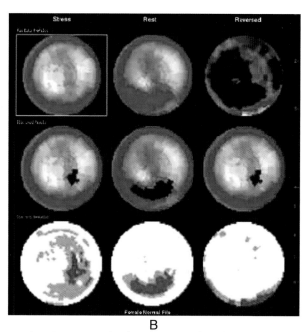

A

B

COLOR FIGURE 6.16 (*A*) In resting tomographic slices, intense subdiaphragmatic activity is noted to lie adjacent to the inferior wall of the left ventricle (in the x-plane). Because of the ramp-filter, count density is subtracted from the adjacent inferior wall of the left ventricle, creating an artifactual defect in resting tomographic slices and also (*B*) the resting polar plot, creating an artifact mimicking "reverse distribution."

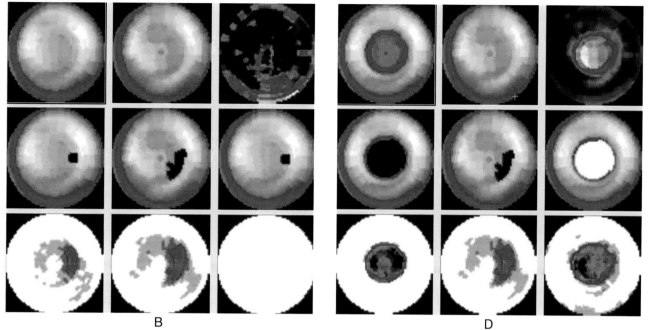

B   D

COLOR FIGURE 6.17 (A) With apical and basal slice limits correctly positioned, (B) polar plots in a normal individual demonstrate normal tracer distribution. (C) When the stress apical limit is positioned too far distally, an artifactual apical defect is created in (D) the reconstructed stress polar plot. In this case example, only the stress apical limit is positioned incorrectly, mimicking stress-induced ischemia. (See 6.17 A and C in text.)

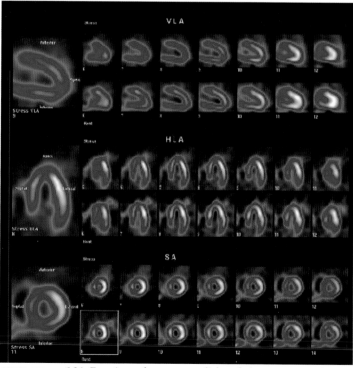

COLOR FIGURE 6.21 Exercise and rest myocardial perfusion tomograms in a patient with left bundle branch block but normal coronary arteries. An artifactual decrease in tracer concentration in the septum is present.

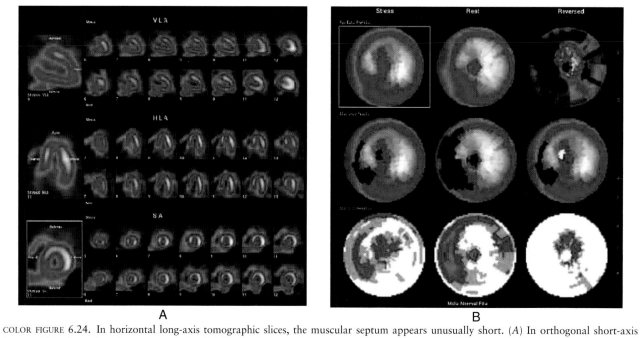

COLOR FIGURE 6.24. In horizontal long-axis tomographic slices, the muscular septum appears unusually short. (*A*) In orthogonal short-axis tomographic slices, there is an apparent fixed defect in the base of the septum. This normal variant is incorrectly identified as a basal septal perfusion defect in quantitative (*B*) polar plots.

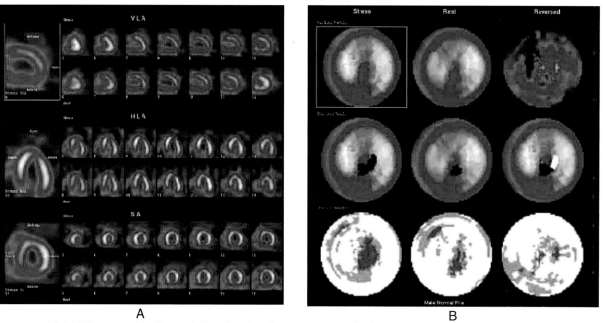

COLOR FIGURE 6.25 (*A*) Tomographic slices and (*B*) polar plots demonstrate a small, "linear," fixed apical defect, representing "apical thinning."

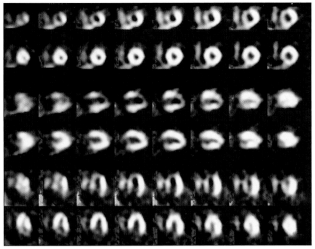

COLOR FIGURE 9.10 Perfusion abnormality in distribution of left anterior descending coronary artery.

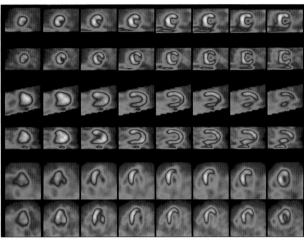

COLOR FIGURE 9.11 Perfusion abnormality in distribution of left circumflex coronary artery.

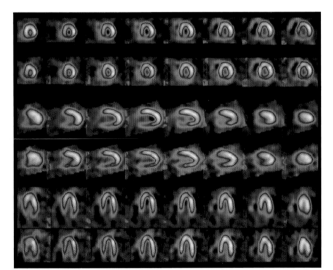

COLOR FIGURE 9.12 Perfusion abnormality in distribution of right coronary artery.

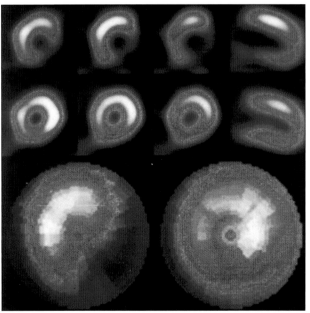

COLOR FIGURE 9.13 SPECT images obtained with sestamibi after the tracer was injected during temporary balloon occlusion of the left circumflex artery. The rest images were acquired a day later.

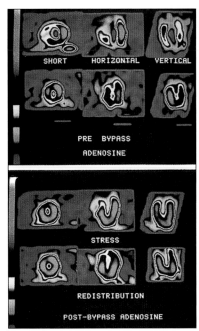

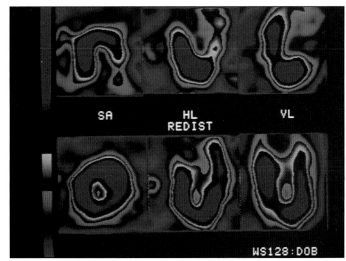

COLOR FIGURE 10.9 Dobutamine thallium SPECT image. (From Hays et al. [41]. Reprinted with permission from the American College of Cardiology.)

COLOR FIGURE 10.6 *(Top panel)* Adenosine Tl-201 single-photon emission computed tomography (SPECT) images in a patient with three-vessel coronary artery disease before coronary bypass surgery (prebypass). Representative initial tomographic slices *(top row)* demonstrate perfusion defects in the anterior wall and septum (short axis); apex and septum (horizontal long axis); and anterior wall, apex, and posterior wall (vertical long axis). Tomographic slices 4 hours later *(bottom row)* show complete redistribution indicating myocardial ischemia. Notice the presence of left ventricular dilation in the initial tomograms. *(Bottom panel)* Adenosine Tl-201 SPECT images in the same patient after three-vessel coronary artery bypass surgery (postbypass). The images are displayed in a format identical to those in top panel. No perfusion defects are seen in the initial *(top row)* or 4-hour redistribution *(bottom row)* tomographic slices. (Reproduced with permission from Verani et al. [89].)

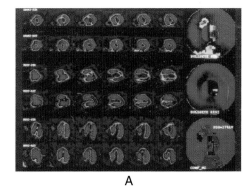

A

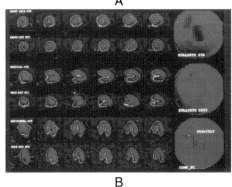

B

COLOR FIGURE 11.52 Adenosine technetium-99m-sestamibi myocardial perfusion tomography (SPECT) images *(left)* and polar maps *(right)* of a 41-year-old man who received thrombolytic therapy for acute myocardial infarction. Once stabilized, the patient underwent a baseline SPECT (A) on day 2 after admission. The baseline study shows a predominantly ischemic perfusion defect in the left anterior descending and right coronary artery vascular territories with a large total perfusion defect size (PDS) of 27%. The patient was treated medically with aspirin, long-acting nitrates, beta-blockers, and calcium antagonists. Simvastatin was given to treat hyperlipidemia. The patient returned for a repeat SPECT (B) 6 weeks later, which showed an almost entirely normal study. The patient is still asymptomatic 18 months later.

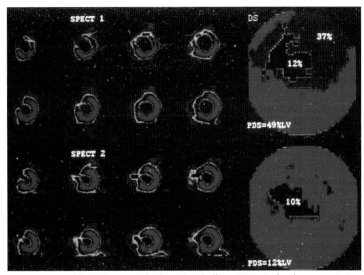

COLOR FIGURE 11.49 Sequential adenosine thallium-201 single-photon emission computed tomography (SPECT) images *(left)* and polar maps *(right)* in a patient following acute myocardial infarction. On initial baseline SPECT (1), the polar map shows a large (49%) primarily ischemic (37%) left ventricular (LV) perfusion defect size (PDS) (green) in the left anterior descending (LAD) coronary artery vascular territory with minimal scar (12%) (black). Following angioplasty of the LAD, the ischemic defect is no longer present (SPECT 2) with only a small residual scar (10%).

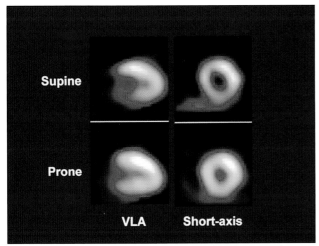

COLOR FIGURE 14.5 In a patient who presented to the ED with symptoms suspicious for ischemia but a nondiagnostic ECG, initial resting Tc-99m-sestamibi imaging (*top row*) demonstrated a possible inferobasal defect, consistent with either acute ischemia in that territory or diaphragmatic attenuation artifact. Prone imaging (*bottom row*) was performed, and inferobasal perfusion appeared normal, suggesting that the initial study represented diaphragmatic attenuation artifact and not ischemia. VLA, vertical long axis.

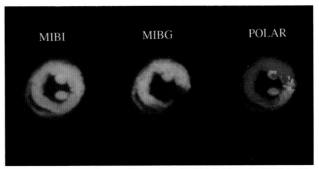

COLOR FIGURE 15.8 Autoradiographs of MIBI (*left*) and MIBG (*middle*) from a rabbit heart with regional denervation produced by the application of phenol to the epicardial surface. A defect is present in the MIBG image in a region that is well perfused in the MIBI image. The color funcional map shows the reduced MIBG relative to perfusion as yellow to green. Normally innervated myocardium is shown in red.

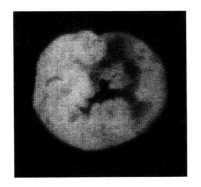

MIBI

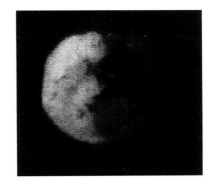

MIBG

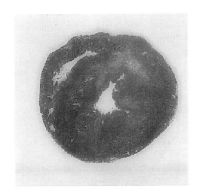

H & E

AAR

COLOR FIGURE 15.10 MIBI and MIBG autoradiographs (*above*) from a rabbit with a chronic myocardial infarction studied 3 days after coronary occlusion and reperfusion. An H&E stained adjacent tissue section shows the area of chronic infarction that corresponds to the MIBI perfusion defect above. The lower right image is a photograph of the tissue section showing blue dye (perfused tissue), and absence of blue dye delineating the area at risk (AAR) or ischemic region during coronary occlusion. The MIBG defect is similar to the distribution of the ischemic bed.

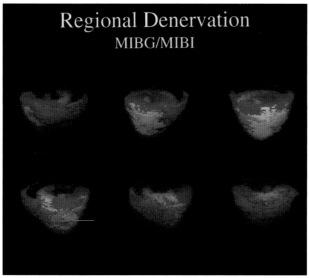

COLOR FIGURE 15.11 3-D color functional maps of regionally denervated myocardium from serial images of slices as illustrated in Figure 15.8.

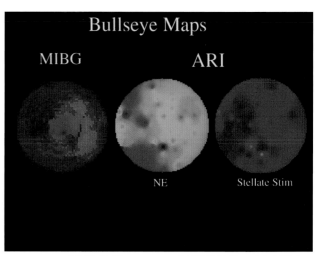

COLOR FIGURE 15.12 Bull's-eye maps of MIBG (*left*) and Δ ARI during norepinephrine (NE) infusion (*middle*) and stellate stimulation (*right*). Green represents denervation in the MIBG map. In ARI maps, green represents shortening, purple represents prolongation, and red represents little change in ARI.

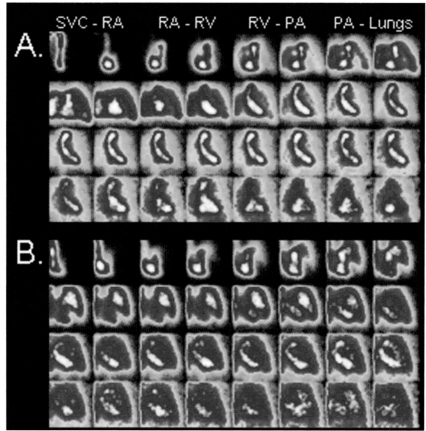

COLOR FIGURE 17.2 Serial resting FPRNA images obtained on the same patient with Tc-99m-DTPA (*A*) and Tc-99m-teboroxime (*B*) demonstrate the usual sequence of tracer transit, from SVC to RA, RV, PA, and lungs, followed by the levophase (*A*, second and third rows). However, there is significant extraction and retention of Tc-99m-teboroxime in the pulmonary parenchyma (*B*), which markedly increases the level of background during the levophase (see text), which impairs background subtraction (see Fig. 17.8).

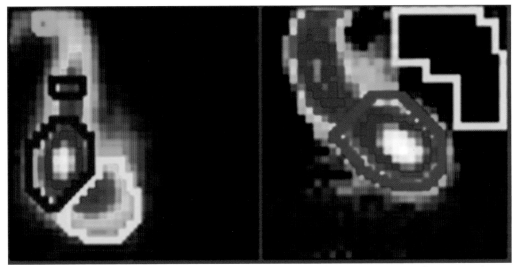

COLOR FIGURE 17.3 Raw FPRNA images of the dextrophase (*left image*) and levophase (*right image*) with typical regions of interest drawn, including upper entry to the SVC from the right axillary vein (*green*), mid-SVC (*red*), RA (*dark blue*), and RV (*yellow*) on the dextrophase, and the left lung (*yellow*) and LV (*royal blue*).

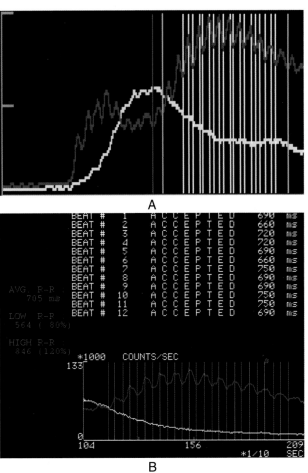

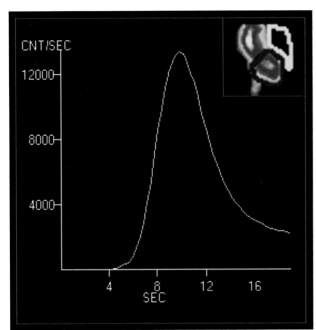

COLOR FIGURE 17.5 A pulmonary histogram derived from a paraventricular region of interest is shown, with a pulmonary mean transit time of 5.1 seconds. Although this is usually measured using a gamma variate fit, the pulmonary mean transit time can be quickly estimated by the time from peak RV counts to the time of peak LV counts, or by a FWHM of the lung transit curve. The normal range is usually taken as 6.6 ± 2.2 seconds, decreasing to less than half the resting value with exercise.

COLOR FIGURE 17.6 FPRNA levophase time–activity curves are shown based on regions of interest in Figure 17.3, with the LV histogram (*in royal blue*) and the end of the pulmonary histogram (*in yellow*) in two patients with severe LV dysfunction due to coronary artery disease. In the upper frame, the operator selected background frame is shown in red, and the limits for frame selection are in green. In the processing stage depicted in the lower frame, the selected beats can be carefully edited in order to exclude arrhythmias. ED selections are in green, and the selected ES frames are in red.

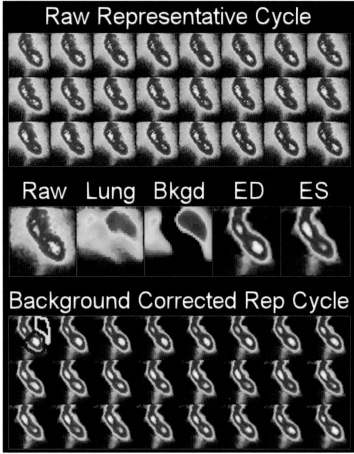

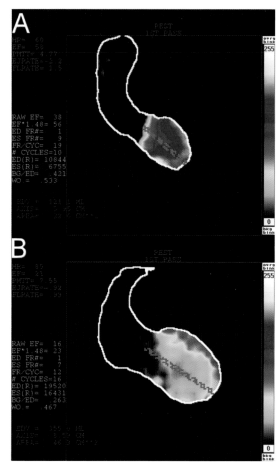

COLOR FIGURE 17.7 The representative cycle is formed by combining the beats selected as in Figure 17.6. The raw images are background corrected using one pulmonary/RV frame for each beat in the representative cycle, beginning at the operator chosen inflection point (as in Figure 17.6), and moving backward (to subtract more RV counts). This composite lung (Lung) frame is shown in the middle panel. An ED mask image is subtracted from the lung frame prior to its application to the raw representative cycle, producing the final background matrix (Bkgd). A fraction of this image, calculated to obtain a zero value in one pixel (usually left lung or RV), is substracted from the raw representative cycle to produce the background corrected representative (Rep) cycle.

COLOR FIGURE 17.9 LV ED volume is calculated in two patients with the Sandler and Dodge equation for the anterior projection (see text), in which the area is obtained by a region of interest placed over the LV portion of a regional ejection fraction image, and the long axis of the ventricle is marked from apex to midaortic valve plane. In (A), the patient has normal LV size and function. In (B), there is marked LV dilatation with regional (inferior, inferobasal, inferoapical, and apical) and global LV dysfunction in a patient with severe CAD.

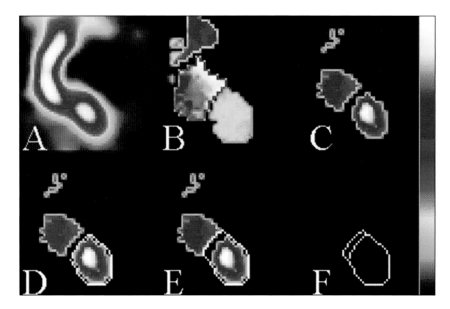

COLOR FIGURE 17.10 Anterior projection FPRNA images are shown. The background corrected representative cycle ED frame (A), Fourier phase (B), and amplitude (C) are shown. Note the presence of amplitude in both the left ventricle and aorta, which are easily distinguished by the opposite values on the phase image, and are separated by a low amplitude region. The valve plane of end-systolic region of interest (ROI) is drawn using the inferior margin of this amplitude image (D). The end-diastolic ROI is obtained by tracing the end-systolic ROI, except for the valve plane, which is drawn using the upper margin of the low amplitude region (E). These dual-ROIs are shown comparatively in (F). From Holman et al. [43] with permission.

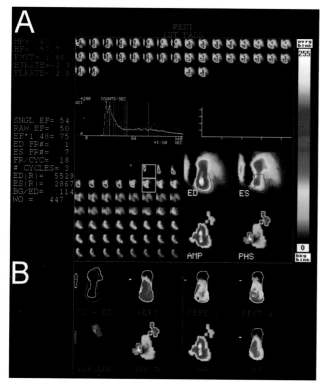

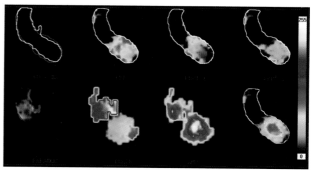

COLOR FIGURE 17.13 Functional images utilized for the assessment of regional function are shown, including ED-ES perimeter image, regional EF index (REFI), REFI first half of systole (REFI 1), REFI second half of systole (REFI 2), paradox (ES-ED), Fourier phase and amplitude, and SV (ED-ES) images. The ED-ES perimeter shows reduced global LV function, with regional impairment of apical function, depicted by the lack of excursion from ED to ES. The REFI images also show poor global function, but most severely abnormal at the apex, with more of the function in the apical and lateral apical regions occurring in the second half of systole (REFI 2). The paradox image is faintly positive at the apex, indicating a small count increase during systole, which defines this myocardial segment as dyskinetic (aneurysmal). Fourier transformation of the frames in the representative cycle gives the timing (phase) and absolute value (amplitude) of pixel count changes during the cardiac cycle. The phase image is read on the 0–255 color scale expanded to represent 0° to 360°. The LV should be uniform in timing, and 180° out of phase with the aorta and left atrium. In this example, the apical segment is delayed (tardokinetic) with decreased amplitude. The SV image also shows decreased apical performance.

COLOR FIGURE 17.11 Resting RV images are shown on the same patients from Figure 17.9, with normal (upper panel) and abnormal global RV function, respectively. The background frame for correction uses the RA frames just prior to tracer crossing the tricuspid valve, which is identified as the peak in the RA time activity curve (yellow histograms). RV beat selection is shown (blue histogram), with ED (lavender) and ES (green) frames. Raw representative cycles (A, upper right quadrant) can be used to obtain an EF without correction (50% and 26%, respectively). The background corrected representative cycles (A, upper left quadrant) have "historical" single ROI method of EFs of 54% and 28%, respectively, which increased to 58% and 35% using the dual ROI method to track valve plane movement. In (B) functional images utilized for the assessment of regional function are shown, including ED − ES perimeter images, regional EF index (REFI), REFI first half of systole (REFI 1), REFI second half of systole (REFI 2), paradox (ES − ED), Fourier phase and amplitude (redisplayed), and SV (ED-ES) images. See text and Figure 17.13 for details.

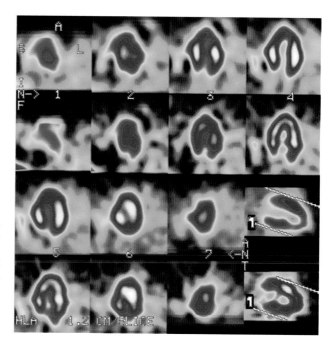

COLOR FIGURE 17.14 Four quadrant display of FPRNA (*top*) and SPECT perfusion (*bottom*) performed with a same-day low-dose–high-dose (8 and 24 mCi) rest and exercise Tc-99m-sestamibi protocol in a patient with a high-grade stenosis of the mid-left anterior descending coronary artery. Resting SPECT (below slice numbers) and FPRNA (upper two quadrants) are normal, with an LV EF of 60%. With exercise, the patient demonstrated distal septal, apical, and inferoapical reversible ischemia as evidenced by regional wall motion (perimeter) and perfusion images, with an LV EF of 39%.

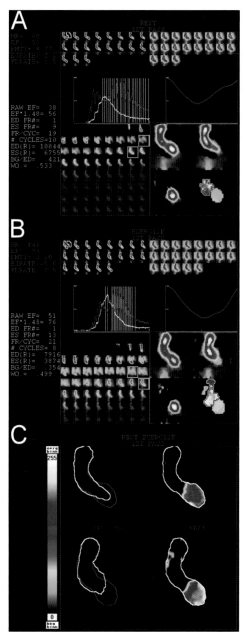

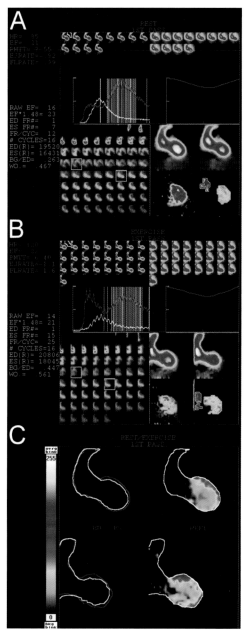

COLOR FIGURE 17.15 Clinical FPRNA data are shown at rest (A) and exercise (B), with functional images (C) in a patient with no evidence of significant reversible myocardial ischemia. The LV EF increased from 58% at rest to 70% with exercise. Bolus appearance on serial images (lower left images), pulmonary curves and histograms, beat selection, background correction, Fourier phase and amplitude, raw representative cycle, and background corrected representative cycles are appropriate and within normal limits at rest. With exercise, the bolus is slightly degraded and persists on the serial images from several frames, but this does not affect the remainder of the analysis, which is normal by all parameters, including a rise in the ejection fraction and a decline in pulmonary mean transit time (consistent with increased cardiac output with exercise).

COLOR FIGURE 17.16 Same schema as Figure 17.15, with clinical FPRNA data at rest (A) and exercise (B), with functional images (C) in a patient with severe coronary artery disease and prior myocardial infarction, with evidence for significant reversible myocardial ischemia in the lateral-apical and anterolateral segments. The LV EF increased from 21% at rest to 22% with exercise. The LV chamber is dilated (quantitated in Figure 17.9). There is global and regional dysfunction at rest, which worsens with stress. The failure of the significant decline in pulmonary mean transit time is consistent with poor cardiac output with exercise. These images were obtained using low-dose rest and high-dose exercise Tc-99m-sestamibi. Note that the counting statistics are high with this gamma camera at rest and stress (20,000 at ED), obtained with 25 frames per cycle with stress, but only 16 frames per cycle with the lower dose resting study.

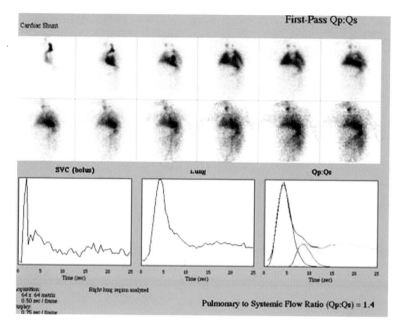

COLOR FIGURE 17.18 An 11-year-old male with question of partial anomalous pulmonary return. Pulmonary-to-systemic flow ratio = 1.4 confirms clinical impression of a hemodynamically insignificant left-to-right shunt. (Reprinted from http://nucmedweb.tch.harvard.edu/Patient/Cardiovascular/lrshunt.html, accessed on 7/1/01, with permission of Dr. Ted Treves.)

COLOR FIGURE 21.2 Newer myocardial perfusion tracers. Patient with previous inferior myocardial infarction and LV dysfunction (inferior akinesia and septal hypo-akinesia). SPECT imaging shows concordance in the detection of viable myocardium between rest-redistribution ^{201}T1 (two upper rows) and rest ^{99m}Tc-furifosmin (bottom row) studies. The images demonstrate presence of hibernated myocardium in the inferior and septal walls. (Courtesy of Dr. A. Cuocolo, Università Federico II, Napoli, Italy.)

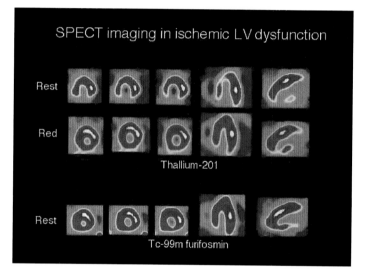

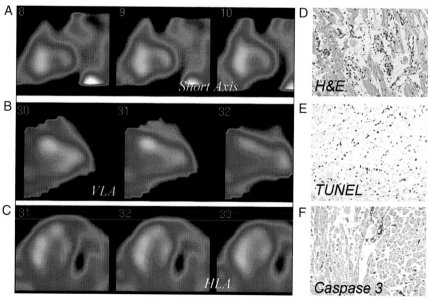

COLOR FIGURE 21.4 Noninvasive detection of apoptosis by ^{99m}Tc-annexin-V imaging (A–C) in a cardiac allograft recipient with histologic evidence of vascular rejection (D–F), 8 months after heart transplantation. SPECT imaging performed 3 hr after intravenous injection of radiolabeled annexin-V demonstrated multifocal myocardial uptake of radiotracer. Smoothening of the images and cardiac SPECT processing in the short axis (A), vertical long axis (B), and horizontal (C) long axis views revealed myocardial perfusion scan-like images with diffuse uptake in whole myocardium, suggesting apoptosis in the myocardium. Endomyocardial biopsy interpretation was consistent with severe vascular rejection. H&E stained histologic sections revealed spreading apart of myocytes with interstitial edema, interstitial lymphomononuclear cell infiltration and endothelial cell swelling ([D], ×20). Positive TUNEL staining was observed in almost every endothelial cell in the field and occasional myocytes (brown color product, [E]) with corresponding caspase-3 staining (red color product, [F]) in endothelial cells (arrows) and myocytes (arrowheads).

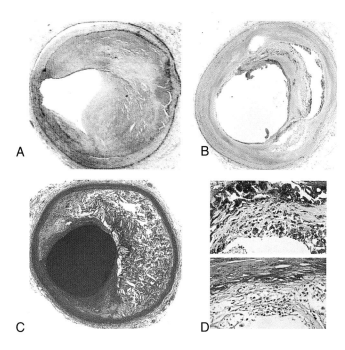

COLOR FIGURE 21.7 Morphologic characteristics of vulnerable plaques. Photomicrographs of coronary arteries show stable plaque (A), vulnerable plaque (C & D), and plaque rupture (B). A shows stable plaque that consist almost exclusively of fibrous tissue. Vulnerable plaque (C) comprises all characteristics of plaque rupture except that site of rupture is absent; characteristics include necrotic lipid core, thin (<65 μm) overlying fibrous cap, and heavy infiltration of fibrous cap by macrophages. The macrophages are stained brown after immunohistochemical staining with antimacrophage KP-1 antibody (D). (B) is a photomicrograph of plaque rupture with nonocclusive luminal thrombus. Note large necrotic core that occupies large portion of plaque and thin fibrous cap with rupture and overlying thrombus. (Courtesy of Dr. Renu Virmani, Armed Forces Institute of Pathology, Washington, DC.)

COLOR FIGURE 21.9 Morphologic characteristics of postangioplastic restenosis (A) and stent placement (B). Photomicrograph (A) is a section of coronary artery from patient who underwent angioplasty 3 months before death; note neointima (inside arrowheads). The neointimal growth consits of smooth muscle cells in proteoglycan-collagen matrix and surrounding plaque. Photomicrograph (B) is a section from a right coronary artery of a 59-year-old man who died suddenly 4 months after balloon angioplasty and Palmaz-Schatz stent placement. (B) demonstrates cross-section of artery (empty spaces represents sites of stent struts) with neointimal thickening or restenosis developing inside stent. (Courtesy of R. Virmani, Armed Forces Institute of Pathology, Washington, DC.)

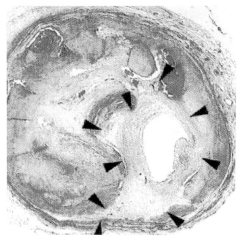

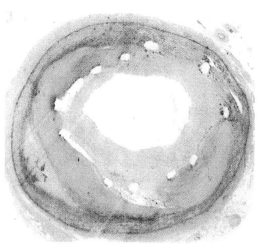

A

B

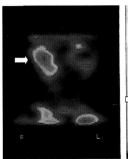 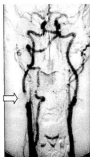 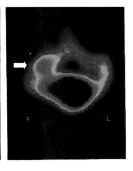

Coronal view   **Angio**   **Transverse view**

COLOR FIGURE 21.11 Atheroma imaging in human. SPECT images showing focal Z2D3 uptake at the site of a right carotid plaque. The coronal image shows focal antibody uptake on the right carotid artery with absent uptake in the contralateral side. The transverse image shows focal uptake on the right carotid artery anterior to the nonspecific uptake in the bone marrow. The carotid arteriogram shows the stenotic region corresponding to the uptake in atherosclerotic plaque.

12 | Use of nuclear techniques in the assessment of patients before and after cardiac revascularization procedures

TIMOTHY M. BATEMAN, JAMES A. CASE, AND S. JAMES CULLOM

Mechanical myocardial revascularization using the standard techniques of percutaneous coronary interventions (PCI) and coronary artery bypass graft (CABG) surgery has become a mainstay for the treatment of selected patients with coronary artery disease (CAD). According to the American Heart Association, there were approximately 650,000 PCI and 600,000 CABG procedures performed in the United States in 1996 [1]. Radionuclide myocardial perfusion imaging is well suited for identifying patients who may benefit from these revascularization procedures, for documenting adequacy of the selected method, and for predicting both short- and long-term outcomes. Because all patients who have undergone a revascularization procedure have a chronic disease process, they are at higher likelihood for further complications of CAD than the general population. It should not be surprising therefore that a significant percentage of clinically indicated myocardial perfusion studies are focused on addressing issues pertinent to coronary revascularization.

Furthermore, the past half-decade has witnessed the introduction of an increasing number of alternative medical and mechanical ways to achieve myocardial revascularization. Radionuclide techniques have emerged as a scientific standard for critically evaluating the merits of these newer techniques.

ASSESSMENT BEFORE REVASCULARIZATION

Radionuclide imaging is frequently useful in selecting patients for and planning of revascularization procedures. Although the most extensive data relate to single-photon emission computed tomography (SPECT) myocardial perfusion imaging, there is also sufficient information to indicate selective utility of both radionuclide ventriculography and positron emission tomography (PET). The major applications are to document the presence, extent, severity, and location of ischemia; to quantitate left ventricular function; to determine the viability of dysfunctioning myocardium; and to stratify risk for major cardiac events such as death or myocardial infarction in the absence of revascularization (Table 12.1). This information can be helpful in deciding between alternative forms of therapy including continued medical management, PCI, or CABG.

Identification of Appropriate Candidates for Revascularization

Perhaps the most important application of radionuclide imaging prior to revascularization is to identify those patients who are at increased risk of cardiac death. CABG has been shown to reduce the risk of cardiac death in several subsets, including those with three-vessel or left main disease, proximal left anterior descending disease, and those with significant ischemia in the setting of reduced left ventricular function [2–6]. While assessment of cardiac risk and decisions about the potential benefit of a revascularization technique are daily occurrences in cardiology practice, the exercise remains challenging. Clinical indexes alone are frequently insufficient: 1-year mortality for patients with stable, progressive, and unstable angina varies by only a few percentage points, and many patients with mild or even no symptoms have severe CAD. A prior chap-

TABLE 12.1 *Indications for SPECT Myocardial Perfusion Imaging before Revascularization Procedures*

Objective demonstration of presence, site, extent, and severity of ischemia
Stratification of risk for cardiac death: low (< 1%); intermediate; high (> 3%)
Identification of the culprit artery
Determination of viability of dysfunctioning myocardium
In some cases, recommendation for type of therapy (medical, PCI, CABG, transplant)

PCI, percutaneous coronary interventions; CABG, coronary artery bypass grafts.

ter has documented the ability of radionuclide techniques to identify patients with low, intermediate, or high risk of subsequent cardiac events. In addition, it is known that prognosis using myocardial perfusion indexes is superior to that provided by both clinical and angiographic information. For the applications under consideration here, the rationale is to identify patients in whom coronary angiography and subsequent revascularization might improve survival.

Randomized trials of CABG compared to medical therapy have shown that patients randomized to CABG had a lower mortality only if they were at substantial risk. Those with a 5-year survival rate of about 95% with medical therapy (equivalent to an annual mortality rate of 1%) did not have a lower mortality rate with CABG. Indexes from a stress myocardial perfusion study that would categorize a patient at < 1% annual mortality have been previously discussed, and include normal or near normal scans with normal left ventricular size and function. Most patients with abnormalities in a single vascular territory also appear to be at low mortality risk, even though the angiographic extent of CAD may be greater than the scan appearances might imply [7]. In contrast, patients with a survival advantage with CABG, such as those with three-vessel disease, have an annual mortality rate > 3%.

As shown in Table 12.2, myocardial perfusion imaging can be effectively employed as a risk-based gatekeeper to migrating from medical therapies for CAD to revascularization techniques. For example, referral to coronary angiography after normal or near normal scans is rarely undertaken [8–10], and the American Society of Nuclear Cardiology has emphasized the clinical and economic importance of this strategy in a published statement [11]. A large multicenter comparison of clinical outcomes and costs associated with coronary angiography versus perfusion imaging first and subsequent referral to angiography dependent on the findings demonstrated that the latter approach provided similar event-free clinical outcomes but at substantial economic savings [12].

Coronary angiography with a view to revascularization is appropriate for patients whose annual mortality risk exceeds at least 1%, and based on anticipated postprocedural mortality in the range of 1%–2%, would ideally be > 3%. Perfusion correlates of high annual risk include large defects involving a substantial amount of the left ventricular mass, summed stress scores in the moderate-to-high range, any size reversible or partially reversible perfusion defect in the presence of reduced left ventricular ejection fraction (LVEF), perfusion defects in multiple coronary distributions, and perfusion defects in conjunction with abnormal thallium-201 (Tl-201) lung uptake or left ventricular enlargement. Currently recognized scintigraphic findings that identify high-risk patients are listed in Table 12.2. Patients identified as high risk are generally referred for coronary angiography independent of their symptomatic status. In general and when appropriately used, perfusion imaging is less costly than direct coronary angiography, especially when the pretest probability of severe CAD is low. When the pretest probability of severe CAD is high, direct referral for coronary angiography has been shown to be most cost-effective, because the total number of tests is reduced.

Many perfusion studies categorize risk as in between the extremes of normal or near normal scans (< 1% annual mortality) and findings suggesting high (> 3%) annual mortality. In general, this would apply to pa-

TABLE 12.2 *Scintigraphic Findings Helpful in Risk-Stratifying Patients into Low, Intermediate, and High Risk for Major Cardiac Events**

Low-Risk (< 1%)
 Normal or near normal perfusion
 Normal LVEF with normal or near normal perfusion will be an exceptionally low-risk group
Intermediate-Risk (< 1% for cardiac death; ~ 1% for nonfatal MI)
 Small perfusion defect (< 15% of LV volume; low summed stress score) with normal LVEF and absence of nonperfusion markers of LV decompensation with exercise
High-Risk (> 3% for cardiac death)
 Severe resting LV dysfunction
 Severe exercise LV dysfunction
 Large stress-induced PD
 Moderate stress-induced PD with abnormal Tl-201 lung uptake
 Multiple moderate stress-induced PD
 Large fixed PD with abnormal lung uptake or LV dilation

LVEF, left ventricular ejection fraction; MI, myocardial infarction; PD, perfusion defect.
*Low-risk patients can be followed medically; high-risk patients are ideal candidates for revascularization; and intermediate-risk patients can be followed medically except for special circumstances such as intolerability of symptoms or for occupational reasons.

tients with mild-moderate perfusion defects restricted to one or two vascular territories, involving a small amount of total left ventricular myocardium ($< 15\%$), and with normal LV function [13–16]. Furthermore, an investigation showed that myocardial perfusion imaging can identify patients who are at low risk of death but increased risk of nonfatal myocardial infarction (MI) [14]. This distinction is important in selecting patients for revascularization on the basis of risk reduction, because neither CABG nor PCI has been shown in prospective randomized trials to reduce the risk of nonfatal myocardial infarction [2,17,18]. Therefore, such patients should preferentially be managed medically unless there are extenuating circumstances such as uncontrolled symptoms.

Several recent prospective trials have compared medical management with revascularization for total hard cardiac events (death and nonfatal infarction) in patients with mild-moderate CAD and normal left ventricular function. Although these trials did not employ nuclear imaging for randomization, considerable data from retrospective clinical databases suggest that the findings may be extrapolatable to patients with mild reversible perfusion defects and normal LVEF by ECG-gated SPECT scintigraphy. Three randomized trials compared PCI with medical management of angina [19–23]. The ACME study [19] randomized 212 patients with single-vessel disease, stable angina, and ischemia on treadmill testing to PCI or medical therapy. This trial demonstrated superior control of symptoms and exercise capacity in patients treated with PCI, but hard events were infrequent and similar in both groups. The Veterans Administration ACME trial investigators also reported 6-month results for an additional 101 randomized patients with double-vessel disease [20]; patients randomized to medical therapy or PCI had similar improvement in exercise duration, freedom from angina, and improvement in quality of life. This small study suggests that PCI is less effective in controlling symptoms in angina patients with double-vessel as compared to single-vessel disease.

The RITA-2 investigators followed 1018 stable angina patients randomized to PCI or medical therapy [21]. Patients who had inadequate control of their symptoms with optimal medical therapy were allowed to cross over to PCI. The combined end point of the trial was all cause mortality and nonfatal MI. Over a mean follow-up of 2.7 years, death and nonfatal infarction occurred in 32 of the 504 PCI patients (6.3%) and in 17 of the 514 medical patients (3.3%), $p = .02$. Of the 18 deaths (11 PCI and 7 medical) only 8 were cardiac. Twenty-three percent of the medical patients required a revascularization procedure during follow-up. Angina improved in both groups but there was a 16.5% absolute excess of grade 2 or worse angina in the medical group at 3 months following randomization ($p < .001$), and the PCI patients also had greater improvement in exercise duration ($p < .001$). During follow-up 40 patients randomized to PCI required CABG surgery (7.9%) as compared to 30 of the medical patients (5.8%). Thus, RITA-2 demonstrated that PCI results in better control of symptoms and improves exercise capacity, but is associated with a higher combined end point of death and periprocedural MI. Importantly, although the patients in this trial were asymptomatic or had only mild angina, most had severe anatomic CAD: 62% had multivessel disease and 34% had significant disease in the proximal left anterior descending coronary artery.

The Asymptomatic Cardiac Ischemia Pilot (ACIP) study randomized 558 asymptomatic CAD patients who had demonstrable ischemia by ambulatory ECG monitoring, and had anatomy suitable for revascularization, to three treatment strategies: angina-guided drug therapy ($n = 183$), angina plus ischemia-guided drug therapy ($n = 183$), and revascularization by PCI or CABG surgery ($n = 192$) [22]. Of the 192 patients that were randomized to revascularization, 102 were selected for PCI and 90 for CABG. At 2 years of follow-up, death or MI had occurred in 4.7% of the revascularization patients as compared to 8.8% of the ischemia-guided group and 12.1% of the angina-guided group ($p < .01$). Because a large portion of the patients underwent CABG surgery instead of PCI in order to achieve complete revascularization, it is not appropriate to directly compare these results with RITA-2. Nonetheless, the ACIP study suggests that outcomes of revascularization with CABG surgery and PCI are very favorable compared to medical therapy in patients with asymptomatic ischemia. It should be emphasized that aggressive lipid-lowering therapy was not widely employed in the medical treatment arm of ACIP.

AVERT [23] randomly assigned 341 patients with stable CAD, normal LV function, and Class I or II angina to PCI or medical therapy with 80 mg daily atorvastatin (mean LDL = 77 mg/dl). At 18-months follow-up, 13% of the medically treated group had ischemic events as compared to 21% of the PCI group ($p = 0.048$); angina relief was greater in those treated with PCI. Although not statistically different when adjusted for interim analysis, these data suggest that in low-risk patients with stable CAD, aggressive lipid-lowering therapy can be as effective as PTCA in reducing ischemic events.

Based on these limited data, it seems prudent to consider medical therapy for the initial management of most patients with Canadian Cardiovascular Society Classification Class I and II angina, limited extent and severity of ischemia, and normal left ventricular function. More symptomatic patients or those who wish to remain physically active with no or minimal symptoms may be candidates for PCI, although the RITA trial suggests that this may be associated with an increased initial risk. The results of the ACIP trial indicate that higher-risk patients with asymptomatic ischemia and significant CAD who undergo complete revascularization with CABG or PCI may have a better outcome than those with medical management, but note that this finding had not been previously demonstrated by multicenter trials comparing medical management with CABG revascularization [2]. In contrast, the results of AVERT indicate revascularization provides no benefit when compared to aggressive lipid-lowering therapy in low-risk patients.

Although most of these studies did not include or report on the results of nuclear imaging as requisites for randomization, there are considerable data, as discussed in earlier chapters, to indicate that perfusion imaging can identify these patients with active CAD but with relatively low risk for major events. In general, such patients have stress perfusion defects involving < 15% of the ventricle, in a single vascular territory, with a low (< 8) summed stress score, and normal or near normal LVEF by gated SPECT.

Assessment of Myocardial Viability

Patients with reduced left ventricular function and demonstrable ischemia are a special subset identifiable by myocardial perfusion imaging who are likely to benefit from surgery [24–28]. In patients with a normal EF, CABG provides little survival benefit. In patients with mild to moderately depressed function, the poorer the LV function, the greater the potential benefit of surgery [29,30]. The relative benefit is similar, but there is greater absolute benefit because of the high-risk profile of these patients. It is important to note that the randomized trials did not include patients with an LVEF < 0.35. Thus, many of the patients operated on today were not well represented in the randomized trials. A major growth in our understanding of the potential reversibility of chronic systolic dysfunction among patients with CAD has occurred in the past few years. Systolic dysfunction that is a result of chronic hypoperfusion ("hibernating") and not a result of infarction can now be identified noninvasively by positron emission tomographic scanning, radioisotope imaging, or dobutamine echocardiography. Patients with large areas of myocardial viability may benefit from revascularization. Small, observational studies of patients with hibernating myocardium who are undergoing coronary revascularization have shown functional and perhaps survival benefit, especially when LV function is particularly poor.

Left ventricular dysfunction is an important negative prognostic marker. Sharir et al. [31] showed that when LVEF is reduced, even moderately extensive perfusion defects are associated with a marked worsening of short-term mortality. As such, it may be particularly important to assess this patient population for the presence of ischemia, with a view to PTCA or CABG if ischemia is found. Because the risk of interventions is higher in these patients, knowing of which vessels are causing flow abnormalities and the extent of myocardial viability is critical to deciding on management.

Identification of Culprit Coronary Arteries

Both PCI and CABG are important therapeutic tools for the relief of disabling angina. Myocardial perfusion imaging is useful in planning revascularization procedures, because it demonstrates whether a specific coronary stenosis is associated with a stress-induced perfusion abnormality [32–34]. Although less critical in CABG, where typically all suitable vessels with significant angiographic stenoses (≥ 50%) are bypassed, myocardial perfusion imaging is particularly helpful in determining the functional importance of single or multiple stenoses when PCI is targeted to the "culprit lesion," that is, the ischemia-provoking stenosis. For this application, it is important that patients achieve 85% of maximum-predicted heart rate (MPHR), in order to "unmask" more than just the most severely ischemic region that could lead to early exercise termination. If a patient cannot achieve this high level of exercise, pharmacologic stress may be superior to detect all regions of stress-induced abnormal perfusion.

Selection of Mode of Revascularization

There has been considerable effort to evaluate the relative effectiveness of CABG versus PCI for coronary revascularization. Subsets that may have improved outcomes with CABG include diabetics with extensive ischemia and patients with viable and ischemic myocardium not completely revascularizable with PCI but where CABG would offer full revascularization. The potential role of nuclear testing in these decisions has not been fully explored, but in selected cases the information provided can be helpful.

Cost-Effectiveness

The findings of the Economics of Noninvasive Diagnosis (END) multicenter trial [12] indicate that selection of patients for angiography based on the results of a screening myocardial perfusion scan can provide cost savings and similar patient outcomes. The majority of the cost savings arose from a reduction in revascularization procedures. Importantly, this study was retrospective and did not have criteria for referral for revascularization regardless of whether perfusion imaging or angiography served as the gatekeeper. The Clinical Outcomes Utilization Revascularization and Aggressive Drug Evaluation (COURAGE) trial, a 3250 patients-based trial, will compare intensive medical therapy with revascularization over 5 to 7 years. It will assess relative hard and soft events, quality of life, and economic implications. A nuclear substudy will address thresholds of ischemia in relation to outcomes of medical therapy versus revascularization.

Assessment after PCI

SPECT myocardial perfusion scintigraphy has excellent utility after PCI for detecting success or failure of the procedure. The ACC/AHA Guidelines on Clinical Cardiac Radionuclide Imaging [35], on the Management of Patients with Chronic Stable Angina [36], and on PCI [37] all cite this as a Class 1 indication for patients with symptoms and for selected asymptomatic patients. Optimal interpretation of the images, however, can be more difficult than in the setting of nonrevascularized suspected or known CAD, as the causes of abnormalities are more varied. Perfusion abnormalities can reflect acute reocclusion, acute and transient procedure-related changes in coronary flow reserve, procedure-related myocardial injury, restenosis, side-branch compromise, new disease, or previously unrecognized disease (Table 12.3). Because subsequent management decisions often depend on how the nuclear cardiologist translates an abnormality, interpretations should always be performed with an understanding of how these different problems may be expressed on a SPECT scan,

TABLE 12.3 *Potential Basis for Abnormal Perfusion Patterns in a Post-PCI SPECT Study*

Prior myocardial injury
New periprocedural myocardial injury
Restenosis
Nonrevascularized CAD
New stenoses
Side-branch compromise (plaque disruption/shift; stent "jailing")

and knowledge of the preprocedure angiogram and what was done during the procedure. Having the procedural report available at the time of interpretation can be invaluable in explaining in the final SPECT report the likely basis for any abnormal findings.

Early after PTCA

There is general agreement that there is no role for routine SPECT testing in the first several weeks after PTCA. However, occasionally SPECT may be helpful and there is no reason to avoid testing if there is a clinical question that requires an answer. Some patients have complicated procedures with electrocardiographic changes and CPK-MB elevations. ECG-gated SPECT myocardial perfusion studies can quantitate LVEF, assess regional wall motion and thickening, and measure the amount of myocardium that has been injured. Other patients may have undergone recent procedures in preparation for a major noncardiac operation. Dependent on the extensiveness of the procedure and the angiographic results, perfusion imaging may be helpful in deciding on the advisability of proceeding with elective surgery. Finally, SPECT may be helpful in determining whether postprocedure chest pain is ischemic in origin. McPherson et al. [38] showed that direct coronary angiography in patients with recurrent chest pain in the first 4–6 weeks after coronary stenting was not very productive: almost half had no restenosis, side-branch compromise, new disease, or previously unrecognized CAD. Several studies have shown advantages of SPECT in this time frame, as compared to treadmill exercise testing. Milan et al. [52] reported on 37 patients with recurrent chest pain and equivocal treadmill tests: SPECT had positive and negative predictive values for angiographic restenosis of 81% and 86%, respectively.

Coronary flow reserve may be impaired very early after PTCA, so that minor reversible perfusion defects may not be diagnostic for acute reocclusion or early restenosis. Using sequential planar thallium-201 studies, Manyari et al. [39] demonstrated mild and transient perfusion defects at 9 days that normalized over the course of about 6 months. Importantly, however, these observations have not been substantiated by others, especially in the current era of PTCA where procedural success is often defined by techniques other than by anatomic catheterization data. On the contrary, Iskandrian et al. [40] studied 25 patients who underwent very early (4 ± 3 days) post-PTCA SPECT testing and had follow-up angiography. Images were normal in 17 and abnormal in 8 patients. Careful examination of the angiograms of the 8 cases with scan abnormalities revealed an anatomic explanation for all: 4 had residual stenosis either in a secondary branch or downstream; 2 had residual stenosis of the dilated region; 1 had local dissection; and 1 had a prior Q-wave infarction with a corresponding fixed defect. Several investigators have demonstrated that despite a reduced concordance of perfusion pattern with angiographic findings very early post-PTCA, the perfusion findings were highly predictive of late clinical and angiographic restenosis [41–46]. Hardoff et al. [41], for example, found that the predictive value of a pacing-induced perfusion defect within the first 24–48 hours after PTCA for ultimate restenosis was 56%, compared to a restenosis rate of only 10% in patients whose scan was normal. Similar results in relation to perfusion findings have been demonstrated for oral dipyridamole [42] in the very early post-PTCA time frame, and during the first few weeks after PTCA with exercise stress [43–46].

3–6 Months after PTCA

A more common time to assess for restenosis is after 3–6 months have passed since PTCA. Nobuyoshi et al. [47] showed that the majority of restenosis occurred by this time, regardless of recurrence of symptoms. Numerous studies and excellent reviews have evaluated myocardial perfusion scintigraphy in this time interval after PTCA [48–60]. The findings support its utility for detecting restenosis, its cost-effectiveness, its incremental value over treadmill testing and angiography, and its value for risk stratification and subsequent management decisions.

Hecht et al. [48] compared treadmill exercise testing and SPECT Tl-201 imaging for detecting restenosis in 116 patients a mean of 6 months after PTCA. About half the patients had multivessel PTCA, and about a quarter were incompletely revascularized. Sensitivity, specificity, and accuracy all favored SPECT: 93% versus 52%, 77% versus 64%, and 86% versus 57%, respectively. Furthermore, SPECT correctly localized restenosis to specific arteries with 86% accuracy.

In a companion study, Hecht et al. [49] examined the relative values of treadmill testing and SPECT in relation to symptom status post-PTCA. In this study, restenosis was angiographically proved in 61% of asymptomatic and 59% of symptomatic patients. SPECT accuracy for detecting restenosis and localizing it to a specific coronary artery was high and similar independent of symptoms. The investigation established what is well recognized today—that restenosis often occurs without angina despite its presence before PTCA, and that the exercise ECG is inaccurate in detecting silent restenosis.

Marie et al. [50] also examined the role of SPECT Tl-201 to detect asymptomatic restenosis. Sixty-two asymptomatic patients who had angina before PTCA were tested with SPECT and coronary angiography 6 months after PTCA. They concluded that asymptomatic restenosis occurs frequently, induces an amount of ischemia equivalent to that of symptomatic restenosis, and is better detected by exercise SPECT than by treadmill testing.

Radionuclides other than Tl-201 have also been assessed. Georgoulias et al. [51] studied 41 patients with technetium-99m (Tc-99m) tetrofosmin 6 months after PTCA. All underwent subsequent angiography: restenosis was present in 39% of patients and 35% of vessels. Sensitivity and specificity were 81% and 88% by patient, and 81% and 90% by specific vessel.

Milan et al. [52] evaluated the accuracy of Tc-99m-sestamibi in predicting restenosis. This study was in 37 patients with an equivocal symptom-limited treadmill test, all of whom had follow-up coronary angiography. It established high sensitivity and specificity for detecting restenosis of patients and specific vessels, even in this cohort with nondiagnostic treadmill tests.

A meta analysis of publications between 1975 and 2000 that examined the relative value of testing modalities at 6 months post-PTCA for the detection of restenosis has recently been reported [53]. This showed that the treadmill test has a poor sensitivity (46%, 95% confidence interval 33% to 58%) and a moderate specificity (77%). Nuclear perfusion imaging was much superior, with sensitivity 87% (95% CI 74% to 100%) and specificity 78% (95% CI 74% to 81%).

Late after PTCA

There has been little written about the value of SPECT imaging beyond approximately 6 months after PTCA. Ho et al. [61] studied the 7-year outcomes of 211 patients who underwent exercise Tl-201 SPECT between 1 and 3 years after PTCA. Events were rare—the 5-year survival was 95%. Univariate associations of cardiac death and nonfatal infarction were the summed stress score, the summed reversibility score, and the Duke Treadmill Score. The authors concluded that when there is an indication for stress testing late after PTCA, perfusion imaging provides superior risk stratification to treadmill testing.

Findings Common after Coronary Stenting

Stents have led to a substantial reduction in restenosis rates and are now very commonly performed. Knowledge that a percutaneous interventional procedure was performed using a stent rather than just balloon angioplasty is important to the interpreter of a myocardial perfusion scan. Side-branch compromise is a well-described occurrence, affecting as many as 20%–30% of procedures. Most often this affects septal perforators or diagonals when stents are placed into the proximal to mid left anterior descending artery (LAD). The appearance on a scan is typical, demonstrating ischemia of the anteroseptum and/or anterior/high lateral walls, but sparing the apex (Fig. 12.1). The apical sparing is the most reliable way to differentiate LAD side-branch "jailing" from stent restenosis. The same phenomenon can occur when the distal right coronary artery (RCA) is stented, such that a posterolateral or posterior descending vessel can be affected. Likewise, an obtuse branch or subbranch may be affected in that circulation. Clearly, specific knowledge of where stents were placed and the recognition during the procedure that side-branches were blocked is helpful to interpreting the meaning of scintigraphic findings. It is helpful to have the procedural report on hand at the time of report generation.

Several recent studies using Doppler flow probes or PET have shown that coronary flow and coronary flow reserve normalize very early after stenting. Kosa et al. [62], for example, showed that resting and hyperemic flows as assessed by PET were the same in stented as compared to remote areas very early after stenting. This may reflect the larger lumens and overall improved results of interventions when stents are used. One im-

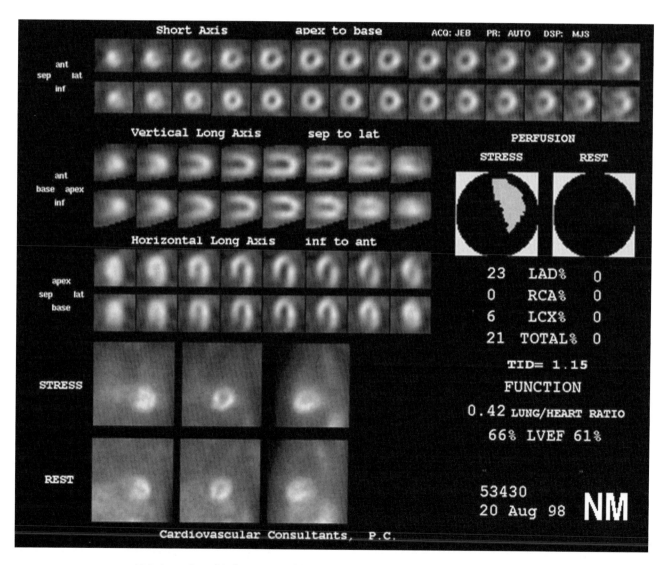

FIGURE 12.1 Anterolateral ischemia caused by diagonal side-branch "jailing" by a proximally placed LAD stent.

portant potential implication is that myocardial perfusion imaging may be more useful in the very early postprocedural time period to detect acute thrombosis after stenting than has been reported after PTCA.

The optimal time to assess for restenosis after stenting is not known. The pathophysiology of restenosis may be different than after balloon angioplasty, so that probably studies need to be undertaken to determine if the same 3–6 month postprocedure time is best. Some data might suggest that earlier imaging could be beneficial, as restenosis beyond 6 months is rare [63]. Milavetz et al. [64] evaluated 209 patients with SPECT, approximately 2.5 months after stenting. Sensitivity, specificity, positive and negative predictive values, and accuracy for stent restenosis (> 70%) were 95%, 73%, 88%, 89%, and 88%, respectively, in 33 patients who had quantitative coronary angiography.

ASSESSMENT AFTER CABG

The effectiveness of CABG as a treatment for extensive and life-threatening CAD is limited by two factors: the continued integrity of the bypass grafts, and the development of new CAD in nonbypassed areas or in the grafts themselves. ACC/AHA guidelines strongly endorse stress imaging as the method to assess appropriately selected patients post-CABG, rather than routine treadmill exercise testing, because of the added information about localizing ischemia and determining its extent [65]. SPECT studies post-CABG should all be interpreted with knowledge of pre-CABG anatomy, the vessels that were bypassed, and optimally with the actual angiographic and operative reports on hand. This information is critical to understanding the reasons for any abnormalities seen on the scan. Post-CABG abnormalities in perfusion may reflect any or a combination of nonrevascularized but diseased vessels; entrapped vessels; new disease; disease at or beyond anastomotic sites; or pathology of the grafts themselves (Table 12.4). The problem of entrapped regions leads to a "classic" SPECT finding of ischemia at the base of the heart in diagonal, septal, or both regions. This occurs when a proximal LAD stenosis limits antegrade flow into the LAD, and a midvessel stenosis limits retrograde flow despite a healthy bypass into the more distal LAD. One study suggests that this common scintigraphic finding is not prognostically worrisome [66].

Saphenous vein closure rates are disturbingly high early and especially late after CABG. Grondin et al. [67] reported that 12%–20% of grafts were closed by 1 year after CABG, that 2%–4% closed each year from

TABLE 12.4 *Potential Basis for Abnormal Perfusion Patterns in a Post-CABG SPECT Study*

Prior myocardial injury
New periprocedural myocardial injury
Graft disease
Stenoses downstream from graft anastomoses
Incomplete revascularization (side-branch disease, entrapped segments)
? Immature arterial conduits during first few weeks post-CABG

year 1 to year 5, and that about 50% of grafts were closed by 5 years after CABG. Others have also published closure rates of similar magnitude in the 5–10-year post-CABG time frame [68–70]. Unfortunately, neither the recurrence of chest pain nor the results of routine treadmill testing are particularly helpful in elucidating the basis or the severity of underlying problems, or the prognosis of patients after CABG [71–73].

Most often, SPECT imaging performed after CABG is for risk stratification, and determining whether coronary angiography would be advisable with a view toward prognostic improvement with further revascularization. However, several studies have addressed whether perfusion imaging could detect bypass graft stenoses or closure [74–79]. This is a potentially important objective of perfusion imaging, as at least one study has shown that patients with ischemia produced by atherosclerotic stenoses in vein grafts are at higher risk with medical therapy than are those whose ischemia is produced by native-vessel disease [80]. Rasmussen et al. [76] studied 41 patients with planar imaging 6 months after CABG, and reported a sensitivity of 71% and a specificity of 94% for graft closure. Pfisterer et al. [77] reported similar results in a second small study. More recently, Lakkis et al. [78] examined exercise SPECT's capability to imply graft patency based upon the perfusion pattern in the distribution of grafts. In 50 patients approximately 4 years after CABG and who had angiography within 3 weeks, 48 of 119 grafts were stenosed at least 50%. Tl-201 detected 40 (83%) of these. The sensitivity was higher than that of the exercise stress test in patients with both typical (84% vs 24%) and atypical (70% vs 50%) symptoms. In addition, sensitivity for individual grafts was 82% for the LAD, 92% for the RCA, and 75% for the left circumflex artery (LCX). Subsequently, Khoury et al. [79] demonstrated similar results using adenosine pharmacologic stress. They concluded that the results of adenosine Tl-201 SPECT were almost always abnormal in patients with late graft stenosis, and that false positive perfusion defects were most often due to either nonbypassed CAD or a previous myocardial infarction.

Early (First 2 Years) after CABG

Few studies have focused on assessing the potential value of myocardial perfusion imaging during the first few years after CABG. Miller et al. [66] followed up 411 patients for 5.8 years who had undergone exercise SPECT Tl-201 within 2 years after CABG. There were 53 cardiac deaths or myocardial infarctions and 22 late revascularization procedures. The only variable in multivariate analyses to show a statistically significant association with all three events was the number of abnormal thallium segments. The 5-year freedom from hard events varied from 93% for patients without angina and a SPECT scan that was normal or near normal, to 71% for those with angina and a medium or large perfusion defect. Additionally, ischemia proximal to bypass graft insertion was not predictive of cardiac death or nonfatal infarction. This study showed that Tl-201 imaging performed relatively early after CABG could provide clinically meaningful risk stratification.

Some observers have commented on false positive scans, although they are clinically infrequent, in the distribution of arterial bypass conduits early after CABG. Kubo et al. [81] recently reported on 23 patients who had SPECT before and within 4 weeks after CABG, and who also had post-CABG angiography that confirmed that all grafts were patent. Stress-induced reversible perfusion defects were present in 64% of segments bypassed by a patent arterial conduit. Clearly, this issue needs further investigation. The author's own clinical experience is not consistent with a high incidence of falsely positive LAD territory reversible perfusion defects early after left internal mammary artery (LIMA) bypass of the LAD.

Years 2 through 5 after CABG

Tc-99m-sestamibi imaging was performed in 75 patients at a mean of 38 months post-CABG in a study reported by Desideri et al. [82]. The summed reversibility score was the strongest scintigraphic predictor of events. The chi-square nearly doubled when this variable was added to clinical and treadmill test information.

Late (beyond 5 years) after CABG

A total of four studies have examined the contribution of SPECT imaging late after CABG to assessment of likelihood of major cardiac events. All have shown useful and incremental information over that of clinical assessment alone.

Palmas et al. [83] assessed the incremental prognostic value of SPECT Tl-201, beyond the information available from clinical and exercise test variables, performed late (> 5 years) after CABG. There were 20 cardiac deaths and 21 nonfatal infarctions in 294 patients, followed for a mean of 2.5 years. Dyspnea and peak exercise heart rate were independently predictive of events, as were two scintigraphic variables: the summed reversibility score and increased lung uptake of Tl-201. The global chi-square for predicting events doubled when the nuclear variables were combined with the clinical variables.

In a similar study by Nallamothu et al. [84], 255 patients a mean of 5 years after CABG underwent SPECT imaging and were then followed for 41 months. The size of any perfusion defects and the presence of abnormal lung uptake were independent predictors of event-free survival and added incrementally to combined clinical and stress test variables.

Lauer et al. [85] reported that SPECT imaging provided important prognostic information even in asymptomatic patients late after CABG. Among 873 patients followed for 3 years, those with perfusion defects were at higher risk for death (9% vs 3%) or major events (11% vs 4%) than were those without. Tl-201 perfusion defects and impaired exercise capacity were strong and independent predictors of subsequent death or nonfatal infarction. This investigation also emphasized that even asymptomatic patients late after CABG were a relatively high risk group: the annual mortality rate was 3%. This important Cleveland Clinic study concluded that current recommendations against routine screening of asymptomatic patients late after CABG should be reconsidered.

Most recently, Zellweger et al. [86] compared the prognostic significance of SPECT in patients early versus late after CABG. Among 1544 patients followed for at least 1 year, there were 53 cardiac deaths. Multivariate analysis identified age, summed difference score, and size of nonreversible defects as independent predictors of cardiac death. When analyzed according to time post-CABG, the study suggested that symptomatic patients < 5 years post-CABG and all patients > 5 years after CABG may benefit from testing.

ASSESSMENT AFTER NEWER METHODS OF REVASCULARIZATION

Despite the tremendous contribution of PCI and CABG to quality of life and longevity of many patients with CAD, a significant percentage of those with advanced CAD are not suitable candidates despite inadequacy of medical management. This reality has spawned efforts

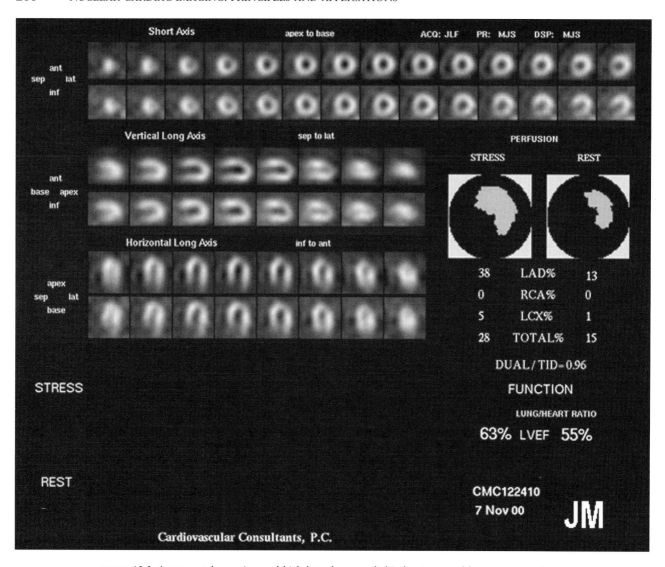

FIGURE 12.2 Anteroseptal, anterior, and high lateral myocardial ischemia caused by an entrapped segment of LAD in a post-CABG patient. Note that the apex is well perfused, implying a patent bypass graft. This pattern is caused by a left main or ostial LAD stenosis, with a second stenosis further downstream but above the attachment of the distal anastomosis. Both antegrade and retrograde perfusion of the entrapped segment is compromised.

to develop new approaches to revascularization. While none of these have yet reached the clinical mainstream, they do need validation both in terms of patient outcomes and scientific demonstration of improved myocardial perfusion. Radionuclide techniques have been called upon to provide data about their impact on perfusion, before and after intervention. Often this contribution begins in animal research and progresses through to Phase III clinical trials. Three examples are transmyocardial laser revascularization, external enhanced counterpulsation, and medical approaches to inducing angiogenesis.

In theory, a radionuclide approach for these purposes is ideal, as these provide the most quantitative information available from noninvasive tests with respect to pertinent variables such as myocardial flow or flow reserve, size and severity of defects, and changes over time. However, much is yet to be defined about the measurement variability of the tests themselves. For example, the ATLANTIC study used SPECT Tl-201 to compare the relative effects of laser therapy with traditional therapies in patients with symptomatic CAD [87]. In the 90 patients who had constant medical therapy, there were no changes in average percentage of ischemic myocardium, but on a patient-by-patient basis there was a variability that averaged 43%–55% of the baseline value. It is unclear how much of this variability relates to the specific radionuclide used, details of the imaging protocol or to the stressor, and to real changes in flow reserve despite no clinically apparent changes.

Transmyocardial laser revascularization (TMLR) appears to improve symptoms of refractory angina in selected patients [88,89]. The basis for its beneficial effects on anginal class is unclear and ranges from neuronal disruption to improved flow through creation of transmural left ventricular channels. Rimoldi et al. [90] used PET with 15-O-labeled water in seven patients to measure myocardial blood flow before, and at 2 and 9 months after TMLR performed with a carbon dioxide laser. Flow was measured at rest and after maximal intravenous dobutamine. Their study found no differences in either baseline or maximal flows in lasered areas despite an improvement in anginal class.

Al-Sheikh et al. [91] confirmed the lack of flow improvement at rest or after hyperemia, in eight patients studied with N-13 ammonia PET. However, they did demonstrate a significant increase in carbon-11 hydroxyephedrine (HED) uptake, suggesting that the benefit of TMLR is not increased perfusion but rather sympathetic denervation.

Hughes at al. [92] compared effects on swine myocardial blood flow before and 6 months after TMLR, using three different types of lasers. Their study suggested that improved perfusion occurred only with either carbon dioxide or holmium lasers, but not with the excimer laser. They concluded that differences in laser energy or wavelength or both may be important in induction of angiogenesis.

The mechanism by which enhanced external counterpulsation (EECP) therapy improves symptoms of chronic angina patients is also unknown. Masuda et al. [93] studied 11 patients who underwent 35 sessions, using N-13 ammonia PET at baseline and after dipyridamole stress. Both resting and hyperemic myocardial perfusion improved with therapy, and these improvements correlated with increased exercise time and time to 1 mm ST depression during exercise.

SPECT was used to assess myocardial perfusion in 14 humans before and at 30 and 60 days after intracoronary administration of recombinant human vascular endothelial growth factor (rhVEGF) [94]. A higher dose, compared to a lower dose, appeared to improve rest but not peak stress summed segmental scores. These results were discordant with those of Vale et al. [95] whose study did demonstrate in selected patients substantial 60-day improvements in both resting and peak perfusion.

CONCLUSIONS

SPECT myocardial perfusion imaging has evolved to become a diagnostic mainstay for assessing patients with known or suspected CAD. It is especially useful for assessing risk for major events, and therefore selecting those patients whose risk–benefit ratio is best served by medical versus interventional procedures. These decisions not only are important clinically they also have large societal cost implications. In those patients who do undergo interventions, follow-up is indicated based on the technique used, patient symptom status, perceived risk for subsequent problems, and time that has passed since the intervention.

REFERENCES

1. American Heart Association. 2000 Heart and Stroke Statistical Update. Dallas, Texas: American Heart Association, 1999.
2. Yusuf S, Zucker D, Peduzzi P, et al. Effect of coronary artery bypass graft surgery on survival: overview of 10-year results from randomized trials by the Coronary Artery Bypass Graft Surgery Trialists Collaboration. Lancet 1994; 344: 563.
3. Chaitman BR, Fisher LD, Bourassa MG, et al. Effect of coronary bypass surgery on survival patterns in subsets of patients with left main coronary artery disease. Am J Cardiol 1981; 48: 765.
4. Caracciolo EA, Davis KB, Sopko G, et al. Comparison of surgical and medical group survival in patients with left main equivalent coronary artery disease. Circulation 1995; 91: 2335.
5. Alderman EL, Bourassa MG, Cohen LS, et al. Ten-year follow-up of survival and myocardial infarction in the randomized CASS. Circulation 1990; 82: 1629.
6. Passami E, Davis KB, Gillespie MJ, et al. A randomized trial of coronary artery bypass surgery: survival of patients with low ejection fraction. N Engl J Med 1985; 312: 1665.
7. Kwok JM, Christian TF, Miller TD, et al. Identification of severe coronary artery disease in patients with a single abnormal coronary territory on exercise thallium-201 imaging: the importance of clinical and exercise variables. J Am Coll Cardiol 2000; 35: 335.
8. Bateman TM, O'Keefe JH Jr, Dong VM, et al. Coronary angiography rates following stress SPECT scintigraphy. J Nucl Cardiol 1995; 2: 217.
9. Nallamothu N, Pancholy SB, Lee KR, et al. Impact of exercise single-photon emission computed tomographic thallium imaging on patient management and outcome. J Nucl Cardiol 1995; 2: 334.
10. Hachamovitch R, Berman DS, Kiat H, et al. Exercise myocardial perfusion SPECT in patients without known coronary artery disease: incremental prognostic value and use in risk stratification. Circulation 1996; 93: 905.
11. Bateman TM. Clinical relevance of a normal stress-rest myocardial perfusion scintigraphic study: ASNC position paper. J Nucl Cardiol 1997; 4: 172.

12. Shaw LJ, Hachamovitch R, Berman DS, et al. The economic consequences of available diagnostic and prognostic strategies for the evaluation of stable angina patients. J Am Coll Cardiol 1999; 33: 661.

13. Iskandrian AS, Chae SC, Heo J, et al. Independent and incremental prognostic value of exercise single photon emission computed tomographic (SPECT) thallium imaging in coronary artery disease. J Am Coll Cardiol 1993; 22: 665.

14. Hachamovitch R, Berman DS, Shaw LJ, et al. Incremental prognostic value of myocardial perfusion single photon emission computed tomography for the prediction of cardiac death: differential stratification for risk of cardiac death and myocardial infarction. Circulation 1998; 97: 535.

15. Vancetto G, Ormezzano O, Fagret D, et al. Long-term prognostic value of thallium-201 myocardial perfusion imaging over clinical and exercise stress test in low to intermediate risk patients: study in 1137 patients with 6-year follow-up. Circulation 1999; 100: 1521.

16. O'Keefe JH, Bateman TM, Ligon RW, et al. Outcome of medical versus invasive treatment strategies for non-high risk ischemic heart disease. J Nucl Cardiol 1998; 5: 28.

17. Hlatky MA, Califf RM, Harrell FEJ, et al. Comparison of predictions based on observational data with the results of randomized controlled clinical trials of coronary artery bypass surgery. J Am Coll Cardiol 1988;11:237.

18. Mulbaier LH, Pryor DB, Rankin JS, et al. Observational comparison of event-free survival with medical and surgical therapy in patients with coronary artery disease. Circulation 1992;86(Suppl II): 198.

19. Parisi AF, Folland ED, Hartigan P. A comparison of angioplasty and medical therapy in the treatment of single vessel coronary artery disease. N Engl J Med 1992; 326: 10.

20. Parisi AF, Hartigan PM, Folland ED. Evaluation of exercise thallium scintigraphy versus exercise electrocardiography in predicting survival outcomes and morbid cardiac events in patients with single and double-vessel disease. Findings from the Angioplasty Compared to Medicine (ACME) Study. J Am Coll Cardiol 1997; 30: 1256.

21. RITA-2 trial participants. Coronary angioplasty versus medical therapy for angina: the second Randomized Intervention Treatment of Angina (RITA-2) trial. Lancet 1997; 350: 461.

22. Bourassa MG, Pepine CJ, Forman SA, et al. Asymptomatic Cardiac Ischemia Pilot (ACIP) study: effects of coronary angioplasty and coronary artery bypass graft surgery on recurrent angina and ischemia. J Am Coll Cardiol 1995; 26: 606.

23. Pitt B, Waters D, Brown WV, et al. Aggressive lipid-lowering therapy compared with angioplasty in stable coronary artery disease. N Engl J Med 1999; 341: 70.

24. Cuocolo A, Nicolai E, Petretta M, et al. One-year effect of myocardial revascularization on resting left ventricular function and regional thallium uptake in chronic CAD. J Nucl Cardiol 1997; 38:1684.

25. Li S, Liu X, Lu Z, et al. Quantitative analysis of technetium-99m-2-methoxyisobutyl isonitrile single photon emission computed tomography and isosorbide dinitrate infusion in assessment of myocardial viability before and after revascularization. J Nucl Cardiol 1996; 3: 457.

26. Califf RM, Harrell FEJ, Lee KL, et al. The evolution of medical and surgical therapy for coronary artery disease: a 15-year perspective. JAMA 1989; 261: 2077.

27. Myers WO, Gersh BJ, Fisher LD, et al. Medical versus early surgical therapy in patients with triple-vessel disease and mild angina pectoris: a CASS registry study of survival. Ann Thorac Surg 1987;44:471.

28. Myers WO, Schaff HV, Gersh BJ, et al. Improved survival of surgically treated patients with triple vessel coronary artery disease and severe angina pectoris: a report from the Coronary Artery Surgery Study (CASS) registry. J Thorac Cardiovasc Surg 1989;97:487.

29. Scott SM, Deupree RH, Sharma GV, et al. VA Study of Unstable Angina: 10-year results show duration of surgical advantage for patients with impaired ejection fraction. Circulation 1994;90 Suppl II:120.

30. Scott SM, Luchi RJ, Deupree RH. Veterans Administration Cooperative Study for treatment of patients with unstable angina: results in patients with abnormal left ventricular function. Circulation 1988;78 Suppl I:113.

31. Sharir T, Germano G, Kavanagh PB, et al. Incremental prognostic value of post-stress left ventricular ejection fraction and volume by gated myocardial perfusion single photon emission computed tomography. Circulation 1999; 100: 1035.

32. Ritchie JL, Narahara KA, Trobaugh GB, et al. Thallium-201 myocardial imaging before and after coronary revascularization. Circulation 1977; 56: 830.

33. Verani MS, Marcus ML, Ehrhardt JC, et al. Thallium-201 myocardial perfusion imaging in the evaluation of saphenous aortocoronary bypass graft surgery. J Nucl Med 1978; 19: 765.

34. Hirzel HO, Nuesch K, Sialer G, et al. Thallium-201 exercise myocardial imaging to evaluate myocardial perfusion after coronary artery bypass surgery. Br Heart J 1980; 43: 426.

35. Ritchie JL, Bateman TM, Bonow RO, et al. ACC/AHA Guidelines for Clinical Use of Cardiac Radionuclide Imaging. J Am Coll Cardiol 1995; 25: 521.

36. Gibbons RJ, Chatterjee K, Daley J, et al. ACC/AHA/ACP-ASIM Guidelines for the Management of Patients with Chronic Stable Angina. J Am Coll Cardiol 1999; 33: 2092.

37. Smith JC, Dove JT, Jacobs AK, et al. ACC/AHA Guidelines for Percutaneous Coronary Intervention. Circulation 2001; 103: 3019.

38. McPherson JA, Robinson PS, Powers ER, et al. Angiographic findings in patients undergoing catheterization for recurrent symptoms within 30 days of successful coronary intervention. Am J Cardiol 1999; 84: 589.

39. Manyari DE, Knudtson M, Kloiber R, et al. Sequential thallium-201 myocardial perfusion studies after successful percutaneous transluminal coronary angioplasty: delayed resolution of exercise-induced scintigraphic abnormalities. Circulation 1988; 77: 86.

40. Iskandrian AS, Lemlek J, Ogilby JD, et al. Early thallium imaging after percutaneous transluminal coronary angioplasty: tomographic evaluation during adenosine-induced coronary hyperemia. J Nucl Med 1992; 33: 2086.

41. Hardoff R, Shefer A, Gips S, et al. Predicting late restenosis after coronary angioplasty by very early (12 to 24 h) thallium-201 scintigraphy: implications with regard to mechanisms of late coronary restenosis. J Am Coll Cardiol 1990; 15: 1486.

42. Jain A, Mahmarian JJ, Borges-Neto S, et al. Clinical significance of perfusion defects by thallium-201 single photon emission tomography following oral dipyridamole early after coronary angioplasty. J Am Coll Cardiol 1988; 11: 970.

43. Lewis BS, Hardoff R, Merdler A, et al. Importance of immediate and very early postprocedural angiographic and thallium-201 single photon emission computed tomographic perfusion measurements in predicting late results after coronary intervention. Am Heart J 1995; 130: 425.

44. Breisblatt WM, Weiland FL, Spaccavento LJ. Stress thallium-201 imaging after coronary angioplasty predicts restenosis and recurrent symptoms. J Am Coll Cardiol 1988; 12: 1199.

45. Pfisterer M, Rickenbacher P, Kiowski W, et al. Silent ischemia

after percutaneous transluminal coronary angioplasty: incidence and prognostic significance. J Am Coll Cardiol 1993; 22: 1446.

46. Wijns W, Serruys PW, Reiber JH, et al. Early detection of restenosis after successful percutaneous transluminal coronary angioplasty by exercise-redistribution thallium scintigraphy. Am J Cardiol 1985; 55: 357.

47. Nobuyoshi M, Kimura T, Nosaka H, et al. Restenosis after successful percutaneous transluminal coronary angioplasty: serial angiographic follow-up of 229 patients. J Am Coll Cardiol 1988; 12: 616.

48. Hecht H, Shaw R, Bruce RT, et al. Usefulness of tomographic thallium-201 imaging for detection of restenosis after percutaneous transluminal coronary angioplasty. Am J Cardiol 1990; 6: 1314.

49. Hecht HS, Shaw RE, Chin HL, et al. Silent ischemia after coronary angioplasty: evaluation of restenosis and extent of ischemia in asymptomatic patients by tomographic thallium-201 exercise imaging and comparison with symptomatic patients. J Am Coll Cardiol 1991; 17: 670.

50. Marie PY, Danchin N, Karcher G, et al. Usefulness of exercise SPECT thallium to detect asymptomatic restenosis in patients who had angina before coronary angioplasty. Am Heart J 1993; 126: 571.

51. Georgoulias P, Demakopoulos N, Kontos A, et al. Tc-99m tetrofosmin myocardial perfusion imaging before and six months after percutaneous transluminal coronary angioplasty. Clin Nucl Med 1998; 23: 678.

52. Milan E, Zoccarato O, Terzi A, et al. Technetium-99m-sestamibi SPECT to detect restenosis after successful percutaneous coronary angioplasty. J Nucl Med 1996; 37: 1300.

53. Garzon PP, Eisenberg MJ. Functional testing for the detection of restenosis after percutaneous transluminal coronary angioplasty: a meta-analysis. Can J Cardiol 2001; 17: 41.

54. Mishra J, Iskandrian AE. Stress myocardial perfusion imaging after coronary angioplasty. Am J Cardiol 1998; 81: 766.

55. Herzel HO, Nuesch K, Gruentzig AR, et al. Short and long-term changes in myocardial perfusion after percutaneous transluminal coronary angioplasty assessed by thallium-201 exercise scintigraphy. Circulation 1981; 63: 1001.

56. Rosing DR, VanRaden MJ, Mincemoyer RM, et al. Exercise, electrocardiographic and functional responses after percutaneous transluminal coronary angioplasty. Am J Cardiol 1984; 53: 36C.

57. Scholl JM, Chaitman BR, David PR, et al. Exercise electrocardiography and myocardial scintigraphy in the serial evaluation of the results of percutaneous transluminal coronary angioplasty. Circulation 1982; 66: 380.

58. Alazraki P, Krawczynska EG. Thallium imaging in management of post-revascularization patients. Q J Nucl Med 1996; 40: 85.

59. Miller DD, Liu P, Strauss HW, et al. Prognostic value of computer-quantitated exercise thallium imaging early after percutaneous transluminal coronary angioplasty. J Am Coll Cardiol 1987; 10: 275.

60. Miller DD, Verani MS. Current status of myocardial perfusion imaging after percutaneous transluminal coronary angioplasty. J Am Coll Cardiol 1994; 24: 260.

61. Ho KT, Miller TD, Holmes DR, et al. Long-term prognostic value of Duke treadmill score and exercise thallium-201 imaging performed one to three years after percutaneous transluminal coronary angioplasty. Am J Cardiol 1999; 84: 1323.

62. Kosa I, Blasini R, Schneider-Eicke J, et al. Early recovery of coronary flow reserve after stent implantation as assessed by positron emission tomography. J Am Coll Cardiol 1999; 34: 1036.

63. Kimura T, Yokoi H, Nakagawa Y, et al. Three-year follow-up after implantation of metallic coronary artery stents. N Engl J Med 1996; 334: 561.

64. Milavetz JJ, Miller TD, Hodge DO, et al. Accuracy of single-photon emission computed tomography myocardial perfusion imaging in patients with stents in native coronary arteries. Am J Cardiol 1998; 82: 857.

65. Eagle KA, Guyton RA, Davidoff R, et al. ACC/AHA Guidelines for Coronary Artery Bypass Graft Surgery. J Am Coll Cardiol 1999; 34: 1262.

66. Miller TD, Christian TF, Hodge DO, et al. Prognostic value of exercise thallium-201 imaging performed within 2 years of coronary artery bypass graft surgery. J Am Coll Cardiol 1998; 31: 848.

67. Grondin CM, Campeau L, Thornton JC, et al. Coronary artery bypass grafting with saphenous vein. Circulation 1989; 79 Suppl I: 24.

68. Lytle BW, Loop FD, Cosgrove DM, et al. Long-term (5 to 12 years) serial studies of internal mammary artery and saphenous vein coronary bypass grafts. J Thorac Cardiovasc Surg 1985; 89: 248.

69. Bourassa MG. Fate of venous grafts: the past, the present and the future. J Am Coll Cardiol 1991; 17: 1081.

70. Fitzgibbon GM, Leach AJ, Kafka HP, et al. Coronary bypass graft fate: long-term angiographic study. J Am Coll Cardiol 1991; 17: 1075.

71. Dubach P, Froelicher V, Klein J, et al. Use of the exercise test to predict prognosis after coronary artery bypass grafting. Am J Cardiol 1989; 63 530.

72. Yli-Mayrry S, Huikuri HV, Airaksinen J, et al. Usefulness of a postoperative exercise test for predicting cardiac events after coronary artery bypass grafting. Am J Cardiol 1992; 70: 56.

73. Weiner DA, Ryan RJ, Parsons L, et al. Prevalence and prognostic significance of silent and symptomatic ischemia after coronary artery bypass surgery: a report from the Coronary Artery Surgery Study (CASS) randomized population. J Am Coll Cardiol 1991; 18: 343.

74. Ritchie JL, Narahara KA, Trobaugh GB, et al. Thallium-201 myocardial imaging before and after coronary revascularization: assessment of regional myocardial blood flow and graft patency. Circulation 1977; 56: 830.

75. Fioretti P, Reijs AE, Neumann D, et al. Improvement in transient and persistent perfusion defects on early and late postexercise thallium-201 tomograms after coronary artery bypass grafting. Eur Heart J 1988; 9:1332.

76. Rasmussen SL, Nielsen SL, Amtorp O, et al. Thallium-201 imaging as an indicator of graft patency after coronary artery bypass surgery. Eur Heart J 1984; 5: 494.

77. Pfisterer M, Emmenegger H, Schmitt HE, et al. Accuracy of serial myocardial perfusion scintigraphy with thallium-201 for prediction of graft patency early and late after coronary artery bypass surgery. Circulation 1982; 66: 1017.

78. Lakkis NM, Mahmarian JJ, Verani MS. Exercise thallium-201 single photon emission computed tomography for evaluation of coronary artery bypass graft patency. Am J Cardiol 1995: 76: 107.

79. Khoury AF, Rivera JM, Mahmarian JJ, et al. Adenosine thallium-201 tomography in evaluation of graft patency late after coronary artery bypass graft surgery. J Am Coll Cardiol 1997; 29: 1290.

80. Lytle BW, Loop FD, Taylor PC, et al. Vein-graft disease: the clinical impact of stenoses in saphenous vein bypass grafts to coronary arteries. J Thorac Cardiovasc Surg 1992; 103: 831.

81. Kubo S, Tadamura E, Kudoh T, et al. Assessment of the effect of revascularization early after CABG using ECG-gated perfusion single photon emission computed tomography. Eur J Nucl Med 2001; 28: 230.

82. Desideri A, Candelpergher G, Zanco P, et al. Exercise technetium-99m sestamibi single-photon emission computed tomography late after coronary artery bypass surgery: long-term follow-up. Clin Cardiol 1997; 20: 779.

83. Palmas W, Bingham S, Diamond GA, et al. Incremental prognostic value of exercise thallium-201 myocardial single photon emission computed tomography late after coronary artery bypass surgery. J Am Coll Cardiol 1995; 25: 403.

84. Nallamothu N, Johnson JH, Bagheri B, et al. Utility of stress single-photon emission computed tomography (SPECT) perfusion imaging in predicting outcome after coronary artery bypass grafting. Am J Cardiol 1997; 80: 1517.

85. Lauer MS, Lytle B, Pashkow F, et al. Prediction of death and myocardial infarction by screening with exercise thallium testing after coronary artery bypass grafting. Lancet 1998; 351: 615.

86. Zellweger MJ, Lewin HC, Lai S, et al. When to stress patients after coronary artery bypass surgery. J Am Coll Cardiol 2001; 37: 144.

87. Burkhoff D, Jones JW, Becker LC. Variability of myocardial perfusion defects assessed by thallium-201 scintigraphy in patients with coronary artery disease not amenable to angioplasty or bypass surgery. J Am Coll Cardiol 2001; 38: 1033.

88. Spertus JA, Jones PG, Coen M, et al. Transmyocardial CO2 laser revascularization improves symptoms, function, and quality of life: 12-month results from a randomized controlled trial. Am J Med 2001; 111: 341.

89. Horvath KA, Aranki SF, Cohn LH, et al. Sustained angina relief 5 years after transmyocardial laser revascularization with a CO2 laser. Circulation 2001; 104: I81.

90. Rimoldi O, Burns SM, Rosen SD, et al. Measurement of myocardial blood flow with positron emission tomography before and after transmyocardial laser revascularization. Circulation 1999; 100: II 134.

91. Al-Sheikh T, Allen KB, Straka SP, et al. Cardiac sympathetic denervation after transmyocardial laser revascularization. Circulation 1999; 100: 135.

92. Hughes GC, Kypson AP, Annex BH, et al. Induction of angiogenesis after TMR: a comparison of holmium YAG, CO2, and excimer lasers. Ann Thorac Surg 2000; 70: 504.

93. Masuda D, Nohara R, Hirai T, et al. Enhanced external counterpulsation improved myocardial perfusion and coronary flow reserve in patients with chronic stable angina: evaluation by (13)N-ammonia positron emission tomography. Eur Heart J 2001; 16: 1451.

94. Hendel RC, Henry TD, Rocha-Singh K, et al. Effect of intracoronary recombinant human vascular endothelial growth factor on myocardial perfusion: evidence for a dose-dependent effect. Circulation 2000; 101: 118.

95. Vale PR, Losordo DW, Milliken CE, et al. Left ventricular electromechanical mapping to assess efficacy of phVEGF (165) gene transfer for therapeutic angiogenesis in chronic myocardial ischemia. Circulation 2000; 102: 965.

13 | Diagnosis and risk assessment in women

LYNNE L. JOHNSON

The status of women in society has changed from decade to decade since the end of the Second World War. While the image of the housewife in ruffled apron has been replaced by the working mom juggling her job with soccer games, dance lessons, and dinner preparation, the perception of women's health and health issues has also changed. The first conference sponsored by the AHA on women and heart disease was 35 years ago. The purpose of the conference was to instruct wives on how to take care of their husbands' hearts. In 1989 the AHA held its first conference dealing with heart disease in women. Over the past decade scientific information on incidence and manifestations of coronary artery disease (CAD) in women has burgeoned as the incidence of coronary heart disease in women has increased [1]. In 1979 cardiovascular disease (CVD) mortality was lower for women than for men [1]. In 1984 the CVD mortality for women exceeded that for men and the difference has continued to grow and is now the leading cause of death in women in the United States. The lifetime mortality risk from CVD is 10 times greater than for breast cancer. Despite these data there continues to be a disconnection between facts and public perceptions. A Gallup poll conducted in 1995 found that four out of five women and one out of three primary care physicians thought that breast cancer was a greater threat to women than CVD [1].

EVALUATION OF CHEST PAIN IN WOMEN

Contributing to the underappreciation of the importance of CAD in women are gender differences in age distribution of disease onset, relative risk factor importance, and nature of chest pain. Because of the antiatherosclerotic effects of endogenous estrogens through the menopause there is about a 10-year delay in onset of disease in women compared to men. However, the relative protection of endogenous estrogens is completely negated by diabetes. From the National Health and Nutrition Examination Survey (NHANES) study of coronary risk factors, diabetes confers a relative risk of 2.4 for women compared to 1.9 for men [2]. The incidence of insulin resistance and impaired glucose tolerance increases with age and with obesity, and since the population is aging and getting heavier the incidence of impaired glucose tolerance has continued to increase in the United States over the past 50 years. These trends will lead to an increasing number of premenopausal women with CAD. From the same epidemiological study, hypertension imparts a similar risk for men and women, hypercholesterolemia a slightly higher risk for men, and cigarette smoking a slightly higher risk for women [2].

In addition to differences in the relative importance of traditional risk factors between men and women there are also differences in presentation of CAD between men and women. Women are more likely to present with chest pain and men with myocardial infarction or sudden death [3]. Although CAD is usually first manifest by chest pain in women, the nature of the pain is frequently not "classic" and can lead to misdiagnosis [4]. Angina in women is more likely to occur with emotional or mental stress or during sleep [5]. Conversely, of the women with classic angina pectoris who underwent coronary angiography in the Coronary Artery Surgery Study (CASS) study, only 72% had documented CAD [6]. Many of these women with typical angina and normal coronary angiograms may have true ischemia without epicardial coronary artery narrowing due to spasm, endothelial dysfunction, or myocardial metabolic abnormalities as demonstrated by magnetic resonance (MR) spectroscopy in the Women's Ischemia Syndrome Evaluation (WISE) study [7].

According to Bayesian principles, disease prevalence determines predictive accuracy. In the evaluation of chest pain, the greatest benefit from the results of an imaging test comes in patients with a moderate pretest probability (20% to 70%). Based on differences in age of disease

271

onset, risk factor importance, and nature of chest pain, different criteria must be applied to women in determining pretest probability for test ordering [8] (Fig. 13.1). A woman with moderate risk will be older than a man, may have more atypical features of chest pain, and hypertension or cigarette smoking. A diabetic woman of any age is at moderate to high risk. For cost-effective patient management the initial test must be the least expensive to provide the highest diagnostic accuracy. In a man with normal resting 12-lead ECG and moderate pretest probability, the treadmill ECG stress test is recommended as the first screening test. In women the choice of the initial test is more problematic. Exercise-induced ST-depression has been reported to have both reduced specificity and sensitivity in women when compared to men [9–12]. Values for sensitivity to detect CAD in women vary from 48% to 89% and for specificity from 63% to 93% [12]. In the AHA/ACC published guidelines for exercise testing the conclusion drawn from meta analysis of 11, 691 patients is that the "true diagnostic value of the exercise ECG lies in its relatively high specificity. Diagnostic accuracy of the treadmill test in women may be increased by using the Duke Treadmill Score, an index based on ST-segment deviation, treadmill time, and presence of angina during exercise [13].

There are several approaches to diagnosing women with chest pain. The first is to perform treadmill testing on all women as a first test and then proceeding to imaging in those with abnormal ECG thought to be false positive—no greater than 1 mm depression at peak with rapid reversion early in recovery. Another approach is to perform stress perfusion imaging as the first test in all women. A third approach would be to go directly to coronary angiography as the first diagnostic test. When compared to coronary angiography the approach of performing stress perfusion imaging as the first screening test to evaluate women with stable chest pain for presence or absence of CAD has been shown to be more cost-effective [14]. Data from seven clinical sites comprising 4638 women were divided into women referred directly to diagnostic coronary angiography and women referred first to stress perfusion imaging followed by diagnostic angiography in those with reversible perfusion defects. Composite cost per patient including follow-up medical care was lower for patients undergoing myocardial perfusion imaging first.

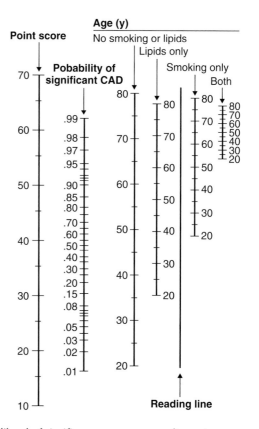

Directions for use

1. Calculate the history–EKG point score and locate score on left-hand scale.

2. Using the appropriate age scale, extrapolate to the reading line.

3. Place a ruler between the point score and age (*moved to the reading line*).

4. Read the probability of significant CAD on the center scale.

History–EKG point score

Chest pain
   Typical 26
   Atypical 10
   Nonanginal 0

Previous myocardial infarction
   History only 26
   EKG Q waves 10
   Both..0
   EKG ST–T wave changes 6
   Diabetes mellitus...................................7

FIGURE 13.1 Nomogram for estimating the likelihood of significant coronary artery disease in women. CAD, coronary artery disease; EKG, electrocardiogram. (Adapted from Pryor DB, Harell FE, Lee KL, et al. Estimating the likelihood of significant coronary artery disease. Am J Med 1983;75:771–780.)

DIAGNOSTIC ACCURACY OF TREADMILL STRESS PERFUSION IMAGING IN WOMEN

Until the mid-1990s reports of the diagnostic accuracy for single-photon emission computed tomography (SPECT) perfusion imaging compared to coronary angiography included relatively small numbers of women [15]. Several studies did, however, focus on the diagnostic accuracy of SPECT thallium imaging in women. Chae and coworkers evaluated the value of exercise thallium imaging to identify women with high-risk coronary anatomy including left main and multivessel disease [16]. By univariate analysis, factors that predicted high-risk anatomy included older age, lower workload, lower peak heart rate achieved, and diabetes. By multivariate analysis, only perfusion defects in multiple vascular territories and low exercise heart rate were predictive. Hansen and coworkers pointed out a technical limitation of thallium SPECT imaging in women [17]. These investigators compared the diagnostic accuracy of stress thallium imaging in men and women. Using receiver operator curve (ROC) analysis they compared both men versus women and small hearts versus large hearts for both sexes. They found that diagnostic accuracy was lower in women than in men and the difference was explained by the smaller heart sizes in women. The authors attributed this reduced accuracy in smaller hearts to spatial resolution, blurring due to cardiac motion, and to filtered backprojection. They also proposed that technetium-based perfusion tracers may have better accuracy because of the higher energy of the technetium photons with less scatter and blurring. A more recent retrospective report on SPECT thallium stress perfusion imaging in women by Iskandrian et al. included 489 women and 727 men who underwent either exercise or adenosine thallium SPECT imaging and coronary angiography plus 117 women and 74 men with low probability [12]. Sensitivity for detecting CAD was significantly lower in women than for men for both exercise (72% vs 92%) and for adenosine stress (84% vs 94%). Explanations given by the authors for these gender differences included undercall of mild defects in the presence of breast artifacts, underappreciation of the true incidence of CAD in women, and lower workloads and heart rates achieved by women compared to men. The smaller hearts of women, as shown by Hansen [17], and the relatively high scatter and attenuation of thallium should also be considered.

These reports of reduced diagnostic accuracy of SPECT thallium in women may be due, at least in part, to the properties of the tracer. This hypothesis is supported by a subsequent study reported by Taillefer and colleagues who compared the diagnostic accuracy of thallium-201 (Tl-201) and Tc-99m-sestamibi SPECT imaging in detecting CAD in women [18] (Fig. 13.2). The study group comprised 85 women who underwent stress perfusion imaging studies with Tl-201 and with Tc-99m-sestamibi and coronary angiography and 30 low-likelihood volunteers. The sensitivity and specificity values for thallium SPECT reported in this study are similar to those reported by Iskandrian et al. [12] (sensitivity 75% vs 72%, specificity 62% vs 69%). In the Taillefer study there was no difference in sensitivity for detected disease between the two tracers; however, the specificity for Tc-99m-sestamibi was higher for detecting lesions > 70% (58.8% for Tl-201 and 82.4% for Tc-99m-sestamibi). When analysis of the gated images was added, the specificity further improved. Breast artifacts when present usually appear as fixed anterior or septal defects. The presence of normal anterior wall motion and wall thickening on the gated images identified defects due to breast attenuation artifact (Figs. 13.3 and 13.4).

Another technical advance that shows promise for further improving the diagnostic accuracy of stress perfusion imaging in women is attenuation correction. Initial efforts to develop the technology to correct for the nonuniform attenuation in the thorax using triple-detector systems and fan beam collimator led to false defects from truncation artifacts. A more successful camera configuration is a two-headed camera with the detectors

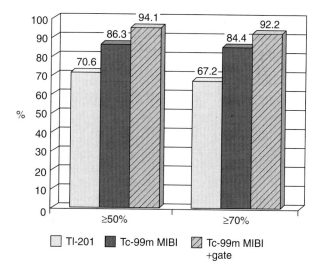

FIGURE 13.2 Specificity for Tl-201 SPECT (speckled bars), Tc-99m-sestamibi SPECT (solid gray bars), and Tc-99m gated SPECT (striped bars) for detecting coronary lesions ≥ 50% (*left*) and ≥ 70% (*right*). (Adapted from Taillefer R, DePuey EG, Udelson J, et al. Comparative diagnostic accuracy of thallium-201 and tc-99m sestamibi (perfusion and gated SPECT) in detecting coronary artery disease in women. J Am Coll Cardiol 1997; 29:69.

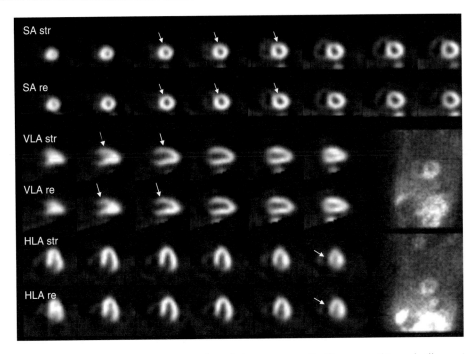

FIGURE 13.3 Reconstructed SPECT images from 2-day stress–rest Tc-99m-sestamibi treadmill exercise in 58-year-old woman with chest pain. The projection images in right lower corner show breast artifact, and reconstructed slices show fixed mild anterior perfusion defect (arrows). SA = short axis; VLA = vertical long axis; HLA = horizontal long axis; str = stress; re = rest.

mounted at right angles and opposite lead-lined moving bars housing solid sources such as gadolinium-153 (Gd-153) [19]. For each step the solid transmission source moves across the field of view. The detectors record simultaneously both emission data from the patient and transmission data from the moving source. This allows generation of a patient-specific attenuation map that can be used to correct the emission data. Scatter correction and depth-dependent resolution compensation algorithms are also applied. One multicenter study describing sensitivity and specificity of this technology using early hardware and software design has been reported [19]. These results should not be applied to more updated systems that have improved the attenuation maps. A sin-

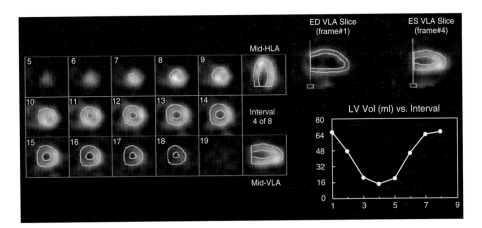

FIGURE 13.4 Gated SPECT data from same patient as in Figure 13.3. Short axis and representative HLA and VLA show normal wall thickening. The white outlines identify end-systole. The presence of normal anterior wall motion in the presence of mild fixed anterior perfusion defect in this woman indicates that the defect is due to breast attenuation artifact and not to anterior scar.

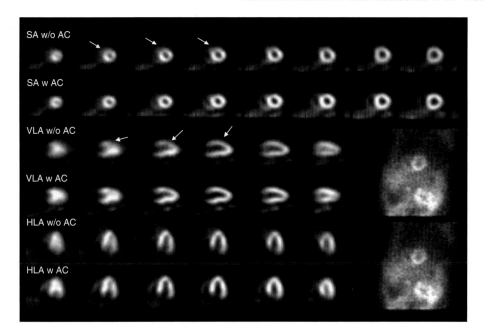

FIGURE 13.5 Reconstructed SPECT images from a 60-year-old woman with risk factors being evaluated for chest pain. She underwent a Tc-99m-sestamibi treadmill stress protocol. Images were acquired with and without attenuation correction. The top row of each pair is from the noncorrected study (without attenuation correction) and the bottom row of each pair is from the corrected study (with attenuation correction). The projection images in the right lower corner show a prominent breast artifact. The uncorrected images show an anterior wall defect (arrows). The study corrected for attenuation shows normal perfusion. Based on these results the patient did not return for the rest study.

gle-site study using attenuation hardware and software (Vantage Pro, ADAC, Milpitas, CA) in a stress-only protocol has been reported recently [20]. In this study 652 medium probability patients (428 females) were referred for chest pain evaluation. They underwent stress sestamibi perfusion imaging using attenuation correction as part of a 2-day protocol, had scans interpreted as normal with the aid of attenuation corection (AC) (correction for breast and diaphragmatic artifacts) and did not return for the second-day rest scan (Fig. 13.5). Clinical follow-up was performed as a surrogate for a determination of normalcy. Over 23 ± 6 months follow-up there were two noncardiac deaths, one nonfatal MI, and three patients with unstable angina, giving the overall cardiac event rate of 0.6%. These results support the safety and usefulness of the stress-only protocol using Tc-99m-sestamibi and attenuation correction as a cost-effective diagnostic tool in women with chest pain.

PHARMACOLOGIC STRESS TESTING IN WOMEN

Because of the clinically important additional information provided by treadmill parameters such as exercise performance, combining perfusion imaging with exer-cise stress is advisable in as many patients as possible. Patients who are unable to exercise longer than several minutes on the treadmill must undergo pharmacologic stress testing. A high percentage of elderly women are unable to exercise due to musculoskeletal disorders, neurological disease, or general debility and therefore comprise many of the patients referred to a nuclear laboratory for pharmacologic stress testing. The choice of drugs include dipyridamole, adenosine, and dobutamine. Until there are further published data available on the diagnostic accuracy of dobutamine perfusion imaging it is recommended that this mode of stress be reserved for patients with reactive airways disease who are unable to walk on the treadmill. The diagnostic accuracy for dipyridamole imaging was compared in 43 consecutive women and 71 consecutive men undergoing planar Tl-201 imaging and coronary angiography by Kong et al. They found a lower sensitivity for detecting single-vessel disease in women than in men but no difference in detecting multivessel disease [21]. In a more recent study looking only at women Amanullah and coworkers evaluated the diagnostic accuracy of dual-isotope adenosine SPECT imaging in 201 women with either low likelihood for disease or with recent coronary angiography [22]. They found a high normalcy rate (93%) and sensitivity, specificity, and diagnostic accuracy for identifying > 50% stenoses of 93%, 78%, and 88%, respectively.

Because elderly women comprise a large number of patients undergoing pharmacologic stress testing and increasing incidence of multivessel disease with age, several groups of investigators looked at the diagnostic accuracy of pharmacologic stress testing to identify left main or multivessel disease. Travin and coworkers found no significant difference in the accuracy of dipyridamole Tc-99m-sestamibi SPECT to identify multivessel disease in men (71%) and women (64%) [23]. Amanullah and coworkers performed univariate and multivariate analysis on clinical and scan data from 130 women who underwent adenosine Tc-99m-sestamibi SPECT to look at the value of the scan to identify extensive CAD [24]. The only independent predictor of severe or extensive CAD was the summed stress score.

PROGNOSTIC VALUE OF STRESS PERFUSION IMAGING IN WOMEN

There are several strategies besides stress imaging for evaluating a female patient with suspected or known CAD including treadmill ECG stress testing for lower probability patients and proceeding directly to coronary angiography for higher-risk patients. In selecting a strategy an important factor to consider is additional information regarding prognosis provided by stress imaging modalities, especially stress perfusion imaging. With a single testing procedure the diagnosis of flow limiting CAD can be confirmed or excluded with a fairly high degree of certainty and at the same time the event-free survival can be estimated based on the severity and extent of the stress defect. These data can provide important additional information to help the clinician decide between medical therapy and revascularization.

The benign prognosis associated with a normal stress perfusion scan has been well documented in studies comprising both males and females and summarized by Brown in a review [25]. Several studies directly compared the incremental prognostic value of stress perfusion imaging in men versus women [26–29]. The event-free survival for a woman with a normal scan is similar in all three of these studies and is in the range of 0.8% to 1% over 2–3 years. The majority of patients reported in these studies underwent sestamibi imaging either as a 1-day or dual-isotope protocol and underwent either treadmill or dipyridamole stress testing. Several studies have examined the prognostic value of a normal scan with pharmacologic stress testing in women. Another study followed 80 women for a mean of 23 months af-

ter 2-day stress–rest sestamibi dobutamine stress perfusion imaging. The cohort included women with low and medium probability as well as documented CAD. The investigators found only two soft events and no hard events [30]. In another study, Amanullah and coworkers followed 462 women with normal dual-isotope adenosine SPECT perfusion imaging for a mean of 26 months and found rates for cardiac death of 0.8% and for nonfatal MI of 0.5% [31]. Although it appears that a normal scan confers a good prognosis for at least 2–3 years it is important to comment that there are insufficient data available in the literature regarding the time warranty for a normal scan in a diabetic woman. The clinician must consider a diabetic woman as a special case in deciding when to repeat a test.

In these same published studies referred to previously, the incremental prognostic value of an abnormal perfusion scan over other clinical and stress variables in women compared to men was also reported [26–30]. Hachamovitch and coinvestigators reported on 4136 patients, including 1394 women who underwent dual-isotope SPECT imaging and who were followed for a mean of 20 months [26]. During this time there were 95 hard events in men (63 myocardial infarctions, 32 cardiac deaths) and 45 hard events in women (31 MIs and 14 cardiac deaths). The nuclear scan data provided 17% additional prognostic information in men and 37% in women over clinical and exercise variables. From the Kaplan-Meier survival curves the event-free survival for a woman with a moderate-to-high pretest likelihood and abnormal scan result was worse than it was for a man with a similar pretest likelihood and abnormal scan result. Travin and coworkers performed a similar study but did not divide patients into pretest likelihood groups. They plotted Kaplan-Meier curves and found the opposite from Hachamovitch et al., that is, event-free survival was lower for men with abnormal scans than for women with abnormal scans [28]. The mean ages for men and women were identical in the two studies. The most likely explanation for the difference in results is difference in patients referred for stress perfusion imaging between the sites. The men reported by Travin had higher incidence of typical angina and prior infarction, raising the likelihood of more severe disease in their high probability patients. That differences in local referral patterns explain differences in the results of these two studies is supported by the results of a large multicenter trial that showed no difference in all-cause mortality between men and women with abnormal scans [27]. In this study, data from six academic centers were combined and included 5009 men and 3402 women. Cardiac mortality over 2.4 years was similar for men and women (RR = 1.04, 95% CI

0.99–1.08). When Kaplan-Meier curves were divided by severity of reversible or fixed defects and plotted separately for men and women, prognostic implications and adjusted relative risks were similar for both genders. From the same database (Economics of Noninvasive Diagnosis) women were placed in one of three risk groups based on presence or absence of diabetes, left ventricular hypertrophy, and reversible perfusion defects. Event-free survival was plotted for the risk groups and the plots were similar for men and women [32] (Fig. 13.6).

The great majority of women included in these studies underwent exercise testing. Amanullah and coworkers looked at the prognostic value of adenosine myocardial perfusion SPECT in women [31]. They followed 923 women who underwent dual-isotope SPECT pharmacologic stress testing with adenosine for a mean of 26 months. There were 77 hard events (46 cardiac deaths, 31 nonfatal MIs). They found that an abnormal scan result added incremental prognostic value over all clinical and stress variables and that the summed stress score further stratified patients into risk subgroups. Annual event rates in the mildly abnormal

and moderately-to-severely abnormal scans were 4.6% and 11.8%, respectively. Hendel and coworkers looked at the perioperative and long-term prognostic value of dipyridamole planar thallium imaging in 380 men versus 187 women undergoing vascular surgery between 1984 and 1991 [33]. They found a higher rate of perfusion defects in men but they found that the scan predicted both perioperative and long-term events equally well in both sexes. A reversible defect was associated with 3.9-fold increase in perioperative cardiac events in men and 5.5-fold increased risk in women. Mean follow-up period from the time of imaging was 50 months. In men there was a 14.8% event rate and for women an 11.8 event rate. An abnormal scan reduced event-free survival to an equal degree for both men and women.

SUMMARY

In evaluating chest pain in women it is important to note that symptoms can be atypical, the relative importance of risk factors is different from men, and age

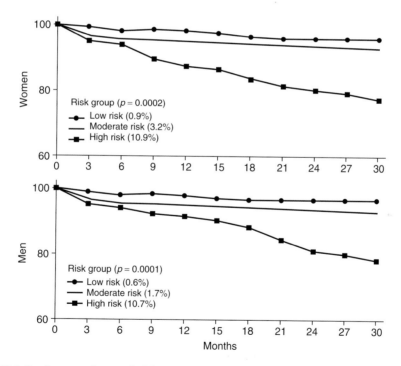

FIGURE 13.6 Cardiac event-free survival for women and for men by risk group. Low risk is defined as normal resting ECG and no diabetes. Moderate risk is defined as ST/T abnormalities on ECG, or LVH, or diabetes. High risk is defined as one of the three following: reversible perfusion defect plus diabetes, or insulin-requiring diabetes in a woman, or a reversible perfusion defect plus one of the ECG or clinical descriptors without diabetes. (Adapted from Shaw LJ, Miller DD, Gillespie KN, et al. A gender-specific clinical and noninvasive coronary risk scoring system for patients with suspected coronary artery disease. Clin Performance Quality Health Care 1995;3:209–217.

of onset of disease is delayed by a decade compared to men. Pretest probability must be assessed using gender-specific algorithms. In a woman with moderate risk, performing a stress perfusion test can be justified for a number of reasons. These reasons include the reduced accuracy of the treadmill ECG response, the prognostic value of a normal scan, and the development of gated SPECT imaging and attenuation correction to correct for breast artifact, which improves accuracy. For a woman of any age with diabetes a stress perfusion test is justified because of the high likelihood for CAD. Because of the documented limitations of thallium imaging in women and improved specificity of Tc-99m-sestamibi over thallium it is recommended that women should undergo imaging with Tc-99m-sestamibi. Frequently, elderly women cannot perform treadmill exercise and must undergo pharmacologic stress testing. From review of the published literature there are no gender differences in the diagnostic accuracy of pharmacologic stress testing to identify CAD and assess severity of disease. Differences between men and women in event-free survival rates predicted from scans noted in individual center studies are probably due to differences in referral. A large multicenter study did not show any significant difference between men and women. An abnormal scan in a woman has the same diagnostic and prognostic implications as it does in a man.

REFERENCES

1. Wenger NK. The natural history of coronary artery disease in women: epidemiology, coronary risk factors, and clinical characteristics. In: *CAD in Women*, edited by P Charney. Philadelphia: Am Coll of Physicians, 1998, pp. 3–38.

2. Centers for Disease Control. Coronary heart disease incidence, by sex—United States 1971–1987. MMWR Morb Mortal Wkly Rep 1992; 41(SS-2):526.

3. Lerner DJ, Kannel WB. Patterns of coronary heart disease morbidity and mortality in the sexes: a 26-year follow-up of the Framingham population. Am Heart J 1986; 111:383.

4. Douglas PS, Ginsburg GS. The evaluation of chest pain in women. N Engl J Med 1996; 334:1311.

5. Pepine CJ, Abrams J, Marks RG, et al. Characteristics of a contemporary population with angina pectoris: TIDES investigators. Am J Cardiol 1994; 74:226.

6. Chaitman BR, Bourassa MG, David K, et al. Angiographic prevalence of high-risk coronary artery disease in patient subsets (CASS). Circulation 1981; 64:360.

7. Buchthal SD, denHollander JA, Merz CNB, et al. Abnormal myocardial phosphorus-31 nuclear magnetic resonance spectroscopy in women with chest pain but normal coronary angiograms. N Engl J Med 2000; 342:829.

8. Shaw LJ, Peterson ED, Johnson LL. Noninvasive testing techniques for diagnosis and prognosis. In: *CAD in Women*, edited by P Charney. Philadelphia: Am Coll of Physicians, 1998, pp. 327.

9. Barolsky SM, Gilbert CA, Faruqui A, et al. Differentials in electrocardiographic responses to exercise of women and men: a non-Bayesian factor. Circulation 1979; 60:1021.

10. Hlatky MA, Pryor DB, Harrell FE Jr, et al. Factors affecting sensitvity and specificity of exercise electrocardiography: multivariable analysis. Am J Med 1984; 77:64.

11. ACC/AHA Guidelines for Exercise Testing: Executive Summary. Circulation 1997;98:345.

12. Iskandrian AE, Heo J, Nallomothu N. Detection of coronary artery disease in women with use of stress single-photon emission computed tomography myocardial perfusion imaging. J Nucl Cardiol 1997;4:329.

13. Mark DB, Shaw L, Harrell FE Jr, et al. Prognostic value of a treadmill exercise score in outpatients with suspected coronary artery disease. N Engl J Med 1991; 325:849.

14. Shaw LJ, Heller GV, Travin MI, et al. Cost analysis of diagnostic testing for coronary artery disease in women with stable chest pain. J Nucl Cardiol 1999;6:559.

15. Johnson LL. Sex specific issues relating to nuclear cardiology. J Nucl Cardiol 1995; 2:339.

16. Chae SC, Heo J, Iskandrian AS, et al. Identification of extensive coronary artery disease in women by exercise single-photon emission computed tomographic (SPECT) thallium imaging. J Am Coll Cardiol 1993; 21:1305.

17. Hansen CL, Crabbe D, Rubin S. Lower diagnostic accuracy of thallium-201 SPECT myocardial perfusion imaging in women: an effect of smaller chamber size. J Am Coll Cardiol 1996; 28:1214.

18. Taillefer R, DePuey EG, Udelson J, et al. Comparative diagnostic accuracy of thallium-201 and Tc-99m sestamibi (perfusion and gated SPECT) in detecting coronary artery disease in women. J Am Coll Cardiol 1997;29:69.

19. Hendel RC, Berman DS, Follansbee WP, et al. Effects of attenuation corrected SPECT myocardial perfusion imaging on diagnostic accuracy: results of a multicenter trial. Circulation 1996; 94:303.

20. Gibson P, Hudson W, Johnson LL. Low event rate for stress only perfusion imaging in patients evaluated for chest pain. J Am Coll Cardiol 2002;39:999.

21. Kong BA, Shaw L, Miller DD, et al. Comparison of accuracy for detecting coronary artery disease and side-effect profile of dipyridamole thallium-201 myocardial perfusion imaging in women versus men. Am J Cardiol 1992; 70:168.

22. Amanullah AM, Kiat H, Friedman JD, et al. Adenosine technetium-99m sestimibi myocardial perfusion SPECT in women: diagnostic efficacy in detection of coronary artery disease. J Am Coll Cardiol 1996; 27:803.

23. Travin MI, Katz MS, Moulton AW, et al. Accuracy of dipyridamole SPECT imaging in identifying individual coronary stenoses and multivessel disease in women versus men. J Nucl Cardiol 2000; 7:213.

24. Amanullah AM, Berman DS, Hachamovitch R, et al. Identification of severe or extensive coronary artery disease in women by adenosine technitium-99m sestamibi SPECT. Am J Cardiol 1997; 80:132.

25. Brown KA. Prognostic value of myocardial perfusion imaging: state of the art and new developments. J Nucl Cardiol 1996;3:516.

26. Hachamovitch R, Berman DS, Kiat H, et al. Effective risk stratification using exercise myocardial perfusion SPECT in women: gender-related differences in prognostic nuclear testing. J Am Coll Cardiol 1996; 28:34.

27. Marwick TH, Shaw L, Lauer MS, et al. The noninvasive prediction of cardiac mortality in men and women with known or suspected coronary artery disease. Am J Med 1999; 106:172.

28. Travin MI, Duca MD, Kline GM, et al. Relation of gender to physician use of test results and to the prognostic value of stress technetium 99m sestamibi myocardial single-photon emission computed tomography scintigraphy. Am Heart J 1997; 134:73.

29. Boyne TS, Koplan BA, Parsons WJ, et al. Predicting adverse outcome with exercise SPECT technetium-99m sestamibi imaging in patients with suspected or known coronary artery disease. Am J Cardiol 1997; 79:270.

30. Geleijnse ML, Elhendy A, vanDomburg RT, et al. Prognostic significance of normal dobutamine-atropine stress sestamibi scintigraphy in women with chest pain. Am J Cardiol 1996; 77:1057.

31. Amanullah AM, Berman DS, Erel J, et al. Incremental prognostic value of adenosine myocardial perfusion single-photon emission computed tomography in women with suspected coronary artery disease. Am J Cardiol 2001; 82:725.

32. Shaw LJ, Miller DD, Gillespie KN, et al. A gender-specific clinical and noninvasive coronary risk scoring system for patients with suspected coronary artery disease. Clin Performance Quality Health Care 1995;3:209.

33. Hendel RC, Chen MH, L'Italien GJ, et al. Sex differences in perioperative and long-term cardiac event-free survival in vascular surgery patients: an analysis of clinical and scintigraphic variables. Circulation 1995; 91:1044.

14 | Evaluation of patients with acute chest pain syndromes: assessment with perfusion imaging in the emergency department

JAMES E. UDELSON, COLIN D. SHAFER, AND DAVID M. VENESY

Each year in the United States, between 5 and 7 million patients present to emergency departments (EDs) with chest pain or other symptoms suggestive of acute cardiac ischemia (ACI) [1]. A partial differential diagnosis of chest pain is listed in Table 14.1. Two-thirds of such patients ultimately are found to have symptoms that are not cardiac in origin [2]. Efficient and appropriate triage of these patients, as customarily based on the clinical presentation and electrocardiogram (ECG), is problematic, as the decision-making ED physicians generally operate at a high sensitivity though low specificity threshold for detecting ACI, so as not to miss any significant cases of acute ischemic heart disease. By necessity, this approach results in many unnecessary admissions of patients without acute cardiac ischemia. Currently, over half of those patients admitted for ACI prove to be false positive admissions, that is, they do not have ACI [2,3], and yet about 4%–7% of those patients *with* ACI, including 2%–4% of those with acute myocardial infarction (AMI), are inadvertently sent home, that is, false negative discharges [2,4,5–7]. Moreover, only about half of those with ACI ultimately are found to rule-in for AMI [4,7,8,9].

Unnecessary hospital and coronary care unit (CCU) admissions for suspected ACI total in the range of 3 million admissions per year, while approximately 60,000 patients with ACI, including 20,000 with AMI, are mistakenly sent directly home from the ED. Thus, ED triage for potential ACI and the associated decision-making process have important implications for individual patient morbidity and mortality, and also for overall health-care costs, including for malpractice litigation. In the United States, where ACI is a leading cause of morbidity and mortality, and an enormous consumer of health-care resources, these unnecessary CCU admissions represent a substantial waste: in this country the direct costs alone may be as much as $3 billion annually [10]. Testing targeted to reduce both false positive and false negative triage could potentially benefit both end points, and do so with substantial economic benefits.

Attempts to improve ED triage accuracy of patients with suspected ACI have included the use of

- identification of high-risk clinical indicators
- rapid determination of cardiac enzymes
- mathematically derived decision instruments
- two-dimensional echocardiography
- thallium-201 (Tl-201) scintigraphy
- technetium-99m (Tc-99m)-based perfusion agents

In reviewing the value of each of these modalities, it is important to bear in mind the *end point* in any given study. While many studies focus on the end point of correct distinction of acute myocardial infarction (AMI) from all other patients, the ED physician facing a triage decision (admit or not admit) is more interested in the separation of those patients with acute cardiac ischemia (ACI), that is, those with AMI *or* unstable angina, from all other patients with noncardiac chest pain. Thus, tests dependent on a degree of myocardial necrosis, such as rapid enzyme subfraction analysis, while useful to detect AMI, may be less so for the ED physician, as patients with unstable angina and no necrosis may not be detected.

280

TABLE 14.1 *Differential Diagnosis of Acute Chest Pain*

Cardiac
    Acute myocardial infarction
    Angina/acute coronary syndrome
    Aortic stenosis
    Pericarditis
    Hypertrophic cardiomyopathy
    Mitral valve prolapse
Vascular
    Aortic dissection
    Pulmonary embolism
    Pulmonary hypertension
Pulmonary
    Pneumonia
    Pleuritis
    Pneumothorax
    Tracheobronchitis
    Tumor
    Mediastinitis
    Pneumomediastinum
Gastrointestinal
    Esophageal reflux
    Esophageal spasm
    Peptic ulcer disease
    Biliary disease
    Pancreatitis
Musculoskeletal
    Costochondritis (Tietze's syndrome)
    Thoracic outlet syndrome
    Cervical disc disease
    Intercostal muscle cramp
Miscellaneous
    Herpes zoster
    Anxiety
    Breast disorder
    Chest wall tumor

STUDIES EVALUATING PATIENTS WITH SUSPECTED ACI IN AN ED SETTING

Numerous methodologies have been proposed to help the ED physician more accurately diagnose acute ischemic heart disease and improve the accuracy of the admission decision. Typically the ED physician relies on the patient's history and the electrocardiogram (ECG) as aids in making this decision. Unfortunately, there are many limitations to the use of the electrocardiogram alone. Many patients have abnormal baseline electrocardiograms or nondiagnostic electrocardiogram changes, which make interpretation imprecise. Various studies have shown that the sensitivity of the resting electrocardiogram for predicting myocardial infarction ranges from 65% to 88% [11–15]. Similar difficulties exist for the accurate diagnosis of acute ischemia in patients who present with symptoms suggestive of unstable angina but with nondefinitive clinical and electrocardiogram criteria.

Risk Stratification by Clinical Indicators

Several investigators have attempted to risk-stratify patients based on clinical and electrocardiographic criteria to determine the likelihood of ischemic heart disease. Lee et al. [13] found that among patients presenting to an ED with chest pain, the presence of a normal electrocardiogram placed such patients in a low-risk group; however, only 19% of patients fit this criterion. Certain characteristics of the chest pain history and the lack of prior cardiac history also placed patients in a low-risk group; however, this again applied to only a small percentage of the study group. Tierney et al. [16] identified several high-risk variables, including ST-segment elevation, new Q waves, diaphoresis with chest pain, and history of prior myocardial infarction. The presence of these factors increased the specificity for predicting myocardial infarction (78%–86%), but they were less sensitive than the ED physicians' independent evaluation (81% vs 87%).

DETERMINATION OF CARDIAC ENZYMES

In the ED, further testing is often sought in the case of patients with chest pain whose clinical history, physical examination, and ECG do not indicate high-risk status. Biochemical markers, in the form of cardiac enzymes that detect myocardial necrosis, have been employed for many years to establish the diagnosis of myocardial infarction, as well as to risk-stratify patients with symptoms suggestive of ACI, but who present with nondiagnostic ECGs. Currently, there is active research investigating several different cardiac enzymes, in addition to the most appropriate utilization of these biochemical markers in the acute setting of the ED. The release kinetics of the major cardiac enzymes are listed in Table 14.2.

Myoglobin

Myoglobin is a heme-carrying protein found in all muscle tissues that can be detected in serum within 1 to 2 hours after myocardial injury. Myoglobin is very sen-

TABLE 14.2 *Release of Cardiac Enzymes after Myocardial Injury*

Enzyme	Rise (hours)	Peak (hours)	Duration (days)
Myoglobin	1–2	4–6	1–2
Creatine kinase-MB band	3–6	12–24	1–3
Troponins	3–6	12–24	7–12

sitive for myocardial necrosis, and can be detected in more than two-thirds of patients with acute myocardial infarction within 3 hours and in nearly all patients at 6 hours [17]. This biochemical marker, however, has low specificity for myocardial damage. False positives can occur in the settings of renal failure, skeletal muscle injury, and shock [15,18]. Myoglobin's rapid-release kinetics can also demonstrate a "staccato" pattern after AMI, whereby myoglobin appears in circulation in multiple short bursts, often lasting only 1–2 hours [19]. These factors diminish the clinical utility of myoglobin as an independent laboratory marker in the ED evaluation of chest pain syndromes [20].

Creatine Kinase-MB Band (CK-MB)

Creatine kinase-MB band (CK-MB), measured in a serial fashion over 24 hours, is the gold-standard of biochemical markers for establishing the diagnosis of myocardial necrosis and is the most widely used cardiac enzyme today. Gibler et al. demonstrated that these serial measurements over a 24-hour period could have sensitivity of up to 100% and a specificity of 98% for detecting AMI [21]. CK-MB analysis at the time of ED presentation has not been helpful, however, with Lee et al. [22] showing only a 38% sensitivity and 80% specificity for predicting myocardial infarction at that time point, which is of course when the initial triage decision needs to take place. A fundamental deficit with CK-MB analysis is its inherent inability to detect non-infarction ACI, which is of great concern to ED physicians deliberating the appropriate triage of patients presenting with chest pain. Also, there are several non-cardiac origins of CK-MB, such as the tongue, diaphragm, small intestine, prostate, and uterus; tumors of these organs can produce measurable amounts of CK subunits, which can potentially confound evaluation of this enzyme measurement. Recently, much attention has been focused on accelerated testing intervals of cardiac enzymes in the ED, some with enzyme determination as frequently as 2 hours [21,23,24]. These protocols appear promising, as they have demonstrated sensitivities and specificities over 90%, but are not widely utilized.

Troponins

The newest biochemical markers to be utilized in the evaluation of potential ACI are the troponins. Troponin I and troponin T are highly sensitive and specific markers of myocardial necrosis, appearing in the serum 3–16 hours after the onset of symptoms. It has been shown recently that measurements of these cardiac-specific contractile proteins are superior to CK-MB for the de-

tection of myocardial injury and are powerful, independent predictors of adverse events in patients with ACI [25–29]. Troponin levels persist in serum for up to 12 days, a feature that can have occasional clinical importance outside of the acute management in the ED but that can confound determination of reinfarction in the patient with recent AMI. More recently, Hamm et al. demonstrated an excellent prognosis in patients with negative troponin levels, utilizing an accelerated protocol of rapid testing for this enzyme in the ED [30].

It has not been established how well troponin detects noninfarction ACI. Several studies suggest that 20%–35% of patients having clinical classified unstable angina will have positive troponin assays, and that these patients are at higher risk for subsequent infarction and death [25–27]. These patients with a clinical syndrome consistent with unstable angina and elevated troponins also appear in retrospective analysis of clinical trials to have a substantial benefit from the use of intravenous platelet inhibitors [31]. The majority of patients with unstable angina, however, will have negative assays; similar to the other markers, troponin is therefore of limited value to *exclude* unstable angina. Thus, although these markers are in wide use already, there remains uncertainty in the clinical practice of ED physicians about the appropriate use of troponin in the *initial* evaluation of patients with chest pain, particularly when they are required to make rapid triage and discharge decisions in the ED. The effectiveness of this enzyme for patient triage decisions has not extensively been evaluated in a prospective, randomized manner.

While the use of these biochemical markers is an important component of a comprehensive ED evaluation strategy in such patients, the data would appear to suggest that they are not sufficiently sensitive for all acute ischemic syndromes to be used independently for ED triage and discharge decisions.

MATHEMATICALLY BASED DECISION AIDS FOR ACI

The goal of mathematically based diagnostic aids for ACI and AMI is to improve physicians' use of clinical information. This may be done by directing attention to important variables, by quantifying risk, and by reassuring physicians in the face of uncertainty [32]. Early work suggests that, of these potential functions, improving physicians' risk estimates may be the most important [33].

Using multivariate logistic regression, "predictive instruments" can be derived that provide ED physicians with a given patient's probability of ACI [2,34–36]. These instruments incorporate clinical and ECG findings of ED patients presenting with symptoms suggestive of ACI, including chest pain or left arm pain, abdominal pain or nausea, shortness of breath, and dizziness or lightheadedness. In controlled prospective trials of the instrument's use, the use of the predictive instrument reduced false positive CCU admissions by 30%, with no increase in false negative discharges to home [2,34].

Despite these encouraging data, the use of this technology has not become widespread. It is possible that ED physicians may not be able to comfortably rely on an abstract unit of information along a spectrum of probabilities (a sophisticated risk assessment) as provided by mathematically based ED decision aids to discharge patients from the ED. In this regard, an imaging procedure evaluating myocardial perfusion or function, if read as normal, in conjunction with knowledge of both a high negative predictive value of the imaging modality for ACI, accompanied by a low incidence of subsequent morbid cardiac events in the setting of a normal image, may allow a more confident possibility of ED discharge.

STUDIES OF MYOCARDIAL PERFUSION AND FUNCTION IN THE ED SETTING

Because of the difficulties inherent in electrocardiography as an aid to optimize ED triage of chest pain patients, more direct methods of assessing abnormalities of regional myocardial perfusion or regional ventricular function as signs of ACI are attractive targets for study (Fig. 14.1).

Noninvasive cardiac imaging is capable of evaluating abnormalities in regional perfusion (by imaging radionuclide myocardial perfusion tracers) as well as abnormalities in regional ventricular function (by

"The Ischemic Cascade"
Myocardial Perfusion Abnormality
→ Supply & Demand Mismatch
→ Diastolic Function Abnormality
→ Regional Wall Motion Abnormality
→ ECG Signs of Ischemia
→ Symptoms of Angina
→ Myocardial Infarction

FIGURE 14.1 The ischemic cascade concept: myocardial ischemia is not a sudden, threshold phenomenon, but rather often represents a pathophysiologic spectrum of events reflecting degrees of imbalance in coronary blood supply and regional myocardial oxygen demand. The earliest phenomenon is an abnormality in myocardial perfusion, followed at further degrees of supply/demand mismatch by regional ventricular functional abnormality, and then ECG signs of ischemia and finally symptoms of angina.

echocardiography, gated SPECT imaging, computed tomography, or magnetic resonance imaging). While both radionuclide and echocardiographic modalities have been explored in the evaluation of ED patients with chest pain (as reviewed later), the most conceptually attractive approach is noninvasive imaging analysis of regional myocardial perfusion. Perfusion imaging provides the most direct assessment of the primary abnormality in patients with acute coronary syndromes (i.e., diminished regional myocardial blood flow), and theoretically may demonstrate abnormalities in regional flow even when symptoms, ECG changes, and regional wall motion abnormalities have not occurred.

Echocardiography in the ED

It has been shown that ventricular wall motion abnormalities are early signs of myocardial ischemia [37], often occurring prior to the onset of definitive electrocardiographic signs of ischemia. Therefore, echocardiographic detection of regional left ventricular dysfunction has been assessed as a tool to improve the diagnosis of acute cardiac ischemia in the ED. In a small study, Peels et al. [38] found echocardiography to be highly sensitive for the detection of myocardial infarction as well as acute ischemia in the ED setting (92% and 88%, respectively). However, this high sensitivity was importantly dependent upon the presence of symptoms *during the echocardiographic study*. The specificity of this approach was limited, at 53% and 78% for infarction and ischemia, respectively. Sasaki et al. [39] demonstrated similar results, in that a poor sensitivity of echocardiographically detected regional ventricular dysfunction was observed in the absence of ongoing symptoms. Echocardiographic analysis was also limited to those patients with normal conduction systems and without prior myocardial infarction, as conduction disturbances and prior areas of infarct can both cause regional wall motion abnormalities in the absence of acute ischemia.

Sabia and coworkers [40] reported a sensitivity of 93% for echocardiographically detected regional wall motion abnormalities to correctly identify acute ischemic heart disease presenting as myocardial infarction. These investigators estimated that the use of echocardiography in the ED could result in a 32% reduction in hospital admissions, though this procedure was not demonstrated to do so in a prospective manner. This study again demonstrated a modest specificity (57%) and was also limited by the requirement of ongoing symptoms at the time of study, as well as the lack of wall motion abnormalities in a small subset of patients ultimately diagnosed as having non-Q-wave infarction. Other investigators have also observed these false negative findings [41,42]. Kontos et al. [43] were able to show a high negative predictive value of normal echocardiographic studies in patients with chest pain, however, which correlated with a benign prognosis at 10 months. Trippi and colleagues [44] demonstrated the possible role of dobutamine stress tele-echocardiography for the evaluation of ED patients with chest pain, reporting a sensitivity of 90% and a specificity of 89%. This technology, however, is not currently in widespread use.

Thus, while these studies demonstrated the feasibility of using echocardiography in the ED setting, they were concordant in demonstrating that optimal sensitivity for this approach required ongoing symptoms during the study and that the specificity was sub optimal. The latter characteristic would suggest limited use for this technique in diminishing the false positive admissions of ED patients with chest pain, and no study has evaluated the actual impact of the use of echocardiography on triage from the ED.

Thallium-201 Myocardial Perfusion Imaging in Patients with Acute Chest Pain

Radionuclide imaging of myocardial blood flow has also been studied as a means of detecting acute abnormalities in regional myocardial perfusion. In the past, Tl-201 was the most widely used agent to trace myocardial blood flow [45]. In 1976, Wackers et al. [46] showed Tl-201 defects in 100% of patients with acute myocardial infarction who were studied within 6 hours of the onset of symptoms. The sensitivity for detecting ischemia diminished as time increased beyond 6 hours from the onset of symptoms. In a later study involving patients with unstable angina, Wackers and coworkers [47] found planar Tl-201 scintigraphy to have 76% sensitivity and 67% specificity for predicting myocardial infarction or severe coronary disease. In addition, in the presence of an abnormal baseline electrocardiogram with transient changes, the sensitivity for a positive Tl-201 scan increased to 94% but with a specificity of only 46%.

While Tl-201 scintigraphy has been widely used since that time as an indicator of myocardial perfusion in stable patients with suspected coronary artery disease (in conjunction with stress testing), its use in the ED setting has in practical terms been limited. The primary reason for its limited use has been the time constraints imposed by its "redistribution" properties, requiring that imaging be completed in a relatively short time after injection. Moreover, this isotope is not always readily available for acute imaging. More recently, both of these significant limitations have been overcome by the use of Tc-99m-based myocardial perfusion imaging agents.

Imaging with Technetium-99m-Based Agents in Patients with Acute Chest Pain

Tc-99m labeled radioisotopes such as Tc-99m-sestamibi and tetrofosmin have also been studied as alternative myocardial perfusion imaging agents [48]. These agents have several distinct advantages over Tl-201: their physical characteristics are better suited to gamma camera imaging, they are less subject to tissue attenuation, they can be used with contemporary electrocardiographic gated SPECT (single-photon emission computed tomography) imaging, and they can be readily available for acute imaging. Most importantly, Tc-99m agents have *minimal redistribution* after their initial flow-related distribution within the myocardium, allowing for imaging up to *several hours after injection* [49], with the resulting images reflecting myocardial regional blood flow *at the time of injection*. These characteristics make Tc-99m-based agents more ideal for perfusion imaging of patients in the ED setting, as injection can be done at rest in the ED and the patient then transported to the nuclear medicine department for high-quality gated SPECT imaging.

The clinical basis for the use of Tc-99m agents in patients with suspected ACI comes from a study by Bilodeau et al. [50] evaluating 45 patients already admitted to a hospital with suspected unstable angina. In this study, all patients underwent coronary angiography, revealing significant coronary artery disease (CAD) in 26 patients. Tc-99m-sestamibi was injected during a spontaneous episode of chest pain, and SPECT imaging demonstrated 96% sensitivity and 79% specificity for the detection of coronary artery disease, while the predictive value of a negative scan to exclude CAD was 94%. An ECG performed simultaneously with the injection of sestamibi had only 35% sensitivity for detecting coronary ischemia. The results of the imaging were blinded from the treating physicians, so prospective testing of this modality to reduce the need for admission or catheterization was not analyzed. Importantly, however, this seminal study showed that the injection of sestamibi during an episode of chest pain was very sensitive for detecting significant coronary disease and had a strong negative predictive value for excluding significant coronary disease if the imaging was negative.

Emergency Department Imaging with Tc-99m-Based Agents for Patients with Acute Chest Pain

Christian and colleagues initially evaluated the use of sestamibi imaging in ED patients by documenting perfusion defects in 13 of 14 patients found to have had an acute myocardial infarction but presenting with chest pain and *nondiagnostic* ECGs [51]. Such studies demonstrated the feasibility of this technique in the ED setting and suggested that this imaging modality could provide important incremental information beyond the clinical and electrocardiographic data to improve ED triage. There is now a substantial body of literature evaluating the performance of rest SPECT perfusion imaging in the ED setting for patients with a clinical suspicion of ACI.

Varetto et al. [52] performed resting Tc-99m-sestamibi SPECT imaging in 64 patients presenting to the ED with suspected ACI and nondiagnostic electrocardiograms. Thirty-four patients had normal scans, none of whom were subsequently found to have significant coronary artery disease by coronary angiography or stress testing. *All of the patients with normal scans remained free of morbid cardiac events up to 18 months after discharge.* Of the 30 patients with perfusion defects, 13 were found to have had an acute myocardial infarction (by enzyme or electrocardiographic criteria), 14 were found to have significant coronary artery disease by angiography, and the remaining 3 patients were considered to have false positive findings. Overall, sensitivity and specificity for the detection of acute myocardial infarction or significant coronary artery disease was 100% and 92%, respectively, while the predictive value of a negative scan to exclude CAD or a subsequent cardiac event was 100% (Table 14.3). While these data strongly support the feasibility of performing acute sestamibi imaging in this population, as well as confirm the earlier study [50] regarding performance characteristics for detecting or ruling out ACI, this study was not

designed to test this imaging modality in a prospective manner. However, it does extend the prior data by demonstrating the important prognostic power of perfusion imaging. These imaging results were blinded from the admitting ED physicians, so the potential impact of sestamibi imaging in this setting on reducing unnecessary admissions (53% of the patients admitted to the CCU in this study) was not tested.

In addition to these important findings, Varetto and colleagues reported that myocardial perfusion defects were identified (and diagnostic sensitivity of the test was maintained) even when sestamibi injection was delayed up to 3–4 hours after resolution of chest pain [52]. These important data suggest that, in contrast to echocardiographic analysis of regional wall motion abnormalities, the detection of myocardial perfusion abnormalities identifying ACI seems possible even after symptoms have abated.

Hilton and coworkers [53] looked specifically at the prognostic significance of sestamibi myocardial perfusion images obtained in ED patients with chest pain. Only one cardiac event (defined as cardiac death, nonfatal myocardial infarction, or need for acute coronary intervention) occurred during short-term hospital follow-up among 102 patients with normal scans (Fig. 14.2). In a multivariate analysis, the presence of an abnormal sestamibi scan was the only independent variable predictive of the occurrence of a cardiac event among multiple clinical and demographic variables. These investigators subsequently extended their previous data regarding the low-risk prognosis associated with a normal sestamibi perfusion image in ED chest pain patients [54]. Among patients with a normal scan

TABLE 14.3 *Summary of Major Clinical Trials Involving Myocardial Perfusion in Acute Chest Pain*

Study	n	Sens	Spec	PPV	NPV	End point
Wackers 1979	203	100	63	55	100	MI
Bilodeau 1991	45	96	79	86	94	CAD (by angiography)
Varetto 1993	64	100	67	43	100	MI
		100	92	90	100	CAD
Hilton 1994	102	100	78	38	99	MI
		94	83	44	99	All events
Tatum 1997	438	100	78	7	100	MI
		82	83	32	98	MI, revasc
Kontos 1997	532	93	71	15	99	MI
		81	76	40	95	MI, revasc
Heller 1998	357	90	60	12	99	MI
Duca 1999	75	100	73	33	100	MI
		73	93	89	81	CAD
Kosnik 1999	69	71	92	50	97	MI, revasc, or cardiac death

Sens, sensitivity; Spec, specificity; PPV, positive predictive value; NPV, negative predictive value; MI, myocardial infarction; CAD, objective evidence for coronary artery disease; revasc, revascularization (coronary artery bypass grafting or percutaneous transluminal coronary angioplasty).

in this setting, there were no subsequent cardiac events [death, nonfatal infarction, thrombolysis, percutaneous transluminal coronary angioplasty (PTCA), or coronary artery bypass graft (CABG) during a 3-month posthospital follow-up.

Since these studies were performed, there have been several larger studies involving similar patients with essentially similar results following perfusion imaging with the Tc-99m-based agents sestamibi or tetrofosmin [55–59] (see Table 14.3). In all of these studies, myocardial perfusion imaging showed a high sensitivity for detecting those patients with ischemia and infarction beyond that found by history or ECG (Fig. 14.3). When one examines the published observational series regarding the relationship between SPECT perfusion imaging results in the ED setting and patient outcomes, the negative predictive value for ruling out an MI in the ED setting is over 99%, and the negative predictive value for ruling out an MI or any follow-up cardiac event is over 97%. Moreover, the imaging data have incremental value over clinical, ECG, and enzymatic data for the prediction of patients going on to have unfavorable cardiac events [55] (Fig. 14.4).

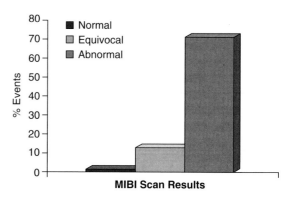

FIGURE 14.2 Cardiac event rate (y-axis) as a function of results of resting Tc-99m-sestamibi imaging (x-axis) in ED patients with suspected ischemia. Patients with a normal scan had a very low event rate, and patients with an abnormal scan a very high event rate. Patients with an "equivocal" scan had an intermediate event rate, likely reflecting some patients whose scans were influenced by artifacts, while others had small areas of ischemia or infarct. (Adapted from Hilton TC, Thompson RC, Williams H, et al. Technetium99m-sestamibi myocardial perfusion imaging in the emergency room evaluation of chest pain. J Am Coll Cardiol 1994; 23:1016–1022.) MIBI, Tc99m-sestamibi. ED, emergency department.

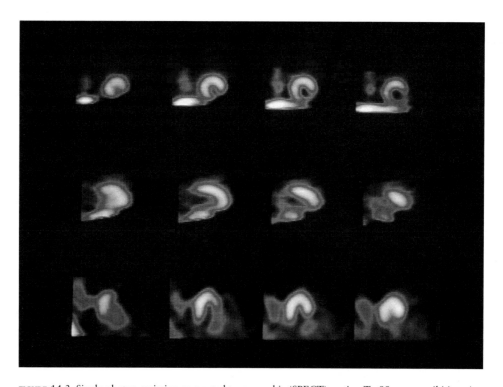

FIGURE 14.3 Single-photon emission computed tomographic (SPECT) resting Tc-99m-sestamibi imaging of a 39-year-old man who presented to the ED at New England Medical Center with chest pain atypical for angina and a near normal initial ECG. The images demonstrate a severe resting perfusion defect in the inferolateral wall. Due to this finding and ongoing symptoms, he was taken to the catheterization laboratory, where an acute left circumflex occlusion was found, treated with primary angioplasty.

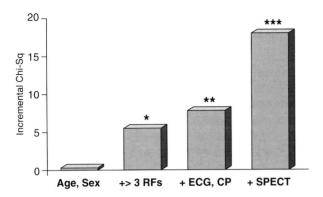

FIGURE 14.4 Analysis of the incremental value of resting perfusion imaging data to predict cardiac events in ED patients with suspected ischemia. The incremental chi-square value (y-axis) measures the strength of the association between individual factors added to the knowledge base in incremental fashion (x-axis) and unfavorable cardiac events. Addition of SPECT perfusion imaging data (SPECT) adds highly statistically significant value even with knowledge of age, sex, risk factors for CAD (RFs), ECG changes, and presence/absence of chest pain (CP). $*p = .02$; $**p = .05$; $***p = <.0001$. (Adapted from Heller GV, Stowers SA, Hendel RC, et al. Clinical value of acute rest technetium-99m tetrofosmin tomographic myocardial perfusion imaging in patients with acute chest pain and nondiagnostic electrocardiograms. J Am Coll Cardiol 1998; 31:1011–1017.)

Based on the negative predictive value with a normal resting perfusion scan and very low event rate on follow-up in this setting, the use of myocardial perfusion imaging appears to be able to rapidly identify patients without ischemia and infarction, and thus has the potential to determine which patients with chest pain and nondiagnostic ECG changes may be eligible for safe discharge.

Randomized Trials Involving ED Patients with Acute Chest Pain and Tc-99m-Based Perfusion Imaging

There is a large body of observational studies involving the use of Tc-99m-based imaging in ED patients presenting with chest pain, which have been consistent in showing that Tc-99m perfusion imaging has a higher sensitivity for detecting myocardial ischemia than either the ECG or initial cardiac enzymes and a high negative predictive value for ruling out an MI or cardiac events in ED patients with suspected ischemia. None of these studies evaluated the impact of incorporating imaging data into the decision-making process, however. There have been two trials in which patients have been randomly assigned to have imaging or not to have imaging data influence subsequent management. These two randomized studies evaluated the benefit of using this modality on health-care costs and length of hospital stay, and for its ability to influence ED physicians' triage decision making.

Stowers and colleagues [60] evaluated 46 patients presenting to the ED with ongoing chest pain and a non-diagnostic ECG who underwent Tc-99m-tetrofosmin imaging before being randomly assigned to a conventional arm (physicians blinded from imaging results) or perfusion imaging–guided arm (imaging results were unblinded to the physician). The study's primary analyses focused on assessing the differences in total in-hospital costs and average lengths of stay between the two study arms. They found that median hospital costs were $1843 less for patients in perfusion-guided strategy compared with costs with conventional management. In addition to these cost differences, the conventional arm had a 2.0-day longer median hospital stay and 1.0-day longer median ICU stay. This study also demonstrated that physicians provided with imaging results ordered fewer cardiac catheterizations without any difference in outcomes by hospital discharge or by 30 days of follow-up. Thus, while the study population was small, there appears to be a cost benefit and shorter lengths of stay for intermediate-risk chest pain patients admitted from the ED when myocardial perfusion imaging results are made available as part of the diagnostic strategy.

A larger prospective, randomized study by Udelson and colleagues—the Emergency Room Assessment of Sestamibi for the Evaluation of Chest Pain trial (ERASE Chest Pain) [61] evaluated the role of myocardial perfusion imaging on the triage decision made by ED physicians. Investigators enrolled 2475 patients with chest pain or other symptoms suggestive of acute cardiac ischemia and a normal or nondiagnostic ECG. Patients were randomly assigned to receive either the usual ED evaluation strategy or the usual strategy supplemented by acute resting Tc-99m-sestamibi SPECT imaging. The study found that there were no differences in the ED triage decision between the two arms for those patients with either an AMI or with unstable angina. However, for those patients *without* cardiac ischemia, hospitalization was reduced from 52% with usual care to 42% with sestamibi imaging ($p < .001$). In their study, the median time from ED presentation to admission or discharge home was 4.7 hours in the usual care arm and 5.3 hours in the sestamibi imaging arm. On 30-day follow-up, there were no differences in outcomes between the usual care and sestamibi imaging groups. Therefore, this study showed that the incorporation of sestamibi imaging into triage decision making provided a clear benefit in reducing unnecessary hospital admissions in patients *without* ischemia, without reducing appropriate admission for patients *with* acute ischemia.

These two prospective, randomized trials have shown that acute rest myocardial perfusion imaging in patients presenting to the ED with low-to-intermediate risk chest pain and nondiagnostic ECGs can provide significant cost savings and improve the overall clinical effectiveness of the ED triage process.

Comparison of Myocardial Perfusion Imaging with Enzymatic Markers for ED Patients with Acute Coronary Syndromes

There are several distinctions between the information provided by SPECT myocardial perfusion imaging in ED patients and that provided by serial cardiac enzyme analysis. The various cardiac enzymes that are generally evaluated mark the presence of myocardial necrosis and will be positive in the vast majority of patients with acute myocardial infarction [62]. Recent data also suggest that among patients with what is traditionally regarded as an unstable angina, approximately 30% will have positive troponin markers [25,63]. This subgroup of patients with unstable angina is at higher risk for adverse cardiac events over time compared to patients with an unstable angina syndrome but normal troponin results [25,64]. However, the majority of patients with an unstable angina syndrome will have enzyme marker levels within the normal range. In contrast, myocardial perfusion imaging should theoretically be abnormal in any patient with an abnormality in myocardial blood flow, including patients with both an acute myocardial infarction and unstable angina. The high sensitivity and negative predictive value of the published studies support the concept that perfusion imaging can provide powerful discriminatory value in this setting.

Another important distinction between perfusion imaging and enzyme results is the significant difference in the *time course* during which results are abnormal in patients with acute coronary syndromes. Perfusion imaging data should be abnormal almost immediately after an abnormality in myocardial blood flow is established. Cardiac enzyme markers, and particularly the troponins, may begin to show abnormal results 4–8 hours after symptom onset with the peak abnormality being evident at 12–18 hours after symptom onset. In a multicenter study of cardiac enzyme markers, optimal sensitivity for troponins T or I to detect an acute MI occurred at 18 hours after symptom onset [65]. Similarly, the most powerful prognostic value for adverse cardiac events using troponin assays also occurs at approximately 18 hours after symptom onset [66].

Consistent with these data are a study from Kontos and colleagues [67] of a large group of patients seen in the Chest Pain ED at the Medical College of Virginia and a smaller study by Duca and colleagues [63]. In these studies, SPECT sestamibi imaging performed in the ED was between 92% and 100% sensitive for detecting acute MI, while cardiac troponin I values drawn *at the same time* had a sensitivity of only 11%–30%. Subsequently, the maximum troponin I over the first 24 hours had sensitivity similar to that of the acute rest sestamibi imaging but at a distinctly later time point. For those patients with an acute coronary syndrome, the sensitivity was higher for acute sestamibi imaging compared with both the initial cardiac troponin and troponin levels at 24 hours. Therefore, there appears to be a benefit in using acute sestamibi imaging over troponin levels for the *earlier* detection of both AMI and ACI in patients who present to the ED with chest pain, which has therapeutic implications regarding the rapidity of reperfusion strategies.

Comparison of Myocardial Perfusion Imaging with Echocardiography for ED Patients with Acute Coronary Syndromes

As described earlier, echocardiography can be useful in identifying patients with acute coronary ischemia. Only one study, by Kontos and colleagues [68], has directly compared the use of myocardial perfusion imaging and echocardiography in patients presenting to the ED with chest pain. This study included 185 patients presenting to the ED with chest pain considered low-to-moderate risk of coronary ischemia based on history and ECG. Acute rest sestamibi injection and echocardiography were performed to evaluate for AMI or ACI. In 90% of the patients, both studies were performed within 1 hour of each other; however, no details were given about the timing of the studies in relation to the patient's chest pain. For the detection of AMI there were equal sensitivities of 100% and similar specificities of 82% and 84% for echocardiography and sestamibi imaging, respectively. For the detection of ACI (MI, significant disease by coronary angiography or a positive stress test) there were equal sensitivities of 71% and specificities of 87% and 89% for echocardiography and sestamibi imaging, respectively. Additionally, patients with negative echocardiograms and imaging studies had no cardiac events at 1 year.

This study shows that there are similarly high sensitivities and specificities for detection of both AMI and ACI in patients presenting to the ED with low-to-moderate chest pain for echocardiography and perfusion imaging. The negative predictive values for these tests were also prognostic for cardiac events over the next year. Further studies are needed to evaluate the impact of symptom resolution on this comparison, as the earlier studies of echocardiography in the ED setting have demonstrated that optimal sensitivity is dependent on the presence of symptoms during the evaluation [38–42].

COST-EFFECTIVENESS OF TC-99-BASED MYOCARDIAL PERFUSION IMAGING IN THE ED

While the incorporation of myocardial perfusion imaging into an ED strategy engenders an added cost, the potential for reduction of inappropriate hospital or observation unit admissions might more than offset the additional costs of imaging. Weissman et al. [69] found that 68% of the physicians' decisions were affected by the perfusion imaging results and estimated a potential cost savings of $786 per patient. Radensky and colleagues [70] calculated similar potential cost savings of $796 per patient using a decision model comparing a scan strategy versus a no-scan strategy. In a report by Ziffer et al. [71] of several thousand patients evaluated in a chest pain center, following the incorporation of perfusion imaging into the algorithm, the "missed MI" rate (that is, the proportion of patients sent directly home from the ED but who were actually having an MI) dropped from 1.8% to 0.1%, while unnecessary hospital admissions were also reduced. They estimated savings (charges) of approximately $1900 per patient.

The prospective, randomized study by Stowers et al. [60] assessed differences in hospital cost between a conventional and perfusion imaging–guided strategy. They found that the median hospital costs per patient were $1843 lower in the perfusion imaging–guided arm compared with the conventional arm. In addition, patients in the perfusion imaging–guided arm had a shorter hospital stay and had fewer diagnostic catheterizations without any change in 30-day outcomes. Heller and coworkers [55] estimated savings in a similar range.

In contrast, an observational study by Kosnik and colleagues [72] evaluated 69 patients already being admitted to the hospital and estimated that the use of sestamibi imaging would hypothetically lead to more appropriate triage in 42% of patients but at an additional cost of $307 per patient.

Overall, the majority of studies, including the only prospective, randomized study, point to a potential cost savings by incorporating the routine use of acute rest myocardial perfusion imaging in patients with low-to-moderate-risk chest pain and nondiagnostic ECGs. When this saving is extrapolated to the 5–7 million patients [1] who present yearly to EDs with chest pain, the yearly potential cost savings for this group would be substantial.

IMAGE INTERPRETATION IN SUSPECTED ACUTE ISCHEMIA PATIENTS

An important goal in the triage of patients seen in the ED setting with suspected acute ischemia is the optimal identification of those who do have an acute ischemic syndrome. To this end, in the interpretation of resting myocardial perfusion images in this setting, it is important to aim for high sensitivity, that is, when confronted with a study that is equivocal for abnormality, to err on the side of interpreting as abnormal. This is supported by one study that reported the prognostic significance of resting perfusion imaging in ED patients with suspected ischemia and also categorized imaging results as normal, equivocal, or abnormal [53]. Patients who had a normal resting sestamibi study had an extremely low risk, while patients with an abnormal study had a substantially higher risk. Patients with a study read as "equivocal," however, had an intermediate (i.e., not low) risk (see Fig. 14.2). These latter studies likely represent a subgroup of patients whose scans have artifacts such as diaphragm or breast attenuation and another subgroup of patients with small territories of ischemia at the time of injection. Given these results, interpretation of perfusion images in this setting should be "aggressive," in order to optimize sensitivity for detecting acute ischemia.

Image interpreters use several methodologies in an attempt to better classify "equivocal" images as truly normal or abnormal. These include incorporating information from gated SPECT imaging of regional function, attenuation correction algorithms, and prone imaging.

In standard stress–rest imaging, fixed defects possibly representing diaphragm or breast attenuation artifact can often be interpreted more correctly as infarct or artifact by incorporating gated SPECT information [73]. Theoretically in ED imaging, this may not be as helpful as there is only one image set, the resting perfusion image. An area of mildly abnormal uptake, such as a mild inferobasal defect that may represent diaphragm attenuation artifact or a small area of ischemia, with preserved regional function may represent not only artifact but could also be an area that was ischemic at the time of injection but which has recovered wall motion by the time of imaging. In this setting, attenuation correction may theoretically be more helpful.

There are as yet few data addressing this point. In a preliminary study, Hendel and colleagues [74] examined the ERASE chest pain trial database in which some centers routinely used attenuation correction and gated

SPECT imaging. In 319 patients, the use of both attenuation correction and gating reduced the number of equivocal scans and increased reader confidence in interpretation. By segmental scoring, scores were more normal in patients ultimately found to not have an acute ischemic syndrome, by both methods. However, attenuation correction slightly reduced the scores of patients with an acute ischemic syndrome (inappropriately). From these data it appears that either method has the potential to be useful, though gating perhaps more so. The comparative usefulness of these modalities will need to be re-evaluated as attenuation correction techniques continue to evolve.

Prone imaging can also be used to assist in the determination of the presence or absence of a true abnormality in the inferior wall, discriminating from diaphragmatic attenuation [75,76]. While this has not been systematically studied in the ED setting, the experience in our laboratory has been that in selected situations prone imaging may be quite effective in this regard (see Color Fig. 14.5 in separate color insert).

SETTING UP AN ED IMAGING SERVICE

Setting up an ED perfusion imaging protocol requires significant contribution and cooperation from many "stakeholders," including ED physicians and support personnel, cardiologists who are often called upon to assist in the decision making, and nuclear medicine and nuclear cardiology physicians who must perform and interpret the imaging with confidence and quality. While a reduction in unnecessary hospitalization with potential associated cost savings is a worthy goal and outcome, in some provider settings there are paradoxical incentives that may work against such a program. For instance, short observation or telemetry unit admissions to rule out myocardial infarction can in some settings be profitable for hospitals based on the local payment system. Thus, sending such patients home directly from the ED may be an important source of lost income for an institution. Adoption of this proven technology into such a setting will often require realigning incentives among payers and providers to allow incorporation of such a potential cost-effective algorithm into the ED setting. When used properly and with expertise, a reduction in unnecessary hospitalization is obviously favorable for patients and for the health-care system.

It is also important to define the ideal patients eligible for an imaging protocol. Patients who report to the ED with symptoms consistent with an acute coronary syndrome and an ECG diagnostic for acute ischemia or infarction do not benefit from acute imaging. Such patients are triaged based on the presence of ST elevation or ST depression into appropriate algorithms for acute myocardial infarction or unstable angina/non-ST-segment elevation infarction, respectively [77]. Ideal patients for imaging are those with nondiagnostic or normal electrocardiograms and symptoms suspicious for acute ischemia. Ideal patients also have no prior history of infarction or significant Q waves on the ECG. Such patients will often have a perfusion defect representative of the old infarction, and thus the data will not be as helpful for discrimination of a new acute ischemic syndrome.

FUTURE DIRECTIONS

While the randomized data from the ERASE Chest Pain trial and the other observational studies provide compelling evidence for incorporation of acute SPECT myocardial perfusion imaging into ED evaluation strategies for patients with suspected acute ischemia, future studies will refine the patient population likely to benefit most from such a procedure. Certain clinical characteristics are likely in such patients, which may on a larger scale be identified by ECG predictive instruments, for example, in which the pretest probability of acute ischemia is so low that imaging is not beneficial. The optimal combination of imaging data, enzyme data, and stress testing and the temporal distribution of such testing also needs to be better defined.

However, given the difficulty that many physicians have in evaluating such patients with confidence, reflected by the very high rate of admission for observation or evaluation in the ED, the incorporation of perfusion imaging has the potential to reduce unnecessary hospitalizations significantly, with potential associated cost savings.

REFERENCES

1. Selker HP, Zalenski RJ. An evaluation of technologies for detecting acute cardiac ischemia in the emergency department: a report of the NIH national heart attack alert program. Ann Emerg Med 1997; 29:1.
2. Pozen MW, D'Agostino RB, Selker HP, et al. A predictive instrument to improve coronary care unit admission practices in acute ischemic heart disease. N Engl J Med 1984; 310:1273.
3. McCarthy BD, Wong JB, Selker HP. Detecting acute cardiac ischemia in the emergency department: a review of the literature. J Gen Intern Med 1990; 5:365.
4. Lee TH, Rouan GW, Weisberg MC, et al. Clinical characteristics and natural history of patients with acute myocardial infarction sent home from the emergency room. Am J Cardiol 1987; 60:219.

5. McCarthy BD, Beshansky JR, D'Agostino RB, et al. Missed diagnoses of acute myocardial infarction in the emergency department: results from a multicenter study. Ann Emerg Med 1993; 22:579.

6. Pope JH, Aufderheide TP, Ruthazer R, et al. Missed diagnoses of acute cardiac ischemia in the emergency department. N Engl J Med 2000; 342:1163.

7. Schor S, Behar S, Modan B, et al. Disposition of presumed coronary patients from an emergency room. A follow-up study. JAMA 1976; 236:941.

8. Goldman L, Weinberg M, Weisberg M, et al. A computer-derived protocol to aid in the diagnosis of ER patients with acute chest pain. N Engl J Med 1982; 307:588.

9. Selker HP, Griffith JL, Dorey FJ, et al. How do physicians adapt when the coronary care unit is full? A prospective multicenter study. JAMA 1987; 257:1181.

10. Fineberg HV, Scadden D, Goldman L. Care of patients with a low probability of acute myocardial infarction: cost-effectiveness of alternatives to coronary-care-unit admission. N Engl J Med 1984; 310:1301.

11. Behar S, Schor S, Kariv I, et al. Evaluation of electrocardiogram in emergency room as a decision-making tool. Chest 1977; 71:486.

12. Goldman L, Cook EF, Brand DA, et al. A computer protocol to predict myocardial infarction in emergency department patients with chest pain. N Engl J Med 1988; 318:797.

13. Lee TH, Cook F, Weisberg M, et al. Acute chest pain in the emergency room: identification and examination of low risk patients. Arch Intern Med 1985; 145:65.

14. Rude RE, Poole WK, Muller JE, et al. Electrocardiographic and clinical criteria for recognition of acute myocardial infarction based on analysis of 3697 patients. Am J Cardiol 1983; 52:936.

15. Vaidga HC. Myoglobin. Lab Med 1992; 23:306.

16. Tierney WM, Roth BJ, Psaty B, et al. Predictors of myocardial infarction in emergency room patients. Crit Care Med 1985;13:526.

17. Gibler WB, Giber CD, Weinshenker E, et al. Myoglobin as an early indicator of acute myocardial infarction. Ann Emerg Med 1987; 16:851.

18. Hoberg E, Katus HA, Diederich KW, et al. Myoglobin, creatine kinase-B isoenzyme, and myosin light chain release in patients with unstable angina pectoris. Eur Heart J 1987; 8:989.

19. Kagen L, Scheidt S, Butt A. Serum myoglobin in myocardial infarction: the "staccato phenomenon." Is acute myocardial infarction in man an intermittent event? Am J Med 1977; 62:86.

20. de Winter RJ, Koster RW, Sturk A, et al. Value of myoglobin, troponin T, and CK-MB-mass in ruling out an acute myocardial infarction in the emergency room. Circulation 1995; 92:3401.

21. Gibler WB, Lewis LM, Erb RE, et al. Early detection of acute myocardial infarction in patients presenting with chest pain and nondiagnostic ECGs: serial CK-MB sampling in the emergency department. Ann Emerg Med 1990; 19:1359-1366; erratum 1991; 20:420.

22. Lee TH, Weisberg MC, Cook EF, et al. Evaluation of creatine kinase and creatine kinase-MB for diagnosing myocardial infarction: clinical impact in the emergency room. Arch Intern Med 1987; 147:115.

23. Gibler WB, Young GP, Hedges JR, et al. Acute myocardial infarction in chest pain patients with non-diagnostic ECGs: serial CK-MB sampling in the emergency department. Ann Emerg Med 1992; 21:504.

24. Marin MM, Teichman SL. Use of rapid serial sampling of creatine kinase MB for very early detection of myocardial infarction in patients with acute chest pain. Am Heart J 1992; 123:354.

25. Antman EM, Tanasijevic MJ, Thompson B, et al. Cardiac-specific troponin I levels to predict the risk of mortality in patients with acute coronary syndromes. N Engl J Med 1996; 335:1342.

26. Hamm CW, Ravkilde J, Gerhardt W, et al. The prognostic value of serum troponin T in unstable angina. N Engl J Med 1992; 327:146.

27. Ohman EM, Armstrong PW, Christenson RH, et al. Cardiac troponin T levels for risk stratification in acute myocardial ischemia. N Engl J Med 1996; 335:1333.

28. Ravkilde J, Nissen H, Horder M, et al. Independent prognostic value of serum creatine kinase isoenzyme MB mass, cardiac troponin T and myosin light chain levels in suspected acute myocardial infarction: analysis of 28 months of follow-up in 196 patients. J Am Coll Cardiol 1995; 25:574.

29. Wu AH, Abbas SA, Green S, et al. Prognostic value of cardiac troponin T in unstable angina pectoris. Am J Cardiol 1995; 76:970.

30. Hamm CW, Goldmann BU, Heeschen C, et al. Emergency room triage of patients with acute chest pain by means of rapid testing for cardiac troponin T or troponin I. N Engl J Med 1997; 337:1648.

31. Heeschen C, Hamm CW, Goldmann B, et al. Troponin concentrations for stratification of patients with acute coronary syndromes in relation to therapeutic efficacy of tirofiban. PRISM Study Investigators. Platelet Receptor Inhibition in Ischemic Syndrome Management. Lancet 1999; 354:1757.

32. Wasson JH, Sox HC, Neff RK, et al. Clinical prediction rules: applications and methodological standards. N Engl J Med 1985; 313:793.

33. Selker HP. Coronary care unit triage decision aids: how do we know when they work? Am J Med 1989; 87:491.

34. Pozen MW, D'Agostino RB, Mitchell JB, et al. The usefulness of a predictive instrument to reduce inappropriate admissions to the coronary care unit. Ann Intern Med 1980; 92:238.

35. Selker HP, D'Agostino RB, Laks MM. A predictive instrument for acute ischemic heart disease to improve coronary care unit admission practices: a potential on-line tool in a computerized electrocardiograph. J Electrocardiol 1988; 88:S11.

36. Selker HP, Griffith JL, D'Agostino RB. A tool for judging coronary care unit admission that is appropriate for both real-time and retrospective use: a time-insensitive predictive instrument (TIPI) for acute cardiac ischemia: a multicenter study. Med Care 1991; 29:610.

37. Hauser AM, Gangadharan V, Ramos R, et al. Sequence of mechanical, electrocardiographic and clinical effects of repeated coronary artery occlusion in human beings: echocardiographic observations during coronary angioplasty. J Am Coll Cardiol 1985; 5:193.

38. Peels CH, Visser CA, Kupper AJF, et al. Usefulness of two-dimensional echocardiography for immediate detection of myocardial ischemia in the emergency room. Am J Cardiol 1990; 65:687.

39. Sasaki H, Charuzi Y, Beeder C, et al. Utility of echocardiography for the early assessment of patients with non-diagnostic chest pain. Am Heart J 1986; 112:494.

40. Sabia P, Afrookteh A, Touchstone D, et al. Value of regional wall motion abnormality in the emergency room diagnosis of acute myocardial infarction. Circulation 1991; 84:I-85.

41. Kaul S, Sabia PJ, Abbott RD. Use of two-dimensional echocardiography in the emergency department. Prim Cardiol 1992; 18:26.

42. Loh IK, et al. Early diagnosis of non-transmural myocardial infarction by two-dimensional echocardiography. Am Heart J 1982; 104:963.

43. Kontos MC, Arrowood JA, Paulsen WHJ, et al. Early echocardiography can predict cardiac events in emergency department patients with chest pain. Ann Emerg Med 1998; 31:550.

44. Trippi JA, Lee KS, Kopp G, et al. Dobutamine stress tele-echocardiography for evaluation of emergency department patients with chest pain. J Am Coll Cardiol 1997; 30:627.

45. Strauss HW, Harrison K, Langan JK, et al. Thallium-201 for myocardial imaging: relation of thallium-201 to regional myocardial perfusion. Circulation 1975; 51: 641.

46. Wackers FJ, Sokole EB, Samson G, et al. Value and limitations of thallium-201 scintigraphy in the acute phase of myocardial infarction. N Engl J Med 1976; 295:1.

47. Wackers FJ, Lie KI, Keon KL, et al. Thallium-201 scintigraphy in unstable angina pectoris. Circulation 1978; 57:738.

48. Beller GA. Radiopharmaceuticals in nuclear cardiology. In: *Clinical Nuclear Cardiology*, edited by GA Beller. Philadelphia: WB Saunders 1995, pp. 37–81.

49. Okada RD, Glover D, Gaffney T, et al. Myocardial kinetics of Tc-99m-hexakis-2-methoxy-2-methylpropylisonitrile. Circulation 1988; 77:491.

50. Bilodeau L, Theroux P, Gregoire J, et al. Tc-99m sestamibi tomography in patients with spontaneous chest pain: correlations with clinical, electrocardiographic and angiographic findings. J Am Coll Cardiol 1991; 18:1684.

51. Christian TF, Clements IP, Gibbons RI. Non-invasive identification of myocardial risk in patients with acute myocardial infarction and nondiagnostic electrocardiogram with Tc-99m sestamibi. Circulation 1991; 83:1615.

52. Varetto T, Cantalupi D, Altieri A, et al. Emergency room Tc-99m sestamibi imaging to rule out acute myocardial ischemic events in patients with nondiagnostic electrocardiography. J Am Coll Cardiol 1993; 22:1804.

53. Hilton TC, Thompson RC, Williams H, et al. Tc-99m sestamibi myocardial perfusion imaging in the emergency room evaluation of chest pain. J Am Coll Cardiol 1994; 23:1016.

54. Hilton TC, et al. Ninety day follow up of emergency department patients with chest pain with normal or non-diagnostic ECG who undergo acute cardiac imaging with Tc-99m sestamibi (abstract). J Am Coll Cardiol 1995; 25:192A.

55. Heller GV, Stowers SA, Hendel RC, et al. Clinical value of acute rest technetium-99m tetrofosmin tomographic myocardial perfusion imaging in patients with acute chest pain and nondiagnostic electrocardiograms. J Am Coll Cardiol 1998; 31:1011.

56. Kontos MC, Jesse RL, Schmidt KL, et al. Value of acute rest sestamibi perfusion imaging for evaluation of patients admitted to the emergency department with chest pain. J Am Coll Cardiol 1997; 30:976.

57. Kontos MC, Kurdziel KA, Ornato JP, et al. A nonischemic electrocardiogram does not always predict a small myocardial infarction: results with acute myocardial perfusion imaging. Am Heart J 2001; 141:360.

58. Kosnik JW, Zalenski RJ, Shamsa F, et al. Resting sestamibi imaging for the prognosis of low-risk chest pain. Acad Emerg Med 1999; 6:998.

59. Tatum JL, Jesse RL, Kontos MC, et al. Comprehensive strategy for the evaluation and triage of the chest pain patient. Ann Emerg Med 1997; 29:116.

60. Stowers SA, Eisenstein EL, Wackers FJ, et al. An economic analysis of an aggressive diagnostic strategy with single photon emission computed tomography myocardial perfusion imaging and early exercise stress testing in emergency department patients who present with chest pain but nondiagnostic electrocardiograms: results from a randomized trial. Ann Emerg Med 2000;35:17.

61. Udelson JE. The ERASE Chest Pain trial. Presented at "Special Session: Clinical Trials" at the 72nd Scientific Sessions of the American Heart Association. Atlanta GA. November 1999.

62. Adams JE III, Bodor GS, Davila-Roman VG, et al. Cardiac troponin I: a marker with high specificity for cardiac injury. Circulation 1993; 88:101.

63. Duca MD, Satyendra G, Wu AHB, et al. Comparison of acute rest myocardial perfusion imaging and serum markers of myocardial injury in patients with chest pain syndromes. J Nucl Cardiol 1999; 6:570.

64. Hamm CW, Heeschen C, Goldmann B, et al. Benefit of abciximab in patients with refractory unstable angina in relation to serum troponin T levels. C7E3 Fab antiplatelet therapy in unstable angina (CAPTURE) study investigators. N Engl J Med 1999; 340:1623.

65. Zimmerman J, Fromm R, Meyer D, et al. Diagnostic marker cooperative study for the diagnosis of myocardial infarction. Circulation 1999; 99:1671.

66. Newby LK, Christianson RH, Ohman EM, et al. Value of serial troponin T measures for early and late risk stratification in patients with acute coronary syndromes. Circulation 1998; 98: 1853.

67. Kontos MC, Jesse RL, Anderson FP, et al. Comparison of myocardial perfusion imaging and cardiac troponin I in patients admitted to the emergency department with chest pain. Circulation 1999; 99:2073.

68. Kontos MC, Arrowood JA, Jesse RL, et al. Comparison between 2-dimensional echocardiography and myocardial perfusion imaging in the emergency department in patients with possible myocardial ischemia. Am Heart J 1998; 136:724.

69. Weissman IA, Dickinson CZ, Dworkin HJ, et al. Cost-effectiveness of myocardial perfusion imaging with SPECT in the emergency department evaluation of patients with unexplained chest pain. Radiology 1996; 199:353.

70. Radensky PW, et al. Potential cost effectiveness of initial myocardial perfusion imaging for assessment of emergency department patients with chest pain. Am J Cardiol 1997; 79:595.

71. Ziffer J, Nateman DR, Janowitz WR, et al. Improved patient outcomes and cost-effectiveness of utilizing nuclear cardiology protocols in an emergency department chest pain center (abstract). J Nucl Med 1998; 39:139P.

72. Kosnik JW, Zalenski RJ, Grzybowski M, et al. Impact of technetium-99m sestamibi imaging on the emergency department management and costs in the evaluation of low-risk chest pain. Acad Emerg Med 2001; 8:315.

73. Taillefer R, DePuey EG, Udelson JE, et al. Comparative diagnostic accuracy of Tl-201 and Tc-99m sestamibi SPECT imaging (perfusion and ECG-gated SPECT) in detecting coronary artery disease in women. J Am Coll Cardiol 1997; 29:69.

74. Hendel RC, Selker HP, Heller GV, et al. The impact of attenuation correction and gating on SPECT perfusion imaging in patients presenting to the emergency department with chest pain (abstract). Circulation 2000; 102:II-543.

75. Kiat H, Van Train KF, Friedman, et al. Quantitative stress-redistribution thallium-201 SPECT using prone imaging: methodologic development and validation. J Nucl Med 1992; 33:1509.

76. Perault C, Loboguerrero A, Liehn JC, et al. Quantitative comparison of prone and supine myocardial SPECT MIBI images. Clin Nucl Med 1995; 20:678.

77. Braunwald E, Antman EM, Beasley JW, et al. ACC/AHA guidelines for the management of patients with unstable angina and non-ST-segment elevation myocardial infarction. A report of the American College of Cardiology/American Heart Association Task Force on Practice Guidelines (Committee on the Management of Patients with Unstable Angina). J Am Coll Cardiol 2000; 36:970.

15 | Fatty acid and MIBG imaging

NAGARA TAMAKI AND MICHEL W. DAE

Part 1

IPPA-BMIPP

NAGARA TAMAKI

Myocardial perfusion imaging has been most widely used for assessing patients with suspected or known coronary artery disease. On the other hand, nuclear medicine has progressed in association with the growth of molecular medicine. Myocardial metabolic imaging is one of the new fields studied with nuclear medicine techniques. Myocardial energy metabolism has long been investigated in experimental models with use of Langendorff's perfusion system and coronary sinus blood sampling. An introduction of a variety of radio-pharmaceutical agents has made it possible to visualize myocardial energy metabolism in vivo.

MYOCARDIAL METABOLISM

The heart is an active organ that needs high oxygen uptake to maintain its mechanical function. The major purpose of oxygen uptake of the heart is to provide sufficient energy to balance the requirement of its mechanical function. Glucose and free fatty acids are major energy sources in the myocardium. The uptake of various substrates by the heart is partially dependent on the arterial concentration of the fuel. In the fasting state, where plasma levels of free fatty acids are high, free fatty acid uptake in the myocardium is also high, with suppression of glucose oxidation. On the other hand, when glucose and/or insulin levels are high such as in postprandial condition, glucose oxidation increases with suppression of fatty acid utilization [1].

Long-chain fatty acids are the principal energy source for the normoxic myocardium and are rapidly metabolized by beta-oxidation. Approximately 60%–80% of ATP produced in aerobic myocardium derives from fatty acid oxidation. Long-chain free fatty acids easily pass through the sarcolemmal membrane to be acti-

vated as acyl-CoA. The extraction of free fatty acids is regulated by chain length, various metabolic substrates, such as plasma glucose and free fatty acid levels, circulating levels of hormones, and cardiac workload [1,2]. The acyl-CoA is carried into mitochondria as acyl carnithine carrier system to enter the beta-oxidation pathway, which cuts off two carbon fractions. This activation of free fatty acids is an energy-dependent process. After beta-oxidation, acetyl-CoA is formed, which enters the tricarbonic acid cycle for further oxidation to become water and carbon dioxide. A fraction of the free fatty acid is not oxidized but is incorporated as triglyceride and myocardial structural lipids and stays in the myocardium for a longer time.

During ischemia, on the other hand, glucose plays a major role for residual oxidative metabolism, while oxidation of long-chain fatty acid is greatly suppressed [2,3]. Lack of oxygen supply rapidly suppresses beta-oxidation, and acyl-CoA increases in the mitochondria. Since beta-oxidation is inhibited, the activated fatty acids are shunted into triglyceride storage pools. The back diffusion of nonmetabolized free fatty acids is also increased.

Thus, alteration of fatty acid oxidation is considered to be a sensitive marker of ischemia and myocardial damage. A number of radiolabeled fatty acid analogs have been introduced to assess myocardial cellular function (Fig. 15.1).

Positron emission tomography (PET) is considered a reliable method to probe myocardial metabolic imaging in vivo. PET has a unique character for in vivo tracing various physiological and biochemical functions using various radiolabeled physiological compounds [4,5]. C-11 palmitate, one of the radiolabeled long-chain saturated fatty acid compounds, is most commonly used for assessing myocardial fatty acid metab-

293

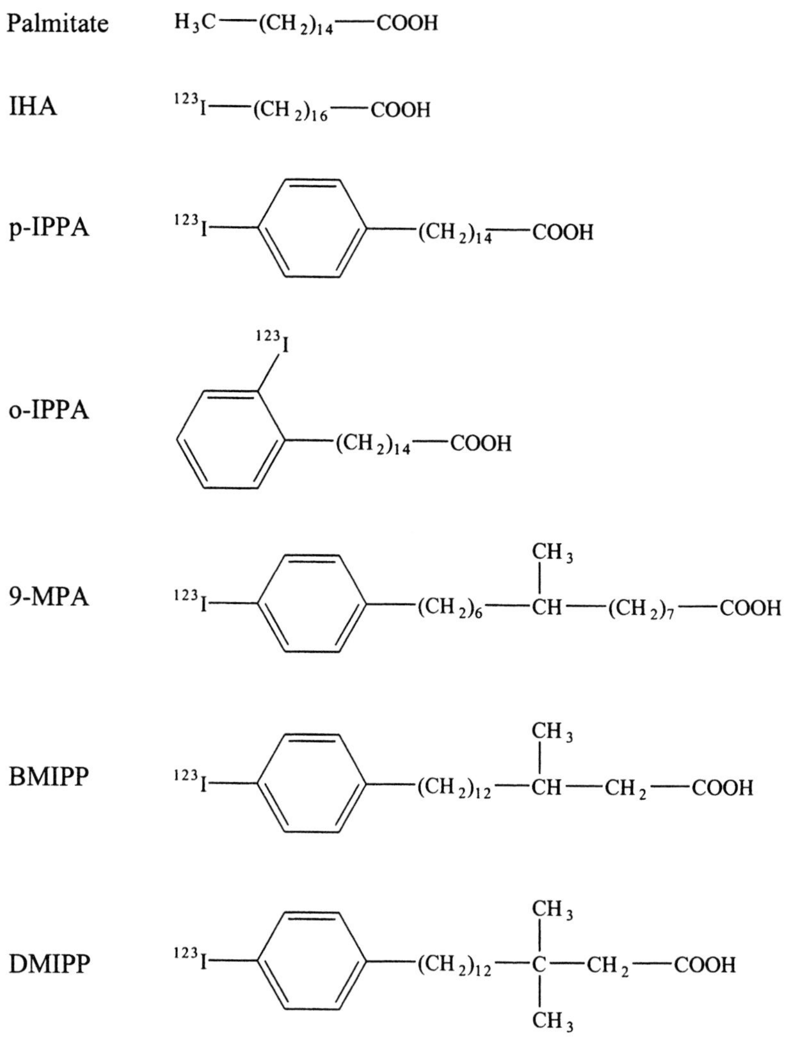

Palmitate H_3C—$(CH_2)_{14}$—COOH

IHA ^{123}I—$(CH_2)_{16}$—COOH

p-IPPA ^{123}I—⬡—$(CH_2)_{14}$—COOH

o-IPPA   [benzene ring with ^{123}I substituent]—$(CH_2)_{14}$—COOH

9-MPA ^{123}I—⬡—$(CH_2)_6$—CH(CH_3)—$(CH_2)_7$—COOH

BMIPP ^{123}I—⬡—$(CH_2)_{12}$—CH(CH_3)—CH_2—COOH

DMIPP ^{123}I—⬡—$(CH_2)_{12}$—C(CH_3)(CH_3)—CH_2—COOH

FIGURE 15.1 Structures of various radioiodinated fatty acid analogs. (Reprinted with permission of the Society of Nuclear Medicine from Tamaki N, et al. The roles of fatty acids in cardiac imaging. J Nucl Med 2000;41:1525.)

olism in PET studies [6–8]. Unfortunately, only a few institutions have PET cameras and a cyclotron that can study myocardial energy metabolism in vivo. There have been a number of attempts to solve this limitation. The introduction of a variety of I-123 labeled fatty acid compounds is one of the promising solutions. There are a variety of iodinated fatty acid compounds to probe myocardial energy metabolism in vivo in routine clinical nuclear medicine facilities. Iodine-123 is an appropriate choice for labeling metabolic substrates, because of its chemical property for synthesis by halogen exchange reaction, replacing a molecular methyl group, thereby allowing wide application in clinical practice. Thus, iodine-123 labeled fatty acids have received a lot of attention for assessing myocardial metabolism in vivo [9–12].

TWO TYPES OF IODINATED FATTY ACID COMPOUNDS

There are two groups of iodinated fatty acid compounds, including straight-chain fatty acids and modified branched fatty acids (Fig. 15.1 and Table 15.1) [9–12]. The straight-chain fatty acids, such as IPPA, are generally metabolized via beta-oxidation and released from the myocardium (Fig. 15.2). Therefore, fatty acid oxidation can be directly assessed by the washout kinetics of the tracer, similar to C-11 palmitate. However, a rapid washout from the myocardium may require a fast dynamic acquisition for imaging following tracer administration (Fig. 15.3). This rapid washout of these tracers may become a critical problem when imaging is done with a rotating tomographic gamma camera.

TABLE 15.1 *Characteristics of Straight-Chain and Branched Fatty Acids*

	Straight-Chain Fatty Acids	Branched Fatty Acids
PET tracers	^{11}C-palmitate	^{11}C-3-(R,S)-methyl heptadecanoic acid
SPECT tracers	^{123}I-16-iodohexadecenoic acid	^{123}I-(p-iodophenyl)-3-(R,S)-methylpentadecanoic acid (BMIPP)
	^{123}I-17-iodoheptadecanoic acid (IHA)	123I-(p-iodophenyl)-3,3-dimethylpentadecanoic acid (DMIPP)
	^{123}I-iodophenylpentadecanoic acid (IPPA)	^{123}I-(p-iodophenyl)-9-(R,S)-methylpentadecanoic acid (9MPA)
Measurement	Uptake and clearance	Uptake (metabolic trapping)
Advantages	beta-oxidation assessment	Suitable for SPECT imaging
		Excellent image quality

Rapid single-photon emission computed tomography (SPECT) acquisition may afford inadequate counts with poor image quality. Besides, delayed SPECT acquisition may result in poor images with low target-to-background ratio. In addition, back diffusion and metabolites should be considered in the kinetic model for quantitative analysis of fatty acid metabolism.

The modified fatty acids, such as BMIPP, were introduced based on the concept of myocardial retention due to metabolic trapping (see Fig. 15.2). The high retention in the myocardium with slow or no washout from the myocardium enables the creation of excellent myocardial images with long acquisition time (see Fig. 15.3). On the other hand, their uptake may not directly reflect fatty acid oxidation. Instead, the uptake is based on the fatty acid uptake and turnover rate of the lipid pool. A combined imaging of the iodinated fatty acid and per-

fusion is required to demonstrate perfusion-metabolism mismatch and to characterize fatty acid utilization.

I-123 LABELED STRAIGHT-CHAIN FATTY ACID COMPOUNDS

Basic Considerations

Introducing radioiodine into the terminal position of a fatty acid has made great progress without altering its extraction efficiency compared to naturally occurring compounds. To eliminate rapid deiodination of the iodinated compounds, stable iodinated fatty acid compounds have been developed with iodide attached to the para or ortho position of the phenyl ring. Machulla et al. [13] introduced the terminally phenylated iodinated straight-chain fatty acid, 15(p-(123I)-iodophenyl) pen-

Kinetics of Fatty Acids

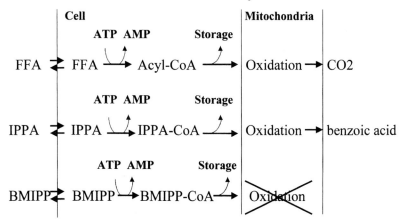

FIGURE 15.2 Tracer kinetics of radiolabeled free fatty acids (FFA), such as C-11 palmitate, iodinated straight-chain fatty acid compounds, such as IPPA, and iodinated branched fatty acid compounds, such as BMIPP. FFA and IPPA are oxidized in the mitochondria and washed out from the myocardium as carbon dioxide and I-123 benzoic acid, respectively. On the contrary, BMIPP is retained in the myocardium without rapid oxidization. (Reprinted with permission of the Society of Nuclear Medicine from Tamaki N, et al. The roles of fatty acids in cardiac imaging. J Nucl Med 2000; 41: 1525–1534.)

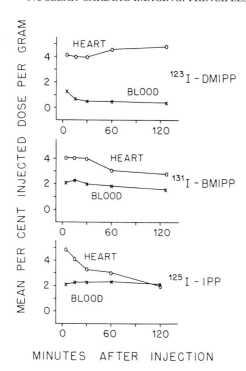

FIGURE 15.3 Tracer kinetics of iodinated compounds over time. DMIPP and BMIPP are examples of branched fatty acid compounds showing slow or no washout from the myocardium. IPPA is an example of straight-chain fatty acid compounds showing rapid washout from the myocardium. (Reprinted with permission of the Society of Nuclear Medicine from Knapp F, et al. Radioiodinated 15-(p-iodophenyl)-3,3 dimethylpentadecanoic acid: a useful new agent to evaluate myocardial fatty acid uptake. J Nucl Med 1986; 27: 521–531.)

tadecanoic acid (IPPA). This agent showed no essential release of free radioiodide into the circulation. Kaiser et al. [14] analyzed the differences in tracer kinetics of the para or ortho position of 15(p-(123I)-iodophenyl) pentadecanoic acid. Ortho 15(p-(123I)-iodophenyl) pentadecanoic acid is readily taken up and retained in the myocardium with a long retention time, similar to branched fatty acid compounds. Para 15(p-(123I)-iodophenyl) pentadecanoic acid is rapidly excreted from the myocardium as I-123 benzoic acid (see Fig. 15.2). Since IPPA is the most widely investigated compound, basic and clinical characteristics of IPPA are discussed in the remaining section.

Reske et al. [15,16] demonstrated rapid accumulation of tracer in the heart following administration of IPPA with fast clearance from the myocardium in biexponential fashion characteristic of C-11 palmitate. While a high myocardial uptake was observed in the normal myocardium, a decreased uptake was noted in the areas supplied with an occluded coronary artery. Yang et al. [17] showed initial reduction of IPPA uptake with fill-in

on the delayed scan (resting redistribution) during sustained low flow with myocardial asynergy. They concluded that serial IPPA imaging may be useful for assessing myocardial viability in low flow ischemia, but they also suggested overestimation of viable myocardium by IPPA in the postreperfusion infarcted myocardium.

Clinical Applications

There are a number of clinical reports using IPPA in the study of patients with coronary artery disease in Europe and the United States. Hansen et al. [18] and Kennedy et al. [19] both showed a segmental reduction of IPPA, which correlated well with regional perfusion defects on thallium scan. Reske et al. [15] showed the IPPA defects were generally more prominent than the thallium defects, probably due to lower extraction fraction of IPPA in ischemic areas. They also indicated that the IPPA study at rest was useful for the detection of myocardial ischemia in patients with coronary artery disease. Besides, Caldwell et al. [20] compared the IPPA uptake with perfusion during exercise to find the linear correlation of IPPA uptake with myocardial blood flow during exercise. They indicated the possibility for detecting areas of reduced flow reserve by exercise IPPA imaging. Interestingly, the image quality and diagnostic values were similar under fasting and nonfasting states with IPPA [21], which may be quite different from fatty acid imaging with C-11 palmitate.

For viability assessment, Kuikka et al. [22] described that IPPA uptake was identified in 39% of the segments with persistent MIBI defect and normalized in 25% of these segments. Although they did not prove that the areas with decreased IPPA uptake represented reversible ischemic myocardium, they indicated a potential clinical value of IPPA imaging over the MIBI perfusion study. Murray et al. [23] compared the dynamic IPPA study data, acquired with a multicrystal camera, with transmural biopsies and thallium scan results to conclude that the IPPA-viable segments corresponded well to biopsy-viable segments and depicted viable myocardium more accurately than the thallium scans. Recent studies indicate the clinical value of IPPA SPECT imaging at rest for viability assessment based on the prediction of functional recovery after revascularization. Hansen et al. [24] identified the areas showing intermediate range IPPA washout (less than the normal range but more than the infarcted areas) as ischemic but viable myocardium. Iskandrian et al. [25] indicated that reversibility on IPPA imaging was more often seen than on the rest-redistribution thallium imaging. They showed advantages of semiquantitative analysis of IPPA kinetics over rest-redistribution thallium imaging.

A recent report by Verani et al. indicated the value of IPPA imaging for the prediction of enhanced left ventricular function after coronary artery bypass grafting [26]. Among clinical and scintigraphic variables, the single most important predictor for improvement of function was the number of IPPA-viable segments. Since IPPA shows differential washout from the myocardium in the normal, ischemic, and infarcted myocardium, IPPA kinetic analysis is considered to be valuable for assessing myocardial viability. Areas with initial reduction of IPPA that fill in on the delayed scan may indicate tracer distribution in the myocardium with decreased fatty acid oxidation, and thus these areas are considered to represent ischemic but viable myocardium (Fig. 15.4).

IPPA imaging has also been studied in various myocardial disorders. Ugolini et al. [27] demonstrated greater heterogeneity of IPPA uptake with faster washout rate in patients with dilated cardiomyopathy than in normal subjects. Wolfe et al. [28] studied stress IPPA imaging in patients with left ventricular hypertrophy secondary to arterial hypertension. Reduced uptake and delayed washout of IPPA from the myocardium, indicating regional myocardial ischemia in hypertrophic myocardium, were noted. Although stress thallium imaging did not show abnormal perfusion, such regional heterogeneity of fatty acid metabolism suggests impaired microcirculation in hypertrophic myocardium. Since many myocardial disorders may be associated with metabolic alterations, IPPA imaging may hold a key role for differential diagnosis and staging of the myocardial disorders.

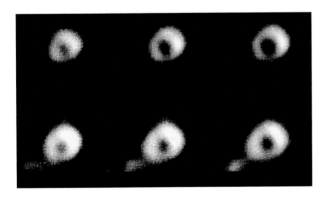

FIGURE 15.4 A series of short-axis slices of early (*top*) and delayed (*bottom*) IPPA SPECT images of a patient with unstable angina. Note initial reduction of IPPA uptake with significant filling in inferior and septal region, indicating delayed washout of IPPA in the ischemic myocardium. (Reprinted with permission of the American Society of Nuclear Cardiology from Tamaki N, et al. Radionuclide assessment of myocardial fatty acid metabolism by PET and SPECT. J Nucl Cardiol 1995; 2: 256–266.) (Courtesy of Dr. Ami Iskandrian.)

In summary, the tracer kinetics of IPPA are well documented, reflecting both fatty acid uptake and oxidation. Its unique properties of probing perfusion and fatty acid turnover have resulted in many important clinical studies. In particular, reduced initial uptake with slow washout of IPPA, so called redistribution, is commonly seen in ischemic but viable myocardium. Such kinetic studies have a key role for assessing myocardial viability. On the other hand, relatively rapid washout from the myocardium may pose some difficulty to kinetic analysis with a conventional SPECT camera. Wider clinical experience is warranted to confirm the clinical utility of these agents for detection of coronary artery disease, assessment of tissue viability, and evaluation of myocardial disorders.

I-123 LABELED MODIFIED FATTY ACIDS

Variety of the Tracers

One of the major characteristics of branched fatty acid compounds is that methyl branching of the fatty acid chain retains the compounds in the myocardium while protecting against metabolism by beta-oxidation (metabolic trapping). Thus, excellent myocardial images are obtained with long acquisition time. Although their uptake may not directly reflect fatty acid oxidation, they retain some of the physiologic properties, such as fatty acid uptake and turnover rate of the triglyceride pool. The degree of branching and the chain length determine the myocardial uptake of these tracers.

A number of iodinated branch-chain fatty acids have been introduced to assess fatty acid utilization. One example is iodine-123-(p-iodophenyl-9-(R,S)-methyl pentadecanoic acid ([123I] 9MPA) for clinical investigation. This tracer is trapped in the myocardium with a similar mechanism as that of free fatty acids. While other branched fatty acid analogs stay in the myocardium for a long time, 9MPA is converted to iodophenyl-3-methylnonanoic acid (3MNA) after three cycles of beta-oxidation. Since 3MNA is a water-soluble intermediate metabolite, it is rapidly washed out from the myocardium. Thus, this agent is designed to trace both fatty acid uptake and to some degree beta-oxidation.

The first clinical study was reported by Chouraqui et al. [29] who showed a high uptake and retention in the myocardium shortly after 9MPA administration. They indicated that the postexercise study of 9MPA may be comparable with a stress thallium study. Unfortunately, they did not evaluate the clinical importance of metabolism beyond a perfusion study. After their initial study, clinical trials of 9MPA were performed in Japan [30–32]. Abnormal uptake of this tracer (less uptake than that of a perfusion marker in most of the cases) was well demonstrated in ischemic regions. The results seem to be comparable or even better than BMIPP findings to identify ischemic myocardium. In addition, there is some washout from the myocardium. Its washout rate seems to differ in various myocardial disorders. Since the washout rate of this compound was slower than the straight-chain fatty acid IPPA, this tracer is more feasible for washout analysis with SPECT.

16-[^{123}I]-iodo-3-methylhexadecanoic acid (MIHA) is another example of a methyl-branched analog that has been used clinically in Europe. Marie et al. [33] showed that a reversible MIHA defect was more often observed than on rest-reinjection thallium imaging, indicating the value for identifying ischemic myocardium. They also indicated that MIHA was a reliable marker of reversible ischemic myocardium after revascularization in patients with a prior myocardial infarction [34]. They concluded that preserved uptake of MIHA in the hypoperfused areas may be a better marker of tissue viability than the conventional thallium imaging.

Another approach for labeling metabolically trapped analog is to use a phenylene substituted fatty acid analog. 13-p-[^{123}I]-3-(p-phenylene)-tridecanoic acid (PHIPA) is considered the most promising tracer for myocardial imaging. PHIPA is extracted by the myocardium in a manner similar to the extraction of the unmodified fatty acid analog IPPA. The retention of the tracer results from the presence of the p-phenylene group, which prevents more than one beta-oxidation cycle [35]. In the human study during cardiac transplantation by Jonas et al. [36], a greater uptake of PHIPA than Tc-99m-sestamibi perfusion was observed in the residual viable myocardium, while a matched defect was associated with myocardial scar. More clinical experience is warranted to confirm the value of this agent for viability assessment.

Basic Considerations of BMIPP

Methyl-branched fatty acid is based on the concept of inhibition of beta-oxidation by the presence of methyl group in the beta-position. Knapp et al. [37] introduced 15-(p-iodophenyl)-3(R,S)-methyl pentadecanoic acid (BMIPP). The animal experiments showed a slow clearance of BMIPP (approximately 25% in 2 hours). The fractional distribution of this compound at 30 minutes after tracer injection in rats indicated 65% to 80% of the total activity resided in the triglyceride pool [38]. Sloof et al. [39] compared BMIPP with another branched fatty acid analog, 15-(para-iodophenyl)-3,3-dimethyl pentadecanoic acid (DMIPP), in human subjects, and concluded that BMIPP was more favorable

due to lower liver uptake. BMIPP has been most widely used to investigate basic kinetics and clinical implications, particularly in Japan and Europe.

A number of experimental studies have been performed to assess the tracer kinetics of BMIPP in the myocardium. Fujibayashi et al. [38] in a canine study indicated that 74% of injected BMIPP dose was extracted from the plasma into the myocardium and about 65% was retained, following an intracoronary injection of BMIPP, with only 8.7% fraction of washout from the myocardium. The slow washout from the myocardium was seen as alpha- and beta-oxidation metabolites [40,41]. Hosokawa et al. [42] showed the enhanced rapid washout from the myocardium by long-chain fatty acid transporter inhibitor, etomoxir, which may produce a similar condition as myocardial ischemia. Fujibayashi et al. [43,44] analyzed the BMIPP uptake in acutely damaged myocardium treated with dinitrophenol or tetradecylglycidic acid, an inhibitor of mitochondrial carnitine acyltransferase I, and found that BMIPP uptake correlated with ATP concentration. Nohara et al. [45] also showed a significant correlation with ATP levels in the occlusion and reperfusion canine model. They concluded that BMIPP may be useful to differentiate ischemic from infarcted myocardium in their model. These results support the importance of ATP levels for the retention of BMIPP, probably due to cytosolic activation of BMIPP into BMIPP-CoA.

The postischemic myocardium often showed higher BMIPP uptake than thallium uptake in both in vivo and ex vivo occlusion-reperfusion model studies [46,47]. These findings (more BMIPP uptake than perfusion) conflicted with the clinical reports, where less BMIPP uptake than perfusion is often observed. Such conflicting results may be partly explained by the fatty acid uptake, which was influenced by both residence time in the capillary bed and the rate of back diffusion from the myocardium. In acute ischemia, the size of the nonoxidized lipid pool is increased. Once BMIPP enters into the myocardium, it goes to this enlarged lipid pool with slower turnover than in the normal myocardium. Thus, BMIPP uptake may possibly be increased in acute ischemic myocardium. During prolonged ischemia, on the other hand, the net extraction fraction of the tracer decreases probably due to shunting into the triglyceride pool and back diffusion into the coronary venous circulation. Thus, regional uptake of this fatty acid analog may be reduced in chronic and severely ischemic myocardium. Such decrease in BMIPP uptake is most often observed in ischemic myocardium due to enhanced back diffusion of BMIPP from the myocardium. In the canine ischemic model, Hosokawa et al. [48] nicely showed an increase in back diffusion of nonmetabolized BMIPP in the coronary sinus sampling after BMIPP administration. Thus, regional uptake of BMIPP may be reduced in the severely ischemic myocardium.

BMIPP is usually injected under fasting conditions. SPECT imaging is obtained about 15–30 minutes after tracer administration. BMIPP uptake in the myocardium was not influenced by the plasma substrate levels in a human study [46]. Approximately 0.2%–1% of all clinical BMIPP studies revealed no accumulation of BMIPP in the myocardium [50]. The comparative studies indicated a reduction of C-11 palmitate uptake with enhanced FDG uptake in the myocardium in these patients, indicating metabolic shifting from free fatty acid to glucose utilization in the fasting state [50]. Absent BMIPP uptake in the myocardium may be related to the absence of membrane fatty acid transporter CD-36, which might possibly relate to the BMIPP uptake in these cases [51].

Clinical Applications of BMIPP

Clinical studies show a rapid and high myocardial uptake with long retention after BMIPP administration with low background and low uptake in the liver and lungs at 15–60 minutes after BMIPP injection. SPECT images of high quality can be obtained by collecting myocardial images for approximately 20 minutes. BMIPP distribution is carefully assessed to identify regional decrease in tracer distribution as an area of altered fatty acid uptake and metabolism. Regional BMIPP uptake may also be compared with regional perfusion to detect presence of perfusion-metabolism mismatch.

Tamaki et al. [52] demonstrated in a study of patients with myocardial infarction that less BMIPP uptake than thallium perfusion was often seen in areas of recent infarction, areas with recanalized arteries, and those with severe wall motion abnormalities (Fig. 15.5). European studies also showed less BMIPP uptake than Tc-99m-sestamibi perfusion in subacute myocardial infarction [53,54]. These studies suggest less BMIPP uptake than perfusion is a result of delayed recovery of metabolism after recovery of perfusion, or stunning.

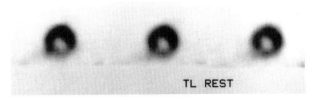

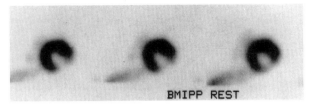

FIGURE 15.5 A series of short-axis slices of thallium and BMIPP at rest in patients with inferior wall myocardial infarction. While similar decrease in tracer uptake was seen in inferior regions, a definite decrease in BMIPP relative to thallium is noted in the lateral region. (Reprinted with permission of the European Society of Nuclear Medicine from Tamaki N, et al. Prognostic value of iodine-123 labeled BMIPP fatty acid analogue imaging in patients with myocardial infarction. Eur J Nucl Med 1996; 2: 272–279.)

Furutani et al. [55] indicated that BMIPP defect size may identify the area at risk in patients with acute myocardial infarction treated with successful revascularization, since in this setting the BMIPP defect was much larger than the thallium perfusion defect. Kawai et al. [56] proved that the BMIPP defect areas in the subacute phase correlated with the areas at risk calculated by the perfusion imaging on admission in the acute phase of myocardial infarction. They suggested that BMIPP may reflect prior severe ischemia after recovery of perfusion, so called ischemic memory. Many investigators showed that areas with less BMIPP uptake than perfusion in acute and subacute phases of myocardial infarction improved wall motion abnormalities on the follow-up study, suggesting these areas contained stunned myocardium [57–60].

Since persistent metabolic alteration is often seen in severe ischemic myocardium, BMIPP at rest has been used for identifying ischemic myocardium [61–65]. Table 15.2 summarizes the diagnostic accuracy of BMIPP imaging at rest for detecting patients with coronary stenosis without a history of myocardial infarction.

TABLE 15.2 *Diagnostic Accuracy of BMIPP Imaging at Rest for Identifying Coronary Lesions*

Study	No. of Patients	DIAGNOSTIC ACCURACY		
		Sensitivity	Specificity	Accuracy
Takeishi [61,62]	68	34/62 (55%)	5/6 (83%)	39/68 (57%)
Tateno [63]	31	27/31 (87%)	NA	27/31 (87%)
Suzuki [64]	28	25/28 (89%)	NA	25/28 (89%)
Yamabe [65]	104	52/83 (63%)	20/21 (96%)	72/104 (69%)
Total	231	138/204 (68%)	25/27 (93%)	163/231 (71%)

The sensitivity of BMIPP imaging for detecting coronary artery lesions ranged from 55% to 89%, which might be slightly inferior to the conventional stress perfusion imaging which provides 80%–90% of sensitivity. On the other hand, this type of imaging does not require a stress test, and therefore is quite suitable for patients with unstable angina or severe coronary artery disease. The sensitivity tended to be higher in the study of patients with unstable angina [62–65]. In addition, decrease in BMIPP uptake was often associated with regional wall motion abnormalities in those without a history of myocardial infarction [63]. Furthermore, metabolic alterations are most often seen in patients with vasospastic angina, probably as a result of repetitive ischemic episodes [66]. On the other hand, a stress perfusion study may not identify regional perfusion abnormalities. Recently Yamabe et al. [67] reported that reduced BMIPP uptake was observed in patients with severe coronary artery disease (without a prior myocardial infarction) who may require subsequent interventional therapy. Thus, BMIPP imaging is considered a method of choice to identify regional abnormalities as persistent metabolic abnormalities ("ischemic memory") in these patients, and may assist in the choice of therapeutic options in patients with chest pain [67B].

The discordance between BMIPP uptake and perfusion may represent reversible, ischemic myocardium. Matsunari et al. [68] and Kawamoto et al. [69] both reported that the areas with reduced uptake of BMIPP showed thallium redistribution on stress-delayed scan (Fig. 15.6). Tamaki et al. [10,70] showed that such discordant BMIPP uptake was observed in areas with increase in FDG uptake as a marker of exogenous glucose utilization. The areas with discordant BMIPP uptake were most likely to show ischemia by PET, whereas a concordant decrease both in BMIPP and thallium reflected myocardial scar by PET. In addition, such areas showed preserved oxidative metabolism, as assessed by C-11 acetate PET studies. In ischemic myocardium, fatty acid oxidation is easily suppressed and glucose metabolism plays a major role as energy source [70]. In addition, the dysfunctional areas corresponding to BMIPP-perfusion mismatch were more likely to have residual inotropic reserve under dobutamine infusion than those with a matched pattern [71]. Furthermore, Kudoh et al. [72] showed that BMIPP-thallium mismatched areas had < 10% fibrosis by histological examination during cardiac surgery. All of these data indicate that such discordant BMIPP uptake (less than thallium) may represent reversible ischemic myocardium that has a potential for improvement.

A number of reports indicate that such discordant BMIPP/thallium uptake is evidence of reversible ischemia that may improve regional function after revascularization (Fig. 15.7). Franken et al. [57] showed that areas with less BMIPP uptake than Tc-99m-sestamibi uptake improved cardiac function shortly after myocardial infarction. Ito et al. [58] also showed recovery of regional dysfunction after myocardial infarction in areas with discordant defect size by BMIPP and thallium images. Furthermore, the degree of perfusion-metabolism mismatch in the acute phase of infarction may correlate with the amount of subsequent improvement after infarction [59]. In addition, Taki et al. [73] showed that the size of discordant BMIPP uptake (less than thallium uptake following thallium reinjection) before revascularization was a good predictor of improvement of ejection fraction. These data indicate that such discordant BMIPP uptake (less than perfusion) may represent reversible ischemic myocardium that will improve regional as well as global dysfunction. Furthermore, the improvement in regional function after revascularization seems to be associated with improvement in BMIPP uptake [73–75].

The combination of BMIPP and perfusion imaging has been used for risk stratification of patients with coronary artery disease. Since discordant BMIPP uptake may represent ischemic and jeopardized myocardium, combined BMIPP and thallium imaging may have potential value for risk stratification of coronary patients. Tamaki et al. [76] surveyed 50 consecutive pa-

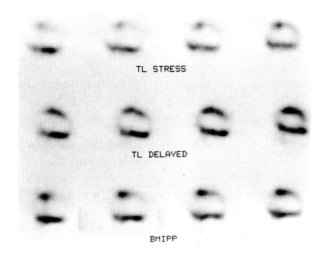

FIGURE 15.6 A series of vertical long-axis slices of stress (*top*) and delayed (*middle*) thallium scans and resting BMIPP scan (*bottom*) of a patient with unstable angina. A reduction of BMIPP at rest is clearly seen in the anterior and apical regions where stress-induced ischemia with redistribution in the anterior region is observed on thallium scan. (Reprinted with permission of the American Society of Nuclear Cardiology from Tamaki N, et al. Radionuclide assessment of myocardial fatty acid metabolism by PET and SPECT. J Nucl Cardiol 1995; 2: 256–266.)

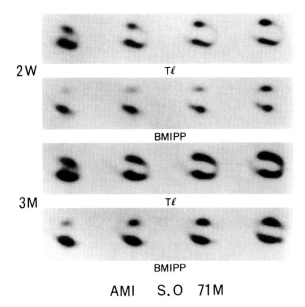

2W   Tℓ

BMIPP

3M   Tℓ

BMIPP

AMI   S.O   71M

FIGURE 15.7 A series of vertical long-axis slices of resting thallium and BMIPP scan at 2 weeks (*top two rows*) and at 3 months (*bottom two rows*) after myocardial infarction. A reduction of thallium with greater decrease in BMIPP uptake relative to thallium is noted in the anterior and apical region in the acute stage. A striking improvement in perfusion with mild improvement in BMIPP uptake is observed in the chronic stage, indicating reversible ischemia in the areas with BMIPP-thallium mismatch. (Reprinted with permission of the Kluwer Academic Publishers from Tamaki N, et al. Future of BMIPP. Int J Card Imaging 1999; 15: 79–89.)

tients with myocardial infarction who received BMIPP and thallium scans and were followed-up for a mean interval of 23 months. Among various clinical, angiographic, and radionuclide indexes, discordant BMIPP uptake was the best predictor of future cardiac events followed by number of coronary stenosis. Nakata et al. [77] in their multicenter study indicated that the BMIPP defect score was the most powerful index for predicting future cardiac events in patients after acute myocardial infarction. In a study of patients with chest pain without a history of myocardial infarction, abnormal BMIPP uptake was often observed in patients with coronary stenosis who required subsequent revascularization on follow-up [67]. These preliminary studies indicate that BMIPP and thallium imaging may hold promise for identifying high-risk subgroups among patients with coronary artery disease.

Assessment of myocardial metabolism may play an important role for assessing pathophysiology in patients with cardiomyopathy. Alterations of fatty acid or oxidative metabolism are frequently observed in patients with hypertrophic cardiomyopathy assessed by PET with C-11 palmitate or C-11 acetate, respectively [78,79]. BMIPP has been extensively studied in patients

with hypertrophic cardiomyopathy in Japan, indicating heterogeneous distribution of BMIPP in hypertrophied myocardium, independent of thallium perfusion findings [80–82]. Although thallium uptake is rather heterogeneous in the hypertrophied septal region, BMIPP uptake is strikingly decreased, indicating perfusion and metabolism mismatch. Thus, BMIPP may permit detection of alteration of fatty acid metabolism independent of perfusion. This finding seems to be an early sign in patients with cardiomyopathy when compared with abnormalities on PET imaging [83]. Since most of the patients with hypertrophic cardiomyopathy showed such discordant BMIPP uptake (less than perfusion) in septal regions, the combined imaging of BMIPP and perfusion tracer may differentiate those with cardiomyopathy from those with other causes of hypertrophic myocardium, such as hypertensive heart disease where no such discordant distribution was observed.

Idiopathic dilated cardiomyopathy has also been investigated with BMIPP imaging. Hashimoto et al. [84] showed a defect of BMIPP uptake in relation to severity of left ventricular dysfunction. The percentage of fractional shortening measured by echocardiography correlated significantly with the BMIPP defect score, but not with the thallium defect score, indicating closer correlation of metabolic information with ventricular function rather than perfusion. Yoshinaga et al. [85,86] suggested that patients with dilated cardiomyopathy with a decrease in BMIPP uptake may respond poorly to beta-blocker therapy. Furthermore, a recent experimental study indicated that myocardial extraction and retention of BMIPP was impaired in dogs with pacing-induced heart failure [87]. Although these data remain preliminary, they may provide new insights into pathophysiology and treatment strategy in patients with poor left ventricular function.

CONCLUSIONS

Basic studies and preliminary clinical results have suggested a number of potential clinical roles for fatty acid imaging. While fatty acid is a major energy source in the normal myocardium, fatty acid oxidation is easily suppressed in ischemic and postischemic myocardium. Thus, assessment of fatty acid metabolism by radionuclide imaging has an important role for early detection of myocardial ischemia and assessment of severity of ischemic heart disease. Reduced utilization of fatty acids at rest was often observed in severely ischemic myocardium and possibly in postischemic myocardium despite normal perfusion at rest. The role of metabolic imaging for identifying postischemic insult as "ischemic memory imaging" has recently been emphasized. Although basic studies and more clinical experience are required to prove this concept, this new idea may expand the utilization of metabolic imaging in the evaluation of coronary artery disease. The segments with discordant BMIPP uptake (less than perfusion), which are often seen in patients with coronary artery disease, may represent ischemic but viable myocardium. Therefore, combined imaging using a fatty acid analog and a perfusion marker permits detection of ischemic but viable myocardium on the basis of alteration of myocardial energy metabolism. Furthermore, iodinated fatty acid compounds hold the promise of demonstrating early alteration of energy metabolism in a variety of myocardial disorders. While these tracers are available only in certain countries at present, they will probably be widely used all over the world soon.

REFERENCES

1. Opie LH. *The Heart; Physiology and Metabolism*, 2nd Edition. New York: Raven Press, 1991.
2. Neely JR, Rovetto M, Oram J. Myocardial utilization of carbohydrate and lipids. Prog Cardiovasc Dis 1972; 15: 289.
3. Liedke AJ. Alterations of carbohydrate and lipid metabolism in the acutely ischemic heart Prog Cardiovasc Dis 1981; 23: 321.
4. Schwaiger M, Hicks R. The clinical role of metabolic imaging of the heart by positron emission tomography. J Nucl Med 1991; 32: 565.
5. Schelbert MR. Cardiac PET: microcirculation and substrate transport in normal and diseased human myocardium. Ann Nucl Med 1994; 8: 91.
6. Goldstein RA, Klein MS, Welch MJ, et al. External assessment of myocardial metabolism with C-11 palmitate. J Nucl Med 1980; 21: 342.
7. Schon HR, Schelbert HR, Robinson G, et al. C-11 palmitate for the noninvasive evaluation of regional myocardial fatty acid metabolism with positron computed tomography. Am Heart J 1982; 103: 532.
8. Schelbert HR, Henze E, Keen R, et al. C-11 palmitate for the noninvasive evaluation of regional myocardial fatty acid metabolism with positron computed tomography. IV. In vivo evaluation of acute demand-induced ischemia in dogs. Am Heart J 1983; 103: 736.
9. Knapp FF Jr, Kropp J. Iodine-123-labelled fatty acids for myocardial single-photon emission tomography: current status and future perspectives. Eur J Nucl Med 1995; 22: 361.
10. Tamaki N, Fujibayashi Y, Magata Y, et al. Radionuclide assessment of myocardial fatty acid metabolism by PET and SPECT. J Nucl Cardiol 1995; 2: 256.
11. Corbett JR. Fatty acids for myocardial imaging. Semin Nucl Med 1999; 29: 237.
12. Tamaki N, Morita K, Kuge Y, et al. The role of fatty acids in cardiac imaging. J Nucl Med 2000; 41: 1525.
13. Machulla HJ, Marsmann M, Dutschka K. Biochemical synthesis of a radioiodinated phenyl fatty acid for in vivo metabolic studies of the myocardium. Eur J Nucl Med 1980; 5: 171.
14. Kaiser KP, Geuting B, Grobmann K, et al. Tracer kinetics of 15-(ortho[123/131]I-phenyl)-pentadecanoic acid (oPPA) and 15-(para-[123/131]I-phenyl)-pentadecanoic acid (pPPA) in animals and man. J Nucl Med 1990; 31: 1608.
15. Reske SN, Biersack HJ, Lackner K, et al. Assessment of regional myocardial uptake and metabolism of ω-(p-123I-iodophenyl)-pentadecanoic acid with serial single-photon emission tomography. J Nucl Med 1982; 23: 249.
16. Reske SN, Sauer W, Machulla HJ, et al. 15-(p-(^{123}I)-iodophenyl)-pentadecanoic acid as a tracer of lipid metabolism: comparison with (1-^{14}C) palmitic acid in murine tissues. J Nucl Med 1984; 25: 1335.
17. Yang JY, Calnon DA, Watson DD, et al. Assessment of myocardial viability using 123I-labeled iodophenylpentadecanoic acid at sustained low flow or after acute infarction and reperfusion. J Nucl Med 1999; 40: 821.
18. Hansen CL, Corbett JR, Pippin JJ, et al. Iodine-123 phenylpentadecanoic acid and single-photon emission computed tomography in identifying left ventricular regional metabolic abnormalities in patients with coronary heart disease: comparison with thallium-201 myocardial tomography. J Am Coll Cardiol 1988; 12: 78.
19. Kennedy PL, Corbett JR, Kulkarni PV, et al. Iodine 123-phenylpentadecanoic acid myocardial scintigraphy: usefulness in the identification of myocardial ischemia. Circulation 1986; 74: 1007.
20. Caldwell JH, Martin GV, Link JM, et al. Iodophenylpentadecanoic acid-myocardial blood flow relationship during maximal exercise with coronary occlusion. J Nucl Med 1990; 31: 99.
21. Heller GV, Iskandrian AE, Orlandi C, et al. Fasting and nonfasting iodine-123-iodophenylpentadecanoic acid myocardial SPECT imaging in coronary artery disease. J Nucl Med 1998; 39: 2019.
22. Kuikka JT, Mussalo H, Hietakorpi S, et al. Evaluation of myocardial viability with technetium-99m hexakis-2-methoxy-isonitrile isonitrile and iodine-123 phenyl-pentadecanoic acid and single photon emission tomoraphy. Eur J Nucl Med 1992; 19: 882.
23. Murray G, Schad N, Ladd W, et al. Metabolic cardiac imaging in severe coronary disease: assessment of viability with iodine-123-iodophenyl-pentadecanoic acid and multicrystal camera, and coronary relation with biopsy. J Nucl Med 1992; 33: 1269.
24. Hansen CL, Heo J, Oliner CM, et al. Prediction of improvement in left ventricular function with iodine-123-IPPA after coronary revascularization. J Nucl Med 1995; 36: 1987.
25. Iskandrian AS, Power J, Cave V, et al. Assessment of myocardial viability by dynamic tomographic 123I-iodophenylpentadecanoic acid imaging: comparison to rest-redistribution thallium imaging J Nucl Cardiol 1995; 2: 101.
26. Verani MS, Taillefer R, Iskandrian AE, et al. 123I-IPPA SPECT for the prediction of enhanced left ventricular function after coronary bypass graft surgery. J Nucl Med 2000; 41: 1299.
27. Ugolini V, Hansen CL, Kulkarni PV, et al. Abnormal myocardial fatty acid metabolism in dilated cardiomyopathy detected by 123I-iodine phenylpentadecanoic acid and tomographic imaging. Am J Cardiol 1988; 62: 923.
28. Wolfe CL, Kennedy PL, Kulkarni P, et al. Iodine-123 phenylpentadecanoic acid myocardial scintigraphy in patients with left ventricular distribution and utilization. Am Heart J 1990; 119: 1338.
29. Chouraqui P, Maddahi J, Henkin R, et al. Comparison of myocardial imaging with iodine-123-iodophenyl-9-methyl pentadecanoic acid and thallium-201 chloride for assessment of patients with exercise-induced myocardial ischemia. J Nucl Med 1991; 32: 447.
30. Hashimoto J, Kubo A, Iwasaki R, et al. Scintigraphic evaluation

of myocardial ischaemia using a new fatty acid analogue; iodine-123-labelled 15-(p-iodophenyl)-9-(R,S)-methylpentadecanoic acid (9MPA). Eur J Nucl Med 1999; 26: 887.

31. Fujiwara S, Takeishi Y, Yamaoka M, et al. Fatty acid imaging with ^{123}I-15-(p-iodophenyl)-9-(R,S)-methylpentadecanoic acid in acute coronary syndrome. J Nucl Med 1999; 40: 1999.

32. Fukuchi K, Hasegawa S, Ito Y, et al. Detection of coronary artery disease by iodine-123 labeled iodophenyl-9-methylpentadecanoic acid SPECT: comparison with thallium-201 and iodine-123 BMIPP SPECT. Ann Nucl Med 2000; 14: 11.

33. Marie PY, Karcher G, Danchin N, et al. Thallium-201 rest-reinjection and iodine-123-MIHA imaging of myocardial infarction: analysis of defect reversibility. J Nucl Med 1995; 36: 1561.

34. Marie PY, Angioni M, Danchin N, et al. Assessment of myocardial viability in patients with previous myocardial infarction by using single-photon emission computed tomography with a new metabolic tracer: [^{123}I]-16-iodo-3-methylhexadecanoic acid (MIHA): comparison with the rest-reinjection thallium-201 technique. J Am Coll Cardiol 1997; 30: 1241.

35. Eisenhut M, Lehmann WD, Hull WE, et al. Trapping and metabolism of radioiodinated PHIPA 3-10 in the rat myocardium. J Nucl Med 1997; 38: 1864.

36. Jonas M, Brandau W, Vollet B, et al. Simultaneous evaluation of fatty acid metabolism and myocardial flow in an explanted heart. J Nucl Med 1997; 37: 1990.

37. Knapp FF Jr, Goodman MM, Callahan AP, et al. Radioiodinated 15-(p-iodophenyl)-3,3-dimethylpentadecanoic acid: a useful new agent to evaluate myocardial fatty acid uptake. J Nucl Med 1986; 27: 521.

38. Fujibayashi Y, Nohara R, Hosokawa R, et al. Metabolism and kinetics of iodine-123-BMIPP in canine myocardium. J Nucl Med 1996; 37: 757.

39. Sloof GW, Visser FC, Lingen AV, et al. Evaluation of heart-to-organ ratios of ^{123}I-BMIPP and the dimethyl-substitued 123I-DMIPP fatty acid analogue in humans. Nucl Med Commun 1997; 18: 1065.

40. Morishita S, Kusuoka H, Yamamichi Y, et al. Kinetics of radioiodinated species in subcellular fractions from rat hearts following administration of iodine-123-labelled 15-(p-iodophenyl)-3-(R,S) methylpentadecanoic acid (^{123}I-BMIPP). Eur J Nucl Med 1996; 23: 383.

41. Yamamichi Y, Kusuoka H, Morishita K, et al. Metabolism of ^{123}I-labeled 15-p-iodophenyl-3-(R,S)-methyl-pentadecanoic acid (BMIPP) in perfused rat heart. J Nucl Med 1995; 36: 1043.

42. Hosokawa R, Nohara R, Fujibayashi Y, et al. Metabolic fate of iodine-123-BMIPP in canine myocardium after administration of etomoxir. J Nucl Med 1996; 37: 1836.

43. Fujibayashi Y, Yonekura Y, Takemura Y, et al. Myocardial accumulation of iodinated beta-methyl-branched fatty acid analogue, iodine-125-15-(p-iodophenyl)-3-(R,S) methylpentadecanoic acid (BMIPP), in relation to ATP concentration. J Nucl Med 1990; 31: 1818.

44. Fujibayashi Y, Yonekura Y, Tamaki N, et al. Myocardial accumulation of BMIPP in relation to ATP concentration. Ann Nucl Med 1993; 7: 15.

45. Nohara R, Okuda K, Ogino M, et al. Evaluation of myocardial viability with iodine-123-BMIPP in a canine model. J Nucl Med 1996; 37: 1403.

46. Miller DD, Gill JB, Livni E, et al. Fatty acid analogue accumulation: a marker of myocyte viability in ischemic-reperfused myocardium. Circ Res 1988; 63: 681.

47. Nishimura T, Sago M, Kihara K, et al. Fatty acid myocardial imaging using ^{123}I-β-methyl-iodophenyl pentadecanoic acid (BMIPP): comparision of myocardial perfusion and fatty acid utilization in canine myocardial infarction (occlusion and reperfusion model). Eur J Nucl Med 1989; 15: 341.

48. Hosokawa R, Nohara R, Fujibayashi Y, et al. Myocardial metabolism of ^{123}I-BMIPP in a canine model of ischemia implication of perfusion-metabolism mismatch on SPECT images in patients with ischemic heart disease. J Nucl Med 1999; 40: 471.

49. Kurata C, Wakabayashi Y, Shouda S, et al. Influence of blood substrate levels on myocardla kinetics of iodine-123-BMIPP. J Nucl Med 1997; 38: 1079.

50. Kudoh T, Tamaki N, Magata Y, et al. Metabolism substrate with negative myocardial uptake of iodine-123-BMIPP. J Nucl Med 1997; 38: 548.

51. Tanaka T, Kawamura K. Isolation of myocardial membrane long-chain fatty acid-binding protein: homology with a rat long-chain fatty acids. J Mol Cell Cardiol 1995; 27: 1613.

52. Tamaki N, Kawamoto M, Yonekura Y, et al. Regional metabolic abnormality in relation to perfusion and wall motion in patients with myocadial infarction: assessment with emission tomography using an iodonated branched fatty acid. J Nucl Med 1992, 33: 659.

53. DeGeeter F, Franken P, Knapp FF Jr, et al. Relationship between blood flow and fatty acid metabolism in subacute myocardial infarction: a study by means of Tc-99m sestamibi and iodine-123-beta-methyl iodophenyl pentadecanoic acid. Eur J Nucl Med 1994; 21: 283.

54. Franken P, DeGeeter F, Dendale P, et al. Abnormal free fatty acid uptake in subacute myocardial infarction after coronary thrombolysis: correlation with wall motion and inotropic reserve. J Nucl Med 1994; 35: 1758.

55. Furutani Y, Shiigi T, Nakamura Y, et al. Quantification of area at risk in acute myocardial infarction by tomographic imaging. J Nucl Med 1997; 38: 1875.

56. Kawai Y, Tsukamoto E, Nozaki Y, et al. Use of ^{123}I-BMIPP single-photon emission tomography to estimate areas at risk following successful revascularization in patients with acute myocardial infarction. Eur J Nucl Med 1998; 25: 1390.

57. Franken PR, Dendale P, DeGeeter F, et al. Prediction of functional outcome after myocardial infarction using BMIPP and sestamibi scintigraphy. J Nucl Med 1996; 37: 718.

58. Ito T, Tanouchi J, Kato J, et al. Recovery of impaired left ventricular function in patients with acute myocardial infarction is predicted by the discordance in defect size on ^{123}I-BMIPP and ^{201}Tl SPECT images. Eur J Nucl Med 1996; 23: 917.

59. Hashimoto A, Nakata T, Tsuchihashi K, et al. Postischemic functional recovery and BMIPP uptake after primary percutaneous transluminal coronary angioplasty in acute myocardial infarction. Am J Cardiol 1996; 77: 25.

60. Naruse H, Arii T, Kondo T, et al. Clinical usefulness of iodine-123-labeled fatty acid imaging in patients with acute myocardial infarction. J Nucl Cardiol 1998; 5: 275.

61. Takeishi Y, Fujiwara S, Atsumi H, et al. Clinical significance of decreased myocardial uptake of 123 I-BMIPP in patients with stable effort angina pectoris. Nucl Med Commun 1995; 16:1002.

62. Takeishi Y, Sukekawa H, Saito H, et al. Impaired myocardial fatty acid metabolism detected by ^{123}I-BMIPP in patients with unstable angina pectoris: comparison with perfusion imaging by 99mTc-sestamibi. Ann Nucl Med 1995; 9: 125.

63. Tateno M, Tamaki N, Kudoh T, et al. Assessment of fatty acid uptake in patients with ischemic heart disease without myocardial infarction. J Nucl Med 1996; 37: 1981.

64. Suzuki A, Takada Y, Nagasaka M, et al. Comparison of resting β-methyl-iodophenyl pentadecanoic acid (BMIPP) and thallium-

201 tomography using quantitative polar maps in patients with unstable angina Jpn Circ J 1997; 61: 133.

65. Yamabe H, Abe H, Yokoyama M, et al. Resting ^{123}I-BMIPP scintigraphy in diagnosis of effort angina pectoris with reference to subsets of the disease. Ann Nucl Med 1998; 12: 139.

66. Nakajima K, Schimizu K, Taki J, et al. Utility of iodine-123-BMIPP in the diagnosis and follow-up of vasospastic angina. J Nucl Med 1995; 36: 1934.

67. Yamabe H, Fujiwara S, Rin K, et al. Resting ^{123}I-BMIPP scintigraphy for detection of organic coronary stenosis and therapeutic outcome in patients with chest pain. Annals Nucl Med 2000; 14: 187.

67B. Kawai Y, Tsukamoto E, Nozaki Y, et al. Significance of reduced uptake of iodinated fatty acid analogue for the evaluation of patients with acute chest pain. J Am Coll Cardiol 2001; 38:1888.

68. Matsunari I, Saga T, Taki J, et al. Kinetics of iodine-123-BMIPP in patients with prior myocardial infarction: assessment with dynamic rest and stress images compared with stress thallium-201 SPECT. J Nucl Med 1994; 35: 1279.

69. Kawamoto M, Tamaki N, Yonekura Y, et al. Combined study with I-123 fatty acid and thallium-201 to assess ischemic myocardium. Ann Nucl Med 1994; 8: 47.

70. Tamaki N, Tadamura E, Kawamoto M, et al. Decreased uptake of iodinated branched fatty acid analog indicates metabolic alterations in ischemic myocardium. J Nucl Med 1995; 36: 1974.

71. Hambye ASE, Vaerenberg MM, Dobbeleir AA, et al. Abnormal BMIPP uptake in chronically dysfunctional myocardial segments: correlation with contractile response to low-dose dobutamine. J Nucl Med 1998; 39: 1845.

72. Kudoh T, Tadamura E, Tamaki N, et al. Iodinated free fatty acid and ^{201}Tl uptake in chronically hyperperfused myocardium. Histologic correlation study. J Nucl Med 2000; 41: 293.

73. Taki J, Nakajima K, Matsunari I, et al. Assessment of improvement of myocardial fatty acid uptake and function after revascularization using iodine-123-BMIPP. J Nucl Med 1997; 38: 1503.

74. Matsunari I, Saga T, Taki J, et al. Improved myocardial fatty acid utilization after percutaneous transluminal coronary angioplasty. J Nucl Med 1995; 36: 1605.

75. Takeishi Y, Fujiwara S, Atsumi H, et al. Iodine-123-BMIPP imaging in unstable angina: a guide for interventional therapy. J Nucl Med 1997; 38: 1407.

76. Tamaki N, Tadamura E, Kudoh T, et al. Prognostic value of io-

dine-123 labelled BMIPP fatty acid analogue imaging in patients with myocardial infarction. Eur J Nucl Med 1996; 23: 272.

77. Nakata T, Kobayashi T, Tamaki N, et al. Prognosis value of impaired myocardial fatty acid uptake in patients with acute myocardial infarction. Nucl Med Commun 2000; 21: 897.

78. Grover-McKey M, Schwaiger M, Krivokapitch J, et al. Regional myocardial blood flow and metabolism at rest in mildly asymptomatic patients with hypertrophic cardiomyopathy. J Am Coll Cardiol 1989; 13: 317.

79. Tadamura E, Tamaki N, Matsumori A, et al. Myocardial metabolic changes in hypertrophic cardiomyopathy. J Nucl Med 1996; 37: 572.

80. Taki J, Nakajima K, Bunko H, et al. ^{123}I-labelled BMIPP fatty acid myocardial scintigraphy in patients with hypertrophic cardiomyopathy. Nucl Med Commun 1994; 14: 181.

81. Takeishi Y, Chiba J, Abe S, et al. Heterogeneous myocardial distribution of iodine-123 15-(p-iodophenyl)-3-R,S-methylpentadecanoic acid (BMIPP) in patients with hypertrophic cardiomyopathy. Eur J Nucl Med 1992; 19: 775.

82. Ohtsuki K, Sugihara H, Kuribayashi T, et al. Impairment of BMIPP accumulation at junction of ventricular septum and left and right ventricular free walls in hypertrophic cardiomyopathy. J Nucl Med 1999; 40: 2007.

83. Tadamura E, Kudoh T, Hattori N, et al. Impairment of BMIPP uptake precedes abnormalities in oxygen and glucose metabolism in hypertrophic cardiomyopathy. J Nucl Med 1998; 39:390.

84. Hashimoto Y, Yamabe H, Yokoyama M, et al. Myocardial defect detected by 123I-BMIPP scintigraphy and left ventricular dysfunction in patients with idiopathic dilated cardiomyopathy. Annals Nucl Med 1996; 10: 225.

85. Yoshinaga K, Tahara M, Torii H. Predicting the effects on patients with dilated cardiomyopathy of beta-blocker therapy by using iodine-123 15-(p-iodophenyl)-3-R,S-methylpentadecanoic acid (BMIPP) myocardial scintigraphy. Ann Nucl Med 1998; 12: 341.

86. Yoshinaga K, Tahara M, Torii H. Myocardial scintigraphy using iodine-123 15-(p-iodophenyl)-3-R,S-methylpentadecanoic acid predicts the reponse to beta-blocker therapy in patients with dilated cardiomyopathy but does not reflect therapeutic effect. J Cardiol 2000; 35: 343.

87. Kataoka K, Nohara R, Hosokawa R, et al. Myocardial lipid metabolism in compensated and advanced stages of heart failure: evaluation by canine pacing model with BMIPP. J Nucl Med 2001; 42: 124.

Part 2

MIBG Imaging

MICHAEL W. DAE

The sympathetic nervous system has profound influences on myocardial function and pathophysiology. The heart is densely innervated with sympathetic nerves, which are distributed on a regional basis. Heterogeneity of myocardial sympathetic innervation, or autonomic imbalance, has long been hypothesized as a major mechanism underlying sudden cardiac death. In addition global activation of myocardial sympathetic nerves is thought to be a major contributor to adverse consequences, especially in congestive heart failure. Recent developments in cardiac imaging have lead to the ability to map abnormalities in heart innervation in vivo, using radiolabeled metaiodobenzylguanidine (MIBG). As a result, the pathophysiologic mechanisms relating alterations in sympathetic nerve activity to disease processess are now being explored.

EXPERIMENTAL FOUNDATION FOR MIBG UPTAKE

Myocardial sympathetic nerves have been shown to take up exogenously administered catecholamines [1–4]. MIBG is thought to localize to myocardial sympathetic nerves due to its structural similarity to norepinephrine [5], but is not metabolized by monoamine oxidase or catechol-o-methyl transferase [5]. Numerous studies have evaluated the characteristics of MIBG uptake and distribution in experimental models designed to alter global and regional function of myocardial sympathetic nerves [6–10]. In regionally denervated myocardium, MIBG uptake is decreased, while myocardial perfusion remains intact (Color Fig. 15.8). Although MIBG is delivered to the myocardium by perfusion, MIBG localization is clearly dependent on the presence of intact sympathetic nerves. Previous studies have shown that the ability of sympathetic nerves to take up radiolabeled catecholamines is a more sensitive indicator of intact neuronal function than myocardial norepinephrine content [11]. Studies in the transplanted human heart have shown an absence of MIBG uptake within the first 4 months after surgery, consistent with global denervation [7]. Subsequent imaging at 1 year following surgery showed a return of MIBG uptake in about 50% of patients, consistent with reinnervation [12] (Fig. 15.9).

SYMPATHETIC INNERVATION IN ISCHEMIC HEART DISEASE

The sympathetic nerves are acutely affected in regions of myocardial ischemia. Enhanced washout of MIBG has been demonstrated from the ischemic territory due to local release from sympathetic nerve endings [13]. Ischemia severe enough to cause myocyte necrosis can also cause necrosis of sympathetic nerves (see Color Fig. 15.10 in separate color insert). It has been shown that transmural myocardial infarction can lead to a partially denervated ventricle [14], which may predispose the heart to arrhythmia [15].

Transmural myocardial infarction produces denervation secondary to necrosis of proximal sympathetic nerve trunks that travel in the subepicardium [14]. Viable myocardium distal to the infarction becomes denervated as a result of loss of proximal nerve input. As opposed to the distal denervation produced by transmural myocardial infarction, nontransmural infarction results in local ischemic damage of sympathetic nerve endings that are present within the ischemic zone [13,16]. Partial denervation has been shown to occur in humans after myocardial infarction [17–19].

SYMPATHETIC INNERVATION IN DIABETES

Recent studies have shown regional myocardial MIBG uptake abnormalities in diabetic neuropathy [20]. Diabetic rats have shown reduced uptake of MIBG, which was reversed with early insulin or aldosereductase inhibitor therapy [21]. The aldosereductase inhibitor improved MIBG uptake without improving glucose regulation, implying a direct neuropathy. In newly diagnosed diabetic patients, 77% have evidence of regionally reduced MIBG uptake, consistent with neuropathy [22]. It is interesting that a partial restoration of MIBG abnormalities were shown at 1 year following intense

MIBG
S/P Transplantation

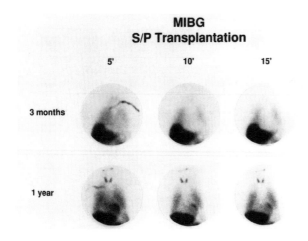

FIGURE 15.9 MIBG images from a patient studied at 3 months and 1 year after transplantation. There is an absence of MIBG myocardial localization at 3 months. One year after transplantation, MIBG uptake is present in the anterior wall of the left ventricle. S/P, status post.

metabolic control [22]. In diabetic patients, MIBG uptake is likely the most accurate and objective measure of autonomic dysfunction [22].

SYMPATHETIC INNERVATION AND ARRHYTHMOGENESIS

Numerous studies lead to the concept that heterogeneity of sympathetic innervation, or "sympathetic imbalance" could adversely affect the electrical stability of the heart [23–26]. Studies that compared MIBG scintigraphy to electrophysiologic responses in dogs with myocardial infarction showed enhanced shortening of effective refractory period in denervated myocardium consistent with denervation supersensitivity [27–29]. Increased susceptibility to induced ventricular fibrillation or ventricular tachycardia in dogs with myocardial infarction and denervation has also been reported [15,28]. We also observed heterogeneous sympathetic innervation in a population of german shepherd dogs with inherited spontaneous ventricular arrhythmias and sudden death [30].

We compared the spatial distribution of sympathetic innervation to the spatial distribution of myocardial repolarization in regionally denervated rabbit hearts [31]. We evaluated the effects of sympathetic stimulation on myocardial repolarization in regions of mild, moderate, and severe denervation created by phenol application to the epicardium in rabbits. Innervation was measured from three-dimensional reconstructions of autoradiographs of MIBG and MIBI (see Color Fig. 15.11 in separate color insert), while repolarization was

measured from activation recovery intervals (ARI) derived from unipolar electrograms at the epicardium. ARI is a measure related to the action potential duration (APD) of cells near the extracellular electrode, and has as its advantage the ability to simultaneously record a large number of sites. More important for our purposes, changes in ARI at a given site during an intervention correlate extremely well with changes in APD meausred with microelectrodes. Imaging results were compared to ARI at 64 epicardial sites in each animal (see Color Fig. 15.12 in separate color insert). Norepinephrine infusion shortened ARI in 95% of the electrodes in the denervated regions and increased dispersion. Left stellate stimulation shortened ARI in 30% of electrodes and prolonged ARI in 70%. The dispersion of repolarization was related to the severity of denervation, as well as the type of stimulation—neural (stellate stimulation) versus humoral (norepinephrine). The differences were likely related to the concentration of norepinephrine released. Our results show that the dispersion of repolarization is significantly influenced by regional changes in autonomic tone.

For clinical studies, the presence or absence of denervated but viable myocardium, the severity of denervation, the underlying level of sympathetic tone, and the subsequent influences on local ventricular repolarization may be important and interactive determinants of arrhythmogenesis. Regional heterogeneity of MIBG uptake has been demonstrated in patients with idiopathic ventricular tachycardia [32–34], and arrhythmogenic right ventricular cardiomyopathy [35].

SYMPATHETIC INNERVATION IN CONGESTIVE HEART FAILURE

One of the early physiologic responses to counteract depressed myocardial function is activation of a number of neurohumoral systems, such as the renin-angiotensin system, the sympathethic nervous system, and the arginine vasopressin system [36]. It is now widely accepted that excessive stimulation of these compensatory systems eventually leads to deterioration of ventricular function and may contribute to sudden cardiac death [36]. Sustained activation of the sympathetic nervous system is thought to play a major role in the etiology of sudden cardiac death [37]. More than 300,000 sudden cardiac deaths occur each year in the United States, accounting for 50% of all cardiac related mortality [38]. The majority of these deaths occur in patients with prior healed myocardial infarctions and left ventricular dysfunction [39]. These deaths are thought to originate as ventricular tachycardia, which may degenerate into ventricular fibrillation. In most instances, there is no associated evidence for either acute infarction or significant ischemia [39]. Arrhythmia and sudden death are also important features of noncoronary cardiomyopathy and heart failure. Approximately 40% of patients with severe heart failure die suddenly, presumably of arrhythmia [40].

Myocardial MIBG imaging has been shown to play a role in detecting sympathetic nervous system activation. Henderson et al. studied the myocardial distribution and kinetics of MIBG in images obtained from patients with congestive cardiomyopathy compared to normal controls [41]. Patients with congestive cardiomyopathy had a 28% washout rate of MIBG from the heart over a period from 15 minutes to 85 minutes following intravenous injection, as compared to a washout rate of 6% in the controls. Imamura et al. demonstrated that the level of myocardial MIBG washout was related to the severity of heart failure, as measured by New York Heart Association classification [42]. In a study by Nakajima et al. [43], patients with various cardiac disorders underwent planar MIBG imaging at 20 minutes and 3 hours after injection. A very high washout rate of more than 25% was seen in a number of cases of dilated cardiomyopathy (5/11), hypertrophic cardiomyopathy (9/24), ischemic heart disease (23/34), essential hypertension (5/13), and hypothyroidism (6/13). Mean washout in control patients was 9.6%. As demonstrated, enhanced MIBG washout can be seen in a number of different diseases. The mechanism in common is most likely activation of the sympathetic nervous system.

Several different patterns of MIBG uptake are detectable in patients with congestive heart failure (CHF) (Fig. 15.13). As shown in Figure 15.13, patients can show good initial uptake and retention of MIBG, good initial uptake and poor retention on delayed images, or poor uptake on the initial and delayed images. The underlying mechanisms resulting in these diverse image patterns have not been well defined to date. However, enhanced washout of MIBG in congestive heart failure due to increased sympathetic tone, and selective damage to sympathetic neurons in advanced disease probably play a role. A number of studies have suggested that the degree of MIBG uptake on the delayed image carries strong prognostic information for outcome in patients with CHF. Merlet et al. [44] reported the results of a prospective study of a group of 112 patients with idiopathic dilated cardiomyopathy and New York Heart Association class II–IV heart failure. They assessed cardiac MIBG uptake, circulating norepinephrine concentration, left ventricular ejection fraction, peak VO$_2$, cardiothoracic ratio on X-ray, M-mode

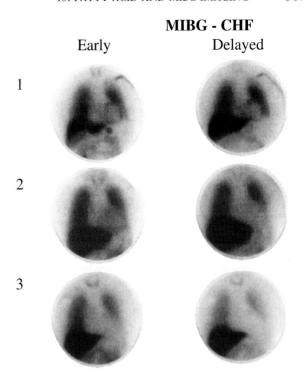

MIBG - CHF

Early   Delayed

FIGURE 15.13 Early (15 minutes) and delayed (3 hours) images of MIBG in three patients with CHF. Patient 1 shows good early uptake and retention on the delayed image. Patient 2 shows good early uptake with poor retention on the delayed image (increased washout). Patient 3 shows poor early and delayed uptake. CHF, congestive heart failure.

echocardiographic end-diastololic diameter, and right heart catheterization parameters. During a mean follow-up period of 27 months, 19 patients had transplants, 25 died of cardiac death (8 sudden deaths), and 2 died of noncardiac causes. MIBG uptake and circulating norepinephrine concentration were the only independent predictors for life duration using multivariate analysis. MIBG uptake on delayed imaging outperformed left ventricular ejection fraction, cardiac index, plasma norepinephrine, and peak VO$_2$ [44]. In a study of 93 patients with moderate heart failure, followed for a mean of 10 months, both MIBG and peak VO$_2$ were predictive of death or transplantation, however, peak VO$_2$ emerged as the strongest predictor on multivariate analysis [45]. Differences between the two studies may relate to the severity of heart failure, with patients studied by Merlet having more severe failure. Exercise testing is often not feasible in patients with severe heart failure.

Nakata et al. evaluated the ability of MIBG imaging to predict cardiac death in failing and nonfailing hearts [46]. They studied 414 consecutive patients—42% with symptomatic heart failure—and followed the patients for a mean period of 22 months. Among an extensive list of clinical variables that were evaluated for each patient, the late heart to mediastinal MIBG uptake ratio was the most powerful predictor of cardiac death. Further, the most powerful incremental prognostic variables were obtained by using MIBG imaging in combination with conventional clinical variables [46]. These interesting results suggest that there may be a significant role for MIBG imaging in the assessment of prognosis in patients with heart failure, particularly those with severe failure.

Other studies have shown the value of MIBG imaging in predicting the response to antiadrenergic therapy in patients with CHF [47–49]. Suwa et al. performed MIBG imaging in 45 patients with dilated cardiomyopathey before the start of bisoprolol [49]. They measured the heart to mediastinal MIBG uptake ratio on initial and delayed images, along with MIBG washout. They showed that the heart to mediastinal ratio at a threshold of 1.7 on delayed images provided a useful indication of whether or not patients with dilated cardiomyopathey would respond to therapy. Choi et al. [50] recently examined the ability of MIBG to predict the improvement in left ventricular function and exercise capacity in patients with heart failure after treatment with carvedilol. Of a total of 18 patients, 11 were randomized to carvedilol, and 7 received placebo. Only the carvedilol-treated patients showed improvement in function. Within the treatment group, washout of MIBG showed a significant inverse correlation with improvement in left ventricular function. Patients who showed a poor ejection fraction (EF) response (increase in EF < 7%) had a washout rate of > 40%, whereas patients with a good EF response (increase > 7%) had a washout of < 40%. The diagnostic accuracy of MIBG washout rate for predicting EF response was 91%. These studies are all provocative and suggest sufficient promise for MIBG to characterize patient prognosis to warrant a large scale randomized clinical trial.

MIBG imaging may find particular utility in aiding the decision to perform transplantation versus antiadrenergic therapy. Figure 15.14 shows a possible strategy for incorporating the results of MIBG imaging in the triage of patients with heart failure. This approach acknowledges the fact that ischemia is the most common cause of heart failure, and revascularization offers the greatest hope for improvement if viable but jeopardiaed myocardium is detected. In situations where underlying ischemia is not present, MIBG imaging may provide a new diagnostic tool for further stratification of patients to allow more optimal selection of therapy.

Future studies to compare functional abnormalities of the sympathetic nerves to myocardial perfusion, metabolism, and adrenergic receptor density may provide

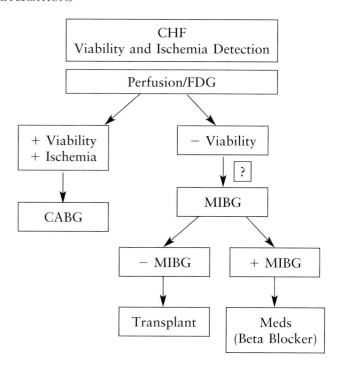

FIGURE 15.14 Clinical paradigm for MIBG imaging in CHF.

a more comprehensive understanding of the action of the autonomic nervous system in disease states. The ability to detect the distribution of innervation scintigraphically and to correlate these imaging findings with electrophysiologic assessment of vulnerability may provide important new understanding of the interaction of the sympathetic nerves and cardiac pathophysiology. In addition, a noninvasive means may be found to detect patients at risk for sudden death, and possibly provide a basis for more rational approaches to therapy. It is very likely that MIBG imaging will become a highly effective tool for obtaining clinically useful information to assess prognosis; however, definitive clinical trials remain to be performed. A limitation to the continued development of MIBG is the lack of FDA approval for the I-123 labeled compound. A further challenge is that the short, 13-hour half-life of I-123 will require daily shipments of the compound—a distribution challenge. The availability of I-123 remains limited as well. Development of Tc-labeled MIBG analogs will likely provide a stimulus for more widespread adoption.

REFERENCES

1. Whitby LG, Axelrod J, Weil-Malherbe H. The fate of 3H-norepinephrine in animals. J Pharm Exp Ther 1961; 132:193.

2. Iversen LL. Role of transmitter uptake mechanisms in synaptic neurotransmission. Br J Pharmac 1971; 41:571.

3. Lightman SL, Iversen LL. The role of uptake in the extraneu-

ronal metabolism of catecholamines in the isolated rat heart. Br J Pharmac 1969; 37:638.

4. Kopin I. False adrenergic transmitters. Ann Rev Pharmacol 1968; 8:377.

5. Wieland DM, Brown LE, Rogers WL, et al. Myocardial imaging with a radioiodinated norepinephrine storage analog. J Nucl Med 1981; 22:22.

6. Sisson JC, Wieland DM, Sherman P, et al. Metaiodobenzylguanidine as an index of the adrenergic nervous system integrity and function. J Nucl Med 1987; 28:1620.

7. Dae, M, De Marco T, Botvinick E, et al. Scintigraphic assessment of MIBG uptake in globally denervated human and canine hearts: implications for clinical studies. J Nucl Med 1992; 33:1444.

8. Dae MW, O'Connell JW, Botvinick EH, et al. Scintigraphic assessment of regional cardiac adrenergic innervation. Circulation 1989; 79:634.

9. Sisson JC, Lynch JJ, Johnson J, et al. Scintigraphic detection of regional disruption of adrenergic neurons in the heart. Am Heart J 1988; 116:67.

10. Mori H, Pisarri T, Aldea G, et al. Usefulness and limitations of regional cardiac sympathectomy by phenol. Am J Physiol 1989; 257:HI523.

11. Tyce GM. Norepinephrine uptake as an indicator of cardiac reinnervation in dogs. Am J Physiol. 1987; 235:H289.

12. De Marco T, Dae M, Yuen-Green M, et al. Iodine-123 metaiodobenzylguanidine scintigraphic assessment of the transplanted human heart: evidence for late reinnervation. J Am Coll Cardiol 1995;25:927.

13. Dae M, O'Connell J, Botvinick E, et al. Acute and chronic effects of transient myocardial ischemia on sympathetic nerve activity, density, and norepinephrine content. Cardiovasc Res 1995; 30:270.

14. Barber MJ, Mueller TM, Henry DP, et al. Transmural myocardial infarction in the dog produces sympathectomy in noninfarcted myocardium. Circulation 1983; 67:787.

15. Herre J, Wetstein L, Lin YL, et al. Effect of transmural versus nontransmural myocardial infarction on inducibility of ventricular arrhythmias during sympathetic stimulation. J Am Coll Cardiol 1988; 11:414.

16. Dae M, Herre J, O'Connell J, et al. Scintigraphic assessment of sympathetic innervation after transmural versus nontransmural myocardial infarction. J Am Coll Cardiol 1991; 17:1416.

17. Stanton MS, Tuli MM, Radtke NL, et al. Regional sympathetic denervation after myocardial infarction in humans detected noninvasively using I-123-metaiodobenzylguanidine. J Am Coll Cardiol 1989; 14:1519.

18. McGhie A, Corbett J, Akers M, et al. Regional cardiac adrenergic function using I-123 meta-iodobenzylguanidine tomographic imaging after acute myocardial infarction. Am J Cardiol 1991; 67:236.

19. Tomoda J, Yoshioka K, Shiina Y, et al. Regional sympathetic denervation detected by iodine 123 metaiodobenzylguanidine in non-W-wave myocardial infarction and unstable angina. Am Heart J 1994;128:452.

20. Langer A, Freeman M, Josse R, et al: Metaiodobenzylguanidine imaging in diabetes mellitus: assessment of cardiac sympathetic denervation and its relation to autonomic dysfunction and silent myocardial ischemia. J Am Coll Cardiol 1995;25:610.

21. Kurata C, Okayama K, Wakabayashi Y, et al. Cardiac sympathetic neuropathy and effects of aldose reductase inhibitor in streptozotocin-induced diabetic rats. J Nucl Med 1997; 38:1677.

22. Schnell O, Muhr D, Dresel S, et al. Partial restoration of scintigraphically assessed cardiac sympathetic denervation in newly diagnosed patients with insulin-dependent (Type 1) diabetes mellitus at one-year follow-up. Diabet Medicine 1997; 14:57.

23. Schwartz PJ, Snebold NG, Brown AM. Effects of unilateral cardiac sympathetic denervation on the ventricular fibrillation threshold. Am J Cardiol 1976;37:1034.

24. Schwartz PJ, Stone HL, Brown AM. Effects of unilateral stellate ganglion blockade on the arrhythmias associated with coronary occlusion. Am Heart J 1976;92:589.

25. Randall WC, Kaye MP, Hageman GR, et al. Cardiac arrhythmias in the conscious dog following sugially induced autonomic imbalance. Am J Cardiol 1976;38:178.

26. Schwartz PJ. Sympathetic imbalance and cardiac arrhythmias. In: *Nervous Control of Cardiovascular Function*, edited by WC Randall. New York: Oxford University Press, pp. 225–252.

27. Minardo JD, Tuli MM, Mock BH, et al. Scintigraphic and electrophysiologic evidence of canine myocardial sympathetic denervation and reinnervation produced by myocardial infarction or phenol application. Circulation 1988; 78:1008.

28. Inoue H, Zipes D. Results of sympathetic denervation in the canine heart: supersensitivity that may be arrhythmogenic. Circulation 1987; 75:877.

29. Newman D, Munoz L, Chin M, et al. Effects of canine myocardial infarction on sympathetic efferent neuronal function: scintigraphic and electrophysiologic correlates. Am Heart J 1993;126:1106.

30. Dae M, Lee R, Ursell P, et al. Heterogeneous sympathetic innervation in german shepherd dogs with inherited ventricular arrhythmia and sudden cardiac death. Circ 1997; 96:1337.

31. Yoshioka K, Gao D, Chin M, et al. Heterogeneous sympathetic innervation influences local myocardial repolarization in normally perfused rabbit hearts. Circ 2000;101:1060.

32. Mitrani R, Klein L, Miles W, et al. Regional cardiac sympathetic denervation in patients with ventricular tachycardia in the absence of coronary artery disease. J Am Coll Cardiol 1993; 22:1344.

33. Gill J, Hunter G, Gane J, et al. Asymmetry of cardiac 123I metaiodobenzylguanidine scans in patients with ventricular tachycardia and a "clinically normal" heart. Br Heart J 1993;69:6.

34. Schafers M, Wichter T, Lerch H, et al. Cardiac ^{123}I-MIBG uptake in idiopathic ventricular tachycardia and fibrillation. J Nucl Med 1999; 40:1.

35. Wichter T, Hindricks G, Lerch H, et al. Regional myocardial sympathetic dysinnervation in arrhythmogenic right ventricular cardiomyopathy-an analysis using 123 I-Meta-Iodobenzylguanidine scintigraphy. Circ 1994;89:667.

36. Farrari R, Ceconi C, Curello S, et al. The neuroendocrine and sympathetic nervous system in congestive heart failure. Eur Heart J 1998;19 Suppl F:F45.

37. Meredith I, Broughton A, Jennings G, et al. Evidence of a selective increase in cardiac sympathetic activity in patients with sustained ventricular arrhythmias. N Engl J Med 1991;325:618.

38. Myerburg R, Kessler K, Castellanos A. Sudden cardiac death: structure, function, and time-dependence of risk. Circ 1992;85:I-2.

39. Hurwitz J, Josephson M. Sudden cardiac death in patients with chronic coronary heart disease. Circ 1992;85:I-43.

40. Francis G. Development of arrhythmias in the patient with congestive heart failure: pathophysiology, prevalence, and prognosis. Am J Cardiol 1986;57:3B.

41. Henderson, EB, Kahn JK, Corbett J, et al. Abnormal I-123 metaidobenzylguanidine myocardial washout and distribution may reflect myocardial adrenergic derangement in patients with congestive cardiomyopathy. Circ. 1988;78:1192.

42. Imamura Y, Ando H, Mitsuoka W, et al. Iodine-123 meta-

iodobenzylguanidine images reflect intense myocardial adrenergic nervous activity in congestive heart failure independent of underlying cause. J Am Coll Cardiol 1995;26:1594.

43. Nakajima K, Taki J, Tonami N, et al. Decreased 123-I MIBG uptake and increased clearance in various cardiac diseases. Nucl Med Commun 1994;15:317.

44. Merlet P, Benvenuti C, Moyse D, et al. Prognostic value of MIBG imaging in idiopathic dilated cardiomyopathy. J Nucl Med 1999; 40(6):917.

45. Cohen-Solal A, Esany Y, Logeart D, et al. Cardiac meta-iodobenylguanidine uptake in patients with moderate chronic heart failure: relationship with peak oxygen uptake and prognosis. J Am Coll Cardiol 1999;33(3):759.

46. Nakata T, Miyamoto K, Doe A, et al. Cardiac death prediction and impaired cardiac sympathetic innervation assessed by MIBG in patients with failing and nonfailing hearts. J Nucl Cardiol 1998; 5: 579.

47. Fukukoa S, Hayashida K, Hirose Y, et al. Use of iodine-123 metaiodobenzylguanidine myocardial imaging to predict the effectiveness of β-blocker therapy in patients with dilated cardiomyopathy. Eur J Nucl Med 1997; 24: 523.

48. Kakuchi H, Sasaki T, Ishida Y, et al. Clinical usefulness of 123I meta-iodobenzylguanidine imaging in predicting the effectiveness of beta blockers for patients with idiopathic dilated cardiomyopathy before and soon after treatment. Heart 1999;81(2): 148.

49. Suwa M, Otake Y, Moriguchi A, et al. Iodine-123 metaiodobenzylguanidine myocardial scintigraphy for prediction of response to β-blocker therapy in patients with dilated cardiomyopathy. Am Heart J; 1997; 133: 353.

50. Choi J, Lee K-H, Hong K, et al. Iodine-123 MIBG imaging before treatment of heart failure with carvedilol to predict improvement of left ventricular function and exercise capacity. J Nucl Cardiol 2001;8:4.

16 | Myocardial perfusion imaging in the assessment of therapeutic interventions

ALBERT J. SINUSAS AND FRANS J. TH. WACKERS

Radionuclide myocardial perfusion imaging is conceptually an attractive modality to monitor the effect of therapeutic interventions. The procedure is noninvasive and can be repeated easily without adverse effects in the elderly population with coronary artery disease. Myocardial perfusion imaging can be accomplished with either single-photon emission tomography (SPECT) or positron emission tomography (PET). Importantly, radionuclide myocardial perfusion imaging effectively visualizes regional changes in myocardial blood flow, a principal target of many therapies in patients with coronary artery disease. This chapter reviews the role of SPECT and PET imaging of regional myocardial perfusion in the evaluation and monitoring of the effects of medical therapy, and mechanical revascularization. The role of perfusion imaging in the evaluation of newer angiogenic therapies is also addressed.

The use of SPECT or PET myocardial perfusion imaging for this purpose requires careful attention to several technical issues. Monitoring the effect of therapeutic interventions assumes that abnormal myocardial perfusion can be imaged reproducibly under unchanged pathophysiologic conditions. Furthermore, improvement of regional myocardial perfusion realistically can be expected to be more an improvement in the degree of abnormality rather than complete normalization. Accordingly, quantitative methods will offer an important advantage over qualitative or even semiquantitative approaches for image analysis. Therefore, in the evaluation of these therapeutic interventions we need to consider the imaging approach, selection of perfusion tracer and imaging protocol, and method of image analysis.

SPECT IMAGING

Reproducibility of SPECT Imaging

Only a limited number of studies have addressed the important issue of reproducibility of stress myocardial perfusion imaging on repeat testing [1,2]. First, one should consider the reproducibility of the stress test itself. Repeat exercise testing may show improved exercise tolerance without demonstrable regression of disease or significant therapeutic intervention. This modest favorable effect is most likely due to the effect of training or greater familiarity of a patient with the test or both. In addition, coronary artery disease is a dynamic process with temporary modest improvement or worsening of symptoms. It is assumed, although not proven, that well-standardized pharmacologic stress with vasodilators (i.e., dipyridamole or adenosine) or adrenergic agonists (dobutamine) may be more reproducible and preferable to monitor the effect of therapeutic interventions. The reproducibility of SPECT imaging was demonstrated in a semiquantitative way by Alazraki et al. [3] and quantitatively by Mahmarian et al. [1]. Both studies showed that in stable patients without intervening cardiac events and change of medications, stress myocardial perfusion imaging is highly reproducible. However, it is also clear that these images are not exactly identical and that subtle differences can be noted.

Quantification of SPECT Imaging

Since the changes in myocardial perfusion defects on SPECT images of patients who had medical interventions can be expected to be modest, such subtle changes may be difficult to identify reproducibly by visual analysis. Radionuclide imaging is an intrinsically digital imaging technique that is ideally suited for quantification. A number of commercially available SPECT quantitative software packages have been validated [4–12]. These programs usually provide a digital analysis of the relative radiotracer uptake in reconstructed slices and compare this to a normal database. Two general approaches are utilized to display the results of this analysis, the polar map, or "bull's-eye," display and the circumferential count profile display. For well over 10 years our laboratory has routinely used quantification with circumferential profiles. This quantification method was validated in experimental animal studies and in phantom studies [6,8,11]. Stress and rest myocardial perfusion abnormalities are expressed as percentage of left ventricular volume. Compared to our method of quantification, the bull's-eye methods tend to overestimate myocardial perfusion abnormalities in particular in larger perfusion defects. This is due to the distortion of the mid- and basal ventricular area on the bull's-eye display. Based on studies of the reproducibility of this quantitative method, a change in myocardial perfusion defect size of greater than 5% (of the left ventricle) represents a true change. Table 16.1 shows a comparison of various methodologies to measure myocardial perfusion defect size [13]. Unfortunately, no accepted standard exists for quantification of SPECT myocardial perfusion defect size, or even for the categorization of perfusion abnormalities as small, moderate, or large. Characterization of defects as small, moderate, or large is probably insufficient when trying to demonstrate small changes in regional myocardial perfusion.

SPECT Imaging Agents and Imaging Protocol

Currently, thallium-201 (Tl-201) and technetium-99m(Tc-99m) labeled tracers, like Tc-99m-sestamibi and Tc-99m-tetrofosmin, are used interchangeably for the detection of coronary artery disease. However, there are substantial differences in myocardial uptake and clearance kinetics and biodistribution among each of the Tc-99m labeled perfusion tracers and Tl-201 [14]. These differences should be considered in the clinical application of perfusion imaging. Myocardial perfusion imaging can be critically affected by the biodistribution of a tracer, particularly in organs adjacent to the heart, especially the lungs and the liver. The relative tracer activity in these organs is relevant for the optimal timing of myocardial imaging. Exercise is performed in conjunction with perfusion imaging to provoke flow heterogeneity in the presence of a subcritical (non-flow-limiting) coronary stenosis. Patients who are unable to exercise are injected with a perfusion tracer during vasodilator stress in order to mimic alterations in flow associated with exercise. The level of exercise, or the type of pharmacologic stress, can also affect the biodistribution [15]. The biodistribution of Tc-99m-sestamibi shows considerable change with stress, suggesting that the kinetics of this tracer are influenced by the level of stress [15]. Adenosine is one of the most commonly used pharmacologic stressors for stress perfusion imaging; however, adenosine causes significant side effects and systemic vascular and hemodynamic effects, which may alter the biodistribution of a radiotracer. Thus, the mode of stress applied has clear implications for the choice of optimal imaging agent [14].

The Tc-99m labeled agents also have lower myocardial extraction fraction than Tl-201, and therefore the uptake of these tracers tends to plateau at higher regional myocardial blood flows often achieved with vasodilators. Thus, reliable detection of mild coronary artery stenosis may be jeopardized with certain stress-tracer combinations because insufficient heterogeneity of radiotracer uptake is created even by moderate regional differences in flow, in the high flow regions. Thus, Tl-201 may represent the imaging agent of choice if adenosine or dipyridamole were used. It should be emphasized that for the purpose of monitoring the effect of interventions, the sensitivity needed to detect changes in perfusion may be higher than that needed merely for the detection of disease. When using Tc-99m

TABLE 16.1 *Characterization of Abnormal SPECT Results*

Defect Size	Small	Medium	Large
Visual territories	< 1/2 of one vascular territory	1 vascular territory only	2 or 3 vascular territories
SSS	4–8	9–13	> 13
Polar maps	< 10% LV	10%–20% LV	> 20% LV
Circumferential profiles	< 5% LV	5%–10% LV	> 10% LV

SSS, sum stress score; LV, left ventricle.

Reprinted with permission of the American Society of Nuclear Cardiology, modified from table 1, Wintergreen Panel Summaries, editors: Beller GA, Zaret BL. J Nucl Cardiol. 1999;6:93–155.

labeled agents, a 2-day imaging protocol would be preferred, as opposed to a same-day imaging protocol that uses a split dose of Tc-99m. In the same-day protocol, one of the two images necessarily has lower count density and requires slightly different filtering. These differences in image quality are subtle and usually of no clinical importance when detection of disease is the issue. However, for the purpose of monitoring the effect of treatment, the detection of relatively small changes in perfusion may be required.

When the aim is to reliably compare defect reversibility, both the rest and stress study should be of optimal and comparable image quality. Serial SPECT studies aimed to detect improvement of stress-induced myocardial ischemia should probably not use a dual-isotope (rest Tl-201, stress Tc-99m-estamibi) protocol, since defect reversibility *may be* less reliably detected due to the physical differences of the two radiotracers [16].

Dynamic SPECT Imaging

The advent of multidetector SPECT imaging systems has enabled the acquisition of rapid serial SPECT images [17–21]. This type of dynamic SPECT imaging can provide an index of absolute myocardial flow or flow reserve. Smith et al. demonstrated that dynamic SPECT imaging of Tc-99m labeled teboroxime has the potential for quantitatively measuring regional myocardial perfusion in experimental models [17,19]. More recently, Iida and Eberl outlined a strategy for quantitative assessment of regional myocardial blood flow in humans using dynamic SPECT Tl-201 [20]. Thus, evidence is accumulating, that high-resolution, accurate measures of absolute flow or flow reserve can be obtained with dynamic SPECT, and may be significantly more valuable than the relative measures of perfusion obtained with conventional SPECT imaging. However, these dynamic imaging approaches will also require the use of radiotracers with high myocardial extraction. Recently, Sugihara et al. reported a potentially simpler approach, which integrates analysis of dynamic planar imaging with static cardiac SPECT using compartmental modeling [22]. However, this technique works only for radiopharmaceuticals that act like "microspheres" [23]. With this approach, it is important that the radiotracer extraction remain constant over a large flow range. The "microsphere" method also relies on not having any washout from the tissue from the time of injection to the time of measurement. It is anticipated that modified SPECT acquisition and processing will be able to routinely provide absolute measures of myocardial perfusion. However, these types of analysis will also need to include attenuation compensation to

provide accurate quantitative images and improved sensitivity for detection of subtle changes in perfusion [24].

PET IMAGING

Quantification of Myocardial Flow Using Positron Emission Tomography

PET imaging provides an accurate noninvasive method for assessment of relative and absolute regional myocardial blood flows [25]. Several blood flow tracers are available, including cyclotron-produced radiopharmaceuticals such as O-15 water and N-13 ammonia and generator-produced rubidium-82 (Rb-82 and copper-62 (Cu-62) pyruvaldehyde-bis-(N-4-methylthiosemicarbazone) (PTSM). Initial comparative studies with Tl-201 SPECT have shown that PET has a higher diagnostic accuracy. Beyond improved diagnostic performance, the quantitative flow measurements provided by PET represent another important advantage. Quantification of blood flow based on tracer kinetic modeling yields blood flow values in close agreement with determinations provided by invasive procedures. Myocardial blood flow at rest and pharmacologic stress can be measured reproducibly with N-13 ammonia PET [26].

Arrighi et al. directly compared the sensitivity of adenosine Tc-99m-sestamibi SPECT with N-13 ammonia PET in a chronic canine model of ischemia, produced by gradual ameroid occlusion [27]. SPECT imaging was performed at 3 and 5 weeks after implantation of an ameroid occluder. PET imaging was performed at 4 weeks, in between the two SPECT studies. In this experimental model adenosine Tc-99m-sestamibi SPECT significantly underestimated ischemia and defect severity compared with N-13 ammonia PET (Fig. 16.1). This difference has been attributed to "rolloff" of Tc-99m-sestamibi at high flows produced by adenosine.

Thus, serial noninvasive quantification of relative or absolute blood flow with PET can be used to quantify the effect of various therapeutic interventions on myocardial flow and vasodilator reserve and may offer advantages over SPECT imaging.

MONITORING MECHANICAL THERAPIES WITH PERFUSION IMAGING

Stress myocardial perfusion imaging is performed not only to detect significant coronary artery disease but also to provide guidance in patient management decisions. Patients with markedly abnormal and high-risk

SPECT ⁹⁹ᵐTc-Sestamibi - 3 WKS

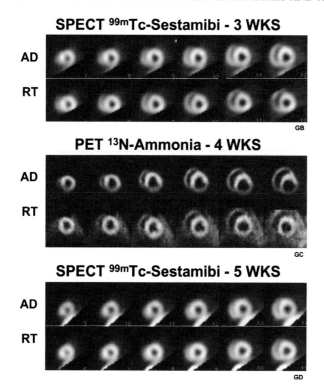

PET ¹³N-Ammonia - 4 WKS

SPECT ⁹⁹ᵐTc-Sestamibi - 5 WKS

FIGURE 16.1 Comparison of Tc-99m-sestamibi SPECT and N-13 ammonia PET imaging in a dog with left circumflex ameroid occluder. Tc-99m-sestamibi SPECT was performed at 3 and 5 weeks after implantation of an ameroid occluder. N-13 ammonia PET imaging was performed at 4 weeks in between the two SPECT studies. SPECT images demonstrate a very subtle perfusion defect in the posterolateral region. Interpretation of the SPECT images was complicated by scatter from extracardiac activity. The PET images demonstrate a large stress-induced defect in the posterolateral region. In this experimental model, adenosine Tc-99m-sestamibi SPECT significantly underestimated ischemia and defect severity compared with N-13 ammonia PET.

stress myocardial perfusion images usually will be considered candidates for coronary revascularization, either by coronary bypass surgery or percutaneous coronary interventions, angioplasty and stenting.

Myocardial Perfusion Imaging before and after Revascularization

Although many patients have stress myocardial perfusion imaging *prior* to revascularization, this imaging is not routinely performed *after* coronary bypass surgery and is, according to guidelines, only indicated when symptoms reoccur. Since many patients have nonspecific ST-T segment changes on the baseline electrocardiogram (ECG) after surgery, myocardial perfusion imaging is preferred over the exercise electrocardiography to evaluate these patients [28,29]. With knowledge of the details of revascularization, tomographic localiza-

tion of perfusion abnormalities allows determination of whether clinical ischemia is likely to be caused by coronary graft closure or by newly developed disease in other coronary arteries [30]. Alazraki et al. followed 336 patients randomized to coronary bypass graft surgery or coronary angioplasty in the EAST study with quantitative Tl-201 SPECT imaging [31]. At 1 year after revascularization, stress-induced ischemia occurred more frequently after angioplasty than after surgery (46% vs 27%, $p < .001$). Quantitative Tl-201 SPECT imaging effectively stratified patients according to the occurrence of subsequent cardiac events at 3-year follow-up.

Percutaneous Coronary Intervention

Stress myocardial perfusion imaging may be particularly useful after coronary intervention of patients with multivessel coronary artery disease. Often the most severe stenosis in the "culprit" vessel is dilated and stented. However, a question often remains whether the stenoses in other vessels are of significance. During interpretation of SPECT images the interpreter can focus on a particular vascular territory. The optimal timing of imaging after percutaneous transluminal coronary angioplasty (PTCA) remains unclear. Initial investigators [32] reported a high incidence of false positive myocardial perfusion abnormalities early after PTCA, presumably because of delayed return of coronary flow reserve within the territory of the dilated artery. Since these data were published, substantial progress has been made with interventional techniques and technology. The general experience now is that most patients have normal myocardial perfusion images within the first week of successful coronary intervention. At approximately 4 weeks after PTCA, a good correlation has been demonstrated between stress-induced myocardial perfusion abnormalities and the presence or absence of restenosis, independent of clinical symptoms [33–36].

Garzon et al. performed a meta analysis of all studies, between the years 1975 and 2000, examining the diagnostic abilities of exercise treadmill testing, stress nuclear imaging, and stress echocardiography at 6 months after PTCA for detection of restenosis [37]. The pooled analysis demonstrated that nuclear perfusion imaging has a sensitivity of 87% and specificity of 78% for detection of restenosis. However, these investigators speculated that the value of routine post-PTCA testing to detect restenosis would decline as the rates of restenosis are substantially reduced with the use of coronary stenting.

In our own laboratory we perform electrocardiographic treadmill stress testing shortly after PTCA to assess functional status and exercise-induced symptoms. Stress myocardial perfusion imaging is performed in patients who develop symptoms suggestive of restenosis, or at 6 months in those who are asymptomatic [34,37]. SPECT imaging allows determination of whether clinical ischemia is caused by restenosis at the site of angioplasty or by progression of disease in other coronary arteries.

Transmyocardial Laser Revascularization

Transmyocardial laser revascularization (TMLR) is a relatively new approach for the management of coronary artery disease. TMLR involves direct laser treatment to the myocardium. This laser treatment has been successfully accomplished with three different types of lasers; carbon dioxide, holmium: YAG, and excimer. TMLR has been shown consistently to provide symptomatic improvement in patients with angina who are not candidates for conventional therapies. While this novel treatment approach provides proven symptomatic relief to patients, the mechanism by which this is achieved remains unclear.

Three major mechanistic hypotheses have been postulated and tested, yet no one has clearly demonstrated legitimacy. The first theory suggests that the laser-produced channels remain patent indefinitely, allowing blood flow from the ventricular chamber and endocardial surface to flow into the ischemic regions. Next, it is possible that production of the laser channels stimulates angiogenesis in the treatment region, again improving flow. Finally, it is possible that laser treatment does not actually improve flow to ischemic tissues, but rather results in a denervation of visceral nerves that transmit the sensation of pain, resulting in the decreased perception of pain. We have postulated an alternative mechanism for the action of TMLR, namely, a mechanical model for the improvement of flow in treated areas. The lasered channels into the myocardium result in the formation of scar tracks as the tissue heals. These scar tracks may change the mechanical properties of the myocardium, resulting in stiffening of ischemic myocardium. Normally there is a component of shear deformation that acts to compress intramyocardial vasculature, predominately during systole. While this phenomenon is present in nondiseased hearts, the abnormal deformation of ischemic tissue with bulging and increased shear may in fact accentuate this vasculature compression and further impair blood flow. This vascular compression affects flow in the ischemic area, as well as remote territories, which must compensate for the abnormal ischemic deformation. With TMLR and the establishment of these reinforcing scar tracks, this shear and bulging are reduced and thus allow for greater patency of intramyocardial vessels, ultimately improving flow to the treated and remote regions of the heart.

A number of experimental studies have demonstrated improvement in regional myocardial perfusion following TMLR. Our group has evaluated excimer laser TMLR-induced changes of myocardial flow and function in a canine model of chronic ischemia produced with an ameroid occluder [38]. Serial gated Tc-99m-sestamibi SPECT and dynamic N-13 ammonia PET imaging were performed before and after TMLR. Under these experimental conditions, Tc-99m-sestamibi SPECT images revealed very small defects, which did not change significantly following TMLR. For the analysis of PET images, absolute regional myocardial blood flow was computed for 24 myocardial segments, using an established PET compartmental analysis. TMLR significantly increased resting PET flow in both the treated ischemic and remote nonischemic regions and tended to increase maximum achievable flow with adenosine in the ischemic region.

Several prospective controlled multicenter trials have been conducted comparing TMLR with medical therapy in patients with refractory angina, demonstrating ischemic regions of myocardium not amenable to conventional coronary revascularization [39–41]. These studies have used a variety of radiotracers and multiple methods of analysis. Frazier et al. employed dipyridamole/redistribution/rest Tl-201 SPECT and qualitative analysis [40]. Patients treated with carbon dioxide TMLR demonstrated an improvement in perfusion, along with a reduction in anginal class and cardiac events. A similar multicenter study was conducted by Schofield et al., although these investigators performed Tc-99m-sestamibi SPECT at 3, 6, and 12 months after randomization to carbon dioxide TMLR or medical therapy [39]. Unlike the previous study, this study did not demonstrate a significant qualitative improvement in regional myocardial perfusion. A single-center study using dipyridamole/redistribution/rest Tl-201 imaging also did not demonstrate an improvement in semiquantitative perfusion score following carbon dioxide TMLR relative to medical therapy [42]. Allen et al. published the first multi-center study evaluating the holmium:YAG laser. They compared TMLR to medical therapy in patients with demonstrable ischemia and refractory angina [41]. Serial dipyridamole/redistribution/rest Tl-201 SPECT imaging was performed in these patients, and studies were analyzed using a quantitative algorithm. There was no significant quantitative improvement in perfusion associated with TMLR over medical therapy. These results are summarized in Figure 16.2. In addition there was no

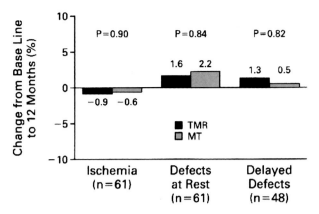

FIGURE 16.2 Changes in quantitative perfusion scores from serial dipyridamole/redistribution/rest Tl-201 SPECT imaging performed as part of a multicenter study evaluating holmium:YAG transmyocardial laser revascularization (TMR) compared to medical therapy (MT) in patients with demonstrable ischemia and refractory angina. Shown are changes in ischemia and in rest and redistribution scores from baseline for patients treated with either TMR or MT. There was no significant quantitative improvement in perfusion associated with TMR over medical therapy. (Reprinted with permission from Allen KB, et al. Comparison of transmyocardial revascularization with medical therapy in patients with refractory angina. N Engl J Med 1999;341:1029–1036.)

correlation of perfusion results with observed changes in anginal class. Burkhoff conducted a similar multicenter study evaluating holmium:YAG TMLR [43]. This study also utilized dipyridamole Tl-201 scintigraphy. Again no difference was observed in Tl-201 perfusion between TMLR and medical therapy. Only one pilot multicenter study has been conducted evaluating TMLR using an excimer laser [44]. Unlike most of the other multicenter studies that evaluated TMLR, this study evaluated patients receiving TMLR as an adjunctive procedure to coronary artery bypass grafting. Changes in perfusion were evaluated with quantitative analysis of Tc-99m-sestamibi SPECT images obtained before, and 1 and 6 months after combined bypass grafting and TMLR. Improvements in stress perfusion were seen in territories treated with both TMLR and bypass grafting, but not in untreated segments.

Rimoldi et al. evaluated the effect of TMLR using quantitative PET O-15 labeled water analysis of regional myocardial flow [45]. This study demonstrated only a slight improvement in coronary flow reserve in the region remote from the TMLR treatment, but not in the treated segments. This observation would be consistent with our own experimental observations, and might be related to an improvement in myocardial mechanics associated with TMLR.

TMLR has complex effects on the myocardial microvasculature, as well cardiac mechanics. The clinical

and experimental studies have demonstrated that TMLR has variable effects on myocardial perfusion. The ideal approach for assessing the changes in perfusion post-TMLR is not established, nor is the sensitivity of SPECT perfusion imaging for detecting these changes if they exist.

MONITORING MEDICAL THERAPY WITH PERFUSION IMAGING

In the routine serial evaluation of patients with coronary artery disease it is important to consider the potential effects of medical therapy on myocardial perfusion. Studies have demonstrated that the extent and severity of coronary artery disease can be underestimated in patients on antianginal therapy [46]. Therefore, some investigators have recommended holding antianginal therapy prior to stress perfusion imaging. Several studies have demonstrated the potential of myocardial SPECT perfusion imaging for monitoring the efficacy of medical therapy for coronary artery disease [47]. Although symptoms have proved to be unreliable for guiding management of patients with coronary artery disease, quantitative perfusion imaging may provide a useful tool for optimizing medical management, and may even lead to improvement in long-term outcome [48]. Studies in which perfusion imaging was used to monitor medical therapy are summarized below. These studies are segregated based on several general classes of medical therapy.

Nitroglycerin Therapy

Several studies have demonstrated the effect of nitroglycerin therapy on myocardial perfusion in patients with ischemic heart disease [49–53]. A study by Mahmarian et al. demonstrated an improvement in myocardial perfusion in patients with stable angina treated with transdermal nitroglycerin for 6 days compared to a placebo control group [52]. More recently, Lewin et al. demonstrated a sustained reduction in the extent and severity of the exercise SPECT perfusion defect with long-term nitroglycerin therapy in patients with chronic stable angina assessed at 5 days and 6 weeks after initiation of therapy [53]. This study employed both semiquantitative assessment of perfusion as well as quantitative analysis of defect size (Fig. 16.3). However, these types of SPECT analysis can provide only an index of changes in relative myocardial perfusion, even if a quantitative index is employed. PET imaging of patients before and after nitroglycerin therapy has provided information regarding absolute changes in

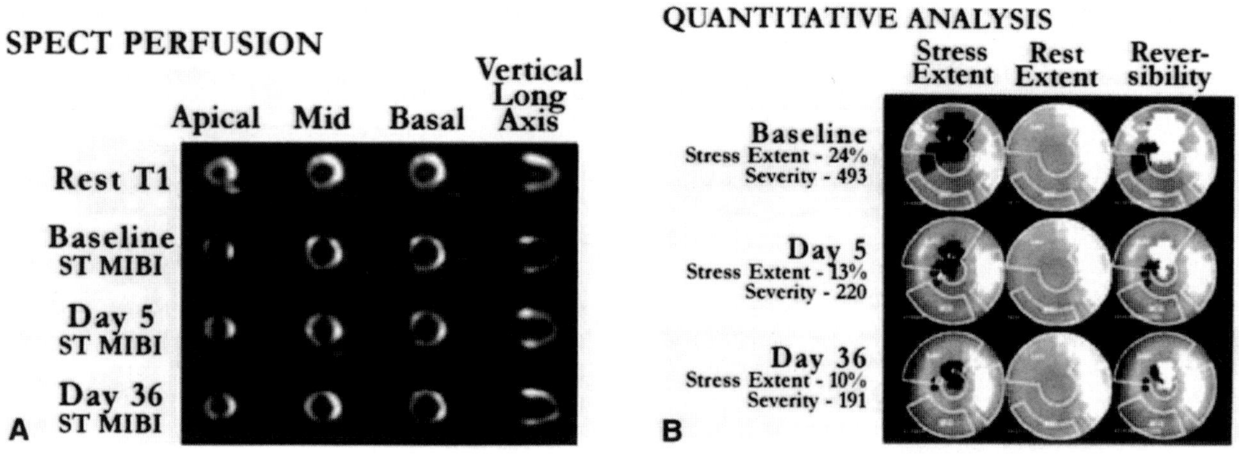

SPECT PERFUSION

QUANTITATIVE ANALYSIS

FIGURE 16.3 Perfusion-defect size (or extent) and perfusion-defect severity were assessed using quantitative rest Tl-201/exercise stress Tc-99m-sestamibi SPECT in patients with chronic stable angina pectoris before and after treatment with extended release isosorbide-5-mononitrate (Imdur). Shown are an example of SPECT perfusion (A), and quantitative analysis results of a patient completing the study protocol (B). Short-axis slices of the apical, mid, and basal left ventricle are displayed, as well as the mid-ventricular vertical long axis (to assess the apex) for the SPECT images (A). The rest Tl-201 SPECT from the baseline study is shown in the top row, with normal resting perfusion. Just below are the stress Tc-99m-sestamibi SPECT for the studies at baseline, day 5, and day 36. At baseline, there is a defect in the distal anterior wall and apex. By means of quantitative analysis, this defect represents 24% of the left ventricular myocardium and has a severity of 493. After 5 days of treatment, the defect is significantly reduced, both visually and quantitatively. On the final study, the defect is without change visually, whereas there is a slight improvement in the quantitative extent and severity. (Reprinted with permission of the American Society of Nuclear Cardiology from Lewin HC, et al. Sustained reduction of exercise perfusion defect extent and severity with isosorbide mononitrate (Imdur) as demonstrated by means of technetium 99m sestamibi. J Nucl Cardiol 2000;7:342–353.)

blood flow associated with nitroglycerin therapy [50]. In patients with documented coronary artery disease and stress-induced ischemia, 3 hours of transdermal nitroglycerin therapy was shown to specifically improve blood flow, as determined by N-13 ammonia PET imaging, in the ischemic region without significantly affecting systemic hemodynamics [50].

Lipid-Lowering Therapies

High cholesterol levels are associated with abnormal endothelial vasodilator capacity [54]. Cholesterol lowering has been shown to improve endothelial dependent vasodilation [55,56] and myocardial perfusion on both SPECT [57] and PET [58] imaging. Mostaza et al. performed a recent randomized placebo-controlled study with cross-over design to evaluate if cholesterol lowering in patients with coronary artery disease and normal cholesterol improved relative myocardial perfusion as assessed by dipyridamole Tl-201 SPECT imaging [59]. Lipid lowering with an HMG-CoA reductase inhibitor resulted in an improvement in both semiquantitative summed stress score and quantitative defect size compared to placebo [59].

Beta-Adrenergic Receptor Blockade

Analysis of absolute blood flow with N-13 ammonia PET has demonstrated that beta-receptor blockade reduces resting flow, increases coronary vasodilator capacity, and thereby increases myocardial flow reserve [60]. Conversely, beta-adrenergic stimulation will increase resting myocardial flow as assessed by N-13 ammonia PET [61], and may impair myocardial flow reserve. During dobutamine stress Tc-99m-sestamibi SPECT perfusion imaging, beta-blocker therapy attenuates and in some cases eliminates inducible flow heterogeneity in patients with coronary artery disease [62].

Combined Medical Therapies versus Revascularization

Dakik et al. employed serial quantitative adenosine SPECT imaging to monitor changes in perfusion in patients following myocardial infarction, who were randomly assigned to be treated with either aggressive combination medical therapy or percutaneous coronary angioplasty (PTCA) [63]. Combination medical therapy included nitroglycerin, beta-blockers, aspirin, lipid-lowering agents, and a calcium channel blocker (Dilti-

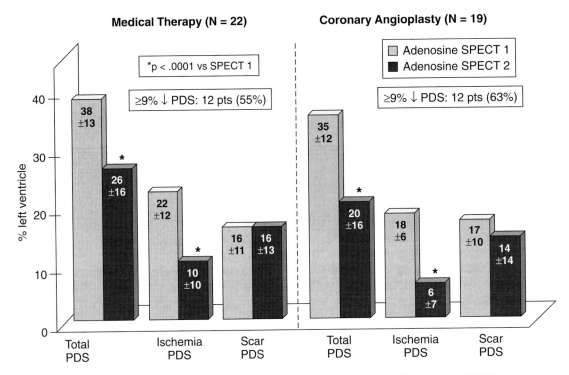

FIGURE 16.4 Changes in perfusion defect score (PDS) in 41 patients studied with sequential SPECT, randomized to medical therapy or PTCA. The total left ventricular (LV) PDS significantly decreased after anti-ischemic therapy ($p < .0001$). The reduction in ischemic PDS from $20 \pm 10\%$ to $8 \pm 9\%$ ($p < .0001$) accounted entirely for the decrease observed in total PDS. The scar size did not significantly change with therapy. Total and ischemic PDS were also significantly reduced in patients randomized to either medical therapy or PTCA. The magnitude of the absolute reduction in ischemic ($-12 \pm 10\%$ versus $-12 \pm 9\%$) PDS was similar ($p =$ ns) in both groups. (Reprinted with permission of the American Heart Association from Dakik HA, et al. Intensive medical therapy versus coronary angioplasty for suppression of myocardial ischemia in survivors of acute myocardial infarction: a prospective, randomized pilot study. Circulation 1998;98:2017–2023.)

azem) in patients with normal left ventricular function. In this pilot study, intensive medical therapy and PTCA were comparable at suppressing ischemia postmyocardial infarction (Fig. 16.4).

MONITORING NOVEL GENE THERAPY WITH PERFUSION IMAGING

New therapies for ischemic heart disease are directed at stimulation of angiogenesis, which represents the formation of new capillary blood vessels from existing microvessels, by cellular outgrowth. Angiogenesis has been demonstrated conclusively in a variety of animal models and in patients with coronary artery disease [64–66]. Preclinical studies have demonstrated the efficacy of angiogenic therapy in animal models, using relatively invasive measures to assess efficacy [65,67,68]. However, preliminary clinical trials of stimulated angio-

genesis in patients with severe coronary artery disease have demonstrated a minimal benefit over placebo, when evaluated using standard clinical SPECT perfusion imaging [69–72]. Figures 16.5 and 16.6 summarize the results from two of these early clinical trials. An expert panel has evaluated the role of perfusion imaging for the assessment of newer therapies directed at stimulating coronary angiogenesis [73]. This panel raised several important issues relevant to this specific population. First, the usefulness of perfusion imaging for the detection of improved perfusion associated with enhanced collateral supply has not been established. Patients entered into these trials often have multivessel disease, depressed left ventricular function, and frequently have undergone prior coronary revascularization. Therefore, these patients may not be able to achieve maximal exercise, which would be required to optimize detection of ischemia. These patients may also develop only small improvements in endocardial flow with these therapies, and

SPECT imaging may not have the necessary sensitivity or resolution to detect these subtle changes in flow. The effect of ischemic dysfunction on remote coronary flow reserve has been raised by several experimental studies [74,75]. Thus, analyses of only relative coronary flow reserve or perfusion may be inadequate.

Many early clinical trials of therapeutic angiogenesis used perfusion imaging to investigate whether these therapies actually increase myocardial blood flow. Only limited data are currently available, which have been obtained primarily from small uncontrolled trials or registries [73]. Unfortunately, no perfusion imaging strategies have proved uniformly effective in evaluation of cardiac angiogenesis. The development of more sensitive and specific imaging strategies for the evaluation of myocardial angiogenesis and tracking this process noninvasively will be critical in evaluation of angiogenic therapy for the heart.

Therefore, at this time no definite conclusions can be reached regarding the reliability of perfusion imaging as a primary end point for future clinical trials of angiogenic therapies. If myocardial perfusion imaging is to be utilized, clearly a quantitative approach will be necessary. Because Tl-201 demonstrates the best linearity of uptake with flow, we would favor its use from among the currently approved SPECT radiotracers. Initial single-site pilot studies might be best accomplished using quantitative PET imaging. Unfortunately, application of this technology in a large multicenter study has proven to be difficult.

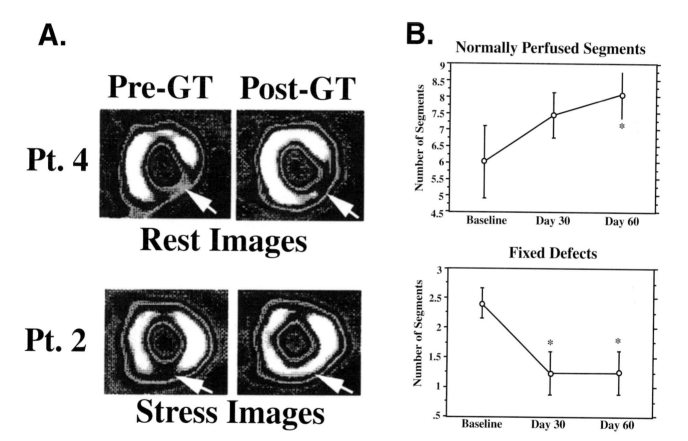

FIGURE 16.5 SPECT Tc-99m-sestamibi perfusion imaging in patients treated with direct myocardial injection of phVEGF165 as sole therapy for myocardial ischemia. Two patient image examples are shown (A), before (Pre-GT) and after gene therapy (Post-GT). Graphic summary of semiquantitative image findings in five treated patients (B). Short-axis views were divided into a total of 13 segments and graded as normal (no perfusion defect), reversible (perfusion defect during stress that partially or completely reversed at rest), or fixed (perfusion defect during stress that persists at rest). Values represent mean ± SEM for all five patients at baseline, 30 days, and 60 days postgene therapy (*$p < .05$ compared with baseline). (Reprinted with permission of the American Heart Association from Losordo DW, et al. Gene therapy for myocardial angiogenesis initial clinical results with direct myocardial injection of phVEGF165 as sole therapy for myocardial ischemia. Circulation 98:2800–2804, 1998.)

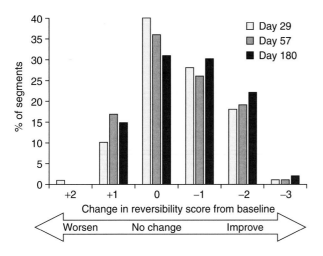

FIGURE 16.6 Effect of recombinant fibroblast growth factor-2 on inducible ischemia as assessed by semiquantitative analysis of dual-isotope gated SPECT Tl-201/Tc-99m-sestamibi, in patients with advanced coronary artery disease. Shown is the segmental distribution of the change from baseline in segmental reversibility score, a measure of the magnitude of inducible ischemia. (Reprinted with permission of the American Heart Association from Udelson JE, et al. Therapeutic angiogenesis with recombinant fibroblast growth factor-2 improves stress and rest myocardial perfusion abnormalities in patients with severe symptomatic chronic coronary artery disease. Circulation 2000;102:1605–1610.)

CONCLUSIONS

Ischemic heart disease has a complex pathophysiology that cannot be fully characterized by simple identification of epicardial coronary obstructions angiographically [48]. The management of ischemic heart disease can also not be simply limited to mechanical revascularization. The effects of coexisting diseases like hypertension, hypercholesterolemia, and diabetes must also be considered, along with changes in myocardial metabolism and mechanics. The entire coronary vasculature is involved in the ischemic process, including the microcirculation. Accordingly, the evaluation of myocardial perfusion and perfusion reserve with SPECT or PET imaging may provide additional important insight regarding the underlying pathophysiology, and lead to improved clinical outcome by allowing more directed therapy and follow-up.

For the purpose of the topic of discussion in this chapter, that is, monitoring the effects of interventions, the importance of standardization of the stressor, the imaging protocol, and the method of image analysis should be emphasized. Quantitative PET perfusion imaging offers some clear advantages for evaluation of therapeutic interventions, which may have complicated physiological effects on regional flow. However, after careful review of the available literature, adenosine SPECT Tl-201 imaging with quantitative analysis may represent the most practical methodology of choice for monitoring therapeutic interventions, whether they be mechanical, medical, or genetic.

REFERENCES

1. Mahmarian JJ, Moye LA, Verani MS, et al. High reproducibility of myocardial perfusion defects in patients undergoing serial exercise thallium-201 tomography. Am J Cardiol 1995;75:1116.
2. Golub RJ, Ahlberg AW, McClellan JR, et al. Interpretive reproducibility of stress Tc-99m sestamibi tomographic myocardial perfusion imaging. J Nucl Cardiol 1999;6:257.
3. Alazraki NP, Krawczynska EG, DePuey EG, et al. Reproducibility of thallium-201 exercise SPECT studies. J Nucl Med 1994;35:1237.
4. Van Train KF, Areeda J, Garcia EV, et al. Quantitative same-day rest-stress technetium-99m-sestamibi SPECT: definition and validation of stress normal limits and criteria for abnormality. J Nucl Med 1993;34:1494.
5. Van Train KF, Garcia EV, Maddahi J, et al. Multicenter trial validation for quantitative analysis of same-day rest-stress technetium-99m-sestamibi myocardial tomograms. J Nucl Med 1994;35:609.
6. Liu YH, Sinusas AJ, Shi CQ, et al. Quantification of technetium 99m-labeled sestamibi single-photon emission computed tomography based on mean counts improves accuracy for assessment of relative regional myocardial blood flow: experimental validation in a canine model. J Nucl Cardiol 1996;3:312.
7. Kang X, Berman DS, Van Train KF, et al. Clinical validation of automatic quantitative defect size in rest technetium-99m-sestamibi myocardial perfusion SPECT. J Nucl Med 1997;38:1441.
8. Liu YH, Sinusas AJ, DeMan P, et al. Quantification of SPECT myocardial perfusion images: methodology and validation of the Yale-CQ method. J Nucl Cardiol 1999;6:190.
9. Sharir T, Germano G, Waechter PB, et al. A new algorithm for the quantitation of myocardial perfusion SPECT. II: validation and diagnostic yield. J Nucl Med 2000;41:720.
10. Santana CA, Garcia EV, Vansant JP, et al. Three-dimensional color-modulated display of myocardial SPECT perfusion distributions accurately assesses coronary artery disease. J Nucl Med 2000;41:1941.
11. Kirac S, Wackers FJ, Liu YH. Validation of the Yale circumferential quantification method using 201Tl and 99mTc: a phantom study. J Nucl Med 2000;41:1436.
12. Van Train KF, Garcia EV. New algorithm for quantification of myocardial perfusion SPECT. J Nucl Med 2001;42:391.
13. American Society of Nuclear Cardiology. Wintergreen Panel Summaries. In: Fourth Invitational Wintergreen Conference, edited by G Beller and B Zaret. Wintergreen, VA, J Nucl Cardiol 1999; 6:93.
14. Kailasnath P, Sinusas A. Technetium-99m-labeled myocardial pefusion agents: are they better than thallium-201. Cardiol Rev 2001;9:160.
15. Wackers FJ, Berman DS, Maddahi J, et al. Technetium-99m hexakis 2-methoxyisobutyl isonitrile: human biodistribution, dosimetry, safety, and preliminary comparison to thallium-201 for myocardial perfusion imaging. J Nucl Med 1989;30:301.
16. Siebelink HM, Natale D, Sinusas AJ, et al. Quantitative comparison of single-isotope and dual-isotope stress-rest single-photon emission computed tomographic imaging for reversibility of defects. J Nucl Cardiol 1996;3:483.

17. Smith AM, Gullberg GT, Christian PE, et al. Kinetic modeling of teboroxime using dynamic SPECT imaging of a canine model. J Nucl Med 1994;35:484.

18. Chiao P-C, Ficaro E, Dayanikli F, et al. Compartmental analysis of technetium-99m-teboroxime kinetics employing fast dynamic SPECT at rest and stress. J Nucl Med 1994;35:1265.

19. Smith AM, Gullberg GT, Christian PE. Experimental verification of technetium 99m-labeled teboroxime kinetic parameters in the myocardium with dynamic single-photon emission computed tomography: reproducibility, correlation to flow, and susceptibility to extravascular contamination. J Nucl Cardiol 1996; 3:130.

20. Iida H, Eberl S. Quantitative assessment of regional myocardial blood flow with thallium-201 and SPECT. J Nucl Cardiol 1998; 5:313.

21. Di Bella E, Ross S, Kadrmas D, et al. Compartmental modeling of technetium-99m-labeled teboroxime with dynamic single-photon emission computed tomography: comparison to static thallium-201 in a canine model. Inv Radiol 2001;36:178.

22. Sugihara H, Yonekura Y, Kataoka K, et al. Estimation of coronary flow reserve using dynamic planar and SPECT images of Tc99m tetrofosmin. J Nucl Cardiol 2001;(in press).

23. Gullberg G, Di Bella E, Sinusas A. Estimation of coronary flow reserve: can SPECT compete with other modalities? J Nucl Cardiol 2001;(in press).

24. Tsui BM, Frey EC, LaCroix KJ, et al. Quantitative myocardial perfusion SPECT. J Nucl Cardiol 1998;5:507.

25. Schwaiger M, Muzik O. Assessment of myocardial perfusion by positron emission tomography. Am J Cardiol 1991;67:35D.

26. Nagamachi S, Czernin J, Kim AS, et al. Reproducibility of measurements of regional resting and hyperemic myocardial blood flow assessed with PET. J Nucl Med 1996;37:1626.

27. Arrighi J, Dione D, Condos S, et al. Adenosine Tc99m-sestamibi SPECT underestimates ischemia compared with N-13 ammonia PET in a chronic canine model of ischemia. J Nucl Med 1999; 40:6P.

28. Nallamothu N, Johnson J, Bagheri B, et al. Utility of stress single-photon emission computed tomography (SPECT) perfusion imaging in predicting outcome after coronary artery bypass grafting. Am J Cardiol 1997;80:1517.

29. Palmas W, Bingham S, Diamond G, et al. Incremental prognostic value of exercise thallium-201 myocardial single-photon emission computed tomography late after coronary artery bypass surgery. J Am Coll Cardiol 1995;25:403.

30. Khoury A, Rivera J, Mahmarian J, et al. Adenosine thallium-201 tomography in evaluation of graft patency late after coronary artery bypass graft surgery. J Am Coll Cardiol 1997;29: 1290.

31. Alazraki NP, Krawczynska EG, Kosinski AS, et al. Prognostic value of thallium-201 single-photon emission computed tomography for patients with multivessel coronary artery disease after revascularization (the Emory Angioplasty versus Surgery Trial [EAST]). Am J Cardiol 1999;84:1369.

32. Manyari D, Knudtson M, Kloibar R, et al. Sequential thallium-201 myocardial perfusion studies after successful percutaneous transluminal coronary artery angioplasty: delayed resolution of exercise-induced scintigraphic abnormalities. Circulation 1988; 77:86.

33. Miller DD, Liu P, Strauss HW, et al. Prognostic value of computer-quantitated exercise thallium imaging early after percutaneous transluminal coronary angioplasty. J Am Coll Cardiol 1987;10:275.

34. Jain A, Mahmarian J, Borges-Neto S, et al. Clinical significance of perfusion defects by thallium-201 single photon emission tomography following oral dipyridamole early after coronary angioplasty. J Am Coll Cardiol 1988;11:970.

35. Hecht H, Shaw R, Bruce T, et al. Usefulness of tomographic thallium-201 imaging for detection of restenosis after percutaneous transluminal coronary angioplasty. Am J Cardiol 1990;66:1314.

36. Miller DD, Verani MS. Current status of myocardial perfusion imaging after percutaneous transluminal coronary angioplasty. J Am Coll Cardiol 1994;24:260.

37. Garzon PP, Eisenberg MJ. Functional testing for the detection of restenosis after percutaneous transluminal coronary angioplasty: a meta-analysis. Can J Cardiol 2001;17:41.

38. Bedair H, Dione D, Arrighi J, et al. Transmyocardial excimer laser revascularization results in improvement of resting myocardial flow. J Nucl Cardiol 2001;8:S112.

39. Schofield PM, Sharples LD, Caine N, et al. Transmyocardial laser revascularisation in patients with refractory angina: a randomised controlled trial [see comments] [published erratum appears in Lancet 1999 May 15;353(9165):1714]. Lancet 1999; 353:519.

40. Frazier OH, March RJ, Horvath KA. Transmyocardial revascularization with a carbon dioxide laser in patients with end-stage coronary artery disease. N Engl J Med 1999;341:1021.

41. Allen KB, Dowling RD, Fudge TL, et al. Comparison of transmyocardial revascularization with medical therapy in patients with refractory angina [see comments]. N Engl J Med 1999;341: 1029.

42. Landolfo CK, Landolfo KP, Hughes GC, et al. Intermediate-term clinical outcome following transmyocardial laser revascularization in patients with refractory angina pectoris. Circulation 1999; 100:II128.

43. Burkhoff D, Schmidt S, Schulman SP, et al. Transmyocardial laser revascularisation compared with continued medical therapy for treatment of refractory angina pectoris: a prospective randomised trial. ATLANTIC Investigators. Angina Treatments-Lasers and Normal Therapies in Comparison [see comments]. Lancet 1999;354:885.

44. Sinusas A, Gundry S, Verrier E, et al. Adjunctive transmyocardial laser revascularization improves regional SPECT perfusion during coronary bypass grafting: a multicenter trial. J Nucl Med 1999;40:84P.

45. Rimoldi O, Burns SM, Rosen SD, et al. Measurement of myocardial blood flow with positron emission tomography before and after transmyocardial laser revascularization. Circulation 1999;100:II134.

46. Sharir T, Rabinowitz B, Livschitz S, et al. Underestimation of extent and severity of coronary artery disease by dipyridamole stress thallium-201 single-photon emission computed tomographic myocardial perfusion imaging in patients taking antianginal drugs. J Am Coll Cardiol 1998;31:1540.

47. Cerqueira MD. Monitoring medical management of coronary artery disease: patient selection, optimal management, and potential problems for diagnosis. [letter; comment]. J Nucl Cardiol 2000;7:392.

48. Pepine CJ, Deedwania PC. How do we best treat patients with ischemic heart disease? Circulation 1998;98:1985.

49. Liu P, Houle S, Burns RJ, et al. Effect of intracoronary nitroglycerin on myocardial blood flow and distribution in pacing-induced angina pectoris. Quantitative assessment by single-photon emission tomography. Am J Cardiol 1985;55:1270.

50. Fallen EL, Nahmias C, Scheffel A, et al. Redistribution of myocardial blood flow with topical nitroglycerin in patients with coronary artery disease. Circulation 1995;91:1381.

51. Aoki M, Sakai K, Koyanagi S, et al. Effect of nitroglycerin on

coronary collateral function during exercise evaluated by quantitative analysis of thallium-201 single photon emission computed tomography. Am Heart J 1991;121:1361.

52. Mahmarian JJ, Fenimore NL, Marks GF, et al. Transdermal nitroglycerin patch therapy reduces the extent of exercise-induced myocardial ischemia: results of a double-blind, placebo-controlled trial using quantitative thallium-201 tomography. J Am Coll Cardiol 1994;24:25.

53. Lewin HC, Hachamovitch R, Harris AG, et al. Sustained reduction of exercise perfusion defect extent and severity with isosorbide mononitrate (Imdur) as demonstrated by means of technetium 99m sestamibi. J Nucl Cardiol 2000;7:342.

54. Creager MA, Cooke JP, Mendelsohn ME, et al. Impaired vasodilation of forearm resistance vessels in hypercholesterolemic humans. J Clin Invest 1990;86:228.

55. Egashira K, Hirooka Y, Kai H, et al. Reduction in serum cholesterol with pravastatin improves endothelium-dependent coronary vasomotion in patients with hypercholesterolemia. Circulation 1994;89:2519.

56. Treasure CB, Klein JL, Weintraub WS, et al. Beneficial effects of cholesterol-lowering therapy on the coronary endothelium in patients with coronary artery disease. N Engl J Med 1995;332:481.

57. Eichstadt HW, Eskotter H, Hoffman I, et al. Improvement of myocardial perfusion by short-term fluvastatin therapy in coronary artery disease. Am J Cardiol 1995;76:122A.

58. Gould K, Martucci J, Goldberg D, et al. Short-term cholesterol lowering decreases size and severity of perfusion abnormalities by positron emission tomography after dipyridamole in patients with coronary artery disease. A potential noninvasive marker of healing coronary endothelium. Circulation 1994;89:1530.

59. Mostaza JM, Gomez MV, Gallardo F, et al. Cholesterol reduction improves myocardial perfusion abnormalities in patients with coronary artery disease and average cholesterol levels. J Am Coll Cardiol 2000;35:76.

60. Bottcher M, Czernin J, Sun K, et al. Effect of beta 1 adrenergic receptor blockade on myocardial blood flow and vasodilatory capacity. J Nucl Med 1997;38:442.

61. Sun KT, Czernin J, Krivokapich J, et al. Effects of dobutamine stimulation on myocardial blood flow, glucose metabolism, and wall motion in normal and dysfunctional myocardium. [see comments]. Circulation 1996;94:3146.

62. Shehata AR, Gillam LD, Mascitelli VA, et al. Impact of acute propranolol administration on dobutamine-induced myocardial ischemia as evaluated by myocardial perfusion imaging and echocardiography. Am J Cardiol 1997;80:268.

63. Dakik HA, Kleiman NS, Farmer JA, et al. Intensive medical therapy versus coronary angioplasty for suppression of myocardial ischemia in survivors of acute myocardial infarction: a prospective, randomized pilot study. [see comments]. Circulation 1998;98:2017.

64. Sasayama S, Fujita M. Recent insights into coronary collateral circulation. Circulation 1992;85:1197.

65. Giordano FJ, Ping P, McKirnan MD, et al. Intracoronary gene transfer of fibroblast growth factor-5 increases blood flow and contractile function in an ischemic region of the heart [see comments]. Nat Med 1996;2:534.

66. Wolf C, Cai WJ, Vosschulte R, et al. Vascular remodeling and altered protein expression during growth of coronary collateral arteries. J Mol Cell Cardiol 1998;30:2291.

67. Unger E, Banai S, Shou M, et al. Basic fibroblast growth factor enhances myocardial collateral flow in a canine model. Am J Physiol 1994;266:H1588.

68. Lazarous DF, Scheinowitz M, Shou M, et al. Effects of chronic systemic administration of basic fibroblast growth factor on collateral development in the canine heart. Circulation 1995;91:145.

69. Losordo DW, Vale PR, Symes JF, et al. Gene therapy for myocardial angiogenesis: initial clinical results with direct myocardial injection of phVEGF165 as sole therapy for myocardial ischemia. Circulation 1998;98:2800.

70. Rosengart TK, Lee LY, Patel SR, et al. Angiogenesis gene therapy: phase I assessment of direct intramyocardial administration of an adenovirus vector expressing VEGF121 cDNA to individuals with clinically significant severe coronary artery disease. Circulation 1999;100:468.

71. Hendel RC, Henry TD, Rocha-Singh K, et al. Effect of intracoronary recombinant human vascular endothelial growth factor on myocardial perfusion: evidence for a dose-dependent effect. Circulation 2000;101:118.

72. Udelson JE, Dilsizian V, Laham RJ, et al. Therapeutic angiogenesis with recombinant fibroblast growth factor-2 improves stress and rest myocardial perfusion abnormalities in patients with severe symptomatic chronic coronary artery disease. Circulation (Online) 2000;102:1605.

73. Simons M, Bonow R, Chronos N, et al. Clinical trials in coronary angiogenesis: issues, problems, consensus: an expert panel summary. Circulation (Online) 2000;102:E73.

74. Wu JC, Yun JJ, Dione DP, et al. Severe regional ischemia alters coronary flow reserve in the remote perfusion area. J Nucl Cardiol 2000;7:43.

75. Daher E, Dione DP, Heller EN, et al. Acute ischemic dysfunction alters coronary flow reserve in remote nonischemic regions: potential mechanical etiology identified in an acute canine model. J Nucl Cardiol 2000;7:112.

17 | Radionuclide angiography

KIM A. WILLIAMS, JEFFREY S. BORER, AND PHYLLIS SUPINO

Part 1

First-Pass

KIM A. WILLIAMS

FIRST-PASS RADIONUCLIDE ANGIOGRAPHY: A HISTORICAL PERSPECTIVE

The first recorded first-pass radionuclide study of the human circulation was performed in 1927 by Herman Blumgart and his colleagues who used a diluted solution of radon injected in one arm, and measured the transit time to the contralateral arm [1]. Since that time there has been steady progress in the development of imaging hardware, computer techniques, and radiopharmaceuticals, which have propelled first-pass into a mature field, with clinically relevant and accurate imaging of cardiac function.

The development of first-pass imaging required the development of high-count-rate-capable imaging devices, such as the multicrystal cameras (e.g., Baird System-Seventy Seven, and Scinticor). First-pass radionuclide angiography (FPRNA) utilizes rapidly acquired images on a high-count-rate gamma camera with high temporal resolution to track a tracer bolus through the venous system into the right atrium (RA), right ventricle (RV), pulmonary arteries (PA), lungs, left atrium (LA), left ventricle (LV), and finally, the aorta. Several cardiac cycles are sampled continuously. The change in radiotracer content over time is used to calculate functional information, such as ejection fraction, cardiac output, and transit times, as well as to assess regional wall motion by comparison of end-diastolic (ED) and end-systolic (ES) images. The first-pass approach is uniquely suited for the detection of intracardiac left to right shunting, by mathematical analysis of time-activity curves generated by a region of interest placed over the lung. The first-pass approach can be applied to patients both at rest and during exercise stress.

First-pass is commonly used for determination of right and left ventricular ejection fraction, regional wall motion, shunts, and pulmonary transit times [2]. It is particularly useful for determining prognosis in ischemic heart disease [3], and can be performed with myocardial perfusion imaging [4], especially since the advent of Tc-99m labeled myocardial perfusion agents in the late 1980s.

COMPARISON WITH OTHER TECHNIQUES FOR VENTRICULAR FUNCTION: A PRACTICAL PERSPECTIVE

The evaluation of LV systolic function has become one of the most common applications of nuclear imaging, using FPRNA, planar gated equilibrium radionuclide angiography (GERNA), and, more recently, gated tomographic perfusion and equilibrium blood pool imaging. Among these techniques, FPRNA has some distinct advantages (Table 17.1). These include (1) the acquisition of data in less than 30 seconds; (2) RV function with less overlap of activity in other chambers; (3) the use of multiple radiopharmaceuticals including bone, renal, and myocardial scintigraphic agents; (4) the ability to obtain high-quality studies in even morbidly obese individuals; (5) a proven robust measurement of stress ventricular function at true peak exercise; and (6) the presence of a wealth of prognostic information available for management of patients with ischemic heart disease based on stratification by FPRNA exercise ejection fractions (EF).

Relative to FPRNA, echocardiography is less easily quantified. Gated blood pool imaging gives less accu-

323

TABLE 17.1 *Comparison of First-Pass Radionuclide Angiography with Other Scintigraphic Techniques for Ventricular Function*

Technique	FPRNA	Gated Planar Blood Pool	Gated SPECT Blood Pool	Gated Planar Perfusion	Gated SPECT Perfusion
Multiple views or projections	Only with biplane camera or multiple injections	Yes	Yes	Yes	Yes
Camera	High-count-rate capable	Any	SPECT capable	Any	SPECT capable
Radiopharmaceuticals	Most water-soluble (e.g., bone, blood pool, hepatobiliary, etc.)	Red cells or serum agents only	Red cells or serum agents only	Perfusion only	Perfusion only
Stress ejection fraction	Yes	Yes, but not precisely at peak exercise	Dobutamine or arbutamine only	Yes, but not precisely at peak exercise	Dobutamine or arbutamine only
ECG required	No	Yes	Yes	Yes	Yes
Acquisition time	30 sec	10 min	15 min	5 min	15 min
Combined perfusion and function	Yes	No	No	Yes	Yes
Clinical value in assessing valvular disease	Yes (tricuspid regurgitation and stroke counts for regurgitant fraction)	Yes (stroke counts for regurgitant fraction)	No	No	No
Intravenous line	Rapid bolus through central, external jugular or large bore medial arm veins only)	Any	Any	Any	Any
RV function	Yes	Poor	Yes	No	Yes

FPRNA, first-pass radionuclide angiography; RV, right ventricle.

rate measures of RV function due to overlap of this chamber with the RA and scatter from and a small degree of overlap of the LV. The three-dimensional techniques, computed tomography and magnetic resonance, are both more time consuming. None of these techniques can isolate the actual peak of exercise, as obtained with a 10 to 15-second acquisition using FPRNA. However, because of the demands for meticulous bolus injection technique for tracer administration and an especially high-count-rate-capable gamma camera, FPRNA is less commonly performed.

INSTRUMENTATION

Multicrystal Cameras

The development of first-pass imaging was augmented by the development of high-count-rate-capable imaging devices, such as the multicrystal cameras (e.g., Baird and Scinticor) [5,6]. The multicrystal camera has lower resolution but is a more sensitive device and is best used for FPRNA studies. These gamma cameras use standard Anger camera electronics, including the thallium activated sodium iodide crystals.

The older version of the multicrystal camera (Baird System-Seventy Seven) had 294 individual 1-inch thick and 1-centimeter square crystals (21 columns and 14 rows), which were individually coupled to two photomultiplier tubes, one for the *x*-axis position and one for the *y*-axis position. This allows very high count rates (up to 500,000 counts per second, open energy window, see Fig. 17.1), since no position information is collected. The usual nuclear imaging system with a single sodium iodide crystal would count no more than 150,000 counts per second prior to decreasing count recovery due to pulse pile-up and increasing dead-time loss.

The newer version used a similar concept with a partitioned or optically divided single 1-inch thick crystal (e.g., Scinticor SIM-400). This camera is capable of even higher count rates (up to 1 million counts per second, open energy window), but shares the poorer spatial resolution with the prior version.

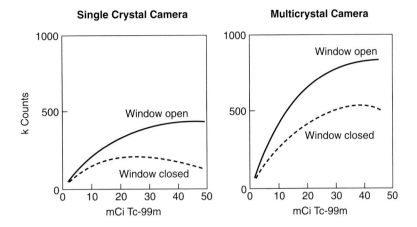

FIGURE 17.1 Comparison of counting rates achieved using a single-crystal camera (Elscint) and a multicrystal camera (Scinticor) with open and closed energy windows, documenting the total count rates attained using Tc-99m pertechnetate. (Edited with permission from Jones RH. Radionuclide angiocardiography. In: Marcus M, Schelbert H, Skorton D, Wolf G, eds. Cardiac imaging. Philadelphia: WB Saunders, 1991.)

Single-Crystal Gamma Cameras

FPRNA can also be performed with a single-crystal high-count-rate gamma camera fitted with a high-sensitivity parallel-hole collimator. One particular model of single-crystal camera (Elscint, Haifa, Israel) was designed with high-count-rate capability [7,8]. This camera can count up to 500,000 counts per second. This high count rate is obtained by opening the energy window and sacrificing the usual spatial resolution associated with a single-crystal camera.

Other single-crystal camera systems (e.g., General Electric, Milwaukee, WI) have software for determination of EF, and have been validated despite the theoretical limitations of poor-count-rate linearity [9,10], but are most commonly used for RV assessment during injection of tracer for gated equilibrium blood pool imaging. Some of these devices have the advantage of having two camera heads with a 90° orientation. This feature allows acquisition of simultaneous biplane FPRNA, in either the anterior and left lateral positions, or the right anterior oblique and left anterior oblique positions.

Multiwire Proportional Chamber Gamma Cameras

One imaging detector has been developed that does not use the principle of scintillation crystal/photomultiplier combination described above. Multiwire proportional chambers (MWPCs) have been used as position-sensitive charged particle detectors in nuclear and high-energy physics, and have recently been adapted to cardiac imaging. MWPCs are large-area gas-filled ionization chambers, in which large arrays of fine wires are used to measure the position of ionization produced in the gas by the passage of charged particles. Key features of MWPCs include high spatial resolution, large-area, and high-count-rate imaging at a potentially lower cost. MWPCs can have a charged particle resolution of 0.4 mm at a count rate of several million per second [11].

Since gamma rays or X-rays cannot be detected directly by the MWPC, they must be converted into photo- or Compton scatter electrons for detection or nuclear isotope imaging. This is accomplished by use of high atomic number materials in the body of the chamber, such as pressurized xenon [12]. This high-pressure xenon gas MWPC is the key to a highly competitive system that can outperform scintillator-based systems. The count rate performance is close to a million counts per second and the intrinsic spatial resolution is better than the best scintillator-based camera.

Although the MWPC gamma camera produces high-quality ejection fraction and wall motion information [12–14], it is optimal only for the detection of gamma rays at energies below 100 keV, such as tantalum-178 (see Radiopharmaceuticals section below). The detection of higher-energy gamma rays will require the development of a solid photon–electron convertor to be incorporated into the chamber.

RADIOPHARMACEUTICALS FOR FIRST-PASS RADIONUCLIDE ANGIOGRAPHY

Radiation dosimetric estimates for several pharmaceuticals are listed in Table 17.2. One significant advantage

TABLE 17.2 *Estimates of Radiation Absorbed Dose (in millirads) for 30 mCi of ^{99m}Tc-MIBI, TETRO and DTPA, 30 mCi of ^{99m}TcO$_4^-$, 1 mCi of ^{178}W, and 100 mCi of ^{178}Ta for a 70 kg Subject*

Organ of Interest	^{99m}Tc-DTPA	^{99m}TcO$_4^-$	^{99m}Tc-MIBI	^{99m}Tc-TETRO	^{178}Ta	^{178}W
Breasts	—	—	200	210	—	—
Gall bladder wall	—	—	2000	5400	—	—
Urinary bladder wall	3450	2550	2000	2130	600	990
Blood	—	—	—	—	300	—
Heart wall	—	—	500	450	—	27
Small intestine	—	—	3000	1890	—	63
Upper large intestine wall	—	3600	5400	3390	—	120
Lower large intestine wall	—	3300	3900	2460	—	280
Kidneys	2700	—	2000	1380	520	88
Liver	—	—	600	450	540	74
Lungs	—	—	300	240	490	23
Ovaries	330	900	1500	1050	66	64
Red marrow	—	510	500	450	760	110
Skeleton	—	—	700	630	680	140
Spleen	—	—	—	420	—	32
Stomach wall	—	1530	600	510	—	—
Testes	225	270	300	330	560	39
Thyroid	—	3900	700	660	—	—
Whole body	180	330	500	—	530	48

DTPA, diethylenetriaminepentaacetic acid; W, tungsten; MIBI, sestamibi; TETRO, tetrofosmin; TcO$_4^-$, pertechnetate; Ta, tantalium.

of the FPRNA technique over other scintigraphic methods of determining cardiac function is the ability to use multiple radiopharmaceuticals. These tracers can subsequently localize in a targeted organ system, resulting in the addition of clinical information on the performance of the heart to a variety of nuclear medical studies. The basic requirements for a tracer to be appropriate for first-pass imaging are (*1*) that it pass from the venous system through the central circulation and into an arterial phase without significant trapping of the tracer in the pulmonary vasculature or pulmonary parenchyma; and (*2*) that it can be injected in high enough specific activity to provide a high count rate in a small volume of fluid for a compact bolus. This excludes very few tracers that are routinely used in clinical nuclear medicine. Examples include thallium-201 (Tl-201), which has a low specific activity, a small administered dose (3 to 4 mCi), and is avidly extracted by the lungs on first-pass, especially in smokers and patients with an increased pulmonary capillary wedge pressure.

Technetium-99m (Tc-99m) labeled macroaggregated albumin, commonly used for pulmonary perfusion studies, is trapped by the pulmonary capillary system and can only be used for the assessment of RV EF.

Tc-99m-teboroxime, a myocardial perfusion agent with avid pulmonary and rapid myocardial uptake and washout, was originally thought to be suitable for combined perfusion and FPRNA imaging [15]. However, Tc-99m-teboroxime was found to have prominent first-pass extraction in the lungs, which resulted in impor-

tant differences in the results of FPRNA [16]. These include prolongation of the mean pulmonary transit time (and therefore an increase in the calculated pulmonary blood volume index, the product of mean pulmonary transit time and cardiac index), and an increased level background activity during the levophase of tracer transit. The latter finding results in lower raw and background subtracted LV EF values, an increase in the percentage of the lung background matrix needed for subtraction of pulmonary activity from the background corrected representative cycle, and interference with interpretation of FPRNA images (see Color Fig. 17.2 in separate color insert).

Tracers that are obtained from generators, for example, such as rubidium-82 from its strontium-82 parent [17], are only suitable for first-pass imaging when the generator is fresh enough to allow rapid bolus injection of a small volume of high activity.

Technetium-99m Labeled Agents

The standard tracers for FPRNA are Tc-99m-sodium pertechnetate (NaTcO$_4$) and Tc-99m-diethylenetriaminepentaacetic acid (DTPA). NaTcO$_4$ can be bolus injected directly as eluted from the molybdenum generator, requiring no kit preparation. If gated planar or tomographic blood pool images are desirable (e.g., for myocardial topography postinfarction or regional wall motion assessment in multiple views), NaTcO$_4$ can be bolus injected after administration of stannous pyrophosphate (Sn-PYP). This results in red blood cell labeling due to the chemical reduction of hemoglobin by the tin. The reduced hemoglobin then avidly binds the Tc-99m-pertechnetate ions. The optimum method of "in vivtro" (i.e., combination of in vivo and in vitro) labeling is to withdraw 20 to 30 ml of the patient's blood into a syringe containing 1.5 mg of stannous pyrophosphate, mixing for several seconds (not long enough to allow clotting), and reinfusing the blood. Resting FPRNA is performed after a 10-minute delay, to allow further red blood cell uptake of stannous ion. Tc-99m-pertechnetate (25 to 30 mCi) in a volume of less than 1 ml is given by rapid flushing with at least 30 ml of normal saline through the indwelling catheter. Stannous pyrophosphate may result in poor red cell tagging in patients undergoing heparin infusion or chemotherapy. An alternative to red cell labeling is Tc-99m labeled human serum albumin (HSA).

Tc-99m-DTPA, a renal function imaging agent, is often used if no gated images are required, because it has a lower radiation dosimetry profile due to rapid excretion of the tracer from normal kidneys, up to 90% in the first 2 hours. Tc-99m-diphosphonates are useful for FPRNA in patients who require simultaneous evaluation of bone scintigraphy and prechemotherapy EF.

In recent years, many of the FPRNA studies have been performed in the setting of rest or stress myocardial perfusion imaging, which can add both diagnostic and prognostic information (see Clinical Applications). Of the three currently FDA-approved perfusion agents, Tc-99m-sestamibi (an isonitrile) and Tc-99m-tetrofosmin (a diphosphine) have been utilized successfully, while the use of Tc-99m-teboroxime has been limited, as described before.

On-Site Generator-Produced Agents

Tungsten-178–tantalum-178

FPRNA with any Tc-99m labeled agent is limited to one or two injections, for example, resting and peak exercise, due to considerations of radiation exposure to the patient (see Table 17.2). Serial studies, for example, during incremental doses of inotropic or vasodilator therapy, or in multiple stages of a graded exercise test, have not been feasible using these agents. By contrast, because of its 9.3-minute physical half-life, tantalum-178 (Ta-178) has been used as a research tool for FPRNA with a multiwire gamma camera (see above). This tracer can be injected at 20 times the quantity of Tc-99m but with a low radiation burden to the patient. Ta-178 is readily available by elution from a shielded tungsten-178 generator (W-178, half-life 21.7

days), with minimal breakthrough of the parent (less than 1%) [13,18]. The relatively low energy of the gamma rays of Ta-178 (55 to 64 keV) is optimally imaged with the multiwire camera. Recent developments in this technology include a completely self-contained, shielded, and computerized elution system within the housing of the multiwire camera [11]. This system has been used extensively in the invasive cardiac laboratory, detailing regional and global RV and LV dysfunction during coronary arterial occlusion during balloon angioplasty [14].

Rubidium-81–krypton-81m

The noble gas, krypton-81m (Kr-81m) is produced from a rubidium-81 (Rb-81)–Kr-81m generator. Kr-81m decays by isomeric transition, with a gamma emission of 191 keV and has a physical half-life of only 13 seconds. Because it is not a nuclear byproduct material and it decays so rapidly to relatively stable Kr-81, it is not considered to be an environmental hazard and avoids the need for storage/collecting devices. After intravenous injection, this tracer can be used to image the RV only, since it is excreted by the lungs prior to reaching the left heart [20]. Because the parent isotope Rb-81 has a physical half-life of about 4.5 hours, the use of this generator is usually one working day (about 12 hours), which makes it impractical for most clinical laboratories.

Osmium-191–iridium-191m

Iridium-191m is another generator-produced, short-lived tracer, which has been used for FPRNA, both in evaluation of ventricular function and quantitation of left to right shunts [21–24]. The original description of the osmium-191 generator [21] had a 2-week shelf life, which has recently been improved, with greater yields of the daughter iridium-191m [22]. Iridium-191m has a very short half-life (4.96 sec), allowing low radiation exposures up to 100 mCi of injection. The dual photopeaks of Ir-191m (65 and 129 keV), make it a suitable tracer for either the multiwire gamma camera (MWGC) or conventional imaging techniques. Although the half-life is short enough to question the use of this tracer for determination of LV EF, it has been shown that results comparable to Tc-99m agents are obtained for both RV and LV EFs [23,24].

Mercury-195m–gold-195m

A fourth generator-produced, short-lived tracer (half-life = 30.6 seconds) is gold-195m (Au-195m). This tracer is eluted from its Hg-195m parent, which has a 41-hour half-life [25]. Au-195 has a 262 keV gamma emission. This is higher than the optimal range of imaging with standard gamma camera electronics, but not problematic for the 1-inch thick crystals of the multicrystal cameras [26]. This tracer has been used for measurement of LV EF in canine model and in humans, correlating excellently with Tc-99m labeled agents [26–29].

Positron-Emitting Agents

Although positron-emitting agents such as fluorine-18 (F-18) deoxyglucose and Rb-82 have been imaged with positron emission tomography (PET) and in planar mode with specially shielded single-crystal and multicrystal cameras [30–32], there have been no clinical studies of comparative ventricular performance published of FPRNA with these tracers or devices in single-photon (planar) mode.

However, in a study by Chen et al. [33], determination of cardiac output during Rb-82 with PET has been compared with the Tc-99m labeled red blood cell method on the same patients, giving similar results. Rb-82 is another generator-produced agent with a short (76 second) half-life, obtained by the decay of strontium-82 (Sr-82, half-life 25 days). This suggests that FPRNA may be performed three-dimensionally, in a combined perfusion/function study using PET imaging with high sensitivity and temporal resolution.

PERFORMANCE ASPECTS OF FIRST-PASS RADIONUCLIDE ANGIOGRAPHY

Image Acquisition

The keys to high-quality FPRNA image acquisition are careful patient positioning, setting acquisition parameters that allow an adequate sampling rate, and tracer delivery in a compact bolus [34].

Patient positioning

Optimal patient positioning in front of the camera can be ensured by obtaining a transmission image using: (1) sheet source (e.g., cobalt-57) behind the patient; or (2) aiming the open end of the lead pig containing the patient's FPRNA dose at the patient from 6 to 10 feet behind. The latter results in a slightly collimated point source. The contrast between the lung density and the myocardium should allow confirmation that the cardiac chambers are within the field of view of the camera. An alternative method is to inject a small "tracer dose" of 1 mCi of the patient's dose prior to a resting study. If images are acquired in a rest–stress or stress–rest sequence, the prior dose's localization (e.g., Tc-99m-tetrofosmin in the myocardium) can be used to confirm the patient's position.

Laboratories differ on whether the anterior or the right anterior oblique (RAO) projection should be acquired. The anterior position is very reproducible, while the RAO projection is best performed with a foam wedge in order to reproduce the patient's position between acquisitions. The RAO completely obscures the circumflex territory but allows maximal separation of the atria from the ventricles. During exercise, the anterior position provides optimal stabilization of the chest in front of the camera by laboratory personnel (a "holder" or technologist) applying pressure from behind the patient into the camera.

Acquisition parameters

Images are generally acquired in a 32 × 32 pixel matrix or less, sacrificing spatial resolution for a high count rate. The frame rate should be set after measuring the heart rate by ECG gating or measuring the pulse rate, at 24 (± 8) frames per cardiac cycle. Higher frame rates improve the accuracy of diastolic filling parameters but sacrifice image quality if counting statistics are weak. The acquisition duration should be set for at least 30 seconds, in order to allow for complete transition through the central circulation. Longer acquisition times may be needed in patients with severe congestive heart failure or valvular regurgitation.

Tracer injection with bolus technique

Adequate bolus delivery of the tracer requires some expertise and is the single issue that precludes the routine use of FPRNA in many laboratories. Intravenous access should be obtained using a large-bore indwelling polyethylene catheter. If central venous access is not present, many laboratories prefer placement of either an 18- or 20-gauge catheter in an external jugular vein, or a 14- or 16-gauge in a medial antecubital vein. The median and lateral arm veins drain through the deltopectoral groove and may result in a poor bolus in the presence of an ipsilateral pacemaker pocket or with exercise. The patient's aversion to either the external jugular approach or the large-bore arm vein approach can be assuaged with a small-needle (27-gauge tuberculin or insulin) intradermal injection of lidocaine over the anticipated venipuncture site.

The catheter should be connected to a saline-loaded 20 to 30 ml syringe using tubing that has a 3 to 5 ml capacity and a three-way stopcock. The tracer is then loaded into the tubing and subsequently forced through this system using maximal hand pressure on the syringe after starting the acquisition.

Exercise studies

When the patient is undergoing physical exercise, careful attention should be paid to minimizing and correcting for motion artifacts. Motion correction can be performed prior to image processing either intrinsically, using the peak LV phase counts (usually aortic root) to align the frames, or extrinsically, using a point source (e.g., Americium-241 at 59 keV, or Tc-99m) attached to the skin as a reference for frame realignment. This point source is more important for treadmill FPRNA acquisitions, since there is a greater degree of vertical motion than with upright bicycle exercise, the usual and standard method of exercise with FPRNA. The appearance of the point source in each frame of the study should be confirmed prior to motion correction.

Treadmill exercise gives similar ventricular function information as upright leg cycle exercise FPRNA [35]. However, the incidence of angina pectoris and ischemic ST-segment depression is far greater with treadmill than with leg cycling [36].

Image Processing

The bolus

Placing a region of interest over the superior vena cava (see Color Fig. 17.3 in separate color insert) on the acquired frames, and obtaining a time-activity curve will examine the adequacy of the bolus. This time-activity curve should have a single peak, with a full-width at half-maximum of less than 1 second, and preferably less than 0.5 seconds (Fig. 17.4). A slightly less vigorous bolus velocity may be used if the study is being performed primarily for the assessment of RV function, as a rapid and tight bolus may clear the RV in 1 to 2 cycles in a normal subject, especially if injected through the external jugular approach.

A split bolus is problematic and may preclude accurate data processing. Identification of a delayed or split bolus alerts the physician to the possibility of oversubtraction of RV background and the resultant spurious increase in LV EF, decrease in LV volume, and overestimation of regional wall motion in regions overlapping the RV.

Lung curve analysis

A region of interest should be placed over the left lung for analysis of pulmonary flow characteristics and mean transit time. Since the transit time depends upon bolus quality, the absence of shunts, cardiac output, and both valvular and ventricular function, this serves as a quality control (see Color Fig. 17.5 in separate color insert).

Frame method for RV and LV ejection fraction

FPRNA data are analyzed using the frame method for RV or LV EF (see Fig. 17.8 and Color Figs. 17.6 and 17.7 in separate color insert), which creates a representative ventricular volume cycle by summing frames of several (usually 2 or 4 for RV and 5 to 15 for LV) cardiac cycles, aligned by matching their ED frames (histogram peaks) and ES frames (histogram valleys) during the operator defined levophase of tracer transit. If the acquisition is obtained using ECG gating, the R-wave triggers are used to align the frames into a representative cycle.

The background corrected representative cycle is then interrogated with a fixed region of interest (ROI) in order to obtain the final first-pass time-activity curve. This region of interest is usually drawn over the RV or LV as defined by a first harmonic Fourier transformation phase image, which clearly distinguishes the ventricle from atrial or great vessel counts. ED is taken as the first frame of the representative cycle, and ES is defined as the frame with the minimum counts in the histogram. Historically, the EF was taken as the ED counts minus the ES counts, divided by the background subtracted ED counts.

Background correction for final LV ejection fraction and volume determination

For the LV EF, the pulmonary frame background method is utilized to correct the raw representative cycle, after determination of the background fraction [7,8,16] (see Color Fig. 17.9 in separate color insert). The pulmonary background subtraction factor is derived after selection of one pulmonary background frame for each cardiac cycle in the raw representative cycle to comprise a summed background frame. The initial background frame, or "inflection point," is operator defined at the ES frame prior to tracer entry into the LV. The summed ED image is then subtracted from the summed pulmonary frame in order to obtain a lung mask image, which is then applied to both the background and the ED frames. The background frame to ED frame count ratio in the masked (lung background) area is calculated, in order to determine the fraction of the pulmonary background frame which will be subtracted from the raw representative cycle to create the final background subtracted representative cycle. This factor is the background subtraction factor.

The background corrected representative cycle is then used to determine the final LV EF, as well as the end-diastolic volume (EDV) using the Sandler and

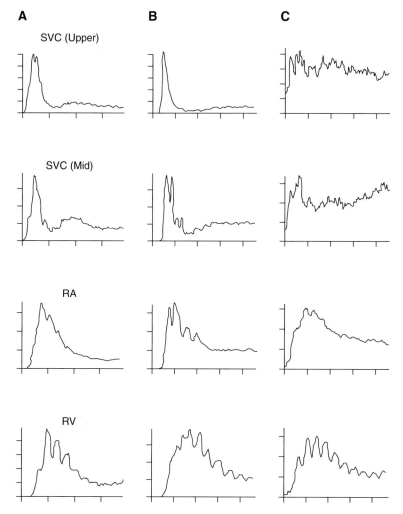

FIGURE 17.4 FPRNA dextrophase time-activity curves are shown for three patients, obtained with regions of interest over the SVC (upper inflow from subclavian vein, *top row*), the mid-SVC (*second row*), the RA (*third row*), and RV (*lower row*). *Patient A* has a good bolus, characterized by a full-width at half maximum (FWHM) of 1 second. There is only a trivial degree of tricuspid regurgitation (TR), noted by the small increases in RA tracer activity during RV systole. *Patient B* has an excellent bolus (FWHM 0.7 seconds), but in the mid-SVC and RA tracings, marked increases in tracer activity are noted during RV systole, consistent with significant TR, with an RA injection fraction of 25%. *Patient C* has a fragmented bolus, but with rapid enough inflow to allow assessment of both LV and RV function. The SVC curves are contaminated by pulmonary tracer flow in the later frames. The RA outflow is delayed, with no TR; the incrased RA tracer activity during RV systole after the initial RA peak is due to bolus fragmentation.

Dodge area-length equation [37] for the volume of and ellipsoid of revolution:

$$EDV = 8A^2/3\pi L$$

where A = LV area and L = the long-axis length in the anterior projection, which are measured directly. This formula is often shortened to:

$$EDV = 0.85A^2/L$$

Alternatively, ventricular volumes can be calculated with the count-proportional method of Massardo et al. [38]. For this method, the required data are the total counts in the LV, the counts in the hottest pixel in the LV, and the area of a pixel (m) in centimeters. The EDV is calculated as:

$$EDV = 1.38 \ m^{3/2} \times R^{3/2}$$

where R = total LV counts/counts in the hottest pixel.

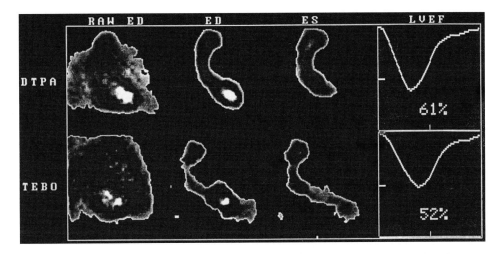

FIGURE 17.8 The usual result from the frame method of background correction is shown in the same patient depicted in Figure 17.2, using Tc-99m-DTPA. With Tc-99m-teboroxime (TEBO), however, the increased pulmonary activity impairs the background correction, such that pulmonary activity is present lateral to the apex (giving the appearance of an LV aneurysm), and the LV EF is artificially lowered, as shown on the histogram of the background corrected representative cycles.

Dual regions of interest for LV ejection fraction

It has been shown by other imaging techniques, including echocardiography and magnetic resonance imaging [39–42] that the base of the heart, including the aortic valve plane, moves toward the apex during systole (see Color Fig. 17.10 in separate color insert). The extent of this motion is an index of systolic function, as it is more pronounced in vigorously contracting ventricles. In patients with a normal LVEF, the descent of the base of heart exceeds 10 mm [40]. Thus, the standard method of FPRNA analysis with a fixed ROI drawn ED region of interest is likely to have substantial contamination from the ES counts within the aortic root and sinuses of Valsalva. Using a single ROI drawn at ES would exclude the counts in the basal portion of the ventricle. Both of these types of errors would result in a lowering of the EF.

A dual ROI correction for valve plane motion was published by Williams et al. [43]. This correction resulted in a mean increase of 0.06 in LV EF measurements (i.e., 6 EF units, a 13% increase), to a range of values that was equivalent to that obtained with GERNA, a technique that similarly utilizes a variable ROI analysis. This increase in the measured EF should be applicable to any scintigraphic device that employs a single ROI throughout the cardiac cycle.

Unfortunately, a large body of literature has been developed using the older single ROI technique. Despite good correlation coefficients between FPRNA and other EF techniques [44–48], it has been reported that the single ROI technique for FPRNA underestimates invasively and noninvasively derived EFs by as much as 12% to 25% [44–47]. The dual ROI technique has improved the "substitutability" (i.e., agreement between actual values) of FPRNA EFs for those obtained with other techniques [43]. This technique has high levels of inter- and intraobserver reproducibility (r = 0.98 and 0.99, respectively), and narrow limits of agreement.

RV ejection fraction

Quantitation of RV EF has been validated with and without background correction, since the RA results in the only significant background for the RV phase of first-pass tracer flow. The degree of overlap of the RA and RV depends upon positioning of the patient, with minimal overlap in the RAO position [49]. In the anterior position, the "inflection point" or initial background frame should be taken as the frame prior to tracer flow across the tricuspid valve into the RV (see Color Fig. 17.11 in separate color insert). Similar to the LV technique described above, the fraction of the background frame subtracted depends upon the fraction required to result in a single pixel of zero counts in the RA.

The effects of background RA counts on the RV time-activity curve can be lessened by the use of two ROIs, one drawn for the ED image and one for the ES image, similarly to the LV EF technique described above. Johnson et al. [50] have validated three methods of RV EF determination with FPRNA, and GERNA, versus the reference standard cine-MRI of the RV. In that study, the methods used to calculate RV

EF from FPRNA were a single ROI method, a dual ROI method, and a method in which a single ROI is applied to RA subtracted first-pass dynamic data. They found that the most accurate methods were the dual ROI method and the first-pass RA subtracted single ROI. The FPRNA single ROI method underestimated RV EFs, and the RV EF values measured from GERNA were less accurate.

Pitfalls of Acquisition and Processing

Count-poor studies, whether from tracer hang-up in the venous system, syringe, or tubing, will lessen the accuracy of the EF and wall motion analyses. A fragmented bolus will result in biventricular activity, which makes optimal inflection point selection difficult, and in some cases, impossible.

Atrial and or ventricular arrhythmias cannot be easily filtered out with FPRNA. However, software that performs "frame cycle addition" can easily average the systolic and diastolic time intervals, and adjust each beat in the cycle by interpolation, provided that there is only a twofold increase or decrease in the cycle lengths. Short or long cycles that vary from the mean by a greater degree (< 50% or > 200% of the R-R interval) should be rejected from the analysis.

Significant tricuspid regurgitation (TR) can degrade the tracer bolus, since a fraction of the tracer will re-enter the RA during each RV systole (see Fig. 17.4). This feature can be used to detect and evaluate the severity of TR using FPRNA analysis of RA time-activity curves and calculation of the RA injection fraction from the RV [51]. With moderate or severe TR, the RA tracer counts oscillate enough to markedly increase the pulmonary transit time and result in significant biventricular activity, rendering inflection point selection difficult to impossible. With tracer lingering in the RV and pulmonary artery (PA), the background correction will often produce an oversubtraction artifact, removing counts from the LV phase in the inferior and septal regions and from the aorta.

Image Interpretation

Optimal image interpretation is performed using a display that incorporates both quality control and clinical aspects of the examination. Interpretation should be performed in a consistent, methodical manner with careful attention to the quality of the data, due to the large number of variables that can affect the final result. This is unlike GERNA, in which a quick inspection of the cinematic display of the cardiac cycle is sufficient to reassure the interpreter that the data are adequately acquired and processed. The final FPRNA representative cardiac cycle that is used to generate both the EF and wall motion assessment is dependent upon many factors, including the adequacy of the bolus injection, the acquired count rate, the number and type of beats chosen for inclusion in the analysis, the background activity, and patient motion. Most commercial software packages routinely store enough of this processing data for display during final interpretation.

Serial image inspection

A serial image compacts the 20 to 30-second FPRNA acquisition into summed images of 1-second duration (see Fig. 17.2). This display allows visual inspection of the bolus and the tracer flow. Cinematic display of this serial image of tracer transit through the heart and great vessels is useful in the analysis of any alterations of tracer transit occurring in patients with congenital anomalies, or acquired abnormalities, such as obstruction of or collateralization of flow around the superior vena cava (SVC), or asymmetric pulmonary regional blood flow. The count rate per second (cps) should also be noted, with optimum being over 250,000 cps for a multicrystal camera, and over 150,000 in a single-crystal camera. The presence of chamber enlargement, cardiac malposition, and aortic enlargement can also be ascertained by inspection of these images.

Time–activity curves, pulmonary transit time, and representative cycles

Ventricular and pulmonary ROIs should be placed in order to evaluate cardiac rhythm and pulmonary mean transit time (PMTT). The PMTT is a reflection of the central circulation time, which can be affected by any abnormality within the circuit. This includes cardiac output, ventricular function, valvular function, and pulmonary vascular resistance (Figs. 17.4–17.8) [52–54]. The pulmonary blood volume index (the product of mean pulmonary transit time and cardiac index) is routinely measured during FPRNA. A change in pulmonary blood volume index with exercise has been correlated with exercise-induced symptoms of dyspnea [55], and an increase in pulmonary capillary wedge pressure [56].

The raw and background corrected representative cycles should be inspected and compared to ensure the adequacy and accuracy of background subtraction. The background counts in the pulmonary and RV regions should be minimized in the LV corrected representative cycle. The adequacy of counts in the representative cycle attests to the quality of the study. In general, the ED counts in the representative cycle should exceed 4000 counts.

During interpretation, the histogram used to confirm appropriate beat selection may be used to confirm that an appropriate frame was chosen for background subtraction. This inflection point may be altered in order to optimize background subtraction. A frame as close to the beginning of the LV phase but not including any LV activity is usually adequate, but moving several frames earlier in the acquisition may correct for RV undersubtraction. Viewing the summed background frame may be useful in ensuring that LV activity is not included, and detecting excessive activity in the RV that could result in oversubtraction of background. In some instances, the lung frame method of background correction described earlier may not be accurate due to simultaneous RV and LV tracer activity. In such cases wall motion may be assessed on the raw representative cycle. This uncorrected representative cycle may be viewed after manually windowing out of some background counts, which may allow adequate assessment of regional wall motion.

As described above, the dual ROI approach for analysis is preferred for both RV and LV representative cycles. These regions and the resulting time-activity curves, corresponding to changes in ventricular volume, should be inspected for continuity, which can be compromised by arrhythmias.

The final ventricular volume curve contains information on heart rate, systolic ejection period, peak ejection rate, EF, the isovolume relaxation period, peak filling rate, time to peak filling, filling in the first third of diastole, and the fractional atrial contribution to ventricular filling (Fig. 17.12).

Display of the final representative cycle should be in a time-smoothed cinematic, endless loop format. Most software packages use a color display for this cine as well as for the functional images. Spatial smoothing is optional, depending upon the system and the robustness of the counts in the final representative cycle.

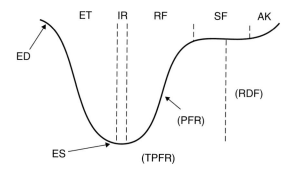

FIGURE 17.12 Ventricular volume curve from a background corrected representative cycle, showing the end-diastolic counts (ED), end-systolic counts (ES), ejection time (ET), isovolumic relaxation period (IR), rapid filling wave (RF), slow filling wave (SF), atrial kick, time-to-peak filling rate (TPFR), peak filling rate in end-diastolic volumes per second (PFR), and rapid diastolic filling fraction (RDF).

Interpretation of the data will be influenced by the intrinsic cardiac rhythm during the acquisition. Premature ventricular contractions (PVCs), ventricular bigeminy, and atrial fibrillation may affect the EF or regional wall motion. Ventricular bigeminy, for example, may necessitate the reporting of the PVC EF (often lower than a normal beat EF), and the post-PVC EF (10 to 15 EF units higher than a normal sinus beat). With atrial fibrillation, the representative cycle may consist of beats with widely varying R-R intervals, each with different EDVs and EFs. RV pacing causes septal asynchrony, similar to left bundle branch block, but the mechanical activation sequence begins at the apex and moves toward the base, which is easily recognized using the Fourier phase images, which describe the timing of wall motion.

Systolic function

It should be recalled that EF is an afterload sensitive ejection phase index of LV function, and may not reflect the true inotropic state of the myocardium. EF will underestimate the inotropic state in conditions with markedly elevated afterload, such as systemic hypertension or aortic stenosis (LV EF), or pulmonary hypertension or stenosis (RV EF). The RV EF may decrease acutely with stress if there is LV failure, mitral regurgitation, or mitral stenosis.

It should be borne in mind that the EF is not a fixed number, and will vary with cardiac rhythm, heart rate, circulating catecholamines, preload (e.g., upright vs supine position), and medications. The normal LV EF ranges from 55% to 75% (with the dual ROI technique), while normal LV EF range with the older single ROI technique would be 50% to 70%. The normal RV EF is typically 7 to 15 EF units lower, consistent with the greater RV EDV, but equivalent stroke volume (SV, which equals EDV × EF).

A more precise reflection of systolic function could be obtained using pressure-volume analysis [57–59], or analysis of ES wall stress [60]. But these techniques have not been routinely applied in clinical studies, in favor of the more clinically validated, rigorously measured, and quality controlled, though less physiologically pure, EF.

Diastolic function

Diastole is defined as the period of the cardiac cycle during which the LV fills [61–67]; it comprises four phases:

1. Early isovolumic relaxation (IR)
2. Rapid filling (passive atrial emptying, RF)
3. Slow filling (diastasis, SF)
4. Atrial systolic filling (atrial kick, AF).

Diastolic filling has both active (i.e., energy-dependent) and passive components. Several factors determine the filling properties of the LV during diastole. Intrinsic factors that can influence diastolic (also called "lusitropic") function of the LV include:

1. Inotropic state (e.g., adrenergic state)
2. Nonuniformity of relaxation (e.g., regional ischemia)
3. LV dimensions
4. LV wall thickness
5. Intrinsic mechanical properties (chamber stiffness)

Extrinsic, or nonmyocardial factors that can influence diastolic function include:

1. Loading conditions (affect ventricular "suction" or restoring forces)
2. Gradient across mitral valve (from atrium to ventricle)
3. RV dimensions
4. Pericardial properties (constriction or tamponade)
5. Extrinsic compression (e.g., pleural effusion or tumors)
6. Coronary vascular turgor (erectile effect)

In addition to these factors, diastolic filling properties can be altered pharmacologically by calcium channel blockers [64], and by increased adrenergic tone.

It has long been recognized that many patients with the syndrome of congestive heart failure, as evidenced by symptoms of dyspnea and often X-ray evidence for pulmonary edema, have adequate LV systolic function but poor indexes of diastolic filling. Several diagnoses occur frequently in such patients:

1. Hypertensive heart disease with LV hypertrophy
2. Ischemic heart disease with regional dysfunction due to scarring or acute ischemia [62,63,66]
3. Hypertrophic cardiomyopathy [64]
4. Diabetes mellitus with small vessel ischemia
5. Infiltrative diseases of the LV myocardium (amyloidosis, iron overload) [61]
6. Early or "healed" myopathic disorders (e.g., daunorubicin toxicity, viral cardiomyopathy, alcoholic cardiomyopathy)

As noted before, the representative cycle is derived from multiple LV or RV beats, comprising of net tracer inflow and outflow from the ventricle. The inflow beats typically overestimate filling of the ventricle (counts on the way up), and underestimate emptying (counts on the way down). The outflow beats overestimate emptying and underestimate filling. Thus, in order to evaluate diastolic filling parameters, the best possible balance between inflow and outflow is needed when the software or operator selects beats for inclusion into the representative cycle. Similarly, the accuracy of the evaluation of diastolic indexes is dependent upon matching beats with a stable cardiac rhythm during FPRNA.

To measure the phases of diastole, a technique must provide a relative left ventricular volume curve with high temporal resolution. Changes in volume are assessed by analyzing alteration from the normal filling pattern, in terms of timing of filling phases and relative contribution of early and late (atrial systolic) filling. Atrial systole should contribute no more than 25% of the ventricular filling.

The parameters most frequently utilized for assessment of diastolic relaxation are (with normal values as established with GERNA by Bonow et al. [67]):

1. Time to peak filling rate (TPFR, normally less than 180 msec)
2. Peak diastolic filling rate (PDFR, normally greater than 2.5 EDV/second)
3. Fraction of filling during the rapid filling phase (RDF, normally at least 69% of SV)

Diastolic filling is difficult to assess during exercise or during resting heart rates over 100 beats per minute, due to the simultaneous occurrence of rapid filling and atrial systole.

Wall motion analysis

Analysis of regional wall motion can be performed either with visual inspection of a cine loop of the representative cycle or analysis of functional images (see Color Fig. 17.13 in separate color insert). Functional images have the advantage of using computer-enhanced mathematics, which allow rapid visual assessment of wall motion in a static image. The commonly utilized functional images include Fourier phase and amplitude, regional EF index (REFI), REFI first half of systole (REFI1), REFI second half of systole (REFI2), paradox (ES-ED), and SV (ED-ES) images. Fourier transformation of the frames in the representative cycle gives the timing (phase) and absolute value (amplitude) of pixel count changes during the cardiac cycle. Fourier phase and amplitude analysis has additive value in detecting conditions that can alter the timing of mechanical activity, such as myocardial ischemia [68]. Although these wall motion images are highly specific for ischemic heart disease, they can be affected by electrical or conduction system abnormalities, such as left bundle branch block or RV pacing resulting in septal hypokinesis. Right bundle branch block has no effect on the LV contraction pattern. FPRNA is limited in regional wall motion analysis by the use of a single projection, such as the RAO, which cannot evaluate the circumflex coronary artery territory.

A cinematic display and functional images of the representative cycle should be used to grade myocardial segments for the presence of mild, moderate, or severe hypokinesis, akinesis, dyskinesis, or tardokinesis (late contraction), for each region. Aneurysm formation can be identified by the presence of a dyskinetic segment, which has phase aligned with the great vessels (i.e., filling during systole, emptying during diastole).

Chamber volumes

LV volumetric analysis, as noted previously, can be performed with either geometric equations using an area-length equation [37], or with count-proportional non-geometric methods, which employ measurement of the total counts within the LV ROI, the area of the ROI and the maximum pixel count [38].

Prior to reporting, it should be ascertained that the value for the EDV is physiologically reasonable simply by calculating the cardiac index (CI), that is, EDV × EF = SV, SV × heart rate = cardiac output (CO), and CO/body surface area = CI. Normal subjects (e.g., prechemotherapy patients with no prior heart disease) should consistently have normal values (> 3.0 liters/minute/m^2). An EDV index of more than 110 ml/m^2 would be considered evidence for LV dilatation. However, normal values should be established within each laboratory, since they will vary with the type of processing used, and the patient's position during the acquisition, that is, supine, semisupine, or upright. The ESV (EDV × EF) is a particularly useful measurement, since it incorporates ventricular function as well as ventricular size.

Detection of enlargement of the right heart chambers and PA relies upon visual inspection of serial images, since there are no well-validated or reliable RV or RA volume algorithms for FPRNA. RV EDV can be estimated in patients with no significant valvular regurgitation as the LV EDV × (LV EF/RV EF), since the SVs should be similar between the two chambers.

Enlargement of the left atrium (LA) can be discerned by inspection of the LV representative cycle, looking for an increase in tracer activity in the region of the LA appendage.

Exercise studies

For detailed wall motion comparison, the representative cycles of both rest and exercise studies should be viewed in a simultaneous cinematic display (see Color Fig. 17.14 in separate color insert). During exercise or dobutamine infusion, for example, global function and regional wall motion should increase. Regional wall motion abnormalities at rest that improve with stress indicate viable myocardium without inducible ischemia (e.g., after a non-Q-wave infarction, with an open in-farct related artery). A fall in global function may reflect either global ischemia or a marked alteration in loading conditions, such as sudden isometric or sudden strenuous aerobic exercise, or a marked hypertensive response to stress. However, wall motion abnormalities that appear or worsen with exercise, with no discernible other cause (e.g., exercise-induced left bundle branch block, or uncorrected patient motion artifact) indicate myocardial ischemia.

The pulmonary mean transit time may become prolonged during exercise, because of the appearance of inducible LV ischemia, RV ischemia, or papillary muscle dysfunction resulting in ischemic tricuspid or mitral valvular insufficiency. However, this finding may also reflect prolongation of the bolus due to a Valsalva maneuver performed with the strain of peak exercise.

LV EDV tends to increase with upright bicycle exercise. The magnitude of the increase is typically in the 10%–20% range although larger increases do occur in normal subjects with high exercise levels. Larger volume increases may indicate coronary disease, especially when associated with a significant drop in EF. When geometric approaches to EDV calculation are utilized, motion artifacts can result in higher values, due to a "smearing" effect on the image. This factor may account for the lack of prognostic values obtained with indexes of volume obtained using this approach [3].

The majority of the data accumulated over the past two decades on GERNA and FPRNA have revolved around the LV EF at rest and exercise. The EF response to upright exercise of gradually increasing intensity should be an increase of 5 EF units. The LV EF with stress depends upon a large number of physiologic factors, and is highly variable in patients with and without coronary artery disease (CAD) [69–71]. A low resting EF limits the fall in ejection fraction [70]. The EF may decrease if the patient is presented with a sudden workload [72,73]. In any case, an absolute value of an exercise LV EF of 56% or greater is inconsistent with the development of significant myocardial ischemia [74,75]. However, a flat or abnormal EF response may occur in patients with hyperdynamic resting function, systemic hypertension, prior myocarditis or cardiomyopathy, and mitral valve prolapse; and in elderly patients, obese patients, women, and diabetics, especially those with autonomic insufficiency [60,76–78].

CLINICAL APPLICATIONS OF FIRST-PASS RADIONUCLIDE ANGIOGRAPHY

Diagnosis of Ischemic Heart Disease

The reported sensitivity and specificity of rest–stress RNA for the diagnosis of ischemic heart disease vary widely, depending upon whether GERNA or FPRNA is employed, which population is studied, and the criteria used for detection of CAD [78–81]. As described before, the hallmarks of CAD with inducible myocardial ischemia that are demonstrable by FPRNA include development or worsening of regional or global ventricular dysfunction. The functional data derived are robust, reproducible, and reliably exclude significant CAD when normal [78–80]. Examples of normal and abnormal FPRNA are shown in Color Figures 17.15 and 17.16 (in separate color insert).

The LV EF response to exercise was originally suggested as a diagnostic parameter for ischemic heart disease in 1978 by Borer et al. [79] using ERNA. The first use of FPRNA EFs and volumes for diagnosis of CAD was reported in 1978 by Rerych et al. [80], who measured these parameters in 30 normal subjects and 30 patients with CAD. The normal response was characterized by an increase in EF, a decrease in pulmonary transit time, a modest increase in pulmonary blood volume, a decrease in ESV, and an increase in SV. In patients with ischemic heart disease, however, a fall in EF was noted, associated with large increases in EDV, ESV, and pulmonary blood volume, as the Starling mechanism was used to maintain SV. The magnitude of these exercise-induced ischemic functional abnormalities and wall motion abnormalities was directly related to the anatomic extent and severity of the ischemic disease, with the most severe exercise LV dysfunction observed in patients with three-vessel and left main disease.

There were many overoptimistic reports about the use of the LV EF and its dramatic decrease with exercise in patients with CAD, some containing small numbers of subjects, and some containing patients with very severe CAD who were compared with very healthy, young volunteers. This led to a perception that this parameter had very high diagnostic accuracy. However, the physiologic complexity of this variable became apparent as the population to whom these tests were applied expanded [81].

A higher degree of specificity is expected from regional wall motion abnormality at rest or induced by exercise than from the EF response, although global ischemia may be represented by a fall in EF without appreciable regional differences in wall motion. For this reason, FPRNA has largely become an adjunctive technique in the era of high-quality SPECT perfusion imaging with Tc-99m labeled agents.

Prognosis in Ischemic Heart Disease

The noninvasive assessment of resting LV performance has become an integral part of the evaluation of patients with known or suspected cardiac disease, having important diagnostic, therapeutic, and prognostic significance [2,3,82–89]. In particular, the exercise LV EF has greater prognostic value in patients with ischemic heart disease than many other clinical, noninvasive and invasively derived variables [3,85–88]. An exercise EF of 0.50 (50%) has been identified as the inflection point, below which patients with CAD demonstrate a probability of cardiac death, which increases as the EF decreases [3,86].

Although the EF response to exercise varies in individual patients, studies that have examined groups of patients with CAD have found a consistent relationship between the extent and severity of coronary stenoses, the degree of exercise-induced ventricular dysfunction, and the likelihood of future cardiac events (cardiac death or myocardial infarction). Investigators at Duke University [3,86–88,90], using multivariate analysis of FPRNA, examined clinical and arteriographic variables to identify those related to future cardiac events in several hundred patients receiving medical therapy for CAD. The exercise LV EF was the most important variable, containing over 70% of the prognostic information provided by combination of all of the other variables in their model. Other significant determinants of prognosis include resting ESV and resting EF. The relationship between cardiac events and exercise EF was curvilinear, with patients having an exercise EF above 50% having very few events. Patients with progressively lower EFs, demonstrated a marked increase in cardiac events (Fig. 17.17) [3]. This prognostic relationship was confirmed in patients with medical treatment but no arteriography [86,87].

These data indicate that cardiac function during exercise, especially the exercise LV EF, provides a sensitive index of the myocardial ischemic burden, including the effects of myocardial scarring and inducible myocardial ischemia, the main determinant of survival in patients with CAD. The clinical implications of this include the assignment of low-risk CAD patients to medical therapy, while patients who are deemed to be at high risk of future myocardial infarction or death will benefit most from bypass surgery or other interventional therapy.

Evaluation of Ventricular Function Using FPRNA with Perfusion Agents

As described earlier (see Radiopharmaceuticals), Tc-99m labeled perfusion agents provide the possibility of determining both LV and RV function with a bolus injection of the tracer using FPRNA, followed by SPECT perfusion imaging. The widespread use of Tc-99m labeled perfusion agents has led to greater interest in ob-

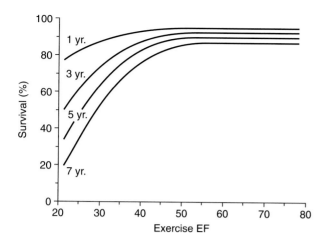

FIGURE 17.17 Curves of survival at 1, 3, 5, and 7 years as a function of exercise ejection fraction (EF). (Reprinted from Lee et al. [3] by permission of authors and the American Heart Association, Inc.)

taining simultaneous perfusion and function information with a single study [4,16,44,91–113], potentially adding both diagnostic and prognostic information. Information from these two modalities could be combined to potentially distinguish ischemic from nonischemic causes of LV dysfunction (Table 17.3).

However, in the absence of widespread use of FPRNA and the requisite high-count-rate gamma camera and impeccable bolus technique, gated SPECT perfusion imaging has become more commonly utilized. Yet the ability to perform imaging at the peak of exercise with perfusion imaging has not been accomplished with any technique other than FPRNA.

The combination of FPRNA with perfusion imaging has also been applied to pharmacologic stress testing with inotropic agents, such as dobutamine [100] and arbutamine [101]. Infusion of beta-adrenergic agonists results in an increment in EF in normals, and a fall in EF with induction of wall motion abnormalities in patients with an ischemic response, similar to the results obtained with exercise.

Because the degree of impairment of left ventricular function is directly related to reversible myocardial ischemia or myocardial necrosis, there is a strong relationship between FPRNA and SPECT perfusion imaging (see Color Fig. 17.14). In a study by Borges-Neto et al., this relationship was confirmed [110]. Both rest EF and stress EF correlated significantly (r = 0.77 and 0.78) with the extent of perfusion abnormalities on quantitative polar maps of rest and stress SPECT.

Comparison with ECG-gated scanning for determination of left ventricular function

One of the major roles for FPRNA in recent years has been in the validation and calibration of techniques for EFs and volumes derived from gated SPECT or planar perfusion imaging [44,93,102–107]. FPRNA has been utilized extensively as a reference standard because of the capacity for determining EF with myocardial perfusion and metabolic agents. Because of its versatility, FPRNA has been used as a convenient simultaneous validation technique for gated perfusion SPECT agents, such as with Tc-99m-sestamibi [44,93,102–105] and Tc-99m-tetrofosmin [106]. With FPRNA, background tracer activity can be either subtracted or overwhelmed by the high-count rate employed. Thus, Tc-99m has been injected soon after imaging with other pharmaceuticals for calibration of the EFs obtained, such as with Tl-201 [105] and the 123-iodinated fatty acid compound, I-123 labeled beta-methyl-p-iodophenyl-pentadecanoic acid (BMIPP) [107].

FPRNA in combination with perfusion imaging: redundant or incremental information?

Diagnosis of coronary artery disease. Although the combined assessment of perfusion and function is uniquely suited to FPRNA with perfusion agents, the question arises whether or not the incremental cost and equipment requirements are justified by any increment in diagnostic accuracy, either for detection of CAD or determination of myocardial viability.

Palmas et al. [108] have demonstrated improved di-

TABLE 17.3 *Simultaneous First-Pass Radionuclide Angiography with Myocardial Perfusion Scintigraphy: A Diagnostic Algorithm*

	Resting Function	Exercise Function	Resting Perfusion	Exercise Perfusion
Normal	−	−	−	−
Attenuation	−	−	+	+
Myopathy*	+	+	−	−
Infarction	+	+	+	+
Ischemia	−	+	−	+

*Myopathic patients will often have subtle perfusion abnormalities consistent with microvascular.

agnostic accuracy for detection of multivessel disease using the combination of FPRNA and perfusion indexes, rather than either test alone, by receiver operating characteristic analysis in 70 patients with CAD. They performed a stepwise addition of scintigraphic data (first perfusion, then function) to the exercise treadmill score, showing significant incremental value for prediction of the angiographic score at each step. Not surprisingly, the exercise LV EF, taken alone, was the strongest independent predictor of angiographic severity. However, the accuracy for detection of multivessel disease was improved by the addition of SPECT perfusion information to the treadmill score, and by the addition of regional wall motion data to both of them. When taken in this sequence, the EF failed to show any further independent value.

However, with infusion of an inotrope, perfusion may be significantly more sensitive than wall motion. Iftikhar et al. [100] compared FPRNA and SPECT perfusion with Tc-99m-sestamibi at rest and with beta-adrenergic stimulation with an infusion of 40 mcg/kg/min of dobutamine in 38 patients who also underwent cardiac catheterization. The sensitivity for CAD detection by myocardial perfusion SPECT was 78% compared with only 33% for FPRNA wall motion. They concluded that changes in myocardial perfusion are more sensitive than changes in left ventricular function for detecting CAD during dobutamine stress.

Detection of viable myocardium. Peix et al. [109] compared rest and nitroglycerin (NTG)-enhanced Tc-99m-tetrofosmin and FPRNA wall motion for detection of viable myocardium in 50 patients after myocardial infarction. In the 26 patients with ventricular dysfunction, they found a 73% agreement between the functional improvement and increased Tc-99m-tetrofosmin uptake post-NTG, indicative of similar data being obtained with each technique.

Prognosis in patients with coronary artery disease. It has been shown that perfusion SPECT and LV EF have incremental prognostic value when combined in the assessment of patients who have undergone thrombolytic therapy for acute myocardial infarction [113]. The addition of resting EF to SPECT indexes and clinical data provided a level correlation with patient outcomes that could not be ascertained by coronary arteriography.

Mast et al. [114] demonstrated that the resting FPRNA LV EF had incremental predictive power in the assessment of risk for future cardiac events (cardiac death or nonfatal acute myocardial infarction) in 240 patients with recent acute myocardial infarction who underwent pharmacologic stress myocardial perfusion

SPECT. Clinical information, perfusion SPECT, and FPRNA LV EF each were significant univariate predictors of patient outcomes ($\chi^2 = 7.4$, 14.0, and 21.8, respectively). The addition of myocardial perfusion findings to clinical information provided incremental prognostic information ($\chi^2 = 15.2$). The addition of FPRNA EF provided further predictive information ($\chi^2 = 22.5$). However, when the LV EF was first added to the clinical information, myocardial perfusion SPECT had no incremental prognostic value.

Although preliminary data (presented in abstract form) have suggested that exercise FPRNA and SPECT could provide even more incremental prognostic information, no published studies confirm this concept.

Evaluation of Ventricular Function Using FPRNA in Nonischemic Conditions

FPRNA to determine the acute effects of an intervention

Because of the ability of FPRNA to rapidly assess ventricular function, and the inherent mobility of the current generation of gamma cameras (i.e., SIM-400), this technique has been employed in the operating room and catheterization suite to monitor cardiac function and to determine the acute effects of medical or surgical interventions and invasive procedures.

Right and left ventricular function can be evaluated during procedures that can significantly alter hemodynamics, such as infusion of the alpha- and beta-blocker labetalol, the calcium channel blocker verapamil, cross clamping the aorta for vascular procedures, or balloon valvuloplasty [57,115–121].

FPRNA for monitoring the effects of chemotherapy

Among the chemotherapeutic agents with cardiotoxic effects, the anthracyclines, of which daunorubicin is the most commonly used, are the most potent. Various analogs of anthracycline (including doxorubicin, carminomycin, detorubicin, epirubicin, esorubicin, idarubicin, marcellomycin, quelamycin, and rodorubicin) have been synthesized. However, none of these agents have any advantage over doxorubicin [122]. Each of these agents can cause myocardial necrosis due to free radical formation, characterized by myocellular vacuolization, with progressive lowering of the LV EF as the cumulative dose of the agent increases. Risk factors for development of more rapid deterioration in LV function may include hypertension, radiation to the chest, CAD, and childhood, elderly, or previous myopathic injury (e.g., ethanol or viral-induced).

The majority of patients undergoing chemotherapy with these agents have been evaluated with GERNA or echocardiography [123–127]. According to Steinherz et al. [127], an echocardiographic evaluation should be performed before every course of doxorubicin up to a total dose of 300 mg per square meter, given with or without concurrent radiation therapy. RNA should also be performed if the patient is receiving more than 400 mg per square meter of the drug in one course. An echocardiogram should be repeated 3, 6, and 12 months after the completion of therapy and every 2 years thereafter, and the RNA should be done after 12 months and then every 5 years. However, many institutions elect to perform a resting RNA for more rigorous quantitation of each EF, rather than echocardiographic estimation of function.

In adults, a 10% decline in LVEF to below the lower limit of normal or an absolute LVEF of 45%, or a 20% decline in LVEF at any level is indicative of deterioration in cardiac function. In children, deterioration in cardiac function during or after the completion of therapy with doxorubicin is indicated by a drop in fractional shortening (FS) by an absolute value of ≥ 10 percentile units or below 29%, and a decline in LVEF of 10 percentile units or an LVEF below 55%. In general, if test results indicate deterioration in cardiac function associated with doxorubicin, the benefit of continued therapy must be carefully evaluated against the risk of producing irreversible cardiac damage.

However, several institutions use FPRNA for EF due to its inherent reproducibility, when intravenous access is not problematic [128,129]. When compared, FPRNA was found to be more sensitive than echocardiography for detection of anthracycline-induced LV dysfunction [129].

Evaluation of valvular heart disease

Stroke count method. In the presence of a single valve regurgitant lesion, a simple comparison of RV and LV stroke counts with either FPRNA or GERNA, can be used to estimate the degree of right- or left-sided valvular regurgitation, or regurgitant fraction [130–134]. This technique reflects only differences between ventricles, will not be useful if valvular regurgitation is present on both sides of the heart, and cannot distinguish aortic from mitral or pulmonic from tricuspid regurgitation.

Tricuspid regurgitation. FPRNA has also been used to detect tricuspid valvular regurgitation (TR), specifically by identification of the regurgitant jet in the RA, brachiocephalic veins, or inferior vena cava during RV

systole as an indication of regurgitation (see Fig. 17.4) [51,135–137]. As described before, significant TR can significantly prolong tracer delivery to the LV, rendering FPRNA difficult to process for LV function [51]. Time-activity curve analysis of a radionuclide bolus injection was initially described from the pulmonary capillary wedge position on FPRNA for the detection of mitral and aortic valvular regurgitation by Metz et al. in an experimental model [138]. Williams et al. [51] applied this principle to RA time-activity curves for the detection and quantitation of the severity of TR in 51 patients, 24 with and 27 without TR by pulsed Doppler echocardiography. They described an RA "injection fraction" (IF) which had 100% sensitivity and 96% specificity, using Doppler as the reference standard:

$$\text{RA IF} = \frac{(\text{RA counts at RV ES}) - (\text{RA counts at RV ED})}{(\text{RA counts at RV ED})} \times 100\%.$$

The RA IF results also correlated well with the pulsed Doppler estimate of severity, with a mean RA IF of 4%, 8%, and 22% in patients with trivial, mild, and moderate-to-severe TR, respectively.

Shunt detection and quantitation

FPRNA can be used to detect and quantitate left-to-right shunts [21,139], but is less precise than magnetic resonance imaging (MRI) in this regard [140], and is far less utilized than echocardiography, particularly with the advent of Doppler imaging of blood flow, microbubble contrast enhancement, and transesophageal imaging [141].

Detection of an intracardiac shunt requires strict adherence to bolus technique, and interrogation of regions of interest placed as widely as possible over both lungs, but carefully excluding the SVC and cardiac chambers. The first frame of the curve should unequivocally represent pulmonary activity rather than any SVC, RA, or RV activity, since the shape of the early part of the curve will determine the shape of the subsequent mathematical fit. The resultant pulmonary curves are analyzed by a gamma variate fit (or exponential fit) to quantitate the initial right ventricular outflow, and the secondary peak caused by pulmonary recirculation (Color Fig. 17.18). The fitted curve is then subtracted from the raw data to leave the shunt component, which can, itself, be fitted with another curve. The shunt ratio Qp:Qs is then calculated as:

$$(A_1 + A_2)/A_1$$

where A_1 = the area under the primary fitted curve, and A_2 = the area under the secondary (shunt) fitted curve. A deconvolution technique has also been described [142], which improves the accuracy of this approach.

Localization of the shunt (i.e., at the atrial, ventricular, ductus arteriosus, or intrapulmonary level) requires comparative analysis of time-activity curves generated from RA, RV, and pulmonary regions of interest [143]. In the absence of right-sided valvular incompetence, these time-activity curves show the greatest abnormality in the cardiac chambers distal to the left-to-right shunt. An atrial septal defect typically alters the RA and RV curves, but the RV curve cannot be relied upon to differentiate a ventricular septal defect from a patent ductus arteriosus [143].

However, the FPRNA quantitation of the pulmonic to system flow ratio (Qp:Qs) can be considered as a reference standard, and may be more accurate than oximetry in ventricular septal defects [144].

GERNA has also been used to detect and quantitate shunts in patients without valvular regurgitation [145,146] using RV to LV SC ratios for left-to-right shunts and LV to RV SC ratios for shunts at the level of the ductus arteriosus. However, this technique is less accurate than FPRNA for quantitation of small shunts, with Qp:Qs of less than 2.0, when compared with invasive oximetric data [146]. The SC ratio technique has also been validated in patients using FPRNA [147], but the incidence of significant valvular regurgitation that could alter these results (e.g., TR in patients with long-standing shunting and pulmonary hypertension) is high in this patient population.

Evaluation of Right Ventricular Function

RV function is less often measured than LV function, but has been shown to hold clinical diagnostic and prognostic importance in many disorders [148–159]. Owing to its accuracy, FPRNA has become a noninvasive reference standard for RV EF, and has often been performed in concert with other measurements of RV function as a calibration method [20,49,50,157–159].

RV hypertrophy and dysfunction are common occurrences in pressure overload (e.g., pulmonic stenosis, severe obstructive pulmonary disease, pulmonary embolism) and volume overload (e.g., tricuspid valvular regurgitation) situations. The combination of RV volume and pressure overload often results in rapid deterioration in clinical status, with peripheral edema, anasarca, and hepatic failure from passive congestion.

Patients with RV dysfunction due to pulmonary hypertension caused by mitral regurgitation have a poorer outcome with both medical and surgical therapy

[148,149]. Improvements in RV function can be used to track the reduction in pulmonary vascular resistance in lung volume reduction surgery for emphysema [150]. In patients with severe LV dysfunction, preserved RV function correlates with improved exercise tolerance, functional capacity, and survival [151,152]. Patients with ischemic heart disease can be noninvasively diagnosed as having proximal right coronary artery disease by an abnormal RV EF response to exercise [153], although this can be affected by exercise-induced pulmonary hypertension from LV dysfunction due to left anterior descending or circumflex stenoses [14,154–156].

One of the major indications for RV FPRNA is the distinction of patients with ventricular tachycardia (VT) due to arrhythmogenic RV dysplasia (ARVD) or complex (ARVC) (Uhl's anomaly, parchment RV) from those with VT originating in the RV outflow tract (RVOT). This disorder is a malformation of the myocardium with altered tissue characteristics (fibrofatty replacement of myocardium), occurring in an estimated 5% of sudden cardiac deaths in people age 35 and younger in the United States [160]. ARVD should be distinguished from other RVOT tachycardias, since they have a more benign course and can be treated with radiofrequency ablation. These RVs are characterized by marked dilatation and depressed EFs. They also have temporal dispersion of electrical and mechanical contractile activation, as evidenced by epsilon waves or localized prolongation (> 110 ms) of the QRS complex in right precordial leads (V1-V3), late potentials on signal averaged ECG, and Fourier phase images of the RV [161]. Although the latter is best demonstrated by GERNA [161], an abnormal result is predictive of sudden arrhythmic cardiac death. Right-sided enlargement and dysfunction in a patient with arrhythmias may lead to the diagnosis of ARVD, but may also indicate acute or chronic pressure overload, as in acute or chronic pulmonary embolism.

REPORTING OF FIRST-PASS RADIONUCLIDE ANGIOGRAPHY

General guidelines for reporting of FPRNA have been developed and published by the American Society of Nuclear Cardiology (ASNC) [74]. A complete report should have sections that list the technical details of the laboratory procedure, which will be used mainly by the nuclear physicians, as well as a clinical section of results and interpretation, which will be directed toward the referring physicians.

The technical section should include demographics (i.e., name, gender, age, date of study, medical record number, height, weight, and body surface area), and acquisition details for example, clinical problem, indication for the study, rest only or rest plus intervention, tracer type and dose, injection location, body position (i.e., upright, semiupright, supine, prone), and study quality.

The clinical results section should include hemodynamic and clinical variables (symptoms, heart rate, blood pressure, ECG rhythm and pattern) at rest and with stress or intervention. Scintigraphic results should include the transit times, chamber size, EF, and regional wall motion at rest and/or with intervention, and itemize the significant changes that occurred.

The conclusion section should interpret these data, indicating whether the findings are normal, abnormal, or equivocal in nature. The severity of any abnormalities should be described. The relationship to perfusion findings (concordance or discordance) should be noted if perfusion images were acquired with FPRNA. Finally, the current data should be compared with previous studies, detailing any alterations in function that have occurred and their clinical implications.

REFERENCES

1. Blumgart HL, Weiss S. Studies on the velocity of blood flow. VII. The pulmonary circulation time in normal resting individuals. J Clin Invest 1927;4:399.
2. Williams KA, Sherwood DF, Fisher KM. The frequency of asymptomatic and electrically silent exercise-induced regional myocardial ischemia during first-pass radionuclide angiography with upright bicycle ergometry. J Nucl Med 1992;33:359.
3. Lee KL, Pryor DB, Pieper KS, et al. Prognostic value of radionuclide angiography in medically treated patients with coronary artery disease. A comparison with clinical and catheterization variables. Circulation 1990;82:1705.
4. Sporn V, Perez-Balino N, Holman BL, et al. Simultaneous measurement of ventricular function and myocardial perfusion using the technetium-99m isonitriles. Clin Nucl Med 1988;13:77.
5. Schad N, Nickel O. Assessment of ventricular function with first-pass angiocardiography. Cardiovasc Radiol 1979;2:149.
6. Nickel O, Schad N. Image analysis of the heart action recorded with a high speed multicrystal gamma camera. Med Prog Technol 1978;5:163.
7. Gal R, Grenier RP, Carpenter J, et al. High count rate first-pass radionuclide angiography using a digital gamma camera. J Nucl Med 1986;27:198.
8. Gal R, Grenier RP, Schmidt DH, et al. Background correction in first-pass radionuclide angiography: comparison of several approaches. J Nucl Med 1986;27:1480.
9. DePuey EG, Salensky H, Melancon S, et al. Simultaneous biplane first-pass radionuclide angiocardiography using a scintillation camera with two perpendicular detectors. J Nucl Med 1994;35:1593.
10. Nichols K, DePuey EG, Gooneratne N, et al. First-pass ventricular ejection fraction using a single-crystal nuclear camera. J Nucl Med 1994;35:1292.
11. Ott RJ. Wire chambers revisited. Eur J Nucl Med 1993;20:348.
12. Lacy JL, LeBlanc AD, Babich JW, et al. A gamma camera for medical applications, using a multiwire proportional counter. J Nucl Med 1984; 25:1003.
13. Holman BL, Harris GI, Neirinckx RD, et al. Tantalum-178—a short-lived nuclide for nuclear medicine: production of the parent W-178. J Nucl Med 1978;19:510.
14. Verani MS, Guidry GW, Mahmarian JJ, et al. Effects of acute, transient coronary occlusion on global and regional right ventricular function in humans. J Am Coll Cardiol 1992;20:1490.
15. Johnson LL, Seldin DW. Clinical experience with technetium-99m teboroxime, a neutral, lipophilic myocardial perfusion imaging agent. Am J Cardiol 1990;66:63E.
16. Williams KA, Taillon LA, Draho JM, et al. First-pass radionuclide angiographic studies of left ventricular function with Tc-99m-teboroxime, Tc-99m-sestamibi and Tc-99m-DTPA. J Nucl Med 1993;34:394.
17. Williams KA, Ryan JW, Resnekov L, et al. Planar positron imaging of rubidium-82 for myocardial infarction: a comparison with thallium-201 and regional wall motion. Am Heart J 1989;118:601.
18. Lacy JL, Layne WW, Guidry GW, et al. Development and clinical performance of an automated, portable tungsten-178/tantalum-178 generator. J Nucl Med 1991;32:2158.
19. Verani MS, Lacy JL, Guidry GW, et al. Quantification of left ventricular performance during transient coronary occlusion at various anatomic sites in humans: a study using tantalum-178 and a multiwire gamma camera. J Am Coll Cardiol 1992;19:297.
20. Wong DF, Natarajan TK, Summer W, et al. Right ventricular ejection fraction measured by first-pass intravenous krypton-81m: reproducibility and comparison with technetium-99m. Am J Cardiol 1985;56:776.
21. Treves S, Cheng C, Samuel A, et al. Iridium-191 angiocardiography for the detection and quantitation of left-to-right shunting. J Nucl Med 1980; 21:1151.
22. Packard AB, Day PJ, Treves ST. An improved 191Os/191mIr generator using a hybrid anion exchanger. Nucl Med Biol 1995;22:887.
23. Hellman C, Zafrir N, Shimoni A, et al. Evaluation of ventricular function with first-pass iridium-191m radionuclide angiocardiography. J Nucl Med 1989;30:450.
24. Heller GV, Treves ST, Parker JA, et al. Comparison of ultra-short-lived iridium-191m with technetium-99m for first pass radionuclide angiocardiographic evaluation of right and left ventricular function in adults. J Am Coll Cardiol 1986;7:1295.
25. Brihaye C, Guillaume M, Lavi N, et al. Development of a reliable Hg-195m—Au-195m generator for the production of Au-195m, a short-lived nuclide for vascular imaging. J Nucl Med 1982;23:1114.
26. Wackers FJ, Giles RW, Hoffer PB, et al. Gold-195m, a new generator-produced short-lived radionuclide for sequential assessment of ventricular performance by first pass radionuclide angiocardiography. Am J Cardiol 1982;50:89.
27. Mena I, Narahara KA, de Jong R, et al. Gold-195m, an ultra-short-lived generator-produced radionuclide: clinical application in sequential first pass ventriculography. J Nucl Med 1983; 24:139.
28. Elliott AT, Dymond DS, Stone DL, et al. A 195mHg-195mAu generator for use in first-pass nuclear angiocardiography. Phys Med Biol 1983;28:139.
29. Fazio F, Gerundini P, Margonato A, et al. Quantitative radionuclide angiocardiography using gold-195m. Am J Cardiol 1984;53:1442.

30. Cochavi S, Goldsmith SJ, Strashun A, et al. Planar imaging of positron-emitting radionuclides with a multicrystal camera. J Nucl Med 1982;23:725.

31. Williams KA, Ryan JW, Resnekov L, et al. Planar positron imaging of rubidium-82 for myocardial infarction: a comparison with thallium-201 and regional wall motion. Am Heart J 1989;118:601.

32. Williams KA, Taillon LA, Stark VJ. Quantitative planar imaging of glucose metabolic activity in myocardial segments with exercise thallium-201 perfusion defects in patients with myocardial infarction: comparison with late (24-hour) redistribution thallium imaging for detection of reversible ischemia. Am Heart J 1992;124:294.

33. Chen EQ, MacIntyre WJ, Fouad F, et al. Measurement of cardiac output with first-pass determination during rubidium-82 PET myocardial perfusion imaging. Eur J Nucl Med 1996;23:993.

34. Imaging guidelines for nuclear cardiology procedures. American Society of Nuclear Cardiology. First-pass radionuclide angiography (FPRNA). J Nucl Cardiol 1996;3:G16.

35. Foster C, Gaeckle T, Braastad R, et al. First-pass radionuclide angiography during bicycle and treadmill exercise. J Nucl Cardiol 1995;2:485.

36. Williams KA, Taillon LA, Carter JE Jr. Asymptomatic and electrically silent myocardial ischemia during upright leg cycle ergometry and treadmill exercise (clandestine myocardial ischemia). Am J Cardiol 1993;72:1114.

37. Sandler H, Dodge HT. The use of single plane angiocardiograms for the calculation of left ventricular volume in man. Am Heart J 1968;75:325.

38. Massardo T, Gal RA, Grenier RP, et al. Left ventricular volume calculation using a count-based ratio method applied to multigated radionuclide angiography. J Nucl Med 1990;31:450.

39. Simonson J, Schiller N. Descent of the base of the left ventricle: an echocardiographic index of left ventricular function. J Am Soc Echocardiogr 1989;2:25.

40. Alam M, Rosenhamer G. Atrioventricular plane displacement and left ventricular function. J Am Soc Echocardiogr 1992;5:427.

41. Arts T, Hunter WC, Douglas AS, et al. Macroscopic three-dimensional motion patterns of the left ventricle. Adv Exper Med Biol 1993;346:383.

42. Qi P, Thomsen C. Stahlberg F, et al. Normal left ventricular wall motion measured with two-dimensional myocardial tagging. Acta Radiol 1993;34:450.

43. Williams KA, Bryant TA, Taillon LA. First-pass radionuclide angiographic analysis with two regions of interest: improved "substitutability" for gated equilibrium ejection fractions. J Nucl Med 1998;39:1857.

44. Williams KA, Taillon LA. Left ventricular function in patients with coronary artery disease using gated tomographic myocardial perfusion images: comparison with contrast ventriculography and first-pass radionuclide angiography. J Am Coll Cardiol 1996;27:173.

45. Nusynowitz ML, Benedetto AR, Walsh RA, et al. First-pass Anger camera radiocardiography: biventricular ejection fraction, flow, and volume measurements. J Nucl Med 1987;28:950.

46. Folland ED, Hamilton GW, Larson SM, et al. The radionuclide ejection fraction: a comparison of three radionuclide techniques with contrast angiography. J Nucl Med 1977;18:1159.

47. Nichols K, DePuey EG, Gooneratne N, et al. First-pass ventricular ejection fraction using a single-crystal nuclear camera. J Nucl Med 1994;35:1301.

48. Vainio P, Jurvelin J, Kuikka J, et al. Analysis of left ventricular function from gated first-pass and multiple gated equilibrium acquisitions. Int J Card Imaging 1992;8:243.

49. Caplin JL, Flatman WD, Dymond DS. Effects of projection and background correction method upon calculation of right ventricular ejection fraction using first-pass radionuclide angiography. Int J Card Imaging 1985;1:171.

50. Johnson LL, Lawson MA, Blackwell GG, et al. Optimizing the method to calculate right ventricular ejection fraction from first-pass data acquired with a multicrystal camera. J Nucl Cardiol 1995;2:372.

51. Williams KA, Walley PE, Ryan JW. Detection and assessment of severity of tricuspid regurgitation using first-pass radionuclide angiography and comparison with pulsed Doppler echocardiography. Am J Cardiol 1990;66:333.

52. Pillay M, Rezvani M, Cox PH. Changes in pulmonary mean transit time demonstrated by the scintigraphic first pass technique in patients receiving radiation therapy. Eur J Nucl Med 1987;13:305.

53. Reichart B, Hemmer W, Markewitz A, et al. Late (11 to 19 years) assessment of hemodynamic and prosthetic valve function in patients with Starr Edwards ball valves: a noninvasive study utilizing 99m-technetium pertechnetate scintigraphy. Thorac Cardiovasc Surg 1985;33:162.

54. Fouad FM, MacIntyre WJ, Tarazi RC. Noninvasive measurement of cardiopulmonary blood volume. Evaluation of the centroid method. J Nucl Med 1981;22:205.

55. Iskandrian AS, Hakki AH, Kane SA, et al. Changes in pulmonary blood volume during upright exercise. Clinical implications. Chest 1982;82:54.

56. Okada RD, Osbakken MD, Boucher CA, et al. Pulmonary blood volume ratio response to exercise; a noninvasive determination of exercise-induced changes in pulmonary capillary wedge pressure. Circulation 1982;65:126.

57. Harpole DH, Skelton TN, Davidson CJ, et al. Validation of pressure-volume data obtained in patients by initial transit radionuclide angiocardiography. Am Heart J 1989;118:983.

58. Purut CM. Sell TL. Jones RH. A new method to determine left ventricular pressure-volume loops in the clinical setting. J Nucl Med 1988;29:1492.

59. Kass DA, Maughan WL. From "Emax" to pressure-volume relations: a broader view. Circulation 1988;77:1203.

60. Borow KM, Jaspan JB, Williams KA, et al. Myocardial mechanics in young adult patients with diabetes mellitus: effects of altered load, inotropic state and dynamic exercise. J Am Coll Cardiol 1990;15:1508.

61. Aroney CN, Ruddy TD, Dighero H, et al. Differentiation of restrictive cardiomyopathy from pericardial constriction: assessment of diastolic function by radionuclide angiography. J Am Coll Cardiol 1989;13:1007.

62. Grossman W. Relaxation and diastolic distensibility of the regionally ischemic left ventricle. In: *Diastolic Relaxation of the Heart,* edited by WH Grossman and BH Lorell. Boston: Martinus-Nijhoff, 1988, p. 196.

63. Bonow RO, Vitale DF, Bacharach SL, et al. Asynchronous left ventricular regional function and impaired global diastolic filling in patients with coronary artery disease: reversal after angioplasty. Circulation 1985;71:297.

64. Bonow RO, Frederick TM, Bacharach SL, et al. Atrial systole and left ventricular filling in hypertrophic cardiomyopathy: effect of verapamil. Am J Cardiol 1983;51:1386.

65. Bonow RO. Radionuclide angiographic evaluation of left ventricular diastolic function. Circulation 1991;84:I208.

66. Bonow RO, Bacharach SL, Green MV, et al. Impaired left ventricular diastolic filling in patients with coronary artery disease: assessment with radionuclide angiography. Circulation 1981; 64:315.

67. Bonow RO. Radionuclide angiographic evaluation of left ventricular diastolic function. Circulation 1991;84:I208.

68. Wu J, Takeda T, Toyama H, et al. Phase changes caused by hyperventilation stress in spastic angina pectoris analyzed by first-pass radionuclide ventriculography. Ann Nucl Med 1999; 13:13.

69. Gibbons RJ, Lee KL, Cobb F, et al. Ejection fraction response to exercise in patients with chest pain and normal coronary arteriograms. Circulation 1981;64:952.

70. Port S, McEwan P, Cobb FR, et al. Influence of resting left ventricular function on the left ventricular response to exercise in patients with coronary artery disease. Circulation 1981;63:856.

71. Gibbons RJ, Lee KL, Cobb FR, et al. Ejection fraction response to exercise in patients with chest pain, coronary artery disease and normal resting ventricular function. Circulation 1982;66: 643.

72. Foster C, Dymond DS, Anholm JD, et al. Effect of exercise protocol on the left ventricular response to exercise. Am J Cardiol 1983;51:859.

73. Foster C, Anholm JD, Hellman CK, et al. Left ventricular function during sudden strenuous exercise. Circulation. 1981;63:592.

74. American Society of Nuclear Cardiology. Imaging guidelines for nuclear cardiology procedures, part 2. J Nucl Cardiol 1999; 6:G47.

75. American Society of Nuclear Cardiology. Updated imaging guidelines for nuclear cardiology procedures, part 1. J Nucl Cardiol 2001;8:G5.

76. Sacher HL, Sacher ML, Landau SW, et al. First-pass radionuclide cineangiography in diagnosis of coronary artery disease in patients older than 75 years: evaluation of sensitivity. J Am Osteopath Assoc 1995;95:415.

77. Murray GL, Cowan GS Jr, Vander-Zwagg R. Exercise-induced wall motion abnormalities and resting left ventricular dysfunction in the morbidly obese as assessed by radionuclide ventriculography. Obes Surg 1991;1:37.

78. Jones RH, McEwen P, Newman GE, et al. Accuracy of diagnosis of coronary artery disease by radionuclide measurement of left ventricular function during rest and exercise. Circulation 1981;64:586.

79. Borer JS, Bacharach SL, Green MV, et al. Real-time radionuclide cineangiography in the noninvasive evaluation of global and regional left ventricular function at rest and during exercise in patients with coronary-artery disease. N Engl J Med 1977;296:839.

80. Rerych SK, Scholz PM, Newman GE, et al. Cardiac function at rest and during exercise in normals and in patients with coronary heart disease: evaluation by radionuclide angiocardiography. Ann Surg 1978;187:449.

81. Rozanski A, Diamond GA, Berman D, et al. The declining specificity of exercise radionuclide ventriculography. N Engl J Med 1983;309:518.

82. Greenberg H, McMaster P, Dwyer EM, et al. Left ventricular dysfunction after acute myocardial infarction: the results of a prospective multicenter study. J Am Coll Cardiol 1984;4:867.

83. Nesto RW, Cohn LH, Collins JJ Jr, et al. Inotropic contractile reserve: a useful predictor of increased 5 year survival and improved post-operative left ventricular function in patients with

84. Ritchie JL, Hallstrom AP, Troubaugh GB, et al. Out-of-hospital sudden coronary death: rest and exercise left ventricular function in survivors. Am J Cardiol 1985;55:645.

85. Muhlbaier LH, Pryor DB, Rankin JS, et al. Observational comparison of event-free survival with medical and surgical therapy in patients with coronary artery disease: 20 years of follow-up. Circulation 1992;86:II198.

86. Jones RH, Johnson SH, Bigelow C, et al. Exercise radionuclide angiocardiography predicts cardiac death in patients with coronary artery disease. Circulation 1991;84:I52.

87. Johnson SH, Bigelow C, Lee KL, et al. Prediction of death and myocardial infarction by radionuclide angiocardiography in patients with suspected coronary artery disease. Am J Cardiol 1991;67:919.

88. Pryor DB, Harrell FE Jr, Lee KL, et al. Prognostic indicators from radionuclide angiography in medically treated patients with coronary artery disease. Am J Cardiol 1984;53:18.

89. Zhu WX, Gibbons RJ, Bailey KR, et al. Predischarge exercise radionuclide angiography in predicting multivessel coronary artery disease and subsequent cardiac events after thrombolytic therapy for acute myocardial infarction. Am J Cardiol 1994; 74:554.

90. Pryor DB, Harrell FE Jr, Lee KL, et al. An improving prognosis over time in medically treated patients with coronary artery disease. Am J Cardiol 1983;52:444.

91. Jones RH, Borges-Neto S, Potts JM. Simultaneous measurement of myocardial perfusion and ventricular function during exercise from a single injection of Tc-99m sestamibi in coronary artery disease. Am J Cardiol 1990;66:68E.

92. Berman DS, Kiat H, Maddahi J. The new 99mTc first-pass radionuclide angiography agents: 99mTc-sestamibi and 99mTc-teboroxime. Circulation 1991;84:I7.

93. Williams KA, Taillon LA. Gated planar technetium-99m-sestamibi myocardial perfusion image inversion for quantitative scintigraphic assessment of left ventricular function. J Nucl Cardiol 1995;2:285.

94. Baillet GY, Mena IG, Kuperus JH, et al. Simultaneous technetium-99m MIBI angiography and first-pass radionuclide angiography. J Nucl Med 1989;30:38.

95. Larock MP, Cantineau R, Legrand V, et al. 99mTc-MIBI (RP-30) to define the extent of myocardial ischemia and evaluate ventricular function. Eur J Nucl Med 1990;16:223.

96. Elliott AT, McKillop JH, Pringle SD, et al. Simultaneous measurement of left ventricular function and perfusion. Eur J Nucl Med 1990;17:310.

97. Villanueva-Meyer J, Mena I, Narahara KA. Simultaneous assessment of left ventricular wall motion and myocardial perfusion with technetium-99m-methoxy isobutyl isonitrile at stress and rest in patients with angina: comparison with thallium-201 SPECT. J Nucl Med 1990;31:457.

98. Bisi G, Sciagra R, Bull U, et al. Assessment of ventricular function with first-pass radionuclide angiography using technetium 99m hexakis-2-methoxyisobutylisonitrile: a European multicentre study. Eur J Nucl Med 1991;18:178.

99. Boucher CA, Wackers FJ, Zaret BL, et al. Technetium-99m sestamibi myocardial imaging at rest for assessment of myocardial infarction and first-pass ejection fraction. Multicenter Cardiolite Study Group. Am J Cardiol 1992;69:22.

100. Iftikhar I, Koutelou M, Mahmarian JJ, et al. Simultaneous perfusion tomography and radionuclide angiography during dobutamine stress. J Nucl Med 1996;37:1306.

101. Borges-Neto S, Curtis MA, Morris EI, et al. Combined Tc-99m sestamibi first-pass radionuclide angiography and cardiac SPECT imaging during arbutamine infusion delivered by a computerized closed-loop system. Clin Nucl Med 1999;24:42.

102. Germano G, Kiat H, Kavanagh PB, et al. Automatic quantification of ejection fraction from gated myocardial perfusion SPECT. J Nucl Med 1995;36:2138.

103. Iskandrian AE, Germano G, VanDecker W, et al. Validation of left ventricular volume measurements by gated SPECT 99mTc-labeled sestamibi imaging. J Nucl Cardiol 1998; 5:574.

104. Vallejo E, Dione DP, Sinusas AJ, et al. Assessment of left ventricular ejection fraction with quantitative gated SPECT: accuracy and correlation with first-pass radionuclide angiography. J Nucl Cardiol 2000, 7:461.

105. He ZX, Cwajg E, Preslar JS, et al. Accuracy of left ventricular ejection fraction determined by gated myocardial perfusion SPECT with Tl-201 and Tc-99m sestamibi: comparison with first-pass radionuclide angiography. J Nucl Cardiol 1999, 6:412.

106. Yoshioka J, Hasegawa S, Yamaguchi H, et al. Left ventricular volumes and ejection fraction calculated from quantitative electrocardiographic-gated 99mTc-tetrofosmin myocardial SPECT. J Nucl Med 1999; 40:1693.

107. Inubushi M, Tadamura E, Kudoh T, et al. Simultaneous assessment of myocardial free fatty acid utilization and left ventricular function using 123I-BMIPP-gated SPECT. J Nucl Med 1999;40:1840.

108. Palmas W, Friedman JD, Diamond GA, et al. Incremental value of simultaneous assessment of myocardial function and perfusion with technetium-99m sestamibi for prediction of extent of coronary artery disease. J Am Coll Cardiol 1995;25:1024.

109. Peix A, Lopez A, Ponce F, et al. Enhanced detection of reversible myocardial hypoperfusion by technetium 99m-tetrofosmin imaging and first-pass radionuclide angiography after nitroglycerin administration. J Nucl Cardiol 1998 5:469.

110. Borges-Neto S, Coleman RE, Potts JM, et al. Combined exercise radionuclide angiocardiography and single photon emission computed tomography perfusion studies for assessment of coronary artery disease. Semin Nucl Med 1991;21:223.

111. Kim Y, Goto H, Kobayashi K, et al. A new method to evaluate ischemic heart disease: combined use of rest thallium-201 myocardial SPECT and Tc-99m exercise tetrofosmin first pass and myocardial SPECT. Ann Nucl Med 1999;13:147.

112. Borges-Neto S, Javid A, Kong D, et al. Prediction of myocardial perfusion abnormalities by quantitative regional function using a radionuclide angiography database: a comparison with wall motion analysis. Clin Nucl Med 2000;25:110.

113. Dakik HA, Mahmarian JJ, Kimball KT, et al. Prognostic value of exercise 201Tl tomography in patients treated with thrombolytic therapy during acute myocardial infarction. Circulation 1996;94:2735.

114. Mast ST, Shaw LK, Ravizzini GC, et al. Incremental prognostic value of RNA ejection fraction measurements during pharmacologic stress testing: a comparison with clinical and perfusion variables. J Nucl Med 2001;42:871.

115. Johnson LL, Cubbon J, Escala E, et al. Hemodynamic effects of labetalol in patients with combined hypertension and left ventricular failure. J Cardiovasc Pharmacol 1988;12:350.

116. D'Agostino HJ Jr. Pritchett EL. Shand DG. Jones RH. Effect of verapamil on left ventricular function at rest and during exercise in normal men. J Cardiovasc Pharm 1983;5:812.

117. Harpole DH, Davidson CJ, Skelton TN, et al. Early and late changes in left ventricular systolic performance after percutaneous aortic balloon valvuloplasty. Am J Cardiol 1990;66:327.

118. Harpole DH, Rankin JS, Wolfe WG, et al. Assessment of left ventricular functional preservation during isolated cardiac valve operations. Circulation 1989;80:III1.

119. Harpole DH, Clements FM, Quill T, et al. Right and left ventricular performance during and after abdominal aortic aneurysm repair. Ann Surg 1989;209:356.

120. Davidson CJ, Harpole DA, Kisslo K, et al. Analysis of the early rise in aortic transvalvular gradient after aortic valvuloplasty. Am Heart J 1989;117:411.

121. Peterson RJ, Young WG Jr, Godwin JD, et al. Noninvasive assessment of exercise cardiac function before and after pectus excavatum repair. J Thorac Cardiovasc Surg 1995;90:251.

122. Singal PK, Iliskovic N. Doxorubicin-induced cardiomyopathy. N Engl J Med 1998;339:900.

123. McKillop JH, Bristow MR, Goris ML, et al. Sensitivity and specificity of radionuclide ejection fractions in doxorubicin cardiotoxicity. Am Heart J 1983;106:1048.

124. Alexander J, Dainiak N, Berger HJ, et al. Serial assessment of doxorubicin cardiotoxicity with quantitative radionuclide angiocardiography. N Engl J Med 1979;300:278.

125. Ritchie JL, Singer JW, Thorning D, et al. Anthracycline cardiotoxicity: clinical and pathologic outcomes assessed by radionuclide ejection fraction. Cancer 1980;46:1109.

126. Piver MS, Marchetti DL, Parthasarathy KL, et al. Doxorubicin hydrochloride (Adriamycin) cardiotoxicity evaluated by sequential radionuclide angiocardiography. Cancer 1985;56:76.

127. Steinherz LJ, Graham T, Hurwitz R, et al. Guidelines for cardiac monitoring of children during and after anthracycline therapy: report of the Cardiology Committee of the Childrens Cancer Study Group. Pediatrics 1992;89:942.

128. Morgan GW, McIlveen BM, Freedman A, et al. Radionuclide ejection fraction in doxorubicin cardiotoxicity. Cancer Treat Rep 1981;65:629.

129. Lahtinen R, Uusitupa M, Kuikka J, et al. Non-invasive evaluation of anthracycline-induced cardiotoxicity in man. Acta Med Scand 1982;212:201.

130. Alderson PO. Radionuclide quantification of valvular regurgitation. J Nucl Med 1982;23:851.

131. Novack H, Machac J, Horowitz SF. Inversion of the radionuclide regurgitant index in right-sided valvular regurgitation. Eur J Nucl Med 1985;11:205.

132. Nicod P, Corbett JR, Firth BG, et al. Radionuclide techniques for valvular regurgitant index: comparison in patients with normal and depressed ventricular function. J Nucl Med 1982;23:763.

133. Hurwitz RA, Treves S, Freed M, et al. Quantitation of aortic and mitral regurgitation in the pediatric population: evaluation by radionuclide angiography. Am J Cardiol 1983;51:252.

134. Ohtake T, Nishikawa J, Machida K, et al. Evaluation of regurgitant fraction of the left ventricle by gated cardiac blood pool scanning using SPECT. J Nucl Med 1987;28:19.

135. Mishkin FS, Mishkin ME. Documentation of tricuspid regurgitation by radionuclide angiocardiography. Br Heart J 1974; 36:1019.

136. Lumia FJ, Patil A, Germon PA, et al. Tricuspid regurgitation by radionuclide angiography and contrast right ventriculography: a preliminary observation. J Nucl Med 1981;22:804.

137. Winzelberg GG, Boucher CA, Pohost GM, et al. Right ventricular function in aortic and mitral valve disease. Relation of gated first-pass radionuclide angiography to clinical and hemodynamic findings. Chest 1981;79:520.

138. Metz CE, Kirch DL, Steele PP. A mathematical model for the determination of cardiac regurgitant and ejection fractions from radioisotope angiocardiograms. Phys Med Biol 1975;20:531.

139. Maltz DL, Treves S. Quantitative radionuclide angiocardiography: Determination of Qp:Qs in children. Circulation 1973; 47:1049.

140. Arheden H, Holmqvist C, Thilen U, et al. Left-to-right cardiac shunts: comparison of measurements obtained with MR velocity mapping and with radionuclide angiography. Radiology 1999;211:453.

141. Brickner ME, Hillis LD, Lange RA. Congenital heart disease in adults—first of two parts. New Engl J Med 2000;342:256.

142. Kuruc A, Treves S, Parker JA. Accuracy of deconvolution algorithms assessed by simulation studies: concise communication. J Nucl Med 1983;24:258.

143. Tian JH, Murray IP, Walker B, et al. First-pass radionuclide angiocardiography in the determination of left-to-right cardiac shunt site in children. Cathet Cardiovasc Diagn 1982;8:459.

144. Baker EJ, Ellam SV, Lorber A, et al. Superiority of radionuclide over oximetric measurement of left to right shunts. Br Heart J 1985;53:535.

145. Brunotte F, Laurens MH, Cloez JL, et al. Sensitivity and specificity of radionuclide equilibrium angiocardiography for detection of hemodynamically significant secundum atrial septal defect. Eur J Nucl Med 1986;12:468.

146. Eterovic D, Dujic Z, Popovic S, et al. Gated versus first-pass radioangiography in the evaluation of left-to-right shunts. Clin Nucl Med 1995;20:534.

147. Kelbaek H, Aldershvile J, Svendsen JH, et al. Evaluation of left-to-right shunts in adults with atrial septal defect using first-pass radionuclide cardiography. Eur Heart J 1992;13:491.

148. Hochreiter C, Niles N, Devereux RB, et al. Mitral regurgitation: relationship of noninvasive descriptors of right and left ventricular performance to clinical and hemodynamic findings and to prognosis in medically and surgically treated patients. Circulation 1986;73:900.

149. Wencker D, Borer JS, Hochreiter C, et al. Preoperative predictors of late postoperative outcome among patients with nonischemic mitral regurgitation with 'high risk' descriptors and comparison with unoperated patients. Cardiology 2000;93:37.

150. Sciurba FC, Rogers RM, Keenan RJ, et al. Improvement in pulmonary function and elastic recoil after lung-reduction surgery for diffuse emphysema. N Engl J Med 1996;334:1095.

151. Di Salvo TG, Mathier M, Semigran MJ, et al. Preserved right ventricular ejection fraction predicts exercise capacity and survival in advanced heart failure. J Am Coll Cardiol 1995;25:1143.

152. Baker BJ, Wilen MM, Boyd CM, et al. Relation of right ventricular ejection fraction to exercise capacity in chronic left ventricular failure. Am J Cardiol 1984;54:596.

153. Johnson LL, McCarthy DM, Sciacca RR, et al. Right ventricular ejection fraction during exercise in patients with coronary artery disease. Circulation 1979;60:1284.

154. Brown KA, Okada RD, Boucher CA, et al. Right ventricular ejection fraction response to exercise in patients with coronary artery disease: influence of both right coronary artery disease and exercise-induced changes in right ventricular afterload. J Am Coll Cardiol 1984;3:895.

155. Berger HJ, Johnstone DE, Sands JM, et al. Response of right ventricular ejection fraction to upright bicycle exercise in coronary artery disease. Circulation 1979;60:1292.

156. Reduto LA, Berger HJ, Cohen LS, et al. Sequential radionuclide assessment of left and right ventricular performance after acute transmural myocardial infarction. Ann Intern Med 1978;89:441.

157. Manno BV, Iskandrian AS, Hakki AH. Right ventricular function: methodologic and clinical considerations in noninvasive scintigraphic assessment. J Am Coll Cardiol 1984;3:1072.

158. Bartlett ML, Seaton D, McEwan L, et al. Determination of right ventricular ejection fraction from reprojected gated blood pool SPET: comparison with first-pass ventriculography. Eur J Nucl Med 2001;28:608.

159. Rezai K, Weiss R, Stanford W, et al. Relative accuracy of three scintigraphic methods for determination of right ventricular ejection fraction: a correlative study with ultrafast computed tomography. J Nucl Med 1991;32:429.

160. McKenna WJ, Thiene G, Nava A, et al. Diagnosis of arrhythmogenic right ventricular dysplasia/cardiomyopathy. Task Force of the Working Group Myocardial and Pericardial Disease of the European Society of Cardiology and of the Scientific Council on Cardiomyopathies of the International Society and Federation of Cardiology. Br Heart J 1994;71:215.

161. Le Guludec D, Gauthier H, Porcher R, et al. Prognostic value of radionuclide angiography in patients with right ventricular arrhythmias. Circulation 2001;103:1972.

Part 2

Equilibrium Imaging

JEFFREY S. BORER AND PHYLLIS SUPINO

Clinical nuclear cardiology began almost 35 years ago with radionuclide angiography. To this day, radionuclide angiography provides the most accurate estimates of prognosis available for most cardiac diseases. In one or another of its forms, this method is employed every day in making management decisions and evaluating therapy. This chapter briefly reviews the history of the technique, some important instrumentation and software issues, and data supporting current clinical applications.

HISTORY AND FUTURE

Radionuclide-based cardiac functional assessment began in 1962 as a nonimaging experiment performed with direct left ventricular (LV) administration of isotope at cardiac catheterization [1]. However, as a modality readily applicable in clinical practice, the direct forerunner of equilibrium radionuclide angiography was introduced in 1968 as a "noninvasive" (that is, isotope administration by vein without additional entry into the body) solution to the problem of defining cardiac function [2]. Information available from this pioneering effort was not strictly "angiographic": photons emitted from the LV were collected by a nonimaging radiation detector (probe) placed appropriately over the patient's chest. The resulting time-activity curve directly paralleled the time-volume relation, defining LV volume variations during the cardiac cycle. The lack of images limited application of this early method. (Nonetheless, images available from later technical developments have been used to confirm positioning of newer probes, allowing probe technology to be applied at the bedside [3], where camera positioning might be logistically difficult, and during ambulatory activity [4].)

Images soon were provided, but only when isotope again was administered via catheter directly into the left ventricular blood pool [5]. Temporal resolution of the images was crude and this, together with the invasive approach, limited the technique only to research applications. However, by 1971, the noninvasive approach and recognizable cardiac images were married

[6]. The enabling technology was a "gating" system, by which information was transmitted from the Anger camera to film only during a predetermined time interval initiated by a specific portion of a simultaneously recorded electrocardiogram (ECG). After collection of data from many cardiac cycles, spatial resolution of the resulting "composite" image was sufficient so that the LV outline could be defined and chamber volume could be calculated geometrically. Images were collected in the anterior position, with the camera face parallel to the anterior chest wall. In this position, the LV and right ventricle (RV) overlap to some extent, but the border of the cardiac silhouette corresponds roughly to that of the LV, to which the standard geometric formulas for ventricular volume could be applied.

Thus, true radionuclide angiography began as an equilibrium technique, that is, with isotope fully mixed in the intravascular blood pool. This approach has the potential advantage that radioactive emissions detected from a cardiac chamber during imaging are directly proportional to the blood volume in that chamber. However, application of this principle in evaluation of radionuclide angiograms would wait several years, until evolution of new technologies, as described below.

Data collection during a prespecified subinterval within the cardiac cycle was critical for quantitative application of radionuclide angiography. To calculate cardiac performance descriptors like ventricular ejection fraction (EF), temporal variations in intraventricular blood volumes must be defined. The accuracy of such calculations depends on the temporal resolution of the images. To enable determination of temporal variations, the early gating devices were designed to detect the ECG QRS complex. Then, after an operator-determined delay, an electrical signal to the radiation detector triggered recording of detected photons on X-ray film for a short and finite interval bracketing end-diastole. Once data were collected from a sufficient number of cardiac cycles so that an interpretable image had been produced, the gating device was reset so that the signal for imaging onset was sent later after the QRS, at a time during which end-systole could be expected to occur. Imaging was continued for an interval tightly bracketing end-systole, after which the data collection stopped. However, the ECG is relatively imprecise in predicting the timing of end-systole; therefore, to ensure that true end-systole would be captured, early devices set the imaging interval at 80 ms. Since true end-systole is shorter than 80 ms, the value estimated from the 80 ms interval is a composite of true end-systole and slightly larger instantaneous ventricular blood volumes present immediately before and after end-systole. The rate of change in ventricular volume with time is directly proportional to heart rate. Therefore, to provide reasonable accuracy in estimating end-systolic volume from an 80 ms interval, studies should be performed only at relatively slow heart rates and, specifically, at heart rates generally achieved at rest [7]. Another limitation of this system was that end-diastolic and end-systolic images were not obtained from the same cardiac cycle but rather from cycles separated by as many as 20 minutes, the time necessary to collect radioactive emissions sufficient to produce two interpretable images; therefore, the accuracy of the calculation depended on reasonably constant heart rate and ventricular functional state during this period. In addition, because the system provided only two images, end-diastole and end-systole, descriptors of ventricular performance other than EF, such as ejection rate, filling rate, etc., could not be obtained.

In 1972, the method of EF calculation from images readopted the approach used with the 1968 probe: the inherent advantage of proportionality between collected emissions and the emitting volume was harnessed [8] by positioning the camera over the patient in the left anterior oblique (LAO) position, isolating the LV and precluding overlap among cardiac chambers, just as the probe had done without images. This positioning freed the operator from the need for the precise outlining of ventricular borders that is necessary for accurate application of geometric volume calculations. Instead, it was possible to define a region of interest (ROI) that contained the entire LV and no other structure, within which radioactive emissions could be quantified by standard counting methods. Selection of another ROI, close to but sufficiently distant from the LV so that cyclic volume fluctuations over time were not apparent, made it possible to define background activity that could be subtracted from the LV ROI to allow calculation of relative LV volume during the imaging interval.

The only impediment that remained was improving temporal resolution by diminishing the duration of the images. Solution to this problem was begun in 1971, when the Anger camera and ECG were married to a computer, and was gradually developed during 5 years of research. As this advance was perfected, images could be collected and immediately stored in computer memory. Now, no guessing was needed to time end-diastole and end-systole: these images could be selected from among an array spanning the entire cardiac cycle. The only limitation on temporal resolution was the total time available for imaging, to ensure sufficient counts within each image so that the heart could be visualized adequately for spatial evaluation. By 1976, the final piece was in place: a computer program was completed allowing collection and simultaneous computer display of radioactive emissions in real time [9–13]. Fundamentally, the system is based on computer capacity to archive continually collected photons in temporally organized files of predetermined duration. These can be displayed as a time-activity curve (Fig. 17.19), paralleling the time-volume curve of a cardiac chamber, or can be displayed visually as a series of movie frames (Fig. 17.20); after the data collection is complete, sequential files can be added, if necessary, to increase counts per movie frame, adding to spatial resolution at the expense of temporal resolution. With minor collimator modification to enhance emission collection rate, this technique was applied during exercise, and a new era in clinical cardiac evaluation was born [13–15]. (Simultaneous with these developments, the spatial and temporal problems of radionuclide angiography were solved by a different approach, employing first-pass collection with a highly sensitive radiation detector [16]. This important step forward is detailed in Part 1 of this chapter.)

Though instrumentation has improved and software enhancements have been added, the approach to radionuclide angiography used today fundamentally is that developed in 1976. However, despite the importance of the achievement, thorny problems remained. First, spatial resolution of individual Anger camera images is inherently limited, precluding precise identification and quantification of regional abnormalities. This problem is potentiated by the overlap of cardiac chambers in all views except the LAO. Therefore, with planar imaging, direct visualization of wall motion is possible only for a limited portion of the heart. Additionally, simultaneous collection of myocardial perfusion scintigrams for optimal diagnosis together with angiographic data for optimal prognostication is cumbersome when blood pool scintigraphy is the angiographic approach. This problem can be mitigated by marrying first-pass radionuclide angiography to myocardial perfusion scintigraphy [17], as described elsewhere in this volume. Another approach is to abandon count-based ejection fraction determinations and employ the perfused myocardium for geometric calcula-

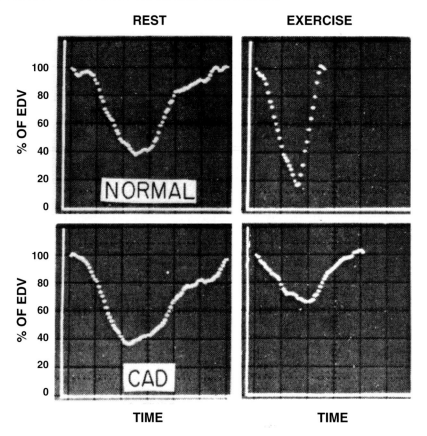

FIGURE 17.19 Time-activity curves for rest and exercise equilibrium radionuclide studies. The top two panels are those in a normal subject and the bottom two panels are in a subject with coronary disease (CAD). Note that ejection fraction (=[end-diastolic volume(EDV) − end-systolic volume]/EDV) increases with exercise in the normal subject, and decreases with exercise in the patient with CAD. (Reproduced with permission: Borer et al. N Engl J Med 1977;286:839–844.)

tion of volumes [18–20]. The latter approach is widely used. Results are described in the sections of this volume devoted to myocardial perfusion scintigraphy.

Because of these limitations, research has proceeded to advance the methodology. Single-photon emission computerized tomography (SPECT) has been employed to overcome the problems inherent in limited spatial resolution and limited views [21–25]. SPECT blood pool scintigraphy has provided some obvious advantages over planar imaging [26,73]. However, these advantages have not yet been sufficient to justify replacing the less expensive, less time-consuming, and less complex planar approach. In particular, acquisition time with SPECT remains excessively long for practical application during peak stress. Moreover, while certainly inferior in precision to LVEF and LV volume determinations by SPECT and planar blood pool scintigraphy, LVEF calculation by geometric formulation with SPECT myocardial perfusion scintigrams (abetted by assessment of regional wall thickening from

the SPECT images) has responded adequately to the need for assessments of ventricular mechanical performance with stress during myocardial perfusion scintigraphy. Ultimately, radiolabeled ligand imaging (Chapter 21) may improve the link between pathobiology and clinical outcome without the need for interposition of stress. However, while development of the newer imaging techniques proceeds, stress remains an important adjunct to clinical evaluation based on cardiac function.

METHODOLOGY

This section presents the methodological considerations specific for equilibrium radionuclide angiography. In addition, the interested reader should refer to the chapters devoted to radiopharmaceutical characteristics and to instrumentation in nuclear cardiology elsewhere in this volume.

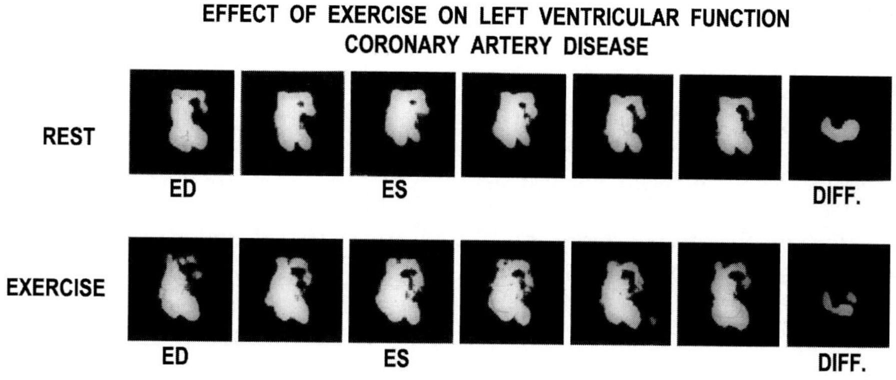

EFFECT OF EXERCISE ON LEFT VENTRICULAR FUNCTION
CORONARY ARTERY DISEASE

FIGURE 17.20 Serial movie frames representing rest and exercise equilibrium radionuclide cineangiograms in a patient with known three-vessel coronary artery disease (CAD). Left ventricular (LV) performance is normal at rest but deteriorates with exercise. ED, end-diastole; ES, end-systole; diff, difference between ED and ES. (Reproduced with permission: Borer et al. N Engl J Med 1977;286:839–844.)

The Radiopharmaceutical and Its Administration

Though several radioisotopes have been employed for radionuclide angiography and particularly for first-pass applications, the physical characteristics [68] of Tc-99m have caused it to predominate for equilibrium studies. The form in which a radiopharmaceutical is administered is dictated by the requirement that the isotope must remain within the intravascular blood pool for an interval sufficient to enable statistical precision of images and time-activity curves while minimizing the development of extravascular backgound activity that would progressively distort functional calculations. To achieve this goal, Tc-99m is bound to a carrier that resides in the intravascular pool at least for several hours without substantial degradation or other elimination. Such carriers have included human serum albumin (suboptimal because its metabolism begins relatively quickly) and red blood cells, currently the standard carrier. Red cell binding is mediated by a reducing agent, stannous pyrophosphate, which binds both to the red cell surface and to Tc-99m. Red cell binding can be achieved in vivo by intravenous administration of stannous pyrophosphate with subsequent spontaneous binding to intravenously administered Tc-99m. Because of the ease of achieving red cell labeling with this method, currently it is the standard approach. In vitro labeling also can be effected if a blood sample from the subject is combined with stannous pyrophosphate and technetium pertechnetate in a test tube. This method is preferred when the patient is receiving drug treatment that might alter in vivo reaction kinetics. A modified in vitro approach ("ex vitro") involves intravenous administration of the binder and its equilibration in the intravascular blood, followed by withdrawal of a blood sample that is mixed with technetium pertechnetate in

a test tube [27–30]. Though in vitro and ex vitro labeling may be slightly more efficient than the in vivo approach, labeling efficiency approaches 90% with all three methods, while the biological half-life of the labeled red cell exceeds the physical half-life of the isotope.

Tracer equilibration in the blood pool is required for equilibrium studies. Therefore, the characteristics of the intravenously administered bolus are of little consequence. However, administration should be directly into the vein from the syringe, since polyethylene intravenous lines adsorb stannous pyrophosphate and may alter the binding of red cells (or albumin) radiolabeled prior to intravenous administration.

Photon Detection Systems

The Anger camera currently is the standard detection implement for equilibrium radionuclide angiography. Fundamentally similar detection equipment is employed for SPECT blood pool studies, though gantry mounting enables data collection through an arc of 180° or more. The Anger camera, equipped with a single thallium-activated sodium iodide crystal, provides relatively high spatial resolution (between 0.5 and 1.0 cm by standardized measures) but suffers from loss of potential efficiency because dead-time after photon capture affects the entire crystal and because a collimator, analogous to a lens, must be placed between the patient and the crystal to maximize the accuracy with which the position of incident photons can be related to the position of their source. The maximal thickness of the crystal is a direct determinant of crystal sensitivity but is inversely proportional to spatial resolution that can be achieved; the thickness selected must provide an acceptable balance between the sensitivity and resolution to permit achievement of the goals of imaging. Today, optimization of crystal thickness and collimation results in near-linear proportionality between photon density incident upon the collimator and photon density transmitted to the computer in the range of 30,000 counts/sec (older models) to 80,000 counts/sec (newer nondigital cameras), though this rate may be exceeded if digital cameras are employed.

By consensus of experienced investigators, acquisition of > 2 million counts from within the field of view (the region of and immediately surrounding the heart), translating to at least 100,000 to 150,000 counts per composite movie frame, is necessary to enable spatial resolution sufficient to allow acceptably accurate visual assessment and statistically stable quantitative calculations. When the patient is at rest, these counting statistics can be achieved within 10 minutes when high-resolution collimation is employed. Therefore, if only resting studies are required, low-energy–high-resolution (LEHR) collimation is appropriate. However, the unique value of radionuclide angiography is its applicability during exercise. It is difficult to maintain stable hemodynamics and other physiologic variables at maximal exercise for 10 minutes; in practice, 2 to 3 minutes is the interval usually available for imaging at peak exercise. Therefore, low-energy–high-sensitivity (LEHS) collimators or the somewhat less sensitive low-energy–all-purpose (LEAP) collimators must be used for exercise studies, and should be used for the paired resting studies, as well, to assure parallel quantitative analyses. When we developed radionuclide cineangiography and applied it during exercise, my coworkers and I determined that, during a 2-minute collection interval employed during exercise in a normal subject (the author), high-sensitivity collimation resulted in only a 15% loss in resolution (FWHM) as compared with a high-resolution collimator, while increasing count detection by 250%. The increased count density of the resulting image more than compensated for the reduction in resolution, both visually and in precision of LVEF calculation.

The characteristics of the Anger camera circumscribe the number of emissions that can be collected per unit time. Therefore, to achieve the count density required for most visual and quantitative analyses, data collected from sequential cardiac cycles are archived and superimposed by a computer to provide a composite series of images (frames) that can be displayed in rapid sequence in endless loop format as a movie (see Fig. 17.20). The frames from sequential beats are collected and maintained in precise registration by referring each frame temporally to the associated QRS complex. Or-

ganization of acquired data into frames can be achieved by several computer algorithms. Maximal information content from radionuclide angiography is provided by list mode data acquisition [7,9–12,14,15]. This approach involves prespecification of frame duration based on the temporal resolution required by the parameter under assessment. The number of frames created is variable, and is determined by the cardiac cycle length. Several computer "addresses" then are assigned to each detected photon: first, a spatial address, identifying its position on a planar surface, second, a heart rate address, identifying the beat length interval at the time the photon was collected, and third, a clock time address, identifying the absolute time at which the photon was collected. Therefore, after data collection is complete, it is possible to delete photons collected during dysrhythmic beats or during heart rates higher or lower than the heart rate desired for evaluation (a distinct advantage when studies are performed during exercise, since collection can begin prior to peak exercise, when the peak achievable level may not be known, and images obtained only truly during peak exercise can be selected for review after the fact). To facilitate identification and rejection of unwanted heart beats, a cycle length histogram is constructed after completion of data collection; the histogram also can be used to define the heart rate range, or series of ranges, to be analyzed in any single study [11]. Also, it is possible to divide an imaging interval into temporally sequential segments, potentially useful for pharmacodynamic studies or for studies during variable exogenous stresses like exercise. Because frame duration is selected a priori based on the needs of the analysis, rather than based on the cardiac cycle length, any functional parameter can be efficiently calculated. Commonly, 10 ms frames are created, allowing precise calculation of ejection rates and filling rates at heart rates achieved during exercise, when particularly high temporal resolution is required [7]. (In contrast, LVEF calculation, even during exercise, seldom requires greater temporal resolution than 40 ms, for which 10 ms frames are more than adequate.)

Many commercially available systems do not offer a list mode option. Instead, data are collected in frame mode. With this approach, the number of frames that span a cardiac cycle generally is constant for all heart rates. Thus, frame duration is a function of heart rate (cycle length). This approach requires prespecification of heart rate prior to data collection so that frame duration can be determined before the fact. If heart rate is markedly different from the predefined value, frames late in the sequence may be relatively devoid of counts, resulting in deformed and often uninterpretable time-activity curves. Dysrhythmic beat rejection is possible with frame mode, based on the deviation of a cycle length from the prespecified target cycle length. However, while list mode allows post-hoc cycle length rejection, with frame mode, cycle rejection is done "on the fly" based on the predetermined target cycle length.

Acquisition Protocols

At equilibrium, all cardiac chambers simultaneously are filled with radiolabeled blood. Therefore, quantitation of ventricular volumes and function can be performed only when the chambers are oriented so that they do not overlap. To separate the RV and LV, the LAO position can be employed. Optimal ventricular separation can be reasonably assured by test imaging prior to collection of a definitive study. Since imaging can be performed for hours after isotope administration and studies require only minutes, malpositioned studies can be repeated. To make use of this option, of course, it is necessary to review the images shortly after they are obtained, a requirement often overlooked in practice. Generally, adequate ventricular separation is achieved in the 45° LAO position. To separate the left atrium (LA) from the LV, a 15° caudal tilt is used to modify the LAO position. The right atrium (RA) cannot be fully separated from the RV in this position but, as noted below, this generally does not present a practical problem. For qualitative wall motion assessment, other positions, including the anterior view (for anterolateral and apical motion, and sometimes adequate for the inferior wall), steep LAO, left lateral, or left posterior oblique views (all for the inferior wall) can be employed. Generally, it is impractical to perform more than one exercise test during a single study session; therefore, since it enables quantitation of functional parameters, most exercise studies are obtained only in the LAO position. Nonetheless, exercise studies have been performed in multiple positions [31] and have been repeated in a single position before and after pharmacologic interventions [32].

Exercise traditionally is employed with the patient supine to facilitate positioning under the camera while minimizing patient motion [14] but upright bicycle exercise also can be used [33]. The problem of maintaining perfect registration on sequential cardiac cycles during the greater patient motion usually associated with treadmill exercise has limited application of the use of this exercise modality during equilibrium studies, though a radiation point source can be applied to the chest wall distant to the heart to facilitate post-hoc reregistration.

Unless a specific question can be best answered with submaximal exercise, most exercise protocols for radionuclide angiography are designed to be symptom-limited (angina, dyspnea, fatigue) or limited by some prespecified event (e.g., arrhythmia). Therefore, to provide standards against which to compare responses of LVEF in patients who cannot exercise to heart rates near those predicted as maximum for their ages, average EF responses have been defined in normal subjects for submaximal exercise heart rates, as well [34]. Stress also has been applied with cold temperature stimulation [35] and with pharmacologic stimuli [36–38], but standards for these procedures are not well established.

Data Analysis and Interpretation

A major advantage of equilibrium radionuclide angiography is the capacity to determine volume irrespective of chamber shape. For this calculation, count density is a primary determinant of precision (i.e., of the variability and reproducibility of the point estimate of the average of the many superimposed cardiac cycles, as well as the accuracy in comparison with an external standard). Thus, while geometric formulations can be applied to volume determination from equilibrium images, volumes and volume changes (as in LVEF) generally are determined by count-based methodology. For LV volumes and LVEF, the region of interest (ROI) can be defined in end-diastole and fixed in this configuration throughout systole. This approach has the potential disadvantage of underestimating LVEF if background structures enter the ROI during systole. The ROI also can be made to vary throughout the cardiac cycle. Manual, semiautomated, and automated edge detection algorithms exist for performing the necessary operation on each image frame [14,39,40]. Either way, the relation between radionuclide angiographic LVEF and the corresponding contrast angiographic value is excellent both at rest and during exercise [41].

The equilibrium approach is more difficult to apply to determination of RVEF. With any camera angle, right heart structures invariably overlap. However, at end-diastole, only minimal blood and, hence, radionuclide, is present in the RA. Therefore, in the LAO view (in which only the RA and RV overlap), the effect of the RA can be disregarded with minimal impact on accuracy. In addition, in this view, any residual radioactivity in the RA delivers relatively few counts to the radiation detector, because the RA is posterior to the RV and therefore more distant from the detector. At end-systole, atrioventricular separation generally is sufficient to permit clear spatial resolution of the two chambers. Consequently, separate end-diastolic and end-systolic ROIs can result in reasonably accurate RVEF calculations [42] as compared with first-pass methodology (the current standard) [42] or with contrast angiography [41]. Complete time-activity/time volume curves would be very difficult to define from equilibrium studies because overlap and RA contribution to RV counts are difficult to eliminate except at end-diastole and end-systole. Therefore, other physiologic parameters cannot be measured unless first-pass techniques are employed. In practice, frequent use of the method is required for consistent identification of RV borders and valve planes to ensure accurate and reproducible RVEF from equilibrium studies.

Background radioactivity accounts for 35%–60% of total counts in equilibrium studies. Therefore, inconsistencies in background determination can result in relatively large variations in calculated EF. When radionuclide cineangiography first was developed, a crescent of pixels close to the periphery of the LV free wall and apex was found generally to produce a time-activity curve that did not vary during the cardiac cycle (i.e., did not include any meaningful contribution from intrachamber blood); when the average counts in each pixel of this ROI were subtracted from the counts in the pixels of the LV ROI, accurate EF could be calculated. Therefore, this method became standard for background region determination. Other background ROIs have been defined for use with automatic or semiautomatic analysis algorithms. The LV background ROI is also used most commonly to determine RVEF, though a separate background can be determined for this purpose.

Count densities achieved at equilibrium are sufficient to provide statistically stable regional time-activity curves for calculation of regional LVEF; temporal asynchrony also can be detected by comparison of regional time-activity curves [43–45]. This determination can be performed only in the LAO position. Therefore, the distributions of two or more coronary arteries often overlap in a single regional ROI, commonly precluding precise assessment of the contribution of any single lesion to myocardial dysfunction when multivessel disease is present. Despite this potential limitation, of course, regional determinations can be used to quantify the effect of therapeutic interventions.

Definition of absolute chamber volumes can be performed using count-based methods in the LAO view. Attenuation correction [46] and normalization for duration of collection must be performed; calculation then is adjusted for counts collected by the camera (and also normalized for duration of counting) from a reference blood sample drawn from the patient at the time of imaging [47]. If the sample is drawn at a time substantially before or after imaging, counts must be corrected for radioactive decay. Volume determination also can be performed without attenuation correction; when the

calculation accounts for the ratio of total-to-peak LV pixel counts (this ratio is a function of LV volume), there is no need for blood sampling [48]. Geometric formulas exist for calculation of absolute LV volume in the lateral view [49], but resulting accuracy can be expected to be inferior to the count-based approach.

With > 2 minute acquisitions after administration of standard (10–25 mCi) doses of Tc-99m, count density usually is sufficient to provide statistically stable time-activity curves throughout the cardiac cycle. When high (10 ms) temporal resolution is achieved with list mode (or with frame mode at relatively high heart rates), accurate ventricular ejection rates and diastolic performance indexes (peak filling rate, time to peak filling rate, all particularly sensitive to temporal resolution) can be obtained. Diastolic assessments are useful in detecting coronary artery disease (detectable diastolic dysfunction precedes detectable systolic dysfunction) and in assessing drug effects [50–52]. Temporal dispersion of cycle length generally increases in inverse relation to heart rate; temporal dispersion is far greater in diastole (primarily in diastasis) than in systole. Therefore, when patients are at rest, registration of the diastolic portion of the curve may preclude accurate filling rate determinations. Conversely, temporal resolution required to accurately characterize diastolic filling *increases* directly with heart rate. The problem of registration can be obviated by "backward framing," which maximizes diastolic temporal registration; however, this method requires list mode data [7,10,50], which, fortuitously, also can solve the temporal resolution problem. Diastolic functional assessments generally cannot be performed with acceptable accuracy with frame mode.

Radionuclide angiography can be used to define intrinsic LV contractility indexes (generally calculated from pressure-volume relations). For some of these calculations, accurate assessment of afterload stress is employed, requiring measurement of LV mass and wall thicknesses. For this purpose, radionuclide angiographic data can be combined with echocardiographic measures. One such approach, involving normalization of EF change from rest to exercise (ΔEF) for end-systolic stress change from rest to exercise, has proven particularly useful for prognosticating in patients with aortic regurgitation [53]. Indexes of pulmonary vascular pressures also have been obtained during equilibrium radionuclide cineangiography, based on activity in ROIs placed over the lung [54]. This approach is little used today, since efficient and accurate noninvasive pulmonary pressure measurement can be achieved with Doppler echocardiography. However, a rough estimate of pulmonary pressure can be inferred from determination of RVEF, which is inversely proportional to pulmonary pressure [55]. RVEF, itself, is more important as a prognosticator in situations where pulmonary pressures are elevated, as in mitral valve disease or heart failure of any cause.

Other analyses enabled by the high count density of equilibrium radionuclide angiograms include "functional" images, which display regional count density data in a single image, simplifying identification of regional abnormalities. These images include (1) "subtraction" image or "stroke volume map" (end-systolic frame subtracted from end-diastolic frame, with resulting pixel amplitude proportional to the change from diastole to systole; a color code can be employed to depict the gradations of absolute change); (2) EF map, created by normalizing the stroke volume map for the end-diastolic image; and (3) Fourier map to help demarcate specific structures that might be unclear in other functional images. Fourier maps are constructed by transforming the raw two-dimensional spatial images into spatial frequency components relating the rapidity of change in counts in each pixel ("Fourier transformation"). These frequency components are defined in terms of their amplitude and phase, transforming spatial information into the frequency domain. The time-activity curve of each pixel can be approximated as a sinusoidal wave, the lowest frequency of which (the "fundamental frequency") is defined by the heart rate [56–58]. Harmonics of this fundamental frequency can be defined mathematically. From this family of harmonics, each pixel within the ROI can be related in terms of amplitude (a function of stroke volume) and alignment, or phase angle, the latter defining the delay in emptying from one pixel to the next. Fourier expressions can characterize contraction patterns, enabling detection of conduction or contraction abnormalities, adding to regional function assessment.

Since the size of the data set in an equilibrium study is limited only by imaging time and by computer memory, it is possible to collect sufficient data so that highly precise calculations can be performed. However, if similar imaging systems are employed, it can be demonstrated mathematically that, even for the temporally limited acquisition during exercise, precision of volume determination with the equilibrium approach is greater than that with the first-pass technique [59]. (Of course, the first-pass approach traditionally has used equipment providing relatively low spatial resolution in order to enhance counting efficiency.)

CLINICAL APPLICATIONS

Equilibrium radionuclide angiography has been applied in virtually every cardiac disease state. This is not surprising since, to date, LVEF remains the most efficient predictor of outcome in patients with coronary artery disease, valvular heart diseases, and various cardiomyopathies. Consequently, the capacity to measure this parameter is critically important in making decisions about patient management. Nuclear methods, as a group, lack the spatial resolution of echocardiography, X-ray contrast angiography, or magnetic resonance imaging. Therefore, nuclear methods have little value when precise anatomic detail is required (e.g., for coronary plaque localization required to plan surgery, for definition of LV mass, for diagnosis of complex congenital heart defects, for etiologic assessment of valvular diseases, etc.). Nonetheless, particularly during the stress of exercise, assessments of ventricular volumes and their changes arguably can be performed more accurately, efficiently, and expeditiously by equilibirum radionuclide angiography than by any other method currently available.

Early after its development, the primary application of radionuclide cineangiography involved patients with coronary artery disease, both for diagnosis and for prognostication. In recent years, application in this area has declined precipitously as use of geometric methods for LVEF determination has allowed prognostic inferences from LVEF to be obtained from the same scintigram that provides primary diagnostic information from perfusion assessment. Development of the combined approach was facilitated by development of technetium-based perfusion agents, providing count densities adequate for ventricular wall definition even in most infarcted regions. (Today, improving camera and computer technology has allowed application of these same geometric methods to thallium-based perfusion images, as well, though with diminished precision relative to technetium-based imaging.) Though lacking the precision and accuracy of count-based blood pool radionuclide angiographic EF, the functional information available from the perfusion scintigram is adequate to guide most clinical decisions while having the advantage of cost- and time-efficiency compared with the performance of two separate studies, or of combined first-pass blood pool plus perfusion scintigraphy. Nonetheless, diagnostic information available from blood pool radionuclide angiograms is accurate and, in certain cases (e.g., balanced ischemia) superior to that available from perfusion scintigrams. More important, EF-based prognostication from radionuclide angiograms is unsurpassed in patients with coronary artery disease, albeit employed relatively infrequently today.

For nonischemic heart diseases, chamber performance and myocardial function indexes remain the standards for decision making. Here again, blood pool scintigraphy is less commonly used than in earlier years, primarily because of the ease of application of echocardiography and the greater accuracy of this method in providing structural and geometric detail. However, echocardiography is essentially a two-dimensional technique that outlines cardiac structures (though three-dimensional reconstructions are possible from views in multiple planes). Thus, functional assessments are based on geometric formulations, resulting in less accuracy and precision than can be achieved with radionuclide angiography, especially when applied during exercise [60]. Consequently, in many centers, blood pool scintigraphy remains an important part of the routine clinical evaluation strategy for patients with a variety of nonischemic heart diseases and, most particularly, for those with regurgitant valvular diseases. Moreover, because of its relative precision, blood pool scintigraphy generally remains the preferred technique for assessments of drug cardiotoxicity and for therapeutic clinical trials, particularly those with pharmacologic agents, when ventricular function measurement is required.

Coronary Artery Disease

Diagnosis

Reported accuracy for diagnosis of chronic, stable coronary occlusive disease varies widely, as a result of differences in study populations and diagnostic criteria. Sensitivity and specificity both have reached 100% in some studies, but a reasonable synthesis of published studies suggests an average sensitivity in the range of 90% and specificity of approximately 85%. Limitations of diagnostic accuracy are attributable in part to lack of pathobiologic specificity of global or regional ventricular dysfunction for coronary artery disease, the lack of spatial resolution needed to identify very small regions of ischemic dysfunction, and the confounding effects of physiologic compensatory mechanisms (collateral coronary flow, intrinsic myocardial metabolic variations), cardioactive and, particularly, anti-ischemic drugs and comorbid conditions. Nonetheless, radionuclide cineangiography remains a viable diagnostic modality when used alone and adds significantly to diagnostic accuracy when used in conjunction with myocardial perfusion scintigraphy [61–63].

Data on diagnostic accuracy have been extensively reviewed within the past 10 years [36,64]. The first demonstration of diagnostic potential, by Borer et al. [13,14], involved a highly selected group of 11 patients with arteriographically demonstrated coronary obstructions and 14 apparently nondiseased controls; it was followed by a more extensive assessment of diagnostic accuracy by the same group [34], which revealed

diagnostic sensitivity of 95% and specificity of 100%. The high specificity was attributable both to reliance on regional dysfunction rather than the less specific global dysfunction for diagnosis and, more importantly, on exclusion of patients with known valvular, myopathic, congenital, or hypertensive disease, all of which can result in myocardial dysfunction. However, while the latter patient selection factor may have exaggerated calculated specificity, another selection factor, not shared by any subsequent investigation, prevented "artifactual" specificity diminution: since the diagnostic accuracy of radionuclide-based methods was not yet known and since no alternative diagnostic test was available at the time except for catheter-based coronary angiography, patients were not excluded from catheterization because of "low probability" of disease based on other objective factors. This study characteristic would be impossible today if the accuracy of a new diagnostic method were to be assessed. Indeed, as explained by Bayes theorem [65], the current practice of "selection bias" by exclusion from catheterization of patients with normal noninvasive assessments, and substitution of noncatheterized patients with clinically determined "low probability" of disease [66,67] as the "normal" reference population for specificity determination, assures that calculated specificities will underestimate values based on catheterizing consecutive patient series selected only for suggestive symptoms. A reasonable estimate of radionuclide cineangiographic diagnostic accuracy for chronic stable disease was provided by Gibbons [69], who pooled data from eight early peer-reviewed reports (involving 657 catheterized patients, including 495 with coronary disease and 162 without, though these were not necessarily free from heart disease) published through 1981, when selection bias was likely at its minimum. However, this analysis is not strictly relevant to equilibrium studies: six of the eight studies used first-pass methodology and the final estimates were heavily weighted by the largest study of the eight, which employed first-pass methodology and reported the lowest specificity. Despite this limitation, the results were reasonably good: sensitivity averaged 88% (range: 82% to 100%) and specificity averaged 81% (range: 55% to 100%, the latter reported in five of the eight studies). In comparison with other diagnostic methods, the pooled data suggested that, when commonly employed diagnostic criteria are applied for both methods, radionuclide angiography is considerably more sensitive than the exercise ECG, though somewhat less specific, and slightly more sensitive than planar myocardial perfusion scintigraphy with thallium, though slightly less specific. No large-scale comparison has been performed with SPECT perfusion scintigraphy, a test that is more sensitive than the planar modality but seems to maintain the specificity of the planar modality.

The most specific diagnostic finding for coronary artery disease with radionuclide angiography is regional dysfunction [14,34,70], detection of which may be enhanced by use of Fourier transformations [70,71]. However, even this abnormality can be found in association with nonischemic diseases such as dilated cardiomyopathy and aortic regurgitation; in the latter, hypokinesia characteristically appears at the apex, the site at which subendocardial blood flow is limited due to variations in wall stress even when coronary arteries are normal [72]. Global function, inherently nonspecific for ischemia, can be affected by valvular disease [73,74], congenital anomalies [75,76], hypertension [74,77], mitral valve prolapse [78], cardiomyopathy [79,80], certain cardiotoxic drugs [81], extrinsic loads including, perhaps, even those associated with exercise, itself [82], etc. Nonetheless, enhanced diagnostic accuracy has been associated with measurement of a variety of global performance indexes other than LVEF, including a single point contractility descriptor [83], diastolic filling characteristics [7,50,71,84,85], and combinations of descriptors [86]. Pharmacologic stress has been applied to blood pool scintigraphy to unmask ischemia, using both dipyridamole and dobutamine [87–91], but application has been limited and, therefore, a useful reference database for diagnostic and prognostic evaluation is lacking.

Descriptors of ventricular function and volume cannot descriminate between recent and remote impairment. Therefore, radionuclide angiography has little value for diagnosis of acute myocardial infarction (MI). However, the regional impairment associated with MI can be well delineated [92] and functional assessment can be useful in identifying RV involvement when an acute insult is inferred from other data [93]; indeed, despite recent improvements in echocardiographic imaging, radionuclide angiography may be unexcelled in RVMI diagnosis by functional assessment.

Prognosis and management decision making: chronic stable disease

The prognostic value of radionuclide angiography [36] is based on the empirical observation that, when coronary obstructions are present, the effect of exercise on LV function provides a valid index of the likelihood of subsequent ischemic events. Indeed, currently there is no superior method for prognostication, including anatomic definition of the coronary lesion by contrast angiography [36,94]. However, abnormalities unmasked by exercise identify patients at high risk *relative to those who lack the abnormalities*; the accuracy of *absolute* risk determination in any individual is modest [36], though adequate for making rational decisions about the appropriateness of management with or without specific therapies, as discussed below. The reason for this apparent discrepancy is that the relation between exercise-induced cardiac dysfunction and ischemic events is largely fortuitous. Patients do not die or sustain infarction because of ischemia measured during exercise testing but rather because of sudden structural change in a lesion that may or may not have caused the exercise-induced dysfunction. The biological relation between test result and event is, at best, tenuous. Indeed, improvement in prognostication and management decision making probably will require application of radiolabeled metabolites or ligands that enable identification of unstable plaques imminently likely to rupture [95].

Nonetheless, until interrogation of lesion biology becomes a reality, radionuclide angiography provides the most accurate and precise noninvasive prognostication in patients with coronary artery disease. Early demonstration of prognostic utility was made with the first-pass technique [96], an important observation, since, as noted previously, first-pass studies can be obtained immediately after isotope is injected for myocardial perfusion scintigraphy so that both types of data can be obtained in a single study. However, equilibrium studies inherently are more precise than first-pass [59] and, in recent years, have provided considerable prognostic information based on studies involving more than 2500 patients [94,97–109] (Table 17.4). In patients with coronary artery disease, prognosis varies directly with LVEF whether measured at rest (LVEF$_{rest}$), during maximal, symptom-limited exercise (LVEF$_{exercise}$), or as ∆LVEF. However, prognostic efficiency of these parameters differs in a manner that affects their applicability in specific situations. Thus, when LVEF$_{rest}$ is < 30%, markedly restricted life expectancy can be inferred (> 10% per year mortality risk); below this value mortality risk varies inversely with LVEF$_{rest}$ and also with LVEF$_{exercise}$, which tends to track directly and closely with LVEF$_{rest}$ in this low range. ∆LVEF has little discriminatory capacity below the 30% cutpoint. Risk is considerably less, though still greater than that expected in an unselected age-matched population, when LVEF$_{rest}$ is > 30% but less than normal. LVEF$_{rest}$ has little prognostic discriminatory capacity within the very wide normal range. In contrast, LVEF$_{exercise}$ maintains prognostic utility throughout its range. However, when LVEF$_{rest}$ is > 30%, the *most* potent prognosticator is ∆LVEF, which is significantly more pre-

TABLE 17.4 *Prognostic Value of Equilibrium Radionuclide Angiography in Chronic Stable Coronary Artery Disease*

Study	Population (No. Pts)	End Points	Results
Bonow et al. [98]	(117) Med Rx FCa I-II; EFr > 40% Documented CAD V = ≥ 1, ≥ 50% LDN	Sudden death Sudden death or ↑ AP	*AMR* ΔEF < 0%(no rise), ↓ ST, ex cap ≤ 120W ⇒ 7.5% (3V only) ΔEF < 0%, ↓ ST ⇒ 4.5% Ex cap ≤ 120 W ⇒ 2.0% ↓ ST ⇒ 2.0% ΔEF < 0% ⇒ 1.75% ΔEF ≥ 0% ⇒ 0% ↓ ST ⇒ 0% Ex cap > 120 W ⇒ 0%
Bonow et al. [97]	(131) Med Rx; FCa ≤ I EFr > 40% Documented CAD V ≥ 1, ≥ 50% LDN	Sudden death	All Sudden deaths were in pts with 3V + ΔEF < 0% + ↓ ST Risk stratification/prognostic implication of silent inducible ischemia & symptomatic ischemia were similar ΔEF and ↓ ST correlated with anatomic severity of CAD
Clements et al. [99]	(93) Med Rx EFr < 50%; FCa = 0-IV CAD = suspected	Cardiac death Cardiac events	*AMR* TPFR < 167 ms ⇒ 27% EFr < 35% ⇒ 24% PFR ≥ 1.67 ⇒ 18% PFR < 1.67 ⇒ 10% EFr ≥ 35% ⇒ 5% TPFR ≥ 167 ms ⇒ 2%
Mazotta et al. [100]	(53) FCa ≤ II; EFr = 20-40% Documented CAD V ≤ 2, LDN ≥ 50%	Cardiac death Cardiac events	*AMR* EF$_x$ ≤ 30% ⇒ 6.3%; EFx > 30% ⇒ 0.5%; RR = 12.6, p < .05 ΔEF ≤ 0% (no rise) ⇒ 4.3%; ΔEF > 0% (rise) ⇒ 0.0%; p < .005 *Annual Cardiac Event Risk* EF$_x$ ≤ 30% ⇒ 8.8%; EFx > 30% ⇒ 3.2%; RR = 2.75, p < .005 ΔEF ≤ 0% ⇒ 6.7%; ΔEF > 0% ⇒ 2.4%; RR = 2.79, p < .005
Miller et al. [101]	(65) FCb ≥ 0;EFr < 50% Documented CAD	Death (all causes) Cardiac events	*Mortality Risk Through 18 Months:by Univariate Cox Model* EF$_r$ ⇒ x^2 = 12.72, p < 0.005 EF$_x$ ⇒ x^2 = 11.71, p < 0.005, V ≤ 2, LDN ≥ 70% Cardiac Event Risk Through 18 months +Severely ischemic RNCA ⇒ 27%; − ⇒ 8%;RR = 3.38, p < .05
Supino et al. [102]	(41) Post-CABG ≥65 yrs V ≥ 1; LDN ≥ 50%	Death (all causes) Cardiac events	*AMR* EFr ≤ 45% ⇒ 7.8%; EFr > 45% ⇒ 2.3%; RR = 3.39; p < .04 RI = incompl ⇒ 6.0%; RI = compl ⇒ 1.7%; RR = 3.53; p < .06 *AAR Major Nonsurgical Cardiac Events* 3V ⇒ 5.6%; 1-2V ⇒ 1.0; RR = 5.6; p < .08
Taliercio et al. [103]	(424) Documented CAD V ≥ 1; FC$_a$ < II	Cardiac events	*AAR for Cardiac Events* EFr < 30% ⇒ 11%; EFr > 50% ⇒ 1%; RR = 11% Only EFr, V and age were independently related to CE
Wallis et al. [104]	(265) CAD documented byCath in 161 EFr < 30% 227 Med Rx; 38 Surg	Death (all causes)	*AMR* Med (n = 227) Surg (n = 38) EFr ≤ 15% ⇒ 23.3% 22.5% EFx < 20% ⇒ 19.9% 10.0% Overall mortality ⇒ 14.8% 3.3% EFr > 15% ⇒ 10.0% 3.3% EFx ≥ 20% ⇒ 6.7% 0%
Wallis et al. [105]	(192) Post-CABG FC$_b$ ≥ 1;EFr ≥ 30%	Cardiac death Cardiac events	*AMR* *Death Death/MI Death/MI/CABG/PTCA* ΔEF: fall ≥ 10% ⇒ 8.5% 11.3% 17.0% ΔEF: −9% to 0% ⇒ 2.3% 3.8% 6.2% ΔEF > 0% (rise) ⇒ 0.8% 2.0% 4.2% (ΔEF independently (p < 0.0001) predicted death, death/MI and death/MI/reCABG/PTCA rates

TABLE 17.4 (*Continued*)

Study	Population (No. Pts)	End Points	Results
Iqbal et al. [106]	(536) CAD: Suspected	Cardiac events	*4 Year MI-free Survival (Independent Predictors)*

Iqbal et al. [106] — (536) CAD: Suspected — Cardiac events

4 Year MI-free Survival (Independent Predictors)

	Hazard Ratio	(95% CI)	p
EF < 58% (vs ≥ 58%)	⇒ 0.5	(0.4–0.7)	< .001
HRx > 122 bpm (vs ≤ 122 bpm)	⇒ 0.4	(0.3–0.6)	< .001
Hx MI vs no MI hx	⇒ 0.2	(1.1–3.5)	< .01
Age > 65 yrs (vs ≤ 65 yrs)	⇒ 1.5	(1.1–2.2)	< .04

Moriel et al. [107] — (419) ΔEF, Med Rx, 52% Hx MI — Cardiac events

5 Yr Cardiac Event Rates (Independent Predictors)

Prior MI

ΔWMS ≥ 2 ⇒ ~62%; ΔWMS < 2 ⇒ ~25%; RR ~ 2.5, p = .0001

No Prior MI

EFx < 55% ⇒ ~45%; EFx ≥ 55% ⇒ ~27%; RR ~ 1.7, p = .04

Shapira et al. [108] — (100) post-CABG — Cardiac death, Cardiac events

6 Yr Cardiac Death/Event Rates (Independent Predictors)

Cardiac death	⇒ ΔEF (cutpoint NA, p = .03)
MI	⇒ EFr (cutpoint NA, p = .05)
reCABG/PTCA	⇒ ΔEF (cutpoint NA, p = .002)
All events	⇒ ΔEF (cutpoint NA, p = .009)
	⇒ EFr (cutpoint NA, p = .02)

Shaw et al. [109] — (863) documented CAD by Cath symptomatic, Med Rx — Cardiac death

RR of Cardiac Death during 5 Yr Followup

	RR	95%CI	p
EFr	⇒ 1.2	1.1–1.5	<.0001
EFx	⇒ 1.4	1.2–1.6	<.0001
Peak workload	⇒ 1.9	1.1–1.4	.0002
"Clinical index"	⇒ 1.6	1.4–1.8	.0006

Supino et al. [94] — (167) documented CAD by Cath, V = 3; LDN ≥ 50% — Cardiac death, Cardiac events

AAR of Events Among Patient Sub-groups

	Med Rx	Early CABG	Late CABG	All CABG
Cardiac Death				
ΔEF > 0%(rise)	⇒ 0.0%	0.0%	0.0%	0.0%
ΔEF:0 to −7%	⇒ 1.4%	0.0%	2.7%	1.5%
ΔEF:rise/fall < −8%	⇒ 0.8%	0.0%	2.3%	1.3%
ΔEF:fall ≥ −8%	⇒ 4.3%	0.5%	1.7%	1.2%
all patients	⇒ 1.9%	0.3%	1.9%	1.2%
Cardiac Death or MI				
ΔEF > 0% (rise)	⇒ 0.9%	0.0%	0.0%	0.0%
ΔEF 0 to −7%	⇒ 2.8%	0.0%	2.7%	1.5%
ΔEF:rise/fall < −8%	⇒ 1.9%	0.0%	2.3%	1.3%
ΔEF: fall ≥ −8%	⇒ 6.9%	1.4%	3.0%	2.3%
all patients	⇒ 3.5%	0.9%	2.7%	2.0%

ΔEF was strongest independent predictor (p = .003) of cardiac events among medical patients; preop ΔEF also predicted magnitude of CABG benefit (p = .04)

AAR, average annual risk; AMR, annual mortality risk; BPM, beats per minute; CABG, coronary artery bypass grafting; CAD, coronary artery disease; Cath, coronary angiography; CHF, congestive heart failure; compl, complete revascularization; EDP, end-diastolic pressure; EF, left ventricular ejection fraction; ex cap, exercise capacity; ΔWMS, exercise wall motion worsening score; FCa, Canadian Heart Association functional class; FCb, New York Heart Association functional class; HTN, hypertension; Hx, history; incompl, incomplete revascularization; LDN, luminal diameter narrowing; MI, nonfatal myocardial infarction; NA, not available; PFR, peak filling rate; PTCA, percutaneous transluminal coronary angioplasty; r, rest; revasc, revascularization; RI, revascularization index; RNCA, radionuclide cineangiogram; RR, relative risk; surg, surgical; ↓ ST, ST segment depression ≥ 1 mm; TPFR, time to peak filling rate; V, number of stenotic arteries; W, watts; WMA, wall motion abnormality; WMS, wall motion score; x, exercise; Δ, change from r to x; +, present; −, absent. Cardiac events may include cardiac death or MI, CHF, nonfatal arrest, CABG, or PTCA.

*Medications not held for RNCA.

dictive than LVEFexercise for the more than 90% of patients who fall into this category [94]. Specific prognostic cut points vary among reported studies (see Table 17.4). However, in general, risk of events (death or MI) is > 5% per year when ΔLVEF is at least −5% and can be significantly improved by surgical therapy [94]; parallel risks can be inferred when LVEFexercise is < 30% [109]. The prognostic utility of radionuclide angiography applies whether or not bypass grafting or angioplasty have been performed prior to testing [105].

Most important, prognostication with radionuclide angiography lends itself to selection among competing therapeutic/management options for patients with chronic, clinically stable ischemic heart disease. To optimize management decisions, the physician should know the effect on prognosis of all possible management options. To provide this information, studies must involve populations with relatively similar primary disease characteristics who are evaluated by the chosen prognostic test prior to randomized application of all available management strategies. Though such optimal information is not available for any cardiovascular disease, reasonable estimates of the relative prognostic benefit of coronary artery bypass grafting plus medical therapy versus medical therapy alone recently has been developed for patients who, prior to therapy, had three-vessel coronary artery disease and $LVEF_{rest} > 30\%$. In this study, management was not assigned on a randomized basis; rather, surgery was undertaken because of worsening symptoms or because of the belief of the primary physician that long-term outcome could be improved by this strategy. Therefore, in general, patients who underwent surgery were likely to have been more severely ill than those who did not, causing underestimation of any benefits of surgery. Nonetheless, from among 167 patients with three-vessel coronary artery disease who were followed an average of 9 years if event-free, it was possible to relate index $\Delta LVEF$ to subsequent relative risk of death or infarction when surgery was or was not added to medical therapy [94] (Fig. 17.21). When $\Delta LVEF$ rose during exercise, no advantage accrued to those undergoing surgical therapy. As $\Delta LVEF$ fell in the population, the benefit of surgery gradually increased, reaching a fivefold advantage at 9 years when index $\Delta LVEF$ was $\geq 20\%$.

Prognosis and management decision making: early postmyocardial infarction

Equilibrium radionuclide angiography also can be applied to prognosticate during the acute and early recovery phases of myocardial infarction (Table 17.5). $LVEF_{rest}$ is a primary determinant of survival both during hospitalization [36,110] and after discharge [36,111,112,117] irrespective of whether thrombolysis or angioplasty is applied, though, of course, the absolute relation of LVEF to mortality risk has been altered by the use of early revascularization. As a corollary, radionuclide-based regional $LVEF_{rest}$ can confirm sustained reperfusion of the infarct-related artery after thrombolysis [113]. $LVEF_{exercise}$ improves predictive accuracy for posthospital survival in the absence or presence of throm-

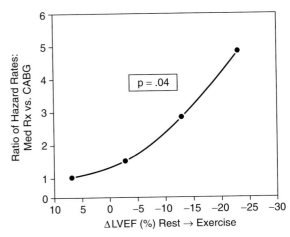

FIGURE 17.21 Relation of baseline ischemia severity to benefit of coronary artery bypass grafting (CABG) among 167 patients with three-vessel coronary artery disease. *P* value reflects differences among cardiac event hazard ratios (H/R) for death or myocardial infarction [MI] derived from non-CABG (medically treated) vs CABG-treated patients, stratified according to sequential 10% increments of change in left ventricular ejection ($\Delta LVEF$) fraction from rest to exercise at initial study ($+3\%$ to $+12\%$ [midpoint = $+7.5\%$, H/R $\approx$ 1]; $+2\%$ to -7% [midpoint = -2.5%, H/R = 1.60]; -8% to -17% [midpoint = -12.5%, H/R = 2.94], -18% to -27% [midpoint = -22.5%, H/R = 4.95]). MED Rx = medical treatment. (Reproduced with permission of the American Heart Association, Dallas, TX: Supino et al. Circulation 1999;100:924–932.)

bolysis or primary angioplasty [114–116,118–127], while tomographic imaging with SPECT allows prognostication among patients undergoing LV aneurysmectomy, a complication of MI [26].

Assessment of pharmacologic and mechanical interventions. By quantifying ventricular volumes and systolic and diastolic performance at rest and during exercise, equilibrium radionuclide angiography provides useful data for assessing the effects of drugs, surgery, and angioplasty in patients with CAD [e.g.,36,105, 116,32,128].

Valvular Heart Diseases

Recent epidemiological data indicate that valvular heart diseases (Table 17.6) affect substantially more than 10 million individuals in the United States alone; hemodynamically severe valvular abnormalities, which may be appropriate for surgical therapy to prevent heart failure or sudden death in asymptomatic patients, are present in as many as 4 million Americans, and are increasing in prevalence as the population ages [129]. Management of patients with valvular heart diseases represents a particularly challenging problem for clinicians. Diagnosis and quantification of hemodynamic severity are best made with echocardiography. How-

TABLE 17.5 *Prognostic Value of Equilibrium Radionuclide Angiography after Acute Myocardial Infarction*

Study	Population (No. Pts)	End Points	Results
Abraham et al. [117]	(75)	Cardiac death or major nonfatal events	*2-Year Cumulative Risk of Cardiac Death or Major Nonfatal Events* EFx < 50% ⇒ 58%; EFx ≥ 50% ⇒ 17%, RR = 3.41, $p < .05$ EFr < 50% ⇒ 46%; EFr ≥ 50% ⇒ 16%, RR = 2.88, NS
Candell-Riera et al. [116]	(115)	Death or major nonfatal events	*1 Yr Probability of Death or Major Nonfatal Events* (Echo) EFr < 45%, aneurysm ⇒ 88% (Tl201) # of ischemic segments > 1 ⇒ 86% (RNCA) EFx < 40% ⇒ 82% Load × < 75 W ⇒ 79% Cath: aneurysm ⇒ 75%
Corbett et al. [118]	(61)	Cardiac death or major nonfatal events	*Cardiac Death or Major Nonfatal Events During Avg 9.6 Mos* 　　　　　　　　SENSITIVITY　　SPECIFICITY ΔESVI: increase > 5% ⇒　95%　　96% ΔEF: rise < 5% ⇒　95%　　96% P/VI × < 35% ⇒　97%　　88% ΔWMS (↓) ⇒　81%　　88%
Corbett et al. [119]	(117)	Sudden death or major nonfatal events	*Predictive Accuracy for Sudden Death or Major Nonfatal Events Through 6 Mos* ΔEF: rise < 5% ⇒ 93% ΔESVI: increase > 5% ⇒ 91% EFr ≤ 40% vs EFr > 40% differentiated pts with events from event-free pts ($p < 0.001$)
Dewhurst and Muir [120]	(100)	Sudden death Major cardiac events	*Predictive Value for Sudden Death ≤ 2 yrs* EFr < 35% ⇒ 40%; EFx < 35% + Δ EF: fall > 5% ⇒ 88% *Predictive Value for Sudden CHF ≤ 1yr* EFr < 35% ⇒ 100%
Kuchar et al. [121]	(153)	Cardiac death Major nonfatal events	*Cardiac Death Risk During Median 14 Mos* EFr < 40% ⇒ 11%; EFr > 40% ⇒ 1%; RR = 11.0, $p < .05$ *Major Cardiac Event Risk During Median 14 Mos* EFx < 30% ⇒ 31%; EFx ≥ 30% ⇒ 5%; RR = 6.2%, $p < 0.001$
Morris et al. [122]	(106)	Cardiac death Nonfatal MI UAP AP → CABG	*CV Death Risk Through 2 Yrs* EFx < 40% ⇒ ≈ 30%; EFx > 40% ⇒ ≈ 10%, RR = ≈ 3.0 (p value not given) EFx : strongest multivariate predictor of cardiac death ($p < .001$)
Nicod et al. [123]	(42)	Cardiac death or major nonfatal events	*Predictive Accuracy for Cardiac Death or Major Nonfatal Events During 8 Mos* 　　　　　　In 1-V　　In Multi-V 　　　　　　Disease Pts　Disease Pts EFr < 55% ⇒　44%　　77% EFr ≤ 40% ⇒　50%　　50% ΔEF: rise < 5% ⇒　81%　　96% ΔESVI: increase > 5% ⇒　69%　　77%
Roig et al. [124]	(93)	Cardiac death or major nonfatal events	*For Future Cardiac Events During Avg 16 Mos* 　　　　　SENSITIVITY　SPECIFICITY ΔEF: fall > 5% ⇒　43%　　90% WMAr ⇒　64%　　72% ΔEF: rise < 5% ⇒　79%　　58% Event risk best predicted by baseline ΔEF < 5% ($p < .03$), 　ΔEF < −5% ($p < .01$)
Mazotta et al. [125]	(183)	Cardiac death or major nonfatal events Cardiac death or CHF	*4 Yr Probability of Cardiac Death or Major Nonfatal Events* ΔEF < 0% + ↓ ST + x-inducible angina ⇒ 74% ΔEF < 0% + ST ↓ only ⇒ 33% x-inducible angina only ⇒ 30% none of the above ⇒ 17% *4 Yr Probability of Cardiac death or CHF* EFx ≤ 35% ⇒ 48%; EFx > 35% ⇒ 16.6%, RR = 2.89, 　$p < .0001$

(Table continues on next page)

TABLE 17.5 *Prognostic Value of Equilibrium Radionuclide Angiography after Acute Myocardial Infarction (Continued)*

Study	Population (No. Pts)	End Points	Results
Zhu et al. [126]	(94)	Cardiac death or major nonfatal events	*3 Yr Event Rates: death, MI or nonfatal arrest* EFx < 40% ⇒ 26%; EFx ≥ 40% ⇒ 2%; RR = 13.0; p = .003 *3 Yr Event Rates: death, MI, nonfatal arrest or late CABG/PTCA* EFx < 40% ⇒ 31%, EFx ≥ 40% ⇒ 9%; RR = 3.44; p = .003 EFx independent (p = .003) predictor of cardiac death or nonfatal events
Gosselink et al. [127]	(272)	Cardiac death Cardiac death or MI	*Cardiac Death Risk During Avg 30 Mos* EFr < 40% ⇒ 16%; EFr ≥ 40% ⇒ 2%; RR = 8, p = .0004 *Cardiac Event Risk During Avg 30 Mos* X Risk Score ≥ 2 ⇒ 10%, X Risk Score < 2 ⇒ 1%; RR = 10.0, p = .0008

Cath, cardiac catheterization; CHF, congestive heart failure; CV, cardiovascular; echo, echocardiography; r, rest; MI, myocardial infarction; NS, not significant; MI, myocardial infarction (reinfarction); P/VI, pressure-volume index; r, rest; RNCA, radionuclide cineangiography; ↓ ST, ECG ST segment depression ≥ 1 mm; UAP, unstable angina pectoris; WMA, wall motion abnormality; V, vessel; WMS, wall motion score; x, exercise; ↓, worsening; Δ, change from r to x. Major nonfatal events may include MI, CHF, angina pectoris (AP), unstable AP, resuscitated arrest, coronary artery bypass grafting, percutaneous transluminal coronary angioplasty, or arrhythmia.

ever, prognosis, on which selection of patients for surgical amelioration of the valvular lesion depends, is more appropriately based on the myocardial response to the pressure or volume loads induced by the disease than on the magnitude of the loads, themselves. Equilibrium radionuclide angiography is more precise than echocardiography for this purpose, both at rest and, particularly, during exercise [60], when myocardial contractile abnormalities are unmasked to optimize prognostication in the asymptomatic patient [53,130, 131].

Stenotic lesions

Though the pathophysiology of aortic stenosis and the effects of surgery on LVEF have been clarified with equilibrium radionuclide cineangiographic studies [74,131–133], as yet there is no role for this method in identifying patients most appropriate for valve surgery. In patients with mitral stenosis, too, pathophysiology and effects of surgery have been elucidated [131], but criteria for surgery do not require radionuclide-

based investigations. However, the primary shock organ in mitral stenosis is the RV, uniquely assessable by radionuclide angiography, though the first-pass approach is the method of choice. Nonetheless, as in mitral regurgitation (see below), RV volume and performance from equilibrium studies have prognostic value [134,135] that may be useful in management decisions.

Regurgitant lesions

Radionuclide-based measures of ventricular performance, size, and function are of well-established value in identifying patients for prophylactic valve surgery if either aortic or mitral regurgitation is present [131]. LVEF$_{rest}$ is a primary determinant of prognosis for aortic regurgitation (AR) [149,151]; subnormal LVEF$_{rest}$, even in the absence of symptoms, is accepted by consensus as a basis for "prophylactic" operation to prolong life. The strategy is based in part on preoperative radionuclide angiographic evaluations and subsequent postoperative follow-up of symptomatic patients who

TABLE 17.6 *Prognostic Value of Equilibrium Radionuclide Angiography in Valvular Heart Diseases*

Study	Population (No. Pts)	End Points	Results
Bonow et al. [149]	80 Post AVR	Death (all causes)	*Death Risk Through 5.5 Years Post AVR* Preop LVEF$_r$ ≤ 45% ⇒ 37%; LVEF > 45% ⇒ 4%; RR = 9.25, p < .01 Preop LVEF$_r$ ≤ 45% + x time < 22.5mins or preop + postop LV dysfunction > 18 mos⇒ 48%; other pts ⇒ 3%; RR = 16.0, p < .005 Preop LVEF$_x$ (p < .02), FS (p < .001) and LVIDs (p < .01) also predicted death as continuous variables

TABLE 17.6 *Prognostic Value of Equilibrium Radionuclide Angiography in Valvular Heart Disease (Continued)*

Study	Population (No. Pts)	End Points	Results
Hochreiter et al. [55]	(53) Chronic severe MR 35 Med Rx, 21 VS* (*incl 3 cross-overs from MED Rx)	Sudden or CHF death	*Death During Avg 28 mos (Med Patients)* $RVEF_r \leq 30 + /-LVEF_r \leq 45 \Rightarrow 62.5\%$; $RVEF_r > 30 + LVEF_r > 45 \Rightarrow 0\%$; $RR = N/C$ $p < .001$ $+ VT \Rightarrow 11\%$; $- VT$ Preop FC_b 4 4%; $RR = 16.0$, $p < .005$ $LVEF_{r,x}$; $RVEF_{r,x}$; FS ($p \leq .001$); $LVIDs$ ($p < .01$); $\Delta RVEF$ ($p < .05$) also predict death as continuous variables
Furer et al. [150]	(18) Post MVR	Persistent postop Sx	*Predictive Accuracy of Preop Predictors For Persistent Postop Sx Post MVR* $ESS/ESVI < 1.9 \Rightarrow 94\%$ $ESS/ESVI \times LVEF < .80 \Rightarrow 94\%$ $FS < 31\% \Rightarrow 89\%$ Preop FC 4 $\Rightarrow 89\%$ $RVEF \leq 30\% \Rightarrow 83\%$ $LVEF < 45\% \Rightarrow 72\%$ $LVIDsi > 2.6/m^2 \Rightarrow 89\%$
Rosen et al. [130]	(31) Chronic severe MR asx/min sx nl RV/LVEF_r	Operable Sx	*AAR of Op Sx During Avg 5 Yrs* $\Delta RVEF \leq 0$ (no change or fall) $\Rightarrow 14.8\%$; $\Delta RVEF > 0$ (rise) $\Rightarrow 4.9\%$; $RR = 3.02$ $\Delta RVEF$ also independently predicts ($p < .03$) operable sx as continuous variable)
Borer et al. [53]	(104) Chronic severe AR asx/min sx, nl LVEF	Operable Sx, LV dysfunction or cardiac death	*AAR of All Cardiac Endpoints During Avg 7 Yrs* $\Delta LVEF$-ESS Index -17 to $-33 \Rightarrow 13.3\%$; $\Delta LVEF$-ESS Index -1 to $-11 \Rightarrow 1.8\%$; $RR = 7.39$, $p = .0001$ $\Delta LVEF$: fall $> 5\% \Rightarrow 12.5\%$; $\Delta LVEF$: rise $> 3\% \Rightarrow 1.9\%$; $RR = 6.58$, $p = .001$ $\Delta LVEF$-ESS Index independently predicted ($p < .001$) all endpoints
Tornos et al. [151]	(85) Post AVR	Postop CHF	*RR of CHF During Avg 6 Postop Yrs* $LVEF_r < 40$:RR vs. $LVEF > 40 = 10.6$ (95% CI: 2.3-50) $ESD > 50$: RR vs. $ESD \leq 50 = 7.4$ (95% CI: 2-27) Age > 50: RR vs. age $\leq 50 = 10.4$ (95% CI: 2.3-49) $LVEF_r$ ESD and age independently predicted CHF in multivariate model
Borer et al. [140]	(43) Post AVR	Death (all causes) or persistent Sx	*Deaths or Persistent Sx During Avg 12 Postop Yrs* $\Delta LVEF$-ESS -13.7 or more negative $\Rightarrow 59.1\%$; $\Delta LVEF$-ESS 0 to $-13.7 \Rightarrow 28.6\%$; $RR = 2.07$ $p = .04$ $\Delta LVEF$-ESS was sole outcome predictor in univariate analysis
Supino et al. [144]	(61) Chronic severe AR asx/min sx, nl LVEFr	Sudden death, CHF or subnl LVEF_r ($< 45\%$)	*AAR of Death or Persistent Sx* $\Delta LVEF$: fall $\geq 5\%$ at baseline $+$ at 5 yrs $\Rightarrow 22\%$ $\Delta LVEF$: fall $\geq 5\%$ at 5 yrs only $\Rightarrow 11\%$ $\Delta LVEF$: fall $\geq -5\%$ at baseline only $\Rightarrow 4\%$ $\Delta LVEF$: fall $\geq -5\%$ absent: $\Rightarrow 3\%$; p (global) $= .0004$ $\Delta LVEF$ at 5 yrs, best independent predictor ($p = .01$)
Hochreiter et al. [152]	(52) Post MVR	Sudden death	*5 Yr Rates of Sudden Death* Consistent VT $\Rightarrow 13\%$ ($p = .01$ vs. no [or inconsistent] VT: no deaths) Consistent VT $+$ subnl $LVEF_r$ and/or $RVEF_r \Rightarrow 17\%$ Consistent VT, nl $LVEF_r$ and/or $RVEF_r \Rightarrow 8\%$ Inconsistent (or no VT) with/without subnl $LVEF_r/RVEF_r \Rightarrow$ no deaths
Wencker et al. [143]	(14) "High risk" post MVR	Death (all causes)	*Avg Survival Time 9 Years Post MVR* $RVEF_r \leq 20\% \Rightarrow 6.9$ yrs; $RVEF_r > 20\% \Rightarrow 14$ yrs; $RST = 0.49$, $p = .03$ $RVEF_x \leq 20\% \Rightarrow 7.7$ yrs; $RVEF_x > 20\% \Rightarrow 14$ yrs; $RST = 0.55$, $p = .05$

AAR, average annual risk; AR, aortic regurgitation; asx, asymptomatic; AVR, aortic valve replacement; CHF, congestive heart failure; d, at diastole; EDV, end-diastolic volume; EF, ejection fraction; ESD, end systolic diameter; ESS, end systolic stress; ESV, end systolic volume; FC, New York Heart Association Functional Class; FS, fractional shortening; i, index/indexed; LV, left ventricular; ID, internal dimension; Med Rx, unoperated; min, minimally; MR, mitral regurgitation; MV, mitral valve; nl, normal; preop, preoperative; postop, postoperative; RR, relative risk; r, rest; RST, relative survival time; RV, right ventricular; s, at systole; sx, symptoms/ symptomatic; VS, valve surgery; VT, ventricular tachycardia; x, exercise; Δ, change from rest to exercise; $+$, present; $-$, absent

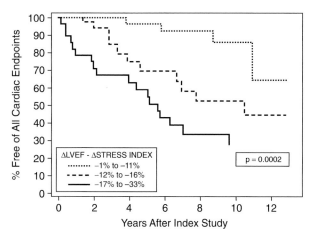

FIGURE 17.22 Relation of a myocardial contractility descriptor (ΔLVEF-ΔESS) to occurrence of any cardiac end point (death, operable symptoms, and/or subnormal LV performance at rest) during follow-up. Population has been divided statistically into 3 terciles. ΔLVEF-ΔESS index boundaries for each tercile are boxed. ΔLVEF = change in left ventricular ejection fraction from rest to exercise, ΔESS = change in end-systolic wall stress from rest to exercise. (Reproduced with permission of the American Heart Association, Dallas, TX: Borer et al. Circulation 1998;97:525–534.)

underwent aortic valve replacement for aortic regurgitation [136,137]. However, study of unoperated *asymptomatic* patients with *normal* LVEF$_{rest}$ indicates that ΔLVEF from equilibrium radionuclide cineangiography is efficient in predicting heart failure, subsequent development of subnormal LVEF$_{rest}$ or sudden death and is even more accurate when adjusted for echocardiographically defined wall stress to form a myocardial contractility index [53] (Fig. 17.22). This measure is more predictive than other radionuclide-based or echocardiographic measures alone, efficiently predicts long-term postoperative survival [140], and can be used to select asymptomatic patients for prophylactic surgery [53]. In addition, progression to a surgical end point or sudden death is predicted by the rate at which ΔLVEF deteriorates over time [144]. Equilibrium studies also have provided unique information about the natural history of LV recovery after surgery [138] contributing to pathophysiologic observations now being further evaluated with cellular and molecular studies [139].

Unlike aortic regurgitation, for which the LV is the primary shock organ, mitral regurgitation (MR) affects both ventricles, imposing a volume overload on the LV and, eventually, a pressure load on the RV. Because it allows measurement of both LVEF and RVEF, radionuclide angiography is particularly well adapted for application in MR [55,130,131]. LVEF is a potent predictor of outcome in patients with MR [141,150], but

radionuclide cineangiographic data suggest that RVEF is a more sensitive indicator of prognostically important cardiac dysfunction [55,130]. RVEF is inversely related to pulmonary artery pressure [55]; when RVEF is subnormal, pulmonary hypertension of at least mild-to-moderate severity is present. Subnormal RVEF$_{rest}$ also indicates relatively high imminent mortality risk, predominantly sudden [55], even in the absence of symptoms. When both LVEF and RVEF are normal at rest in asymptomatic patients, failure of the normal augmentation of RVEF$_{exercise}$ predicts accelerated progression to heart failure; the rate of progression is related to the negative magnitude of ΔRVEF [130]. Finally, both LVEF and RVEF are useful in predicting the long-term outcome of mitral valve surgery (Fig. 17.23), and can be particularly useful in identifying those who will benefit from surgery despite severe biventricular dysfunction [131,143] and severe arrhythmia [152]; parallel data have been reported for combined MR/AR [142].

Cardiomyopathies, Heart Failure, Congenital Heart Disease

Serial LVEF determinations by radionuclide angiography have been used to select patients with heart failure for cardiac transplantation [136] (a situation in which the common occurrence of regional dysfunction renders geometric determinations of LVEF problematic), to assess pathophysiology [80,146] (potentially useful for treatment selection), and to evaluate treatment [79] in patients with cardiomyopathy, to titrate doses of cardiotoxic drugs [81,145] (e.g., doxorubicin)

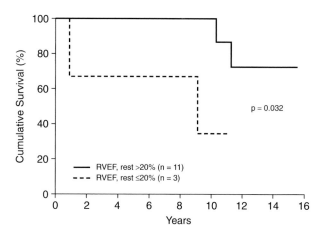

FIGURE 17.23 Survival in operated patients with mitral regurgitation (MR) and left ventricular ejection fraction (LVEF) $\leq$ 30% as a function of right ventricular ejection fraction (RVEF). (Reproduced with permission: Wencker et al. Cardiology 2000;93:37–42.)

used for comorbid conditions, to assess efficacy of new therapies for patients with heart failure or acute ischemic syndromes [148], and to evaluate pathophysiology and treatment effects in patients with congenital heart diseases [75,147].

ACKNOWLEDGMENTS

Preparation of this material was supported in part by The Howard Gilman Foundation, New York, NY, and The Gladys and Roland Harriman Foundation, New York, NY.

REFERENCES

1. Folse R, Braunwald E. Determination of fraction of left ventricular volume ejected per beat and of ventricular end-diastolic and residual volumes. Circulation 1962;25:674.

2. Hoffmann G, Kleine N. Die methode der radiokardiographischen funktions analyse. Nuklearmedizin 1968;7:350.

3. Bacharach SL, Green MV, Borer JS, et al. ECG-gated scintillation probe measurement of left ventricular function. J Nucl Med 1977;18:1176.

4. Tamaki N, Yasuda T, Moore RH, et al. Continuous monitoring of left ventricular function by an ambulatory radionuclide detector in patients with coronary artery disease. J Am Coll Cardiol 1988;12:669.

5. Mason DT, Ashburn WL, Harbert JC, et al. Rapid sequential visualization of the heart and great vessels in man using the wide-field Anger scintillation camera. Circulation 1969;39:19.

6. Strauss WH, Zaret BL, Hurley PJ, et al. A scintigraphic method for measuring left ventricular ejection fraction in man without cardiac catheterization. Am J Cardiol 1971;28:575.

7. Bacharach SL, Green MV, Borer JS, et al. Left ventricular peak ejection rate, filling rate and ejection fraction: frame rate requirements at rest and exercise. J Nucl Med 1979;20:189.

8. Parker JA, Secker-Walker R, Hill R, et al. A new technique for the calculation of left ventricular ejection fraction. J Nucl Med 1972;13:649.

9. Green MV, Ostrow HG, Doulas MA, et al. Scintigraphic cineangiography of the heart. Proceedings MEDINFO 74, North Holland Publishing Co. (Amsterdam) 1974;pp 827.

10. Green MV, Bailey JJ, Ostrow HG, et al. Computerized EKG-gated radionuclide angiocardiography: a non-invasive method for determining left ventricular volumes and focal myocardial dyskinesia. Comput Cardiol (IEEE) 1975; pp. 137.

11. Green MV, Bacharach SL, Douglas MA, et al. The measurement of left ventricular function and the detection of wall motion abnormalities with high temporal resolution ECG-gated scintigraphic angiocardiography. IEEE Trans Nucl Sci 1976;23: 1257.

12. Bacharach SL, Green MV, Borer JS, et al. Real-time scintigraphic cineangiography. Comput Cardiol (IEEE) 1976; pp. 45–48.

13. Borer JS, Bacharach SL, Green MV, et al. Rapid evaluation of left ventricular function during exercise in patients with coronary artery disease. Circulation 1976;54:Suppl II;II–6 (abstract).

14. Borer JS, Bacharach SL, Green MV, et al. Real-time radionuclide cineangiography in the noninvasive evaluation of global and regional left ventricular function at rest and during exercise in patients with coronary artery disease. N Engl J Med 1977;296:839.

15. Bacharach SL, Green MV, Borer JS, et al. A real-time system for multi-image gated cardiac studies. J Nucl Med 1977;18:79.

16. Rerych SK, Scholz PM, Newman GE, et al. Cardiac function at rest and during exercise in normals and in patients with coronary heart disease. Ann Surg 1979;187:449.

17. Borges-Neto S, Coleman RE, Jones RH. Perfusion and function at rest and treadmill exercise using technetium-99m-sestamibi: comparison of one- and two-day protocols in normal volunteers. J Nucl Med 1990;31:1128.

18. Verzijlbergen JF, Suttorp MJ, Ascoop CAPL, et al. Combined assessment of technetium-99m SESTA-MIBI planar myocardial perfusion images at rest and during exercise with rest/exercise left ventricular wall motion studies evaluated from gated myocardial perfusion studies. Am Heart J 1992;123:59.

19. DePuey EG, Nichols K, Dobrinsky C. Left ventricular ejection fraction assessed from gated technetium-99m-sestamibi SPECT. J Nucl Med 1993;34:1871.

20. Szulc M, Herrold EM, Zanzonico P, et al. Left ventricular ejection fractions from technetium MIBI perfusion scintigrams: computer based method and validation. Comput Cardiol 1995;IEEE Publication #0276-6547/95:521.

21. Barat J-L, Brendel J, Colle J-P, et al. Quantitative analysis of left ventricular function using gated single-photon emission tomography. J Nucl Med 1984;25:1167.

22. Maublant J, Bailly P, Mestas D, et al. Feasibility of gated single-photon emission transaxial of the cardiac blood pool. Radiology 1983;146:837.

23. Moore ML, Murphy PH, Burdine JA. ECG-gated emission computed tomography of the cardiac blood pool. Radiology 1980;134:233.

24. Tamaki N, Mukai T, Ishii Y, et al. Multiaxial tomography of heart chambers by gated blood-pool emission computed tomography using a rotating gamma camera. Radiology 1983; 147:547.

25. Corbett JR, Jansen DE, Lewis SE, et al. Tomographic gated blood pool radionuclide ventriculography: analysis of wall motion and left ventricular volumes in patients with coronary artery disease. J Am Coll Cardiol 1985;6:349.

26. Lu P, Liu X-J, Shi R, et al. Comparison of tomographic and planar radionuclide ventriculography in assessment of regional left ventricular function in patients with LV aneurysm before and after surgery. J Nucl Cardiol 1994;1:537.

27. Pavel DG, Zimer AM, Patterson VN. In vivo labeling of red blood cells with 99mTc: a new approach to blood pool visualization. J Nucl Med 1977;18:305.

28. Thrall JH, Freitas JE, Swanson D, et al. Clinical comparison of cardiac blood pool visualization with technetium-99m red blood cells labeled in vivo and with technetium 99m human serum albumin. J Nucl Med 1978:19:796.

29. Hegge FN, Hamilton GW, Larson SM, et al. Cardiac chamber imaging: a comparison of red blood cells labelled with technetium-99m in-vitro and in-vivo. J Nucl Med 1978;19:129.

30. Callahan RJ, Froelich JW, McKusick KA, et al. A modified method for the in vivo labeling of red blood cells with Tc-99m: concise communication. J Nucl Med 1982;23:315.

31. Morris DD, Rozanski A, Berman DS, et al. Non-invasive prediction of the angiographic extent of coronary artery disease following myocardial infarction; comparison of clinical, exercise electrocardiographic and ventriculographic parameters. Circulation 1984;70:192.

32. Borer JS, Bacharach SL, Green MV, et al. Effect of nitroglycerin on exercise-induced abnormalities of left ventricular re-

gional function and ejection fraction in coronary artery disease: assessment by radionuclide cineangiography in symptomatic and asymptomatic patients. Circulation 1978;57:314.

33. Manyari DE, Kostuk WJ. Left and right ventricular function at rest and during bicycle exercise in the supine and sitting positions in normal subjects and patients with coronary artery disease. Am J Cardiol 1983;51:36.

34. Borer JS, Kent KM, Bacharach SL, et al. Sensitivity, specificity and predictive accuracy of radionuclide cineangiography during exercise in patients with coronary artery disease: comparison with exercise electrocardiography. Circulation 1979;60:572.

35. Wainwright RJ, Brennand-Roper DA, Cucni TA, et al. Cold-pressor test in detection of coronary heart-disease and cardiomyopathy using technetium-99m gated blood-pool imaging. Lancet 1979;2:320.

36. Borer JS, Supino P, Wencker D, et al. Assessment of coronary artery disease by radionuclide cineangiography: an evolving role. History, current applications and future directions. Cardiol Clin 1994;12:333.

37. Freeman ML, Palac R, Mason J, et al. A comparison of dobutamine infusion and supine bicycle exercise for radionuclide cardiac stress testing. Clin Nucl Med 1984;9:251.

38. Cates CU, Kronenberg MW, Collins HW, et al. Dipyridamole radionuclide ventriculography: a test with high specificity for severe coronary artery disease. J Am Coll Cardiol 1989;13:841.

39. Bourguignon MH, Douglass KH, Links JM, et al. Fully automated data acquisition processing and display in equilibrium radioventriculography. Eur J Nucl Med 1981;6:343.

40. Hains ADB, Al-Khawaja I, Hinge DA, et al. Radionuclide left ventricular ejection fraction: a comparison of three methods. Br Heart J 1986;57:242.

41. Goldberg HL, Herrold EM, Hochreiter C, et al. Videodensitometric determination of right ventricular and left ventricular ejection fraction. Am J Non-Invasive Cardiol 1987;1:18.

42. Maddahi J, Berman D, Matsuoka DT, et al. A new technique for assessing right ventricular ejection fraction using rapid multiple gated equilibrium cardiac blood pool scintigraphy. Circulation 1979;60:581.

43. Holman BL, Wynne J, Idoine J, et al. Disruption in the temporal sequence of regional ventricular contraction. I. Characteristics and incidence in coronary artery disease. Circulation 1980;61:1075.

44. Maddox DE, Wynne J, Uren R, et al. Regional ejection fraction: a quantitative radionuclide index of regional left ventricular performance. Circulation 1979;59:1001.

45. Vitale DF, Green MV, Bacharach SL, et al. Assessment of regional left ventricular function by sector analysis: a method for objective evaluation of radionuclide blood pool studies. Am J Cardiol 1983;52:1112.

46. Starling MR, Dell'Italia LJ, Walsh RA, et al. Accurate estimates of absolute ventricular volumes from equilibrium radionuclide angiographic count data using a simple geometric attenuation correction. J Am Coll Cardiol 1984;3:789.

47. Links JM, Becker LC, Shindledecker JG, et al. Measurement of absolute left ventricular volume from gated blood pool studies. Circulation 1982;65:82.

48. Massardo T, Gal RA, Grenier RP, et al. Left ventricular volume calculation using a count-based ratio method applied to multigated radionuclide angiography. J Nucl Med 1990;31:450.

49. Ashburn WL, Kostuk WJ, Karliner JS, et al. Left ventricular volume and ejection fraction determination by radionuclide angiography. Semin Nucl Med 1973;3:165.

50. Bonow RO, Bacharach SL, Green MV, et al. Impaired left ventricular diastolic filling in patients with coronary artery disease: assessment with radionuclide cineangiography. Circulation 1981;64:315.

51. Bonow RO, Leon MB, Rosing DR, et al. Effect of verapamil and propranolol on left ventricular systolic function and diastolic filling in patients with coronary artery disease: radionuclide angiographic studies at rest and exercise. Circulation 1982;65:1337.

52. Perrone Filardi P, Bacharach SL, Dilsizian V, et al. Impaired left ventricular filling and regional diastolic asynchrony at rest in coronary artery disease and relation to exercise induced myocardial ischemia. Am J Cardiol 1991;67:356.

53. Borer JS, Hochreiter C, Herrold EM, et al. Prediction of indications for valve replacement among asymptomatic or minimally symptomatic patients with chronic aortic regurgitation and normal left ventricular performance. Circulation 1998;97:525.

54. Okada RD, Osbakken MD, Boucher CA, et al. Pulmonary blood volume ratio response to exercise: a non-invasive determination of exercise induced changes in pulmonary capillary wedge pressure. Circulation 1982;65:126.

55. Hochreiter C, Niles N, Devereux RB, et al. Mitral regurgitation: relationship of non-invasive descriptors of right and left ventricular performance to clinical and hemodynamic findings and to prognosis in medically and surgically treated patients. Circulation 1986;73:900.

56. Bacharach SL, Green MV, Vitale D, et al. Optimum Fourier filtering of cardiac data: a minimum error method. J Nucl Med 1983;24:1176.

57. Links JM, Douglas KH, Wagner HN. Patterns of ventricular emptying by Fourier analysis of gated blood pool studies. J Nucl Med 1980;21:978.

58. Brateman L, Buckley K, Keim SG, et al. Left ventricular regional wall motion assessment by radionuclide ventriculography: a comparison of cine display with Fourier imaging. J Nucl Med 1991;32:777.

59. Green MV, Bacharach SL, Borer JS, et al. A theoretical comparison of first pass and gated equilibrium methods in the measurement of systolic left ventricular function. J Nucl Med 1991;32:1801.

60. Van Royen N, Jaffe CC, Krumholz HM, et al. Comparison and reproducibility of visual echocardiographic and quantitative radionuclide left ventricular ejection fractions. Am J Cardiol 1996;77:843.

61. Berman DS, Kiat H, Germano G, et al. 99m-Tc-sestamibi SPECT. In: Cardiac SPECT Imaging, edited by DePuey, Berman, and Garcia, New York: Raven Press, 1995, pp. 121–146.

62. Iskandrian AS, Heo J, Kong B, et al. Use of technetium-99m isonitrile (RP-30A) in assessing left ventricular perfusion and function at rest and during exercise in coronary artery disease, and comparison with coronary arteriography and exercise thallium-201 SPECT imaging. Am J Cardiol 1989;64:270.

63. Wallis JB, Borer JS. Identification of "surgical" coronary anatomy by exercise radionuclide cineangiography. Am J Cardiol 1991;68:1150.

64. Borer JS. Measurement of ventricular function and volume. In: Nuclear Cardiology: State of the Art and Future Directions, 2nd Edition. edited by BL Zaret and GA Beller. St. Louis: Mosby 1999, pp. 201–215.

65. Redwood DR, Borer JS, Epstein SE. Whither the ST segment during exercise? Circulation 1976;54:703.

66. DePace NL, Iskandrian AS, Hakki AH, et al. Value of left ventricular ejection fraction during exercise in predicting the extent of coronary artery disease. J Am Coll Cardiol 1983;1:1002.

67. Gibbons RJ, Lee KL, Pryor D, et al. The use of radionuclide angiography in the diagnosis of coronary artery disease: a logistic regression analysis. Circulation 1983;68:740.

68. Hauser W, Alkins HL, Nelson KG, et al. Technetium 99m DTPA: a new radiopharmaceutical for brain and kidney scanning. Radiology 1970;94:679.

69. Gibbons RJ. Rest and exercise radionuclide angiography for diagnosis in chronic ischemic heart disease. Circulation 1991;84(Suppl I):I-93.

70. Ratib O, Henze E, Schon H, et al. Phase analysis of radionuclide ventriculograms for the detection of coronary artery disease. Am Heart J 1982;104L:1.

71. Villari B, Betocchi S, Pace L, et al. Assessment of left ventricular diastolic function: comparison of contrast ventriculography and equilibrium radionuclide angiography. J Nucl Med 1991;32:1849.

72. Herrold EM, Goldfine SM, Magid NM, et al. Myocardial blood flow in aortic regurgitation: computer-based predictions from wall stress compared with fluorescent microsphere measurements. Comput Cardiol 1994;IEEE Publication #0276-6547/94:729.

73. Borer JS, Bacharach SL, Green MV, et al. Exercise-induced left ventricular dysfunction in symptomatic and asymptomatic patients with aortic regurgitation: assessment by radionuclide cineangiography. Am J Cardiol 1978;42:351.

74. Borer JS, Jason M, Devereux RB, et al. Function of the hypertrophied left ventricle at rest and exercise: hypertension and aortic stenosis. Am J Med 1983;75(suppl III):III-34.

75. Bonow RO, Borer JS, Rosing DR, et al. Left ventricular functional reserve in adult patients with atrial septal defect: pre- and postoperative studies. Circulation 1981;63:1315.

76. Burow RD, Strauss HW, Singleton R, et al. Analysis of left ventricular function from multiple gated acquisition cardiac blood pool imaging. Circulation 1977;56:1024.

77. Borer JS, Jason M, Devereux RB, et al. Left ventricular performance in the hypertensive patient: exercise-mediated noninvasive separation of loading influences from intrinsic muscle dysfunction. Chest 1983;83(5):314.

78. Gottdiener JS, Borer JS, Bacharach SL, et al. Left ventricular function in mitral valve prolapse: assessment with radionuclide cineangiography. Am J Cardiol 1981;47:7.

79. Borer JS, Bacharach SL, Green MV, et al. Effect of septal myotomy and myectomy on left ventricular systolic function at rest and during exercise in patients with IHSS. Circulation 1979;60(suppl I):I-82.

80. Iskandrian AS, Heifeld H, Lemlek I, et al. Differentiation between primary dilated cardiomyopathy and ischemic cardiomyopathy based on right ventricular performance. Am Heart J 1991;123:768.

81. Gottdiener JS, Mathisen DJ, Borer JS, et al. Doxorubicine cardiotoxicity: assessment of late left ventricular dysfunction by radionuclide cineangiography. Ann Intern Med 1981;94:430.

82. Gibbons RJ, Lee KL, Cobb F, et al. Ejection fraction response to exercise in patients with chest pain and normal coronary arteriograms. Circulation 1981;64:952.

83. Dehmer GJ, Lewis SE, Hillis LD, et al. Volumes and the pressure-volume relationship: a sensitive indicator of left ventricular dysfunction in patients with coronary artery disease. Circulation 1981;63:1008.

84. Mancini GBJ, Slutsky RA, Norris SL, et al. Radio-nuclide analysis of peak filling rate, filling fraction, and time to peak filling rate. Am J Cardiol 1983;51:43.

85. Poliner LR, Farber SH, Glaeser DH, et al. Alteration of diastolic filling rate during exercise radionuclide angiography: a highly sensitive technique for detection of coronary artery disease. Circulation 1984;70:942.

86. Pace L, Bacharach SL, Bonow RO, et al: Diagnosis of coronary artery disease by radionuclide angiography: effect of combining indices of left ventricular function. J Nucl Med 1989;30:1966.

87. Cates CU, Kronenberg MW, Collins HW, et al. Dipyridamole radionuclide ventriculography: a test with high specificity for severe coronary artery disease. J Am Coll Cardiol 1989;13:841.

88. Freeman ML, Palac R, Mason J, et al. A comparison of dobutamine infusion and supine bicycle exercise for radionuclide cardiac stress testing. Clin Nucl Med 1984;9:251.

89. Klein HO, Ninio R, Eliyahu S, et al. Effects of the dipyridamole test on left ventricular function in coronary artery disease. Am J Cardiol 1992;69:482.

90. McGillem MJ, DeBoe SF, Friedman MZ, et al. The effects of dopamine and dobutamine on regional function in the presence of rigid coronary stenoses and subcritical impairments of reactive hyperemia. Am Heart J 1988;115:970.

91. Van Rugge FP, van der Wall EE, Bruschke AVG. New developments in pharmacologic stress imaging. Am Heart J 1992;124:468.

92. Underwood SR, Walton S, Laming PJ, et al. Differential sensitivity of radionuclide ventriculography for the detection of anterior and inferior infarction. Br Heart J 1988;60:411.

93. Starling MR, Dell'Italia LJ, Chaudhuri TK, et al. First transit and equilibrium radionuclide angiography in patients with inferior transmural myocardial infarction: criteria for the diagnosis of associated hemodynamically significant right ventricular infarction. J Am Coll Cardiol 1984;4:923.

94. Supino PG, Borer JS, Herrold EM, et al. Prognostication in 3-vessel coronary artery disease based on left ventricular ejection fraction during exercise: influence of coronary artery bypass grafting. Circulation 1999;100:924.

95. Borer JS. Atherosclerosis imaging: pathophysiological assessment for a new era. J Nucl Med 1993;34:1321.

96. Jones RH, Floyd RD, Austin EH, et al. Role of radionuclide angiography in the preoperative prediction of pain relief and prolonged survival following coronary artery bypass grafting. Ann Surg 1983;197:743.

97. Bonow RO, Bacharach SL, Green MV, et al. Prognostic implications of symptomatic vs asymptomatic (silent) myocardial ischemia induced by exercise in mildly symptomatic and in asymptomatic patients with angiographically documented coronary artery disease. Am J Cardiol 1987;60:778.

98. Bonow RO, Kent KM, Rosing DR, et al. Exercise-induced ischemia in mildly symptomatic patients with coronary artery disease and preserved left ventricular function. N Engl J Med 1984;311:1339.

99. Clements IP, Brown ML, Zinsmeister AR, et al. Influence of left ventricular diastolic filling on symptoms and survival in patients with decreased left ventricular systolic function. Am J Cardiol 1991;67:1245.

100. Mazotta G, Bonow RO, Pace L, et al. Relation between exertional ischemia and prognosis in mildly symptomatic patients with single- or double-vessel coronary artery disease and left ventricular function at rest. J Am Coll Cardiol 1989;13:567.

101. Miller TD, Taliercio CP, Zinsmeister AR, et al. Risk stratification of single- or double-vessel coronary artery disease and impaired left ventricular function using exercise radionuclide angiography. Am J Cardiol 1990;65:1317.

102. Supino PS, Wallis JB, Chlouoverakis G, et al. Risk stratification in the elderly patient after coronary artery bypass grafting: the prognostic value of radionuclide cineangiography. J Nucl Cardiol 1994;1:159.

103. Taliercio CP, Clements IP, Zinsmeister AR, et al. Prognostic value and limitations of exercise radionuclide angiography in medically treated coronary artery disease. Mayo Clin Proc 1988;63:573.

104. Wallis JB, Holmes JR, Borer JS. Prognosis in patients with coronary artery disease and low ejection fraction at rest: impact of exercise ejection fraction. Am Cardiol Imaging 1990;4:1.

105. Wallis JB, Supino PG, Borer JS. Prognostic value of left ventricular ejection fraction response to exercise during long-term follow-up after coronary bypass graft surgery. Circulation 1993;88[part 2]:99.

106. Iqbal A, Gibbons RJ, Zinsmeister AR, et al. Prognostic value of exercise radionuclide angiography in a population-based cohort of patients with known or suspected coronary artery disease. Am J Cardiol 1994;74:119.

107. Moriel M, Rozanski A, Klein J, et al. The differing prognostic utility of exercise radionuclide ventriculography in coronary artery disease patients with and without prior myocardial infarction. Int J Card Imaging 1997;13:403.

108. Shapira I, Heller I, Isakov A, et al. Impact of early exercise radionuclide cineangiography on long-term prognosis after CABG. Ann Thorac Surg 1997;64:473.

109. Shaw LJ, Heinle SK, Borges-Neto S, et al. Prognosis by measurements of left ventricular function during exercise. J Nucl Med 1998;39:140.

110. Griffin BP, Shah PK, Diamond GA, et al. Incremental prognostic accuracy of clinical, radionuclide and hemodynamic data in acute myocardial infarction. Am J Cardiol 1991;68:707.

111. The Multicenter Post Infarction Research Group. Risk stratification and survival after myocardial infarction. N Engl J Med 1983;309:331.

112. Rogers WJ, Papapietro SE, Wackers FJT, et al. Variables predictive of good functional outcome following thrombolytic therapy in the Thrombolysis in Myocardial Infarction Phase II (TIMI II) Pilot Study. Am J Cardiol 1989; 63:503.

113. Wackers FJT, Terrin ML, Kayden DS, et al. Quantitative radionuclide assessment of regional ventricular function after thrombolytic therapy for acute myocardial infarction: results of Phase I Thrombolysis in Myocardial Infarction (TIMI) trial. J Am Coll Cardiol 1989;13:998.

114. Cerqueira MD, Maynard C, Ritchie JL, et al. Long-term survival in 618 patients from the Western Washington Streptokinase in Myocardial Infarction Trials. J Am Coll Cardiol 1992; 20:1452.

115. Borer JS, Miller D, Schreiber T, et al. Radionuclide cineangiography in acute myocardial infarction: role in prognostication. Semin Nucl Med 1987;42:89.

116. Candell-Riera J, Permanyer-Miralda G, Castell J, et al. Uncomplicated first myocardial infarction: strategy for comprehensive prognostic studies. J Am Coll Cardiol 1991;18:1207.

117. Abraham RD, Harris PJ, Roubin GS, et al. Usefulness of ejection fraction response to exercise one month after acute myocardial infarction in predicting coronary anatomy and prognosis. Am J Cardiol 1987;60:225.

118. Corbett JR, Dehmer GJ, Lewis SE, et al. The prognostic value of submaximal exercise testing with radionuclide ventriculography before hospital discharge in patients with recent myocardial infarction. Circulation 1981;64:535.

119. Corbett JR, Nicod P, Lewis SE, et al. Prognostic value of submaximal exercise radionuclide ventriculography after myocardial infarction. Am J Cardiol 1983;52:82A.

120. Dewhurst NG, Muir AL. Comparative prognostic value of radionuclide ventriculography at rest and during exercise in 100 patients after first myocardial infarction. Br Heart J 1983;49: 111.

121. Kuchar DL, Freund J, Yeates M, et al. Enhanced prediction of major cardiac events after myocardial infarction using exercise radionuclide ventriculography. Aust NZ J Med 1987;17:228.

122. Morris KG, Palmeri ST, Califf RM, et al. Value of radionuclide angiography for predicting specific cardiac events after acute myocardial infarction. Am J Cardiol 1985;55:318.

123. Nicod P, Corbett JR, Firth BG, et al. Prognostic value of resting submaximal exercise radionuclide ventriculography after acute myocardial infarction in high-risk patients with single and multivessel disease. Am J Cardiol 1983;52:30.

124. Roig E, Magrina J, Armengol X, et al. Prognostic value of exercise radionuclide angiography in low-risk acute myocardial infarction survivors. Eur Heart J 1993;14:213-218.

125. Mazotta G, Camerini A, Scopinaro G, et al. Predicting severe ischemic events after uncomplicated myocardial infarction by exercise testing and rest and exercise radionuclide ventriculography. J Nucl Cardiol 1994;1:246.

126. Zhu WX, Gibbons RJ, Bailey KR, et al. Predischarge exercise radionuclide angiography in predicting multivessel coronary artery disease and subsequent cardiac events after thrombolytic therapy for acute myocardial infarction. Am J Cardiol 1994; 74:554.

127. Gosselink AT, Liem AL, Reiffers S, et al. Prognostic value of predischarge radionuclide ventriculography at rest and exercise after acute myocardial infarction treated with thrombolytic therapy or primary angioplasty. Clin Cardiol 1998;21:254.

128. Kent KM, Borer JS, Green MV, et al. Effects of coronary artery bypass on global and regional left ventricular function during exercise. N Engl J Med 1978;298:1434.

129. Supino PG, Borer JS. The epidemiology of valvular heart disease: an emerging public health problem. Adv Cardiol 2002; 39:1.

130. Rosen S, Borer JS, Hochreiter C, et al. Natural history of the asymptomatic/minimally symptomatic patient with normal right and left ventricular performance and severe mitral regurgitation due to mitral valve prolapse. Am J Cardiol 1994; 74:374.

131. Borer JS, Wencker D, Hochreiter C. Management decisions in valvular heart disease: the role of radionuclide-based assessment of ventricular function and performance. J Nucl Cardiol 1996;3:72.

132. Harpole DH, Jones RH. Serial assessment of ventricular performance after valve replacement for aortic stenosis. J Thorac Cardiovasc Surg 1990;99:645.

133. Clyne CA, Arrighi JA, Maron BJ, et al. Systemic and left ventricular responses to exercise stress in asymptomastic patients with valvular aortic stenosis. Am J Cardiol 1991;68:1469.

134. Henze E, Schelbert HR, Wisenberg G, et al. Assessment of regurgitant fraction and right and left ventricular function at rest and during exercise: a new technique for determination of right ventricular stroke counts from gated equilibrium blood pool studies. Am Heart J 1982;104:953.

135. Morise AP, Goodwin C. Exercise radionuclide angiography in patients with mitral stenosis: value of right ventricular response. Am Heart J 1986;112:509.

136. Borer JS. Prognostication strategies in heart failure and valvular heart diseases: current concepts and their support. In: Annual of Cardiac Surgery, 1989, edited by M Yacoub. London: Current Science, Ltd. 1989, pp. 115–124.

137. Bonow RO. Asymptomatic aortic regurgitation: indications for operation. J Cardiac Surg 1994;9 (Suppl):170.

138. Borer JS, Herrold EM, Hochreiter C, et al. Natural history of left ventricular performance at rest and during exercise after aortic valve replacement for aortic regurgitation. Circulation 1991;84(Suppl III):III-133.

139. Borer JS, Herrold EM, Hochreiter CA, et al. Pathophysiology of heart failure in regurgitant valvular diseases: relation to ventricular dysfunction and clinical debility. In: *Molecular Cardiology in Clinical Practice*, edited by MR Sanders and JB Kostis. Boston: Kluwer Academic, 1999, pp. 43–56.

140. Borer JS, Hochreiter C, Herrold EM, et al. Prediction of outcome late after aortic valve replacement for aortic regurgitation using pre-operative wall stress-adjusted change in ejection fraction from rest to exercise. Circulation 1998;98(Suppl I):I-475.

141. Phillips HR, Levine FR, Carter JE, et al. Mitral valve replacement for isolated mitral regurgitation: analysis of clinical course and late post-operative left ventricular ejection fraction. Am J Cardiol 1981;48:647.

142. Niles N, Borer JS, Kamen M, et al. Pre-operative left and right ventricular performance in combined aortic and mitral regurgitation and comparison with isolated mitral or aortic regurgitation. Am J Cardiol 1990;65:1372.

143. Wencker D, Borer JS, Hochreiter C, et al. Preoperative predictors of late post-operative outcome among patients with non-ischemic mitral regurgitation with "high risk" descriptors, and comparison with unoperated patients. Cardiology 2000;93:37.

144. Supino PG, Borer JS, Hochreiter C, et al. Chronic aortic regurgitation: natural history of rest and exercise ejection fraction and relation to outcome. Circulation 1999;100(Suppl I):I-519.

145. Gerling B, Gottdiener J, Borer JS. Cardiovascular complications of the treatment of Hodgkin's disease. In: *Hodgkin's Disease: The Consequences of Survival,* edited by Lacher and Redman. Philadelphia: Lea and Febiger, 1989, pp. 267–295.

146. Leon MB, Borer JS, Bacharach SL, et al. Detection of early cardiac dysfunction in patients with severe beta thalassemia and chronic iron overload. N Engl J Med 1979;301:1143.

147. Hochreiter C, Snyder M, Borer JS, et al. Right and left ventricular performance 10 years after Mustard repair of transposition of the great arteries. Am J Cardiol 1994;74:478.

148. Zaret BL, Wackers FJT, Terrin ML, et al. Value of radionuclide rest and exercise left ventricular ejection fractions in assessing survival of patients after thrombolytic therapy for acute myocardial infarction: results of Thrombolysis in Myocardial Infarction (TIMI) phase II study. J Am Coll Cardiol 1995;26:73.

149. Bonow RO, Picone AL, McIntosh CL, et al. Survival and functional results after valve replacement for aortic regurgitation from 1976 to 1983: impact of preoperative left ventricular function. Circulation 1985;72:1244.

150. Furer J, Hochreiter C, Niles NW, et al. Prediction of symptom status following mitral valve replacement for mitral regurgitation by preoperative echocardiographic measurement of the end-systolic stress to end-sytolic volume ratio. Am J Noninvasive Cardiol 1987;1:321.

151. Tornos MP, Olona M, Permanyer-Miralda G, et al. Heart failure after aortic valve replacement for aortic regurgitation: prospective 20-year study. Am Heart J 1998;136:681.

152. Hochreiter CA, Borer JS, Supino PG, et al. Ventricular arrhythmias and sudden death after surgery for chronic nonischemic mitral regurgitation Circulation 2000:102(suppl II):II-369.

18 | Positron emission tomography

HEINRICH R. SCHELBERT

Long considered the domain of research institutions, positron emission tomography (PET) has now entered the mainstream of nuclear medicine. Reasons for this change include approval of positron-emitting radiopharmaceuticals and acknowledgment of PET's clinical efficacy by regulatory agencies, broader reimbursement for clinical PET services, a growing infrastructure in support of clinical PET, and, most important, an already extensive but continuously growing body of scientific knowledge in support of PET not only as an investigative but also as a clinically relevant and cost-effective imaging tool. As an integral component of the diagnostic armamentarium in nuclear medicine, PET at the same time has already and continues to expand the scope of investigational and clinical imaging capabilities. This chapter describes technical and methodological features distinguishing PET from conventional radionuclide imaging but expanding its imaging capabilities. The chapter then focuses on imaging approaches specific to the noninvasive study of the cardiovascular system and closes by exploring past accomplishments and future possibilities for probing and characterizing the function of the human heart in health and disease.

TECHNICAL FEATURES OF PET

Imaging Instrumentation

Fundamental to PET is the uniqueness of the physical decay of positron emitters. Once deposited in tissue and after losing their kinetic energy, positrons—equal in mass to electrons but with a positive charge—combine with electrons. The total mass "annihilates," that is, mass converts into energy, leaving the site of annihilation in the form of two high energetic 511 keV photons in exactly opposite directions. Captured by two diametrically opposed photon detectors at virtually the same time or "in coincidence" they are registered as an annihilation event. The site of the annihilation event can be located, as it must have occurred within the field between the two photon detectors. The site along this

path can be localized in space through a series of multiple, circular rays of photon detectors. Positron-emitting radiopharmaceuticals deposited in an organ or organ region are localized within the image plane described by the circular array of photon detectors or within the three-dimensional space defined by the series of circular detector arrays. Because the image data are gathered as "coincident events," tomographic images of the distribution of positron-emitting radionuclides in the body are formed through image reconstruction algorithms analogous to those employed in X-ray computed tomography (CT). In fact, the application of these algorithms provided the solution during the early stages of positron imaging for generating truly tomographic images, a solution considered a milestone in the development of today's PET [1].

A second feature of PET entails correction of the emission images for photon attenuation. It is accomplished by measuring the photon attenuation with external sources of 511 keV photons. Positron-emitting rods rotate about the patient while transmission images, resembling low-resolution X-ray CT images, are acquired and used for correcting subsequently or already acquired emission images. Depending on the type of correction algorithm, transmission images are acquired for time periods ranging from 5 to 20 minutes. Correction of the emission images for measured photon attenuation produces truly quantitative images that theoretically reflect true tissue activity concentrations in mCi per cm^3 tissue (Figs. 18.1 and 18.2). Current PET systems acquire from 47 to 63 contiguous transaxial images at a plane separation of 2.4 and 3.1 mm over a 15 to16 cm axial field of view. The intrinsic isotropic resolution (e.g., the in-plane and z-axis resolution) of these imaging systems approaches about 4.5 mm equaling a volume resolution of about 0.13 cm^3. Image filtering causes some loss in spatial resolution so that the effective isotropic resolution amounts to about 10 mm full-width half-maximum. The temporal resolution, that is, sampling rates or the speed of acquiring serial images, can be as high as one frame per second although for practical reasons, that is, acquisition of im-

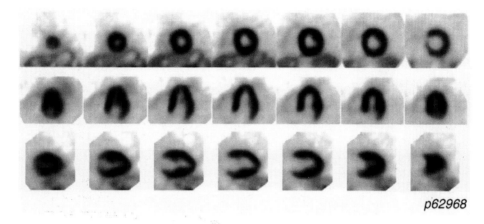

p62968

FIGURE 18.1 Reoriented myocardial images of F-18 deoxyglucose uptake in a normal volunteer.

ages with acceptable count rates, serial images most frequently are acquired at rates of 5 or 10 seconds per frame.

Positron-Emitting Radiopharmaceuticals

A second, equally important component of PET is the long list of radiotracers (exceeding 500), affording noninvasive assays of a broad range of functional processes of the cardiovascular system in humans. Responsible for the large number of radiopharmaceuticals are positron-emitting isotopes of key elements of living matter. Among these are oxygen-15, nitrogen-13, carbon-11, and fluorine-18; they are inserted into natural fuel substrates, receptor ligands, hormones, amino acids, or peptides without necessarily modifying their biological properties. Essential to the design of these radiopharmaceuticals is their retention in the target tissue and their clearance from blood so that images of high signal to noise ratios are recorded. This is true, for example, for carbon-11 labeled palmitate (C-11 palmitate) or acetate (C-11 acetate) or nitrogen-13 labeled ammonia (N-13 ammonia), but not, for example, for C-11 labeled glucose. Because the low myocardial extraction of glucose (about 2% to 5%) and its rapid metabolism and participation in multiple metabolic pathways, myocardial images obtained with carbon-11 labeled glucose are of suboptimal quality. This limitation has been overcome with a modified glucose molecule, 2-deoxyglucose that is metabolically trapped in the myocardium. Labeled with fluorine-18, the glucose analog accumulates in the myocardium in proportion to the rate of uptake of glucose from blood into the myocardium.

The physical half-life of most positron-emitting radionuclides used with PET ranges from only 75 seconds to about 2 hours. Accordingly, imaging studies can be repeated at relatively short time intervals of, for example, every 10 minutes. This then allows assessment of functional responses to physiological or pharmacological interventions during the same study or imaging session. The short physical half-life requires specifically designed techniques for rapid synthesis of high specific activity radiopharmaceuticals. Appropriate and now

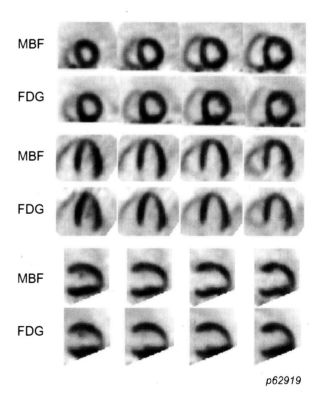

p62919

FIGURE 18.2 Selected reoriented images of myocardial blood flow with N-13 ammonia and of glucose uptake with F-18 deoxyglucose in a patient with idiopathic dilated cardiomyopathy.

largely automated synthesis approaches have become widely available. The cyclotron-produced isotope is automatically transferred to a desktop PC controlled synthesis module producing a sterile, ready for injection radiopharmaceutical. Radiopharmaceuticals produced in this fashion include O-15 labeled water and carbon monoxide, N-13 ammonia, C-11 labeled palmitate, acetate, and hydroxyephedrine, and F-18 2-deoxyglucose. Further, the short physical half-life of most radiopharmaceuticals necessitates on-site production and, thus, an on-site cyclotron. Exceptions include fluorine-18 with a 2-hour physical half-life. Radiopharmaceuticals labeled with this isotope are now available through regional PET radiopharmaceutical distribution centers. Therefore, PET studies are now also possible at medical institutions without a cyclotron and radiopharmacy, commonly referred to as satellite PET. Besides tracers of glucose metabolism as, for example, deoxyglucose, fluorine-18 is also a radiolabel for tracer substances of myocardial blood flow, fatty acid metabolism, or amino acid metabolism so that a new, relatively broad range of radiopharmaceuticals is now available for satellite PET facilities. Finally, other radiopharmaceuticals are already or will be available through generator systems as, for example, rubidium-82 or copper-62, and expand further the scope of studies available through satellite PET imaging centers.

Application of Tracer Kinetic Principles

Tracer kinetic principles, an important assay tool in the biological sciences for measuring regional functional processes in units of micromoles substrates or milliliters blood per minute per gram myocardium, are employed with PET. The approach combines the imaging capabilities of PET with specific properties of positron-emitting radiotracers. Fundamental to quantifying functional processes with this approach are tracer kinetic models. They describe the kinetics of the radiotracer in tissue and in blood in the form of functional pools or compartments. Such compartments may represent anatomical compartments as, for example, the blood pool or vascular space, but may also combine different anatomical spaces or compartments into one functional pool. As an example, the flow tracer O-15 water rapidly exchanges between blood and myocardial tissue. Accordingly, capillary and cell membranes do not exert a barrier effect to the exchange of water so that radiolabeled water in blood and in tissue can be considered as a single functional pool [2,3]. As another example, carbon-11 as a radiolabel for palmitate traverses a series of metabolite pools. These include a pool of the initially activated acyl-CoA, a pool for

mono-, di- and triglycerides, a pool for carbon-11 incorporated into lipids or a pool for carbon-11 labeled 2-carbon fragments as metabolites of beta-oxidation [4]. These pools usually differ in size or their volume of distribution, which in turn determines the rate of equilibration of radiotracer within and its rate of clearance from each pool. Rate constants describe the forward and reverse exchange of the tracer label between pools.

Tracer kinetic models are established through biochemical tissue assays of the radiotracer distribution and their chemical form at various times after tracer administration [4,5]. Other, often complementary approaches include external monitoring of the rate of tracer accumulation in tissue and its clearance from it or, more specifically, its characteristic clearance pattern [6–8]. As an example, monoexponential clearance of radiotracer from the myocardium implies that the tracer has equilibrated within a single functional pool from which it then clears. The rate of clearance depends on the rate of substrate flux through that pool and its size. In contrast, biexponential clearance patterns of tracer from the myocardium indicate that the tracer label has entered at least two different functional pools of markedly different sizes (volumes of distribution) and clearance rates.

A detailed description of the metabolic fate of the tracer label and its incorporation into different metabolites and the changes of the chemical form containing the tracer label on its passage through a metabolic pathway requires multiple pools or compartments all connected by rate constants for exchange of tracer. For example, biochemical assays of the metabolic fate of radiolabeled acetate as a tracer of oxidative metabolism identified at least six pools, all connected by forward and reverse transport constants [5]. While accurately describing the tissue kinetics of radiolabeled acetate during its metabolism in the tricarboxylic acid (TCA) cycle, use of complex, multicompartment tracer kinetic models renders estimates of the functional process to be measured sensitive to errors. As reported for C-11 acetate, for example, this then required simplification of the initial compartment configuration into a model with only two pools, which renders more robust estimates of myocardial oxidative metabolism [9,10].

Number of pools and their respective volumes of distribution together with the rate constants form the underpinning of operational equations that describe the tissue kinetics in mathematical terms. Applied to the tracer kinetics in blood and in tissue as observed with PET, quantitative estimates of the functional process are derived. The operational equation must also take into account differences between tracer and tracee and its concentration in blood. If, for example, the metabolic rate of glucose is to be measured with the glucose analog F-18 deoxyglucose, then a so-called lumped constant corrects for metabolic differences between natural glucose as the tracee and 2-deoxyglucose as the tracer [11,12]. Further, because fluorine-18 2-fluoro 2-deoxyglucose is administered in true tracer amounts, so that its mass is essentially negligible, the rate of glucose uptake in myocardium is adjusted to the arterial plasma concentration of glucose and to differences in the biological behavior of the tracer.

Time-activity curves derived through regions of interest assigned on the serially acquired images to the left ventricular blood pool and the myocardium define the arterial input function of the tracer, while the myocardial tissue time-activity curve reflects the response to it [13,14]. Fitting the time-activity curve with the operational equations derived from the tracer compartment model yields estimates of regional functional processes as, for example, of myocardial blood flow, glucose metabolism, uptake and metabolism of free fatty acid, myocardial oxygen consumption, and oxidative metabolism. Development of tracer kinetic models has matured to a point where they now can be employed routinely for investigational and clinical studies. Computationally less complex are graphical analysis approaches [15]. Based on tracer kinetic models, they allow rapid and convenient calculation of regional functional processes from serially acquired PET images [16]. As an additional benefit, they form the base for generating parametric images and parametric polar maps [17–20]. These depict the geographic distribution of functional processes like blood flow or glucose metabolism in absolute units throughout the left ventricular myocardium [21]. Values of absolute units are encoded along a color scale. From these parametric polar maps, quantitative estimates of functional processes can readily be derived for any region of the myocardium.

POSITRON-EMITTING RADIOPHARMACEUTICALS

Foremost among the functional processes being evaluated and measured with PET are myocardial blood flow, glucose utilization, metabolism of free fatty acid, oxygen consumption, and oxidative metabolism. Other processes include adrenergic neuronal activity and beta-receptor densities.

Tracers of Myocardial Blood Flow

Several positron-emitting tracers are available. Used most widely are O-15 water, Rb-82, and N-13 ammo-nia, but also potassium-38 and, as more recent additions, Cu-62 PTSM and C-11 acetate.

Oxygen-15 water

Oxygen-15 water perhaps most closely meets criteria of an ideal flow tracer. Its myocardial extraction fraction approaches unity and does not decline with higher flows so that the myocardial tracer net uptake as the product of the first-pass tracer extraction fraction tracks myocardial blood flow in a linear fashion [2,3,22]. As a disadvantage, O-15 water equilibrates with blood and adjacent water spaces leading to myocardial perfusion images of low target to background ratios. Blood pool activity can be subtracted from the images by labeling arterial blood pool with O-15 carbon monoxide. Nevertheless, images of the relative distribution of myocardial blood flow are frequently of low count densities for which the short, 120-second physical half-life of oxygen is also responsible. Consequently, the tracer is used mostly for measurements of myocardial blood flow. The short physical half-life further necessitates tracer production at an on-site cyclotron, but conversely permits repeat evaluation and flow measures at time intervals of only 10 minutes. Initial complexities related to the need for blood pool labeling and blood pool corrections appear now to have been largely overcome by novel analytical approaches as, for example, separation of blood pool from myocardial radiotracer activity with the factor analysis [23–25]. Table 18.1 summarizes estimates of myocardial blood flow in the normal heart obtained with the O-15 water technique.

N-13 ammonia

N-13 ammonia is retained metabolically in the myocardium in proportion to myocardial blood flow [8,26]. Its first capillary transient retention fraction (or the fraction of tracer retained in myocardium during a single transit of tracer through the coronary circulation) approaches about 85% for myocardial blood flows at rest (about 0.8 ml $\cdot$ min^{-1} $\cdot$ g^{-1}) but progressively and nonlinearly declines with increasing flows (Fig. 18.3) [8]. Accordingly, the net tracer retention as the product of the first-pass retention fraction and flow increases nonlinearly with myocardial blood flow so that myocardial blood flow in the hyperemic range is associated with disproportionately lower tracer net uptakes or myocardial N-13 ammonia concentrations. Because the tracer is retained in myocardium, but rapidly clears from blood, high diagnostic quality images of the relative distribution of myocardial blood

TABLE 18.1 *Estimates of Myocardial Blood Flow at Rest and during Stress*

Study	N	Age (years)	Technique	Stress	MBF Rest (ml · min⁻¹ · g⁻¹)	MBF Stress (ml · min⁻¹ · g⁻¹)	MF Reserve
Bergmann et al. 1989 [3]	11	25.5	O-15-water	Dipyr	0.90 ± 0.22	3.55 ± 1.15	4.1 ± 1.2
Araujo et al. 1991 [128]	11	26–67	O-15-water	Dipyr	0.84 ± 0.09	3.52 ± 1.12	4.2 ± 1.3
Pitkänen et al. 1996 [112]	20	31 ± 8	O-15-water	Dipyr	0.83 ± 0.13	4.49 ± 1.27	5.4 ± 15
Yokoyama et al. 1998 [129]	13	56 ± 7	O-15-water	Dipyr	0.80 ± 0.39	2.92 ± 1.66	3.7 ± 1.4
Tadamura et al. 2001 [130]	20	23 ± 3	O-15-water	Dipyr	0.67 ± 0.16	4.33 ± 1.23	NA
			O-15-water	Dob + Atr	NA	5.89 ± 1.58	NA
Krivokapich et al. 1989 [13]	13	24 ± 8	N-13-ammonia	Exercise	0.75 ± 0.43	1.50 ± 0.74	2.2 ± 0.7
Hutchins et al. 1990 [27]	7	24 ± 4	N-13-ammonia	Dipyr	0.88 ± 0.17	4.17 ± 1.12	4.8 ± 1.3
Chan et al. 1992 [17]	20	35 ± 16	N-13-ammonia	Dipyr	1.1 ± 0.2	4.3 ± 1.3	4.0 ± 1.3
			N-13-ammonia	Adenosine	NA	4.4 ± 0.9	4.3 ± 1.6
Senneff et al. 1991 [108]	11	25 ± 4	O-15-water	Dipyr	1.16 ± 0.32	4.25 ± 1.54	3.9 ± 1.5
	15	55 ± 9	O-15-water	Dipyr	1.17 ± 0.33	3.12 ± 1.09	3.0 ± 1.4
Czernin et al. 1993 [104]	18	31 ± 9	N-13-ammonia	Dipyr	0.76 ± 0.25	3.0 ± 0.8	4.1 ± 0.9
	22	64 ± 9	N-13-ammonia	Dipyr	0.92 ± 0.25	2.7 ± 0.25	3.0 ± 0.7

MBF, myocardial blood flow; MF, myocardial flow; Dipyr, dipyridamole; Dob + Atr, dobutamine and atropine.

flow are obtained (see Fig. 18.2). N-13 ammonia is therefore preferred to O-15 water for qualitative evaluations of myocardial perfusion. The relatively short, 10-minute physical half-life of nitrogen-13, although longer than that for oxygen-15, permits repeat evaluations of myocardial blood flow at relatively short time intervals of about 40 to 50 minutes, that is 4 to 5 physical half-times during which about 94% to 97% of the initially injected tracer activity has physically decayed.

Tracer kinetic models, one with two and the other with three compartments and both validated in canine myocardium, are used for measurements of myocardial blood flow [13,14,27,28]. These tracer kinetic models correct for the nonlinear net uptake response of N-13 ammonia to flow so that estimates of myocardial blood flow with N-13 ammonia correlate linearly with those obtained simultaneously with the microsphere technique for flows as high as 5.0 ml · min⁻¹ · g⁻¹ [14,28].

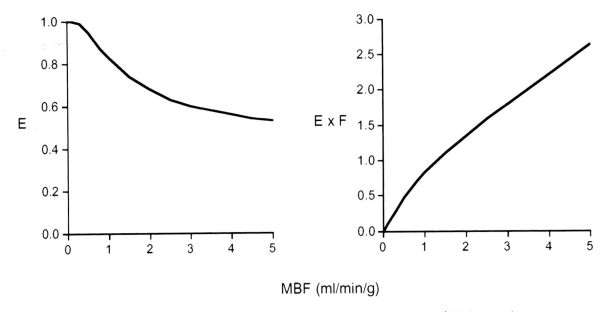

MBF (ml/min/g)

FIGURE 18.3 First-pass retention fraction (E) and myocardial net retention (E·F) of N-13 ammonia as a function of myocardial blood flow (MBF). The net retention of the tracer follows the increase in myocardial blood flow in a curvilinear fashion. Because the relationship between the first-pass retention fraction and myocardial blood flow is constant and is independent of changes in the myocardium state, this fixed relationship allows corrections of the curvilinear flow response of the tracer so that estimates of myocardial blood flow in absolute units can be obtained.

For values of myocardial blood flow in humans see Table 18.1.

Rubidium-82

Rubidium-82, another tracer of blood flow, is available through a generator system [29]. Strontium-82, the parent isotope, has a physical half-life of 28 days so that a generator system can be used clinically for as long as 4 to 5 weeks. Pushbutton-operated infusion systems are available for the generator so that preselected radioactivity doses can be administered at preselected intravenous infusion rates. The 78-second physical half-life of rubidium-82 requires activity doses of as high as 50 to 60 mCi so that sufficient counts for imaging the retention of tracer in myocardium remain after allowing one to two tracer half-lives for clearance of the radiotracer from blood. As a potassium analog, the ^{82}Rb$^+$ cation substitutes for K$^+$ on the sodium/potassium dependent ATPase system. It is actively transported and retained in myocardium in proportion to myocardial blood flow. The first-pass retention fraction of Rb-82 amounts to 65% for myocardial blood flows at rest but declines with higher flows so that again the net retention increases nonlinearly with myocardial blood flows. Acquisition of the Rb-82 myocardial retention images commences 60 to 120 seconds after tracer injection and continues for about 6 minutes [29]. The images are of good diagnostic quality and afford detection of flow abnormalities with an accuracy equal to that of N-13 ammonia [29,30].

More challenging has been the measurement of myocardial blood flow in absolute units. Tracer kinetic models adequately describe the kinetics of Rb-82 cations in myocardium; difficulties relate to the ultrashort physical half-life of the tracer. High activity doses needed to attain statistically adequate images of the tracer retention in the myocardium are associated with high count rates during the tracer input function that exceed the count rate capabilities of many current PET imaging systems and lead to substantial dead-time losses. Nevertheless, measurements of myocardial blood flow in absolute units have become possible [31]. Resulting estimates of myocardial blood flow with Rb-82 have been reported to correlate with those by the microsphere technique in dogs and with those by O-15 water in humans [31,32].

Potassium-38

Potassium-38, another tracer of flow, exhibits properties similar to those of Rb-82 [33]. Its physical half-life is 7.7 minutes and thus requires production at on-site cyclotrons. At myocardial blood flows at rest, its first-pass retention fraction is similar to that of potassium cations but again declines with higher flows so that tracer net retentions are again correlated nonlinearly with myocardial blood flow. Techniques for estimating regional myocardial blood flow in absolute units have not been developed yet.

Copper-62 labeled PTSM

Copper-62 labeled PTSM (pyruvaldehyde bis(N4-methylthiosemicarbazonato)-copper(II) is retained in myocardium in proportion to blood flow but again in a nonlinear fashion [34]. For resting myocardial blood flows, the first-pass retention fraction averages about 50% but again declines with higher myocardial blood flows [35–37]. The physical half-life of Cu-62 is 9.7 minutes; it is available through a generator system with Zinc-62 as the parent isotope. With a 9.2-hour physical half-life of the parent isotope, the generator system is expected to have about 1 to 2 days clinical use. The agent therefore can be used in PET imaging centers without an on-site cyclotron. Based on animal experimental and human investigations, Cu-62 PTSM provides images of myocardial perfusion of high signal to noise ratios and, thus, of high diagnostic quality [35,37–39]. Measurements of myocardial blood flow seem possible with this agent but estimates of hyperemic blood flow have remained unsatisfactory [40,41].

Carbon-11 labeled acetate

Carbon-11 labeled acetate, known as a tracer of myocardial oxidative metabolism, also lends itself as an agent for evaluating the relative distribution and, as reported more recently, for measuring myocardial blood flow [10,42,43]. The initial retention of the tracer in myocardium depends on myocardial blood flow; for blood flows at rest the first-pass retention fraction averages about 60% [44]. As demonstrated in humans, the agent accurately identifies regional flow defects in patients with coronary artery disease [43]. Applied with an appropriate tracer kinetic model, C-11 acetate affords quantitative estimates of myocardial blood flow at rest, but also for hyperemic blood flows [9,45]. Further, and as discussed later, it affords assessments of the myocardium's TCA cycle activity so that myocardial blood flow and oxidative metabolism can be measured simultaneously.

The choice of flow tracer frequently depends on practical and logistical factors but also on specific clinical and investigational needs. At a PET center fully equipped with PET imaging systems, a cyclotron, and a radiopharmacy with radiotracer synthesis capabilities, either O-15 water or N-13 ammonia can be used. Cyclotron production runs and radiopharmaceutical needs for other than cardiac studies may favor use of one flow tracer over the other. Use of O-15 water affords measurements of myocardial blood flow and of its responses to pharmacological and physiological interventions at about 10 to 15 minute time intervals so that as many as three to four measurements can readily be performed during one study session. Conversely, if the main goal is to evaluate the relative distribution of myocardial blood flow, then N-13 ammonia will be preferable because of its "static images" of high diagnostic quality. Generator-based tracers like Rb-82 or Cu-62 PTSM will be an obvious choice for PET imaging laboratories without on-site cyclotron production capabilities.

There has been some debate on the relative merits of the O-15 water and the N-13 ammonia technique for measurements of myocardial blood flow. Comparison studies in animal and in human myocardium indicate that both approaches yield similarly valid and comparable estimates of blood flow in the normal myocardium [46,47]. This, however, does not necessarily apply to diseased myocardium. Disparities between flow estimates by both approaches relate to fundamental differences in methodology. For the N-13 ammonia approach, blood flow is averaged over the entire myocardial region including normal and diseased or ischemically injured myocardium and scar tissue. Resulting flow estimates therefore describe the average transmural myocardial blood flow. In contrast, the O-15 water technique provides estimates of flow only for myocardium capable of rapidly exchanging water [22,48]. Fibrosis, scar tissue, and possibly severely injured myocardium are therefore excluded from the analysis. The O-15 water technique measures flow only in "water perfusable myocardium." This is why in patients with coronary artery disease and transmural reductions in blood flow in myocardial perfusion images, the transmural N-13 ammonia technique indicates flow estimates substantially lower than those observed with "water perfusable tissue fraction" O-15 water approach [49].

Tracers of Substrate Metabolism

Positron-emitting tracers of metabolism cover a broad range of the myocardium's substrate metabolism including that of glucose, free fatty acid, and oxygen.

F-18 2-fluoro 2-deoxyglucose

F-18 2-fluoro 2-deoxyglucose, a glucose analog, traces the initial steps of glucose metabolism [11,12,50]. As a key feature, the phosphorylated glucose analog is a poor substrate for glycogen synthesis, glycolysis, or the fructose-pentose shunt. Initial transmembrane exchange and subsequent hexokinase mediated phosphorylation closely follow those of glucose. Because dephosphorylation of the labeled deoxyglucose-6-phosphate and, thus, return of tracer from myocardium to blood, are essentially negligible, the relative distribution of F-18 activity throughout the myocardium as depicted on static images, or the rate of tracer incorporation into the myocardium as determined from serially acquired images reflect the rate of myocardial glucose utilization (subsequently referred to as myocardial metabolic rate of glucose or MMRGlc; see Figures 18.2 and 18.4) The 120-minute physical half-life of fluorine-18 affords a supply of tracer through regional radiopharmaceutical distribution centers and thus eliminates the need for an on-site cyclotron. Static images of the myocardial uptake of F-18 deoxyglucose are acquired for about 20 minutes beginning at 30 to 40 minutes after intravenous tracer administration. At that time, the tracer has sufficiently cleared from blood with about 80% of the tracer retained in the myocardium in the form of F-18 deoxyglucose-6-phosphate [7].

The first-pass retention fraction of F-18 deoxyglucose is less than 10% so that the myocardial tracer concentrations are independent of blood flow. F-18 deoxyglucose uptake, however, depends on the prevailing substrate selection of the myocardium at the time of the study. Myocardium derives its energy from several fuel substrates including glucose, lactic acid, and free fatty acid. Utilization of each depends on its availability to the myocardium and, thus, on its concentration in arterial blood. Plasma substrate levels, in turn, are governed among other factors by the dietary state, the hormonal milieu, and the physical work. Fasting for more than 4 to 5 hours is associated with high free fatty acid and low glucose and insulin concentrations in blood. Consequently, the myocardium resorts to free fatty acid as its predominant fuel substrate and utilizes less glucose. Accordingly, the F-18 deoxyglucose images reveal little if any tracer retention in the myocardium (Fig. 18.4) [51,52].

Interventions for shifting the myocardium's substrate selection to glucose are therefore important. One intervention is oral administration of glucose [53]. Analogous to glucose tolerance testing, it stimulates insulin secretion and enhances the rate of disposal of glucose from plasma, including greater uptake of glucose and, thus, of F-18 deoxyglucose in the myocardium. A second intervention for enhancing myocardial tracer uptake is the hyperinsulinemic–euglycemic clamp [54–56]. Following a loading dose of glucose and insulin, a 20%

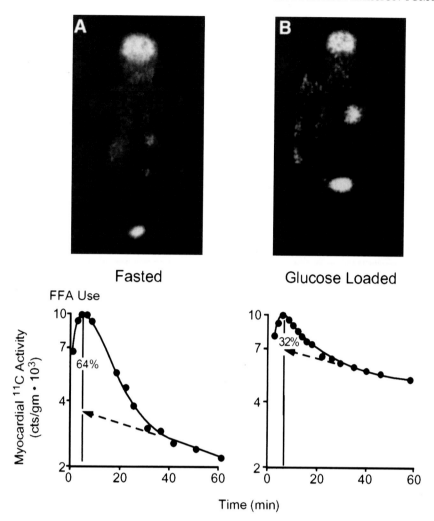

FIGURE 18.4 Myocardial F-18 deoxyglucose uptake and C-11 palmitate clearance patterns as a function of changes in substrate availability and in the myocardium substrate selection. The panels on the left depict studies during fasting conditions when myocardial glucose utilization is low (no F-18 oxyglucose uptake is observed in the myocardium) and free fatty acids serve as the dominant fuel substrate for oxidation. Accordingly, the relative size of the rapid clearance curve component and its clearance rate are high. Both, however, decline after glucose loading, as shown on the right, consistent with reduced free fatty acid utilization and oxidation, which, as shown in the upper right panel, is compensated for by a shift of the myocardium to glucose utilization as evidenced by myocardial F-18 deoxyglucose uptake.

dextrose solution is infused continuously while titrating plasma glucose concentration to normal levels with concomitant insulin infusions. Although labor intensive, the approach produces myocardial F-18 deoxyglucose images of high diagnostic quality and has proved to be especially useful in patients with insulin resistance or with type 2 diabetes. A third intervention reduces with nicotinic acid or its derivatives circulating levels of free fatty acid with the aim of diminishing their inhibitory effect on myocardial glucose utilization. This substrate manipulation has been shown to yield myocardial F-18 deoxyglucose images of high diagnostic quality [57,58].

MMRGlc can be quantified with a three-compartment tracer kinetic model [12,59]. Beginning at the time of F-18 deoxyglucose administration, images are acquired serially for 60 minutes followed by fitting the blood pool and myocardial time-activity curve with the operational equation derived from the tracer kinetic model [59]. Computationally more convenient is the Patlak graphical analysis approach now used almost exclusively for measurement of MMRGlc. Values of myocardial glucose metabolic rates determined noninvasively with F-18 deoxyglucose and PET correlate linearly with estimates by the Fick principle in canine myocardium [15,16,59]. In humans, myocardial metabolic

TABLE 18.2 *Myocardial Glucose and Free Fatty Acid Utilization Estimated with F-18 deoxyglucose and with F-18 fluoro-6-thia-heptadecanoic acid (^{18}FTHA)*

Dietary State*	Glucose $mmol \cdot L^{-1}$	FFA† $mmol \cdot L^{-1}$	Utilization $\mu mol \cdot min^{-1} \cdot 1g^{-1}$	Study
Glucose				
Fasting	4.8 ± 0.3	0.30 ± 0.25	0.24 ± 0.17	Choi et al. 1993 [51]
	5.7 ± 0.05	1.07 ± 0.46	0.13 ± 0.09	Ohtake et al. 1995 [132]
Post glucose	8.6 ± 1.8	0.19 ± 0.14	0.69 ± 0.11	Choi et al. 1993 [51]
	10.2 ± 0.4	N/A	0.69 ± 0.03	Knuuti et al. 1992 [131]
	7.0 ± 0.13	0.31 ± 0.20	0.52 ± 0.05	Ohtake et al. 1995 [132]
Clamp	5.1 ± 0.2	N/A	0.74 ± 0.02	Knuuti et al. 1992 [131]
	5.4 ± 0.13	0.34 ± 0.20	0.54 ± 0.11	Ohtake et al. 1995 [132]
FFA				
Fasting	5.3 ± 0.4	0.560 ± 0.080	5.8 ± 1.7	Mäki et al. 1998 [73]
Clamp	5.4 ± 0.8	0.110 ± 0.030	1.4 ± 0.5	

*Fasting = studies performed after an overnight fast; post glucose = 1 hour after 75 g glucose orally; clamp = study performed during hyperinsulinemic–euglycemic glucose clamping.

†Values for free fatty acid (FFA) uptake are given in $\mu mol \cdot min^{-1} \cdot 100g^{-1}$. N/A, data not reported.

rates of glucose average about 0.70 $\mu mol \cdot min^{-1} \cdot g^{-1}$ in the glucose loaded state, that is, during preferential myocardial glucose utilization and only about 0.20 $\mu mol \cdot min^{-1} \cdot g^{-1}$ during fasting, that is, when free fatty acid is utilized preferentially (Table 18.2) [51,56].

Myocardial ischemia or ischemia-related regional alterations interfere with the normal substrate competition and control. Increased expression of the relatively insulin independent glucose transporter GLUT1 [60] and, possibly, upregulated activities of enzymes controlling the glycolytic pathway may account for the selective increase in glucose utilization and thus in F-18 deoxyglucose uptake in acutely ischemic but also in chronically dysfunctional but viable myocardium [61]. Therefore, local factors apparently override systemic determinants of myocardial substrate regulation and account for the blood flow–glucose metabolism mismatch pattern observed with F-18 deoxyglucose and tracers of blood flow as the hallmark of myocardial viability [53,62].

There are limitations to the information obtained with F-18 deoxyglucose because the agent measures only the initial step of glucose metabolism beginning with extraction from blood up to the branch point of glucose-6-phosphate. Hence, the approach does not offer information on the fraction of glucose entering glycolysis or oxidation or glycogen synthesis. Nor does it provide information on the contribution of glycogen to glycolysis. It would seem, however, that under steady-state conditions, estimates of the myocardial metabolic rate of glucose can provide a measure of the overall glucose metabolism. Moreover, under extreme conditions as, for example, after depletion of glucose storage pools during ischemia when myocardium largely depends on exogenous glucose, more accurate estimates

of the true glycolytic activity seem likely with F-18 deoxyglucose.

Carbon-11 labeled palmitate

Carbon-11 labeled palmitate traces the myocardial metabolism of free fatty acid. Because of first-pass retention fractions in the range of 50% to 60%, the tracer accumulates initially in the myocardium in proportion to myocardial blood flow [63,64]. It then clears from the myocardium. The biexponential clearance pattern reflects, according to tracer kinetic principles, the distribution of tracer label between at least two metabolic pools of different sizes and turnover rates (Fig. 18.4). The rapid clearance curve component represents the fraction of tracer that immediately becomes metabolized through beta-oxidation and the TCA cycle and its flux rate through these oxidative pathways [4]. The slow clearance curve component, in contrast, corresponds to fraction of the tracer label incorporated into larger pools of metabolites with lower turnover rates as, for example, glycerides or lipids.

The morphology of the tissue clearance curve depends on the prevailing pattern of substrate utilization and on the oxidative rate [65]. For example, when glucose dominates as oxidative substrate, the relative size of the rapid clearance curve component and its clearance rate are low. Conversely, a shift in the myocardium selection from glucose to free fatty acid as its preferred substrate for oxidation as, for example, during fasting, increases the relative size of the rapid clearance curve component, consistent with an increase in fraction of free fatty acid proceeding immediately to oxidation (Fig. 18.4). Because the rate of flux through beta-oxidation may also increase, the slope of the rapid clearance face may increase in steepness. Liberation of the tracer label from palmitate and, further, from its 2-carbon fragments and release from myocardium in the form $^{11}O_2$ occurs in the TCA cycle. This then implies that the slope of the rapid clearance phase increases in steepness only if the contribution of free fatty acid derived 2-carbon units to the TCA cycle increases markedly relative to that of glucose.

Ischemia is known to impair beta-oxidation but also the TCA cycle activity. Consequently, less C-11 palmitate enters the immediate oxidation and more is diverted into the slow turnover metabolite pools [66–68]. The clearance curve reflects this response. The relative size of the slow clearance curve component increases paralleled by a decline in the slope of the rapid clearance curve component.

Global and regional changes in free fatty acid metabolism of the myocardium can thus readily be identified from the clearance pattern of C-11 palmitate from the myocardium. The tracer is injected intravenously while acquisition of serial images for 30 to 40 minutes commences. The myocardial time-activity curve is submitted to least square biexponential fitting routines, and relative sizes and slopes of the two major clearance curve components are measured. Besides an evaluation of the myocardial free fatty acid metabolism, more recent studies in animals suggested the possibility of measurements of myocardial free fatty acid including uptake and oxidation in absolute units [69].

Fluorine-18 labeled FTHA

Fluorine-18 labeled FTHA or 14(R,S)-[18F]fluoro-6-thia-heptadecanoic acid has recently been introduced as a tracer of myocardial free fatty acid utilization and, presumably, beta-oxidation. Findings in isolated arterially perfused hearts and in intact animals suggest that the agent provides an index of the rate of beta-oxidation [70–72]. After exchanging into the myocardium, FTHA is sequestered metabolically. Images of the myocardial retention of the tracer in experimental animals and in humans are of high diagnostic quality. A tracer compartment model, comparable to that of F-18 deoxyglucose, together with a graphical analysis approach have been developed and afford measurements of regional myocardial free fatty acid metabolism. Noninvasively obtained metabolic rates of free fatty acid in human myocardium average about 5.8 μmol · min^{-1} · g^{-1} in the fasted state and about 1.5 μmol · min^{-1} · g^{-1} after suppression of circulating free fatty acid concentrations through hyperinsulinemic–euglycemic clamping (Table 18.2) [73].

Carbon-11 labeled acetate

Carbon-11 labeled acetate, already mentioned as a tracer blood flow, has proved useful for measuring noninvasively myocardial oxidative metabolism [74–77]. Upon reaching the myocardium, acetate becomes esterified to acetyl-CoA and engages in the TCA cycle [5]. During its second turn through the cycle, the carbon-11 label is liberated and released from myocardium in the form of $^{11}CO_2$. The tracer clears biexponentially from myocardium (Fig. 18.5). The slow clearance curve component corresponds to retention of tracer label in glutamate and glutamine pools, while the rapid clearance phase corresponds to the rate of substrate flux through the TCA cycle. Estimates of the TCA cycle activity are obtained from the slope of the rapid clearance curve component either by biexponential least square curve fitting routines or through monoexponential fitting of the early downslope of the time-activity curve. Both clearance rate constants, k_1 (obtained by exponential fitting) and k_{mono} (obtained by monoexponential fitting of the early curve portion), have been found to correlate well with the rate of release of $^{11}CO_2$ from the myocardium in animal experiments and, further, because of the close link between TCA cycle activity and oxidative phosphorylation, with myocardial oxygen consumption [76–78].

Both k_1 and k_{mono} reflect only rates of flux but not the mass flux as the product of the rate constant and the substrate concentration. Because mass flux can be

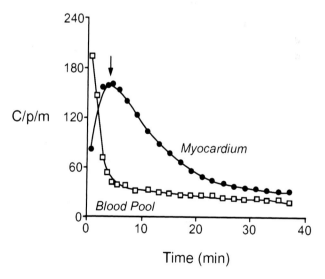

FIGURE 18.5 Myocardial uptake and clearance of C-11 acetate together with the arterial blood concentrations as determined in normal volunteer from serially acquired images. Note the rapid tracer clearance from blood and the biexponential decline in myocardial C-11 activity. C/p/m, counts per nixel per minute.

estimated from the rate constant for clearance of substrate from a metabolite pool and its size or distribution volume, a tracer compartment model has been established through biochemical tissue assays [5,9]. Assuming that the distribution volumes for metabolites of C-11 acetate in myocardium of humans are comparable to those in rodents and, second that pool sizes of metabolites are constant over a wide range of metabolic conditions, the TCA cycle activity and, in turn, myocardial oxygen consumption can be measured. Initial studies in intact dogs and subsequently in humans have confirmed this possibility. With the tracer compartment model, estimates of regional oxygen consumption of 10.5 ml $O_2 \cdot min^{-1} \cdot 100g^{-1}$ have been obtained in normal human volunteers [10]. The tracer compartment model also provides estimates of myocardial blood flow so that both can be measured simultaneously. This offers the opportunity to relate oxygen consumption to blood flow, to derive values of oxygen extraction, and to explore compensatory mechanisms in cardiac disease as, for example, in myocardial ischemia [79].

Molecular oxygen-15

Molecular oxygen-15 has also been employed for measurements of myocardial extraction of oxygen and, when combined with measurements of myocardial blood flow, of the myocardial oxygen consumption [80,81]. Myocardial blood flow is determined with oxygen-15 labeled water and the oxygen extraction after inhalation of molecular oxygen-15. Oxygen extraction values estimated with this approach average in normal volunteers about 60% and are similar to values determined in normal volunteers through the invasive coronary sinus catheter technique (63%) [80,82,83].

Tracers of Neuronal Control

Besides positron-emitting tracers of blood flow and substrate metabolism, interest has increased in other tracers as, for example, of myocardial neuronal control. Radiotracers in this group include receptor ligands as, for example, C-11 MQNB for visualizing myocardial muscarinic receptors or C-11 labeled CGP-12177, an investigational compound binding to myocardial beta-receptors. Investigations in experimental animals and in humans with the latter compound have demonstrated the possibility of quantitative determinations of beta-receptor densities and receptor binding affinities [84–86]. Foremost among radiotracers of myocardial neuronal control have been agents for probing the function of the adrenergic neurons in the myocardium.

Carbon-11 labeled hydroxyephedrine

Carbon-11 labeled hydroxyephedrine (HED), a catecholamine analog, traces the uptake 2 mechanism of adrenergic nerve terminals [87]. This mechanism is responsible for recovery of norepinephrine from the cleft between the neuron terminal and the adrenergic receptor and for its storage in the terminal vesicles. Administered intravenously, the agent rapidly accumulates in the myocardium and promptly clears from blood so that images of the relative myocardial uptake of C-11 hydroxyephedrine are acquired from 40 to 60 minutes after tracer administration. To account for the flow-dependent regional variations in tracer retention, images of myocardial C-11 hydroxyephedrine uptake are frequently compared to images of myocardial blood flow. Striking disparities exist between perfusion and C-11 hydroxyephedrine uptake in myocardial regions with functionally abnormal adrenergic neurons or in denervated myocardial regions [88,89]. Invasive studies in humans similarly have demonstrated a correlation between the extraction of catecholamine across the myocardium and the net retention of C-11 hydroxyephedrine [90]. Estimates of the absolute uptake of tracers in the myocardium are available from serially acquired images. The myocardial tracer activity concentration at 60 minutes after injection is normalized to the integral of the blood pool time-activity curve or the arterial tracer input function. The resulting tracer net retention is also referred to as "volume of distribution."

Observations made with this tracer are important because they (1) uncovered adrenergic neural abnormalities in a number of cardiovascular disorders; and (2) contributed to an understanding of signaling pathways of, for example, coronary circulatory control and of substrate metabolism.

Abnormalities in adrenergic neuronal function. Early studies uncovered reduced tracer retention in ischemic and postischemic myocardium. Despite recovery of myocardial blood flow at rest following an acute myocardial infarction, retention of C-11 hydroxyephedrine remained regionally reduced [91]. In extent, these reductions exceeded those of the flow reductions in postinfarction patients with persistent flow defects, suggesting that the ischemic injury had imparted greater injury to adrenergic neurons than to myocytes. Striking reductions in regional C-11 hydroxyephedrine retention were also observed in normally perfused myocardium in type 2 diabetes [92–95]. The observed abnormalities in tracer retention were found to be correlated with the presence of diabetic neuropathy. Fur-

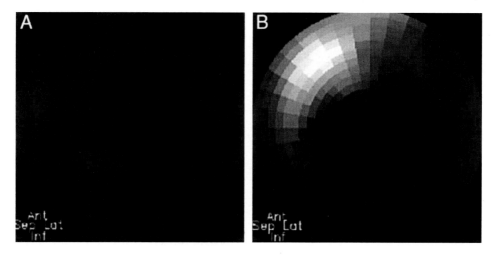

FIGURE 18.6 Polar map displays of C-11 hydroxyephedrine uptake in a cardiac transplant patient early (*A*, 0.3 years) and again 3 years (*B*) following cardiac transplantation. Note the absent tracer uptake on the initial study but the return of uptake in the anterior wall of the left ventricle consistent with reinnervation. (Reproduced from Bengel et al. [97], with permission of the American Heart Association.)

ther, while C-11 hydroxyephedrine distributed homogeneously throughout the left ventricular myocardium in patients with idiopathic dilated cardiomyopathy, the net retention of tracer was significantly reduced [96]. As subsequent investigations reported, the severity of reduced PET tracer uptake was related to the long-term survival of such patients, and thus semiquantitative measurements of tracer concentrations promise to be predictive of cardiac events. In cardiac allografts, retention of C-11 hydroxyephedrine was, as anticipated for the denervated heart, markedly diminished, while myocardial blood flow at rest was normal [88]. Other studies conclusively demonstrated progressive reinnervation of cardiac transplants [97] (Fig. 18.6). Further, adrenergic reinnervation had implications for the response of left ventricular function to exercise [98,99].

Elucidation of signaling pathways. Invasive and noninvasive investigations of the coronary circulatory function, including studies with positron-emitting tracers of myocardial blood flow in PET, have demonstrated perfusion abnormalities in patients with type 2 diabetes [100]. One such functional abnormality entails an absent or attenuated flow response to cold pressor testing. Findings with intracoronary flow velocity probes and with quantitative coronary angiography implicated this provocative test as a probe of endothelial function [101]. In type 2 diabetic patients, regionally absent or reduced C-11 hydroxyephedrine retention was significantly correlated with an absent or diminished flow response to cold, confirming the role of efferent adrenergic neurons for signaling the coronary va-

somotor response [100]. Comparable observations have been made with C-11 hydroxyephedrine in cardiac allografts when the severity of coronary circulatory dysfunction was correlated with the reduction in C-11 hydroxyephedrine retention [102]. Finally, myocardial regions of cardiac allografts with absent or markedly reduced tracer retention exhibit moderately, though statistically significant, higher rates of glucose metabolism, implicating adrenergic neuronal control as a determinant of regional myocardial substrate metabolism [103].

FINDINGS WITH PET IN THE HUMAN HEART

The following section briefly reviews a number of observations made with PET. An attempt is made to synthesize these findings with the aim for demonstrating how the combination of various noninvasive PET-based assay techniques can lead to a more comprehensive characterization of the human myocardium's function.

Myocardial Blood Flow

The ability to measure myocardial blood flow has emerged as a major asset of PET. Estimates of myocardial blood flow at rest can vary considerably between individuals; several investigations have convincingly demonstrated the dependency of such estimates addressed on cardiac work as assessed by the rate-pressure product [104,105]. According to several studies, myocardial blood flow at rest is correlated with the rate-pressure product. Increases in cardiac work in response to supine bicycle exercise or to inotropic stimulation are accompanied by proportionate increases in myocardial blood flow (see Table 18.1) [13,106,107]. Pharmacologic stress with either adenosine or dipyridamole is equally effective in raising myocardial blood flow. Both agents serve to define the total vasodilator capacity, as the ratio of hyperemic to rest myocardial blood flow as determined with PET ranges from 3.5 to 4.5 in young individuals but may decline with age (see also Table 18.1) [104,105,108]. These noninvasively determined values are indeed comparable to those measured by invasive techniques employing intracoronary flow velocity probes and quantitative angiography [109,110].

Coronary risk factors, including plasma lipid abnormalities, diabetes, hypertension, or a family history of premature coronary artery disease attenuate maximum pharmacologically induced hyperemic blood flow and myocardial flow reserve [111–114]. Such measurements may therefore serve as an index of coronary vasomotor abnormalities. Conversely, they may also prove useful for exploring beneficial effects of pharmacologic interventions, as, for example, lipid lowering with HMG-CoA reductase inhibitors. Several investigations report improvements in hyperemic blood flow and myocardial flow reserve after HMG-CoA reductase inhibitor treatment so that improvements in hyperemic myocardial blood flow could serve as surrogate end points of drug interventions [115–117]. Equally exciting are reports on correlations between genetic defects and their severity as, for example, in myotonic dystrophy and the vasodilator capacity of the coronary circulation [118].

Myocardial Substrate Metabolism and Regulation

No less important are findings on the myocardium's substrate metabolism and substrate selection. As had been known from isolated heart preparations, and, later from human investigations using the coronary sinus catheter technique, the myocardical selection of substrate fuel largely depends on the availability in blood. Responses of the myocardium by changing its substrate selection can, as described earlier in this chapter, clearly be demonstrated with positron-emitting tracers of myocardial substrate metabolism. These observations convincingly demonstrate the operation of Randle's cycle in humans while described initially in isolated heart preparations [119]. The changes in the myocardium's substrate selection occur in response to systemic changes. They are, thus, fully synchronized with and are part of a general response system to, for example, changes in

physical activity or nutritional state. At the same time, cardiovascular disease may override or counter these "system-wide" coordinated responses as evidenced, for example, in poorly functioning left ventricular myocardium by a paradoxical response of the free fatty acid metabolism to glucose administration [120], or in chronically dysfunctional myocardium by a disproportionate increase in glucose utilization, now the metabolic hallmark of myocardial viability [62,121].

Myocardial Work and Efficiency

Finally, the ability of PET to measure myocardial oxygen consumption and rates of oxidative metabolism affords estimates of the myocardium's mechanical efficiency, that is, how effectively chemical energy is converted into mechanical energy. Internal mechanical work is difficult to measure. Estimates of the external work can, however, be derived noninvasively and with relative ease. For example, left ventricular volumes in end-diastole and in end-systole are available through gated PET image acquisition itself [122–124] but are also available through gated cardiac radionuclide imaging, echocardiography, and gated MRI. Stroke work can thus be calculated from the left ventricular volume and systolic arterial blood pressure. The majority of studies thus far have employed echocardiographically measured left ventricular volumes and wall thickness and comparisons to oxidative metabolism determined with C-11 acetate or with the molecular oxygen-15 approach. These studies related the stroke work index as a measure of mechanical work to myocardial oxidative metabolism or directly to myocardial oxygen consumption. In normal volunteers, for example, inotropic stimulation with dobutamine significantly raised the external work efficiency [125]. Mechanical efficiency was reduced in left ventricular hypertrophy [83] but also in patients with idiopathic dilated cardiomyopathy [126,127]. Left ventricular unloading with nitroprusside in one of these investigations led to an improvement in the mechanical efficiency [126]. Consistent with this finding are observations in cardiac transplant patients describing an inverse correlation between afterload, as defined by peripheral vascular resistance, but also with pre-load or the end-diastolic volume and the stroke volume [98].

CONCLUSIONS AND FUTURE DEVELOPMENTS

This chapter describes the advantages of PET over more conventional nuclear medicine imaging approaches including SPECT. In many instances, features unique to

PET including those related to instrumentation and to radiopharmaceuticals relate directly to currently and widely used radionuclide approaches to the diagnosis, characterization, and therapy monitoring of coronary artery disease. This applies particularly to the identification of fluid dynamically significant coronary stenosis and to the assessment of myocardial viability as described in more detail in other chapters of this book. Based on the available evidence, PET is likely to enhance the diagnostic accuracy of these particular radionuclide approaches. At the same time, a substantial body of scientific knowledge points to observations that are entirely unique to PET as, for example, the noninvasive quantification of myocardial blood flow of substrate metabolism or neuronal function of the human myocardium. Application of PET to these processes will likely provide new mechanistic insights into cardiovascular disease but also expand possibilities for characterizing disease and its responses to therapy. These applications further hold promise for detection of preclinical disease. Implicit in the ability of early disease detection is the promise of reversal of disease most likely through pharmacologic means. Beyond this, PET promises new tools for designing strategies of gene therapy or myocardial repair as evidenced by early animal experimental studies as well as in humans.

ACKNOWLEDGMENTS

The author thanks Rita Rubins for her assistance in preparing this manuscript and Diane Martin for preparing the illustrations.

REFERENCES

1. Phelps ME, Hoffman EJ, Mullani NA, et al. Application of annihilation coincidence detection to transaxial reconstruction tomography. J Nucl Med 1975;16:210.
2. Bergmann SR, Fox KA, Rand AL, et al. Quantification of regional myocardial blood flow in vivo with H215O. Circulation 1984;70:724.
3. Bergmann SR, Herrero P, Markham J, et al. Noninvasive quantitation of myocardial blood flow in human subjects with oxygen-15-labeled water and positron emission tomography. J Am Coll Cardiol 1989;14:639.
4. Rosamond TL, Abendschein DR, Sobel BE, et al. Metabolic fate of radiolabeled palmitate in ischemic canine myocardium: implications for positron emission tomography. J Nucl Med 1987;28:1322.
5. Ng CK, Huang SC, Schelbert HR, et al. Validation of a model for [1-11C]acetate as a tracer of cardiac oxidative metabolism. Am J Physiol 1994;266:H1304.
6. Armbrecht JJ, Buxton DB, Brunken RC, et al. Regional myocardial oxygen consumption determined noninvasively in humans with [1-11C]acetate and dynamic positron tomography. Circulation 1989;80:863.
7. Krivokapich J, Huang SC, Selin CE, et al. Fluorodeoxyglucose rate constants, lumped constant, and glucose metabolic rate in rabbit heart. Am J Physiol 1987;252:H777.
8. Schelbert HR, Phelps ME, Huang SC, et al. N-13 ammonia as an indicator of myocardial blood flow. Circulation 1981;63:1259.
9. Sun KT, Chen K, Huang SC, et al. Compartment model for measuring myocardial oxygen consumption using [1-11C] acetate. J Nucl Med 1997;38:459.
10. Sun KT, Yeatman LA, Buxton DB, et al. Simultaneous measurement of myocardial oxygen consumption and blood flow using [1-carbon-11]acetate. J Nucl Med 1998;39:272.
11. Huang SC, Williams BA, Barrio JR, et al. Measurement of glucose and 2-deoxy-2-[18F]fluoro-D-glucose transport and phosphorylation rates in myocardium using dual-tracer kinetic experiments. Febs Letters 1987;216:128.
12. Phelps ME, Hoffman EJ, Selin C, et al. Investigation of [18F]2-fluoro-2-deoxyglucose for the measure of myocardial glucose metabolism. J Nucl Med 1978;19:1311.
13. Krivokapich J, Smith GT, Huang SC, et al. 13N ammonia myocardial imaging at rest and with exercise in normal volunteers. Quantification of absolute myocardial perfusion with dynamic positron emission tomography [see comments]. Circulation 1989;80:1328.
14. Kuhle WG, Porenta G, Huang SC, et al. Quantification of regional myocardial blood flow using 13N-ammonia and reoriented dynamic positron emission tomographic imaging. Circulation 1992;86:1004.
15. Patlak CS, Blasberg RG. Graphical evaluation of blood-to-brain transfer constants from multiple-time uptake data. J Cereb Blood Flow Metab 1985;5:584.
16. Gambhir SS, Schwaiger M, Huang SC, et al. Simple noninvasive quantification method for measuring myocardial glucose utilization in humans employing positron emission tomography and fluorine-18 deoxyglucose. J Nucl Med 1989;30:359.
17. Chan SY, Brunken RC, Czernin J, et al. Comparison of maximal myocardial blood flow during adenosine infusion with that of intravenous dipyridamole in normal men. J Am Coll Cardiol 1992;20:979.
18. Choi Y, Hawkins RA, Huang SC, et al. Parametric images of myocardial metabolic rate of glucose generated from dynamic cardiac PET and 2-[18F]fluoro-2-deoxy-d-glucose studies. J Nucl Med 1991;32:733.
19. Choi Y, Huang SC, Hawkins RA, et al. A refined method for quantification of myocardial oxygen consumption rate using mean transit time with carbon-11-acetate and dynamic PET. J Nucl Med 1993;34:2038.
20. Choi Y, Huang SC, Hawkins RA, et al. A simplified method for quantification of myocardial blood flow using nitrogen-13-ammonia and dynamic PET [see comments]. J Nucl Med 1993;34:488.
21. Blanksma PK, Willemsen AT, Meeder JG, et al. Quantitative myocardial mapping of perfusion and metabolism using parametric polar map displays in cardiac PET. J Nucl Med 1995;36:153.
22. Iida H, Kanno I, Takahashi A, et al. Measurement of absolute myocardial blood flow with H215O and dynamic positron-emission tomography. Strategy for quantification in relation to the partial-volume effect. Circulation 1988;78:104.
23. Hermansen F, Ashburner J, Spinks TJ, et al. Generation of myocardial factor images directly from the dynamic oxygen-15-water scan without use of an oxygen-15-carbon monoxide blood-pool scan. J Nucl Med 1998;39:1696.
24. Wu HM, Hoh CK, Buxton DB, et al. Quantification of myocardial blood flow using dynamic nitrogen-13-ammonia PET

studies and factor analysis of dynamic structures. J Nucl Med 1995;36:2087.

25. Wu HM, Hoh CK, Choi Y, et al. Factor analysis for extraction of blood time-activity curves in dynamic FDG-PET studies. J Nucl Med 1995;36:1714.

26. Schelbert HR, Phelps ME, Hoffman EJ, et al. Regional myocardial perfusion assessed with N-13 labeled ammonia and positron emission computerized axial tomography. Am J Cardiol 1979;43:209.

27. Hutchins GD, Schwaiger M, Rosenspire KC, et al. Noninvasive quantification of regional blood flow in the human heart using N-13 ammonia and dynamic positron emission tomographic imaging. J Am Coll Cardiol 1990;15:1032.

28. Muzik O, Beanlands RS, Hutchins GD, et al. Validation of nitrogen-13-ammonia tracer kinetic model for quantification of myocardial blood flow using PET. J Nucl Med 1993;34:83.

29. Gould KL, Schelbert HR, Phelps ME, et al. Noninvasive assessment of coronary stenoses with myocardial perfusion imaging during pharmacologic coronary vasodilatation. V. Detection of 47 percent diameter coronary stenosis with intravenous nitrogen-13 ammonia and emission-computed tomography in intact dogs. Am J Cardiol 1979;43:200.

30. Demer LL, Gould KL, Goldstein RA, et al. Assessment of coronary artery disease severity by positron emission tomography. Comparison with quantitative arteriography in 193 patients. Circulation 1989;79:825.

31. Herrero P, Markham J, Shelton ME, et al. Noninvasive quantification of regional myocardial perfusion with rubidium-82 and positron emission tomography. Exploration of a mathematical model. Circulation 1990;82:1377.

32. Lin JW, Sciacca RR, Chou RL, et al. Quantification of myocardial perfusion in human subjects using 82Rb and wavelet-based noise reduction. J Nucl Med 2001;42:201.

33. Mélon P, Brihaye C, Degueldre C, et al. Myocardial kinetics of potassium-38 in humans and comparison with Copper-62-PTSM. J Nucl Med 1994;35:1116.

34. Green MA, Mathias CJ, Welch MJ, et al. Copper-62-labeled pyruvaldehyde bis(N4-methylthiosemicarbazonato)copper(II): synthesis and evaluation as a positron emission tomography tracer for cerebral and myocardial perfusion. J Nucl Med 1990;31:1989.

35. Beanlands RS, Muzik O, Mintun M, et al. The kinetics of copper-62-PTSM in the normal human heart. J Nucl Med 1992;33:684.

36. Shelton ME, Green MA, Mathias CJ, et al. Kinetics of copper-PTSM in isolated hearts: a novel tracer for measuring blood flow with positron emission tomography. J Nucl Med 1989;30:1843.

37. Shelton ME, Green MA, Mathias CJ, et al. Assessment of regional myocardial and renal blood flow with copper-PTSM and positron emission tomography. Circulation 1990;82:990.

38. Tadamura E, Tamaki N, Okazawa H, et al. Generator-produced copper-62-PTSM as a myocardial PET perfusion tracer compared with nitrogen-13-ammonia. J Nucl Med 1996;37:729.

39. Wallhaus TR, Lacy J, Stewart R, et al. Copper-62-pyruvaldehyde bis(N-methyl-thiosemicarbazone) PET imaging in the detection of coronary artery disease in humans. J Nucl Cardiol 2001;8:67.

40. Herrero P, Markham J, Weinheimer CJ, et al. Quantification of regional myocardial perfusion with generator-produced 62Cu-PTSM and positron emission tomography. Circulation 1993;87:173.

41. Herrero P, Hartman JJ, Green MA, et al. Regional myocardial perfusion assessed with generator-produced copper-62-PTSM and PET. J Nucl Med 1996;37:1294.

42. Chan SY, Brunken RC, Phelps ME, et al. Use of the metabolic tracer carbon-11-acetate for evaluation of regional myocardial perfusion. J Nucl Med 1991;32:665.

43. Wolpers HG, Burchert W, van den Hoff J, et al. Assessment of myocardial viability by use of 11C-acetate and positron emission tomography. Threshold criteria of reversible dysfunction. Circulation 1997;95:1417.

44. Armbrecht JJ, Buxton DB, Schelbert HR. Validation of [1-11C]acetate as a tracer for noninvasive assessment of oxidative metabolism with positron emission tomography in normal, ischemic, postischemic, and hyperemic canine myocardium. Circulation 1990;81:1594.

45. Sciacca RR, Akinboboye O, Chou RL, et al. Measurement of myocardial blood flow with PET using 1-11C-acetate. J Nucl Med 2001;42:63.

46. Bol A, Melin JA, Vanoverschelde JL, et al. Direct comparison of [13N]ammonia and [15O]water estimates of perfusion with quantification of regional myocardial blood flow by microspheres. Circulation 1993;87:512.

47. Nitzsche EU, Choi Y, Czernin J, et al. Noninvasive quantification of myocardial blood flow in humans. A direct comparison of the [13N]ammonia and the [15O]water techniques. Circulation 1996;93:2000.

48. Iida H, Rhodes C, de Silva R, et al. Myocardial tissue fraction—correction for partial volume effects and measure of tissue viability. J Nucl Med 1991;32:2169.

49. Gerber BL, Melin JA, Bol A, et al. Nitrogen-13-ammonia and oxygen-15-water estimates of absolute myocardial perfusion in left ventricular ischemic dysfunction. J Nucl Med 1998;39:1655.

50. Sokoloff L, Reivich M, Kennedy C, et al. The [14C]-deoxyglucose method for the measurement of local cerebral glucose utilization: theory, procedure and normal values in the conscious and anesthetized albino rat. J Neurochem 1977;28:897.

51. Choi Y, Brunken RC, Hawkins RA, et al. Factors affecting myocardial 2-[F-18]fluoro-2-deoxy-D-glucose uptake in positron emission tomography studies of normal humans. Eur J Nucl Med 1993;20:308.

52. Takahashi N, Tamaki N, Kawamoto M, et al. Glucose metabolism in relation to perfusion in patients with ischaemic heart disease. Eur J Nucl Med 1994;21:292.

53. Marshall RC, Tillisch JH, Phelps ME, et al. Identification and differentiation of resting myocardial ischemia and infarction in man with positron computed tomography, 18F-labeled fluorodeoxyglucose and N-13 ammonia. Circulation 1983;67:766.

54. DeFronzo RA, Tobin JD, Andres R. Glucose clamp technique: a method for quantifying insulin secretion and resistance. Am J Physiol 1979;237:E214.

55. Hicks R, von Dahl J, Lee K, et al. Insulin-glucose clamp for standardization of metabolic conditions during F-18 fluorodeoxyglucose PET imaging. J Am Coll Cardiol 1991;17:381A.

56. Mäki M, Luotolahti M, Nuutila P, et al. Glucose uptake in the chronically dysfunctional but viable myocardium. Circulation 1996;93:1658.

57. Nuutila P, Knuuti M, Raitakari M, et al. Effect of antilipolysis on heart and skeletal muscle glucose uptake in overnight fasted humans. Am J Physiol 1994;267:E941.

58. Stone C, Holden J, Stanley W, et al. Effect of nicotinic acid on exogenous myocardial glucose utilization. J Nucl Med 1995;36:996.

59. Ratib O, Phelps ME, Huang SC, et al. Positron tomography

with deoxyglucose for estimating local myocardial glucose metabolism. J Nucl Med 1982;23:577.

60. Schwaiger M, Sun D, Deeb G, et al. Expression of myocardial glucose transporter (GLUT) mRNAs in patients with advanced coronary artery disease (CAD). Circulation 1994;90:I-113.

61. Lopaschuk G, Stanley W. Glucose metabolism in the ischemic heart. Circulation 1997;95:313.

62. Tillisch J, Brunken R, Marshall R, et al. Reversibility of cardiac wall-motion abnormalities predicted by positron tomography. N Engl J Med 1986;314:884.

63. Schön HR, Schelbert HR, Najafi A, et al. C-11 labeled palmitic acid for the noninvasive evaluation of regional myocardial fatty acid metabolism with positron-computed tomography. II. Kinetics of C-11 palmitic acid in acutely ischemic myocardium. Am Heart J 1982;103:548.

64. Schön HR, Schelbert HR, Robinson G, et al. C-11 labeled palmitic acid for the noninvasive evaluation of regional myocardial fatty acid metabolism with positron-computed tomography. I. Kinetics of C-11 palmitic acid in normal myocardium. Am Heart J 1982;103:532.

65. Schelbert HR, Henze E, Sochor H, et al. Effects of substrate availability on myocardial C-11 palmitate kinetics by positron emission tomography in normal subjects and patients with ventricular dysfunction. Am Heart J 1986;111:1055.

66. Schelbert HR, Henze E, Keen R, et al. C-11 palmitate for the noninvasive evaluation of regional myocardial fatty acid metabolism with positron-computed tomography. IV. In vivo evaluation of acute demand-induced ischemia in dogs. Am Heart J 1983;106:736.

67. Schwaiger M, Brunken R, Grover-McKay M, et al. Regional myocardial metabolism in patients with acute myocardial infarction assessed by positron emission tomography. J Am Coll Cardiol 1986;8:800.

68. Schwaiger M, Schelbert HR, Keen R, et al. Retention and clearance of C-11 palmitic acid in ischemic and reperfused canine myocardium. J Am Coll Cardiol 1985;6:311.

69. Bergmann SR, Weinheimer CJ, Markham J, et al. Quantitation of myocardial fatty acid metabolism using PET. J Nucl Med 1996;37:1723.

70. DeGrado TR, Wang S, Holden JE, et al. Synthesis and preliminary evaluation of (18)F-labeled 4-thia palmitate as a PET tracer of myocardial fatty acid oxidation. Nucl Med Biol 2000;27:221.

71. Renstrom B, Rommelfanger S, Stone CK, et al. Comparison of fatty acid tracers FTHA and BMIPP during myocardial ischemia and hypoxia. J Nucl Med 1998;39:1684.

72. Stone CK, Pooley RA, DeGrado TR, et al. Myocardial uptake of the fatty acid analog 14-fluorine-18-fluoro-6-thia-heptadecanoic acid in comparison to beta-oxidation rates by tritiated palmitate. J Nucl Med 1998;39:1690.

73. Mäki MT, Haaparanta M, Nuutila P, et al. Free fatty acid uptake in the myocardium and skeletal muscle using fluorine-18-fluoro-6-thia-heptadecanoic acid. J Nucl Med 1998;39:1320.

74. Brown M, Marshall DR, Sobel BE, et al. Delineation of myocardial oxygen utilization with carbon-11-labeled acetate. Circulation 1987;76:687.

75. Brown MA, Myears DW, Bergmann SR. Validity of estimates of myocardial oxidative metabolism with carbon-11 acetate and positron emission tomography despite altered patterns of substrate utilization. J Nucl Med 1989;30:187.

76. Buxton DB, Nienaber CA, Luxen A, et al. Noninvasive quantitation of regional myocardial oxygen consumption in vivo with [1-11C]acetate and dynamic positron emission tomography. Circulation 1989;79:134.

77. Buxton DB, Schwaiger M, Nguyen A, et al. Radiolabeled acetate as a tracer of myocardial tricarboxylic acid cycle flux. Circ Res 1988;63:628.

78. Brown MA, Myears DW, Bergmann SR. Noninvasive assessment of canine myocardial oxidative metabolism with carbon-11 acetate and positron emission tomography. J Am Coll Cardiol 1988;12:1054.

79. Czernin J, Porenta G, Brunken R, et al. Regional blood flow, oxidative metabolism, and glucose utilization in patients with recent myocardial infarction. Circulation 1993;88:884.

80. Iida H, Rhodes CG, Araujo LI, et al. Noninvasive quantification of regional myocardial metabolic rate for oxygen by use of 15O2 inhalation and positron emission tomography. Theory, error analysis, and application in humans. Circulation 1996;94:792.

81. Yamamoto Y, de Silva R, Rhodes CG, et al. Noninvasive quantification of regional myocardial metabolic rate of oxygen by 15O2 inhalation and positron emission tomography. Experimental validation. Circulation 1996;94:808.

82. Holmberg S, Serzysko W, Varnauskas E. Coronary circulation during heavy exercise in control subjects and patients with coronary heart disease. Acta Med Scand 1971;190:465.

83. Laine H, Katoh C, Luotolahti M, et al. Myocardial oxygen consumption is unchanged but efficiency is reduced in patients with essential hypertension and left ventricular hypertrophy. Circulation 1999;100:2425.

84. Choudhury L, Guzzetti S, Lefroy DC, et al. Myocardial beta adrenoceptors and left ventricular function in hypertrophic cardiomyopathy. Heart 1996;75:50.

85. Schafers M, Lerch H, Wichter T, et al. Cardiac sympathetic innervation in patients with idiopathic right ventricular outflow tract tachycardia. J Am Coll Cardiol 1998;32:181.

86. Wichter T, Schafers M, Rhodes CG, et al. Abnormalities of cardiac sympathetic innervation in arrhythmogenic right ventricular cardiomyopathy: quantitative assessment of presynaptic norepinephrine reuptake and postsynaptic beta-adrenergic receptor density with positron emission tomography. Circulation 2000;101:1552.

87. DeGrado TR, Hutchins GD, Toorongian SA, et al. Myocardial kinetics of carbon-11-meta-hydroxyephedrine: retention mechanisms and effects of norepinephrine. J Nucl Med 1993;34:1287.

88. Schwaiger M, Hutchins GD, Kalff V, et al. Evidence for regional catecholamine uptake and storage sites in the transplanted human heart by positron emission tomography. J Clin Invest 1991;87:1681.

89. Schwaiger M, Kalff V, Rosenspire K, et al. Noninvasive evaluation of sympathetic nervous system in human heart by positron emission tomography [see comments]. Circulation 1990;82:457.

90. Odaka K, von Scheidt W, Ziegler SI, et al. Reappearance of cardiac presynaptic sympathetic nerve terminals in the transplanted heart: correlation between PET using (11)C-hydroxyephedrine and invasively measured norepinephrine release. J Nucl Med 2001;42:1011.

91. Allman KC, Wieland DM, Muzik O, et al. Carbon-11 hydroxyephedrine with positron emission tomography for serial assessment of cardiac adrenergic neuronal function after acute myocardial infarction in humans. J Am Coll Cardiol 1993;22:368.

92. Allman KC, Stevens MJ, Wieland DM, et al. Noninvasive assessment of cardiac diabetic neuropathy by carbon-11 hydroxyephedrine and positron emission tomography. J Am Coll Cardiol 1993;22:1425.

93. Stevens MJ, Dayanikli F, Raffel DM, et al. Scintigraphic assessment of regionalized defects in myocardial sympathetic innervation and blood flow regulation in diabetic patients with autonomic neuropathy. J Am Coll Cardiol 1998;31:1575.

94. Stevens MJ, Raffel DM, Allman KC, et al. Cardiac sympathetic dysinnervation in diabetes: implications for enhanced cardiovascular risk. Circulation 1998;98:961.

95. Stevens MJ, Raffel DM, Allman KC, et al. Regression and progression of cardiac sympathetic dysinnervation complicating diabetes: an assessment by C-11 hydroxyephedrine and positron emission tomography. Metab Clin Exp 1999;48:92.

96. Hartmann F, Ziegler S, Nekolla S, et al. Regional patterns of myocardial sympathetic denervation in dilated cardiomyopathy: an analysis using carbon-11 hydroxyephedrine and positron emission tomography. Heart 1999;81:262.

97. Bengel FM, Ueberfuhr P, Ziegler SI, et al. Serial assessment of sympathetic reinnervation after orthotopic heart transplantation. A longitudinal study using PET and C-11 hydroxyephedrine. Circulation 1999;99:1866.

98. Bengel FM, Ueberfuhr P, Schiepel N, et al. Myocardial efficiency and sympathetic reinnervation after orthotopic heart transplantation: a noninvasive study with positron emission tomography. Circulation 2001;103:1881.

99. Bengel FM, Ueberfuhr P, Schiepel N, et al. Effect of sympathetic reinnervation on cardiac performance after heart transplantation. [Comment In: N Engl J Med. 2001 Sep 6;345(10): 762-4 UI: 21410622]. N Engl J Med 2001;345:731.

100. Di Carli MF, Bianco-Batlles D, Landa ME, et al. Effects of autonomic neuropathy on coronary blood flow in patients with diabetes mellitus. Circulation 1999;100:813.

101. Zeiher AM, Drexler H, Wollschlager H, et al. Endothelial dysfunction of the coronary microvasculature is associated with coronary blood flow regulation in patients with early atherosclerosis. Circulation 1991;84:1984.

102. Di Carli MF, Tobes MC, Mangner T, et al. Effects of cardiac sympathetic innervation on coronary blood flow. N Engl J Med 1997;336:1208.

103. Bengel FM, Ueberfuhr P, Ziegler SI, et al. Non-invasive assessment of the effect of cardiac sympathetic innervation on metabolism of the human heart. Eur J Nucl Med 2000;27:1650.

104. Czernin J, Müller P, Chan S, et al. Influence of age and hemodynamics on myocardial blood flow and flow reserve. Circulation 1993;88:62.

105. Uren NG, Camici PG, Melin JA, et al. Effect of aging on myocardial perfusion reserve. J Nucl Med 1995;36:2032.

106. Krivokapich J, Czernin J, Schelbert HR. Dobutamine positron emission tomography: absolute quantitation of rest and dobutamine myocardial blood flow and correlation with cardiac work and percent diameter stenosis in patients with and without coronary artery disease. J Am Coll Cardiol 1996;28:565.

107. Krivokapich J, Stevenson LW, Kobashigawa J, et al. Quantification of absolute myocardial perfusion at rest and during exercise with positron emission tomography after human cardiac transplantation. J Am Coll Cardiol 1991;18:512.

108. Senneff MJ, Geltman EM, Bergmann SR. Noninvasive delineation of the effects of moderate aging on myocardial perfusion [published erratum appears in J Nucl Med 1992 Feb;33(2):201] [see comments]. J Nucl Med 1991;32:2037.

109. Shelton ME, Senneff MJ, Ludbrook PA, et al. Concordance of nutritive myocardial perfusion reserve and flow velocity reserve in conductance vessels in patients with chest pain with angiographically normal coronary arteries. J Nucl Med 1993;34: 717.

110. Wilson R, Laughlin D, Ackell P. Transluminal subselective measurement of coronary artery blood flow velocity and vasodilator reserve in man. Circulation 1985;72:82.

111. Dayanikli F, Grambow D, Muzik O, et al. Early detection of abnormal coronary flow reserve in asymptomatic men at high risk for coronary artery disease using positron emission tomography. Circulation 1994;90:808.

112. Pitkänen OP, Raitakari OT, Niinikoski H, et al. Coronary flow reserve is impaired in young men with familial hypercholesterolemia. J Am Coll Cardiol 1996;28:1705.

113. Pitkänen OP, Nuutila P, Raitakari OT, et al. Coronary flow reserve is reduced in young men with IDDM. Diabetes. 1998;47:248.

114. Yokoyama I, Ohtake T, Momomura S, et al. Reduced coronary flow reserve in hypercholesterolemic patients without overt coronary stenosis. Circulation 1996;94:3232.

115. Baller D, Notohamiprodjo G, Gleichmann U, et al. Improvement in coronary flow reserve determined by positron emission tomography after 6 months of cholesterol-lowering therapy in patients with early stages of coronary atherosclerosis. Circulation 1999;99:2871.

116. Guethlin M, Kasel AM, Coppenrath K, et al. Delayed response of myocardial flow reserve to lipid-lowering therapy with fluvastatin. Circulation 1999;99:475.

117. Yokoyama I, Momomura S, Ohtake T, et al. Improvement of impaired myocardial vasodilatation due to diffuse coronary atherosclerosis in hypercholesterolemics after lipid-lowering therapy. Circulation 1999;100:117.

118. Annane D, Merlet P, Radvanyi H, et al. Blunted coronary reserve in myotonic dystrophy. An early and gene-related phenomenon. Circulation 1996;94:973.

119. Randle RJ, Garland BP, Hales CN, et al. The glucose fatty acid cycle: its role in insulin sensitivity and the metabolic disturbances in diabetes mellitus. Lancet 1963;1:785.

120. Sochor H, Schelbert H, Schwaiger M, et al. Studies of fatty acid metabolism with positron emission tomography in patients with cardiomyopathy. Eur J Nucl Med 1986;12:S66.

121. Tamaki N, Yonekura Y, Yamashita K, et al. Positron emission tomography using fluorine-18 deoxyglucose in evaluation of coronary artery bypass grafting. Am J Cardiol 1989;64:860.

122. Porenta G, Kuhle W, Sinha S, et al. Parameter estimation of cardiac geometry by ECG-gated PET imaging: validation using magnetic resonance imaging and echocardiography. J Nucl Med 1995;36:1123.

123. Boyd HL, Gunn RN, Marinho NV, et al. Non-invasive measurement of left ventricular volumes and function by gated positron emission tomography. Eur J Nucl Med 1996;23:1594.

124. Hattori N, Bengel FM, Mehilli J, et al. Global and regional functional measurements with gated FDG PET in comparison with left ventriculography. Eur J Nucl Med 2001;28:221.

125. Porenta G, Cherry S, Czernin J, et al. Noninvasive determination of myocardial blood flow, oxygen consumption and efficiency in normal humans by carbon-11 acetate positron emission tomography imaging. Eur J Nucl Med 1999;26:1465.

126. Beanlands RS, Armstrong WF, Hicks RJ, et al. The effects of afterload reduction on myocardial carbon 11-labeled acetate kinetics and noninvasively estimated mechanical efficiency in patients with dilated cardiomyopathy. J Nucl Cardiol 1994;1:3.

127. Bengel FM, Permanetter B, Ungerer M, et al. Non-invasive estimation of myocardial efficiency using positron emission tomography and carbon-11 acetate—comparison between the normal and failing human heart. Eur J Nucl Med 2000;27:319.

128. Araujo L, Lammertsma A, Rhodes C, et al. Noninvasive quan-

tification of regional myocardial blood flow in coronary artery disease with oxygen-15-labeled carbon dioxide inhalation and positron emission tomography. Circulation 1991;83:875.

129. Yokoyama I, Ohtake T, Momomura S, et al. Altered myocardial vasodilatation in patients with hypertriglyceridemia in anatomically normal coronary arteries. Arterioscler Thromb Vasc Biol 1998;18:294.

130. Tadamura E, Iida H, Matsumoto K, et al. Comparison of myocardial blood flow during dobutamine-atropine infusion with that after dipyridamole administration in normal men. J Am Coll Cardiol 2001;37:130.

131. Knuuti M, Nuutila P, Ruotsalainen U, et al. Euglycemic hyperinsulinemic clamp and oral glucose load in stimulating myocardial glucose utilization during positron emission tomography. J Nucl Med 1992;33:1255.

132. Ohtake T, Yokoyama I, Watanabe T, et al. Myocardial glucose metabolism in noninsulin-dependent diabetes mellitus patients evaluated by FDG-PET. J Nucl Med 1995;36:456.

19 | Myocardial viability/hibernation

JEROEN J. BAX, FATHY F. WAHBA, AND ERNST E. VAN DER WALL

CLINICAL RELEVANCE OF HEART FAILURE

Heart failure is becoming the number one problem in clinical cardiology in terms of patients affected. Over the past decade the number of patients presenting with heart failure has increased exponentially [1]. Recent estimations have indicated that 4.7 million patients in the United States have chronic heart failure, with 400,000 new cases each year, resulting in 1 million hospitalizations [1]. The diagnostic and therapeutic costs involved with heart failure are estimated to be more than $11 billion per year [1].

The underlying cause of heart failure may predominantly be coronary artery disease. Gheorghiade and Bonow pooled 13 randomized, multicenter heart failure trials (> 20,000 patients) published in the *New England Journal of Medicine* between 1986 and 1997 and came to the conclusion that coronary artery disease was the underlying etiology in almost 70% of the patients. Possibly this figure is even higher, since many patients in these trials did not undergo coronary angiography. Thus, heart failure is becoming an enormous problem with coronary artery disease being the most frequent cause.

Long-term prognosis of patients with heart failure remains poor, despite advances in different therapies [2]. Data from the Framingham study demonstrated a 5-year mortality rate of 75% for men and 62% for women [3]. More recent data from Cowie et al. [4] showed a a 6- and 12-month mortality of 30% and 38%, respectively; extrapolation of these results demonstrated a comparable 5-year mortality of that observed in the Framingham study [2].

THERAPEUTIC OPTIONS FOR ISCHEMIC CARDIOMYOPATHY

What are the different therapies for heart failure in the presence of coronary artery disease and depressed left ventricular (LV) function (or ischemic cardiomyopathy)? Currently, three main options of treatment are available, including medical treatment, heart transplantation, and revascularization.

Many recent improvements of medical therapy have been obtained over the past years. ACE inhibitors have been demonstrated in large heart failure trials (SAVE, SOLVD) to improve survival [5,6]. In patients with ischemic heart failure, the survival benefit of ACE inhibition is likely due to prevention (reversal) of LV remodeling and hypertrophy, but also a significant reduction in acute ischemic events. Angiotensin-II receptor blockers have been evaluated recently in patients with heart failure; in a direct comparison with ACE inhibitors (ELITE II Trial), both drugs exhibited a similar reduction in mortality [7]. Beta-adrenergic blocking agents have also been proven useful in the treatment of patients with heart failure [8]. Four major trials have all demonstrated a reduction in overall mortality and sudden death with the use of beta-blockers [8]. Spironolactone has been useful in the treatment of heart failure [9], and amiodarone has been demonstrated to reduce sudden death in patients with heart failure [10]. Despite these new drugs, mortality of patients with severe heart failure remains high [2].

Heart transplantation is another therapeutic option with an excellent long-term prognosis, but the limited number of donor hearts is largely exceeded by the demand [11].

Revascularization is a third option in patients with heart failure. However, revascularization is associated with a high periprocedural morbidity and mortality [12]. On the other hand, a substantial survival benefit after surgical revascularization compared with medical therapy has been shown [13]. Moreover, Elefteriades et al. [14] demonstrated that surgical revascularization was associated with an improvement in LV ejection fraction (EF), although not in all patients. Since LVEF is an important prognostic parameter [15], improvement in LVEF may, at least in part, contribute to the improved survival. Moreover, in patients with advanced heart failure the main cause of mortality is progression of heart failure [16], and thus, improvement of pump function may improve survival. It has been estimated that 25%–40% of the patients with chronic coronary artery disease and LV dysfunction have the potential for significant improvement in LV function postrevascularization [17]. Thus, in view of the higher morbidity/mortality of revascularization procedures, on the one hand, and the potential of improvement in LVEF and survival, on the other hand, a careful selection of patients who may benefit from revascularization procedures appears warranted.

THE CONCEPT OF MYOCARDIAL VIABILITY

Since the early works of Tennant and Wiggers, it has been known that total ischemia leads to an acute cessation of contraction, resulting in cell damage and irreversible myocardial necrosis [18]. Accordingly, it was thought that dysfunctional myocardium, related to coronary artery disease, was equivalent to myocardial necrosis. However, from the observational studies by Rahimtoola [19] it became clear that many patients with LV dysfunction exhibited improvement of function after revascularization. This has led to the hypothesis that some dysfunctional myocardium in patients with chronic coronary artery disease may not be irreversibly damaged but may still be viable, although not functioning properly, and may recover in function following adequate restoration of blood flow. To explain the phenomenon of recovery of function postrevascularization, the term *hibernation* was introduced [19].

MYOCARDIAL HIBERNATION

Hibernation refers to a condition of chronic sustained abnormal contraction due to chronic underperfusion in patients with coronary artery disease in whom revascularization causes recovery of function [19]. Indeed, some clinical studies have demonstrated a reduction in resting blood flow in patients with chronic LV dysfunction, with, however, (relatively) preserved glucose utilization [20]. Tawakol and colleagues [21] have recently evaluated patients with chronic LV dysfunction with N-13 ammonia positron emission tomography (PET) (to assess perfusion) and fluorodeoxyglucose (FDG) PET, who underwent subsequent revascularization. In these patients, perfusion in normally contracting areas was 1.14 ± 0.52 ml/min/g, whereas perfusion in dysfunctional but viable areas (as assessed by preserved FDG uptake) was significantly reduced: 0.48 ± 0.15 ml/min/g. Comparable results were observed in four other studies [22]. Other studies, however, have demonstrated that resting perfusion was (near-)normal in chronic dysfunctional myocardium [22]. Vanoverschelde

et al. [23] observed almost similar levels of perfusion in regions with normal contraction and regions with chronic dysfunction: 85 ± 14 ml/min/100 g versus 77 ± 25 ml/min/100 g. Similar results were obtained by other groups who demonstrated that 80% to 90% of the hibernating segments exhibited resting flow almost comparable to resting flow in normally contracting myocardium [22]. In addition, flow reserve appeared abnormal in the hibernating segments. Vanoverschelde et al. [23] used dipyridamole to induce hyperemia in patients with chronic LV dysfunction and observed a blunted flow reserve in the hibernating segments as compared to the normally contracting segments. These findings have led to the hypothesis that repeated ischemic attacks may result in chronic dysfunction, with flow remaining normal or mildly reduced; a situation referred to as *repetitive stunning* [23].

Animal models of hibernation have revealed the following results. Several studies were unable to demonstrate a significant reduction in resting flow in abnormally contracting myocardium [22]. Bolukoglu and colleagues [24] and Liedtke et al. [25] have both failed to demonstrate a reduction in flow in a 1-week hibernation model. Shen and Vatner [26], using a pig model, were also unable to demonstrate reduced flow following 20 ± 3 days of hibernation. Thus, these models, with a short duration of hibernation, consistently showed normal flow in dysfunctional myocardium, and likely represent *chronic stunning*. Firoozan et al. [27] have developed a 6-weeks model of hibernation in dogs using ameroid constrictors on proximal left coronary arteries. Dysfunction occurred early after instrumentation, while flow remained (near-)normal (consistent with stunning) and postmortem histopathologic examination of these regions did not show evidence of necrosis. Later in time, however, some dysfunctional segments developed a gradual decrease in resting flow. Three studies (from different centers) have employed a long-term hibernation model, up to 8 months, and all demonstrated a substantial reduction in resting flow in the dysfunctional areas. Finally, Fallavolita and Canty [28,29] have shown in a pig model of chronic hibernation that in dysfunctional myocardium flow was normal at 1–2 months (indicative of chronic stunning), but was reduced at 3–4 months (hibernation). The initial normal flow at 1–2 months was, however, accompanied by a reduced flow reserve. These observations suggest a temporal progression of chronic stunning, characterized by (near-)normal flow, with reduced flow reserve to hibernation, with also reduced resting flow. Therefore, the chronic reductions in flow are likely to be a consequence, rather than the cause of chronic hibernation. The conflicting findings in patients may well be explained by this hypothesis. Moreover, in the clinical setting different situations may coexist in the same patient. For these reasons, the term "jeopardized myo-cardium" may include the entire spectrum from (repetitive) stunning to chronic stunning to hibernation.

CLINICAL RELEVANCE OF VIABILITY

Assessment of viability in dysfunctional myocardium is important in patients with chronic ischemic LV dysfunction, since recovery of function may be anticipated. The exact incidence of viable myocardium in patients with chronic ischemic LV dysfunction is not entirely clear, but a few studies have suggested that 30% to 50% of the patients may have dysfunctional but viable myocardium. Schinkel and coworkers [30] evaluated 89 patients with ischemic cardiomyopathy with dobutamine echocardiography and demonstrated that 57% of the patients exhibited a substantial amount of dysfunctional but viable myocardium. Currently, 105 studies (using different techniques, see below) have focused on the prediction of improvement of regional function postrevascularization [20]. A total of 3003 patients was studied, and the mean sensitivity and specificity to predict improvement of *regional* function postrevascularization were 84% and 69%, respectively (Fig. 19.1). Is it important to differentiate between chronic stunning and hibernation?

From a clinical point of view it may not be that important to differentiate between these two phenomena, since both need to be revascularized. However, differences in time course of recovery of function may occur [31]. Recent data, using FDG imaging, have demonstrated that stunned myocardium improves in function early postrevascularization, whereas hibernating myocardium may need longer time to (fully) recover in function [31]. Besides improvement of function, a significant reduction in heart failure symptoms occurred more frequently postrevascularization in patients with viable myocardium as compared to patients without viable myocardium [32]. Furthermore, exercise capacity improved in patients with viable myocardium [33], and long-term prognosis appeared favorable if patients with viable myocardium underwent revascularization [32].

AVAILABLE TECHNIQUES FOR ASSESSMENT OF JEOPARDIZED BUT VIABLE MYOCARDIUM

Jeopardized, viable myocardium has unique characteristics and these form the basis for the different imaging modalities that are currently available for the assessment of myocardial viability (Table 19.1). These characteristics include cell membrane integrity, intact mitochondria, preserved glucose and (possibly) fatty acid metabolism, intact resting perfusion, and inotropic reserve [34] (see Table 19.1). Not all viable myocardium exhibits all characteristics; the presence or absence of the different characteristics may be related to the severity of ultrastructural damage at the myocyte level [35]. All these characteristics can be evaluated by scintigraphic techniques (using PET or SPECT) and various radioactive tracers. Cell membrane integrity can be evaluated by thallium-201 (Tl-201); intact mitochondria can be probed by technetium-99m (Tc-99m)-sestamibi or Tc-99m-tetrofosmin; preserved glucose and free fatty acid metabolism can be assessed by FDG and radiolabeled fatty acids such as 123I-IPPA and 123I-BMIPP, respectively, and intact perfusion can be evaluated by both Tl-201 and Tc-99m labeled agents. Contractile reserve, however, has most frequently been evaluated by echocardiography (or more recently by magnetic resonance imaging) using dobutamine stress. However, various studies have recently demonstrated the feasibility of evaluating contractile reserve by gated single-photon emission computed tomography (SPECT) (using Tc-99m labeled agents) during the infusion of dobutamine [36]. The next part of this chapter discusses stepwise the use of the different techniques for assessing viability and the clinical results that are available with this technique.

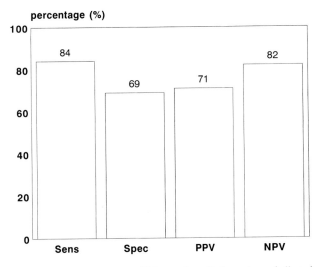

FIGURE 19.1 Sensitivity, specificity, and predictive values of all studies using prerevascularization viability testing to predict improvement of function (regional) postrevascularization (*n* = 105 studies, 3003 patients, data from Bax et al. [20]). Sensitivity is higher than specificity to predict improvement of region LV function postrevascularization.

TABLE 19.1 *Viability Features, Viability Techniques, and Their Viability Criteria*

Feature	Technique	Viability Criteria
Glucose metabolism	FDG PET/SPECT	Normal perfusion/FDG uptake
		Perfusion-FDG mismatch
Intact cell membrane	Thallium-201	Redistribution
		Activity > 50%
Intact mitochondria	Technetium-99m-sestamibi	Activity > 50%
		Improved tracer uptake postnitrates
Contractile reserve	Dobutamine echo (MRI)	Improved contraction during infusion of low-dose dobutamine

FDG, fluorodeoxyglucose; PET, positron emission tomography; SPECT, single-photon emission computed tomography; MRI, magnetic resonance imaging.

CELL MEMBRANE INTEGRITY/ PERFUSION—TL-201 CHLORIDE

Rationale, Protocols, Viability Markers

The initial uptake of Tl-201 is mainly determined by regional perfusion, whereas sustained uptake over longer time is dependent on integrity of the cell membrane and thus viability [37]. Different protocols for the assessment of myocardial viability by Tl-201 are available; the most frequently used are stress-redistribution-reinjection [37] and rest-redistribution [37]. The first provides information on both stress-inducible ischemia and viability, whereas the latter only provides information on viability. Markers of viability are (1) normal Tl-201 uptake (normal perfusion) at stress; (2) stress defects with redistribution (reversible defects) on the 3–4-hour delayed images; (3) redistribution in fixed defects at redistribution following reinjection or delayed rest images (frequently a threshold of 10% increase in tracer uptake is used); (4) tracer uptake > 50% at the redistribution-reinjection images or the delayed rest images [37]. The first three markers appear to adequately reflect jeopardized but viable myocardium, whereas the fourth marker is more complex. Frequently, segments with > 50% tracer uptake do not improve in function; the reason for this observation is the presence of nontransmural infarction, rather than jeopardized, hibernating myocardium (assuming adequate revascularization). Segments with nontransmural infarction contain viable tissue (and thus frequently exhibit > 50% tracer uptake) but are not capable of improving function postrevascularization. Still, the higher the level of Tl-201 uptake, the higher the likelihood of recovery of function postrevascularization, indicating that the amount of viable tissue also determines potential functional recovery [38].

Prediction of Functional Recovery

Thirty-three studies (22 rest-redistribution, 11 reinjection protocol) with a total of 858 patients have focused on prediction of improvement of *regional* function postrevascularization [20]. The mean sensitivity and specificity of these studies were 86% and 59% (Fig. 19.2) [20]. The lower specificity may be related to the definition of viable myocardium; as stated earlier, segments with > 50% tracer uptake are classified as viable but may not improve in function postrevascularization. A higher accuracy for prediction of improvement of function was obtained when inducible ischemia was present in the segments with > 50% tracer uptake [39]. Also, the 33 studies were not uniform in precise protocols and viability markers [20].

Improvement of global LV function was evaluated in five studies, with 96 patients; on average, the LVEF improved from 30% to 38% in patients with viable myocardium. In patients without viable myocardium, the LVEF remained unchanged (29% vs 31%) (Fig. 19.3).

Prediction of Heart Failure Symptoms/Exercise Capacity and Long-Term Prognosis

There are no studies employing Tl-201 imaging focusing at prediction of improvement of heart failure symp-

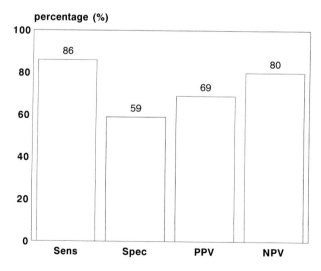

FIGURE 19.2 Accuracy of 33 Tl-201 studies to predict improvement of regional function postrevascularization (data from Bax et al. [20]).

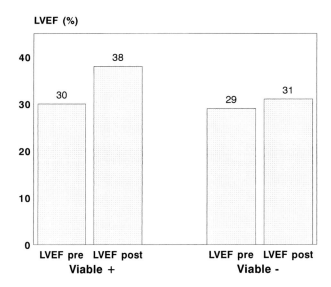

FIGURE 19.3 Change in LVEF postrevascularization in patients with and without viability on Tl-201 imaging (data from Bax et al. [20]).

toms in relation to viability. Long-term prognosis was evaluated in patients with Tl-201 imaging [40–43]; these studies were uniform in demonstrating that a superior long-term survival was present in patients with viable myocardium who underwent revascularization. Pagley et al. [40] studied 70 patients with multivessel disease and depressed LVEF; the patients were divided into two groups, according to the presence or absence of a substantial amount of viable myocardium. All underwent surgical revascularization; cardiac death rate was significantly lower in patients with viable myocardium as compared to patients without viable myocardium (18% vs 41%).

INTACT MITOCHONDRIA, CELL MEMBRANE/ PRESERVED PERFUSION—TC-99M LABELED AGENTS

Rationale, Protocols, Viability Markers

Myocardial uptake of Tc-99m-sestamibi parallels regional perfusion and provides adequate information for the detection of coronary artery disease [20]. The uptake and retention of sestamibi is also dependent on cell membrane integrity and mitochondrial function (membrane potential) [20] and is therefore also a marker of viable tissue. The role of sestamibi for the detection of viable myocardium has been a matter of debate, since several studies observed underestimation of viable myocardium as compared to other imaging modalities, whereas others reported excellent agreement between sestamibi and other modalities [20]. To improve the detection of viability with sestamibi, several modifications

of the imaging protocol have been proposed [20]. Originally, a resting image was performed. Dilsizian et al. [44] compared Tl-201 stress-redistribution-reinjection imaging with rest–stress sestamibi SPECT (1-day protocol) and demonstrated that agreement between the two could be improved by acquiring either an additional redistribution image (4 hours following the initial resting image) or by quantitative analysis of the sestamibi activity in irreversible defects. Levine and colleagues [45] have used gated sestamibi SPECT and combined the information of tracer uptake with the functional (wall motion) information; this approach improved sensitivity to detect viability, but at the cost of a lower specificity. Several groups have performed studies with sestamibi SPECT following administration of nitrates (either orally or intravenously) [46]. It is thought that nitrates enhance blood flow (and tracer uptake) to myocardial regions that are subtended by severely stenosed arteries. In most of these studies, two sets of images are obtained: a resting image and a nitrate-enhanced image and these results are compared. Bisi and coworkers [46] have demonstrated excellent results with nitrate-enhanced sestamibi SPECT imaging for the detection of viable myocardium. Currently, with most of the protocols used, the following criteria are used for assessment of viable myocardium with sestamibi imaging: > 50%–60% tracer uptake (or a somewhat lower uptake in the inferior regions, since attenuation may falsely "lower" activity in this region [20]) or defect reversibility after nitrate administration.

Prediction of Functional Recovery

Twenty studies (seven following nitrate administration) with a total of 488 patients have focused on prediction of improvement of *regional* function post-revascularization [20]. The mean sensitivity and specificity of these studies were 81% and 66% (Fig. 19.4) [20]. Most of the studies used a resting image, and segments were classified as viable when activity exceeded a certain threshold (frequently 50%–60%). Similarly to the Tl-201 studies, these cutoff levels cannot differentiate between jeopardized, viable myocardium and nontransmural infarction, resulting in overestimation of recovery of function and lower specificity. Still, various studies have demonstrated a strong relation between the histologic extent of fibrosis and the level of Tc-99m sestamibi uptake [47,48].

When the nitrate-enhanced studies were analyzed separately (n = 7; 180 patients), a sensitivity of 86% and a specificity of 83% were obtained. In these studies, defect reversibility following nitrate administration was used as a criterion for viability; this criterion may be more ideal for assessment of jeopardized but viable myocardium.

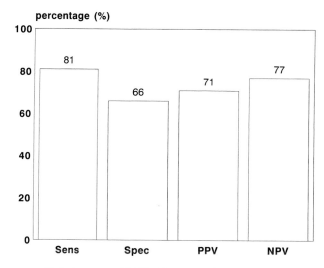

percentage (%)

FIGURE 19.4 Accuracy of 20 Tc-99m-sestamibi studies to predict improvement of regional function postrevascularization (data from Bax et al. [20]).

Improvement of global LV function was evaluated in four studies, with 75 patients; on average, the LVEF improved from 47% to 53% in patients with viable myocardium. In patients without viable myocardium, the LVEF remained unchanged (40% vs 39%) (Fig. 19.5).

Prediction of Heart Failure Symptoms/Exercise Capacity and Long-Term Prognosis

There are no studies employing sestamibi imaging focusing at prediction of improvement of heart failure

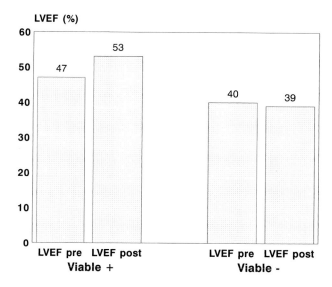

LVEF (%)

FIGURE 19.5 Change in LVEF postrevascularization in patients with and without viable myocardium on Tc-99m sestamibi imaging (data from Bax et al. [20]).

symptoms in relation to viability. Thus far, one study with sestamibi imaging has been published evaluating long-term prognosis in patients with ischemic cardiomyopathy [49]. Sciagra and coworkers [49] evaluated 105 patients with chronic coronary artery disease and LV dysfunction; all underwent nitrate-enhanced sestamibi imaging. The patients were accordingly divided into three groups: medical treatment, complete revascularization, or incomplete revascularization. Superior survival was shown in the patients with complete revascularization, as compared to the other two groups. The most important prognostic predictor of future cardiac events was the number of nonrevascularized dysfunctional regions with viable tissue on sestamibi imaging. Thus, these data also indicate the poor prognosis of patients with viable myocardium who are not revascularized adequately.

PRESERVED GLUCOSE METABOLISM— F18 FLUORODEOXYGLUCOSE

Rationale, Protocols, Viability Markers

FDG closely resembles glucose, with the exception that one OH group has been replaced by an F-18 atom. The initial transsarcolemmal uptake of FDG is identical to that of glucose. Following phosphorylation of FDG, however, no further metabolism is possible and the phosphorylated FDG remains trapped in the myocyte (physical half-life 110 min), providing a strong signal for imaging. To allow optimal identification of jeopardized viable myocardium, information on perfusion and FDG uptake needs to be combined. Dysfunctional segments with preserved perfusion and FDG uptake are thought to represent (repetitively) stunned myocardium, and segments with reduced perfusion but preserved FDG uptake (perfusion-FDG mismatch) are considered hibernating myocardium [20]. In contrast, segments with reduced perfusion and concordantly reduced FDG uptake are considered scar tissue. With FDG imaging, the metabolic conditions during the test are extremely important, since myocardial glucose (and FDG) uptake are highly influenced by these conditions [50]. The two most important factors influencing glucose (and thus FDG) uptake are the plasma levels of free fatty acids and insulin [50]. Low plasma levels of free fatty acids and high levels of insulin allow maximal glucose (and FDG) uptake. This situation can be realized using oral glucose loading and hyperinsulinemic–euglycemic clamping [51]. Oral glucose loading is a simple approach that is effective in the majority of patients. However, this approach results frequently (up to 25% of patients) in suboptimal image quality, particularly in patients with (sub-)clinical insulin resistance or diabetes mellitus [51]. Hyperinsulinemic–euglycemic clamping allows perfect regulation of metabolic conditions, resulting in excellent image quality in all subsets of patients [51].

The clamp, however, is a time-consuming approach and will be impractical for routine FDG imaging, although Martin et al. have demonstrated a rather attractive "shortened clamp" [52]. A recently proposed alternative is imaging following oral administration of Acipimox, a nicotinic acid derivative. Acipimox effectively reduces plasma levels of free fatty acids, but does not increase insulin levels [53]. To increase insulin levels, Acipimox is administered in combination with a small meal [54]. Studies in small numbers of patients have demonstrated good image quality using Acipimox [53,54].

Since FDG is a positron emitter, FDG imaging is performed with PET; PET, however, has limited availability for clinical routine. Driven by the increasing demand for viability studies, much effort has been invested in the development of 511 keV collimators to permit FDG imaging with SPECT [55]. The comparative studies between FDG SPECT and FDG PET demonstrated excellent agreement for assessment of viability between the two techniques [55]. More recently, gamma cameras with the option of coincidence imaging have been developed; this approach enhances resolution of the system, but necessitates the use of attenuation correction [55]. Initial studies demonstrated suboptimal agreement between coincidence imaging and FDG PET. While coincidence imaging (with possibilities for image fusion with computed tomography [CT]) may be preferred in oncology, SPECT imaging with 511 keV collimators may be preferred for cardiac studies [55].

Prediction of Functional Recovery

Twenty studies with FDG PET (total of 598 patients) have focused on prediction of improvement of *regional* function postrevascularization [20]. The mean sensitivity and specificity of these studies were 93% and 58% (Fig. 19.6) [20]. Most of these studies relied on combined information of perfusion and FDG uptake. Moreover, when the studies that used FDG alone (without a flow tracer) were excluded from the pooled analysis, a sensitivity of 88% and a specificity of 74% were obtained.

Also, the metabolic circumstances differed among the 20 studies: 10 were performed following oral glucose loading, 5 during clamping, and 5 during fasting. Studies with FDG SPECT have shown a sensitivity

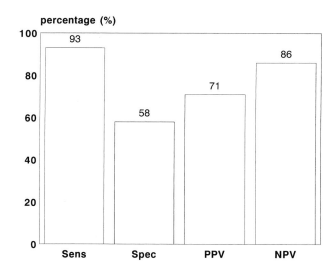

FIGURE 19.6 Accuracy of 20 FDG PET studies to predict improvement of regional function postrevascularization (data from Bax et al. [20]).

of 85% with a specificity of 75% to predict improvement of regional LV function postrevascularization [55], data very similar to the pooled FDG PET results.

Improvement of global LV function was evaluated in 12 FDG PET studies, with 333 patients; on average, the LVEF improved from 37% to 47% in patients with viable myocardium. In patients without viable myocardium, the LVEF remained unchanged (39% vs 40%) (Fig. 19.7). Similarly, FDG SPECT studies demonstrated that patients with viable myocardium improved the LVEF (from $27 \pm 8\%$ to $34 \pm 9\%$, $p <$

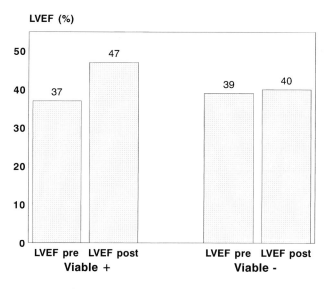

FIGURE 19.7 Change in LVEF postrevascularization in patients with and without viable myocardium on FDG PET (data from Bax et al. [20]).

.01), whereas patients without viable tissue did not improve (31 ± 8% vs 31 ± 8%, NS) [55].

Prediction of Heart Failure Symptoms/Exercise Capacity and Long-Term Prognosis

DiCarli et al. [32] and Eitzman et al. [56] have evaluated the relation between the presence of viability before revascularization and improvement of symptoms postrevascularization. Both studies indicated that improvement in heart failure symptoms postrevascularization predominantly occurred in patients with viable myocardium (Fig. 19.8). These studies have employed the New York Heart Association (NYHA) guidelines to evaluate heart failure symptoms. Similarly, Bax et al. [57], employing FDG SPECT, demonstrated a substantial improvement in NYHA class postrevascularization in patients with viable myocardium (from 3.4 ± 0.5 to 1.7 ± 0.8). DiCarli et al. [33] and Marwick et al. [58] have also determined exercise capacity before and after revascularization in patients with and without viable myocardium on FDG PET. Both studies demonstrated that patients with viable myocardium had a significant improvement of exercise capacity postrevascularization. In addition, DiCarli demonstrated that the magnitude of improvement in exercise capacity was related to the extent of viable tissue.

Seven FDG PET studies (619 patients) have evaluated long-term prognosis in relation to treatment (medical, revascularization) and viability (absent/present) [32,55,59–63]. The patients were divided into four

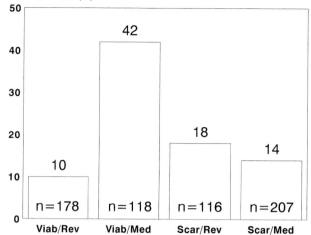

FIGURE 19.9 Prognosis of patients with and without viability on FDG PET and mode of treatment (rev = revascularization; med = medical treatment) (based on pooled data from references 32,56,59–63). The highest event-rate is observed in patients with viable myocardium who underwent medical therapy.

groups: medical viability+, medical viability−, revascularization viability+, revascularization viability− (Fig. 19.9). Pooled analysis of these data demonstrated that the highest event-rate (42%) was observed in patients with viable myocardium who were treated medically, and that the lowest event-rate (10%) was observed in patients with viable myocardium who underwent revascularization (Fig. 19.9). These data strongly suggest that viable myocardium is an unstable substrate and that revascularization is needed to prevent future events. Still, it should be emphasized that all studies used retrospective analyses, and that a prospective, "treatment-randomized" trial is needed before definitive conclusions can be drawn.

CONTRACTILE RESERVE—DOBUTAMINE STRESS ECHOCARDIOGRAPHY

Rationale, Protocols, Viability Markers

Infusions of low-dose dobutamine (5 to 10 mcg/kg/min) have been demonstrated to increase contractility (without a substantial increase in heart rate) in dysfunctional but viable myocardium; this phenomenon has been referred to as "contractile reserve." Segments without viable myocardium do not exhibit this contractile reserve. More recently, a so-called low–high dose protocol has been used for evaluation of viability [20]. This protocol (with infusions up to 40 mcg/kg/min with addition of atropine if needed) permits detection of both viabil-

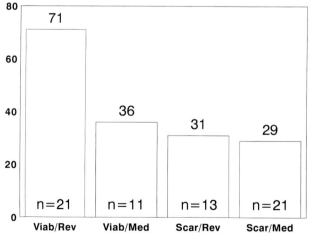

FIGURE 19.8 Percentages of patients with improvement of heart failure symptoms in relation to viability on FDG PET and treatment (rev = revascularization; med = medical treatment) (data from DiCarli et al. [32]).

ity and ischemia. With this protocol four response patterns are possible: (1) biphasic reponse (initial improvement followed by worsening of wall motion); (2) worsening (direct deterioration of wall motion without initial improvement); (3) sustained improvement (improvement of wall motion without subsequent deterioration); and (4) no change (no change in wall motion during the entire study). All patterns except pattern 4 (which represents scar tissue) are related to the presence of viable myocardium. However, not all patterns are related to jeopardized myocardium: pattern 1 represents viability with superimposed ischemia, pattern 2 represents ischemia (probably myocardium perfused by a critical stenosed vessel), and pattern 3 is probably related to subendocardial necrosis. As a consequence, not all patterns are equally predictive of improvement of function postrevascularization [64]. Pattern 1 is strongly related to improvement of function, whereas segments with patterns 2 and 3 less frequently exhibit improvement of function postrevascularization [64]. The safety of the low–high dose protocol in patients with severely depressed LVEF was demonstrated recently by Poldermans et al. [65].

Prediction of Functional Recovery

Thirty-two studies have used dobutamine echocardiography (three used magnetic resonance imaging instead of echocardiography), with a total of 1090 patients, to predict improvement of *regional* function postrevascularization [20]. The mean sensitivity and specificity of these studies were 82% and 79% (Fig. 19.10) [20].

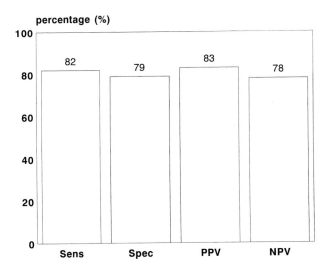

FIGURE 19.10 Accuracy of 32 dobutamine stress echocardiography studies to predict improvement of regional function postrevascularization (data from Bax et al. [20]).

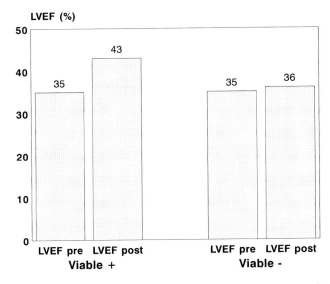

FIGURE 19.11 Change in LVEF postrevascularization in patients with and without viability on dobutamine stress echocardiography (data from Bax et al. [20]).

Most of these studies used low-dose dobutamine echocardiography, whereas four studies used a low–high dose protocol [20]. When the studies with low–high dose were analyzed separately, a mean sensitivity of 79% and a specificity of 85% were obtained [20]. Thus, a slight loss in sensitivity with a small gain in specificity were obtained when low–high dose dobutamine was compared to low-dose dobutamine echocardiography for the prediction of improvement of function postrevascularization.

Improvement of global LV function was evaluated in seven studies, with 254 patients; on average, the LVEF improved from 35% to 43% in patients with viable myocardium. In patients without viable myocardium, the LVEF remained unchanged (35% vs 36%) (Fig. 19.11).

Prediction of Heart Failure Symptoms/Exercise Capacity and Long-Term Prognosis

Two studies have evaluated functional status before and after revascularization in relation to the absence or presence of viable myocardium [58,66]. Bax et al. [66] demonstrated that the majority of patients with viable myocardium improved in NYHA class following revascularization. Marwick and colleagues [58], however, failed to demonstrate a relation between the extent of viability and the improvement of exercise capacity postrevascularization. Six studies (686 patients) have evaluated long-term prognosis in relation to treatment (medical, revascularization) and viability (absent or present) [66–71]. The patients were divided into four

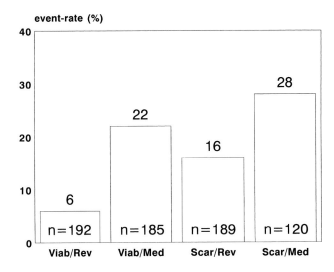

event-rate (%)

FIGURE 19.12 Prognosis of patients with and without viability on dobutamine stress echocardiography and treatment (rev, revascularization; med, medical treatment) (based on pooled data from references 66–71). The lowest event-rate is observed in patients who underwent revascularization and had viable myocardium.

groups, similar to the FDG PET studies (Fig. 19.12); pooled analysis of these data demonstrated that the lowest event-rate (6%) was observed in patients with viable myocardium who underwent revascularization, whereas the event-rates were similar in the other three groups (Fig. 19.12).

NOVEL TECHNIQUES

Besides the aforementioned techniques, several new techniques are currently being developed for the evaluation of viable myocardium. Magnetic resonance imaging (MRI) and MR spectroscopy will probably become important tools in the future. MRI has an excellent resolution, making differentiation between the epi- and endocardium possible. Kim et al. have recently demonstrated that contrast-enhanced MRI allows highly accurate identification of viable myocardium [72].

Myocardial contrast echocardiography allows simultaneous assessment of LV function and perfusion and has already been successfully applied in studies [73].

Radionuclides evaluating free fatty acid metabolism have also been used to detect viable myocardium, in particular 123I-BMIPP and 123I-IPPA [74,75]. These agents have been discussed in Chapters 15 and 21. Finally, gated SPECT in combination with dobutamine infusion permits assessment of perfusion, resting function, and contractile reserve in a single study [36], and is a potentially useful new method.

UNRESOLVED QUESTIONS

By pooling the data of the studies focusing on prediction of improvement of function, heart failure symptoms, and long-term prognosis, it became clear that a lot of information is still missing. First, the exact relation between viability and recovery of function is not clear. Most of the viability studies focusing on prediction of function have a somewhat lower specificity (see Fig. 19.1), indicating that some segments with viable myocardium do not improve in function postrevascularization. Most studies have performed the functional evaluation within 3 months postrevascularization. However, more severely damaged myocardium may need longer than 3 months to (fully) recover in function [31]. Second, the exact amount of viable tissue that is needed to result in improvement of LVEF postrevascularization is unclear. Several studies have demonstrated that patients with viable myocardium exhibit improvement of LVEF postrevascularization, but the criteria to classify a patient as viable varied substantially among the different studies, ranging from 8% of the LV being viable to 50% of the LV being viable. It is clear, however, that the extent of viable tissue is related to the change in LVEF postrevascularization [57,76]. Third, the relation between viability and improvement of heart failure symptoms has been demonstrated in several studies. However, a substantial number of patients without viable tissue also improved in symptoms. Moreover, the exact relation between viability, improvement in LVEF, and improvement in heart failure symptoms is also unclear [77]. Fourth, long-term prognosis may depend on more than improvement of function; Samady et al. demonstrated that absence of improvement of function was not necessarily associated with a poor prognosis [78]. It is conceivable that revascularization of viable tissue, although not resulting in improvement of function, may still have beneficial effects including prevention of LV remodeling and arrhythmias, which may result in improved prognosis [79]. Further studies are needed to address these issues, preferably multicenter, prospective, randomized trials.

CONCLUSIONS

Heart failure secondary to chronic coronary artery disease is a major problem in clinical cardiology. In patients with viable myocardium, revascularization may be an alternative treatment. Currently, a variety of adequate techniques is available for the assessment of viable myocardium. Patients with viable myocardium who undergo revascularization are likely to show improvement in LV function, heart failure symptoms, and prognosis. For these reasons, prerevascularization testing is an important part of the diagnostic workup of patients with ischemic cardiomyopathy and may help to guide optimal treatment.

REFERENCES

1. Gheorghiade M, Bonow RO. Chronic heart failure in the United States. A manifestation of coronary artery disease. Circulation 1998;97:282.

2. Khand A, Gemmel I, Clark A, et al. Is the prognosis of heart failure improving? J Am Coll Cardiol 2000;36:2284.

3. Ho KKL, Anderson KM, Kannel WB, et al. Survival after the onset of congestive heart failure in Framingham Heart Study subjects. Circulation 1993;88:107.

4. Cowie MR, Wood DA, Coats AJ, et al. Incidence and aetiology of heart failure; A population-based study. Eur Heart J 1999; 20:421.

5. Pfeffer MA, Braunwald E, Moye LA, et al. Effect of captopril on mortality and morbidity in patients with left ventricular dysfunction after myocardial infarction: results of the Survival and Ventricular Enlargement Trial. N Engl J Med 1992;327:669.

6. The SOLVD investigators. Effect of enalapril on survival in patients with treduced left ventricular ejection fractions and congestive heart failure. N Engl J Med 1991;325:293.

7. Pitt B, Poole-Wilso PA, Segal R, et al. Effect of losartan compared with captopril on mortality in patients with symptomatic heart failure: randomized trial—The Losartan Heart Failure Study ELITE II. Lancet 2000;355:1582.

8. Braunwald E. Expanding indications for beta-blockers in heart failure. N Engl J Med 2001;344:1711.

9. Pitt B, Zannad F, Remme WJ, et al. The effect of spironolactone on morbidity and mortality in patients with severe heart failure. N Engl J Med 1999;341:709.

10. Caims JA, Connolly SJ, Roberts R, et al. Randomized trial of outcome after myocardial infarction in patients with frequent or repetitive premature depolarizations. Lancet 1997;349:675.

11. Evans RW, Manninen DL, Garrison LP, et al. Donor availability as the primary determinant of the future of heart transplantation. JAMA 1986;255:1892.

12. Baker DW, Jones R, Hodges J, et al. Management of heart failure. III. The role of revascularization in treatment of patients with moderate or severe left ventricular systolic dysfunction. JAMA 1994;272:1528.

13. Pigott JD, Kouchoukos NT, Oberman A, et al. Late results of surgical and medical therapy for patients with coronary artery disease and depressed left ventricular function. J Am Coll Cardiol 1985;5:1036.

14. Elefteriades JA, Tolis G, Levi E, et al. Coronary artery bypass grafting in severe left ventricular dysfunction: excellent survival with improved ejection fraction and functional state. J Am Coll Cardiol 1993;22:1411.

15. White HD, Norris RM, Brown MA, et al. Left ventricular end-systolic volume as the major determinant of survival after recovery from myocardial infarction. Circulation 1987;76:44.

16. Uretsky BF, Sheahan RG. Primary prevention of sudden cardiac death in heart failure: will the solution be shocking? J Am Coll Cardiol 1997;30:1589.

17. Bonow RO, Dilsizian V. Thallium-201 for assessing myocardial viability. Semin Nucl Med 1991;21:230.

18. Tennant R, Wiggers CJ. The effects of coronary occlusion on myocardial contraction. Am J Physiol 1935;112:351.

19. Rahimtoola SH. The hibernating myocardium. Am Heart J 1989;117:211.

20. Bax JJ, Poldermans D, Elhendy A, et al. Sensitivity, specificity, and predictive accuracies of various noninvasive techniques for detecting hibernating myocardium. Curr Probl Cardiol 2001;26: 142.

21. Tawakol A, Skopici HA, Abrahmam SA, et al. Evidence of reduced resting blood flow in viable myocardial regions with resting asynergy. J Am Coll Cardiol 2000;36:2146.

22. Canty JM Jr, Fallavolita JA. Resting myocardial flow in hibernating myocardium: validating animal models of human pathophysiology. Am J Physiol 1999;276:H417.

23. Vanoverschelde JLJ, Wijns W, Depre C, et al. Mechanisms of chronic regional postischemic dysfunction in humans. New insights from the study of noninfarcted collateral-dependent myocardium. Circulation 1993;87:1513.

24. Bolukoglu H, Liedtke JA, Nellis SH, et al. An animal model of chronic coronary stenosis resulting in hibernating myocardium. Am J Physiol 1992;263:H20.

25. Liedtke AJ, Renstrom B, Nellis SH, et al. Mechanical and metabolic functions in pig hearts after 4 days of chronic coronary stenosis. J Am Coll Cardiol 1995;26:815.

26. Shen YT, Vatner SF. Mechanism of impaired function during progressive coronary stenosis in conscious pigs: hibernation or stunning? Circ Res 1995;76:479.

27. Firoozan S, Wei K, Linka A, et al. A canine model of chronic ischemic cardiomyopathy: characterization of regional flow-function relations. Am J Physiol 1999;276:H446.

28. Fallavolita JA, Perry BJ, Canty JM Jr. ^{18}F-2-deoxyglucose deposition and regional flow in pigs with chronically dysfunctional myocardium. Evidence for transmural variations in chronic hibernating myocardium. Circulation 1997;95:1900.

29. Fallavollita JA, Canty JM Jr. Differential ^{18}F-2-deoxyglucose uptake in viable dysfunctional myocardium with normal resting perfusion. Evidence for chronic stunning in pigs. Circulation 1999;99:2798.

30. Schinkel AFL, Bax JJ, Boersma E, et al. How many patients with ischemic cardiomyopathy exhibit viable myocardium? Am J Cardiol 2001; in press.

31. Bax JJ, Elhendy A, Poldermans D, et al. Time course of improvement of left ventricular function post revascularization: repetitive stunning vs hibernation. J Am Coll Cardiol 2001;37: 424A.

32. DiCarli M, Davidson M, Little R, et al. Value of metabolic imaging with positron emission tomography for evaluating prognosis in patients with coronary artery disease and left ventricular dysfunction. Am J Cardiol 1994;73:527.

33. DiCarli MF, Asgarzadie F, Schelbert HR, et al. Quantitative relation between myocardial viability and improvement in heart failure symptoms after revascularization in patients with ischemic cardiomyopathy. Circulation 1995;92:3436.

34. Bax JJ, Van Eck-Smit BLF, Van der Wall EE. Assessment of tissue viability: clinical demand and problems. Eur Heart J 1998;19:847.

35. Pagano D, Townend JN, Parums DV et al. Hibernating myocardium: morphological correlates of inotropic stimulation and glucose uptake. Heart 2000;83:456.

36. Leoncini M, Marcucci G, Sciagra R, et al. Nitrate-enhanced gated technetium 99m sestamibi SPECT for evaluating regional wall motion at baseline and during low-dose dobutamine infusion in patients with chronic coronary artery disease and left

ventricular dysfunction: comparison with two-dimensional echocardiography. J Nucl Cardiol 2000;7:426.

37. Dilsizian V, Bonow RO. Current diagnostic techniques of assessing viability in patients with hibernating and stunned myocardium. Circulation 1993;87:1.

38. Perrone-Filardi P, Pace L, Prastaro M, et al. Assessment of myocardial viability in patients with chronic coronary artery disease. Rest-4-hour-24-hour ^{201}Tl tomography versus dobutamine echocardiography. Circulation 1996;94:2712.

39. Kitsiou AN, Srinivasan G, QQuyyumi AA, et al. Stress-induced reversible and mild-to-moderate irreversible thallium defects: are they equally accurate for predicting recovery of regional left ventricular function after revascularization? Circulation 1998;98:501.

40. Pagley PR, Beller GA, Watson DD, et al. Improved outcome after coronary bypass surgery in patients with ischemic cardiomyopathy and residual myocardial viability. Circulation 1997;96:793.

41. Cuocolo A, Petretta M, Nicolai E, et al. Successful coronary revascularization improves prognosis in patients with previous myocardial infarction and evidence of viable myocardium at thallium-201 imaging. Eur J Nucl Med 1998;25:60.

42. Zafrir N, Leppo JA, Reinhardt CP, et al. Thallium reinjection versus standard stress/delay redistribution imaging for prediction of cardiac events. J Am Coll Cardiol 1998;31:1280.

43. Gioia G, Powers J, Heo J, et al. Prognostic value of rest-redistribution tomographic thallium-201 imaging in ischemic cardiomyopathy. Am J Cardiol 1995;75:759.

44. Dilsizian V, Arrighi JA, Diodati JG, et al. Myocardial viability in patients with chronic coronary artery disease. Comparison of 99mTc-sestamibi with thallium reinjection and [18F]fluorodeoxyglucose. Circulation 1994;89:578.

45. Levine MG, McGill CC, Ahlberg AW, et al. Functional assessment with electrocardiographic gated single-photon computed tomography improves the ability of technetium-99m sestamibi myocardial perfusion imaging to predict myocardial viability in patients undergoing revascularization. Am J Cardiol 1999;83:1.

46. Bisi G, Sciagra R, Santoro GM, et al. Rest technetium-99m sestamibi tomography in combination with short-term administration of nitrates: feasibility and reliability for prediction of postrevascularization outcome of asynergic territories. J Am Coll Cardiol 1994;24:1282.

47. Medrano R, Lowry RW, Young JB, et al. Assessment of myocardial viability with ^{99m}Tc sestamibi in patients undergoing cardiac transplantation. A scintigraphic/pathological study. Circulation 1996;94:1010.

48. Dakik HA, Howell JF, Lawrie GM, et al. Assessment of myocardial viability with ^{99m}Tc-sestamibi tomography before coronary bypass graft surgery. Correlation with histopathology and postoperative improvement in cardiac function. Circulation 1997;96:2892.

49. Sciagra R, Pellegri M, Pupi A, et al. Prognostic implications of Tc-99m sestamibi viability imaging and subsequent therapeutic strategy in patients with chronic coronary artery disease and left ventricular dysfunction. J Am Coll Cardiol 2000;36:739.

50. Gropler RJ. Methodology governing the assessment of myocardial glucose metabolism by positron emission tomography and fluorine 18-labeled fluorodeoxyglucose. J Nucl Cardiol 1994;1:S1.

51. Knuuti J, Nuutila P, Ruotsalainen U, et al. Euglycemic hyperinsulinemic clamp and oral glucose load in stimulating myocardial glucose utilization during positron emission tomography. J Nucl Med 1992;33:1255.

52. Martin WH, Jones RC, Delbeke D, et al. A simplified intravenous glucose loading protocol for fluorine-18 fluorodeoxyglucose cardiac single-photon emission tomography. Eur J Nucl Med 1997;24:1291.

53. Knuuti MJ, Yki-Järvinen H, Voipio-Pulkki LM, et al. Enhancement of myocardial [fluorine-18] fluorodeoxyglucose uptake by a nicotinic acid derivative. J Nucl Med 1994;35:989.

54. Bax JJ, Veening MA, Visser FC, et al. Optimal metabolic conditions during fluorine-18 fluorodeoxyglucose imaging; a comparative study using different protocols. Eur J Nucl Med 1997;23:35.

55. Bax JJ, Patton JA, Poldermans D, et al. 18-Fluorodeoxyglucose imaging with PET and SPECT: cardiac applications. Semin Nucl Med 2000;30:281.

56. Eitzman D, Al-Aouar ZR, Kanter HL, et al. Clinical outcome of patients with advanced coronary artery disease after viability studies with positron emission tomography. J Am Coll Cardiol 1992;20:559.

57. Bax JJ, Visser FC, Poldermans D, et al. Relationship between preoperative viability and postoperative improvement in LVEF and heart failure symptoms. J Nucl Med 2001;42:42:79.

58. Marwick TH, Zuchowski C, Lauer MS, et al. Functional status and quality of life in patients with heart failure undergoing coronary bypass surgery after assessment of myocardial viability. J Am Coll Cardiol 1999;33:750.

59. Lee KS, Marwick TH, Cook SA, et al. Prognosis of patients with left ventricular dysfunction, with and without viable myocardium after myocardial infarction. Relative efficacy of medical therapy and revascularization. Circulation 1994;90:2687.

60. Vom Dahl J, Altehoefer C, Sheehan FH, et al. Effect of myocardial viability assessed by technetium-99m-sestamibi SPECT and fluorine-18-FDG PET on clinical outcome in coronary artery disease. J Nucl Med 1997;38:742.

61. Yoshida K, Gould KL. Quantitative relation of myocardial infarct size and myocardial viability by positron emission tomography to left ventricular ejection fraction and 3-year mortality with and without revascularization. J Am Coll Cardiol 1993;22:984.

62. Tamaki N, Kawamoto M, Takahashi N, et al. Prognostic value of an increase in fluorine-18 deoxyglucose uptake in patients with myocardial infarction: comparison with stress thallium imaging. J Am Coll Cardiol 1993;22:1621.

63. Pagano D, Lewis ME, Townend JN, et al. Coronary revascularization for postischemic heart failure: how myocardial viability affects survival. Heart 1999;82:684.

64. Cornel JH, Bax JJ, Elhendy A, et al. Biphasic response to dobutamine predicts improvement of global left ventricular function after surgical revascularization in patients with stable coronary artery disease. Implications of time course of recovery on diagnostic accuracy. J Am Coll Cardiol 1998;31:1002.

65. Poldermans D, Rambaldi R, Bax JJ et al. Safety and utility of atropine addition during dobutamine stress echocardiography for the assessment of viable myocardium in patients with severe left ventricular dysfunction. Eur Heart J 1998;19:1712.

66. Bax JJ, Poldermans D, Elhendy A, et al. Improvement of left ventricular ejection fraction, heart failure symptoms and prognosis after revascularization in patients with chronic coronary artery disease and viable myocardium detected by dobutamine stress echocardiography. J Am Coll Cardiol 1999;34:163.

67. Chaudhry FA, Tauke JT, Alessandrini RS, et al. Prognostic implications of myocardial contractile reserve in patients with coronary artery disease and left ventricular dysfunction. J Am Coll Cardiol 1999;34:730.

68. Senior R, Kaul S, Lahiri A. Myocardial viability on echocardiography predicts long-term survival after revascularization in patients with ischemic congestive heart failure. J Am Coll Cardiol 1999;33:1848.

69. Williams MJ, Odabashian J, Laurer MS, et al. Prognostic value of dobutamine echocardiography in patients with left ventricular dysfunction. J Am Coll Cardiol 1996;27:132.

70. Afridi I, Grayburn PA, Panza J, et al. Myocardial viability during dobutamine echocardiography predicts survival in patients with coronary artery disease and severe left ventricular systolic dysfunction. J Am Coll Cardiol 1998;32:921.

71. Meluzin J, Cerny J, Frelich M, et al. Prognostic value of the amount of dysfunctional but viable myocardium in revascularized patients with coronary artery disease and left ventricular dysfunction. J Am Coll Cardiol 1998;32:912.

72. Kim RJ, Wu E, Rafael A, et al. The use of contrast-enhanced magnetic resonance imaging to identify reversible myocardial dysfunction. N Engl J Med 2000;343:1445.

73. Kaul S. Myocardial contrast echocardiography. 15 Years of research and development. Circulation 1997;96:3745.

74. Knapp FF Jr, Franken P, Kropp J. Cardiac SPECT with Iodine-123-labeled fatty acids: evaluation of myocardial viability with BMIPP. J Nucl Med 1995;36:1022.

75. Verani MS, Taillefer R, Iskandrian AE, et al. 123I-IPPA SPECT for the prediction of enhanced left ventricular function after coronary bypass graft surgery. Multicenter IPPA Viability Trial Investigators. 123I-iodophenylpentadecaonic acid. J Nucl Med 2001;41:1299.

76. Pagano D, Bonser RS, Townend JN, et al. Predictive value of dobutamine echocardiography and positron emission tomography in identifying hibernating myocardium in patients with postischaemic heart failure. Heart 1998;79:281.

77. Tawakol A, Gewirtz H. Does CABG improve left ventricular ejection fraction in patients with ischemic cardiomyopathy and does it matter? J Nucl Med 2001;42:87.

78. Samady H, Elefteriades JA, Abbott BG, et al. Failure to improve left ventricular function after coronary revascularization is not associated with worse outcome. Circulation 1999;100:1298.

79. Bonow RO. Identification of viable myocardium. Circulation 1996;94:2674.

20 | Other heart diseases

GAVIN I.W. GALASKO AND AVIJIT LAHIRI

CONGESTIVE HEART FAILURE

Epidemiology

Heart failure is one of the commonest chronic diseases of the Western world with high associated morbidity and mortality and high and increasing prevalence and cost [1–13]. In the United Kingdom heart failure affects up to 2% of the population, accounts for over 5% of adult hospital admissions, and costs up to 2% of all National Health Service expenditure [5,7]. It affects a similar number in continental Europe [11,12] and the United States [13], with heart failure now estimated to affect over 3 million Americans [13], costing over $10 billion per year [14]. Mortality is high, even in the modern therapeutic era, with recent community-based 1-year and 5-year survival rates after the onset of heart failure of 76% and 35%, respectively [15]. Once a diagnosis of heart failure has been made, however, it is often poorly managed [16]. Those with clinical heart failure and associated left ventricular systolic dysfunction benefit from ACE-inhibitor, beta-blocker, and spironolactone therapy [17–19], while for those with clinical heart failure but normal left ventricular systolic function (diastolic dysfunction) best therapy is unclear and still under investigation [20,21]. Furthermore, many subjects with ischemic cardiomyopathy, the commonest underlying cause of heart failure, occurring in 60%–70% of cases [22,23], have a significant degree of viable but dysfunctional myocardium ("hibernating myocardium"), where akinetic or severely hypokinetic myocardium retains the ability to contract should perfusion improve [24,25]. This "reawakening" of noncontractile myocardium after restoration of blood flow was noted as early as 1978 by Diamond et al. [26], who referred to such myocardium as "hibernating," a term popularized later by Rahimtoola [27] in a seminal article. Coronary revascularization in such subjects improves both cardiac function and prognosis, with subjects lacking sufficient "hibernating" or "viable" myocardium showing deleterious outcome following surgery [28–37].

Nuclear cardiology may not only play a role in assessing the presence or absence of underlying coronary artery disease in congestive cardiac failure using myocardial perfusion SPECT imaging, but may simultaneously offer an accurate assessment of hibernating myocardium and by means of ECG-gating an assessment of left ventricular systolic function. Positron emission tomography (PET) imaging and novel imaging modalities including fatty acid imaging offer alternative diagnostic modalities for hibernating myocardium, while radionuclide ventriculography provides a highly reproducible and accurate alternative assessment of both left and right ventricular systolic and diastolic function.

Diagnosing Coronary Artery Disease in Congestive Heart Failure

Subjects with ischemic cardiomyopathy have a worse prognosis than those with nonischemic cardiomyopathy [38,39], and respond differently to therapy (Table 20.1). Patients with ischemic cardiomyopathy show a different response to beta-blockade therapy compared with those with nonischemic cardiomyopathy, obtaining less benefit at higher dosages [40–42] as well as obtaining no benefit from calcium antagonist therapy [43]. In one study of 3787 patients with left ventricular systolic dysfunction, those with ischemic cardiomyopathy had a 59% 5-year survival as compared to 69% for those with nonischemic cardiomyopathy when diagnosed on coronary angiography [39]. A formal test is required, however, with a third of subjects with nonischemic cardiomyopathy having typical anginal symptoms, and many subjects with ischemic cardiomyopathy having no anginal symptoms on clinical assessment [39].

Myocardial perfusion imaging using either thallium (Tl-201) or technetium (Tc-99m) based agents has been known for many years to accurately assess the presence or absence of coronary artery disease in subjects with normal or near normal ventricular function [44–47]. Less evidence has been collected in subjects with significant left ventricular systolic dysfunction

TABLE 20.1 *Effect of Therapy on Mortality in Congestive Heart Failure Due to Ischemic or Nonischemic Cardiomyopathy in Large Controlled Studies*

Improves Mortality in ICM 1 NICM	Improves Mortality in NICM only	No Effect on Mortality	Increases Mortality
Nitrates + hydralazine	Amiodarone	Prazosin	Milrinone
ACE-inhibitors	Amlodipine	Digoxin	Amrinone
Carvedilol	Felodipine	Bucindolol	Vesnarinone
Bisoprolol			Dobutamine
Metoprolol			Enoximone
Warfarin			Ibupamine
			Flosequanan
			Xamoterol
			Nifedipine

ICM, ischemic cardiomyopathy; NICM, nonischemic cardiomyopathy.

where fixed perfusion abnormalities may occur despite normal coronary arteries [48,49]. Nitrate-enhanced rest imaging, however, where nitrates are administered sublingually prior to injecting the perfusion agent, has been shown to dramatically improve the accuracy in diagnosing reversible ischemic areas and thus coronary artery disease in such subjects as compared to standard rest imaging, by reducing the proportion of fixed perfusion defects. This has been shown for a variety of perfusion agents including Tl-201, Tc-99m labeled-sestamibi, Tc-99m labeled teboroxime, and Tc-99m labeled tetrofosmin [50–55]. Bisi et al. [51] found that intravenous isosorbide dinitrate given as a 20-minute infusion for 15 minutes prior to and 5 minutes during a Tc-99m-sestamibi rest scan led to a reduction in the global uptake defect of 37.4% in those subjects showing postrevascularization regional function recovery and only a 5.8% increase in those showing no post-revascularization recovery ($p < .0005$) in 19 patients with ischemic cardiomyopathy. Similarly, Thorley et al. [52] compared stress, rest, and glyceryl trinitrate (GTN) enhanced rest Tc-99m-tetrofosmin perfusion images in 30 patients chosen at random from their routine referrals, 19 (63%) with a prior history of coronary artery disease and 8 with previous myocardial infarction. They found stress defects in 43 of the 90 coronary artery territories assessed. Of these, 33 (77%) were reversible using traditional rest imaging, while 37 (86%) were reversible using GTN-enhanced rest imaging. He et al. [55], in a randomized study of 96 subjects with fixed defects at the 4-hour redistribution image following a Tl-201 stress image, found that 33% of patients randomized to reinjection following placebo showed significant reversibility, compared with 58% of patients randomized to reinjection following GTN ($p < .05$). Peix et al. [54], using Tc-99m-tetrofosmin imaging, found that in 50 patients

with previous myocardial infarction, and thus likely left ventricular systolic dysfunction, undergoing stress, rest, and GTN rest Tc-99m-tetrofosmin imaging, of the 186 segments with severe stress defects, 41 of the 74 (55%) segments that improved at rest did so only after administration of GTN.

Mechanism of nitrate action

Nitrates, first used to treat angina pectoris in 1867 [56], with glyceryl trinitrate (GTN) first used in 1879 [57], were first conclusively shown to increase blood flow to regions of poorly perfused myocardium in patients with coronary artery disease in 1971 [58], and first shown to aid detection of viable myocardium in 1974 [59]. Since then, nitrates have been shown to increase perfusion and thus tracer delivery in poorly perfused but viable myocardium in a number of ways. First, they act by vasodilating arteries, arterioles, veins, and venules to reduce both cardiac preload and afterload [60–63], reducing oxygen demand and thus ischemic burden. Second, their arterial vasodilating properties are most profound in the coronary circulation and again especially at sites of stenosis [61], directly improving flow. Third, they improve collateral flow beyond such stenoses [55,64], and improve subendocardial perfusion by reducing left ventricular end-diastolic pressure and thus subendocardial compressive forces. Indeed, they have been shown to improve regional myocardial perfusion at rest [65,66] and during exercise [64,67] as well as global and regional left ventricular function [68,69]. Only during the mid-1990s, however, has this property of increasing myocardial blood flow to poorly perfused but viable myocardium been used to improve the sensitivity, specificity, and diagnostic accuracy for myocardial perfusion imaging of both coronary artery disease per se as well as hibernating myocardium [51–53, 55, 70–72].

TABLE 20.2 *Sensitivities and Specificities for Predicting Functional Recovery after Revascularization (Hibernating Myocardium) Using a Variety of Techniques*

Technique	No. Studies	No. Patients	Sensitivity (%)	Sensitivity (%)
PET imaging	12	332	88	73
Tl-201 stress-redistribution-reinjection	7	209	86	47
Tl-201 rest-redistribution	8	145	90	54
Tc-99m-sestamibi	7	152	81	60
Low-dose dobutamine echocardiography	17	504	84	81
Nitrate-enhanced Tc-99m-sestamibi	5	95	85	83
Nitrate-enhanced Tl-201 rest- redistribution	1	22	92	78

Data from refs. 73–75.

Diagnosing Myocardial Viability

Several noninvasive techniques have been developed to identify dysfunctional but viable or "hibernating" myocardium. These include positron emission tomography (PET) with fluorine-18 fluorodeoxyglucose (F-18 FDG), traditionally the most sensitive and specific technique for predicting recovery of left ventricular function after coronary revascularization, but with limited availability and high cost precluding widespread use; single-photon emission computed tomography (SPECT) with Tl-201 stress-redistribution-reinjection or rest-redistribution imaging, traditionally showing high sensitivity but low specificity for predicting left ventricular functional recovery; SPECT imaging with Tc-99m-sestamibi or Tc-99m-tetrofosmin, and assessment of inotropic reserve using dobutamine echocardiography, a highly operator-dependent technique that may lose sensitivity in cases of severe left ventricular dysfunction. A potential future noninvasive technique currently under evaluation is fatty acid metabolic imaging. Table 20.2 summarizes the overall mean sensitivity and specificity of these various noninvasive techniques in predicting functional improvement following revascularization, with data taken from 43 studies involving almost 1500 patients [73–75]. It can be seen that nitrate-enhanced perfusion imaging with Tc-99m-sestamibi or Tl-201 agents improves sensitivity and specificity dramatically, with the techniques now as good as dobutamine echocardiography and PET imaging. Chapter 19 discusses in further detail the relative merits of these techniques in the assessment of viable or hibernating myocardium.

Revascularization for Viable Myocardium

Ragosta et al. [32] using Tl-201 planar rest-redistribution imaging in 21 subjects with ischemic cardiomyopathy (mean left ventricular ejection fraction 27%) prior to surgical revascularization found that if 8 or more segments in a 15-segment model of the left ventricle had significant myocardial viability then left ventricular ejection fraction rose significantly following revascularization (29% to 41%, $p = .002$), while 7 or fewer viable, asynergic segments led to no significant change in ejection fraction (27% to 30%, $p = NS$). Pagley et al. [28] went on to show a survival benefit in these 21 plus a further 49 subjects where the degree of myocardial viability was greatest. They showed that those with a viability index (mean viability score per segment assessed, with 2 scored for normal viability, 1 scored for "mildly reduced viability," and 0 for no viability in each of the 15 segments assessed) of > 0.67 were significantly freer of cardiac death or transplantation than those with less viability (viability index ≤ 0.67) at 3 years follow-up, with better in-hospital outcome. One criticism of this study, however, is that the vast majority of these patients had presented to hospital with unstable angina or myocardial infarction prior to assessment and revascularization and so are not typical heart failure subjects.

Senior et al. [33], using dobutamine echocardiography to diagnose hibernating myocardium, found similar improvements in left ventricular dysfunction in subjects with chronic stable ischemic cardiomyopathy recruited from the outpatient setting, furthermore showing a survival advantage on long-term follow-up compared with medical therapy of the time [37]. They recruited 87 patients with chronic stable ischemic cardiomyopathy (mean left ventricular ejection fraction 25%), all of whom underwent dobutamine stress echocardiography. Thirty-seven subjects went on to undergo revascularization (33 by multiple coronary artery bypass grafts and 4 by percutaneous coronary angioplasty). At a mean follow-up of 40 months, those

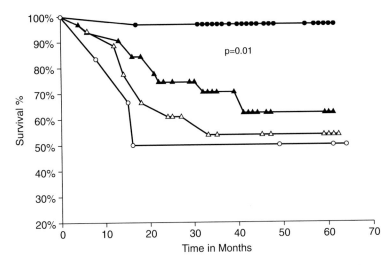

FIGURE 20.1 Cardiac event-free survival for subjects with ischemic cardiomyopathy undergoing surgical revascularization or medical therapy with or without significant myocardial viability. Solid circle = revascularization with myocardial viability; solid triangle = medical therapy with myocardial viability; open triangle = medical therapy without myocardial viability; open circle = revascularization without myocardial viability. (From Senior et al. [37].)

with significant viable myocardium (5 or more viable myocardial segments in a 12-segment model) treated with revascularization had a distinct survival advantage with improved systolic function and New York Heart Association (NYHA) class as compared with those revascularized without significant myocardial viability, or those treated with medical therapy whether or not significant myocardial viability was present (Fig. 20.1). Those who underwent surgical revascularization had a 40-month cardiac mortality of only 3%, compared with 31% for those with myocardial viability treated with medical therapy, 44% for those without myocardial viability treated with medical therapy, and 50% for those without significant viable myocardium treated with revascularization.

Afridi et al. [36] found similar results in 318 patients with ischemic cardiomyopathy (mean left ventricular ejection fraction 27%) who had undergone dobutamine echocardiography assessment of myocardial viability. At a mean follow-up of 18 months, mortality rates were 6%, 20%, 20%, and 17%, respectively for the equivalent groups described above. Again, those with myocardial viability who underwent revascularization, whether surgical or percutaneous, had significantly increased survival as compared to the other three groups. In this study a patient was considered to have significant myocardial viability if 4 or more segments of a 16-segment model demonstrated improvement, worsening, or a biphasic response to low-dose dobutamine. Similar results have also been seen when using positron

emission tomography to diagnose viable myocardium. [29–31].

All of these studies, however, predated the widespread use of beta-blocker therapy in heart failure, a new therapy that may potentially improve outcome in those medically treated for viable myocardium. The carvedilol hibernation reversible ischemia trial, marker of success (CHRISTMAS study) [76] is a double-blind, randomized, placebo-controlled study designed to assess this by looking at the effect of the beta-blocker carvedilol on left ventricular ejection fraction in subjects with ischemic cardiomyopathy with or without significant hibernating myocardium. Myocardial viability is being assessed by use of a combination of resting echocardiography and resting nitrate enhanced Tc-99m-sestamibi SPECT. Carvedilol is being used as the beta-blocker in this study, being the only beta-blocker thus far to show survival advantage in mild, moderate, and severe heart failure [77,78], as well as preventing adverse remodeling following acute myocardial infarction [79], and causing regression of remodeling in chronic heart failure [80,81]. None of these imaging studies looking at revascularization in subjects with congestive heart failure and significant viable myocardium were randomized in study design to aggressive medical therapy versus revascularization, allowing potential although unlikely bias. This is currently being assessed in the Heart-UK (Heart Revascularisation Trial-United Kingdom) study [82], where any validated noninvasive assessment of myocardial viability may be used for the diagnosis of viable myocardium prior to randomization to either best medical therapy, including beta-blockade, or surgical revascularisation plus best medical therapy.

Cardiac Remodeling

Congestive heart failure is a progressive disorder where a vicious cycle of neurohumoral activation occurs, initially providing support for the failing heart, but ultimately producing progressively worsening cardiac function following excessive vasoconstriction, fluid retention, and direct toxic effects, which in turn lead to worsening prognosis [83–85]. Activated systems include the renin-angiotensin-aldosterone system and the sympathetic nervous system. Remodeling involves altered genome expression including molecular, cellular, and interstitial changes that are manifested clinically as alterations in cardiac size, shape, and function [86]. Macroscopically, remodeling consists of progressive left ventricular dilatation, increased end-systolic and end-diastolic volumes, even in the absence of a decrease in left ventricular ejection fraction [87], left ventricular hypertrophy, and increased cardiac sphericity leading to progressive systolic and diastolic dysfunction and ultimately progressive heart failure. Indeed, left ventricular end-systolic volume has been shown to be a more important predictor of survival following acute myocardial infarction than left ventricular ejection fraction [88,89]. Microscopically, both myocyte degeneration and the development of fibrosis occur. Even in the absence of myocyte loss, a disproportionate accumulation of mainly fibrillar collagen occurs producing increased diastolic stiffness, disturbed cardiac filling, and elevated left ventricular filling pressures [90]. This in turn increases diastolic wall stress, reduces coronary flow, and may result in ischemia, further encouraged by increased perivascular fibrosis and thus increased oxygen dissociation distances, leading to further myocyte degeneration and cell death [91]. Furthermore, disruption of the extracellular matrix with upregulation of matrix metalloproteinases and simultaneous downregulation of tissue inhibitors of metalloproteinases results in fibrillar collagen degradation, with myocyte slippage and chamber dilatation [91]. It is hoped that in the future nuclear cardiology may address some of these molecular/cellular changes.

By inhibiting this neurohumoral activation, ventricular remodeling can be favorably altered by use of angiotensin-converting enzyme inhibitors [92] and beta-blockers [80, 81], agents also shown to reduce morbidity and mortality in patients with both chronic congestive heart failure as well as acute myocardial in-

farction, where cardiac remodeling often occurs [19, 77, 78, 93, 94]. Recent studies, using both nitrate-enhanced Tc-99m-sestamibi SPECT and dobutamine stress echocardiography have shown that regression of remodeling occurs following revascularization in those with significant viable myocardium, while progressive remodeling occurs in those treated medically or those undergoing revascularization without significant viable myocardium at mean follow-ups of 17 and 21 months, respectively, in subjects with ischemic cardiomyopathy and congestive cardiac failure [95,96].

Assessing Left Ventricular Systolic Function

An assessment of left ventricular systolic function in all cases of heart failure is important, as it not only stratifies prognosis [97,98] but also dictates best therapy [17–19]. In acute heart failure following myocardial infarction, the GISSI-2 database [98] has shown that mortality rises exponentially as ejection fraction falls, with a sharp upturn in mortality as ejection fraction falls below 40%. In chronic heart failure, again mortality increases as ejection fraction falls, with Gradman et al. finding that those with cardiomyopathy and left ventricular ejection fraction < 20% had a cardiac event rate of 27% at 16 months, compared with 7% for ejection fraction ≥ 30% [97], with left ventricular ejection fraction the variable most closely associated with mortality on multivariate analysis. However, left ventricular systolic dysfunction is often misdiagnosed clinically, and so a formal assessment of left ventricular function is required. Davie et al. [99] found that only 41 of 259 (16%) patients referred from primary care with suspected chronic heart failure to a direct access echocardiography service had evidence of left ventricular systolic dysfunction and so may benefit from ACE-inhibitor, beta-blocker, and spironolactone therapy.

Radionuclide ventriculography

Radionuclide ventriculography, first used clinically in 1976 [100], is an accurate and highly reproducible technique for the assessment of both left ventricular systolic and diastolic function. Both first-pass and, now more usually, blood pool equilibrium techniques can be used. It has a mean inter- and intraobserver variability of measuring ejection fraction (EF) of 2% and a mean interstudy variability of 5% [101–104]. As a result of its impressive reproducibility, along with reasonable cost and availability as compared to magnetic resonance imaging, an alternative gold-standard measure of ejection fraction, it has been and is still being used as a baseline test in many clinical trials of heart failure therapy [19,76,82,93,105] and as a way to assess the effect of a variety of medical therapies on left ventricular dimensions, volumes, remodeling, and ejection fraction [106–113]. Therapies studied in this way have included the beta-blockers carvedilol [106] and metoprolol [107] in subjects with heart failure; enalapril following acute myocardial infarction [108, 109]; both nifedipine and isosorbide dinitrate separately in subjects with significant mitral regurgitation [110]; interferon-α in chronic viral hepatitis [111]; radiofrequency ablation of accessory pathways in Wolff-Parkinson-White syndrome [112], and even left ventricular pacing in subjects with congestive cardiac failure [113].

Although single-center studies assessing variability in echocardiographic assessment of left ventricular ejection fraction, an alternating meaning of ejection fraction, have generally shown good accuracy and reproducibility [114,115], multicenter studies have found the accuracy of echocardiographic assessment to be less satisfactory [116].

ECG-gated myocardial perfusion SPECT

Quantitative electrocardiogram (ECG)-gated perfusion SPECT imaging, with either Tl-201 or more usually Tc-99m-based radioisotopes, allows a well-validated assessment of left ventricular ejection fraction at the same time as the myocardial perfusion image [117]. Over 29 studies have now been performed in over 1000 patients, including those with large perfusion defects or severe left ventricular dysfunction or both, finding good-to-excellent agreement between quantitative gated SPECT techniques and a variety of gold-standards, with excellent interobserver and intraobserver reproducibility [117]. The gold-standards used in these studies have included: two- and three-dimensional echocardiography, first-pass ventriculography, multiple gated acquisition ventriculography, magnetic resonance imaging, and thermodilution techniques, finding good-to-excellent agreement and an overall correlation coefficient of 0.87 [117].

Furthermore, quantitative gated SPECT by allowing visualization of myocardial wall movement further improves the sensitivity, specificity, and accuracy of diagnosing ischemic heart disease, by reducing the effect of attenuation artifact, in turn reducing the number of borderline normal or borderline abnormal scans [118, 119]. Indeed, DePuey et al. [118] demonstrated a decrease in false positive results for myocardial scar (and thus, for coronary artery disease) from 16% to 3% when Tc-99m-sestamibi perfusion tomograms were in-

terpreted with a gated approach rather than a static or ungated approach. The greatest benefit being in women with large breasts and apparent fixed anterior perfusion defects and in men with fixed inferior defects caused by diaphragmatic attenuation.

ECG-gated myocardial perfusion imaging also improves the accuracy in assessing hibernating myocardium, with Levine et al. [120] showing in 50 patients with ischemic cardiomyopathy 1 week prior to revascularization that the additional use of wall motion assessment by use of ECG-gated SPECT improved the sensitivity, specificity, and accuracy in predicting recovery of function from 86%, 55%, and 85%, respectively, to 95%, 55%, and 91%, respectively, using an improvement of $\geq 20\%$ in perfusion or function or both as a measure of myocardial viability.

Assessing Left Ventricular Diastolic Function

Although left ventricular systolic dysfunction often underlies the development of congestive heart failure, with proven therapeutic intervention it is becoming increasingly apparent that abnormal left ventricular filling or "diastolic dysfunction" may also lead to the development of congestive heart failure with or without left ventricular systolic abnormalities. As such, the first therapeutic studies in patients with purely diastolic heart failure are currently underway randomizing subjects to an angiotensin-converting enzyme inhibitor or placebo [20] and an angiotensin-II receptor antagonist or placebo [21]. Common causes for diastolic dysfunction include ischemic heart disease, left ventricular hypertrophy, hypertensive cardiomyopathy of the elderly, constrictive pericarditis, restrictive cardiomyopathy, and familial hypertrophic cardiomyopathy. Recent studies have found that 40%–50% of all cases of congestive heart failure have normal systolic function, especially in females and the elderly [121–123]. Aurigemma et al. [123] have performed the largest prospective study consisting of 2671 subjects aged 65+ years initially free of coronary artery disease and congestive heart failure followed-up for a mean of 5.2 years during which time 170 subjects (6.4%) developed congestive heart failure. Of these, only 45% had significant left ventricular systolic dysfunction (ejection fraction $< 45\%$); 16% borderline left ventricular systolic function (ejection fraction $\geq 45\%$ and $< 55\%$), and 39% normal left ventricular systolic function (ejection fraction $\geq 55\%$) at the time of hospitalization with congestive heart failure. Furthermore, they found that both echocardiographic evidence of altered diastolic filling and altered systolic function at the initial screening echocardiogram, when the subjects were symptom free, independently predicted future incident congestive heart failure.

Although echocardiographic Doppler assessment of mitral and pulmonary venous flow is the technique most commonly used clinically in analyzing diastolic function [124,125], diastolic function may also be assessed by radionuclide ventriculography (RNV) by analyzing the time-activity curve [126]. Measures of diastolic function from this curve include: the peak filling rate, time-to-peak filling, early filling rate, and first one-third and first one-half filling fractions (Fig. 20.2). The peak filling rate (PFR) is the most widely used parameter of diastolic function, assessing rapid early filling. It measures the greatest increase in ventricular counts in early-to-mid diastole and thus the fastest early filling rate. It is typically normalized to end-diastolic volume (EDV) and expressed as EDV per second, normal range ≥ 2.5 EDV/s (lower in the elderly). A second useful marker of diastolic function is the time-to-peak filling (the time interval from the lowest LV count (end-systole) to the occurrence of the PFR (normal < 180 ms). A third measure is the filling fraction, the percentage of filling (normalized to stroke volume) that had occurred at one-third, one-half, and two-thirds of diastole. Atrial filling can also be assessed. To generate the time-activity curve, Fourier transform fits to high temporal resolution data are performed using at least 24 frames and preferably 32 frames per cardiac cycle.

Studies to assess the effects of medical therapies on left ventricular diastolic function have been undertaken using serial RNV examinations. Agents studied in this way have included anthracycline prior to and following chemotherapy [127], erythropoietin prior to and following treatment for anemia in chronic dialysis patients [128], and alteplase reopening of infarct-related arteries following acute myocardial infarction [129].

Metaiodobenzylguanidine (I-123 MIBG) Imaging in Congestive Heart Failure

It has become increasingly apparent that sympathetic nervous system activation plays a major role in the pathophysiology and progression of heart failure. It exerts an initial beneficial inotropic effect, helping to maintain the circulation, but this soon becomes blunted due to progressive downregulation and desensitization of the beta-receptors [130,131]. Simultaneously it activates deleterious secondary messenger cascades including the renin-angiotensin system, both directly and indirectly promotes deleterious vasoconstriction increasing afterload, has a direct toxic effect on the myocardium affecting ventricular mechanical performance, and increases automaticity, the substrate for life-threatening arrhythmias [132]. Indeed, Cohn et al. [133] have shown that plasma norepinephrine concentration is inversely related to survival in patients with heart failure.

Metaiodobenzylguanidine (I-123 MIBG), first developed in the early 1980s as an imaging agent for pheochromocytoma, is a structural analog of norepinephrine that shares similar uptake and storage mechanisms, but unlike norepinephrine is not metabolized by monoamine oxidase or catechol-o-methyl transferase [134,135]. It is taken up and stored in myocardial sympathetic neurones and represents cardiac beta-adrenergic receptor density, which can be imaged by radiolabeling with Iodine-123 [136]. Several authors have shown that initial I-123 MIBG uptake is reduced and I-123 MIBG washout is increased in patients with both idiopathic dilated cardiomyopathy [137–139] and ischemic cardiomyopathy [140–141], suggestive of deranged sympathetic myocardial supply and receptor downregulation. Indeed, Schoefer et al. [138] have shown in 28 subjects with idiopathic cardiomyopathy that I-123 MIBG activity reflects myocardial sympathetic innervation rather than plasma norepinephrine levels by finding a significant correlation between myocardial I-123 MIBG activity and left ventricular ejection fraction and myocardial norepinephrine content, but not with plasma catecholamine levels.

Since myocardial sympathetic activity does not necessarily reflect generalized sympathetic activity, and yet is likely to reflect disease progression in congestive cardiac failure being related to myocardial norepinephrine

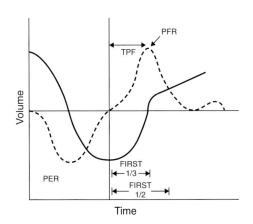

FIGURE 20.2 Left ventricular time-volume curve obtained during radionuclide ventriculography showing measurements obtained from volume (*solid*) curve and the first derivative (*dashed*) curve. PER = peak ejection rate; TPFR = time to peak filling; First 1/3 = first one-third filling fraction; First $^1/_2$ = first one-half filling fraction. (Adapted from Follansbee et al. [163].)

content and left ventricular ejection fraction, it has been postulated that myocardial I-123 MIBG activity may be an important marker of prognosis in congestive cardiac failure. Merlet et al. [142] compared the prognostic value of I-123 MIBG myocardial uptake to other traditional prognostic markers in heart failure including clinical, radiological, echocardiographic, and radionuclide parameters and found that myocardial I-123 MIBG uptake was the most powerful predictor of survival over a 1–27 month follow-up in 90 patients with both ischemic ($n = 24$) and idiopathic ($n = 66$) cardiomyopathy. They found that a reduced heart to mediastinum I-123 MIBG uptake ratio ($< 120\%$) was more discriminatory than a left ventricular ejection fraction $< 20\%$ versus $> 20\%$, with ejection fraction previously shown to be a very powerful marker of prognosis [97,143–145] (Fig. 20.3). They have recently repeated this work in 112 patients with idiopathic cardiomyopathy, incorporating further invasive and noninvasive assessments previously shown to discriminate outcome in congestive cardiac failure, including plasma norepinephrine levels, cardiopulmonary testing, and right heart catheterization data [146]. Again, they found MIBG uptake to be the most powerful independent predictor of mortality over a mean follow-up of 27 months, with left ventricular ejection fraction the only other independent predictor. Thus cardiac MIBG uptake, and by implication beta-adrenergic receptor density, predicts outcome more effectively than any of the standard noninvasive measurements of left ventricular function in patients with congestive heart failure.

A potential future role of MIBG imaging may be in stratifying the requirement for and monitoring the response to specific heart failure therapies. It may be possible to streamline certain therapeutic regimens to patients with the greatest degree of sympathetic down-regulation resultant from greatest neurohormonal activation. Two studies have now shown improved myocardial MIBG uptake and thus sympathetic receptor activity following the long-term use of angiotensin-converting enzyme inhibitors [147] and spironolactone [148], disease modifying drugs. Recently [149,150], MIBG imaging has been proposed as a useful tool in predicting the response of subjects with congestive heart failure to beta-blocker therapy, too. Certainly patients with congestive heart failure have differing responses to beta-blocker therapy as a result of genetic variability [151,152], differing underlying etiologies, concomitant drug therapy, and marked variation in beta-adrenergic receptor expression and function and cardiac adrenergic innervation [137]. For example, patients with congestive heart failure harboring the Ile164 2 adrenergic receptor polymorphism, which significantly alters the function of the receptor by reducing catecholamine and certain beta-receptor antagonists binding affinities, demonstrate a more rapid disease progression and so may be more appropriate for beta-blocker therapy [150]. In a small double-blind, placebo-controlled study, Choi et al. [149] found that MIBG imaging may be useful in predicting response to

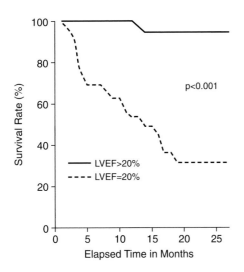

FIGURE 20.3(a) Survival curve, using life table analysis, with a threshold value of 20% for LVEF. A large difference is seen for survival between patients with a LVEF lower (dotted line) or greater (unbroken line) than 20% ($p < .001$). LVEF = left ventricular ejection fraction.

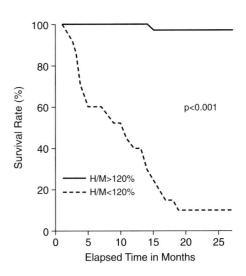

FIGURE 20.3(b) Survival curve, using life table analysis, with a threshold value of 120% for H/M activity ratio. A striking difference is seen for survival between patients with H/M lower (dotted line) or greater (unbroken line) than 120% ($p < .001$). When compared to (a), this graph shows that survival is much poorer in patients with an H/M below 120% than in those with a LVEF below 20%. (From Merlet et al. [142].)

carvedilol therapy in patients with congestive heart failure. They found that in those subjects randomized to carvedilol, the MIBG washout rate prior to randomization was inversely proportional to the increase in left ventricular ejection fraction at 1 year follow-up ($r = -0.74$, $p = .02$), with a diagnostic accuracy of MIBG washout rate of 91% for predicting significant improvement in ejection fraction following carvedilol therapy, with similar results seen for the 3-hour heart to mediastinum ratio, too.

CARDIOMYOPATHY

Congestive heart failure due to left ventricular dysfunction is generally classified into two groups—those with cardiomyopathy due to ischemic heart disease and those with cardiomyopathy due to nonischemic causes. Nonischemic cardiomyopathy can be classified into dilated, hypertrophic, and restrictive. As stated earlier, those with ischemic cardiomyopathy generally have a higher mortality, may respond differently to therapy, and may receive benefit from revascularization therapy as compared to nonischemic cardiomyopathy. Unfortunately, clinical symptoms or risk factor assessment is unhelpful in differentiating ischemic from nonischemic cardiomyopathy. In one study, one-third of patients found to have nonischemic cardiomyopathy by angiography still gave typical anginal symptoms, and 48% gave at least one risk factor for heart disease [39]. By use of ECG-gated myocardial perfusion SPECT, it may be possible to discriminate ischemic from nonischemic cardiomyopathy [49,153].

Dilated Cardiomyopathy

Differentiating ischemic from nonischemic dilated cardiomyopathy

Radionuclide ventriculography assessment of left and right ventricular size and function is a useful technique in diagnosing dilated cardiomyopathy [154,155]. However, although biventricular dysfunction is common, left ventricular dysfunction is usually more advanced, making differentiation from ischemic cardiomyopathy more difficult. Furthermore, although large perfusion defects on myocardial perfusion imaging strongly favors a diagnosis of ischemic cardiomyopathy, large fixed defects (especially apical) have been reported in patients with dilated cardiomyopathy, making the diagnosis less certain. Danias et al. [49] used a quantitative assessment of both fixed and reversible myocardial perfusion defects and wall motion variability using ex-

ercise and rest Tc-99m-sestamibi gated SPECT imaging in 37 subjects, 13 with ischemic cardiomyopathy, to attempt to differentiate ischemic from nonischemic cardiomyopathy. They found that the summed stress, rest, and reversibility scores of patients with ischemic cardiomyopathy were significantly greater than the corresponding scores of patients with nonischemic cardiomyopathy, as diagnosed on coronary angiography (Fig. 20.4a), with no overlap between the two groups in summed stress scores or summed rest defect scores. The summed stress score was greater than or equal to 21 in all ischemic patients and less than or equal to 14 in all nonischemic patients. Furthermore, the addition of gated SPECT analysis of ventricular function improved discrimination further, with greater regional wall motion variability in patients with ischemic cardiomyopathy as compared to those with nonischemic cardiomyopathy (1.08 ± 0.77 vs 0.27 ± 0.28, respectively, $p < .01$) (Fig. 20.4b,c), with variability in regional wall motion score alone able to correctly classify 36 of 37 patients (97%). Similar data have also been published in abstract form in 119 consecutive patients with a left ventricular ejection fraction $\leq 40\%$ undergoing stress–rest Tc-99m-sestamibi gated SPECT imaging and coronary angiography. They found that a combined assessment of regional wall motion variability using gated SPECT along with the summed stress score on perfusion imaging gave a sensitivity, specificity, and diagnostic accuracy of 92%, 82%, and 90%,

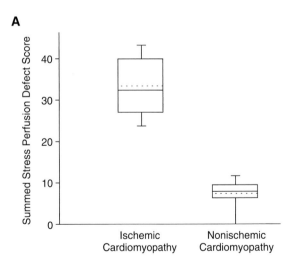

FIGURE 20.4(*a*) Summed stress perfusion defect scores for ischemic and nonischemic cardiomyopathy groups. The solid horizontal lines inside the boxes represent the median values. The dotted horizontal lines represent the mean group values. The upper and lower box borders indicate the 75th and 25th percentiles, respectively. The whisker caps represent the 95th and 5th percentiles. The wide separation between patients with ischemic and nonischemic cardiomyopathy is apparent.

B

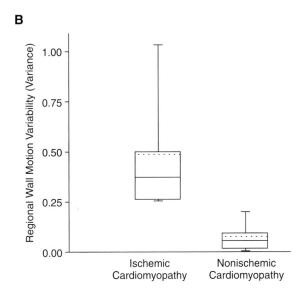

FIGURE 20.4(*b*) Individual patient wall motion variance among vascular territories, for ischemic and nonischemic cardiomyopathy groups. The horizontal solid lines inside the boxes represent the median values. The dotted lines represent the mean group values. The upper and lower box borders indicate the 75th and 25th percentiles, respectively. The whisker caps represent the 95th and 5th percentiles.

respectively, in the identification of ischemic or nonischemic cardiomyopathy [153].

Monitoring adriamycin therapy and preventing adriamycin cardiotoxicity

Adriamycin (doxorubicin), an anthracycline glycoside, is a potent chemotherapeutic agent used in the treatment of a variety of cancers. Cardiotoxicity, the most serious adverse effect, is a well-recognized clinical entity limiting its usage. In extreme cases, cardiotoxicity is manifested by progressive left ventricular dysfunction and heart failure, which is generally irreversible or minimally reversible only. The incidence and severity of adriamycin toxicity increases with increasing dose, being rare below a cumulative dose of 350 mg/m^2 but affecting up to 20% of patients with doses above 700 mg/m^2. However, there is considerable variability in individual susceptibility. Schwartz et al. [156] in following-up 1487 patients over a 7-year period have shown that cardiomyopathy is predated by a gradual progressive fall in left ventricular ejection fraction, and is more likely with abnormal baseline ejection fraction. They have further shown that by using radionuclide ventriculography prior to initiating therapy to exclude unexpected cardiac diseases and then for longitudinal follow-up, the incidence of overt cardiac failure could be reduced by over fourfold, and, moreover, if congestive heart failure did develop, it was mild and responsive to routine therapy. The approach being advocated is that patients with a baseline ejection fraction below 30% should not be started on adriamycin; for patients with a baseline ejection fraction below 50%, repeat ventriculography is recommended prior to each adriamycin dose, and for patients with a normal baseline ejection fraction ($\geq 50\%$) a second study should be performed after 250–300 mg/m^2 dosage, a third study after 400 mg/m^2 dosage in those with other risk factors and after 450 mg/m^2 in those without, and then prior to each subsequent dose. Toxicity is then indicated by a fall in absolute ejection fraction of $> 10\%$

C

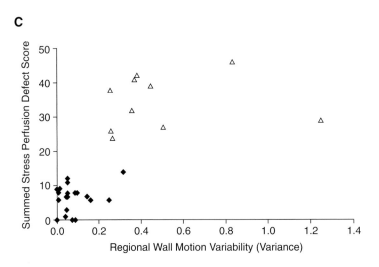

FIGURE 20.4(*c*) Combined assessment of myocardial perfusion and regional wall otion clearly separated patients with ischemic cardiomyopathy (open triangles) from those with nonischemic cardiomyopathy (black circles). (From Danias et al. [49].)

(to a level below 50% if starting from a normal ejection fraction), or a fall in ejection fraction to below 30%. Radionuclide ventriculography has been suggested as the best serial technique to use in this assessment owing to its highly reproducible nature.

Hypertrophic Cardiomyopathy

The diagnosis of hypertrophic cardiomyopathy is usually made on the basis of clinical examination, ECG, and echocardiography, with radionuclide studies usually not required. However, radionuclide ventriculography if performed in selected subjects often demonstrates hyperdynamic left ventricular systolic function, disproportionate upper septal thickening, and impaired diastolic function [157,158]. Furthermore, asymmetrical septal hypertrophy may be detected by myocardial perfusion imaging, by comparing septal thickness with that of the posterior free wall [159]. The left ventricular cavity is generally small, with marked myocardial uptake by hypertrophied myocardium. Exercise-induced perfusion abnormalities are often seen in the absence of epicardial coronary artery stenosis [160], although still imparting a worse prognosis [161]. A worse prognosis is also seen with depressed left ventricular systolic function.

Restrictive Cardiomyopathy

A variety of diagnostic procedures including echocardiography and cardiac catheterization are usually necessary to diagnose restrictive cardiomyopathy. Radionuclide ventriculography generally shows normal or decreased left ventricular end-diastolic volume, normal or mildly depressed left ventricular ejection fraction, dilated atria, and diastolic dysfunction. Myocardial uptake of gallium-67 citrate or Tc-99m pyrophosphate or both is often seen but can be caused by a variety of underlying conditions including: amyloidosis, sarcoidosis, systemic sclerosis, and cardiac tumors. Fixed defects in myocardial Tl-201 perfusion imaging may occur in subjects with sarcoidosis, systemic sclerosis, and cardiac tumors [162,163]. Due to the highly reproducible nature of radionuclide ventriculography, it has found a role in monitoring the progression and therapy of hemochromatosis, thalassemia, and hemosiderosis induced restrictive cardiomyopathy.

Monitoring thalassemia and hemosiderosis

Patients with thalassemia often require regular blood transfusions. Over a period of years this may lead to myocardial hemosiderosis and ultimately cardiac failure. Exercise radionuclide ventriculography can be used as a highly sensitive test for detecting preclinical myocardial dysfunction in these patients. In one study, Leon et al. [164] showed that although resting ejection fraction was normal in 21 of 24 patients (87.5%) with transfusion-dependent beta-thalassemia (mean ejection fraction 53% ± 2%, SEM), exercise ejection fraction was normal in only 11 patients, including all 8 patients who had had fewer than 100 transfusions. In a similar study, Aldouri et al. [165] in performing radionuclide ventriculography in 60 subjects with beta-thalassemia major receiving regular blood transfusions and subcutaneous desferrioxamine chelation, found that 22 subjects (37%) had a resting ejection fraction < 45% at rest or a drop of > 12% on stress, while 19 (32%) were normal and 19 (32%) showed only mild abnormalities. Although no correlation was found this time with the number of units transfused, non-desferrioxamine-compliant patients had worse cardiac function, and repeat studies on 17 patients 6–28 months after better compliance showed a significant overall improvement in ejection fraction. This suggests that those with poor left ventricular function as assessed both at rest and stress should be offered more intense chelation therapy or an alteration in chelation therapy to improve cardiac function. Indeed, adequate iron chelation therapy as assessed thus has led to a striking improvement in survival in this condition, reducing cardiac mortality at age 15 years from 14% to 3%.

Antimyosin Antibody Imaging

Myosin, an insoluble component of contractile myofibrils, is only exposed to the extracellular milieu following membrane disruption as occurs in ischemic, inflammatory and toxic myocardial diseases. Indium-111 radiolabeled antimyosin antibodies, produced by immunizing mice with human myosin, binds to exposed cardiac myosin allowing imaging of regions of cell membrane disruption. This allows a noninvasive evaluation of the site, extent, and quantitation of myocardial necrosis, allowing monitoring of cardiac transplantation as a useful noninvasive marker for rejection.

Assessment of transplant rejection

Allograft rejection accounts for almost one-third of mortality after cardiac transplantation, with clear evidence of rejection required before treatment with high-dose immunosuppressive therapy. Right ventricular biopsy, the gold-standard for detecting and monitoring transplant rejection, is a costly and invasive procedure, associated with a 0.3% mortality. Furthermore, as only a few myocardial areas are biopsied, rejection may be missed. In a comparative study of In-111 antimyosin and cardiac biopsy in the first year after transplantation, Scheutz et al. found a sensitivity of 91% (20 of 22) and specificity of 98% (40 of 41) between the extent of antimyosin uptake and the severity of rejection by biopsy in 63 patients studied [166]. Lower specificities are seen in the first year after transplantation where active myocardial damage without rejection is often seen on biopsy, producing a false positive image. Antimyosin imaging also gives prognostic information, potentially allowing the number of right heart biopsies to be reduced in low-risk individuals and targeted to high-risk individuals, with Ballaster et al. [167] finding that 67% of patients with a heart-lung ratio of above 1.55 and 80% of patients with a heart-lung ratio greater than 1.75 at their 1-year image experienced a subsequent episode of rejection on biopsies taken every 4 months over an 18-month mean follow-up period.

Myocarditis

The diagnosis of myocarditis can generally be established on the basis of a careful history, physical examination, ECG, and chest X-ray. As previously described, right ventricular biopsy, the gold-standard for diagnosing myocarditis, is a costly and invasive procedure, associated with a 0.3% mortality, and is not 100% sensitive. Noninvasive assessment of myocardial inflammation can be performed by use of a number of radionuclides including: gallium-67 citrate [168], Tc-99m pyrophosphate, and In-111 antimyosin [169] imaging. Radionuclide ventriculography may play a further role in both diagnosing myocarditis by showing both left and right ventricular dysfunction and thus generalized myocardial involvement in the majority of cases, as well as being a marker of disease severity and prognosis, with morbidity and mortality felt to depend largely on ventricular function in both the acute and chronic phase.

VALVULAR HEART DISEASE

Valvular heart disease is another important cause of heart failure and sudden death, with measures of ventricular size and performance required to guide further management. Thus, although other noninvasive techniques such as echocardiography and magnetic resonance imaging are used in preference to nuclear techniques in diagnosing valve disease and assessing severity, radionuclide ventriculography is an established technique in assessing prognosis and need for surgery due to its low inter- and intraobserver variability and very low interstudy variability [101–104], its ability to be undertaken during exercise, when functional abnormalities are often unmasked [170], its independence from chamber geometry, often disordered in valvular diseases, and its ability to assess both left and right ventricular function [171, 172]. Although this has given radionuclide ventriculography a role in assessing the prognosis and need for surgical intervention in mitral and aortic regurgitation, currently no role exists in assessing prognosis or disease progression in mitral or aortic stenosis or other valvular disease where the decision to operate is based on symptom status.

Aortic Regurgitation

Resting left ventricular ejection fraction is a major determinant of postoperative outcome in aortic regurgitation, with poor long-term survival seen in those subjects who have developed significant left ventricular dysfunction prior to surgery [173]. Change in left ventricular ejection fraction over time is another major determinant of outcome in subjects with chronic asymptomatic severe aortic regurgitation and normal left ventricular function [174]. Bonow et al. [174] showed in 104 such subjects followed up serially with echocardiography and radionuclide ventriculography for a mean follow-up of 8 years (range 2–16 years) that age, end-systolic diameter, and importantly, the rate of change in ejection fraction and end-systolic dimension over time were the only multivariate predictors of outcome. This finding implies that serial long-term changes in left ventricular ejection fraction in subjects with severe asymptomatic aortic regurgitation identify patients likely to develop symptoms and require aortic valve replacement. They further found that even without a need for long-term follow-up, those subjects with a fall in left ventricular ejection fraction of > 5% with exercise had a 12% per year risk of death, symptoms, or left ventricular dysfunction, compared with a 4% risk for those with a 0%–5% fall in ejection fraction and 1% risk for those with an increase in ejection fraction on their initial assessment. Similar results have been found by Borer et al. [175], who found that the greater the fall in left ventricular ejection fraction with exercise, normalized for change in end-systolic wall stress as assessed on echocardiography, the greater the risk of death, development of symptoms requiring valve replacement surgery, or abnormal left ventricular function on mean follow-up of 7.3 years in 104 patients with asymptomatic severe aortic regurgitation, with change in left ventricular ejection fraction on exercise unadjusted for change in end-systolic wall stress almost as good a predictor on multivariate analysis.

Mitral Regurgitation

Mitral regurgitation affects both left and right ventricular performance prior to symptom development. Only radionuclide ventriculography enables accurate repeatable determination of left and right ventricular ejection fraction at rest and during exercise. Thus radionuclide ventriculography, by assessing both right and left ventricular performance, is ideally suited to assess disease severity even in asymptomatic subjects, defining best management [176,177]. These studies have shown that the risk of mortality is high in asymptomatic subjects with benefit gleaned from surgical repair/replacement when either right ventricular or left ventricular ejection fraction is abnormal at rest [176] and that future heart failure is best predicted by the absence of an increase in right ventricular ejection fraction during exercise [177]. Hochreiter et al. [176] found in 53 subjects with chronic hemodynamically severe mitral regurgitation that asymptomatic subjects thus treated medically with a resting left ventricular ejection fraction $\leq 45\%$ or resting right ventricular ejection fraction $\leq 30\%$ had far higher mortality, usually from sudden death or progressive heart failure, than symptomatic subjects thus treated surgically with similar ejection fractions ($p < .05$) (Fig. 20.5). Rosen et al. [177] similarly found in 31 subjects with asymptomatic or minimally symptomatic severe mitral regurgitation secondary to mitral valve prolapse that those subjects with no change in or a fall in right ventricular ejection fraction on exercise had a 14% per year rate of symptom development compared with a 4% per year rate for those with a rise in right ventricular ejection fraction on exercise ($p = .041$) (Fig. 20.6). Both left ventricular ejection fraction [178] and right ventricular ejection fraction [179] are useful in predicting the long-term outcome of mitral valve surgery. Phillips et al. [178] found in 105 patients undergoing mitral valve replacement for isolated mitral regurgitation that preoperative age > 60 years and left ventricular ejection fraction < 40% were the only independent predictors of decreased survival at 3 to 5-year follow-up ($p < .05$) (Fig. 20.7). Similarly, Furer et al. [179] found that although echocardiographic parameters were more predictive of postoperative symptoms (preoperative end-systolic stress to end-systolic volume index, fractional shortening, and left ventricular end-systolic diameter), a resting right ventricular ejection fraction $\leq 30\%$ had an 83% predictive accuracy in predicting postoperative symptoms.

KAWASAKI DISEASE

Kawasaki disease (mucocutaneous lymph node syndrome) first described by Kawasaki in 1967 is a systemic vasculitic syndrome of unknown etiology found

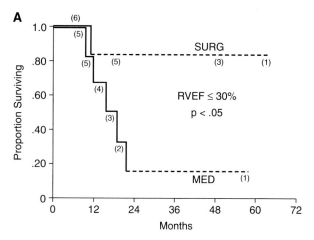
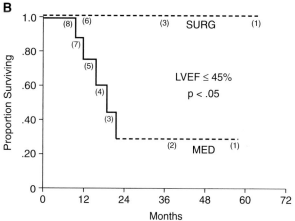
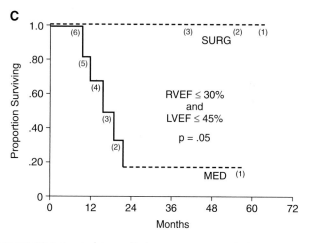

FIGURE 20.5 Survival in medical group versus surgical group as a function of (A) right ventricular ejection fraction (RVEF), (B) left ventricular ejection fraction (LVEF), and (C) combined RVEF and LVEF criteria. (From Hochreiter et al. [176].)

in young children presenting as an acute febrile illness, mucosal inflammation, skin rash, and cervical lymphadenopathy, most commonly before the age of 4 [180]. Early cardiovascular effects may include myocarditis, pericardial effusion, and valvular involve-

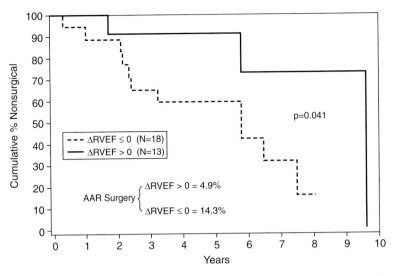

FIGURE 20.6 Natural history of the development of surgical indications in subjects classified according to their change in right ventricular ejection fraction (ΔRVEF) from rest to exercise at study entry. AAR Surgery = average annual risk of developing indications for surgery. Curves were constructed by Kaplan-Meier product limit estimates and compared by the log-rank test. (From Rosen et al. [177].)

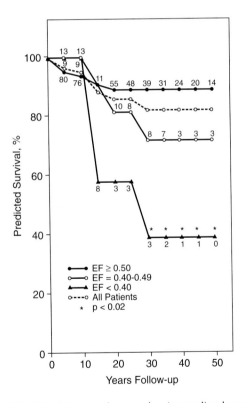

FIGURE 20.7 Life table survival curves showing predicted survival of the overall study population and the study population stratified according to left ventricular ejection fraction (EF). The overall 5 year predicted survival was 82% and survival was significantly reduced in patients with an ejection fraction below 0.40. (From Phillips et al. [178].)

ment [181]. Although Kawasaki disease is generally self-limiting, 15%–25% of children with the disease may develop significant cardiovascular sequelae [182], including persisting coronary artery aneurysms and the development of coronary artery stenoses producing myocardial ischemia and even myocardial infarction [183], especially if early therapy is delayed. Although echocardiography is the most useful method to detect coronary artery aneurysms at the time of diagnosis, obstructive coronary lesions, which often develop over time as aneurysms often regress [184–186], are difficult to evaluate often requiring invasive coronary angiography. Indeed, the coronary artery sequelae of Kawasaki disease are now known to be an important cause of coronary artery disease in young adults often occurring many years after disease onset [187]. Coronary angiography to assess such stenoses carries a higher risk than usual, however, both due to the child's young age in the majority of cases, as well as the fact that all systemic arteries may be affected and inflamed, increasing the risk of arterial occlusion or pseudoaneurysm formation at the catheterization site. This has led to a number of studies to assess the role of myocardial perfusion imaging to screen for silent coronary stenoses in Kawasaki disease and to assess disease severity.

Kondo et al. [188], in 1989, using dipyridamole-stress Tl-201 SPECT imaging found sensitivities of 91% and 88% and specificities of 60% and 93%, respectively, for visual and quantitative analyses of the SPECT images in detecting significant coronary artery stenoses in 49 subjects with Kawasaki disease. Fukunda et al. [189] went on to confirm these results finding a sensitivity of 80% and specificity of 100% for dipyridamole-stress rest Tl-201 SPECT imaging to detect significant coronary artery stenoses in 38 subjects (age 4 to 21 years) who had developed Kawasaki disease a mean of 7 years earlier. They went on to show that treadmill exercise stress electrocardiography had a much lower sensitivity of only 33% in detecting such lesions (*p* < .001). Similar results have also been seen with Tl-99m agents [190, 191]. Schillaci et al. [190] found a sensitivity and specificity for rest and dipyridamole-stress Tc-99m-sestamibi SPECT imaging in detecting coronary lesions in 15 children aged from 1 to 6 years old of 88% and 93%, respectively. Karasawa et al. [191] found a sensitivity of 90% and specificity of 85% for stress–rest Tc-99m-tetrofosmin perfusion imaging to detect significant coronary artery stenoses in 46 subjects with Kawasaki disease, 20 with and 26 without significant coronary artery stenoses. Ogawa et al. [192] have gone on to show that dobutamine stress Tc-99m perfusion imaging is not only useful in detecting silent myocardial ischemia in asymptomatic subjects with Kawasaki disease but also accurately estimates the need for percutaneous transluminal coronary angioplasty (PTCA) and assesses the effectiveness of the PTCA procedure itself. Miyagawa et al. [193] have further shown in 90 consecutive patients with both Kawasaki disease and coronary aneurysms on echocardiography (from 459 consecutive patients with Kawasaki disease) that abnormal dipyridamole-thallium stress-redistribution SPECT perfusion imaging was by far the best independent predictor of long-term cardiac events with the number of aneurysms detected on coronary angiography only minimally adding to the multivariate model.

REFERENCES

1. McKee PA, Castelli WP, McNamara PM, et al. The natural history of congestive heart failure: the Framingham Study. N Engl J Med 1971;285:1441.
2. Stewart AL, Greenfield S, Hays RD, et al. Functional status and well-being of patients with chronic conditions: results from the Medical Outcomes Study. JAMA 1989;262:907.
3. Ho KKL, Anderson KM, Karmel WB, et al. Survival after the onset of congestive heart failure in the Framingham Heart Study subjects. Circulation 1993;88:107.
4. McMurray J, McDonagh T, Morrison CE, et al. Trends in hospitalization for heart failure in Scotland 1980–1990. Eur Heart J 1993;14:1158.
5. McMurray J, Hart W, Rhodes G. An evaluation of the cost of heart failure to the National Health Service in the UK. Br J Med Econ 1993;6:91.
6. Rodríguez-Artalejo F, Guallar-Castillón P, Banegas JR, et al. Trends in hospitalization and mortality for heart failure in Spain, 1980–1993. Eur Heart J 1997;181771.
7. McMurray JJV, Petrie MC, Murdoch DR, et al. Clinical epidemiology of heart failure: public and private health burden. Eur Heart J 1998;19 (Suppl P): P9.
8. Key Health Statistics from General Practice 1996, Analyses of morbidity and treatment data, including time trends, England and Wales, Series MB6 No.1, 1998.
9. Mair FS, Crowley TS, Bundred PE. Prevalence, aetiology and management of heart failure in general practice. Br J Gen Pract 1996;46:77.
10. Clarke KW, Gray D, Hampton JR. How common is heart failure? Evidence from PACT (Prescribing Analysis and Cost) data in Nottingham. J Public Health Med 1995;17:459.
11. Mosterd A, Hoes AW, deBruyne MC, et al. Prevalence of heart failure and left ventricular dysfunction in the general population. The Rotterdam Study. Eur Heart J 1999;20:447.
12. Eriksson H, Svardsudd K, Larsson B, et al. Risk factors for heart failure in the general population: the study of men born in 1913. Eur Heart J 1989:10;647.
13. O'Connell J, Bristow M. Economic impact of heart failure in the United States: time for a different approach. J Heart Lung Transpl 1994;13(Suppl 4): S107.
14. Abraham WT, Bristow MR. Specialized centers for heart failure management. Circulation 1997;96:2755.
15. Senni M, Tribouilloy CM, Rodeheffer RJ, et al. Congestive heart failure in the community: a study of all incident cases in Olmsted County, Minnesota, in 1991. Circulation 1998;98: 2282.
16. McMurray J. Why we need new strategies in CHF management. JRAAS 2000;1 (suppl 1): 12.
17. Packer M, Bristow MR, Cohn JN, et al. The effect of carvedilol on morbidity and mortality in patients with chronic heart failure. N Engl J Med 1996;334:1349.
18. Pitt B, Zannad F, Remme WJ, et al. The effect of spironolactone on morbidity and mortality in patients with severe heart failure. Randomized Aldactone Evaluation Study Investigators. N Engl J Med 1999;341:709.
19. The SOLVD Investigators. Effect of enalapril on survival in patients with reduced left ventricular ejection fractions and congestive heart failure. N Engl J Med 1991;325:293.
20. Cleland JG, Tendera M, Adamus J, et al. Perindopril for elderly people with chronic heart failure: the PEP-CHF study. The PEP investigators. Eur J Heart Fail 1999;1:211.
21. Swedberg K, Pfeffer M, Granger C, et al. Candesartan in heart failure—assessment of reduction in mortality and morbidity (CHARM): rationale and design. J Cardiac Fail 1999;5:276.
22. Cleland JGF, McGowan J. Heart failure due to ischemic heart disease: epidemiology, pathophysiology and progression. J Cardiovasc Pharmacol 1999;33 (Suppl 3); S17.
23. Terrlink J, Goldhaber S, Pfeffer M. An overview of contemporary etiologies of congestive heart failure. Am Heart J 1991; 121:1852.
24. Rahimtoola SH. The hibernating myocardium. Am Heart J 1989;117:211.
25. Bonow RO, Dilsizian V, Cuocolo A, et al. Identification of viable myocardium in patients with chronic coronary artery disease and left ventricular dysfunction. Comparison of thallium scintigraphy with reinjection and PET imaging with ^{18}F-fluorodeoxyglucose. Circulation 1991;83:26.
26. Diamond A, Forrester JS, de Luz PL, et al. Patient extrasystolic potentiation of ischemic myocardium by atrial stimulation. Am Heart J 1978;95:204.

27. Rahimtoola SH. A perspective of the three multicentre randomised clinical trials of coronary bypass surgery for chronic stable angina. Circulation 1985;72:V123.

28. Pagley PR, Beller GA, Watson DD, et al. Improved outcome after coronary artery bypass surgery in patients with ischemic cardiomyopathy and residual myocardial viability. Circulation 1997;96:793.

29. Eitzman D, Al-Aouar Z, Kanter H, et al. Clinical outcome of patients with advanced coronary artery disease after viability studies with positron tomography. J Am Coll Cardiol 1992;20:559.

30. Di Carli MF, Davidson M, Little R, et al. Value of metabolic imaging with positron emission tomography for evaluating prognosis in patients with coronary artery disease and left ventricular dysfunction. Am J Cardiol 1994;73:527.

31. Lee KS, Marwick TH, Cook SA, et al. Prognosis of patients with left ventricular dysfunction, with and without viable myocardium after myocardial infarction: relative efficacy of medical therapy and revascularization. Circulation 1994;90:2687.

32. Ragosta M, Beller GA, Watson DD, et al. Quantitative planar rest-redistribution 201Tl imaging in detection of myocardial viability and prediction of improvement in left ventricular function after coronary artery bypass surgery in patients with severely depressed left ventricular function. Circulation 1993;87:1630.

33. Senior R, Glenville B, Basu S, et al. Dobutamine echocardiography and thallium-201 imaging predict functional improvement after revascularisation in severe ischemic left ventricular dysfunction. Br Heart J 1995;74:358.

34. di Carli MF, Asgarzadie F, Schelbert HR, et al. Quantitative relation between myocardial viability and improvement in heart failure symptoms after revascularisation in patients with ischemic cardiomyopathy. Circulation 1995;92:3436.

35. Meluzin J, Cerny J, Frelich M, et al. Prognostic value of the amount of dysfunctional but viable myocardium in revascularized patients with coronary artery disease and left ventricular dysfunction. J Am Coll Cardiol 1998;32:912.

36. Afridi I, Grayburn PA, Panza JA, et al. Myocardial viability during dobutamine echocardiography predicts survival in patients with coronary artery disease and severe left ventricular dysfunction. J Am Coll Cardiol 1998;32:921.

37. Senior R, Kaul S, Lahiri A. Myocardial viability on echocardiography predicts long term survival after revascularisation in patients with ischemic congestive heart failure. J Am Coll Cardiol 1999;33:1848.

38. Cleland JGF, Swedberg K, Poole-Wilson PA. Successes and failures of current treatment of heart failure. Lancet 1998;352 (Suppl 1):19.

39. Bart BA, Shaw LK, McCants CB Jr, et al. Clinical determinants of mortality in patients with angiographically diagnosed ischemic or nonischemic cardiomyopathy. J Am Coll Cardiol 1997;30:1002.

40. Woodley SL, Gilbert EM, Anderson JL, et al. Beta-blockade with bucindolol in heart failure caused by ischemic versus idiopathic dilated cardiomyopathy. Circulation 1991;84:2426.

41. Bristow MR, O'Connell JB, Gilbert EM. Dose-response of chronic beta-blocker treatment in heart failure from either idiopathic dilated or ischemic cardiomyopathy. Circulation 1994;89:1632.

42. Bristow MR, Gilbert EM, Abraham WT, et al. Carvedilol produces dose-related improvement in left ventricular function and survival in subjects with chronic heart failure. Circulation 1996;94:2807.

43. Lahiri A, Senior R. Evolving therapeutic concepts and imaging in ischemic cardiomyopathy. J Nucl Cardiol 1998;5:598.

44. Fintel DJ, Links JM, Brinker JA, et al. Improved diagnostic performance of exercise thallium-201 single photon emission computed tomography over planar imaging in the diagnosis of coronary artery disease: a receiver-operating characteristic analysis. J Am Coll Cardiol 1989;13:600.

45. Beller GA. Myocardial perfusion imaging with thallium-201. J Nucl Med 1994;35:674.

46. Maddahi J, Rodrigues E, Berman DS, et al. State-of-the-art myocardial perfusion imaging. Cardiol Clin 1994;12:199.

47. Levine MG, Ahlberg A, Mann A, et al. Comparison of exercise, dipyridamole, adenosine, and dobutamine stress with the use of Tc-99m tetrofosmin tomographic imaging. J Nucl Cardiol 1999;6:389.

48. Mody VF, Brunken RC, Warner Stevenson L, et al. Differentiating cardiomyopathy of coronary artery disease from nonischemic dilated cardiomyopathy utilizing positron emission tomography. J Am Coll Cardiol 1991;17:373.

49. Danias PG, Ahlberg AW, Clark BA III, et al. Combined assessment of myocardial perfusion and left ventricular function with exercise technetium-99m sestamibi gated single-photon emission computed tomography can differentiate between ischemic and non-ischemic dilated cardiomyopathy. Am J Cardiol 1998;82:1253.

50. Bisi G, Sciagra R, Santoro GM, et al. Sublingual isosorbide dinitrate to improve technetium-99m-teboroxime perfusion defect reversibility. J Nucl Med 1994;35:1274.

51. Bisi G, Sciagra R, Santoro GM, et al. Rest technetium-99m sestamibi tomography in combination with short term administration of nitrates: Feasibility and reliability for prediction of postrevascularization outcome of asynergic territories. J Am Coll Cardiol 1994;24:1282.

52. Thorley PJ, Bloomer TN, Sheard KL, et al. The use of GTN to improve the detection of ischemic myocardium using Tc-99m-tetrofosmin. Nucl Med Commun 1996;17:669.

53. Thorley PJ, Sheard KL, Wright DJ, et al. The routine use of sublingual GTN with resting 99Tcm-tetrofosmin myocardial perfusion imaging. Nucl Med Commun 1998;19:937.

54. Peix A, Lopez A, Ponce F, et al. Enhanced detection of reversible myocardial hypoperfusion by technetium 99m-tetrofosmin imaging and first pass radionuclide angiography after nitroglycerin administration. J Nucl Cardiol 1998;5:469.

55. He Z-X, Medrano R, Hays JT, et al. Nitroglycerin-augmented 201Tl reinjection enhances detection of reversible myocardial hypoperfusion. A randomized, double-blind, parallel, placebo-controlled trial. Circulation 1997;95:1799.

56. Brunton TL. On the use of nitrite of amyl in angina pectoris. Lancet 1867;2:97.

57. Murrel W. Nitroglycerin as a remedy for angina pectoris. Lancet 1879;1:80,113,151,225.

58. Horwitz LD, Gorlin R, Taylor WJ, et al. Effects of nitroglycerin on regional myocardial blood flow in coronary artery disease. J Clin Invest 1971;50:1578.

59. Helfant RH, Pine R, Meister SG, et al. Nitroglycerin to unmask reversible asynergy: correlation with post coronary bypass ventriculography. Circulation 1974;50:108.

60. Abrams J. Hemodynamic effects of nitroglycerin and long-acting nitrates. Am Heart J 1985;110:216.

61. Brown BG, Bolson E, Petersen RB, et al. The mechanisms of nitroglycerin action: stenosis vasodilation as a major component of the drug response. Circulation 1981;64:1089.

62. Fam WM, McGregor M. Effect of nitroglycerin and dipyridamole on regional coronary resistance. Circ Res 1968;22:649.

63. Brown BG. Response of normal and diseased epicardial coronary arteries to vasoactive drugs: quantitative arteriographic studies. Am J Cardiol 1985;56:23E.

64. Aoki M, Sakai K, Koyanagi S, et al. Effect of nitroglycerin on coronary collateral function during exercise evaluated by quantitative analysis of thallium-201 single photon emission computed tomography. Am Heart J 1991;121:1361.

65. Cohn PF, Maddox D, Holman BL, et al. Effect of sublingually administered nitroglycerin on regional myocardial blood flow in patients with coronary artery disease. Am J Cardiol 1977; 39:672.

66. Fallen EL, Nahmias C, Scheffel A, et al. Redistribution of myocardial blood flow with topical nitroglycerin in patients with coronary artery disease. Circulation 1995;91:1381.

67. Mahmarian JJ, Fenimore NL, et al. Transdermal nitroglycerin patch therapy reduces the extent of exercise-induced myocardial ischaemia: results of a double-blind, placebo-controlled trial using quantitative thallium-201 tomography. J Am Coll Cardiol 1994;24:25.

68. Borer JS, Bacharach SL, Green MV, et al. Effect of nitroglycerin on exercise-induced abnormalities of left ventricular function and ejection fraction in coronary artery disease: assessment by radionuclide cineangiography in symptomatic and asymptomatic patients. Circulation 1978;57:314.

69. Lahiri A, Crawley JCW, Sonecha TN, et al. Acute and chronic effects of sustained action buccal nitroglycerin in severe congestive heart failure. Int J Cardiol 1984;5:39.

70. He ZX, Darcourt J, Guignier A, et al. Nitrates improve detection of ischemic but viable myocardium by thallium-201 reinjection SPECT. J Nucl Med 1993;34:1472.

71. Bisi G, Sciagra R, Santoro GM, et al. Technetium-99m sestamibi imaging with nitrate infusion to detect viable hibernating myocardium and predict post revascularisation recovery. J Nucl Med 1995;36:1994.

72. Galli M, Marcassa C, Imperato A, et al. Effects of nitroglycerin by technetium-99m sestamibi tomoscintigraphy on resting regional myocardial hypoperfusion in stable patients with healed myocardial infarction. Am J Cardiol 1994;74:843.

73. Bax JJ, Wijns WW, Cornel JH, et al. Accuracy of currently available techniques for prediction of functional recovery after revascularisation in patients with left ventricular dysfunction due to chronic coronary artery disease: comparison of pooled data. J Am Coll Cardiol 1997;30:1451.

74. He Z-X, Verani MS. Evaluation of myocardial viability by myocardial perfusion imaging: should nitrates be used? J Nucl Cardiol 1998;5:527.

75. Senior R, Lahiri A. Role of dobutamine echocardiography in detection of myocardial viability for predicting outcome after revascularization in ischemic cardiomyopathy. Am Soc Echocardiogr 2001;14:240.

76. Pennel DJ, Ray SG, Davies G, et al. The carvedilol hibernation reversible ischaemia trial, marker of success (CHRISTMAS) study. Methodology of a randomised, placebo controlled, multicentre study of carvedilol in hibernation and heart failure. Int J Cardiol 2000;72:265.

77. Packer M, Bristow MR, Cohn JN, et al. The effect of carvedilol on morbidity and mortality in patients with chronic heart failure. N Engl J Med 1996;334:1349.

78. Packer M, Coats AJS, Fowler MB, et al. Effect of carvedilol on survival in severe chronic heart failure. N Engl J Med 2001; 344:1651.

79. Senior R, Basu S, Kinsey C, et al. Carvedilol prevents remodeling in patients with left ventricular dysfunction after acute myocardial infarction. Am Heart J 1999;137:646.

80. Doughty RN, Whalley GA, Gamble G, et al. Left ventricular remodeling with carvedilol in patients with congestive heart failure due to ischemic heart disease. J Am Coll Cardiol 1997; 29:1060.

81. Khattar RS, Senior R, van der Does R, et al. Regression of left ventricular remodeling in chronic heart failure: comparative and combined effects of captopril and carvedilol. Am Heart J 2001;142:704.

82. Cleland JG, Alamgir F, Nikitin NP, et al. What is the optimal medical management of ischemic heart failure? Prog Cardiovasc Dis 2001;43:433.

83. Sabbah HN, Goldstein S. Ventricular remodelling: consequences and therapy Eur Heart J 1993;14(Suppl C):24.

84. Mancia G. Sympathetic activation in congestive heart failure. Eur Heart J 1990;11(Suppl A):3.

85. Francis GS, Benedict C, Johnstone DE, et al. Comparison of neuroendocrine activation in patients with left ventricular dysfunction with and without congestive heart failure: a substudy of the studies of left ventricular dysfunction (SOLVD). Circulation 1990;82:1724.

86. Cohn JN, Ferrari R, Sharpe N. Cardiac remodelling—concepts and clinical implications: a consensus paper from an international forum on cardiac remodelling. J Am Coll Cardiol 2000; 35:569.

87. Gaudron P, Eilles C, Kugler I, et al. Progressive left ventricular dysfunction and remodeling after myocardial infarction. Potential mechanisms and early predictors. Circulation 1993;87:755.

88. Hammermeister KE, DeRouen TA, Dodge HT. Variables predictive of survival in patients with coronary disease: selection by univariate and multivariate analyses from the clinical, electrocardiographic, exercise, arteriographic and quantitative angiographic evaluations. Circulation 1979;59:421.

89. White HD, Norris RM, Brown MA, et al. Left ventricular end-systolic volume as the major determinant of survival after recovery from myocardial infarction. Circulation 1987;76:44–51

90. Mandinov L, Eberli FR, Seiler C, et al. Diastolic heart failure. Cardiovasc Res 2000; 45: 813.

91. Hein S, Schaper J. The extracellular matrix in normal and diseased myocardium. J Nucl Cardiol 2001;8:188.

92. Sharpe N, Smith H, Murphy J, et al. Early prevention of left ventricular dysfunction after myocardial infarction with angiotensin-converting-enzyme inhibition. Lancet 1991;337:872.

93. Pfeffer MA, Braunwald E, Moye L. Effect of captopril on mortality and morbidity in patients with left ventricular dysfunction after myocardial infarction. N Engl J Med 1992;327;669.

94. Basu S, Senior R, Raval U, et al. Beneficial effects of intravenous and oral carvedilol treatment in acute myocardial infarction: a placebo-controlled, randomized trial. Circulation 1997;96:183.

95. Senior R, Kaul S, Lahiri A. Nitrate enhanced Tc-99m-sestamibi SPECT predicts regression of remodelling following revascularisation compared to medical therapy in ischemic cardiomyopathy. J Nucl Cardiol 2001;8(Suppl):S47.

96. Senior R, Lahiri A, Kaul S. Effect of revascularization on left ventricular remodeling in patients with heart failure from severe chronic ischemic left ventricular dysfunction. Am J Cardiol 2001;88:624.

97. Gradman A, Deedwanra P, Cody R, et al. Predictors of total mortality and sudden death in mild to moderate heart failure. J Am Coll Cardiol 1989;14:564.

98. Volpi A, De Vita C, Franzosi MG, et al. Determinants of 6-month mortality in survivors of myocardial infarction after thrombolysis. Results of the GISSI-2 data base. Circulation 1993;88:416.

99. Davie AP, Francis CM, Caruana L, et al. Assessing diagnosis in heart failure: which features are any use? Q J Med 1997; 90:335.

100. Borer JS, Bacharach SL, Green MV, et al. Rapid evaluation of left ventricular function during exercise in patients with coronary artery disease. Circulation 1976; 54(Suppl II); II-6 (abstract).

101. Wackers FJ, Berger HJ, Johnstone DE, et al. Multiple gated cardiac blood pool imaging for EF: validation of the technique and assessment of variability. Circulation 1979;43:1159.

102. Upton MT, Rerych SK, Newman GE, et al. The reproducibility of radionuclide angiographic measurements of left ventricular function in normal subjects at rest and during exercise. Circulation 1980;62;126.

103. Hecht HS, Josephson MA, Hopkins JM, et al. Reproducibility of equilibrium radionuclide ventriculography in patients with coronary artery disease: response of left ventricular ejection fraction and regional wall motion to supine bicycle exercise. Am Heart J 1982;104:567.

104. van Royen N, Jaffe CC, Krumholz HM, et al. Comparison and reproducibility of visual echocardiographic and quantitative radionuclide left ventricular ejection fractions. Am J Cardiol 1996;77:843.

105. Waldo AL, Camm AJ, deRuyter H, et al. Survival with oral d-sotalol in patients with left ventricular dysfunction after myocardial infarction: rationale, design, and methods (the SWORD trial). Am J Cardiol 1995;75:1023.

106. Lahiri A, Rodrigues EA, DasGupta P, et al. Effects of carvedilol in patients with impaired left ventricular function due to ischemic heart disease. Z Kardiol 1989;78(Suppl 3):21.

107. Goldstein S, Kennedy HL, Hall C, et al. Metoprolol CR/XL in patients with heart failure: a pilot study examining the tolerability, safety, and effect on left ventricular ejection fraction. Am Heart J 1999;138:1158.

108. Schulman SP, Weiss JL, Becker LC, et al. Effect of early enalapril therapy on left ventricular function and structure in acute myocardial infarction. Am J Cardiol 1995;76:764.

109. The EDEN Study Investigators. Effects of enalapril on left ventricular function and exercise performance after a first acute myocardial infarction. Int J Cardiol. 1997;59:257.

110. Kelbëk H, Aldershville J, Skagen K, et al. Pre- and afterload reduction in chronic mitral regurgitation: a double-blind randomized placebo-controlled trial of the acute and 2 weeks' effect of Nifedipine or isosorbide dinitrate treatment on left ventricular function and the severity of mitral regurgitation. Br J Clin Pharmacol 1996;41:493.

111. Sartori M, Andorno S, La Terra G, et al. Assessment of interferon cardiotoxicity with quantitative radionuclide angiocardiography. Eur J Clin Invest 1995;25:68.

112. Chevalier P, Bontemps L, Fatemi M, et al. Gated blood-pool SPECT evaluation of changes after radiofrequency catheter ablation of accessory pathways. J Am Coll Cardiol 1999;34:1839.

113. Le Rest C, Couturier O, Turzo A, et al. Use of left ventricular pacing in heart failure: evaluation by gated blood pool imaging. J Nucl Cardiol 1999;6:651.

114. Senior R, Sridhara BS, Basu S, et al. Comparison of radionuclide ventriculography and 2D echocardiography for the measurement of left ventricular ejection fraction following acute myocardial infarction. Eur Heart J 1994;15:1235.

115. Galasko GIW, Lahiri A, Senior R. Portable echocardiography: an innovative tool in the assessment of heart failure in the community. Heart 2001;85(Suppl I):27.

116. Bellenger NG, Burgess MI, Ray SG, et al. Comparison of left ventricular ejection fraction and volumes in heart failure by echocardiography, radionuclide ventriculography and cardiovascular magnetic resonance. Are they interchangeable? Eur Heart J 2000;21:1387.

117. Germano G, Berman DS. Quantitative gated perfusion SPECT. In: Clinical Gated Cardiac SPECT. edited by G Germano and DS Berman. Armonk, NY: Futura Publishing Company, 1999, pp. 115–146.

118. DePuey EG, Rozanski A. Using gated technetium-99m-sestamibi to characterize fixed myocardial defects as infarct or artefact. J Nucl Med 1995;36:952.

119. Smanio PEP, Watson DD, Segalla DL, et al. Value of gating of technetium-99m sestamibi single-photon emission computed tomographic imaging. J Am Coll Cardiol 1997;30:1687.

120. Levine MG, McGill CC, Ahlberg AW, et al. Functional assessment with electrocardiographic gated single-photon emission computed tomography improves the ability of technetium-99m sestamibi myocardial perfusion imaging to predict myocardial viability in patients undergoing revascularisation. Am J Cardiol 1999;83:1.

121. Vasan RS, Benjamin EJ, Levy D. Prevalence, clinical features and prognosis of diastolic heart failure: an epidemiologic perspective. J Am Coll Cardiol 1995;26:1565.

122. Vasan RS, Larson MG, Benjamin EJ, et al. Congestive heart failure in subjects with normal versus reduced left ventricular ejection fraction. J Am Coll Cardiol 1999;33:1948.

123. Aurigemma GP, Gottdiener JS, Shemanski L, et al. Predictive value of systolic and diastolic function for incident congestive heart failure in the elderly: the cardiovascular health study. J Am Coll Cardiol 2001;37:1042.

124. Yellin EL, Nikolic S, Frater RWM. Left ventricular filling dynamics and diastolic function. Prog Cardiovasc Dis 1990;32:247.

125. Cohen GI, Pietrolungo JF, Thomas JD, et al. A practical guide to assessment of ventricular diastolic function using Doppler echocardiography. J Am Coll Cardiol 1996;27:1687.

126. Aggarwal A, Brown KA, LeWinter MM. Diastolic dysfunction: pathophysiology, clinical features, and assessment with radionuclide methods. J Nucl Cardiol 2001;8:98.

127. Cottin Y, Touzery C, Coudert B, et al. Diastolic or systolic left and right ventricular impairment at moderate doses of anthracycline? A 1-year follow-up study of women. Eur J Nucl Med 1996;23:511.

128. Topuzovic N. Worsening of left ventricular diastolic function during long-term correction of anemia with erythropoietin in chronic hemodialysis patients—an assessment by radionuclide ventriculography at rest and exercise. Int J Card Imaging 1999;15:233.

129. Levy WC, Cerqueira MD, Weaver WD, et al. Early patency of the infarct-related artery after myocardial infarction preserves diastolic filling. Am J Cardiol 2001;87:955.

130. Bristow MR, Ginsberg W, Minobe RS, et al. Decreased catecholamine sensitivity and -adrenergic receptor density in failing human hearts. N Engl J Med 1982;307:205.

131. Bristow MR, Minobe WA, Raynolds MV, et al. Reduced 1 receptor messenger RNA abundance in the failing human heart. J Clin Invest 1993;92:2737.

132. Packer M. The neurohumeral hypothesis: a theory to explain the mechanism of disease progression in heart failure. J Am Coll Cardiol 1992;20:248.

133. Cohn JN, Levine TB, Olivari MT, et al. Plasma norepineph-

rine as a guide to prognosis in patients with chronic congestive heart failure. N Engl J Med 1984;311:819.

134. Sisson JC, Frager MS, Valk TW, et al. Scintigraphic localisation of phaeochromocytoma. N Engl J Med 1981;305:12.

135. Shapiro B, Copp JE, Sisson JC, et al. Iodine-131 metaiodobenzylguanidine for the locating of suspected phaeochromocytoma: experience in 400 cases. J Nucl Med 1985;26:576.

136. Dae MW. Imaging of myocardial sympathetic innervation with metaiodobenzylguanidine. J Nucl Cardiol 1994; 1: S23.

137. Henderson EB, Kahn JK, Corbett JR, et al. Abnormal I-123 metaiodobenzylguanidine myocardial washout and distribution may reflect myocardial adrenergic derangement in patients with congestive cardiomyopathy. Circulation 1988;78:1192.

138. Schoefer J, Spielman R, Schuchert A, et al. Iodine 123 MetaIodobenzylGuanidine scintigraphy: a noninvasive method to demonstrate myocardial adrenergic system disintegrity in patients with idiopathic dilated cardiomyopathy. J Am Coll Cardiol 1988;12:1252.

139. Lotze U, Kober A, Kaepplinger S, et al. Cardiac sympathetic activity as measured by myocardial 123-I-Metaiodobenzylguanidine uptake and heart rate variability in idiopathic dilated cardiomyopathy. Am J Cardiol 1999;83:1548.

140. Imamura Y, Ando H, Mitsuoka W, et al. Iodine-123 metaiodobenzylguanidine images reflect intense myocardial adrenergic nervous activity in congestive heart failure independent of underlying cause. J Am Coll Cardiol 1995;26:1594.

141. Somsen GA, Szabo BM, van Veldhuisen DJ, et al. Comparison between iodine 123 metaiodobenzyl-guanidine scintigraphy and heart rate variability for the assessment of cardiac sympathetic activity in mild to moderate heart failure. Am Heart J 1997;134:456.

142. Merlet P, Valette H, Rande JLD, et al. Prognostic value of cardiac Metaiodobenzylguanidine imaging in patients with heart failure. J Nucl Med 1992;33:471.

143. Cohn JN, Rector TS. Prognosis of congestive heart failure and predictors of mortality. Am J Cardiol 1988;62:25A.

144. Rector TS, Cohn JN. Prognosis in congestive heart failure. Annu Rev Med 1994;45:341.

145. Galasko GIW, Basu S, Lahiri A, et al. A prospective comparison of echocardiographic wall motion score index and radionuclide ejection fraction in predicting outcome following acute myocardial infarction. Heart 2001;86:271.

146. Merlet P, Benvenuti C, Moyse D, et al. Prognostic value of MIBG imaging in idiopathic dilated cardiomyopathy. J Nucl Med 1999;40:917.

147. Takatsu H, Scheffel U, Fujiwara H. Modulation of left ventricular iodine-125-MIBG accumulation in cardiomyopathic Syrian hamsters using the renin-angiotensin system. J Nucl Med 1995;36:1055.

148. Barr CS, Lang CC, Hanson J, et al. Effects of adding spironolactone to an angiotensin-converting enzyme inhibitor in chronic congestive heart failure secondary to coronary artery disease. Am J Cardiol 1995;76:1259.

149. Choi JY, Lee K-H, Hong KP, et al. Iodine-123 MIBG imaging before treatment of heart failure with carvedilol to predict improvement of left ventricular function and exercise capacity. J Nucl Cardiol 2001; 8: 4.

150. Baliga RR, Narula J, Dec GW. The MIBG tarot: is it possible to predict the efficacy of β-blockers in congestive heart failure? J Nucl Cardiol 2001;8:107.

151. Liggett SB, Wagoner LE, Craft LL. The Ile164β2-adrenergic receptor polymorphism adversely affects the outcome of congestive heart failure. J Clin Invest 1998;102:1534.

152. Wagoner LE, Craft LL, Singh B, et al. Polymorphisms of the 2-adrenergic receptor determine exercise capacity in patients with heart failure. Circ Res 2000;86:834.

153. de Groot MC, Marini D, Cyr G, et al. Technetium-99m (Tc-99m) sestamibi gated SPECT imaging can differentiate between nonischemic (NI) and ischemic (I) origins of dilated cardiomyopathy. J Nucl Cardiol 2000;7:S10.

154. Bulkley BH, Hutchins GM, Bailey I, et al. Thallium-201 imaging and gated blood pool scans in patients with ischemic and idiopathic congestive cardiomyopathy: a clinical and pathologic study. Circulation 1977;55:753.

155. Greenberg JM, Murphy JH, Okada RD, et al. Value and limitations of radionuclide angiography in determining the cause of reduced left ventricular ejection fraction: comparison of idiopathic dilated cardiomyopathy and coronary artery disease. Am J Cardiol 1985;55:541.

156. Schwartz RG, McKenzie WB, et al. Congestive heart failure and left ventricular dysfunction complicating doxorubicin therapy. Seven-year experience using serial radionuclide angiocardiography. Am J Med 1987;82:1109.

157. Pohost GM, Vignola PA, McKusick KE, et al. Hypertrophic cardiomyopathy: evaluation by gated cardiac blood pool scanning. Circulation 1977; 55: 92.

158. Bonow RO, Rosing DR, Bacharach SL, et al. Effects of verapamil and left ventricular systolic function and diastolic filling in patients with hypertrophic cardiomyopathy. Circulation 1981;64:787.

159. Bulkley BH, Rouleau J, Strauss HW, et al. Idiopathic hypertrophic subaortic stenosis: detection by thallium 201 myocardial perfusion imaging. N Engl J Med 1975;293:113.

160. O'Gara PT, Bonow RO, Maron BJ, et al. Myocardial perfusion abnormalities assessed by thallium-201 emission computed tomography in patients with hypertrophic cardiomyopathy. Circulation 1987;76:1052.

161. Dilsizian V, Bonow RO, Epstein SE, et al. Myocardial ischaemia is a frequent cause of cardiac arrest and syncope in young patients with hypertrophic cardiomyopathy. J Am Coll Cardiol 1993;22:796.

162. Forman MB, Sandler MP, Sacks GA, et al. Radionuclide imaging in myocardial sarcoidosis: demonstration of myocardial uptake of technetium pyrophosphate-99m and gallium. Chest 1983;83:570.

163. Follansbee WP, Curtis EJ, Medsger TA Jr, et al. Physiologic abnormalities of cardiac function in progressive systemic sclerosis with diffuse scleroderma. N Engl J Med 1984;310:142.

164. Leon B, Borer JS, Bacharach SL, et al. Detection of early cardiac dysfunction in patients with severe beta-thalassemia and chronic iron overload. N Engl J Med 1979;301:1143.

165. Aldouri MA, Wonke B, Hoffbrand AV, et al. High incidence of cardiomyopathy in beta-thalassaemia patients receiving regular transfusion and iron chelation: reversal by intensified chelation. Acta Haematol 1990;84:113.

166. Scheutz A, Fritsch S, Kemkes BM, et al. Antimyosin monoclonal antibodies for early detection of cardiac allograft rejection. J Heart Transplant 1990;9:654.

167. Ballaster M, Obrador D, Carrio I, et al. Indium-111 monoclonal antimyosin antibody studies after the first year of heart transplantation: identification of risk groups for developing rejection during long-term follow-up and clinical implications. Circulation 1990;82:2100.

168. O'Connell JB, Henkin RE, Robinson JA, et al. Gallium-67 imaging in patients with dilated cardiomyopathy and biopsy-proven myocarditis. Circulation 1984;70:58.

169. Dec GW, Palacois I, Yasuda T, et al. Antimyosin antibody cardiac imaging: its role in the diagnosis of myocarditis. J Am Coll Cardiol 1990;16:97.

170. Borer JS, Bacharach SL, Green MV, et al. Exercise-induced left ventricular dysfunction in symptomatic and asymptomatic patients with aortic regurgitation: assessment by radionuclide cineangiography. Am J Cardiol 1979;42:351.

171. Maddahi J, Berman DS, Matsouka DT, et al. A new technique for assessing right ventricular ejection fraction using rapid multiple gated equilibrium blood pool scintigraphy. Circulation 1979;60:581.

172. Goldberg HL, Herrold EM, Hochreiter C, et al. Videodensitometric determination of right ventricular and left ventricular ejection fraction. Am J Noninvasive Cardiol 1987;1:18.

173. Bonow RO. Asymptomatic aortic regurgitation: indications for operation. J Card Surg 1994;9(2 Suppl): 170.

174. Bonow RO, Lakatos E, Maron BJ, et al. Serial long-term assessment of the natural history of asymptomatic patients with chronic aortic regurgitation and normal left ventricular systolic function. Circulation 1991;84:1625.

175. Borer JS, Hochreiter C, Herrold EM, et al. Prediction of indications for valve replacement among asymptomatic or minimally symptomatic patients with chronic aortic regurgitation and normal left ventricular performance. Circulation 1998;97:525.

176. Hochreiter C, Niles N, Devereux RB, et al. Mitral regurgitation: relationship of non-invasive descriptors of right and left ventricular performance to clinical and hemodynamic findings and to prognosis in medically and surgically treated patients. Circulation 1986;73:900.

177. Rosen SE, Borer JS, Hochreiter C, et al. Natural history of the asymptomatic/minimally symptomatic patient with severe mitral regurgitation secondary to mitral valve prolapse and normal right and left ventricular performance. Am J Cardiol 1994;74:374.

178. Phillips HR, Levine FH, Carter JE, et al. Mitral valve replacement for isolated mitral regurgitation: analysis of clinical course and late post-operative left ventricular ejection fraction. Am J Cardiol 1981;48:647.

179. Furer J, Hochreiter C, Niles NW, et al. Prediction of symptom status following mitral valve replacement for mitral regurgitation by preoperative echocardiographic measurement of the end-systolic stress to end-systolic volume ratio. Am J Noninvasive Cardiol 1987;1:321.

180. Kawasaki T, Kosaki F, Okawa S, et al. A new infantile febrile mucocutaneous lymph node syndrome [MLNS] prevailing in Japan. Pediatrics 1974;54:271.

181. Gersony WM. Diagnosis and management of Kawasaki disease. JAMA 1991;265:2699.

182. Koren G, Lavi S, Rose V, et al. Kawasaki disease: a review of risk factors for coronary aneurysm. J Pediatr 1986;108:388.

183. Shaukat N, Ashraf S, Mebewu A, et al. Myocardial infarction in a young adult due to Kawasaki disease: a case report and review of the late cardiological sequelae of Kawasaki disease. Int J Cardiol 1993;39:222.

184. Takahashi M, Mason W, Lewis AB. Regression of coronary aneurysms in patients with Kawasaki syndrome. Circulation 1987;75:387.

185. Akagi T, Rose V, Benson LN, et al. Outcome of coronary artery aneurysms after Kawasaki disease. J Pediatr 1992;121:789.

186. Kato H, Sugimura T, Akagi T, et al. Long-term consequences of Kawasaki disease: a 10-to-21-year follow-up study of 594 patients. Circulation 1996;94:1379.

187. Kato H, Inoue O, Kawasaki T, et al. Adult coronary artery disease probably due to childhood Kawasaki disease. Lancet 1992;340:1127.

188. Kondo C, Hiroe M, Nakanishi T, et al. Detection of coronary artery stenosis in children with Kawasaki disease. Usefulness of pharmacologic stress 201Tl myocardial tomography. Circulation 1989;80:615.

189. Fukunda T, Akagi T, Ishibashi M, et al. Noninvasive evaluation of myocardial ischemia in Kawasaki disease: comparison between dipyridamole stress thallium imaging and exercise stress testing. Am Heart J 1998;135:482.

190. Schillaci O, Banci M, Scopinaro F, et al. Myocardial scintigraphy with 99mTc-sestamibi in children with Kawasaki disease. Angiology 1995;46:1009.

191. Karasawa K, Ayusawa M, Noto N, et al. Optimum protocol of technetium-99m tetrofosmin myocardial perfusion imaging for detection of coronary stenosis lesions in Kawasaki disease. J Cardiol 1997;30:331.

192. Ogawa S, Fukazawa R, Ohkubo T. Silent myocardial ischemia in Kawasaki disease: evaluation of percutaneous transluminal coronary angioplasty by dobutamine stress testing. Circulation 1997;96:3384.

193. Miyagawa M, Mochizuki T, Murase K, et al. Prognostic value of dipyridamole-thallium myocardial scintigraphy in patients with Kawasaki disease. Circulation 1998;98:990.

21 | Development of newer radiotracers for evaluation of myocardial and vascular disorders

JAGAT NARULA, ALBERT FLOTATS, ADRIAN D. NUNN, AND IGRASI CARRIÓ

Like any pathologic state, myocardial and vascular diseases are also characterized by specific histopathologic alterations, and over- or underexpression of various molecular moieties. All such specific alterations can be potentially targeted by peptides, ligands, or antibodies. If these targeting agents are labeled with appropriate radioisotopes, all pathologic states may become potentially amenable to radionuclide imaging. Radiotracers possess the unique property of accessibility to extra- and intracellular milieus and even intranuclear targets. They are trapped at the specific binding sites, whereas the unbound or free radiotracers are washed out of the cells to render an appropriate target-to-background ratio. Better understanding of the pathophysiology of disease, elucidation of the molecular basis of pathology, and the use of DNA chip technology and computer modeling for development of novel drug allow simultaneous evolution of radionuclide targeting agents. Identification of unique targets (that are exclusively expressed in the disease state), development of designer targeting agents (that possess high specificity and affinity to the unique antigens), and skillful use of radiotracers (that are easy to label, and have a short half-life and ideal imaging characteristics) constitute the most important tenets of molecular nuclear cardiology—a specialty that promises to acquire burgeoning proportions in the next one to two decades.

IMAGING OF MYOCARDIAL ISCHEMIA/HYPOXIA

The functioning of a piece of myocardial tissue is governed by the laws of supply and demand. For short periods demand can exceed supply at the cost of producing a nutrient debt that must be paid back. If the debt becomes too large the viability of the tissue is jeopardized and further reductions in supply lead to cell death. When supply and demand are coupled and the tissue is stable, perfusion—a crude measure of supply in the sense that it records bulk flow but not the nutrient content of that flow—can be used to indirectly assess the status of the tissue on a regional basis.

The patterns of flow distribution, as recorded by thallium or the technetium myocardial perfusion agents, can be read to advantage in many clinical situations despite the fact that these single-photon perfusion agents cannot as yet provide regional flow in quantitative terms. An array of new perfusion tracers is under various stages of evaluation. However, the new tracers may only contribute to improve the imaging characteristics and convenience of imaging procedures (see below), but do not necessarily add significantly to pathophysiologic assessment of myocardial ischemia. When the normal functioning of the tissue is changed or is inherently unknown (as in the case of severely compromised tissue), such that we cannot interpret what the demand is, perfusion becomes of insufficient value and we need instead a measure of the potential for recovery (viability), of the tissue. In these cases a more direct measure of metabolism such as using the currently available fluorodeoxyglucose (FDG) may be more accurate.

Oxygen consumption is at the root of all energy production except in those cases where the tissue goes into oxygen debt. One such situation is anaerobic glycolysis, the extreme of which is the use of glycolysis to maintain sarcolemmal membrane integrity as a last act of survival. FDG measures total glycolysis, both aerobic and anaerobic. The myocardium, of course, prefers to burn fatty acids and must be prompted to use glucose. There are a number of other issues with FDG that must be acknowledged. First, it is taken up, like glucose, by the glucose transporter resident in the cell membrane and further metabolized by the hexokinase system. Various insults to the tissue including ischemia cause changes in the regulation of the glucose transporters in the myocardial cells [1], but it is assumed that in all cases the hexokinase activity is faster and therefore dominant in determining the signal intensity. Second, FDG is taken up by leukocytes, and some of the signal may derive from this source rather than the myocardial cells. This is particularly pertinent to tissue soon after an ischemic insult or reperfusion injury or remodeling at which times there can be high numbers of tissue leukocytes. Thus, there is a danger of interpreting uptake as viable myocardial tissue when in fact it could represent tissue under "demolition." Ideally, then, a direct image of tissue oxygen concentration is most desirable. Use of O-15 is technically feasible for this purpose, but it is not routinely or widely practiced.

Hypoxia-Seeking Agents

In principle, any compound that is permeable through the cell membrane contains a moiety that has a reduction potential within the range of cellular reductases, is reduced to a compound that has lower permeability through the cell membrane, and can be reoxidized to a permeable species by molecular oxygen—it has biochemistry suitable for a hypoxic tissue-imaging agent. Nitroimidazole derivatives are by far the largest group of compounds with some or all of these characteristics that have been investigated as a means of imaging tissue oxygen concentration for two decades. Almost all the knowledge we have on the metabolism of nitroimidazoles has been obtained at the therapeutic doses used for their antibacterial or radiosensitizer effects. It is not at all obvious that the same metabolism occurs or is dominant at the very low doses used for imaging. Indeed, it has been shown that the pharmacokinetics of nitroimidazoles are dose dependent [2]. Nevertheless, from these studies it appears that once inside cells, nitroimidazoles are reduced by an enzyme-mediated single electron reduction of the nitro group to a free radical that is an anion at neutral pH. Thus after this first step, there is a change in the permeability of the radioactive species that is sufficient to cause its retention inside the cell. The oxygen sensitivity rises because the first reduction product is capable of being reoxidized by oxygen within the cell. The rate of reoxidation is proportional to the concentration of oxygen. Thus

nitroimidazoles are initially reduced by all cells with functioning reductases but are rapidly reoxidized in normoxic cells so that little or no net retention of radioactivity occurs. In the cells with reduced oxygen concentration, the retention is inversely proportional to the oxygen concentration.

Although several enzymes have been shown in vitro to be capable of the reduction, the specific enzyme responsible for the reduction of nitroimidazoles in vivo has not been identified and, of course, may differ from cell to cell or may be a variety of enzymes in a given cell. Mello et al. [3] have shown that cells transfected with NADPH:cytochrome P450 reductase exhibit increased retention of BRU5921, a technetium labeled nitroimidazole. Alternatively, xanthine oxidoreductase (XOD) has been commonly used as a representative enzyme and is found in many mammalian cells. There are differences in the abundance of this particular enzyme both between species and in different tissues of the same species. In particular, it has been shown to be much less abundant in human myocardium than in the rat, so caution must be exercised in giving it too prominent a role [4,5]. XOD can reduce nitroimidazoles contained in technetium complexes without reducing the technetium itself [6–8]. As stated earlier, the ability to be reduced by enzymes such as XOD is not of itself the only requirement for efficacy in vivo. The compound must be able to reach the enzymes which appear to be intracellular. Thus the nitroimidazoles based upon the BATO core do not work even in isolated rat cardiomyocytes [6], because the core is poorly permeable [9] and does not allow the nitroimidazole access to the intracellular enzymes. The same is true for an impermeable technetium nitroimidazole complex based upon a bis amino-phenol core (BAPN) [8] and is most likely the reason for the poor performance of HNBAHP [10] and the gadolinium, gallium, and indium complexes of Norman et al. [11].

The issue of species differences is very important when dealing with biochemical probes such as the nitroimidazoles. As reported before, XOD is useful in vitro model but it is present in different concentrations in the myocardium in different species. One must expect to observe species differences and there is already some evidence that they occur. Cowan [12] examined the uptake of a technetium nitroimidazole BMS-181321 in human and animal cancer cell lines in culture, the simplest system avoiding all pharmacokinetic issues. They found increased uptake of radioactivity in the MCF-7 and HeLa human cell lines compared to four rodent cell lines (Chinese Hamster Ovary and rat mammary carcinoma).

Besides technetium nitroimidazole complexes a large number of radiohalogenated nitroimidazoles have been made, the most prominent of which are fluoromisonidazole (FMISO) [13] and IAZA [14] both of which have been tested in humans, although only the FMISO has been examined in the human myocardium [15]. A nitroimidazole per se is not a requisite for the localizing group sensitive to ambient oxygen concentrations inside living cells. A minimal modification of this moiety is to use a nitrofuran rather than a nitroimidazole, provided that the reduction potential is in the appropriate region. The nitro group can be substituted by other suitable species, the most extreme of which may be the use of the metal center itself. This has been done in the case of HL-91 a technetium complex that contains no prosthetic groups apart from those of the chelating agent itself [16]. Although the exact reaction products have not been identified it is reasonable to believe that the active center is the technetium atom modulated by the surrounding ligand. A similar approach has been taken with the technetium and copper thiosemicarbazides [17,18].

Assuming that each of these approaches achieves the same level of biochemical efficacy they still represent as yet unresolved issues concerning their overall efficacy. The technetium-based agents are attractive because of their potential for widespread availability, but the physical half-life may not be ideal in that there is some indication from HL-91 or FMISO imaging in dogs that later imaging times are beneficial [15,19]. Iodine-123 derivatives may be beneficial in this case along with Cu-64. The PET-based compounds have more restricted availability, but the recent proliferation of PET centers and increasing familiarity with manufacturing and distributing short-lived (PET) radiopharmaceuticals have resolved some of the issues. The potential for absolute quantitation and the increasing use of image fusion and hybrid machines with the PET-based compounds may not be as much of an advantage for the myocardium as for oncology. In the case of trapping by a nonnitroimidazole mechanism it appears that at least in tumor tissue the reaction of Cu-ATSM is quite rapid and allows for early imaging [20].

Freshly isolated rat cardiac myocytes and various tumor cell lines have been used to examine the uptake characteristics of hypoxic tissue localizing agents. The use of cardiac myocytes [21] seems to be obvious given that the myocardium is the target organ. However, as noted previously, there are differences in enzyme abundance between species. Human tumor cell lines can be used but the relevance of these transformed cells to those in situ and the different cell types raises issues of validity, and, as noted above, there may be differences in response between human and rodent derived cells. In vivo results in various species may also mislead.

As a result of the dominance of perfusion imaging,

much of the biological work performed with the nitroimidazoles has been to demonstrate at what flow retention increases. Whereas this provides a useful link with a means of interpreting the data, it assumes that perfusion data are a true gold-standard. That this is not the case is evident from the discussions about stunning and hibernating myocardium and from a rudimentary analysis of the relationship between bulk flow and metabolism, as outlined earlier. An examination of the oxygen sensitivity of endothelial cells and cardiomyocytes shows that they are surprisingly resistant to low oxygen concentrations [22]. The biological work that has been done with the radiolabeled hypoxic tissue imaging agents has been to establish two groups of relationships; between the retention of radioactivity and the physiology or biochemistry of the tissue and those between the retention and the subsequent clinical outcome or management of the patient. Much of the latter work has been done in animal models, as clinical work has in most cases only just begun, especially when it comes to the myocardium.

Stone [23] used an extracorporeally perfused coronary model in swine to determine the relationship between flow and retention of BMS-181321 derived radioactivity. In this model the heart is left in the body and supplies blood to the body but the coronary flow is precisely provided to each coronary vessel independently using an extracorporeal pump. Radioactivity is administered into the mixing chamber of the pump and as such is equivalent to an arterial injection with negligible distribution to the other body tissues. The normal flow in the whole heart was approximately 1.2 ± 0.1 ml/min/g. The flow to the left anterior descending artery (LAD) was reduced by 60% for a 40-minute period during which they administered the BMS-181321 as a bolus. The low flow was maintained for 10 minutes after administration of the BMS-181321 before it was returned to normal and reperfused for 70 minutes. A comparison of radioactivity retention, measured after sacrifice, to tissue blood flow just prior to injection of the technetium tracer, measured using microspheres, shows an inverse linear relationship for the LAD bed but no correlation with flow in the normally perfused beds. As expected there were flow and uptake differences between the endocardial and epicardial tissues with the former having lower flows and greater uptake. Similar data on uptake/retention versus flow were obtained for HL91 [19] and for iodovinylmisonidazole [24].

The potential of hypoxic tissue imaging in chronic heart failure has also been examined [25]. They used a technetium nitroimidazole derivative and showed uptake correlated to the histopathology with increased uptake at the myocytolytic stage. Uptake was uniform throughout the myocardium even though the histological changes were multifocal. The imaging of chronic heart failure is obviously going to be difficult both if it is of ischemic origin because there may well be local areas of ischemia-induced hypoxia, and if it is not of ischemic origin, because it may present as a uniform increase in retention. A similar issue confronts MIBG imaging and it remains to be seen if hypoxic tissue imaging presents any advantage.

Hot Spot Imaging of Myocardial Hypoxia

One of the issues with imaging hypoxic tissue in the myocardium is that in the case of ischemia one expects that there will be regional intense uptake in the jeopardized tissue, but in the remainder of the normally perfused myocardium there will be low or no uptake. This poses problems in single-photon emission computed tomography (SPECT) reconstruction and interpretation, because of difficulty in determining the cardiac coordinates. To this end there is a paucity of SPECT images of the myocardium with hypoxic tissue imaging agents; planar images are usually provided [19]. Even when reconstruction is performed the interpretation of the images is not as straightforward as those routinely imaged for perfusion. The "hot spot" is seen with limited reference marks in the chest [26,27].

A related problem occurs in oncology imaging with FDG where the exact placement of the metabolic image on a morphological one has prompted image fusion and the development of hybrid machines. It is unclear if hybrid PET/CT (computed tomography) or SPECT/CT machines will benefit myocardial imaging; the myocardium is of course moving in the chest and registration is inherently more difficult. At early times, the cardiac coordinates can be determined by the radioactivity in the initial bolus or perfusion image, provided there has been no movement of the heart. At later times, this is, of course, not possible and other means of determining the cardiac coordinates must be employed. The attenuation map derived from sealed source imaging can be used for positron emission tomography (PET) and presumably can also be used for SPECT, or a simultaneously imaged long-lived perfusion tracer such as thallium can be used. The latter has been employed with BRU5921 [28] and thus provides both the perfusion and metabolism image at the same time.

To evaluate the relative merits of hypoxia and perfusion imaging, DiRocco [29] compared the retention of BMS-181321 derived radioactivity with that of misonidazole (MISO) or 2-deoxyglucose (2DG) in a rabbit model having an occluded LAD. Twenty minutes after occlusion, 20–30 mCi of Tc-99m labeled BMS-181321 was coinjected with 150 μCi of either C-14-

2DG or C-14-MISO. Thirty minutes later the animals were sacrificed, the hearts removed and sectioned for autoradiography. All three metabolic markers were preferentially retained at the lateral border zone of the ischemic territory as defined by the flow marker teboroxime. Other workers have established this lateral border zone as a region of hypoxic tissue with decreased ATP and creatinine phosphate levels and increased lactate levels. The patterns of retention of the BMS-181321, MISO, or 2DG-derived radioactivity were virtually superimposable. The normal tissue retained some radioactivity, whereas the lack of delivery of the tracers to the central zone precluded any such retention. The BMS-181321-derived radioactivity had essentially the same regional distribution in the lateral border zone as MISO or 2DG. The ratio of the border zone radioactivity to the normal tissue radioactivity in the same animals was 2.7 for MISO and 3.14 for BMS-181321 and was not significantly different. Similarly, the ratio was 4.19 for 2DG and 3.10 for BMS-181321 in a different group of animals and was also not significantly different. The high concordance between the regional distribution of BMS-181321 and 2DG-derived radioactivity in this model suggests that images obtained using the technetium agent will be very similar to those obtained using FDG. However, the information content will be different in that the nitroimidazole compounds will provide an image of hypoxic tissue with intact enzymes at the time of injection, whereas the FDG will provide images of total glycolysis.

Future Directions

The development of nuclear medicine–based hypoxic tissue imaging agents has taken about two decades so far. There are invasive electrode-based methods and various efforts to achieve the same aims by magnetic resonance imaging (MRI) or light imaging. Although there have been both academic and commercial efforts in both the SPECT and PET fields for the myocardium, progress has been slow. More progress has been made in the oncology field with a larger clinical base and attempts to change patient management based on the results. Whether this reflects different biochemistry, different technical problems, or different needs is debatable, but what is not debatable is that the measurement of tissue oxygen on a regional basis is a worthwhile goal.

NEWER MYOCARDIAL PERFUSION TRACERS

At the present time, there are four approved myocardial perfusion agents: T1-201, Tc-99m-sestamibi, Tc-99m-teboroxime, and Tc-99m-tetrofosmin. Additionally there are several PET pharmaceuticals available for perfusion imaging, including rubidium-82. The reader is referred to Chapters 4 and 18 for a comprehensive discussion on their biochemical and kinetic characteristics. This chapter describes the newer Tc-99m-based perfusion agents still not approved by the Food and Drug Administration (FDA), and reviews the scientific literature currently available. Myocardial perfusion studies with radionuclides started using rubidium-86 and potassium-43 in the early 1970s. Soon thereafter, with the introduction of Tl-201, these studies became an integral component of the clinical evaluation of patients with known or suspected coronary artery disease, but the search for better myocardial perfusion imaging agents has never ceased. In the 1990s, Tc-99m myocardial perfusion agents became available. Their use increased rapidly and now has surpassed that of Tl-201. All Tc-99m myocardial perfusion agents benefit from physical characteristics of the radioisotope, which allow injection of higher doses, with higher photon energy, resulting in better image quality compared to Tl-201, and chemical characteristics, which permit its incorporation into a wide range of organic as well as inorganic molecules [30]. It has not been clearly established that Tc-99m-based agents will eventually replace Tl-201, since the latter has the highest and most linear myocardial extraction across the full range of achievable flow rates, only surpassed by Tc-99m-teboroxime (Fig. 21.1), and it is also considered the single-photon tracer of choice for the assessment of myocardial viability.

New Perfusion Tracers

The characteristics of the ideal perfusion tracer consist of a high first-pass extraction and stable myocardial retention, with a myocardial distribution in a linear proportion to blood flow over the wide range values experienced in health and disease, and with minimal pulmonary and splanchnic uptake (Fig. 21.1). The tracer should remain within the myocardium sufficient time for data acquisition, followed by a rapid elimination from the body to allow repeat studies under different conditions. Tracers that redistribute in a predictable and reliable manner and allow a clinically viable imaging protocol are also potentially useful. Other desirable properties include a high photon flux at an energy between 100 and 200 keV (which results in optimal images and the possibility of simultaneous

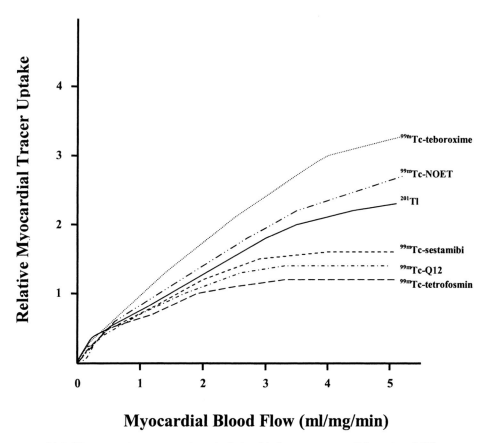

FIGURE 21.1 Diagrammatic representation of relationship between myocardial uptake of different myocardial perfusion agents and myocardial blood flow.

assessment of myocardial perfusion and function), low radiation burden to the patient, easy availability (easy to prepare and based on a generator rather than cyclotron-produced isotope), and low cost [30,31].

Current Tc-99m myocardial perfusion agents can be divided into two broad categories: first, lipophilic cationic agents, consisting of isonitriles (sestamibi), diphosphines (tetrofosmin), and Q complexes (Q3, Q4, Q12, Q63, and Q64); and second, lipophilic neutral agents, consisting of teboroxime and N-NOET [30,31]. Table 21.1 outlines the important properties of major myocardial perfusion agents.

Tc-99m-Q complexes are cationic, nonreducible Tc-99m (III) mixed-ligands. The octahedral coordination sphere of Tc-99m (III) complexes comprises a tetradentate Schiff base ligand and two monodentate phosphine ligands that are situated trans to one another. The cationic Tc-99m (III) core is configured so that it cannot suffer in vivo reduction to a neutral Tc-99m (II) form, which has been shown to wash out of the myocardium. Hence, this resistance to in vivo reduction enables these compounds to be retained in the myocardium for long periods of time [30–36].

Among Q complexes only Tc-99m-Q12 or Tc-99m-furifosmin (trans (1,2-bis (dihydro-2,2,5,5-tetramethyl-3 (2H) furanone-4-methyleneimino) ethane) bis (tris (3-methoxy-1-propyl) phosphine) Tc-99m (III)) has been prepared as an "instant kit," which yields a quality product with a radiochemical purity > 95%. Radiolabeling requires boiling in a water bath for 15 min with sodium pertechnetate. The preparation should be used within 6 hr of reconstitution. Radiochemical purity may be assessed by using a Sep-Pak cartridge [36].

Tc-99m-Q3, the prototypical member of Q complexes (trans (N,N'-ethylene bis acetylacetoneimine) bis (tris (3-methoxy-1-propyl) phosphine) Tc-99m (III)), and Tc-99m-Q12 have identical monophosphine ligands, but Tc-99m-Q3 Schiff base lacks the pair of furanone rings of Tc-99m-Q12. Tc-99m-Q4 derives from Tc-99m-Q3 by the addition of an ester group to the Schiff base ligand, which promotes its myocardial washout [37]. Tc-99m-Q64 shares a common Schiff base with Tc-99m-Q3 but includes different phosphine ligands. Tc-99m-Q63, from its part, shares common phosphine ligands with Tc-99m-Q64, but the Schiff base contains t-butyl groups [36,38].

TABLE 21.1 *Characteristics of Major Myocardial Perfusion Agents*

	Tl-201	Tc-99m-sestamibi	Tc-99m-teboroxime	Tc-99m-tetrofosmin	Tc-99m-Q12	Tc-99m-NOET
Class	Element	Isonitrile	BATO	Diphosphine	Mixed ligand	Nitrido dithiocarbamate
Charge	Cation	Cation	Neutral	Cation	Cation	Neutral
Preparation	Cyclotron	Kit boiling	Kit boiling	Kit room temperature	Kit boiling	Kit boiling
Cellular uptake	Active	Passive	Passive	Passive	Passive	Passive
Average first pass extraction fraction	0.73	0.39	0.88	0.24	0.29	0.55–0.76
Myocardial uptake at rest (%)	4	1	3–4	1.2	1.2-2.2	3
Flow limitation (ml/g/min)	3	2	4.5	1.5	2	>3
Myocardial clearance	$1/2 \sim 6$ hr	Minimal at 5 hr	$t^{1/2} \sim 10$ min	Minimal at 3 hr	Minimal at 3 hr	$t^{1/2} \sim 4$ hr
Redistribution	Significant	Minimal	Significant	None	None	Sig nificant
Blood pool, initial $t^{1/2}$ (min)	5	2.2	<2	<5	1.8	<5
Excretion	Renal	Hepatobiliar +renal	Hepatobiliar	Hepatobiliar +renal	Hepatobiliar +renal	Hepatobiliar +renal
Liver uptake	+	+++	++++	++	+ +	++
Heart-to-liver ratio at exercise (20 min p.i.)	2.6	0.65	Negligible	1.2	1.41.19	
Heart-to-liver ratio at rest (20 min p.i.)	1.4	0.5	Negligible	0.78	0.750.84	
Heart-to-lung ratio at exercise (30 min p.i.)	2.3	2.3	Negligible	5.9	1.71.5	
Start imaging time (min)	<15	>30	<3	15	15	>30
Gated SPECT	+/−	+	−	+	+	+
Viability assessment	Yes	Yes	?	Yes	?	?
Effective dose equivalent	1.6 rem/2 mCi	1.1 rem/30 mCi	1.8 rem/30 mC	i0.8 rem/30 mCi	0.9 rem/30 mCi	0.6 rem/30 mCi

BATO, boronic acid adduct; p.i., postinjection.

Tc-99m-N-NOET is a Tc-99m labeled nitrido dithio-carbamate complex, chemically called bis (N-ethoxy, N-ethyl dithiocarbamato) nitrido Tc-99m (V) and characterized by a Tc-99m-N triple-bond group (Tc $\equiv$ N)$^{2+}$ [39]. It is prepared following a two-step reaction. The first step involves boiling Tc-99m pertechnetate with an acidic solution containing an admixture of trisodium tri (m-sulfophenyl) phosphine and S-methyl N-methyl dithiocarbazoate for 20 min. The second step mixes this intermediate compound that bears the (Tc $\equiv$ N)$^{2+}$ core with dithiocarbamate ligand to obtain neutral Tc-99m-N-NOET. Thin-layer chromatography is used to verify the radiochemical purity of the resultant compound [30].

The cellular uptake of all cationic agents is similar, and according to their lipophilicity in presence of preserved cellular metabolic activity, it is mediated by a nonspecific electrochemical charge-dependent diffusion across the sarcolemma and mitochondrial membranes [30]. Unlike Tl-201, the uptake is unrelated to cation channel transport, and therefore it is not affected by cation channel inhibitors (e.g., ouabain, amiloride, bumetanide, nifedipine) [40,41], but it is inhibited by the metabolic inhibitors iodoacetic acid and 2,4-dinitrophenol, which interfere with potential across the sarcolemma. Studies in isolated mitochondrial preparations show rapid mitochondrial uptake of Tc-99m cationic agents in the presence of oxidative substrate, with release of most of the activity when the mitochondrial uncoupler 2,4-dinitrophenol is added. Mitochondrial uptake of Tc-99m cationic agents requires integrity of their oxidative metabolism, which promotes the potential use of these agents for myocardial viability assessment. Mitochondrial localization of Tc-99m cationic agents seems to be related to a high negative charge (-165 mV) across the mitochondrial membrane compared with other intracellular organelles. Washout of activity from myocytes loaded with Tc-99m cationic agents has been studied by transferring these cells to a Tc-99m free medium. Washout is found to be much slower than the uptake and is biexponential with two compartments (approximately 20% and 80%), having the second compartment long half-lives, resulting in the apparent lack of or minimal redistribution [30].

The cellular uptake of the neutral agents is related to their lipophilicity, regardless of the presence of cellular metabolic activity [30]. Differential centrifugation techniques in homogenized rat heart tissue showed that sarcolemmal proteins are the predominant site of localization of Tc-99m-N-NOET, with no specific concentration in the cytosolic and mitochondrial components [42]. Tc-99m-N-NOET appears to have particular affinity for binding to membrane L-type calcium channels in an energy independent process [43]. Unlike cationic agents, neutral agents show considerable redistribution and differential washout, partly explained by their relatively loose binding to the cell membrane and their interaction with the blood components [44]. Tc-99m-N-NOET has a high myocardial retention in isolated perfused canine and rabbit hearts, and undergoes increased clearance after severe cell membrane damage [45–49].

Preclinical Studies of New Perfusion Agents

First-pass extraction of myocardial perfusion agents is studied in experimental animal models by simultaneous injection of known activities of the perfusion tracer and a nonextractable radiotracer (e.g., I-131 or In-111 labeled albumin), in the left atrium with continuous coronary sinus blood sampling. The ratio of the two agents in coronary sinus blood provides an index of first-pass extraction [30]. Neutral agents have the highest first-pass extraction fraction, which may be related with their lipophilic properties [45] (see Table 21.1).

The relationship between myocardial flow and tracer uptake has been studied in canine models of coronary artery occlusion and pharmacologic-induced hyperemia by simultaneous left atrial injection of the radiotracer and radiolabeled microspheres of adequate size, which are fully extracted in the first encountered capillary bed [30]. Ideally, the perfusion tracer would display a linear correlation with microsphere, with a slope of 1.0 and a 0.0 y-intercept, enhancing, therefore, image contrast between high- and low-flow areas when vasodilation occurs. A tracer displaying a lower slope or a positive y-intercept would, in theory, be less sensitive in discriminating normal from ischemic myocardium [50], overestimating myocardial blood flow in segments with very low flows (positive y-intercept), and underestimating it in segments with very high flow rates (low slope). This may result in a significant underestimation of perfusion abnormalities with mild coronary stenosis, especially when pharmacologic vasodilator stress is used. The threshold at which this so-called roll-of phenomenon occurs varies among different tracers (Fig. 21.1).

Tc-99m-Q complexes

In an open-chest canine model, Tc-99m-Q12 has shown rapid myocardial uptake and blood clearance, which is biexponential, with an initial rapid phase (t^1/$_2$ = 1.8 ± 0.01 min) followed by a late slow phase (t^1/$_2$ = 69 ± 8.2 min). The blood clearance was 1.83 ± 0.13 ml/kg/min, with <5% activity seen in blood 20 min postinjection at rest. Myocardial uptake linearly correlated with myocardial blood flow over a physiologically relevant ranges of flows (from 0.3 to 2 ml/min/g) [33]. The percentage of the injected dose retained in canine myocardium has compared favorably with other cationic perfusion tracers. After initial uptake, myocardial activity remains stable with no evidence of redistribution over a period of the next 4 to 5 hr [33]. The tracer is cleared by both renal and hepatobiliary routes, more rapidly than the other perfusion agents [33].

In an isolated rat heart model, Okada et al. [51] showed that ischemic myocardium (30 min of no-flow followed by 60 min reflow) maintained normal Tc-99m-Q12 kinetics, whereas irreversibly injured myocardium (60 min of no-flow followed by 60 min of reflow) accelerated the early rapid clearance phase. These results support the potential role of Tc-99m-Q12 in the assessment of myocardial viability.

McGoron et al. [41], in isolated rat heart, described ouabain reduction of Tl-201 maximum extraction but not of that of Tc-99m-Q12, suggesting that the cellular extraction mechanisms for these two tracers are different. Furthermore, they observed that net extraction of Tc-99m-Q12 was reduced in the presence of high doses of ouabain while maximum extraction was unchanged, indicating that Tc-99m-Q12 extraction and retention may be metabolism-dependent but controlled by different processes. In addition, late phase washout of Tc-99m-Q12 appeared to be accelerated by high doses of ouabain. However, kinetics of Tc-99m-Q12 were not changed with the human therapeutic levels of ouabain. The same investigators, in a similar model, compared uptake and retention of Tc-99m-Q12, Tc-99m-sestamibi, and Tl-201 during baseline perfusion and during perfusion with a moderately acidotic crystalloid solution containing red cell suspension, to model the acidemia associated with ischemia. They found acidemia to significantly reduce Tl-201 uptake, but not Tc-99m-Q12 or Tc-99m-sestamibi uptake, and, on the other hand, to decrease Tl-201 and Tc-99m-sestamibi retention, with no effect on Tc-99m-Q12 retention, suggesting that Tc-99m-Q12 is less sensitive to metabolic stress than either Tl-201 or Tc-99m-sestamibi.

Tc-99m-Q3, in an open-chest canine model, has shown rapid myocardial uptake and a biexponential blood disappearance, with an initial $t^1/_2$ of 1.7 ± 0.3 min, and a late $t^1/_2$ of 195 ± 26 min. The blood clearance was 0.25 ± 0.07 ml/kg/min. Myocardial uptake linearly correlated with myocardial blood flow from 0 to 6.1 ml/min/g, with no evidence of myocardial redistribution over a 4 hr period [34].

The greatest strength of Q complexes in myocardial perfusion imaging rests with tracers such as Q3, Q63, and Q64, with highly favorable myocardial uptake versus flow relation over a wide range of flows in experimental models [38,50]. This suggests the potential for improved detection of mild coronary artery stenosis compared with the other Tc-99m tracers. The limitations of these promising tracers include lack of a kit allowing instant preparation and the current lack of experience with Tc-99m-Q63 and Q64 in humans.

Tc-99m-N-NOET

Tc-99m-N-NOET exhibits a rapid and moderate-to-high myocardial extraction in animal studies [39,45]. After the initial injection of the radiotracer, its clearance from the blood pool is slower compared with Tl-201 and the cationic agents. Blood activity at 30 min after injection decreased to 20% of the peak activity at 2 min, but thereafter it decreased very slowly with 19% activity at 90 min and 14% at 240 min. Myocardial uptake of the complex in dogs has been found to correlate with the regional coronary blood flow, with little plateauing at high flow rates. Myocardial activity experiences a moderate clearance over time, which results in redistribution, with a faster washout in normoperfused myocardial segments as compared with the hypoperfused ones [45]. Redistribution hastens if flow is normalized after the initial uptake, and it is almost complete within 90 min [45,48,49,52]. Images obtained after intravenous injection of the radiotracer in dogs have shown a high initial lung uptake, which washes out faster than the cardiac uptake, such that the heart/lung ratio increases with time.

Studies performed to determine the cellular binding mechanisms of Tc-99m-N-NOET indicate that the tracer binds to cell membranes [52]. It has also been reported that, in newborn rat cardiomyocytes in primary culture, Tc-99m-N-NOET uptake is reduced in the presence of L-type calcium channel inhibitors (verapamil and diltiazem) and increased in the presence of an activator of these channels, Bay K 8644 [53]. Hence, cellular tracer uptake would involve an energy-independent mechanism with approximately 40% of the tracer binding to L-type calcium channels in an open configuration at a different binding site from that of the calcium channel inhibitors, whereas the remaining 60% of uptake would be distributed nonspecifically in the membranes [54]. Recently, these same investigators reported that, on isolated perfused rat hearts, calcium channel inhibition has no effect on the myocardial uptake and retention of the radiotracer, suggesting that the effect of calcium inhibitors in vitro would not necessarily affect the whole organ or in vivo myocardial uptake [53]. These authors have hypothesized, as Johnson et al., that it is possible that Tc-99m-N-NOET uptake occurs primarily on vascular endothelial cell membranes, where unlike cardiomyocytes and smooth muscle cells, there are no L-type voltage-dependent calcium channels.

The investigations by Johnson et al. [44,46] in isolated nonrecirculating perfused rat hearts showed that tracer retention was very high. There was virtually no myocardial clearance for as long as 1 hr of washout with Krebs-Henseleit buffer perfusion in control hearts or in hearts that underwent 30 or 60 min of no-flow ischemia followed by reperfusion. Only when adding to the perfusate a detergent or cyanide (with induction of severe membrane disruption) [46] or blood elements (erythrocytes with or without albumin) [44], myocardial washout of the tracer was observed. In a separate protocol, these authors observed that erythrocytes incubated with Tc-99m-N-NOET extracted significant amounts of the radiotracer, which was subsequently extracted by the myocardium when these cells were infused into hearts [44]. This was evidence of protein binding as the specific mechanism of uptake for Tc-99m-N-NOET. Thus, Tc-99m-N-NOET appears to have high binding affinity to erythrocytes and albumin and transfers bidirectionally between these and myocardium, providing a residual circulating pool activity, which may represent a potential mechanism of Tc-99m-N-NOET redistribution.

Holly et al. [54] have reported that although Tc-99m-N-NOET is less sensitive than Tl-201 to identify mild ischemic injury, its myocardial extraction and retention are decreased in severe ischemic isolated rabbit hearts (45 min of no-flow) contrasting with the observations of Johnson et al. [46] indicating that the tracer may not be a sensitive marker of cell injury. Similarly, Vanzetto et al. [48] have shown that initial Tc-99m-N-NOET defects on quantitative planar scintigraphy during sustained coronary low flow or transient coronary occlusion in open-chest dogs reflect the myocardial blood flow disparity at the time of tracer injection, and that, in both models, the tracer undergoes significant redistribution over time. The redistribution of Tc-99m-N-NOET and Tl-201 were similar, except in those segments with significant low-flow ischemia (> 80% reduction), in which relative myocardial Tl-201 uptake normalized more than that of Tc-99m-N-NOET. Moreover, Johnson and associates [49] have reported, after their previous study in isolated perfused rat hearts, that resting ischemia caused by moderate-to-severe stenosis (90% reduction in resting flow) in open-chest dogs can be detected with Tc-99m-N-NOET. Redistribution, which principally occurs as a result of differential clearance from normal to ischemic zones, was nearly complete by 90 to 120 min. It is probable that Tc-99m-N-NOET binding affinity to blood elements as well as differences in the amount of reduction of coronary blood flow between different studies, or species-specific differences may account for the discordant data regarding tracer extraction and retention in isolated car-

diac myocytes and different perfused animal hearts. In relation with this, Meleca et al. [50] have studied myocardial flow kinetics of six Tc-99m-labeled perfusion agents (Tc-99m-Q3, Tc-99m-Q4, Tc-99m-Q12, Tc-99m-sestamibi, Tc-99m-tetrofosmin and Tc-99m-N-NOET) and Tl-201 in a canine model of myocardial ischemia. Tl-201 showed the closest to ideal relationship between tracer uptake and myocardial blood flow, followed by Tc-99m-Q3. This relationship was maintained regardless of the normalization technique used.

Although myocardial retention of Tc-99m-N-NOET appears to depend on structural membrane integrity, it may be affected both by the mechanism and by the extension of myocyte injury [56]. The role of Tc-99m-N-NOET in the detection of myocardial viability has been recently analyzed in reperfused acute myocardial infarction in dogs [55]. In this setting, Tc-99m-N-NOET uptake was significantly higher than that of simultaneously administered Tl-201, thus reflecting myocardial blood flow restoration at the time of tracer injection, rather than the extent of myocardial salvage. This feature would differentiate Tc-99m-N-NOET from the other myocardial perfusion imaging agents and may preclude its use to assess the degree of salvage very early after coronary reperfusion. In reperfused, acutely infarcted myocardium, Tc-99m-N-NOET might bind to cell membranes, even if the myocytes are irreversibly injured by ischemia and reperfusion. It is also possible that Tc-99m-N-NOET binds to neutrophils that aggregate in reperfused myocardium, ultimately contributing to the no-reflow phenomenon. These findings do not contradict the decreased Tc-99m-N-NOET uptake observed in patients with chronic myocardial infarction, where fibrosis and scar have substituted myocardiocytes, with no membranes available for Tc-99m-N-NOET binding [57]. Clinically, it remains unknown whether Tc-99m-N-NOET imaging performed 15 to 20 min after injection in the setting of thrombolysis in acute myocardial infarction can prove useful in assessing vessel patency. Likewise, although Tc-99m-N-NOET has been shown to redistribute over time, its role in the detection of hibernating myocardium remains unknown.

Petruzella et al. [52], in a model of vasodilator stress in dogs with critical coronary stenoses, have recently reported that the optimal Tc-99m-N-NOET imaging time may be immediately after the tracer injection for initial poststress images, and as soon as 2 hr later for delayed redistribution images. These data differ from those reported by Ghezzi and colleagues using a canine model of low flow, who did not obtain quality images until 60 min after tracer injection, but they used an early, different Tc-99m-N-NOET formulation [45].

In a study in canine models of coronary ischemia [56], Tc-99m-N-NOET and Tl-201 myocardial uptake was favorable during both adenosine and dobutamine stress, suggesting that both tracers may be superior to Tc-99m-sestamibi for the detection of coronary stenoses during dobutamine stress perfusion imaging. Consequently, dobutamine-induced attenuation of myocardial Tc-99m-sestamibi uptake [57,58] seems a tracer-specific phenomenon rather than a generalized effect.

Clinical Studies of Feasibility of New Perfusion Tracers

Tc-99m-Q complexes

Tc-99m-Q12 has completed Phase III clinical trials [59]. No clinically significant drug-related alterations have been reported (see Color Fig. 21.2 in separate color insert) [32,59,60]. The biexponential clearance of Tc-99m-Q12 shows whole-blood pool peak activity at 2 min (40% of the injected dose), followed by a rapid decay, with <5% of the injected activity at 20 min postinjection. The cardiac activity remains substantially constant after 5 min of injection, and at 1 hr is higher (2.2%) than the other cationic agents, without evidence of redistribution during 5 hr, requiring therefore separate exercise and rest injections for the detection of reversible ischemia [32]. Similarly to other myocardial perfusion agents, heart-to-liver and heart-to-lung ratios improve at stress in relation to those observed at rest, presumably resulting from the higher blood-flow rates encountered during exercise. Excretion is via hepatobiliary and renal systems, faster than that of Tc-99m-sestamibi. After 1 hr liver activity falls to less than myocardial activity, with no improvement in heart-to-liver ratio following the ingestion of a fatty meal. The tracer is maximally concentrated in the gallbladder (peak activity at 35 min postinjection). Urinary excretion at 24 hr (17%–26% of the administered activity) is comparable to that seen with Tc-99m-sestamibi [32,60]. Tc-99m-Q12 appears to combine the relatively high myocardial uptake and prolonged myocardial retention of Tc-99m-sestamibi with the relatively rapid hepatobiliary clearance of Tc-99m-tetrofosmin. Radiation dosimetry studies indicate that critical organs are the gallbladder, large and small intestines, kidneys, heart, and liver [32,60].

Tc-99m-Q3 showed an effective dose equivalent (1.08/30 mCi), comparable to the values of the other Tc-99m labeled myocardial perfusion tracers [35] (see Fig. 21.1). Cardiac activity at 1.5 hr of tracer injection was 1.4% of the injected activity, and the average biologic $t^1/_2$ for the myocardium was 26.4 hr. The highest uptake values of the injected activity were for the gallbladder (5.5%) and the liver (4.1%) at 1.5 hr after stress injection. Overall gastrointestinal tract uptake was 18.8% of the injected activity at 6.5 hr after stress injection. Urinary elimination at 24 hr was 17.1% of the injected activity. The critical organs were the gallbladder and upper large intestine [35].

Gerson and coworkers [60] compared Tc-99m-Q12 rest–stress short protocol with Tl-201 stress-redistribution-reinjection imaging in 20 patients with CAD and 10 patients with a very low likelihood for CAD or without the disease. Sensitivities (Tc-99m-Q12 = 85%, Tl-201 = 90%, p = ns) and normalcy rates (Tc-99m-Q12 = 80%, Tl-201 = 90%, p = ns) between both tracers were comparable, as were sensitivities for the detection of disease in individual coronary arteries. There was excellent agreement between both tracers (89%) for detection of regional perfusion defects, but there was a trend toward detection of reversible ischemia in fewer segments with Tc-99m-Q12 compared with Tl-201. Agreement between tracers for detection of reversibility in abnormal segments was poor. Heart-to-liver and heart-to-lung ratios, both with exercise and rest, were more favorable for Tl-201 compared to Tc-99m-Q12. No relationship between Tc-99m-Q12 heart-to-lung ratios and the number of diseased coronary arteries was found.

Gerson et al. [61] reported, in another study with 27 subjects (19 with and 8 without CAD), comparable diagnostic accuracy with Tc-99m-Q3 rest–stress short protocol and Tl-201 rest-redistribution-reinjection SPECT imaging for overall CAD detection (89% vs 78%, respectively, p = ns) and detection of individual coronary stenoses (83% vs 75%, respectively, p = ns). In addition, there was good interobserver agreement in the interpretation of Tc-99m-Q3 images, comparable to that obtained with Tl-201. The overall agreement between both tracers regarding the presence of a perfusion defect was 86%. Resting heart-to-liver ratios tended to be lower for Tc-99m-Q3 compared to Tl-201, but the differences were not significant. The postexercise mean heart-to-liver ratio was significantly greater for Tl-201 compared to Tc-99m-Q3. Heart-to-lung ratios between the two tracers were similar both at rest and postexercise.

Once more, the same investigators reported similar diagnostic accuracy between Tc-99m-Q12 and Tc-99m-Q3 SPECT rest–stress short protocol imaging in 10 patients with CAD [62]. The presence of disease was correctly determined in all 10 patients with Tc-99m-Q12 and in 9 patients with Tc-99m-Q3. The detection of individual coronary vessel stenosis > 50% was correctly performed in 26/30 vessels (87%) with Tc-99m-Q12 and in 27/30 (90%) vessels with Tc-99m-Q3 (p = ns). In addition, there was good concordance (80%) in the detection of segmental perfusion defects with both tracers. Heart-to-liver ratio was higher for Tc-99m-Q12 compared to Tc-99m-Q3, which, in turn, showed a higher ratio of heart-to-lung activity [62].

Because of the low hepatic activity associated with Tc-99m-Q12, it was believed to be the most favorable Q complex and was selected for testing in Phase III clinical trials. Hendel et al. [59] have reported the results of the largest series to date using Tc-99m-Q12 SPECT imaging in humans. A total of 150 patients with CAD and 39 volunteers with a low likelihood of CAD were studied in seven centers, comparing stress-redistribution Tl-201 imaging with Tc-99m-Q12 stress-rest short protocol. High concordance between both tracers was obtained for detection of myocardial perfusion abnormalities (86%), for the diagnostic categories of normal, ischemia, scar, or mixed defect (67.3%), for the characterization of perfusion defects as reversible or fixed (78% and 86%, respectively), and for detection of CAD within coronary regions considered (range 78%–87.3%), with the highest agreement noted in the anterior wall and the lowest concordance at the apex. Similarly, no systematic differences were noted in regional agreement for ischemia or scar. Patients with a history of a prior myocardial infarction had a high level of concordance between both tracers (94.9%), which substantially decreased in patients without prior infarction (76.1%). Only a reduced level of agreement was observed in women with a fixed perfusion defect (72.5%) when compared with the level of agreement in men with this same finding (86.4%), probably related to differences in the degree of soft tissue attenuation between the two tracers. Perfusion studies in all volunteers yielded a normalcy rate of 100%. Hence, the levels of agreement between Tc-99m-Q12 and Tl-201 noted in this study are similar to those noted for other Tc-99m-based perfusion agents [59].

Although heart-to-lung ratio of Tc-99m-Q12 continues to improve from 15 min to 50 min after injection [60], 15 min images have resulted in sufficient diagnostic quality [32,59,60]. Subjective comparison of the image quality, between Tc-99m-Q12 and Tl-201 studies has given better results for Tc-99m-Q12 images more frequently (34% vs 25%), which may result in more uniform perfusion image interpretation. Naruse et al. [63] quantitatively compared normal exercise planar and SPECT data files obtained with Tl-201, Tc-99m-sestamibi, Tc-99m-tetrofosmin, and Tc-99m-Q12. They found differences between normal planar data files between Tl-201 and Tc-99m-tracers, and among various Tc-99m-tracers, but not between normal SPECT data files, probably as a result of the differential effect of extracardiac radiopharmaceutical accumulation.

First attempts to define the role of Tc-99m-Q12 in identifying viable myocardium have recently been reported by Cuocolo et al. [64]. They compared rest-redistribution Tl-201 with rest Tc-99m-Q12 quantitative SPECT imaging in 21 patients with chronic myocardial infarction and left ventricular dysfunction. Concordance in the detection of viable myocardium between both techniques was observed in 82% of hypokinetic regions and in 83% of akinetic or dyskinetic regions, suggesting that both of them may provide similar information in the detection of myocardial viability.

Thus far, there are no data regarding the use of Tc-99m-Q12 in patient triage in the setting of acute coronary syndromes and nondiagnostic electrocardiograms, but it seems that it may be useful, as no myocardial redistribution of the radiotracer has been described after several hours. It is also probable that pharmacologic stress perfusion imaging with Tc-99m-Q12 would provide comparable results as obtained with exercise, since the physical characteristics do not suggest the potential for any problems unique to Tc-99m-Q12.

Gerson et al. [37] published comparative results of a Phase I study with Tc-99m-Q4 stress-delayed-reinjection and Tl-201 stress-reinjection SPECT imaging in 12 subjects (6 with CAD and 6 normal volunteers). No clinically significant drug-related alterations were reported; the effective dose equivalent was 1.54/30 mCi and the critical organs were the gallbladder and large intestine. Heart-to-liver and heart-to-lung activity ratios remained constant after tracer injection Tc-99m-Q4 imaging yielded perfusion defects in the distribution of most angiographically documented coronary artery stenoses and was associated with uniform myocardial distribution in normal volunteers. Overall agreement between Tc-99m-Q4 and Tl-201 for detection of segmental myocardial perfusion defects was 80%. In both normals and subjects with CAD, significant global washout of TC-99m-Q4 was observed over 4 hr. Moreover, in 5 subjects with CAD the ischemic to normal zone count ratio significantly increased at 4 hr postexercise, suggesting occurrence of differential washout. Nevertheless, image quality was not optimal for clinical testing, and demonstration of perfusion defect reversibility with comparable frequency to that observed with Tl-201 stress-reinjection required separate injections of Tc-99m-Q4, at peak stress and at rest.

Tc-99m-N-NOET

Early trials with Tc-99m-N-NOET have already started in Europe [47,65] but experience is very limited. Biodistribution, safety, and dosimetry have been studied in 10 healthy volunteers (5 at rest and 5 during exercise). Safety parameters measured 48 hr after injection revealed no clinically significant changes. Although initial lung uptake (20% of injected activity at rest and 10% after exercise) was higher than myocardial uptake, on average, biologic $t^{1}/_{2}$ was shorter (51–77 min), and it was possible to image the heart properly at 30–45 min from tracer injection. This delay in the optimum imaging time may pose a problem in certain clinical cases in which rapid redistribution would decrease the ability to identify the presence or degree of ischemia, although the first clinical study using Tc-99m-N-NOET [47] did not reveal the existence of rapid redistribution phenomenon. The blood clearance was as rapid as in all myocardial perfusion-imaging agents, with 95% clearing within 5 min. However, whole-body clearance was slow, comparable with that of Tl-201, but much slower than Tc-99m-sestamibi and Tc-99m-tetrofosmin, with an excretion equally divided between hepatobiliary and renal paths. As with all myocardial perfusion tracers, better heart-to-liver ratios were observed during exercise than when administered at rest. Radiation dosimetry calculations indicated that the upper large intestine, kidneys, liver, and heart were the organs receiving the highest absorbed dose.

The diagnostic concordance in a preliminary clinical trial that compared Tl-201 stress-redistribution-reinjection with Tc-99m-N-NOET stress-delayed (2, 4, and 6 hr postinjection) and rest-delayed (4 hr postinjection) SPECT imaging in 25 subjects (19 with and 6 without CAD) [47] was 88%, with a sensitivity of 74% for Tc-99m-N-NOET and 68% for Tl-201 (p = ns), and specificity of 100% for both tracers. The agreement between these tracers for disease in individual coronary arteries was 96%, with identical sensitivity and specificity for the detection of diseases vessels. Although the severity of defects was lower with Tc-99m-N-NOET than with Tl-201, concordance between both tracers for segmental analysis in stress images was 94%, and concordance for patient classification in the 4 hr images was observed in 21/23 patients. Additionally, rest redistribution of Tc-99m-N-NOET was noted in 4/7 patients. Image quality was "good" in 19/25 patients for Tc-99m-N-NOET, and 24/25 for Tl-201. Despite 30 min imaging delay following Tc-99m-N-NOET administration, pulmonary activity remained relatively high in some patients, and it seemed to be more persistent at rest than during exercise. Therefore, in spite of lower image quality with Tc-99m-N-NOET, diagnostic accuracy for detection of CAD was comparable for both tracers.

Future Directions

To date, clinical experience with newer Tc-99m-based perfusion agents is limited, although early studies suggest that when used in conjunction with exercise testing, Tc-99m-Q12 and Tc-99m-N-NOET provide comparable diagnostic accuracy to that obtained with exercise testing using Tl-201. More studies are needed to determine whether these new agents are different or better than the other Tc-99m agents available now, or if they simply provide an alternative to them. Moreover, there remains a general need for myocardial perfusion tracers with improved myocardial extraction and improved tracer kinetics. Therefore, future research should focus on the development of myocardial flow tracers with the ideal characteristics previously mentioned.

Newer perfusion agents should be developed that improve our ability to accomplish absolute quantitation and allow better detection of the presence and extent of CAD. Development of attenuation and scatter correction would further eliminate some of the current limitations of myocardial perfusion imaging. In the meanwhile, the outstanding tracer uptake versus blood flow of Tc-99m-Q3, Tc-99m-Q63, Tc-99m-Q64, and Tc-99m-N-NOET in animal studies suggests improved detection of mild coronary artery stenosis compared with the other Tc-99m tracers in humans, but further clinical investigations are needed.

It is important to realize that Tc-99m-N-NOET is neither a Tc-99m labeled version of Tl-201 nor behaves like Tc-99m cationic agents; therefore, efforts should be directed to find its particular use, rather than compete for an application that already exists. In this setting, studies comparing radionuclide imaging using Tc-99m-N-NOET with other noninvasive techniques, such as contrast echocardiography and contrast MRI imaging, for accurate assessment of the degree of reflow after reperfusion in acute myocardial infarction appear warranted. Further analysis of myocardial clearance kinetics of Tc-99m-N-NOET may render possible quantitative assessment of regional myocardial blood flow in humans using dynamic SPECT [66].

IMAGING OF MYOCARDIAL NECROSIS

Myocardial necrosis plays an important role in the pathogenesis of various cardiovascular disorders and can result from different insults on the myocardium; therefore, its noninvasive identification and localization may help in the diagnosis of these disorders, as well as in prognostication and answer of treatment response.

First attempts for direct visualization of the area of myocardial necrosis were confined to initial recognition of myocardial infarction (MI) in patients with chest pain. This diagnosis may be difficult despite the number of diagnostic procedures available, with only 2.1% of patients with acute MI discharged from the emergency department [67], but increasing the percentage of patients with acute chest pain who are unnecessarily hospitalized. On the one hand, although most patients with acute MI present with electrocardiogram (ECG) abnormalities, correlation of serial ECG changes with pathological findings indicates that the accuracy of diagnosis by this method is <80% [68]. Limitations include the size and specific location of infarction, previous MI, conduction disturbances, acute pericarditis, electrolyte abnormalities, and cardioactive drugs. On the other hand, biochemical markers of myocardial injury may be missed in very early presenting patients after the onset of symptoms. Likewise, the sensitivity for acute MI of single values on these biomarkers is limited, as is its determination in the assessment of the extent of MI in patients following cardiac resuscitation, thrombolysis, bypass surgery, or coronary angioplasty, and in the assessment of those MIs resulting of intermittent coronary occlusion. Moreover, although detectable increases in the biomarkers of myocardial injury are indicative of damage to the myocardium, they are not synonymous with an ischemic mechanism of damage. Contrarily, direct depiction of myocardial necrosis with infarct-avid agents may provide this additional information when tracer uptake is localized to a specific coronary territory. Infarct-avid imaging agents would have an additional clinical role in measuring infarct size, since clinical data have demonstrated the importance of final infarct size as a major determinant of subsequent patient survival and quality of life. The study of myocardial necrosis with gamma imaging agents has gone beyond the detection of MI, and attempts have been made to diagnose other cardiovascular disorders associated with cardiac cell death such as heart transplant rejection and myocarditis.

Infarct-Avid Agents and Their Unique Characteristics

Imaging of myocardial necrosis with infarct-avid agents started with the use of Tc-99m-tetracycline. Shortly thereafter the utility of imaging acute MI with Tc-99m-pyrophosphate was reported. In the late 1970s, imaging of myocardial necrosis with myosin-specific labeled antibody was described. Detailed discussion of Tc-99m-pyrophosphate is not appropriate in this chapter on

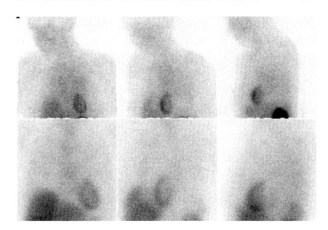

FIGURE 21.3 Imaging of myocardial necrosis. Anterior and 45°–70° LAO images of a patient with extensive anteroseptal and apical myocardial infarction showing matched uptake of ^{99m}Tc-glucarate (upper row) and ^{111}In-antimyosin (lower row) in these regions. Septal uptake of both tracers shines through into inferior wall in the anterior view.

newer developments in nuclear cardiology, but antimyosin scintigraphy requires a detailed description considering the limited period of time that this technique has been commercially available in the United States. Recently, Tc-99m-glucarate has been shown to identify early cell death, although it is still in its initial clinical trial stages.

Tc-99m-pyrophosphate is a polyphosphate derivative, first introduced for bone scanning. The mechanisms by which radiophosphates are bound to the necrotic myocardium are not fully understood, but factors determining their accumulation in MI comprise the presence of residual blood flow or the redevelopment of blood flow to the infarcted region, predominantly targeting the sequestered calcium in the infarcted or severely injured myocardium [69]. Thus, this process can take place within a few hours of the acute event if the infarct-related artery is patent, or later (≥12 hr) if the vessel remains occluded. Maximum infarct uptake occurs 24–72 hr later, and usually lasts for 6–10 days [69]. Therefore, in the early phase of acute MI, Tc-99m-pyrophosphate imaging is more appropriate for confirmation of successful thrombolytic therapy (Fig. 21.3).

Initially, imaging with In-111 labeled murine monoclonal antimyosin Fab antibody fragments (R11D10-Fab) was described as an alternative to Tc-99m-pyrophosphate infarct-avid scintigraphy [70,71]. In-111-antimyosin targets specifically and with high affinity the intracellular heavy chain of cardiac myosin exposed to extracellular fluid by loss of cell membrane integrity. The small dimensions of antimyosin Fab

(65 × 35 Å, molecular weight of 30,000 d) enable it to enter the myocyte membrane gaps created either by ischemia or direct damage via complementing the cell membrane or inflammatory mediators that may subsequently result in myocyte necrosis. The use of Fab fragments has less immunogenicity and a more favorable biodistribution than the whole antibody. Labeling with In-111 is done by transchelation using a bifunctional chelating agent, diethyleneaminopenta-acetic acid (DTPA).

Acute MI is the field where the greatest experience has been achieved, with sufficient experimental and clinical evidence demonstrating specific In-111 antimyosin targeting of necrotic myocardial cells. Sensitivity comparisons between Tc-99m-pyrophosphate and In-111-antimyosin imaging in the diagnosis of acute MI have generally provided similar results (87%–98% for Q wave MI, and 78%–84% for non-Q wave MI) [69], the latter being more specific (85%–96%) [69,72]. False positive results may be obtained when imaging < 24 hr after tracer injection, due to persisting blood pool activity. In contrast to Tc-99m-pyrophosphate, In-111-antimyosin uptake is maximum in areas with severe flow impairment [69]. This difference may be explained considering that antimyosin antibodies remain in the plasma much longer than pyrophosphate does, which is rapidly cleared from the blood due to bone uptake and renal clearance. Thus, antimyosin would have a greater opportunity to interact with necrotic tissue. However In-111-antimyosin uptake is more intense in MI with reperfusion than in MI with persistent coronary occlusion. The time interval between tracer administration and effective visualization of the target necrotic myocardial region has been a major concern in potential clinical applicability of the technique. In reperfused canine models, the experimental MI could be visualized relatively soon after the administration of In-111-antimyosin, although visualization of nonreperfused infarcts took longer. The delay in imaging results from long circulation half-life of the antibody (4–6 hr), which precludes development of optimum target-to-background ratio early after antibody administration. Therefore, a genetically engineered sFv of the monoclonal antimyosin antibody was developed in an attempt to reduce the residence time of the antibody in blood [73]. The antimyosin sFv labeled with Tc-99m enabled earlier visualization of cute reperfused canine MI. However, sFv (protein with a molecular weight of ~20,000 d) may not be able to rapidly localize in sufficiently high concentration in nonreperfused infarcts.

The uptake of In-111-antimyosin by infarcted myocardium may persist for as long as 9 months after an acute event [74], although the intensity of uptake tends to decrease with time. Slow clearance of such a large and insoluble molecule as myosin by granulocytes may account for this persistent uptake. Thus, the use of In-111-antimyosin scintigraphy to differentiate acute from old myocardial injury occurring within 1 year should be interpreted using all available clinical information.

In-111-antimyosin images reflect the normal biodistribution of the Fab protein fragment, with renal, hepatic, splenic, and bone marrow uptake. When there is myocardial damage, focal or diffuse cardiac uptake is apparent, which can be semiquantified by calculating heart-to-lung count density ratio from dividing average counts per pixel in the cardiac region of interest by average counts per pixel in an area of interest drawn on the lungs on the anterior view.

The high sensitivity and specificity of In-111-antimyosin for the detection of necrotic myocardium in ischemic heart disease led to attempts to investigate its role in the diagnosis of various cardiac disorders, also characterized by myocyte necrosis, other than from MI.

In the assessment of heart transplant rejection, comparison of In-111-antimyosin studies with those of endomyocardial biopsy reveals that (1) uptake correlates directly with biopsy score; (2) sensitivity of In-111-antimyosin to detect rejection approximates 100%; and (3) positive scans often coexist with normal biopsies; this discrepancy likely representing biopsy sampling errors [75]. Consequently, In-111-antimyosin imaging may provide the most sensitive means to detect rejection [76]. Nevertheless, this exquisite sensitivity precludes its use as the only diagnostic test for patient management during the first year after transplantation (80% of patients show a positive result), when endomyocardial biopsies are mandatory. After the first year of surgery, In-111-antimyosin studies have revealed that rejection is seldom detected in patients with normal scans. On the contrary, when abnormal uptake is noted, rejection appears at some stage during follow-up, with an increased probability of detecting rejection at biopsy with increasing intensities of the antibody uptake. Thus, at this time, patients can be withdrawn from biopsy, with individual management adjusted on the basis of the In-111-antimyosin study. Anyway, the combination of In-111-antimyosin studies with biopsies during the first trimester after the operation provides additional information to that contained solely in biopsies. A decrease of antibody uptake during this early period appears to be related to absence of severe rejection-related complications during the first year, whereas a persistent In-111-antimyosin uptake alerts against the presence of such complications during that interval [75]. Additionally, the sensitivity and noninvasiveness of In-111-antimyosin imaging allows its use as a research tool in the assessment of the efficacy of new immunosuppressive regimens or drugs.

Doxorubicin functional impairment is a consequence of myocardial cell damage caused by administration of the drug. In-111-antimyosin may provide a tool for improved patient management because it provides early detection of cell damage before functional impairment occurs, relates to the cumulative dose, and permits early identification of patients at risk for significant cardiotoxicity [78].

Since myocardial cell damage is a basic component of myocarditis, In-111-antimyosin scintigraphy is a useful screening method in the initial evaluation of patients with heart failure when myocarditis is clinically suspected [79]. The high predictive value of a negative scan (> 92%) rules out the presence of myocardial necrosis and usually obviates the need for endomyocardial biopsy [79,80]. In-111-antimyosin has also been successfully used to recognize myocarditis in patients with unexplained recent onset of dilated cardiomyopathy, unexplained life-threatening ventricular tachyarrhythmias, or chest pain mimicking acute MI [80,81].

Although the clinical relevance of active myocardial cell damage in the context of dilated cardiomyopathies is still uncertain, studies performed with In-111-antimyosin have confirmed the high prevalence of dilated cardiomyopathy. One study in 17 patients with chronic idiopathic dilated cardiomyopathy showed positive In-111-antimyosin images in 71% of the patients. These results could reflect the presence of ongoing myocyte lesion [82]. The antibody uptake was not due to active inflammation (as evaluated through cardiac explants) [83] or heart failure (patients with stable coronary disease and similar degrees of left ventricular dilation and dysfunction did not show uptake) [82]. Therefore, cell damage appears to be associated with a different yet undefined cause, with impact on long-term survival (intense antibody uptake was associated with increased mortality or need for heart transplantation). In alcoholic patients, uptake depends on alcoholic consumption [84]. A reduction of antibody uptake was observed after alcohol abstention, accompanied by an increase in ejection fraction [84]. In-111-antimyosin imaging may also show myocardial damage in HIV-infected patients [85], and in hypertrophic cardiomyopathy, particularly in the dilated phases of the evolution [86].

Antimyosin-Fab-DTPA (0.5 mg, labeled with 74 MBq of In-111 chloride) has been proved to be safe, well-tolerated, and with no hypersensitive reactions. There has been reported only one patient with a low-titer positive human antimurine antibody (HAMA) response from five clinical studies following single and repeat injections of the antibody, with a total number of 914 evaluable sets of HAMA samples. No adverse events were reported in this patient [87]. In-111-antimyosin has been approved by the FDA for commercial marketing, although approved indication restrains its use only to ischemic heart disease. Unfortunately, it is not commercially available.

Preclinical Studies of Tc-99m-Glucarate Uptake

Although both Tc-99m-pyrophosphate and IN-111-antimyosin are effective in localizing MI, the clinical value of an infarct-avid agent resides in the early identification of the occurrence of the acute event by allowing the early use of interventions for myocardial salvage. To fulfill this role, an infarct-avid imaging tracer should reach the infarct area rapidly and in high concentration despite the persistently occluded status of the coronary artery; clear rapidly from the circulation to allow identification of the target area of infarction, and possess high avidity for the necrotic myocardial tissue to attain a high target-to-background ratio for optimal imaging. Neither Tc-99m-pyrophosphate nor In-111-antimyosin accomplish all of these ideal characteristics for an infarct imaging agent, but they may be fitted by Tc-99m-glucarate.

Glucaric acid is a six-carbon dicarboxylic acid sugar, natural endogenous end-catabolite of UDP-glucose, excreted principally via the urinary system [88]. It can be labeled with Tc-99m, and it was initially used as a transchelator of Tc-99m for radiolabeling Fab' antibody fragments, being observed that it localized in canine reperfused MI very quickly after intravenous administration.

Preliminary results assessing infarct size by simultaneus administration of In-111-antimyosin and Tc-99m-glucarate suggested that the latter might identify both areas of reversible and irreversible myocardial injury [89]. Nevertheless, subsequent studies suggested that Tc-99m-glucarate does not accumulate in ischemic or old necrotic tissues. Orlandi et al. [88], studying canine models of myocardial ischemia and infarct reported a high affinity for Tc-99m-glucarate uptake in necrotic myocardial tissue for several days following the injury, with no uptake in ischemic but viable myocardium. Uptake of Tc-99m-glucarate in the necrotic tissue occurred as early as 3 hr of reperfusion after 90 min of LAD coronary artery occlusion, and was significantly higher at 48 hr; but not uptake was seen at 10 days. Yaoita et al. [90] compared myocardial distribution of Tc-99m-glucarate and H-3-deoxyglucose in a rabbit model of left circumflex artery (LCX) marginal artery occlusion (prolonged vs. repetitive). Tc-99m-glucarate was mainly observed in the most severely injured zones, while

H-3-deoxyglucose concentrated in tissue with injury ranging from mild ischemia to transmural infarction. Although mildly damaged myocardium showed Tc-99m-glucarate uptake, only severe myocardial injury could be visualized by in vivo imaging at 1 hr after intravenous administration. Tc-99m-glucarate uptake occurred within 6 hr after coronary occlusion. The study by Ohtani and colleagues [91] in a rat model of 3 hr of persistent LAD coronary artery ligation showed that 17/21 rats with histologic evidence of MI had significant Tc-99m-glucarate uptake within 1 hr of injection. None of the 10 rats without histologic evidence of MI had Tc-99m-glucarate uptake. There was no Tc-99m-glucarate uptake when the radiotracer was reinjected 72 hr after the coronary occlusion. Narula et al. [92] did not observe Tc-99m-glucarate uptake in ischemic rabbit heart model. Tc-99m-glucarate cleared rapidly from circulation (elimination $t^{1}/_{2} = 36$ min). Infarcts were visualized within 10 min in reperfused and within 30 to 60 min in nonreperfused LAD coronary territories after tracer injection. Tc-99m-glucarate uptake in reperfused and nonreperfused infarct centers was 28 and 12 times greater, respectively, than that in normal myocardium. A direct correlation in the localization between Tc-99m-glucarate and In-111-antimyosin was observed. Target-to-nontarget ratios of Tc-99m-glucarate were higher than the corresponding of In-111-antimyosin in the same tissue samples and at the same time period. Tc-99m-glucarate localized predominantly in the nuclear fraction of the infarct, with lesser extents in the mitochondrial and cytoplasmic fractions. The development of a target-to-background ratio that enabled early detectability of MI resulted from the rapid blood clearance and high avidity of Tc-99m-glucarate for the acutely necrotic myocardial tissue.

Beanlands and coworkers have described higher accumulation and retention of Tc-99m-glucarate in myocardial necrosis in comparison to control and postischemic myocardial injury in an isolated perfused rat heart model [93]. Khaw et al., for their part, have reported a very good correlation between Tc-99m-glucarate and In-111-antimyosin uptake in reperfused canine MI, with an insignificant uptake of the former by viable embryonic rat cardiocytes in vitro cell culture studies [94].

In a preliminary cell culture study directed to determine the specificity of Tc-99m-glucarate for necrotic and apoptotic cell death, Blankenberg et al. [95] found a greater than 25-fold increase in the uptake of Tc-99m-glucarate in necrotic (heated at 60°C) cell cultures as compared with controls, whereas apoptotic cell cultures (serum deprived or IgM α-Fas antibody treated) demonstrated no significant increase in Tc-99m-glucarate as compared with controls, even in the late stages of apoptosis (with irreversible membrane damage).

The proposed mechanism of Tc-99m-glucarate localization in the infarcted myocardium is due to its avidity for the positively charged histones within disintegrated nuclei and reduced subcellular organelles proteins in necrotic myocytes [92,94]. Although the sugar transporter system might play a role in myocardial uptake of Tc-99m-glucarate, it is negligible under nonischemic conditions, when fatty acids are the metabolic substrate. Under ischemia, there may be a greater Tc-99m-glucarate uptake, but it does not achieve sufficient concentration for in vivo detection by gamma imaging [94]. In contrast, when acute myocardial necrosis occurs, the sarcolemmal breaches permit entry of Tc-99m-glucarate into the infarcted zone through collateral circulation and/or diffusion.

Tc-99m-glucarate distribution in the central necrotic zone closely parallels the distribution of In-111-antimyosin [92,94], contrarily to Tc-99m-pyrophosphate, which principally accumulates peripherally to the necrosis, where residual blood flow is highest. The flow dependence of Tc-99m-pyrophosphate concentration and the delayed blood pool clearance of In-111-antimyosin explain their limited clinical application during the early phase of acute MI. Tc-99m-glucarate by comparison, because of its small molecular size (molecular weight of 210 d), appears to have less dependence on residual myocardial blood flow for tracer delivery, and a rapid uptake into either reperfused or nonreperfused necrotic myocardium [92,94], with a relative rapid blood flow clearance. However, the positivity of Tc-99m-glucarate for MI persists only during the acute stages. Whether positivity for nonreperfused MI lasts longer than reperfused MI must await additional study.

Clinical Studies of Tc-99m-Glucarate Imaging

Recent preliminary reports in a small number of patients suggest that Tc-99m-glucarate administration within the first hours after onset of AMI symptoms allows very early noninvasive diagnosis of acute MI (Fig. 21.3). Mariani et al. [96] studied 28 patients with suspected acute MI, imaging at about 3 hr after tracer injection. Lesion detection was in relation to the elapsed time from onset of symptoms and Tc-99m-glucarate administration. All 14 patients with acute MI who were injected within 9 hr of onset of chest pain had positive scans, even if persistent occlusion was present (2 patients did not receive recombinant tissue plasminogen activator therapy, although activation of intrinsic thrombolysis by heparin administration could not be rule out). Nine of the remaining 14 patients with negative scans had acute MI, but were injected > 9 hr after onset of chest pain. The remaining 5 patients were finally diagnosed with unstable angina (3 injected < 9 hr and 2 injected > 9 hr after onset of chest pain). Furthermore, none of the 6 patients with initial positive scans who were reinjected with Tc-99m-glucarate 4–6 weeks after the acute scanning showed tracer uptake. Tc-99m-glucarate retention at the site of the infarction remained 24 hr after tracer injection in 2 patients whose scans were obtained at this time. Results of a preliminary study comparing Tc-99m-glucarate and In-111-antimyosin myocardial uptake in 5 patients with acute MI and in 5 patients with heart disorders associated with diffuse ongoing myocardial damage showed no Tc-99m-glucarate uptake in the latter group, suggesting that either very acute occurrence of necrosis is a prerequisite for Tc-99m-glucarate uptake or that Tc-99m-glucarate uptake in positively charged histones in disintegrating nuclei that are lost early after necrosis supports the former explanation [97].

Unlike Tc-99m-pyrophosphate, Tc-99m-glucarate has minimal bone uptake and no resultant interference with cardiac visualization due to overlying ribs [98]. In comparison to In-111-antimyosin, Tc-99m-glucarate imaging has no interference by hepatic activity for the detection of possible myocardial activity adjacent to the liver in the inferior myocardial wall.

The major strengths of Tc-99m-glucarate include its rapid blood pool clearance, a good target-to-background ratio, lack of toxicity or antigenicity, and sensitivity and specificity for detection of early irreversible myocyte injury. However, since Tc-99m-glucarate predominantly targets the positively charged histones, which disintegrate fairly rapidly, the clinical window for Tc-99m-glucarate uptake appears to be limited to 9 hr after the onset of AMI. This time window may allow differentiation of acute from recent MI [96,97]. The proposed mechanism of Tc-99m-glucarate localization in the infarcted myocardium would also explain why it does not apparently occur in diffuse ongoing myocardial damage [97].

Future Directions

Development of noninvasive tests for detection of myocardial necrosis is of paramount importance. Loss of contractile myocardial mass is directly related to prognostic outcomes in numerous cardiac disorders. Loss of sarcolemmal integrity exposes different intracellular components to the extracellular milieu being susceptible of specific targeting. Some examples are heavy-chain human cardiac myosin and histones in disintegrating nuclei. On the other hand, attempts to image the total spectrum of myocardial damage must also be directed toward programmed cell death or apoptosis detection. Apoptosis differs from cellular necrosis, playing an important role in various cardiovascular disorders. Its detection will bring new light in the pathogenesis of these diseases.

Tc-99m-glucarate is not available in the United States or Europe at present, and prospective human trials in the broad spectrum of patients with suspected ischemic syndromes are needed to further document its safety and efficacy. If early Tc-99m-glucarate uptake in acute MI with persistently occluded infarct related coronary artery is confirmed in clinical studies, it may help to direct the use of thrombolytic therapy in patients presenting with equivocal diagnosis, as well as to differentiate acute from recent infarcts.

The advent of new agents to assess acute myocardial necrosis has to come along with the installation of chest pain units in medical centers to improve the triage of patients presenting to the emergency department with ongoing or recent acute chest pain and normal or nondiagnostic resting ECG. There is also a need to improve the spatial resolution of imaging devices so that it becomes possible to detect small subendocardial infarctions, as well as to quantify the infarct size with confidence, which will enhance the evaluation of dysfunctional myocardial states associated with depressed myocardial flow, that is, differentiation between hibernating myocardium and nontransmural infarction.

IMAGING OF MYOCARDIAL APOPTOSIS

Cell death, long considered an undesirable phenomenon, is now appreciated as an integral part of the life of the organism. Survival depends on the orderly and timely death of cells that have completed their useful function(s). Apoptosis, one of the major mechanisms nature has developed for the cells to exit, is programmed cell death. Apoptosis is an orderly, complex series of events that permits the cell to die without inducing an inflammatory response. In this regard, apoptosis is markedly different from necrosis, which is a disorderly process that results in local inflammation. Necrosis is not part of normal homeostasis, and is found only in tissues or organs subjected to nonphysiological insults. The hallmark of necrotic cell death is the early loss of cell membrane integrity followed by cell swelling and chromatin flocculation and the uncontrolled spillage of intracellular contents leading to inflammation. Necrotic cell death occurs in response to a sudden severe nonphysiologic environmental change in which the normal energy-dependent functions of a cell, including apoptosis, cannot occur. On the other hand, *apoptosis* [99] has been described as a controlled deletion of cells by an active, genetically programmed phenomenon, that plays a complementary but opposite role to mitosis or cellular proliferation. Apoptosis is an obligatory component of embryogenesis (such as organ development), physiologic or senescent regression (such as thymic involution, prostatic regression) of tissues, regulation of physiologic processes (such as immune response), and a cause of cell death in viral illness. Either excessive apoptosis or lack of appropriate apoptosis plays a role in many diseases. Loss of normal apoptosis results in excessive cellular proliferation in oncologic and autoimmune diseases, whereas exaggerated apoptosis is likely related to progressive loss of functioning myocytes or neuronal cells in chronic disorders such as CHF or Alzheimer's disease [100–105].

The onset of apoptotic process is preceded by an *initiation* phase [106]. The duration of this initiation phase depends on cell type, the trigger type, and the intensity and exposure time of the trigger. Regardless of the specific induction pathway, a common proteolytic cascade involving the family of cysteine proteases, recently renamed as *caspases* (cysteine aspartic acid-specific proteases), is activated [107]. There are 13 well-characterized members of the caspase family in mammals known as caspases 1 through 13. Once caspases are activated, the cell enters the *execution* phase of apoptosis. Once committed to apoptosis, the cell undergoes a stereotyped series of changes, wherein initial cytoplasmic and nuclear chromatin condensation is followed by the breakup of the cell into a number of membrane-bound fragments called *apoptotic bodies*. These fragmented cellular masses are ingested and degraded by adjacent cells and phagocytes.

Pathogenetic Basis of Apoptosis Imaging

For noninvasive radionuclide imaging, it is mandatory to target extracellular surface alterations. Cell membrane changes predominantly comprise development of evaginations. These changes are brought about by disorderly distribution of phospholipids in the lipid bilayer and cytoskeletal architectural alterations [108]. Some of these phospholipid changes can be tracked for noninvasive identification of apoptosis.

Exposure of phosphatidylserine (PS) on the cell surface constitutes the most important cell membrane alteration during apoptosis [109–112]. PS is a simple constitutive plasma membrane anionic phospholipid found in abundance within the lipid bilayer. It is actively restricted to the inner leaflet of the lipid bilayer by an energy-dependent enzyme called translocase. PS is virtually absent on the surface of normal cells. Translocase in concert with a second ATP-dependent enzyme—floppase—which actively pumps cationic phospholipids such as phosphatidylcholine (PC) and sphingomyelin (SM) to the outer leaflet to the lipid bilayer, maintains an asymmetric distribution of anionic and cationic phospholipids across the plasma membrane.

During apoptosis, the increase in intracellular calcium deactivates translocase and floppase enzymes and also activates the scramblase enzyme. Scramblase facilitates bidirectional movement of phospholipids within the lipid bilayer. These events all serve to evenly redistribute PS, PC, and SM across the lipid bilayer, abolishing normal membrane phospholipid asymmetry. After exposure of PS on the cell surface, there is a generalized, orderly, irreversible breakdown of cellular elements. The cytoskeleton (actin filaments) and nuclear matrix (nuclear laminar proteins that rigidly support chromatin organization) are actively attacked by the proteolytic system. Protein kinase c, an enzyme involved in the assembly of microfilaments needed to form membrane blebs and ultimately apoptotic bodies, is activated. The sum of these processes results in the blebbing of the plasma membrane, condensation of nuclear chromatin with simultaneous internucleosomal fragmentation of nuclear DNA. The cell breaks up into numerous, membrane-bound, ultrastructurally well-preserved apoptotic bodies. The apoptotic bodies are identified by PS receptors on macrophages and the apoptotic cells are removed without spilling intracellular contents or inducing an inflammatory reaction [113].

The ubiquitous exposure of PS during apoptosis makes it an attractive target for radiopharmaceutical imaging. Annexin V, an endogenous human protein with a molecular weight of 35 kDa, has a high affinity (kd = 7 nM) for PS bound to the cell membrane [114,115]. Human annexin V has recently been produced by expression in Escherichia coli [116]; this material retains membrane bound PS binding activity equivalent to that of native annexin V. Annexin V can be conveniently radiolabeled with Tc-99m [117,118]. Three approaches have been tested to couple technetium to the protein. First, direct technetium reduction in a mixture containing stannous ion and protein at a pH of 6; second, precoupling annexin V to N2S2 with subsequent reduction of technetium to label the protein; and precoupling with HYNIC with subsequent incubation of a stannous tricine technetium solution to achieve protein labeling. Each of these approaches is associated with a different biodistribution. Tc-99m-annexin made by direct coupling has a higher concentration in the liver and spleen, and shorter circulating half-time than that made by either the N2S2 or HYNIC techniques. However, the agent also has higher concentration in the thymus, and lower concentration in the kidneys and GI tract. The N2S2 preparation has greater bowel excretion than the direct labeled or HYNIC material [119]. Using Tc-99m labeled annexin V, feasibility of imaging of apoptosis has been demonstrated both in experimental and clinical cardiovascular disease states.

Role of Apoptosis in Cardiovascular Diseases

The role of apoptosis has been well characterized in various organ systems but it has been traditionally believed that apoptosis does not occur in terminally differentiated tissues such as myocardium [101–105]. However, it is being increasingly recognized that although apoptosis may not occur as a physiologic phenomenon in myocytes, numerous pathologic insults induce apoptosis in cardiovascular disorders. Any necrotic insult that results in cell injury, but is not able to induce cell death, may force the myocytes to die by apoptosis. Apoptosis has also been reported secondary to growth stimulation that leads to fetal genes that are expressed in myocardium and lead to cell hypertrophy, and prepare the cell for mitotic division. However, since myocytes are terminally differentiated they are not able to divide and die by apoptosis, such as in CHF. Finally, apoptosis, which occurs normally during embryogenesis of heart, may lead to various morphological diseases if apoptosis becomes deficient or exaggerated.

Apoptosis significantly contributes to the development of heart, remodeling of the cardiac chambers, and correct routing of the great vessels during embryogenesis. Particularly, a large number of apoptotic cells are observed when bulbus cordis establishes ventriculoarterial concordance [120]. A substantial degree of ventricular remodeling occurs postnatally and apoptosis of right ventricular myocytes facilitates adaptation and transition from the fetal to adult circulation. It is conceivable that abnormalities of apoptosis should lead to structural diseases of the heart. Indeed, extensive apoptosis has been described in right ventricular dysplasia and progressive right ventricular failure. Apoptosis also contributes to postnatal maturation of the conduction system [121]. Excessive apoptosis of the conduction system has been reported in life-threatening bradyarrhythmias and high-grade AV block. On the other hand, lack of apoptosis may lead to persistence of intranodal tracts and re-entrant supraventricular tachyarrhythmias.

Although apoptosis is a physiologic phenomenon in embryologic life, it may also be induced in adult myocytes when they suffer sublethal insult from necrotogenic agents. Pathologic stimuli that are capable of inducing necrosis and apoptosis include ischemia, inflammation, cytokines, and toxic agents. Apoptosis has recently been reported in autopsy studies of acute myocardial infarction. Apoptotic cells are found scattered among the normal myocardial cells in the infarct periphery. It has been proposed that induction of nitric oxide synthetase (iNOS) may play an important role during apoptosis in myocardial infarction [122]. iNOS gene transfection of left ventricular myocardium has been shown to induce significant apoptosis in transfected cells and adjacent myocytes by paracrine effect in a time- and dose-dependent manner. Ultrastructural characterization of transfected cells reveals myofibrillar degradation and accumulation of mitochondria, which can be completely abolished by pretreatment with the nitric oxide synthetase inhibitor N-omeganitro-L-arginine methyl ester. In contrast to nonreperfused infarcts, experimental studies have demonstrated that reperfusion decreases the overall extent of apoptosis in ischemic regions of myocardium but accelerates the onset of apoptosis in nonsalvageable cells consequent to reperfusion injury particularly in the infarct center [123]. Reperfusion is known to be associated with an increase in intracellular calcium and free oxygen radicals, which are potent triggers for apoptosis. On the other hand, ischemic preconditioning significantly reduces the extent of apoptosis. It has been proposed that protein kinase C mediated activation of proton ATPase attenuates intracellular acidification during preconditioning and that the beneficial effect of preconditioning is completely abrogated by blockade of vacuolar proton ATPase activity.

The role of apoptosis has also been studied in inflammatory conditions of myocardium [124,125]. In experimental heterotopic abdominal transplantation the number of apoptotic cardiac myocytes increased sharply in a time-dependent manner. The expression of inducible NOS mRNA, protein, and enzyme activity paralleled in time and extent with the apoptosis of cardiac myocytes. The apoptosis of myocytes is also associated with a strong induction of Fas ligand mRNA in allografts. Extensive apoptosis has also been described in cardiac allografts from patients who died of acute rejection. In addition, endomyocardial biopsy specimens from allograft recipients demonstrated evidence of significant apoptosis in more than 50% of patients. Biopsies with higher grades of histological rejection were more likely to show apoptotic myocytes. On the other hand, the role of apoptosis in clinical myocarditis is uncertain due to the limited number of experimental or clinical studies, and myocardial apoptosis has been reported to be minimal in endomyocardial biopsy samples.

The role of apoptosis has also been demonstrated in

induction of chronic loss of myocytes, such as CHF. In the evolution of congestive heart failure, cardiac output is initially maintained by development of compensatory myocardial hypertrophy and dilatation. These early mechanical adaptations to growth stimulus soon fall short of adequate compensation and culminate in cardiac dysfunction. Various mediators of growth response, which upregulate during myocardial hypertrophy, are also known to be associated with apoptosis. During gestation, cardiac myocytes commit to differentiation and withdraw from the cell cycle such that any subsequent stimulus for division is perceived as a contradictory molecular demand and programmed cell death ensues. Slow but constant loss of myocytes by apoptosis contributes to inexorable decline of ventricular systolic function and the development of heart failure.

Compensatory mechanisms in congestive heart failure occur both at local myocardial as well as systemic levels [101–105]. Local homeostatic mechanisms such as those induced by myocyte stretch or pressure overload lead to activation of mitogenic kinases and early response genes, associated with local increase in angiotensin-II, angiotensinogen, AT1 receptor, Bax, p53 and binding of p53 to the promoter region of the angiotensinogen gene, and decreased expression of Bc12. On the other hand, systemic compensatory response in congestive heart failure is predominently mediated by neurohormonal activation wherein hemodynamic balance is initially restored by increase in peripheral vascular resistance, myocardial contractility, and natriuresis. Heart failure is characteristically associated with a compensatory increase in circulating plasma norepinephrine (NE), tumor necrosis factor-alpha (TNF-α), and atrial natriuretic peptide (ANP), all of which may also lead to induction of apoptosis.

Imaging of Apoptosis with Annexin V

Various animal models of apoptosis have been used for demonstration of the feasibility of annexin V imaging. Tissue with significant apoptosis, such as the liver stimulated to undergo apoptosis by administration of Fas antibody to activate hepatic Fas receptors, or rejecting cardiac transplants in experimental animals, achieve imageable concentrations of Tc-99m-annexin in these organs within 60 min of intravenous administration [117].

Detection of fas antibody induced apoptosis

Fas receptors are physiologically expressed on many cells. The liver has an unusually high concentration of Fas receptors. Rapid induction of massive hepatic apoptosis has been demonstrated following administration

of an antibody that binds to Fas receptors in similar fashion to Fas ligand. To determine if Tc-99m-annexin imaging could detect this process, studies were performed in normal mice and in genetically altered knockout 1pr mice that do not express Fas receptors. In the normal (wild type) mice, hepatic uptake of annexin V increased by threefold within 2 hr of antibody administration, while there was no increase in the 1pr animals. The wild type animals had definite evidence of massive apoptosis while the livers of the 1pr animals were normal [117].

Apoptosis in cardiac transplantation

Since apoptosis significantly contributes to myocardial damage in cardiac allograft rejection, the potential utility of Tc-99m-annexin imaging for the detection of transplant rejection was tested in rats with heterotopic heart transplants [117]. The animals were imaged serially for the first 10 days after transplantation. In addition to in vivo imaging the native transplanted hearts were subjected to ex vivo organ counting and histologic analysis. The transplanted heart developed marked uptake on day 4. At that time minimal histologic evidence of apoptosis was present, but routine histologic evidence of rejection was absent. Over the succeeding days, annexin V uptake grew intense, histologic staining for apoptotic cells became increasingly positive, as did conventional histologic evidence of rejection. Immunosuppressive therapy was started with cyclosporine after day 4. The scans became negative within 2 days.

Clinical studies of apoptosis imaging with annexin V

The in vitro observations and experimental studies of annexin V imaging led to the testing of radiolabeled annexin V as clinical marker for apoptosis. We studied a series of 14 consecutive patients (ages 41 to 68 years; M:F 12:2) who had undergone heart transplantation within the year of scintigraphic study using Tc-99m labeled annexin V [126]. SPECT images were obtained at 2–3 hr after the injection of radiotracer. Processing of the SPECT images was performed initially as "chest tomographic" transaxial, coronal, and sagittal slices in order to characterize any cardiac activity present, with regard to overall orientation of the left ventricle in the chest. Once these were defined, "cardiac tomographic" slices in the short, vertical long, and horizontal long axes were reconstructed using filtered back-projection (see Color Fig. 21.4 in separate color insert). A positive study was identified when myocardial uptake was seen in the chest SPECT images and, more importantly, in the cardiac SPECT images if both myocardium and LV cavity were identified during reconstruction. A negative study was otherwise identified, specifically when activity was seen within the cardiac blood pool, or by absence of tracer in the cardiac region. Right ventricular EMB was performed within 1–4 days of imaging. EMB specimens were interpreted for the evidence of transplant rejection and apoptosis for activation of caspase-3. Caspase-3 gets activated in cells just prior to expression of PS, the binding site for annexin V.

Analyses of SPECT images demonstrated no uptake of annexin. V in 9 of the 14 patients. EMB in these 9 patients were unremarkable and interpreted as International Society of Heart & Lung Transplantation grade 0–1A/4. Lack of immunohistochemical evidence of caspase-3 upregulation in EMB confirmed the absence of significant apoptosis and hence allograft rejection in myocardium. The remaining 5 of the 14 patients demonstrated variable degrees of Tc-99m-annexin V uptake in the left ventricular myocardium. Reconstruction of the SPECT images as myocardial perfusion scans revealed predominantly nondiffuse and regional uptake in 3 of 5 patients and diffuse global uptake in the remaining 2 of 5 patients. EMB specimens in the 3 patients with nondiffuse annexin uptake demonstrated ISHLT grade 2/4 rejection with intense caspase-3 staining in scattered myocytes, endothelial, and interstitial cells. On the other hand, 2 of the 5 patients with diffuse positive annexin scans demonstrated ISHLT grade 3A/4 or higher rejection with corresponding caspase-3 upregulation and activation.

Overall, this preliminary patient series confirmed the feasibility of clinical imaging of apoptosis. The study demonstrated that all 9 patients with no histologic evidence of rejection had a negative scan. Similarly, 5 patients with a positive scan had histologically verified transplant rejection of ISHLT grade 2/4 or higher. Caspase-3 upregulation in the patients with positive annexin V scan confirmed the specificity of noninvasive detection of apoptotic process. Histologic evidence of apoptosis was observed in both myocytes and nonmyocytic cells.

Future Directions

Identification of the contribution of apoptosis to various cardiovascular disorders is of paramount importance. Unlike necrosis, the process of apoptosis can be modulated, and therapeutic intervention can therefore help prevent loss of myocardial cells that are not capable of regeneration. Imaging of apoptosis therefore is likely to contribute to development of newer strategies for management of cardiovascular diseases in the next one to two decades.

IMAGING OF DISORDERED CARDIAC NEUROTRANSMISSION

Visualization and quantitation with SPECT and positron emission tomography (PET) of the pathophysiologic processes that take place in the nerve terminals, synaptic clefts, and postsynaptic sites in the heart, can be referred to as cardiac neurotransmission imaging. Nuclear medicine is currently the only imaging modality with sufficient sensitivity to offer in vivo visualization of cardiac neurotransmission at a micromolar level. Such unique capability allows noninvasive classification of dysautonomias, assessment of the adrenergic innervation status in dilated cardiomyopathies, characterization of pathologic myocardial substrate in arrhythmogenic cardiomyopathies, and assessment of neuronal status in coronary artery disease.

Radiopharmaceuticals for Neurotransmission Assessment

Radiotracers for scintigraphic imaging of cardiac neurotransmission have been developed by radiolabeling of the neurotransmitters or their structural analogs or false neurotransmitters. Binding characteristics, selectivity, and binding reversibility determine the suitability of a given agent. Furthermore, radiochemical purity, and specific activity required to minimize occupation of binding sites by nonlabeled molecules, as well as pharmacologic effects in patients, have to be defined in the process of validation of neurotransmission radiopharmaceuticals for in vivo imaging.

From the many radiopharmaceuticals that have been designed and tested to assess cardiac neurotransmission, the most commonly employed are the following: at a presynaptic level, F-18-fluorodopamine is available to assess norepinephrine synthesis; C-11-hydroxiephedrine, C-11-ephedrine, and I-123-metaiodobenzylguanidine (MIBG) are available to assess presynaptic reuptake and storage by PET and SPECT; at a postsynaptic level, beta blockers such as C-11-CGP and C-11-carazolol are available to assess beta-adrenoceptor expression and density. The quantification of neurotransmitter synthesis and transport by PET requires tracer kinetic modeling. Typically presynaptic norepinephrine reuptake function is assessed by calculation of de distribution volume (V_d) of tracers using compartment models and nonlinear regression analysis to calculate influx and eflux rate constants. Myocardial adrenoceptor density (B_{max}) may be measured by injection of different amounts of radioactivity and cold substance, assessment of input function and estimation of metabolites, and graphical analysis.

F-18-fluorodopamine

F-18-fluorodopamine is taken up in sympathetic nerve terminals and transported into axoplasmic vesicles, where it is converted into F-18-fluoronorepinephrine and stored. During sympathetic stimulation F-18-fluoronorepinephrine is released from sympathetic nerve terminals similarly to H-3-norepinephrine, 6-F-18-fluorodopamine can be synthesised from 6-F-18-fluorodopa by enzymatic decarboxylation using an L-amino acid decarboxylase [127]. Reported mean concentration of F-18-fluorodopamine in left ventricular myocardium peaks at 5 to 8 min after infusion, being 10.2 ± 67 mCi.kg/cc.mCi in normal controls [127].

C-11-hydroxyephedrine and C-11-epinephrine

C-11-hydroxyephedrine is a false neurotransmitter that has the same neuronal uptake mechanism as norepinephrine, via neuronal uptake-1, but it is not degraded by monoamine oxidase and catechol-methyl-transferase, the enzymes responsible for the metabolism of norepinephrine in the heart [128]. The storage and release properties, however, seem to differ from those of the physiological neurotransmitters [129]. C-11-epinephrine may be a more physiological tracer for the evaluation of presynaptic sympathetic nerve function regarding uptake mechanism, vesicular storage, and metabolism [130]. C-11-epinephrine is rapidly transported into the presynaptic nerve terminal via uptake-1 and is stored in the vesicles similarly to norepinephrine. Volume distribution for C-11-hydroxyephedrine in controls has been reported to be of 71 ± 19 ml/g of tissue. Myocardial retention fractions of C-11-hydroxyephedrine and C-11-epinephrine in normals at 5 min postinjection have been reported to be 0.24 ± 0.02 and 0.29 ± 0.02, respectively [131,132].

Metaiodobenzylguanidine

Guanethidine is a potent neuron-blocking agent that acts selectively on sympathetic nerve endings [133]. By the modification of this compound into metaiodobenzylguanidine (MIBG), the affinity for neuronal uptake sites is increased. MIBG was labeled with I-123 to enable scintigraphic visualization of the sympathetic nervous system in humans [134], providing the first radiopharmaceutical for the assessment of cardiac neurotransmission by SPECT. The first clinical application of I-123-MIBG

was the imaging of the adrenal medulla and neoplasms originating from the neural crest, such as pheochromocytoma and neuroblastoma [135]. MIBG scintigraphy also showed a striking uptake in the heart, because of its dense sympathetic innervation. In 1980, the potential use of MIBG in myocardial imaging was first suggested, although at that time no information was available on the physiology of cardiac MIBG uptake and its metabolism in humans under different conditions [134]. Much work has been done to elucidate the mechanism by which the sympathetic nerve endings take up MIBG. It has been shown that MIBG and noradrenaline have similar molecular structures and that both utilize the same uptake and storage mechanisms in the sympathetic nerve endings [136–138].

Neuronal uptake of MIBG is mainly achieved through the sodium and energy dependent uptake-1 mechanism, which is characterized by a temperature dependency, a high affinity (K_m (μmolar) of 1.22 ± 0.12 for MIBG and 1.41 ± 0.50 for noradrenaline) and a low capacity (V_m (pmol/10^6 cells/10 min) of 64.3 ± 3.3 for MIBG and 36.6 ± 7.2 for noradrenaline). Sisson et al. [136,137] demonstrated in animal experiments that the kinetics of I-125-MIBG mimicked those of H-3-noradrenaline under different conditions. In these experiments, yohimbine, an alpha-2-adrenoceptor antagonist, was used to increase sympathetic nerve function, while clonidine was used to induce the opposite effect. It has to be noted that the sodium-independent neuronal uptake of MIBG has also been reported. This nonneuronal uptake-2 mechanism dominates at higher concentrations of the substrate, and is probably the result of passive diffusion. The relative role of each uptake mechanism is dependent upon the plasma concentration of MIBG. However, neuronal uptake is predominantly determined by uptake-1 mechanism, since an extremely small quantity of MIBG is usually injected for diagnostic scintigraphy. Typically one standard dose of 185 MBq contains 6.25×10^{-9} gr MIBG. The use of no-carrier-added MIBG has been reported to yield improved image quality [139].

C-11-CGP

Lipophilic antagonists of beta-adrenoceptors such as iodopindolol have been used in in vitro studies. Lipophilic molecules such as C-11-propanolol cannot be used to study the heart in vivo because of its high accumulation in the lungs. CGP-12177 (4-(3-t-butylamino-2-hydroxypropoxy)-benzimidazol-one) is a hydrophilic antagonist that binds to the receptor with high affinity (0.3 nM) [140]. Because of its high hydrophilicity, it selectively identifies cell-surface beta-adrenoceptors which are coupled to adenylate cyclase. CGP can be labeled with C-11 using CGP-17704 as a precursor and C-11 phosgen. The receptor concentration and the kinetic rate constants can be derived from experimental data using a kinetic or a graphical method [140]. With this approach, values of B_{max} have been reported to be of 10 ± 3 pmol/g of tissue in controls, with a dissociation constant of 0.014 ± 0.002 min^{-1} [140–142].

F-18-fluorocarazolol

Carazolol is a lipophilic, nonselective beta-adrenoceptor antagonist to the beta-1 and beta-2 receptors, that can be labeled with C-11 and F-18 [143]. Uptake in the target organs, such as the heart, is substantial and it can be blocked and displaced by propanolol, in such a way that suggests that fluorocarazolol and propanolol compete for binding to the same receptor sites [144]. Myocardial tissue to plasma concentration ratios of fluorocarazolol in normal individuals reach a plateau value of 18 ± 1 in the heart at 45 min. postinjection of the radiotracer. During the slow kinetic phase, maximal concentrations in the heart range from 0.03 to 0.085 pmole/ml [144].

C-11-MQNB

Methylquinuclidinyl benzilate (MQNB) is a highly specific hydrophilic antagonist of muscarinic receptors that can be labeled with C-11 [145,146]. The stimulation of local muscarinic receptors inhibit norepinephrine release from adrenergic nerve terminals. Although muscarinic receptors are present on sympathetic nerve endings in a prejunctional distribution, it is recognized that they play a role in neurotransmission within the intrinsic cardiac sympathetic nervous system. After compartmental modeling, the B_{max} values reported in controls are 25 ± 7.7 pmol/l, with a dissociation constant of 2.2 ± 1 pmol/ml without significant differences in the septal, anterior, and lateral regions of the left ventricle [146].

Imaging of Cardiac Neurotransmission

Planar imaging has commonly been used to determine cardiac MIBG uptake. Myocardial uptake and distribution are visually assessed. A semiquantitative measurement of myocardial MIBG uptake can be obtained by the calculation of a heart-to-mediastinum ratio. However, there are several limitations to this technique: first, the superposition of noncardiac structures such as lung and mediastinum may preclude optimal visualization; second, superposition of various myocardial segments and motion artifacts interfere with the regional assessment of uptake of the radioligand. SPECT imaging may overcome these disadvantages, although it has to be taken into account that in some pathophysiologic conditions myocar-

dial MIBG uptake may be severely reduced, hampering obtainment of tomographic slices of the heart.

Thirty minutes after thyroid blockade by oral administration of 500 mg potassium perchlorate, approx 370 MBq of I-123-MIBG are administered intravenously. Planar scintigraphic images and SPECT studies of the heart are acquired 20 minutes (early image) and 4 hours (delayed image) after injection. A 20% window is usually used centered over the 159 keV I-123 photo-peak. Planar images are acquired in anterior and 45° left anterior oblique views of the thorax and stored in a 128 × 128 matrix. MIBG uptake is semiquantified by calculating a heart-to-mediastinum ratio (HMR), after drawing regions of interest (ROIs) over the mediastinum in the anterior view and over the myocardium in the left anterior oblique view. Average counts per pixel in the myocardium are divided by average counts per pixel in the mediastinum. Intraobserver variability of HMR is < 2% and interobserver variability is < 5%. Heart-to-mediastinum ratio > 1.8 is considered normal. Washout rate from initial to delayed images is < 10% in normal individuals [147,148]. SPECT studies can be obtained by a single pass of 60 steps at 30 seconds per step (64 × 64 matrix), starting at 45° right anterior oblique projection and proceeding anticlockwise to the 45° left posterior oblique projection. The data are reconstructed in short axis, horizontal long axis, and vertical long axis views, and scatter or attenuation correction may be applied. For visual evaluation of SPECT slices, reduction in MIBG concentration in given myocardial segments can be evaluated using a point scale. In addition, polar maps can be constructed from short-axis images and can be compared to those of normal individuals.

The quantitative assessment of the cardiac uptake of MIBG in the heart, by comparing the cardiac count density with that of a reference region such as the mediastinum, is hampered by several variable factors. First, the tissue attenuation is nonuniform for intrathoracic organs, since tissue density and therefore the attenuation coefficient vary. Correction for this nonuniform attenuation can be performed theoretically using an iterative reconstruction algorithm or by constructing individual attenuation maps during acquisition using a line source. Second, photons that scatter within the patient are often indistinguishable from unscattered photons with respect to their photon energy. These scattered photons contribute to a further loss of spatial resolution. For I-123-MIBG SPECT a limiting factor is the number of counts acquired. Therefore, dose and acquisition time should be maximized. Adequate implementation of procedures to limit the effects of these factors will improve image quality, that is, image resolution and contrast.

Somsen et al. [149,150] have developed a method in which the count density (cd) in the left ventricular cavity is used as a reference. Volumes of the myocardium and the left ventricular cavity are reconstructed from SPECT acquisitions. The left ventricular cavity count density is calibrated by the I-123 activity in a venous blood sample (BS), drawn at the time of the acquisition. Subsequently, cardiac I-123-MIBG uptake can be calculated according to the equation: Cardiac I-123-MIBG uptake = (Myocardial cd/Cavity cd) × BS (Bq/ml).

PET imaging protocols of imaging for disordered neurotransmission vary according to the radiotracer characteristics and the available instrumentation. Obtained volumetric data sets are realigned according to standardized axes. Assessment of physiologic parameters can be achieved by applying tracer kinetic models to quantitative data sets. Region of interest analysis of the activity concentration inside the left ventricular cavity yields the time-activity curve of arterial blood, and allows assessment of the arterial input function. Continuous thoracic PET scanning is performed after F-18-fluorodopamine infusion for up to 3 hr. The total scanning time is divided into intervals of 5 to 30 minutes, and the tomographic results of each interval are assessed. Scan sequences may consist of 5 frames × 1 min, 5 × 5 min, 4 × 15 min, and 3 × 30 min. PET scanning of C-11-hydroxyephedrine and C-11-epinephrine usually lasts for 60 min. Scan sequences may consist of 15 frames: 6 × 30 sec, 2 × 60 sec, 2 × 150 sec, 2 × 300 sec, 2 × 600 sec, and 1 × 1200 sec. With C-11-CGP continuous thoracic scanning, recording data in list mode are typically performed for 1 hr after infusion. When using F-18-fluorocarazolol, acquisition protocols after infusion may consist of 8 × 15 sec frames, 4 × 30 sec, 4 × 1 min, 4 × 2 min, 6 × 4 min, and 2 × 10 min. For C-11-MQNB, recording of data is started with the first injection. Sixty sequential images may be acquired, using one of the cross sections, and reconstructing according to the specific protocol used. Scan sequences may consist of 24 time frames: 8 × 15 sec, 4 × 30 sec, 2 × 60 sec, 8 × 150 sec, after each infusion.

Clinical Imaging for Neurotransmission in the Heart

Primary cardioneuropathy

Dysautonomias. Derangements of sympathetic and para-sympathetic nervous system function are frequently encountered in neurology and cardiology. Three forms of primary dysautonomia can be distinguished: pure autonomic failure, defined as a sporadic, idiopathic cause of persistent orthostatic hypotension and other manifestations of autonomic failure that occur without other neurologic features; Parkinson's disease with autonomic failure; and multiple-system atrophy. However, distinguishing Parkinson's disease with autonomic failure from some forms of multiple-system atrophy is difficult, and physiologic and neurochemical tests often fail to properly separate the different forms of dysautonomia.

Goldstein et al. [151] have used PT scanning with F-18-fluorodopamine to examine cardiac sympathetic innervation in patients with different types of dysautonomia. On the basis of their PET findings, they propose a new pathophysiologic classification of dysautonomias in which sympathetic neurocirculatory failure results from peripheral sympathetic denervation or decreased or absent sympathetic signal traffic. Results of PET scanning are related to signs of sympathetic neurocirculatory failure, with orthostatic hypotension and abnormal blood pressure responses associated with the Valsalva maneuver, to central degeneration, and to responsiveness to treatment with levodopa-carbidopa. Patients with pure autonomic failure or parkinsonism and sympathetic neurocirculatory failure have no myocardial F-18-fluorodopamine uptake or cardiac norepinephrine spillover, indicating loss of myocardial sympathetic nerve terminals. Patients with the Shy-Drager syndrome have increased levels of F-18-fluorodopamine activity, indicating intact nerve terminals and absent nerve traffic. Patients with dysautonomia without sympathetic neurocirculatory failure have normal levels of F-18-fluorodopamine activity in the myocardium and normal rates of cardiac norepinephrine spillover. F-18-fluorodopamine PET studies, in combination with neurochemical tests and clinical observations support this new clinical pathophysiologic classification of dysautonomias, with enhanced diagnostic differentiation between multiple-system atrophy, parkinsonism with autonomic failure, and peripheral autonomic failure [151].

Heart transplantation. During orthotopic heart transplantation, the entire recipient heart is excised except for the posterior atrial walls, to which the donor atria are anastomosed. During the process, the allograft becomes completely denervated. Lack of autonomic nerve supply is associated with major physiologic limitations. The inability to perceive pain does not allow symptomatic recognition of accelerated allograft vasculopathy, and heart transplant patients often develop acute ischemic events or left ventricular dysfunction or die suddenly. In addition, denervation of the sinus node does not allow adequate acceleration of heart rate during stress and efficient increase in cardiac output. Furthermore, loss of vasomotor tone may adversely affect the physiologic alterations in blood flow, produce altered hemodynamic performance at rest and during exercise, and decrease exercise capacity.

Scintigraphic uptake of I-123-MIBG and C-11-hydroxyephedrine supports the concept of spontaneous reinnervation taking place after transplantation [152–155]. All studies performed up to 5 years after heart transplantation suggest that reinnervation is likely to be a slow process and occurs only after 1 year post-transplantation [156].

Sympathetic reinnervation, measured by regional distribution and intensity of myocardial MIBG uptake, increases with time after transplantation, with a positive correlation between heart to mediastinum rates and time after transplantation. Serial MIBG studies over time show that reinnervation begins from the base of the heart and spreads toward the apex. MIBG uptake is seen primarily in the anterior, anterolateral, and septal regions. MIBG uptake is usually not apparent in the posterior or inferior myocardial regions, except for some basal posterior localization. Complete reinnervation of the transplanted heart is not seen on scintigraphic studies, even up to 12 years posttransplantation. Early vasculopathy may inhibit the process of sympathetic reinnervation of the transplanted heart. The relationship between reinnervation status and graft vasculopathy deserves further investigation and may help to characterize subsets of transplant patients with different clinical outcomes.

In a recent PET perfusion and sympathetic reinnervation study of heart-transplant patients, Di Carli et al. [155] demonstrated that blood flow increases in response to sympathetic stimulation in the territory of the left anterior descending artery. This territory has the highest uptake of C-11-hydroxyephedrine, whereas in other territories, increase in flow and uptake of C-11-hydroxyephedrine are minor. This study also showed that basal flow in transplant recipients is similar in all coronary territories despite differences in sympathetic reinnervation, suggesting that cardiac-efferent adrenergic signals play an important role in modulating myocardial blood flow during activation of the sympathetic nervous system.

Idiopathic ventricular tachyarrhythmias. In patients presenting with idiopathic ventricular tachycardia and fibrillation, wherein no structural or functional abnormalities of the myocardium can be demonstrated by conventional imaging and clinical testing, early diagnosis and treatment are of clinical importance because ventricular fibrillation is the most common arrhythmia at the time of sudden death [157]. Typical arrhythmias in these patients can be provoked by physical or mental stress or by

catecholamine application. Schafers et al. [158], using I-123-MIBG, C-11-hydroxyephedrine and C-11-CGP, have demonstrated that in patients with idiopathic right ventricular outflow tract tachycardia, both the presynaptic myocardial catecholamine reuptake and the postsynaptic myocardial beta-adrenoceptors density are reduced despite normal blood catecholamine levels. The maximal binding capacity of the beta-adrenoceptor antagonist is reduced in patients with right ventricular outflow tract tachycardia as compared to controls (6.8 ± 1.2 pmol/g vs 10.2 ± 2.9) [159]. These scintigraphic findings represent the only demonstrable myocardial abnormality in patients with idiopathic tachycardia and fibrillation, and suggest that myocardial beta-adrenoceptor downregulation in these patients occurs subsequently to increased local synaptic catecholamine levels caused by impaired catecholamine reuptake [159].

Secondary cardioneuropathy
Dilated cardiomyopathy. After the onset of myocardial failure, enhanced sympathetic nervous system activity plays an important role in supporting the cardiovascular system by increasing heart rate, contractility, and venous return. Blood pressure to preserve organ perfusion is supported by systemic arterial constriction. But, on the other hand, increased sympathetic activity has deleterious effects on the cardiovascular system. Vascular constriction and increased salt and water retention by the kidneys increase myocardial wall energetic requirements. Altered sympathetic cardiac adrenergic function may also cause arrhythmias, desensitization of postsynaptic beta-adrenoceptors, and activation of other neurohumoral systems such as the renin-angiotensin system, which may themselves exert adverse effects and contribute to progression of myocardial dysfunction. In addition, prolonged exposure to norepinephrine may contribute to disease progression by acting directly on the myocardium to modify cellular phenotype and result in myocyte death [160,161].

In patients with dilated cardiomyopathies, because of the increased concentration of circulating catecholamines resulting from heart failure, the myocardial responsiveness to beta-adrenoceptor agonists is blunted. Frequently, alterations of cardiac sympathetic innervation contribute to fatal outcomes in patients with heart failure. Merlet et al. [162–164], studying patients with functional classes II–IV and left ventricular function less than 40%, and using as end points transplantation and cardiac or noncardiac death, have demonstrated that the only independent predictors of mortality are low MIBG uptake and left ventricular ejection fraction. In addition, MIBG uptake and circulating norepinephrine concentration were the only predictors of life duration when using multivariate life table analysis. Therefore, it seems that impaired cardiac adrenergic innervation as assessed by MIBG imaging is strongly related to mortality in patients with heart failure. Along the same line, Maunory et al. [165] have described that cardiac adrenergic neuronal function is impaired in children with idiopathic dilated cardiomyopathy, although in this particular study they did not have sufficient follow-up to assess prognosis. Patients with congestive cardiomyopathy typically have accelerated washout rates (> 25% from 15 to 85 minutes) as compared to controls (< 10%). Momose et al. [166] assessed the prognostic value of washout rate measurements in patients with heart failure and found that a threshold value of washout of 52% clearly separated negative outcome from survival, making the washout rate the most powerful independent predictor of prognosis. Cohen-Solal et al. [167] have shown that MIBG parameters correlate with other predictors of prognosis such as peak VO_2. Cardiac MIBG SPECT has also been used to assess changes in cardiac sympathetic neuronal uptake function due to pharmacologic intervention [168]. Somsen et al. [149] have shown that enalapril improves cardiac sympathetic uptake function but does not affect plasma noradrenaline levels in a group of patients with heart failure, supporting the concept that a restoration of cardiac neuronal uptake of noradrenaline is one of the beneficial effects of enalapril treatment in these patients. Suwa et al. [169] prospectively evaluated whether MIBG myocardial imaging was useful in predicting responses to beta-blocker therapy in patients with dilated cardiomyopathy. Heart-to-mediastinum ratios on early and delayed imaging as well as the percentage of washout rate were evaluated. The heart-to-mediastinum rate on delayed images was seen to be a good predictor of the response to beta-blocker therapy, with a threshold of 1.7 identifying responders to bisoprolol with a sensitivity of 91% and a specificity of 92%. These results indicate that response to beta-blocker therapy may be monitored with sequential quantitative MIBG studies.

The concept that prolonged sympathetic hyperactivity is detrimental in chronic heart failure has been supported by the trials that demonstrated the beneficial effects of angiotensin converting enzyme inhibitors and beta-adrenoceptor antagonists. Therefore, the reduction of sympathetic nervous activity is considered an important target for drug treatment of heart failure. Several mechanisms may contribute to reduced beta-adrenoceptor responsiveness in heart failure, such as downregulation of beta-adrenoceptors, uncoupling of subtypes of beta-adrenoceptors, upregulation of beta-adrenoceptor kinase, increased activity of G protein, decreased activity of adenylyl cyclase, and increased nitric oxide. Myocardial remodeling involves hypertrophy and apoptosis of myocytes, regression to a fetal phenotype, and changes in the nature of the extracellular matrix. It seems that noradrenaline can contribute to many of these changes by direct stimulation of adrenoceptors on cardiac myocytes and fibroblasts. The hypertrophic effect of noradrenaline is associated with the re-expression of fetal genes and the downregulation of several adult genes. Cardiac neurotransmission imaging can play a role in future trials conducted to assess the effect of new forms of medical therapy to improve outcomes in heart failure (Fig. 21.5).

Coronary artery disease. The sympathetic nervous tissue may be more sensitive to the effects of ischemia than the myocardial tissue. It has been shown that the uptake of iodine-123 metaiodobenzylguanidine (MIBG) is significantly reduced in the areas of myocardial infarction, and acute and chronic ischemia [171–173]. A decrease in MIBG uptake in ischemic tissue represents the loss of integrity of postganglionic, presynaptic neurones. It is likely that ischemia induces damage to sympathetic neurones, which may take a long time to regenerate, and that repetitive episodes of ischemia should result in a relatively permanent loss of MIBG uptake. Early after infarction, sympathetic denervation in adjacent noninfarcted regions is frequently observed [172]. Experimental studies have demonstrated that a transmural infarction produces acute sympathetic denervation in noninfarcted sites apical to the necrotic regions as measured by norepinephrine content and response to stellate stimulation. Nontransmural infarction may also lead to regional ischemic damage of sympathetic nerves, but may spare subepicardial nerve trunks that course the region of infarction to provide a source of innervation to distal areas of the myocardium.

Minardo et al. [174] used I-123-MIBG to show that the area of denervation extended beyond the region of infarction. McGhie et al. [172], evaluating patients on day 10 after acute myocardial infarction with MIBG scintigraphy, found reduced uptake and a more extensive area of reduced uptake than the thallium perfusion defect. These regions may be associated with spontaneous ventricular tachyarrhythmias after myocardial infarction [175]. It is known that sympathetic stimulation lowers the threshold of ventricular tachycardia and fibrillation during acute myocardial ischemia. Adrenergic denervation of viable myocardium results in denervation supersensitivity, with exaggerated response of myocardium to sympathetic stimulation. Denervation supersensitivity is related to vulnerability to ventricu-

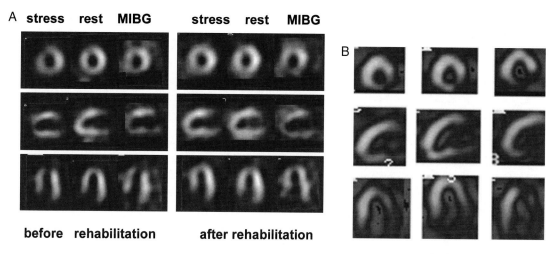

FIGURE 21.5 Imaging of myocardial denervation. (A). Myocardial exercise/rest (a/b) perfusion studies, and sympathetic innervation studies (c) performed before and 6 months after starting exercise rehabilitation in a patient with anterior myocardial infarction. Before the exercise rehabilitation, the myocardial perfusion study shows anterior and apical ischemia with persistence of a little anterior hypoperfusion at rest. The MIBG study shows decreased uptake in the anterior and apical regions, the extent of which is similar to that on the myocardial perfusion study. Six months after the start of exercise rehabilitation, the myocardial perfusion study shows improved perfusion at exercise and the same anterior hypoperfusion at rest, while the MIBG study is similar to the study before exercise rehabilitation. (B) Myocardial exercise (left column)/rest (center) perfusion and sympathetic innervation (right) images of a patient with infero-lateral infarction and residual ischemia. Notice that the extent of the perfusion defect seen on the exercise perfusion images corresponds to the sympathetic innervation defect seen on the MIBG images. (From Estorch, EJNM 2000;27:333, with permission.)

lar arrhythmias. Regional sympathetic denervation is possibly one of the mechanisms that renders patients with coronary artery disease susceptible to ventricular arrhythmias during myocardial ischemia. Reinnervation late after myocardial infarction in peri-infarct regions has also been demonstrated by reappearance of MIBG uptake by 14 weeks after infarction [176,177]. Reinnervation may be in part responsible for the return of function during this period. However, reinnervation may be incomplete as late as 3 month after acute infarction. Hartikainen et al. [176] examined MIBG uptake at 3 and 13 months after a first infarction and found no difference in MIBG activity over time within the infarcted zone, but an increase in activity in the peri-infarcted region without a change in perfusion.

The eventual concordance between the extent of MIBG defect at rest and perfusion defect at exercise in patients with coronary artery disease suggests that mild degrees of ischemia may be injurious to the integrity of myocardial sympathetic neurones [178–181]. Correlation between the MIBG defect and the area at risk and the presence of angina further supports the concept of neuronal damage in the ischemic territory. Although association of MIBG defect with clinical angina can be explained as a consequence of ischemia, it is intriguing that

the perception of pain occurs from the area which lacks sympathetic innervation. Since MIBG defects in the ischemic territory are not absolute, partial neuronal innervation may allow perception of chest pain. The MIBG studies in cardiac allograft recipients also support the finding of both susceptibility of sympathetic neurones to ischemia as well as the adequacy of partial innervation for nociception. Reinnervation in transplant recipients is almost never complete. On the other hand, all patients who sustain episodes of early allograft vasculopathy do not develop reinnervation even up to 12 years after heart transplantation. The latter finding also supports the concept of extreme sensitivity of the sympathetic innervation to ischemic stress, even more sensitive than that of the myocyte [181–184].

Hypertrophic cardiomyopathy. Hypertrophic cardio-myopathy is genetically determined; however, autonomic dysfunction seems to play a role in the phenotypic expression. Several clinical features of hypertrophic cardiomyopathy suggest increased sympathetic outflow. The incidence of chest pain, myocardial hypercontractility, propensity to ventricular arrhythmias and sudden death, and the beneficial effect of beta-blockers suggest increased delivery of norepinephrine to myocardial adrenoceptors. Cardiac presynaptic catecholamine reuptake is impaired in hypertrophic cardiomyopathy, in association with reduced postsynaptic beta-adrenoceptor density, suggesting an increased neurotransmitter concentration in the synaptic cleft. This can be shown by quantitative PET studies using C-11-hydroxyephedrine and C-11-CGP [185,186]. Increased washout rate of $> 25\%$ between initial and delayed images has also been described in hypertrophic cardiomyopathy, secondary to activation of the sympathetic nervous system. The autonomic dysfunction in these patients is probably related to disease progression and ultimately heart failure [187,188]. In patients studies with N-13-ammonia and F-18-fluorodopamine, F-18:N-13 ratio is lower in hypertrophied than in nonhypertrophied regions [188], indicating decreased neuronal uptake of catecholamines in hypertrophied myocardium of patients with hypertrophic cardiomyopathy.

Arrhythmogenic right ventricular dysplasia. Fibrolipomatous degeneration of the right ventricular myocardium is the main structural abnormality in arrhythmogenic right ventricular cardiomyopathy. In these patients, the evidence of provocable ventricular tachyarrhythmias and cardiac arrest during exercise or stress, and the sensitivity to catecholamines strongly suggest an involvement of the sympathetic nervous system in the process of arrhythmogenesis [189,190]. It has been shown, with MIBG SPECT and C-11-hydroxyephedrine PET, that although the left ventricle is not involved in the disease, there is evidence of global and regional denervation in presynaptic catecholamine reuptake and storage of the left ventricle, as well as a reduction in the postsynaptic beta-adrenoceptor density assessed by C-11-CGP PET [191,192]. Patients with arrhythmogenic cardiomyopathy have demonstrated B_{max} values of CGP of 5.9 ± 1.3 pmol/g tissue versus 10.2 ± 2.9 in controls [193]. These findings suggest a reduced activity of the noradrenaline transporter (uptake-1) with subsequent beta-adrenoceptor downregulation, and have potential impact on diagnostic evaluation and therapeutic management of patients with arrhythmogenic right ventricular cardiomyopathy.

Diabetes mellitus. The sympathetic nervous system appears to be activated during the early stages of diabetes, with elevated plasma catecholamine levels. This prolonged exposure to catecholamines leads to downregulation of adrenergic receptors and to alterations in adrenergic nervous fibers in the myocardium. Hyperglycemia and insulin deficiency may also contribute to the abnormalities in cardiac innervation in diabetes.

Kim et al. [194] have shown decreased I-123-MIBG uptake associated with autonomic dysfunction in diabetic patients, and have correlated decreased cardiac MIBG uptake with increased mortality. It seems that MIBG scintigraphy is more sensitive than autonomic nervous function tests for the detection of autonomic neuropathy in diabetes, particularly in early stages of the disease. Scognamiglio et al. [195] have shown that the impairment of cardiac sympathetic innervation, as shown by MIBG studies, correlates with abnormal response to exercise in diabetic patients and may contribute to left ventricular dysfunction before the appearance of irreversible damage and over heart failure. Hattori et al. [196] described diabetic patients in whom there is scintigraphic evidence of severe myocardial denervation who present with hyperreaction to dobutamine stress, which may in part explain the high incidence of sudden death in patients with advanced diabetes mellitus.

Hypertension. Scintigraphy of the cardiac sympathetic innervation may play a role in the assessment of arterial and pulmonary hypertension. Morimoto et al. [197] have investigated the relationship between the regression of hypertensive cardiac hypertrophy and cardiac nervous function, before and after hypertensive therapy in patients with untreated essential arterial hypertension. A regional and global improvement in cardiac sympathetic nervous function, as seen on I-123-MIBG studies, appears to be related to the regression of hypertensive cardiac hypertrophy. Furthermore, in patients with pulmonary hypertension, the uptake ratio of MIBG between the interventricular septum and the left ventricular myocardium correlates with the right ventricular overload [198,199]. Therefore, it is conceivable that scintigraphic assessment of the adrenergic nervous system may play a role in the multidisciplinary assessment and management of hypertension.

Drug-induced cardiotoxicity. MIBG studies have also been used to assess adrenergic innervation impairment due to anthracycline cardiotoxicity. Decreased myocardial MIBG uptake has been observed after adriamycin administration with limited morphological damage [200]. In these studies, decreased myocardial MIBG uptake preceded ejection fraction deterioration. MIBG uptake reveals a dose-dependent decline, which could be due to excessive compensatory hyperadrenergic washout from the myocardium or to direct adrenergic neuron damage. Hyperadrenergism seems unlikely, since myocardial norepinephrine does not decline as plasma norepinephrine levels rise with increasing dose.

This suggests specific adrenergic neuron toxicity rather than a nonspecific response to an impairment in ventricular function. Valdés Olmos et al. [201] reported decreased myocardial MIBG uptake in patients with severely decreased ejection fraction after doxorubicin administration. Correlation with parameters derived from radionuclide angiocardiography suggested a global process of myocardial adrenergic derangement.

A decrease in myocardial MIBG uptake has also been reported regardless of the patient's functional status, suggesting a specific effect. Progressive myocyte necrosis during doxorubicin cardiotoxicity could be associated with cardiac neuroadrenergic tissue necrosis. In fact, the clinical course of doxorubicin cardiotoxicity suggests altered neuroendocrine physiology. This is supported by the observation of a decrease in adrenergic responsiveness and decreased myocardial catecholamine stores with increased plasma catecholamines. The decrease in myocardial MIBG accumulation parallels the evolution of ejection fraction [202]. At intermediate cumulative doses of 240–300 mg/m^2, 25% of patients present with some decrease in MIBG uptake. At maximal cumulative doses, there is a significant decrease in MIBG uptake consistent with impaired cardiac adrenergic activity. A moderate-to-marked decrease in myocardial MIBG uptake at high cumulative doses was observed in all patients but one with decrease in ejection fraction of 10 points [202]. These data suggest that the assessment of drug-induced sympathetic damage could be used to select patients at risk of severe functional impairment and who might benefit from cardioprotective agents or changes in the schedule or administration technique of antineoplastic drugs.

Future Directions

The neuronal function of the heart is altered in many cardiac disorders, such as congestive heart failure, ischemia, cardiac arrhythmias, and certain cardiomyopathies. Cardiac neurotransmission imaging opens many possible ways for improving our understanding of the pathophysiology of the diseases, selection of patients for various treatments, and assessment of the results of therapy. As new additional drugs are shown to be effective for treatment of heart failure, it becomes increasingly important to identify markers predictive of drug efficacy for individual patients. It is clear that neuronal receptor function can be modulated with appropriate treatments, therefore cardiac neurotransmission studies have great potential for impact on clinical decision making if the effectiveness of treatments can be assessed and predicted using SPECT or PET.

IMAGING ATHEROSCLEROTIC LESIONS

Radionuclide imaging of atherosclerotic lesions is expected to target histopathologic substrates of the plaque including lipid cores, macrophage infiltration, or proliferating smooth muscle cells [203]. Since predominance of one of these components determines the behavior of the plaque, it is logical to assume that detection of abundance of a given component will identify the prognostic outcome of plaque [203]. The presence of a large necrotic lipid core contributes to vulnerability of plaque to rupture, in a milieu of intense macrophage infiltration and attendant release of cytokines and matrix metalloproteinases. On the other hand, abundance of smooth muscle cells provides stability to the plaque, but rapid and exaggerated proliferation may lead to progressive luminal stenosis such as in postangioplastic restenosis. It is possible to selectively target any one of these components by radionuclide imaging.

Radiotracers for Potential Imaging of Atherosclerotic Lesions

Atherosclerosis is believed to be an immunoinflammatory process, which is probably initiated by elevated LDL cholesterol and its interaction with the vascular endothelial layer [204,205] (Fig. 21.6). Infiltration of modified LDL through the endothelial layer and consequent expression of adhesion molecules and selectins lead to recruitment of monocytes and their intimal migration. At this time, the growth factors released by dysfunctional endothelium, monocytes, and platelets induce proliferation and migration of medial smooth muscle cells (SMC) to the intimal layer. The neointimal monocyte-macrophages ingest oxidized cholesterol and develop into foam cells. Histomorphologically, the stable atherosclerotic lesion has a thick, multilayer fibrous cap. On the other hand, the vulnerable plaques demonstrate large lipid cores and thin fibrous caps, which harbor intense macrophage infiltration [206] (see Color Fig. 21.7 in separate color insert).

Identification of vulnerable or unstable plaques

Histopathologic characteristics dictate that vulnerable plaques can be identified by targeting either macrophages or large lipid cores. Various constituents of the lipid pool have been radiolabeled and used for noninvasive imaging of atherosclerotic plaques. It is presumed that radiolabeled components should accumulate in the lipid pool similar to unlabeled circulating lipids, lipoproteins, and apolipoproteins, and therefore

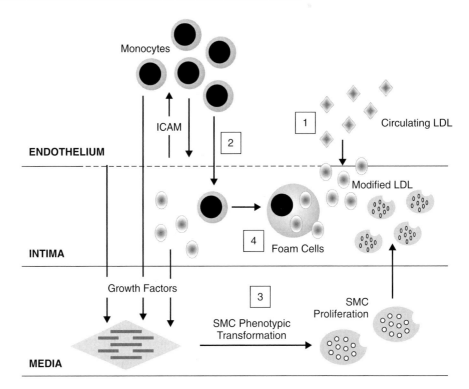

FIGURE 21.6 Evolution of atherosclerotic lesions. Although exact pathogenesis of atherosclerosis is not known, process usually involves oxidation of LDL (1) and endothelial expression of selectins and adhesion molecules, which leads to recruitment of monocytes and their subendothelial migration (2). Growth factors released by altered endothelium, monocytes, and platelets induce phenotypic alteration and proliferation of medial smooth muscle cells and subsequently their migration to intima (3). Subendothelial monocytes (and smooth muscle cells) ingest modified LDL to evolve into foam cells (4). (With permission from Narula et al. [203]).

radiolabeled LDL, cholesteryl ester, and apolipoprotein B have been used for atherosclerotic imaging. Iodine-131 and Tc-99m labeled LDL uptake have been demonstrated in atherosclerotic lesions in patients with carotid and femoral artery disease, as well as in xanthomatous lesions [207,208]. Similarly, iodinated cholesteryl iopanoate has been demonstrated in experimental atherosclerotic lesions in rabbits and subsides after treatment with hypolipidemic drugs [209]. Uptake of apolipoprotein B peptide- SP4 has also been demonstrated in spontaneous atherosclerotic lesions in Watanabe rabbits [210]. To improve the specificity of imaging, it was proposed that only those characteristics of modified lipids need to be targeted that are not expressed in the circulating lipids or lipoproteins. Accordingly, imaging with antibody MDA2, that only recognizes oxidized LDL and does not cross-react with circulating LDL, demonstrates intense uptake in lipid-rich atherosclerotic lesions [211]. Similarly, radiolabeled porphyrins accumulate in the esterified cholesterol deposits [212].

Targeting of macrophages constitutes another important strategy for the imaging of vulnerable plaques (Fig. 21.8). To enhance the specificity of imaging, only those macro-phage epitopes should be targeted that are borne exclusively on the resident macrophages and are not expressed by the circulating monocytes [202]. Numerous selectins and adhesion molecules or their receptors are expressed on monocytes during interaction with endothelium and transfer to subintimal layer (see Fig. 21.8). Development of scavenger receptors on macrophages after their transgression to subintima allows for unlimited ingestion of modified LDL cholesterol; scavenger receptor expression is not suppressed by lipid ingestion. A modest proportion of the scavenger receptors is complementary to the FC component of IgG, and targeting of plaque macrophages has been achieved with nonspecific IgG [213]. On the other hand, chemoattractant receptors and activation-dependent receptors are upregulated during diapedesis of monocytes. Iodinated monocyte chemotactic peptide (MCP-1) has been used for evaluating the intensity of macrophage infiltration in atherosclerotic lesions [214]. Similarly, it is presumed that activation dependent receptors such as Mac-1 can be targeted by radiolabeled LFA or ICAM or VCAM. Furthermore, excessive matrix metalloproteinase release in vulnerable plaques can be targeted with radiolabeled inhibitors of metalloproteinases.

Identification of postangioplastic restenosis

Aggressive proliferation of smooth muscle cells and vascular remodeling lead to restenotic complications of angioplasty [215] (see Color Fig. 21.9 in separate color insert). The likelihood of development of restenosis can be predicted by determining the rate of SMC proliferation by targeting unique antigens expressed by proliferating smooth muscle cells that are not present on quiescent medial cell. Smooth muscle cells are nondividing and maintain a contractile phenotype that contributes to vasoreactivity and vascular tone. These cells have abundant contractile proteins but no protein synthesis machinery. During the process of atherosclerosis or restenosis these cells are transformed, they lose contractile proteins, and

regain their synthetic machinery, to proliferate and migrate to neointima [216]. The transformation is initiated by altered release of vasoactive substances due to endothelial injury and subsequent alteration of extracellular matrix. The altered matrix can be targeted by radiolabeled integrins. The SMC during their phenotypic alteration acquire receptors for tyrosine kinase growth factors (such as PDGF and FGF), or G-protein coupled receptors (such as purinoceptors). Such growth factors can be radiolabeled and used for noninvasive imaging of upregulated receptors. Radiolabeled endothelin derivative [217] as well as diadenosine tetraphosphate [218] have been successfully used for imaging rapidly proliferating SMC. It is also possible to identify the amplified intracellular messenger RNA in proliferating smooth muscle cells. The growth factors lead to activation of a variety of proto-oncogenes and transcription factors such as *c-myb* and *cdk2* kinase, and induce cellular proliferation. It is presumed that radiolabeled antisense oligonucleotides would allow imaging of proliferating smooth muscle cells [219]. During the phenotypic transformation of smooth muscle, some new antigenic moieties are ex-

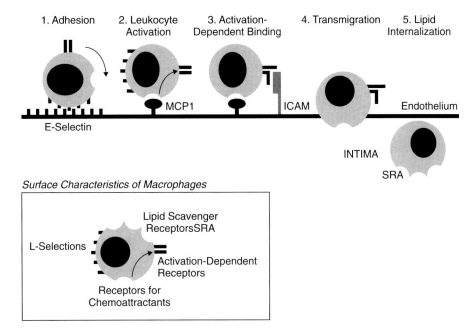

FIGURE 21.8 Model of monocyte-endothelial cell recognition as active phasic process. Monocytes in blood stream slow down and roll along injured endothelial surface because of reversible interaction between selectin molecules. Adherence of monocytes to endothelium is reinforced by endothelial expression of chemoattractants such as MCP-1. Engagement of chemoattractant receptor induces activation-dependent receptors of β1–β2 integrin family (such as LFA-1, VLA-4, Mac-1). Expression of immunoglobulin superfamily adhesion molecules (such as ICAM-1 or 2 and VCAM-1) interact with activation-dependent receptors. Recruited monocytes migrate across to intima through interendothelial cell junction. Subendothelial monocytes in vicinity or oxidized LDL evolve scavenger receptors such as SRA I or II, CD36, CD68 and FcγRII for lipid ingestion. These receptors are distinct from LDL receptors and are not downregulated by intracellular cholesterol contents. (With permission from Narula et al. [203]).

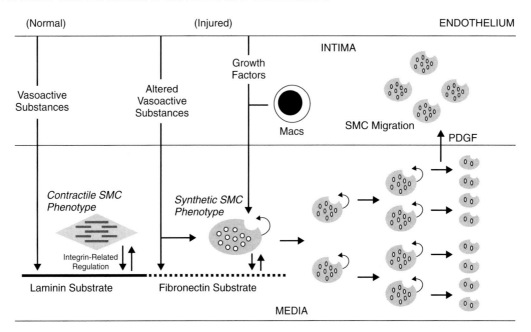

FIGURE 21.10 Phenotypic alteration, proliferation and migration of medical smooth muscle cells. Injured endothelium and altered release of vasoactive substances leads to alteration of extracellular matrix proteins and phenotypic transformation of smooth muscle cells. Smooth muscle cells in adult vasculature are differentiated, contain contractile protein, and do not divide (contractile phenotpe). Integrin-related mechanisms facilitate transformation of these cells into synthetic phenotype, which acquire fetal properties of abundant protein synthesis and proliferation. Transformed cells evolve receptors for growth factors and proliferate under influence of growth factors release from endothelium and accumulation of subendothelial lipids and monocytes. Proliferation of these cells becomes self-perpetuating process as they simultaneously secrete endogenous growth factors. Under influence of growth factors such as PDGF, the cells migrate to intima across internal elastic lamina. Receptors for growth factors expressed by proliferating smooth muscle cells comprise tyrosine kinase and G protein–coupled receptors. (With permission from Narula et al. [203]).

pressed on the cell surface. One such antigen, a heterodimeric protein with a sterol moiety, has been recently identified. The homologous antibody, Z2D3, labeled with In-111 was successfully used for imaging of experimental atherosclerosis in rabbits [220,221] as well as carotid atherosclerotic lesions [222] (see Color Fig. 21.11 in separate color insert) in the patients undergoing carotid endarterectomy (Fig. 21.10). Experimental studies with Z2D3 have demonstrated that the tracer uptake is directly proportional to the rate of SMC proliferation and hence should be able to predict impending restenosis [223].

Future Directions

Development of numerous radiotracers for the targeting of apecific histopathologic characteristics of the atheromatous plaques have raised hopes that prognostic stratification of subocclusive atherosclerotic lesions will become possible in the future. However, with the currently available imaging techniques, noninvasive localization of coronary vessels is difficult. Efforts are being made to develop intravascular imaging devices for possible assignment of *vulnerability score* to atherosclerotic lesions in coronary artery. Further, use of targeting agents based on pathophysiologic alterations should also allow better understanding of the atherogenetic process.

REFERENCES

Hypoxia Agents

1. Tardy-Cantalupi I, Montessuit C, Papgeorgiou I, et al. Effect of transient ischemia on the expression of glucose transporters GLUT-1 and GLUT-4 in rat myocardium. J Mol Cell Cardiol 1999;31:1143.
2. Workman P, Brown JM. Structure-pharmacokinetic relationships for misonidazole analogues in mice. Cancer Chemother Pharmacol 1981;6:39.
3. Mello T, Ballinger JR, Rauth AM. The role of NADPH:Cy-

tochrome P450 reductase in the hypoxic accumulation and metabolism of BRU59-21, a technetium-99m-nitroimidazole for imaging tumour hypoxia. Biochem Pharmacol 2000;60:625.

4. Kooji A, Bosch KS, Frederiks WM, et al. High levels of xanthine oxidoreductase in rat endothelial, epithelial and connective tissues. A relation between localization and function? Virchows Archiv B Cell Pathol 1992;62:143.

5. Podzuweit T, Beck H, Muller A, et al. Absence of xanthine oxidoreductase activity in human myocardium. Cardiovasc Res 1991;25:820.

6. Linder KE, Chan Y-W, Cyr JE, et al. The synthesis, characterisation and in vitro evaluation of nitroimidazole-BATO complexes; new technetium compounds for imaging hypoxia. Bioconjug Chem 1993;4:326.

7. Linder KE, Chan Y-W, Cyr JE, et al. TcO(PnAO-1-(2-nitroimidazole)) [BMS-181321], a new technetium-containing nitroimidazole complex for imaging hypoxia: synthesis, characterisation and xanthine oxidase-catalysed reduction. J Med Chem 1994;37:9.

8. Ramalingam K, Raju N, Nanjappan P, et al. The synthesis and in vitro evaluation of a technetium-99m-nitroimidazole complex based on a bis(amine-phenol) ligand: comparison to BMS-181321. J Med Chem 1994;37:4155.

9. Pirro JP, DiRocco R, Narra RK, et al. The relationship between in vitro transendothelial permeability and in vivo single-pass brain extraction. J Nucl Med 1994;35:1514.

10. Zhang Z, Mannan RH, Wiebe LI, et al. Development of a new technetium complex for hypoxia imaging: a technetium (V) amine nitrophenol complex. In: *Technetium and Rhenium in Chemistry and Nuclear Medicine* 4, edited by M Nicolini, G Bandoli, U Mazzi et al. Padova: SGE Ditorialli, 1995, pp. 307–312.

11. Norman TJ, Smith FC, Parker D, et al. Synthesis and biodistribution of ^{111}In, ^{67}Ga and ^{153}Gd-radiolabelled conjugates of nitroimidazoles with bifunctional complexing agents: imaging agents for hypoxic tissue? Supramolecular Chemistry 1995;4:305.

12. Cowan DSM, Melo T, Park L, et al. BMS181321 accumulation in rodent and human cells: the role of P-glycoprotein. Br J Cancer 1996;74:Suppl XXVII, S264.

13. Rasey JS, Martin GV, Krohn KA. Quantifying hypoxia with radiolabeled fluoromisonidazole: pre-clinical and clinical studies. In: *Imaging of Hypoxia. Tracer Developments*, edited by H-J Machulla. Dordrecht: Kluwer, 1999; pp. 85–117.

14. Wiebe LI. Radiohalogenated nitroimidazoles for single-photon scintigraphic imaging of hypoxic tissues. In: *Imaging of Hypoxia. Tracer Developments*. edited by H-J Machulla. Dordrecht: Kluwer, 1999, pp. 155–176.

15. Martin GV, Caldwell JH, Graham MM, et al. Noninvasive detection of hypoxic myocardium using fluorine-18-fluoromisonidazole and positron emission tomography. J Nucl Med 1992;33:2202.

16. Archer CM, Edwards B, Kelly JD, et al. Technetium labelled agents for imaging tissue hypoxia in vivo. In: *Technetium and Rhenium in Chemistry and Nuclear Medicine*, 4 edited by M Nicolini, G Bandoli, U Mazzi. Padova: SGE Ditorialli, 1995, pp. 535–539.

17. Fujibayashi Y, Cutler CS, Anderson CJ, et al. Comparative studies of Cu-64-ATSM and C-11-acetate in an acute myocardial infarction model: ex vivo imaging of hypoxia in rats. Nucl Med Biol 1999;26:117.

18. Horiuchi K, Tsukamoto T, Saito M, et al. The development of (99m) Tc-analog of Cu-DTS as an agent for imaging hypoxia. Nucl Med Biol 2000;27:391.

19. Okada RD, Johnson G 3rd, Nguyen KN, et al. 99mTC-HL91 "hot spot" detection of ischemic myocardium in vivo by gamma camera imaging. Circulation 1998;97:2557.

20. Chao KS, Bosch WR, Multic S, et al. A novel approach to overcome hypoxic tumour resistance: Cu-ATSM-guided intensity-modulated radiation therapy. Int J Radiat Oncol Biol Phys 2001;49:1171.

21. Rumsey WL, Cyr JE, Raju N, et al. A novel [99m]technetium-labeled nitroheterocyle capable of identification of hypoxia in the heart. Biochem Biophys Res Commun 1993;193:1239.

22. Nunn AD. The biology of technetium based hypoxic tissue localising agents. In: *Imaging of Hypoxia. Tracer Developments*, edited by H-J Machulla. Dordrecht: Kluwer, 1999, pp. 19–45.

23. Stone CK, Mulnix T, Nickles RJ, et al. Myocardial kinetics of a putative hypoxic tissue marker, Tc-99m-labeled nitroimidazole (BMS-181321), after regional ischemia and reperfusion. Circulation 1995;92:1246.

24. Martin GV, Biskupiak JE, Caldwell JH, et al. Characterisation of iodovinylmisonidazle as a marker for myocardial hypoxia. J Nucl Med 1993;34:918.

25. Watanabe Y, Kusuoka H, Fukuchi K, et al. Contribution of hypoxia to the development of cardiomyopathy in hamsters. Cardiovasc Res 1997;35:217.

26. Johnson LL, Schofield L, Mastrofrancesco P, et al. Technetium-99m-nitroimidazole uptake in a swine model of demand ischaemia. J Nucl Med 1998;39:1468.

27. Johnson LL, Schofield L, Donahay T, et al. Myocardial uptake of a 99m-Tc-nitroheterocycle in a swine model of occlusion and reperfusion. J Nucl Med 2000;41:1237.

28. Kuczynski B, Linder K, Patel B, et al. Dual isotope imaging of Tc-99m BMS-194796 and Tl-201 in dog coronary artery stenosis model. J Nucl Cardiol 1995;2:S29 (abstract).

29. DiRocco RJ, Bauer AA, Pirro JP, et al. Delineation of the border zone of ischemic rabbit myocardium by a technetium-labeled nitroimidazole. Nucl Med Biol 1997;24:201.

Newer Perfusion Agents

30. Jain D. Technetium-99m labeled myocardial perfusion imaging agents. Semin Nucl Med 1999;29:221.

31. Dahlberg ST, Leppo JA. Myocardial kinetics of radiolabeled perfusion agents: basis for perfusion imaging. J Nucl Cardiol 1994;1:189.

32. Rossetti V, Vanoli G, Paganelli G, et al. Human biodistribution, dosimetry, and clinical use of technetium-99m-Q12. J Nucl Med 1994;35:1571.

33. Gerson MC, Millard RW, Roszell NJ, et al. Kinetic properties of 99mTc-Q12 in canine myocardium. Circulation 1994;89:1291.

34. Gerson MC, Millard RW, McGoron AJ, et al. Myocardial uptake and kinetic properties of 99mTc-Q3 in dogs. J Nucl Med 1994;35:1698.

35. Rohe RC, Thomas SR, Stabin MG, et al. Biokinetics and dosimetry analysis in healthy volunteers for a two-injection (rest-stress) protocol of the myocardial perfusion imaging agent technetium 99m-labeled Q3. J Nucl Cardiol 1995;2:395.

36. Hendel RC. Technetium 99m furifosmin. In *New Developments in Cardiac Nuclear Imaging*, edited by AE Iskandrian and MS Verani. Armonk, NY: Futura Publishing, 1998, pp. 59–78.

37. Gerson MC, Lukes J, Rosenbaum A, et al. Technetium-99m Q4: a prototype cationic perfusion radiotracer with myocardial washout. Eur J Nucl Med 1998;25:253.

38. McGoron AJ, Biniakiewicz DS, Millard RW, et al. Myocardial kinetics of technetium-99m Q agents: studies in isolated cardiac myocyte, isolated perfused rat heart and canine regional myocardial ischemia models. Invest Radiol 1999;34:704.

39. Pascualini R, Duttani A, Bellande E, et al. Bis(dithiocarbamato) nitrido technetium-99m radiopharmaceuticals: a class of neutral myocardial imaging agents. J Nucl Med 1994;35:334.

40. McGoron AJ, Gerson MC, Biniakiewicz DS, et al. Extraction and retention of technetium-99m Q12, technetium-99m sestamibi, and thallium-201 in isolated rat heart during coronary acidemia. Eur J Nucl Med 1997;24:1779.

41. McGoron AJ, Gerson MC, Biniakiewicz DS, et al. Effects of ouabain on technetium-99m-Q12 and thallium-201 extraction and retention by isolated rat heart. J Nucl Med 1996;37:752.

42. Ucelli L, Giganti M, Duatti A, et al. Subcellular distribution of technetium-99m N-NOET in rat myocardium. J Nucl Med 1995;36:2075.

43. Riou L, Ghezzi C, Mouton O, et al. Cellular uptake mechanism of ^{99m}TcN-NOET in cardiomyocytes from newborn rats: calcium channel interaction. Circulation 1998;98:2591.

44. Johnson G III, Nguyen KN, Pascuallini R, et al. Interaction of technetium 99m N-NOET with blood elements: potential mechanism of myocardial redistribution. J Nucl Med 1997;38:138.

45. Ghezzi C, Fagret D, Arvieux CC, et al. Myocardial kinetics of 99mTcN-NOET: a neutral lipophilic complex tracer of regional myocardial blood flow. J Nucl Med 1995;336:1069.

46. Johnson G III, Allton IL, Nguyen KN, et al. Clearance of technetium 99m N-NOET in normal, ischemic-reperfused, and membrane-disrupted myocardium. J Nucl Cardiol 1996;3:42.

47. Fagret D, Marie PY, Brunotte F, et al. Myocardial perfusion imaging with technetium-99m-Tc NOET: comparison with thallium-201 and coronary angiography. J Nucl Med 1995;36:936.

48. Vanzetto G, Calnon D, Ruiz M, et al. Myocardial uptake and redistribution of 99mTcN-NOET in dogs with either sustained coronary low flow or transient coronary occlusion: comparison with ^{201}Tl and myocardial blood flow. Circulation 1997;96:2325.

49. Johnson G III, Nguyen KN, Liu Z, et al. Planar imaging of ^{99m}Tc-labeled (bis(N-ethoxy, N-ethyl dithiocarbamato) nitrido technetium (V)) can detect resting ischemia. J Nucl Cardiol 1997;4:217.

50. Meleca MJ, McGoron AJ, Gerson MC, et al. Flow versus uptake comparisons of thallium-201 with six technetium-99m perfusion tracers in a canine model of myocardial ischemia. J Nucl Med 1997;38:1847.

51. Okada R, Nguyen K, Lauinger M, et al. Effects of no flow and reperfusion on technetium-99m-Q12 kinetics. J Nucl Med 1995;36:2103.

52. Petruzella FD, Ruiz M, Katsiyiannis P, et al. Optimal timing for initial and redistribution technetium 99m-N-NOET image acquisition. J Nucl Cardiol 2000;7:123.

53. Riou L, Ghezzi C, Pascualini R, et al. Influence of calcium channel inhibitors on the myocardial uptake and retention of technetium 99m N-NOET, a new myocardial perfusion imaging agent: a study on isolate perfused rat hearts. J Nucl Cardiol 2000;7:365.

54. Holly TA, Leppo JA, Gilmore MP, et al. The effect of ischemic injury on the cardiac transport of Tc-99m N-NOET in the isolated rabbit heart. J Nucl Cardiol 1999;6:633.

55. Vanzetto G, Glover DK, Ruiz M, et al. ^{99m}TcN-NOET myocardial uptake reflects myocardial blood flow and not viability in dogs with reperfused acute myocardial infarction. Circulation 2000;101:2424.

56. Calnon DA, Ruiz M, Vanzetto G, et al. Myocardial uptake of ^{99m}TcN-NOET and ^{201}Tl during dobutamine infusion: comparison with adenosine stress. Circulation 1999;100:1653.

57. Calnon DA, Glover DK, Beller GA, et al. Effects of dobutamine stress on myocardial blood flow, ^{99m}Tc-sestamibi uptake and systolic wall thickening in the presence of coronary artery stenoses: implications for dobutamine stress testing. Circulation 1997;96:2353.

58. Wu JC, Yun JJ, Heller EN, et al. Limitations of dobutamine for enhancing flow heterogeneity in the presence of single coronary stenosis: implications for technetium-99m-sestamibi imaging. J Nucl Med 1998;39:417.

59. Hendel RC, Verani MS, Miller DD, et al. Diagnostic utility of tomographic myocardial perfusion imaging with technetium 99m furifosmin (Q12) compared with thallium 201: results of a phase III multicenter trial. J Nucl Cardiol 1996;3:291.

60. Gerson MC, Lukes J, Deutsch E, et al. Comparison of Tc-99m Q12 and Tl 201 imaging for detection of angiographic coronary artery disease. J Nucl Cardiol 1994;1:499.

61. Gerson MC, Lukes J, Deutsch E, et al. Comparison of Tc-99m Q3 and thallium-201 for detection of coronary artery disease in humans. J Nucl Med 1994;35:580.

62. Gerson MC, Lukes J, Deutsch E, et al. Comparison of imaging properties of technetium 99m Q12 and technetium 99m Q3 in humans. J Nucl Cardiol 1995;2:224.

63. Naruse H. Daher D. Sinusas A, et al. Quantitative comparison of planar and SPECT normal data files of thallium-201, technetium-99m-sestamibi, technetium-99m-tetrofosmin and technetium-99m-furifosmin. J Nucl Med 1996;37:1783.

64. Cuocolo A, Rubini G, Acampa W, et al. Technetium 99m furifosmin regional myocardial uptake in patients with previous myocardial infarction: relation to thallium-201 activity and left ventricular function. J Nucl Cardiol 2000;7:235.

65. Vanzetto G, Fagret D, Pascualini R, et al. Biodistribution, dosimetry, and safety of myocardial perfusion imaging agent ^{99m}TcN-NOET in healthy volunteers. J Nucl Med 2000;41:141.

66. Iiada H, Eberl S. Quantitative assessment of regional myocardial blood flow with thallium-201 and SPECT. J Nucl Cardiol 1998;5:313.

Myocardial Necrosis

67. Pope JH, Aufderheide TP, Ruthazer R, et al. Missed diagnosed of acute cardiac ischemia in the emergency department. N Engl J Med 2000;342:1163.

68. Rude PE, Poole WK, Muller JE, et al. Electrocardiographic and clinical criteria for recognition of acute myocardial infarction based on analysis of 3,697 patients. Am J Cardiol 1983;52:936.

69. Khaw BA. The current role of infarct avid imaging. Semin Nucl Med 1999;29:259.

70. Khaw BA, Gold HK, Fallon JT, et al. Scintigraphic quantification of myocardial necrosis in patients after intravenous injection of cardiac myosin specific antibody. Circulation 1986;74:501.

71. Khaw BA, Yasuda T, Gold HK, et al. Acute myocardial infarction imaging with indium-111 labeled monoclonal antimyosin Fab fragments. J Nucl Med 1987;28:1671.

72. Johnson LL, Seldin DW, Becker LC, et al. Antimyosin imaging in acute transmural myocardial infarction: results of a multicenter clinical trial. J Am Coll Cardiol 1989;13:27.

73. Nedelman MA, Shealy DK, Boulin R, et al. Rapid infarct imaging with a technetium-99m-labeled antimyosin recombinant single chain Fv: evaluation in a canine model of acute myocardial infarction. J Nucl Med 1993;34:234.

74. Tamaki N, Yamada T, Matsumori A, et al. Indium-111 antimyosin monoclonal antibody imaging for detecting different stages of myocardial infarction: comparison with tecnetium-99m-pyrophosphate imaging. J Nucl Med 1990;31:136.

75. Ballester M, Obrador D, Carrió I, et al. Early postoperative reduction of monoclonal antimyosin antibody uptake is associated with absent rejection-related complications after heart transplantation. Circulation 1992;85:61.

76. Hosenpud JD. Noninvasive diagnosis of cardiac allograft rejection: another of many searchers for the grail. Circulation 1992;85:386.

77. Ballester M, Obrador D, Carrió I, et al. ^{111}In-monoclonal antimyosin antibody studies after the first year of heart transplantation: identification of risk groups for developing rejection during long-term follow-up and clinical implications. Circulation 1990;82:2100.

78. Carrió I, Lopez-Pousa A, Estorch M, et al. Detection of doxorubicin cardiotoxicity in patients with sarcomas by indium-111 antimyosin monoclonal antibody studies. J Nucl Med 1993;34:1503.

79. Yasuda T, Palacios IF, Dec GW, et al. Indium-111 antimyosin monoclonal antibody imaging in the diagnosis of acute myocarditis. Circulation 1987;76:306.

80. Dec GW, Palacios IF, Yasuda T, et al. Antimyosin antibody cardiac imaging: its role in the diagnosis of myocarditis. J Am Coll Cardiol 1990;16:97.

81. Narula J, Khaw BA, Dec GW, et al. Recognition of acute myocarditis masquerading as acute myocardial infarction. N Engl J Med 1993;3:100.

82. Obrador D, Ballester M, Carrió I, et al. High prevalence of myocardial monoclonal antimyosin antibody uptake in patients with chronic idiopathic dilated cardiomyopathy. J Am Coll Cardiol 1989;13:1289.

83. Obrador D, Ballester M, Carrió I, et al. Active myocardial damage without attending inflammatory response in idiopathic dilated cardiomyopathy. J Am Coll Cardiol 1993;21:1667.

84. Obrador D, Ballester M, Carrió I, et al. Presence, evolving changes, and prognostic implications of myocardial damage detected in idiopathic and alcoholic dilated cardiomyopathy by ^{111}In monoclonal antimyosin antibodies. Circulation 1994;89:2054.

85. Flotats A, Domingo P, Carrió I. Dilated cardiomyopathy in HIV-infected patients. N Engl J Med 1999;340:733.

86. Nishimura T, Nagata S, Uehara T, et al. Assessment of myocardial damage in dilated-phase hypertrophic cardiomyopathy by using indium-111-antimyosin Fab myocardial scintigraphy. J Nucl Med 1991;32:1333.

87. Data on file. Centocor, Inc. Myoscint PLA 94-1210.

88. Orlandi C, Crane PD, Edwards S, et al. Early scintigraphic detection of experimental myocardial infarction in dogs with technetium-99m-glucaric acid. J Nucl Med 1991;32:236.

89. Fornet BB, Yasuda T, Wilkinson R, et al. Detection of acute cardiac injury with technetium-99m glucaric acid [abstract]. J Nucl Med 1989;30:1743.

90. Yaoita H, Fischman AJ, Wilkinson R, et al. Distribution of deoxyglucose and technetium-99m-glucarate in the acutely ischemic myocardium. J Nucl Med 1993;34:1303.

91. Ohtani H, Callahan RJ, Khaw BA, et al. Comparison of technetium-99m-glucarate and thallium-201 for the identification of acute myocardial infarction in rats. J Nucl Med 1992;33:1988.

92. Narula J, Petrov A, Pak KY, et al. Very early noninvasive detection of acute experimental nonreperfused myocardial infarction with ^{99m}Tc-labeled glucarate. Circulation 1995;95:1577.

93. Beanlands RSB, Ruddy TD, Bielawsky L, et al. Differentiation of myocardial ischemia and necrosis by technetium 99m glucaric acid kinetics. J Nucl Cardiol 1997;4:274.

94. Khaw BA, Nakazama A, O'Donell SM, et al. Avidity of technetium 99m glucarate for the necrotic myocardium: in vivo and in vitro assessment. J Nucl Cardiol 1997;4:283.

95. Blankenberg FG, Katsikis PD, Tait JF, et al. Comparison of Tc-99m glucarate uptake in apoptotic (programmed) and necrotic cell death [abstract]. J Nucl Med 1997;38:192P.

96. Mariani G, Villa G, Rossettin PF, et al. Detection of myocardial infarction by ^{99m}Tc-labeled D-glucaric acid imaging in patients with acute chest pain. J Nucl Med 1999;40:1832.

97. Flotats A, Narula J, Santaló M, et al. Myocardial uptake of technetium-99m glucarate occurs in acute regional myocardial necrosis but not in diffuse ongoing myocardial damage [abstract]. J Nucl Cardiol 1999;6(Suppl):S100.

98. Gerson MC, McGoron AJ. Technetium 99m-glucarate: what will be its clinical role? J Nucl Cardiol 1997;4:336.

Myocardial Apoptosis

99. Kerr JF, Wyllie AH, Currie AR. Apoptosis: a basic biological phenomenon with wide-ranging implications in tissue kinetics. Br J Cancer 1972;26:239.

100. Thompson BC. Apoptosis in the pathogenesis and treatment of disease. Science 1995;267:1456.

101. Narula J, Haider N, Virmani R, et al. Apoptosis in myocytes in end-stage heart failure. N Engl J Med 1996;335:1182.

102. Narula J, Hajjar RJ, Dec GW. Apoptosis in heart failure. Cardiol Clin 1998;16:691.

103. Narula J, Pandey P, Arbustin E, et al. Human cardiomyopathy. Proc Natl Acad Sci USA 1999;96:8144.

104. Narula J, Kolodgie F, Virmani R. Apoptosis in cardiomyopathy. Curr Opin Cardiol 2000;53:267.

105. Narula J, Arbustini E, Chandrashekhar Y, et al. Apoptosis in heart failure: a story of apoptosis interruptus and zombie myocytes. Cardiol Clin 2001;19:113.

106. Nagata S, Golstein P. The Fas death factor. Science 1995;267:1449.

107. Thornberry NA, Lazebnik Y, Caspases: enemies within. Science 1998;281:1312.

108. Zwaal RFA, Schroit AJ. Pathophysiologic implications of membrane phospholipid asymmetry in blood cells. Blood 1997;89:1121.

109. Martin SJ, Reutelingsperger CPM, McGahon AJ, et al. Early redistribution of plasma membrane phosphatidylserine is a general feature of apoptosis regardless of the initiating stimulus: inhibition by overexpression of Bcl-2 and Abl. J Exp Med 1995;182:1545.

110. van Engeland M, Kuijpers HJH, Ramaekers FCS, et al. Plasma membrane alterations and cytoskeletal changes in apoptosis. Exp Cell Res 1997;235:421.

111. Allen RT, Hunter WJ, Agrawal DK. Morphological and biochemical characterization and analysis of apoptosis. J Pharmacol Toxicol Methods 1997;37:215.

112. van England M, Mieland LJW, Ramaekers FCS, et al. Annexin V-affinity assay: a review on an apoptosis detection system based on phosphatidylserine exposure. Cytometry 1998;31:1.

113. Fadok VA, Bratton DL, Rose DM, et al. A receptor for phosphatidylserine-specific clearance of apoptotic cells. Nature 2000;405:85.

114. Hofstra L, Liem IH, Dumont EA, et al. Visualization of cell death in vivo in patients with acute myocardial infarction. Lancet 2000;356:209.

115. Dumont EAWJ, Hofstra L, van Heerde WL, et al. Cardiomyocyte death induced by myocardial ischemia and reperfusion. Circulation 2000;102:1564.

116. Wood BL, Gibson DF, Tait JF. Increased phosphatidylserine exposure in sickle cell disease: flow-cytometric measurement and clinical associations. Blood 1996;88:1873.

117. Blankenberg FG, Katsikis PD, Tait JF, et al. In vivo detection and imaging of phosphatidylserine expression during programmed cell death. Proc Natl Acad Sci USA 1998;95:6349.

118. Larsen SK, Solomon HF, Caldwell G, et al. [99mTc]tricine: a useful precursor complex for the radiolabeling of hydrazinonicotinate protein conjugates. Bioconjug Chem 1995;6:635.

119. Brankenberg F, Narula J, Strauss HW. Diagnosis of apoptosis: a measure necessary in myocardial ischemia, infarction and inflammation. J Nucl Cardiol 1999;

120. Takeda K, Yu ZX, Nishikawa T, et al. Apoptosis and DNA fragmentation in the bulbus caordis of the developing rat heart. J Mol Cell Cardiol 1996;28:209.

121. James TN. Complete heart block and fatal right ventricular failure in an infant. Circulation 1996; 1588.

122. Itoh G, Tamura J, Suzuki M, et al. DNA fragmentation of human infarcted myocardial cells demonstrated by the nick and labeling method and DNA agarose gel electrophoresis. Am J Pathol 1995;146:1325.

123. Gottlieb RA, Buresldon KO, Kloner RA, Babior BM, Engler RL. Reperfusion injury induced apoptosis in rabbit cardiac myocytes. J Clin Invest 1994;74:86.

124. Szabolcs M, Michler RE, Yang X et al. Apoptosis of cardiac myocytes during cardiac allograft rejection. Relation to induction of nitric oxide synthase. Circulation 1996;94(7):1665.

125. Puig M, Ballester M, Matias-Guiu X, Bordes R, Carrió I, Aymat MR, Marrugat J, Padró JM, Caralps JM, Narula J. Burden of myocardial damage in cardiac allograft rejection: scintigraphic evidence of myocardial injury and histologic evidence of myocyte necrosis and apoptosis. J Nucl Cardiol 2000;7:132.

126. Narula J, Acio ER, Narula N, Samuels LE, Fyfe B, Wood D, Fitzpatrick JM, Raghunath PN, Tomaszewski JE, Kelly C, Steinmetz N, Green A, Tait JF, Leppo J, Blankenberg FG, Jain D, Strauss HW. Annexin-V imaging for noninvasive detection of cardiac allograft rejection. Nature Medicine 2001;7:1347.

Disordered Neurotransmission

127. Luxen A, Perlmutter M, Vida G, et al. Remote, semiautomated production of 6-F18-fluoro-L-dopa for human studies with PET. Int Appl Rad Isot 1990;41:275.

128. Schwaiger M, Kalff V, Rosenpire K, et al. Noninvasive evaluation of sympathetic nervous system in human heart by positron emission tomography. Circulation 1990;82:357.

129. Rosenpire KC, Haka MS, Jewett DM, et al. Synthesis and preliminary evaluation of 11C-meta-hydroxyephedrine: a false neurotransmitter agent for heart neuronal imaging. J Nucl Med 1990;31:1328.

130. Chakraborty PK, Gildersleeve DL, Jewett DM, et al. High yield synthesis of high specific activity 11C-epinephrine for routine PET studies in humans. Nucl Med Biol 1993;20:939.

131. Münch G, Nguyen N, Nekolla S, et al. Evaluation of sympathetic nerve terminals with 11C-epinephrine and 11C-hydroxyephedrine and positron emission tomography. Circulation 2000;101:516.

132. Ungerer M, Hartmann F, Karoglan M, et al. Regional in vivo and in vitro characterization of autonomic innervation in cardiomyopathic human heart. Circulation 1998;97:174.

133. Short JH, Darby TD. Sympathetic nervous system blocking agents. Derivatives of benzylguanidine. J Med Chem 1967;10:833.

134. Wieland DM, Brown LE, Rogers WL, et al. Myocardial imaging with a radioiodinated norepinephrine storage analog. J Nucl Med 1981;22:22.

135. Wieland DM, Wu JI, Brown LE, et al. Radiolabeled adrenergic neuron-blocking agents: adrenomedullary imaging with 123I-iodobenzylguanidine. J Nucl Med 1980;21:349.

136. Sisson JC, Wieland DM, Sherman P, et al. Metaiodobenzylguanidine as an index of adrenergic nervous system integrity and function. J Nucl Med 1987;28:1620.

137. Sisson JC, Bolgos G, Jhonson J. Measuring acute changes in adenergic nerve activity of the heart in the living animal. Am Heart J 1991;121:1119.

138. Knickmeier M, Matheja P, Wichter T, et al. Clinical evaluation of no-carrier-added meta-(123I)iodobenzylguanidine for myocardial scintigraphy. Eur J Nucl Med 2000;3:302.

139. Gill JS, Hunter GJ, Gane G, et al. Heterogeneity of the human myocardial sympathetic innervation: in vivo demonstration by iodine 123-labeled metaiodobenzylguanidine scintigraphy. Am Heart J 1993;126:390.

140. Delforge J, Syrota A, Lancon JP. Cardiac beta-adrenergic receptor density measured in vivo using PET, CGP 12177, and a new graphical method. J Nucl Med 1991;32:739.

141. Qing F, Rahman S, Hayes M, et al. Effect of long term Ū2-agonist dosing on human cardiac β-adrenoceptor expression in vivo: comparison with changes in lung and mononuclear leukocyte β-receptors. J Nucl Cardiol 1997;4:532.

142. Schaffers M, Schober O, Lerch H. Cardiac sympathetic neurotransmission scitigraphy. Eur J Nucl Med 1998;25:435.

143. Berridge MS, Nelson AD, Zheng LB, et al. Specific beta-adrenergic receptor binding of carazolol measured with PET. J Nucl Med 1994;35:1665.

144. Visser T, vanWaarde A, van der Mark T, et al. Characterization of pulmonary and myocardial beta-adrenoceptors with S-1'-(fluorine-18)fluorocarazolol. J Nucl Med 1997;38:169.

145. Valette H, Deleuze P, Syrota A, et al. Canine myocardial beta-adrenergic muscarinic receptor densities after denervation: a PET study. J Nucl Med 1995;36:140.

146. Le Guludec D, Cohen A, Delforge J, et al. Increased myocardial muscarinic receptor density in idiopathic dilated cardiomyopathy: an in vivo PET study. Circulation 1997;96:3416.

147. Estorch M, Carrió I, Berná L et al. Myocardial iodine-labeled metaiodobenzylguanidine uptake relates to age. J Nucl Cardiol 1995;2:126.

148. Yamazaki J, Muto H, Ishiguro K, et al. Quantitative scintigraphic analysis of 123I-MIBG by polar map in patients with dilated cardiomyopathy. Nucl Med Commun 1997;3:219.

149. Somsen GA, Borm JJ, deMilliano PA, et al. Quantitation of myocardial iodine-123-MIBG uptake in SPECT studies: a new approach using the left ventricular cavity and a blood sample as a reference. Eur J Nucl Med 1995;22:1149.

150. Somsen A. Cardiac neuronal dysfunction in heart failure assessed by 123-Iodine metaiodobenzylguanidine scintigraphy. Thesis, University of Amsterdam, the Netherlands, 1996.

151. Goldstein DS, Holmes C, Cannon RE, et al. Sympathetic cardioneuropathy in dysautonomias. N Engl J Med 1997;336:696.

152. De Marco T, Dae M, Yuen MS, et al. Iodine-123 MIBG scintigraphic assessment of the transplanted human heart: evidence for late reinnervation. J Am Coll Cardiol 1995;25:927.

153. Schwaiger M, Hutchins GB, Kalff V. Evidence for regional catecholamine uptake and storage sites in the transplanted human heart by positron emission tomography. J Clin Invest 1991;87:1681.

154. Dae M, DeMarco T, Botvinick E, et al. Scintigraphic assessment of MIBG uptake in globally denervated human and canine hearts: implications and clinical studies. J Nucl Med 1992;33:1444.

155. DiCarli MF, Tobes MC, Manger T, et al. Effects of cardiac sympathetic innervation on coronary blood flow. N Engl J Med 1997;336:1208.

156. Estorch M, Camprecios M, Flotats A, et al. Sympathetic reinnervation of cardiac allografts evaluated by 123I-MIBG imaging. J Nucl Med 1999;40:911.

157. Lerch H, Wichter T, Schamberger R, et al. Sympathetic myocardial innervation in idiopathic ventricular tachycardia and fibrillation. Eur J Nucl Med 1995;22:805.

158. Schafers M, Lerch H, Wichter T, et al. Cardiac autonomic dysfunction in patients with idiopathic ventricular tachycardia assessed by PET CGP 12177. J Nucl Med 1997;38:171.

159. Schafers M, Lerch H, Wichter T, et al. Cardiac sympathetic innervation in patients with idiopathic right ventricular outflow tract tachycardia. J Am Coll Cardiol 1998;32:181.

160. Ungerer M, Bohm M, Elce JS, et al. Altered expression of beta-adrenergic receptor kinase and beta-adrenergic receptors in the failing human heart. Circulation 1993;87:454.

161. Henderson EB, Kahn JK, Corbet J, et al. Abnormal I-123-MIBG myocardial wash-out and distribution may reflect myocardial adrenergic derangement in patients with congestive cardiomyopathy. Circulation 1988;78:1192.

162. Merlet P, Dubois JL, Adnot S, et al: Myocardial beta-adrenergic desensitization and neuronal norepinephrine uptake function in idiopathic dilated cardiomyopathy. J Cardiovasc Pharmacol 1992;19:10.

163. Merlet P, Valette H, Dubois JL, et al. Prognostic value of cardiac metaiodobenzylguanidine imaging in patients with heart failure. J Nucl Med 1992;33:471.

164. Merlet P, Benvenuti C, Moyse D, et al. Prognostic value of MIBG imaging in idiopathic dilated cardiomyopathy. J Nucl Med 1999;40:917.

165. Maunoury C, Agostini D, Acar PH, et al. Impairment of cardiac neuronal function in childhood dilated cardiomyopathy: an I123-MIBG scintigraphic study. J Nucl Med 2000;41:400.

166. Momose M, Kobayashi H, Iguchi N, et al. The comparison of parameters of I-123-MIBG scintigraphy for predicting prognosis in patients with dilated cardiomyopathies. Nucl Med Commun 1999;20:529.

167. Cohen-Soal A, Esanu Y, Logeart D, et al. Cardiac metaiodobenzylguanidine uptake in patients with moderate chronic heart failure: relationship with peak oxygen uptake and prognosis. J Am Coll Cardiol 1999;33:759.

168. Nakajima K, Taki J, Tonami M, et al. Decreased 123I-MIBG uptake and increased clearance in various cardiac disorders. Nucl Med Commun 1994;15:317.

169. Suwa M, Otake Y, Moriguchi A, et al. Iodine-123 meta-iodobenzylguanidine myocardial scintigraphy for prediction of response to beta-blocker therapy in patients with dilated cardiomyopathy. Am Heart J 1997;133:353.

170. Narula J, Haider N, Virmani R, et al. Programmed myocyte death in end-stage heart failure. N Engl J Med 1996;335:1182.

171. Fagret D, Wolf JE, Comet M. Myocardial uptake of meta-[123I]-iodobenzylguanidine ([123I]-MIBG) in patients with myocardial infarct. Eur J Nucl Med 1989;15:624.

172. McGhie AI, Corbett JR, Akers MS, et al. Regional cardiac adrenergic function using I-123 meta-iodobenzylguanidine tomographic imaging after acute myocardial infarction. Am J Cardiol 1991;67:236.

173. Nishimura T, Oka H, Sago M, et al. Serial assessment of denervated but viable myocardium following acute myocardial infarction in dogs using iodine-123 MIBG and thallium-201 chloride myocardial single photon emission tomography. Eur J Nucl Med 1992;19:25.

174. Minardo JD, Tuli MM, Mock BH, et al. Scintigraphic and electrophysiological evidence of canine myocardial sympathetic denervation and reinnervation produced by myocardial infarction or phenol application. Circulation 1988;78:1008.

175. Hartikainen J, Mäntysaari M, Kuikka J, et al. Extent of cardiac autonomic denervation in relation to angina on exercise test in patients with recent acute myocardial infarction. Am J Cardiol 1994;74:760.

176. Hartikainen J, Kuikka J, Mantsayaari M, et al. Sympathetic reinnervation after acute myocardial infarction. Am J Cardiol 1996;77:5.

177. Hartikainen J, Mustonen J, Kuikka J, et al. Cardiac sympathetic denervation in patients with coronary artery disease without previous myocardial infarction. Am J Cardiol 1997;80:273.

178. Nakata T, Nagao K, Tsuchihashi K, et al. Regional cardiac sympathetic nerve dysfunction and the diagnostic efficacy of metaiodobenzylguanidine tomography in stable coronary artery disease. Am J Cardiol 1996;78:292.

179. Kramer CM, Nicol PD, Rogers WJ, et al. Reduced sympathetic innervation underlies adjacent noninfarcted region dysfunction during left ventricular remodelling. J Am Coll Cardiol 1997;30:1079.

180. Podio V, Spinnler MT, Spandonari T, et al. Regional sympathetic denervation after myocardial infarction: a follow-up study using [123I]MIBG. Q J Nucl Med 1995;39:40.

181. Matsunari I, Schricke U, Bengel FM, et al. Extent of cardiac sympathetic neuronal damage is determined by the area of ischemia in patients with acute coronary syndromes. Circulation 2000;22:2579.

182. Dae MW, O'Connell JW, Botvinik E, et al. Acute and chronic effects of transient myocardial ischemia on sympathetic nerve activity, density, and norepinephrine content. Cardiovasc Res 1995;30:270.

183. Agostini D, Lecluse E, Belin A, et al. Impact of exercise rehabilitation on cardiac neuronal function in heart failure: an iodine-123 metaiodobenzylguanidine scintigraphy study. Eur J Nucl Med 1998;25:235.

184. Estorch M, Flotats A, Serra-grima R, et al. Influence of exercise rehabilitation on myocardial perfusion and sympathetic heart innervation in ischemic heart disease. Eur J Nucl Med 2000;3:333.

185. Lefroy DC, DeSilva R, Choudury L, et al. Myocardial beta-adrenoceptor density is reduced in hypertrophic cardiomyopathy. Circulation 1992;86:I.

186. Lefroy DC, deSilva R, Choudury L, et al. Diffuse reduction of myocardial beta-adrenoceptors in hypertrophic cardiomyopathy: a study with positron emission tomography. J Am Coll Cardiol 1993;22:1653.

187. Schaffers M, Dutka D, Rhodes CG, et al. Myocardial pre and post-synaptic autonomic dysfunction in hypertrophic cardiomyopathy. Circ Res 1998;82:56.

188. Li ST, Tack CJ, Fananapazir L, et al. Myocardial perfusion and sympathetic innervation in patients with hypertrophic cardiomyopathy. J Am Coll Cardiol 2000;7:1867.

189. Choudury L, Guzzeti S, Lefroy DC, et al. Myocardial beta-adrenoceptors and left ventricular function in hypertrophic cardiomyopathy. Heart 1996;75:50.

190. Lerch H, Bartenstein P, Wichter T, et al. Sympathetic innervation of the left ventricle is impaired in arrhythmogenic right ventricular disease. Eur J Nucl Med 1993;20:207.

191. Wichter T, Hindricks G, Lerch H, et al. Regional myocardial sympathetic dysinnervation in arrhythmogenic right ventricular cardiomyopathy. An analysis using ^{123}I-MIBG scintigraphy. Circulation 1994;89:667.

192. Wichter T, Lerch H, Schafers M, et al. Reduction of postsynaptic beta-receptor density in arrhythmogenic right ventricular dysplasia: assessment with positron emission tomography. Circulation 1996;94 Suppl I:I.

193. Wichter T, Schafers M, Rhodes CG, et al. Abnormalities of cardiac sympathetic innervation in arrhythmogenic right ventricular cardiomyopathy: quantitative assessment of presynaptic norepinephrine reuptake and postsynaptic beta-adrenergic receptor density with PET. Circulation 2000;13:1552.

194. Kim SJ, Lee JD, Ryu YH, et al. Evaluation of cardiac sympathetic neuronal integrity in diabetic patients using iodine-123 MIBG. Eur J Nucl Med 1996;23:401.

195. Scognamiglio R, Avogaro A, Casara D, et al. Myocardial dysfunction and adrenergic cardiac innervation in patients with insulin-dependent diabetes. J Am Coll Cardiol 1998;31:404.

196. Hattori N, Tamaki N, Hayasi T, et al. Regional abnormality of iodine-123-MIBG in diabetic hearts. J Nucl Med 1996;37:1985.

197. Morimoto S, Terada K, Keira N, et al. Investigation of the relationship between regression of hypertensive cardiac hypertrophy and improvement of cardiac sympathetic nervous dysfunction using iodine-123-MIBG. Eur J Nucl Med 1996;23:756.

198. Morimitsu T, Miyahara Y, Sinboku H, et al. Iodine-123-metaiodobenzylguanidine myocardial imaging in patients with right ventricular pressure overload. J Nucl Med 1996;37:1343.

199. Sakamaki F, Satoh T, Nagaya N, et al. Correlation between severity of pulmonary arterial hypertension and ^{123}I-metaiodobenzylguanidine left ventricular imaging. J Nucl Med 2000;7:1127.

200. Wakasugi S, Fischman AJ, Babich JW, et al. Metaiodobenzylguanidine: evaluation of its potential as a tracer for monitoring doxorubicin cardiomyopathy. J Nucl Med 1993;34:1282.

201. Valdés Olmos RA, ten Bokkel Huinink WW, ten Hoeve RF, et al. Assessment of anthracycline-related myocardial adrenetgic derangement by ^{123}I-MIBG scintigraphy. Eur J Cancer 1995;31A:26.

202. Carrió I, Estorch M, Berná LI, et al. 111In-antimyosin and ^{123}I-MIBG studies in the early assessment of doxorubicin cardiotoxicity. J Nucl Med 1995:36:2044.

Atherosclerotic Lesions

203. Narula J, Virmani R, Iskandrian AE. Strategic targeting of atherosclerotic lesions [Editorial]. J Nuc Cardiol 1999;6:81.

204. Fuster V, Badimon L, Badimon JJ, et al. The pathogenesis of coronary artery disease. N Engl J Med 1991;326L:242–250, 310.

205. Davies MJ, Woolfe N. Atherosclerosis: what is it and why does it occur? Br Heart J 1993;69:S3.

206. Burke AP, Farb A, Malcom GT, et al. Coronary risk factors and plaque morphology in men with coronary disease who died suddenly. N Engl J Med 1997;17:1859.

207. Lees RS, Lees AM, Strauss HW. External imaging of human atherosclerosis. J Nucl Med 1983;24:154.

208. Lees AM, Lees RS, Schoen FJ, et al. Imaging human atherosclerosis with ^{99m}Tc-labeled LDL. Atherosclerosis 1988;8:461.

209. DeForge LE, Schwendner SW, DeGalan MR, et al. Noninvasive assessment of lipid disposition in treated and untreated atherosclerotic rabbits. Pharm Res 1989;6:1011.

210. Hardoff R, Braegelmann F, Zanzonico P, et al. External imaging of atherosclerosis in rabbits using an 123I-labeled synthetic peptide fragment. J Clin Pharmacol 1993;33:1039.

211. Tsimiakis S, Palinski W, Halpern SE, et al. Radiolabeled MDA 2, an oxidation-specific, monoclonal antibody, identifies native atherosclerotic lesions in vivo. J Nucl Cardiol 1999;6:41.

212. Jain D, Kulkarni P, Kolodgie FD, Narula N, Maini B, Snyder G, Virmani R, Acio ER, Narula J. Noninvasive imaging of atherosclerotic plaques with indium-111-labeled lipid seeking coproporphyrin. J Am Coll Cardiol 2000;35:493.

213. Fischman AJ, Rubin RH, Delvecchio A, et al. Imaging of atheromatous lesions in the illiac and femoral vessels: preliminary expereince '111 In IgG in human subjects [abstract]. J Nucl Med 1989;30:817.

214. Ohtsuki K, Hayase M, Akashi K, Kopiwoda S, Strauss HW. Detection of monocyte chemoattractant protein-1 receptor expression in experimental atherosclerotic lesions: an autoradiographic study. Circulation 2001 Jul 10;104(2):203.

215. Farb A, Virmani R, Atkinson JB, et al. Plaque morphology and pathologic outcome after coronary balloon angioplasty. J Am Coll Cardiol 1990;16:1421.

216. Thyberg J, Heidin U, Sjolund M, et al. Regulation of differentiated properties and proliferation of arterial smooth muscle cells. Arteriosclerosis 1990;10:966.

217. Dinkelborg LM, Duda SH, Hanke H, et al. Molecular imaging of atherosclerosis using a technetium-99m-labeled endothelin derivative. J Nucl Med 1998;39:18100.

218. Elmaleh D, Narula J, Petrov A, et al. Tc-99m-Ap4A for early gamma scintigraphic visualizations of experimental atherosclerotic lesions. Proc Natl Acad Sci 1998;95:691.

219. Dewanjee MK, Narula J. Antinsense mechanism for the diagnosis and treatment of cardiovascular diseases. J Nucl Cardiol 1999;6:345.

220. Narula J, Bianchi C, Petrov A, et al. Noninvasive localization of experimental atherosclerotic lesions with mouse/human chimeric Z2D3 antibody specfic for the proliferating smooth muscle cells of human atheroma. Circulation 1995;92:474.

221. Narula J, Petrov A, Ditlow C, et al. Maximizing radiotracer delivery for scintigraphic localization of experimental atherosclerotic lesions with high-dose negative-charge-modified Z2D3 antibody. J Nucl Cardiol 1997;4:226.

222. Carrio I, Pieri P, Narula J, et al. Noninvasive localization of human atherosclerotic lesions with indium-111-labeled monoclonal Z2D3 antibody specific for proliferating smooth muscle cells. J Nucl Cardiol 1998;5:551.

223. Narula J, Kolodgie FD, Virmani R, Petrov A, Khaw BA. Should assessment of the rate of smooth muscle cell proliferation by indium-111-Z2D3 antibody imaging allow for predicting postangioplastic restenosis? Society of Nuclear Medicine, San Antonio 1997; J Nucl Med 1997;38:3.

22 | Nuclear cardiology compared to other imaging methods

ERNST E. VAN DER WALL, FATHY F. WAMBA, AND JEROEN J. BAX

Noninvasive imaging has become the mainstay in the diagnostic and prognostic workup of patients with known or suspected coronary artery disease. Among the available techniques, four imaging modalities may provide useful clinical information on the presence of coronary artery disease: nuclear imaging, echocardiography, magnetic resonance imaging (MRI), and, recently, electron beam computed tomography (EBCT). The role of the various nuclear imaging techniques has been described elsewhere in this book. This chapter concentrates on the value of nuclear imaging techniques compared to echocardiography, MRI, and EBCT. In particular stress echocardiography has become a major player in the routine use of detecting patients with myocardial ischemia. Although currently restricted by availability, MRI and EBCT also will enter the clinical arena faster than previously envisaged.

STRESS ECHOCARDIOGRAPHY

Detection of Coronary Artery Disease

Methodology

Echocardiographic examination of the myocardium to detect coronary artery disease can be performed under resting circumstances but more preferably following physical exercise or during pharmacologic stress. Resting echocardiography can provide information on regional wall thickness, wall motion and thickening, and on global left ventricular function (LVEF). Hence, in patients with a previous myocardial infarction various markers can be considered as indicators of coronary artery disease: reduced wall thickness, abnormal wall motion and thickening, and reduced LVEF. Many patients with coronary artery disease, however, have a normal LV function, and therefore, when actual ischemia is absent and no previous infarction has occurred, resting echocardiography may not be able to

detect the underlying coronary artery disease. Therefore, the combination of echocardiography and some form of stress has attracted considerable interest during the last 10 years. During or poststress, ischemia is induced and the alterations in wall motion and thickening on echocardiography serve as indicators of stress-inducible ischemia. Several forms of "stress echocardiography" are currently available. If a patient is able to perform physical exercise, the test can be performed with a treadmill or with a supine or upright bicycle. With treadmill exercise, images are obtained immediately before and after exercise and with bicycle exercise the images are obtained before, during, and after the test. Hence, bicycle exercise offers the advantage that images can be obtained at peak stress. For patients who are unable to perform physical exercise, a variety of pharmacologic stressors are available. They can be divided into two groups: adrenergic stimulators and vasodilators.

Among the adrenergic stimulating agents, dobutamine has been used most frequently. Dobutamine is a beta-1-specific agonist that increases myocardial oxygen demand by increasing heart rate, contractility, and arterial blood pressure. Dobutamine is infused intravenously at incremental doses of 5,10,20,30, and 40 mcg $\cdot$ kg^{-1} $\cdot$ min^{-1} at 3–5 min intervals. Atropine (0.25–1.0 mg) can be added if the heart rate response to dobutamine is inadequate. Secknus et al. [1] reported on the side effects in 3011 patients undergoing dobutamine echocardiography. In 7.6% of the patients, the side effects were dose-limiting and resulted in termination of the test prematurely; in 9 patients serious side effects occurred. Beta-blockers can be used as antidote. Dipyridamole and adenosine are the currently available vasodilators. While adenosine is a direct vasodilator, dipyridamole inhibits cellular uptake and breakdown of adenosine. Dipyridamole (0.56 mg $\cdot$ kg^{-1}) is initially administered intravenously over 4 min, followed by a second dose of 0.28 mg $\cdot$ kg^{-1}. The safety profile of dipyridamole echocardiography was evaluated by Picano et al. [2] in 10,451 patients; in 113 (1.2%) patients major complications or dose limiting side-effects occurred. Aminophylline can be used as antidote.

Adenosine has been used in single doses of 0.14 mg · kg^{-1} · min^{-1} and in stepwise infusion protocols (3 min stages of 0.10, 0.14, and 0.18 mg^{-1} · kg^{-1} · min^{-1}) [3,4]. Although side effects are common with adenosine infusion, the use of an antidote is rarely required, since the agent has an extremely short half-life ($<$ 2 sec).

Accuracy of stress echocardiography

All forms of stress echocardiography have been evaluated for their accuracy in the detection of coronary artery disease. For exercise echocardiography, 15 studies have reported on the sensitivity and specificity for the detection of coronary artery disease [5]. Treadmill exercise was used in 11 studies and bicycle exercise in 4. The largest study included 309 patients and showed a sensitivity of 91% with a specificity of 78%. In the other studies, the sensitivities ranged from 71% to 97% and the specificities from 64% to 100%. Dobutamine echocardiography was evaluated in 28 studies; the pooled data of these studies were reviewed by Geleijnse et al. [6]. The authors reported an average sensitivity of 80% with a specificity of 84% (accuracy 81%). Moreover, it was demonstrated that the sensitivity increased with the number of diseased vessels (74% for one-vessel, 86% for two-vessel, and 92% for three-vessel disease). Nineteen studies used vasodilator echocardiography (17 dipyridamole and 2 adenosine) in 2247 patients. The sensitivity ranged from 40% to 96% with a specificity ranging from 87% to 100% [5]. Overall, the sensitivity of vasodilator echocardiography appears somewhat lower as compared to exercise echocardiography and dobutamine echocardiography.

Strengths and limitations of stress echocardiography

In comparison to other imaging modalities, echocardiography has several advantages, including bedside availability, real-time imaging, low costs, absence of radiation. Attenuation problems, as encountered with nuclear imaging, are not present with echocardiography. Besides information on LV function, information on pericardial pathology and valvular (dys-)function can also be derived. Disadvantages of the technique include dropout of the anterior and lateral walls and poor acoustic window, particularly in patients with emphysema. Moreover, analysis of the stress echo data is visual, whereas nuclear imaging permits quantitative (objective) analysis. Also, identification of ischemia superimposed on infarcted myocardium is difficult.

Comparison to nuclear imaging

Various studies have compared some form of stress echocardiography to some form of nuclear imaging for the detection of coronary artery disease. Most of these studies consistently showed a higher sensitivity for nuclear imaging with a higher specificity for stress echocardiography. This is not surprising if one considers the sequence of functional events (referred to as the *ischemic cascade* [7]) taking place when stress is applied to a patient with a flow-limiting stenosis (Fig. 22.1). According to this cascade, perfusion abnormalities due to limited flow reserve precede wall motion abnormalities. Geleijnse and Elhendy have nicely summarized all available studies performing a direct comparison between stress echocardiography and myocardial perfusion imaging [8]. Twenty-one studies, with 1380 patients, performed a head-to-head comparison between stress echocardiography and myocardial perfusion imaging. Pooled data demonstrated a higher sensitivity for perfusion imaging as compared to stress echocardiography (85% vs 75%) and a higher specificity for stress echocardiography (88% vs 79%) (Fig. 22.2). Among these 21 studies, 7 studies employed physical exercise (2 treadmill, 5 bicycle), 8 used dobutamine, 3 adenosine, and 4 dipyridamole. Geleijnse and Elhendy [8] also evaluated sensitivity and specificity for the detection of coronary disease using these different stressors. In the 7 studies (total 397 patients) using

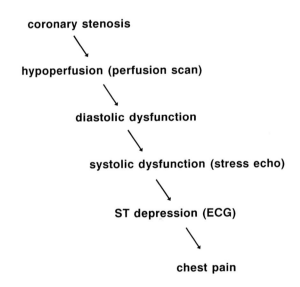

FIGURE 22.1 The sequence of events taking place during ischemia, also referred to as the ischemic cascade. Note: perfusion abnormalities precede wall motion abnormalities. (Based on Nesto and Kowalchuk [7] and Brown et al. [53].)

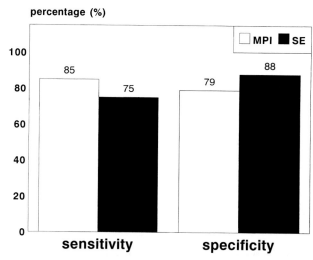

FIGURE 22.2 Sensitivity and specificity for the detection of coronary artery disease: stress echocardiography (SE) vs myocardial perfusion imaging (MPI). Data based only on head-to-head comparisons. Sensitivity was higher for perfusion imaging, whereas specificity was higher for stress echocardiography. (Based on Geleijnse and Elhendy [8].)

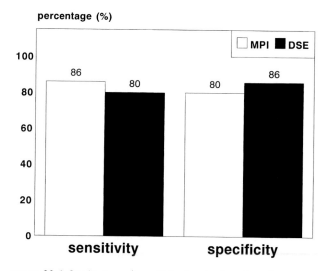

FIGURE 22.4 Sensitivity and specificity for the detection of coronary artery disease: dobutamine stress echocardiography (DSE) vs myocardial perfusion imaging (MPI). Data based only on head-to-head comparisons. Sensitivity was higher for perfusion imaging, whereas specificity was higher for stress echocardiography. (Based on Geleijnse and Elhendy [8].)

physical exercise, myocardial perfusion imaging had a higher sensitivity (83% vs 78%), whereas stress echo had the higher specificity (91% vs 83%) (Fig. 22.3). Similarly, in the 8 dobutamine studies (total 593 patients), the sensitivity was again higher for myocardial perfusion imaging (86% vs 80%) and specificity was higher for stress echocardiography (86% vs 73%) (Fig.

22.4). Also, the 7 studies using vasodilator stress (3 adenosine, 4 dipyridamole) with 390 patients showed the same trends (Fig. 22.5).

When individual vessels were evaluated, myocardial perfusion scintigraphy showed a consistently higher sensitivity as compared to stress echo, whereas specificities were again slightly higher with stress echocar-

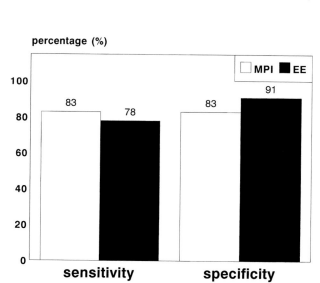

FIGURE 22.3 Sensitivity and specificity for the detection of coronary artery disease: exercise echocardiography (EE) vs myocardial perfusion imaging (MPI). Data based only on head-to-head comparisons. Sensitivity was higher for perfusion imaging, whereas specificity was higher for stress echocardiography. (Based on Geleijnse and Elhendy [8].)

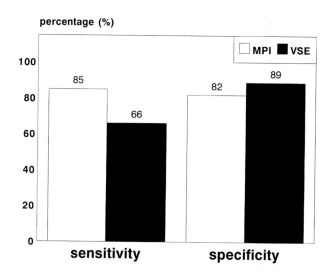

FIGURE 22.5 Sensitivity and specificity for the detection of coronary artery disease: vasodilator stress echocardiography (VSE) vs myocardial perfusion imaging (MPI). Data based only on head-to-head comparisons. Sensitivity was higher for perfusion imaging, whereas specificity was higher for stress echocardiography.

TABLE 22.1 *Detection of Coronary Artery Disease in Different Vessels; Relative Merits of Myocardial Perfusion Imaging and Stress Echocardiography*

	STRESS ECHO		PERFUSION IMAGING	
	Sens (%)	Spec (%)	Sens (%)	Spec (%)
LAD	69	91	73	92
LCX	58	92	43	96
RCA	82	88	69	81
All vessels	62	90	72	91
1-VD	66	—	76	—
MVD	86	—	95	—

Sens, sensitivity; spec, specificity; LAD, left anterior descending artery; LCX, left circumflex artery; RCA, right coronary artery; 1-VD, single-vessel disease; MVD, multivessel disease.

Source: Data based on Geleijnse and Elhendy [8].

diography (Table 22.1). In particular, a large difference in sensitivities for the detection of single-vessel disease was noted.

Prognostic Value in Patients with Known or Suspected Coronary Artery Disease

Besides detection of coronary artery disease, assessment of prognosis is important. Adequate information permits identification of patients with a low risk for future events who can be treated medically and patients with a high risk for subsequent death or infarction in whom more agressive therapy is warranted. Various studies have demonstrated that all different forms of stress echocardiography can provide prognostic information. In patients with known or suspected coronary artery disease, several studies have indicated that a normal or negative stress echocardiogram carries a good prognosis. This has been demonstrated for all forms of stress echocardiography [5]. The negative predictive value in 12 studies (2957 patients) ranged from 67% to 99%; 10 studies demonstrated a negative predictive value of over 90% [5]. It is important to realize that the negative predictive value is influenced by several issues, in particular the pretest likelihood of coronary artery disease in the study population, the events being predicted (hard events vs all events), the stressor, and the definition of a negative test. Poldermans et al. [9] have demonstrated that the annual event-rate was 1.3% in patients with a normal test, whereas a negative test (no ischemia inducible) but with resting regional wall motion abnormalities present was associated with a higher annual event-rate. The positive predictive value varied also among the different studies, ranging from 10% to 68%. Again these values are dependent on the incidence of the disease in the study population, the events, the stressor, and the definition of a

positive test. Poldermans et al. [9], using dobutamine stress echocardiography, studied 1737 patients with known or suspected coronary artery disease and demonstrated that the number of events increased proportionally to the extent and severity of the ischemia present.

Comparison to nuclear imaging

Two studies performed a head-to-head comparison between stress echo and nuclear imaging for assessment of long-term prognosis in patients with known or suspected coronary artery disease [10,11]. Both studies demonstrated comparable value for prediction of future events. Are nuclear imaging and stress echo completely equal, then, for assessment of long-term prognosis in patients with known or suspected coronary artery disease? To answer this question, Brown et al. pooled the available data in the literature and compared the prognostic value of a normal scintigram with that of a normal stress echocardiogram [12]. A total of 3573 patients with known or suspected coronary artery disease had a normal perfusion scintigram. The annual event-rate (death/myocardial infarction) was < 1%. In 1432 patients with a normal stress echocardiogram, however, the annual event-rate was 5% (Fig. 22.6). Similar observations were made when the analysis was restricted to the patients with proven coronary artery disease. This finding is again in line with the is-

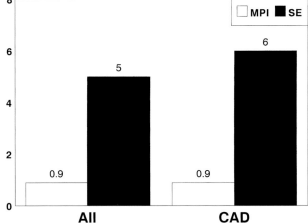

FIGURE 22.6 Annual event-rate (cardiac death/infarction) in patients with a normal stress echocardiogram (SE) as compared to patients with a normal myocardial perfusion study (MPI). All = patients with known or suspected coronary artery disease; CAD = patients with proven coronary artery disease. A normal scan is associated with a lower event-rate as compared to a normal stress echocardiogram. (Based on Brown [12].)

chemic cascade: stress-induced perfusion abnormalities precede stress-induced wall motion abnormalities [7]. These event-rates in the presence of a normal stress echo are too high to classifiy a patient as low risk and, moreover, too high to make the technique serve as a gatekeeper to justify obtaining no further information, as has been demonstrated for nuclear imaging.

Acute Myocardial Infarction

Prediction of spontaneous recovery of function

In patients with acute myocardial infarction who undergo reperfusion (either mechanical or using thrombolysis), stunning may occur to some extent, resulting in regional contractile dysfunction [13]. In these patients, spontaneous recovery may occur over time [13]. However, in patients with dysfunction due to complete infarction, the wall motion abnormalities are irreversible. Both stress echocardiography and nuclear imaging have been preformed for the assessment of stunned, viable myocardium postinfarction, and both techniques have been demonstrated useful in the prediction of improvement of function over time [13]. Marwick summarized the results of five studies using dobutamine stress echocardiography to predict improvement of function postinfarction [5]. In these five studies, with 212 patients, the sensitivities ranged from 72% to 89% with specificities ranging from 68% to 91%. Few studies have directly compared nuclear imaging to stress echocardiography in patients with acute myocardial infarction, aiming at prediction of spontaneous improvement of contractile function (based on the detection of viable, stunned myocardium). Elhendy and coworkers [14] evaluated 30 patients 7 ± 3 days following acute, uncomplicated myocardial infarction with low-dose dobutamine echocardiography and thallium-201 (Tl-201) rest-redistribution imaging. Improvement of function was evaluated by serial echocardiograms obtained at baseline and after 3 months follow-up. A striking difference between the number of dysfunctional but viable segments by dobutamine stress echocardiography and Tl-201 imaging was observed: 35 (31%) of 112 segments were viable by Tl-201 imaging but nonviable by dobutamine echocardiography. Follow-up echocardiography demonstrated improvement of function in 35 (31%) of the segments. This resulted in a sensitivity of 77% for both techniques and a significantly higher specificity for dobutamine echocardiography (84% vs 57%). Thus, a substantial number of segments classified as viable by nuclear imaging but without contractile reserve on stress echocardiography failed to improve in function postrevascularization. The exact mechanism underlying this phe-nomenon is not yet fully understood, and further direct comparisons are needed.

Prognostic value of viability assessment postinfarction

Other studies have evaluated the prognostic value of stress echocardiography following acute myocardial infarction. Not unexpected, most information has been obtained with pharmacologic stress echocardiography [5]. Most of these studies have looked at the prognostic value of inducible ischemia postinfarction; Marwick pooled seven studies (2334 patients) using different stressors (two exercise, one pacing, three dipyridamole, one dobutamine) and demonstrated a high negative predictive value (ranging from 82% to 97%) with a lower positive predictive value (ranging from 14% to 94%). These data are not essentially different from data obtained with nuclear imaging [15]. One direct comparison demonstrated that nuclear imaging and stress echocardiography provided similar prognostic information in patients studied shortly after myocardial infarction [16].

More recent studies have evaluated the value of the presence of viable myocardium on the prediction of long-term prognosis following acute myocardial infarction. Low–high dose dobutamine stress echocardiography permits analysis of both viability (contractile reserve elicited at infusion of low dosages of dobutamine) and ischemia. Picano and colleagues [17]

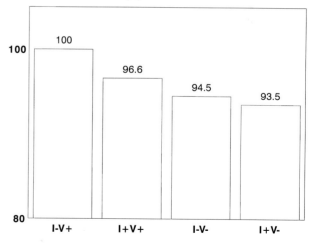

FIGURE 22.7 Long-term survival following acute myocardial infarction according to the presence of viability (V) and/or ischemia (I) on dobutamine stress echocardiography. Viability is associated with a favorable survival, whereas ischemia is associated with a worse survival. (Data based on Picano et al. [17].)

performed a large study in patients ($n = 314$) with recent infarction and analyzed the value of both phenomena for predicting long-term prognosis (follow-up 9 ± 7 months). As can be observed in Figure 22.7, the lowest event-rate was observed in patients with viable myocardium (contractile reserve at low-dose dobutamine), without inducible ischemia. The highest event-rate was observed in patients with inducible ischemia without contractile reserve at low-dose dobutamine (referred to as viable myocardium). Thus, these data suggest a beneficial (protective) effect of viability on long-term prognosis. Available data from nuclear imaging studies are not in line with the findings concerning the presence of viable tissue. Studies with F-18 fluorodeoxyglucose (FDG, a marker of glucose utilization) demonstrated that patients with viable tissue had a higher event-rate as compared to patients with scar tissue only [18]. Huitink and coworkers evaluated 59 consecutive patients with a recent myocardial infarction and showed an event-rate of 49% in patients with viable myocardium over the 47 ± 15 months follow-up period (Table 22.2). It is clear that further research in this field is warranted.

Chronic Ischemic LV Dysfunction

Prediction of outcome postrevascularization

In patients with chronic ischemic LV dysfunction, the presence of viable myocardium has been related to improvement of function following revascularization [19]. In segments exhibiting resting dysfunction, the hallmark of viability on dobutamine echocardiography is the improvement of wall motion during the infusion of low-dose dobutamine (5–10 mcg/kg/min). Data from studies testing this criterion against improvement of function postrevascularization (which is considered the gold-standard for viable myocardium) have demonstrated sensitivities ranging from 52% to 97% and specificities ranging from 62% to 96% [19]. In the more recent

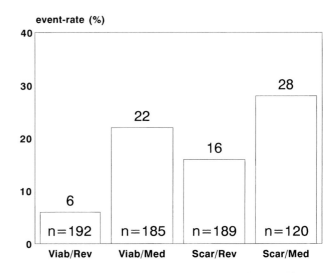

FIGURE 22.8 Prognosis in patients with and without viable myocardium on stress echocardiography, according to treatment (rev = revascularization vs med = medical). The lowest event-rate was observed in patients with viable myocardium who underwent revascularization. (Pooled data from six studies, 686 patients, based on references 21–26.)

dobutamine echocardiography studies, a low–high dose protocol was used. Although Afridi et al. [20] have claimed superior accuracy of this protocol for the prediction of improvement of function, the precise value of both protocols remains to be confirmed in a large patient group. Currently, 30 studies (1048 patients) have evaluated the use of dobutamine echocardiography for the assessment of viable tissue and subsequent prediction of improvement of LV function postrevascularization [19]. Pooling of these data yields a sensitivity of 83% and a specificity of 80% for the prediction of improvement of regional LV function postrevascularization. Improvement of global LV function was evaluated in seven studies, with 254 patients; on average, the LVEF improved from 35% to 43% in patients with viable myocardium. In patients without viable myocardium, the LVEF remained unchanged (35% vs 36%). Six studies (686 patients) have evaluated long-term prognosis in relation to treatment (medical, revascularization) and viability (absent or present) [21–26]. The patients were divided into four groups (Fig. 22.8); pooled analysis of these data demonstrated that the lowest event-rate (6%) was observed in patients with viable myocardium who underwent revascularization, whereas the event-rates were similar in the other three groups.

Comparison to nuclear imaging

Various studies have directly compared some form of nuclear imaging to stress echocardiography. Panza et al.

TABLE 22.2 *Event-Rate in 39 Patients with Viable Myocardium on FDG Imaging as Compared to 14 Patients with Scar Tissue Only*

Event	FDG Viable ($n = 39$)	FDG Scar ($n = 14$)
Cardiac death	5	1
Reinfarction	3	0
Late revascularization	7	0
Unstable AP	4	0
Total	19 (49%)	1 (7%)

FDG, F-18 fluorodeoxyglucose; AP, angina pectoris.
Source: Data based on Huitink et al. [18].

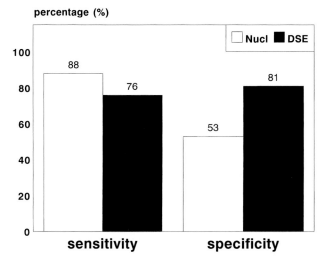

FIGURE 22.9 Sensitivity and specificity of stress echocardiography (DSE) vs nuclear imaging (nucl) to predict improvement of regional function postrevascularization; data based on pooling of 18 studies (563 patients) performing a head-to-head comparison between stress echocardiography and nuclear imaging. Sensitivity was higher for nuclear imaging whereas specificity was higher for stress echocardiography. (Based on Bax et al. [19].)

[27] performed a head-to-head comparison of Tl-201 imaging and dobutamine stress echocardiography in patients with chronic ischemic LV dysfunction. A total of 311 segments were analyzed by both techniques; 84% of these were classified as viable and 16% as nonviable on Tl-201 imaging. The majority of the "Tl-201 nonviable segments" did not exhibit contractile reserve. However, an additional 36% of the "Tl-201 viable segments" also did not exhibit contractile reserve. Similar results were obtained by Cornel et al. comparing FDG imaging with dobutamine echocardiography [28]. Thus, the results indicate that nuclear imaging appears more sensitive than dobutamine echocardiography for the detection of viable tissue. Various studies have compared the predictive accuracy of nuclear imaging with dobutamine echocardiography [19]. Currently, a total of 18 studies (563 patients) have performed a direct comparison between the two modalities: 3 used FDG PET, 5 Tl-201 reinjection, and 10 Tl-201 rest-redistribution. Pooling of these data yielded a higher sensitivity for nuclear imaging (88% vs 76%) and a higher specificity for dobutamine echocardiography (81% vs 53%) (Fig. 22.9).

MAGNETIC RESONANCE IMAGING

Detection of Coronary Artery Disease

Various studies have attempted to validate the use of MRI for the detection of coronary artery disease. As in stress echocardiography, the marker of ischemia is the presence of resting wall motion abnormalities or stress-induced abnormalities. Physical exercise in combination with MRI is difficult; therefore pharmacologic stress has been used. Pennell et al. [29] used MRI in combination with dipyridamole, and compared the results with Tl-201 scintigraphy. The sensitivity of dipyridamole MRI for the detection of coronary artery disease was 62% and the agreement between reversible Tl-201 defects and wall motion abnormalities was 67%. Hence, dipyridamole did not induce wall motion abnormalities in 33% of the regions exhibiting a perfusion defect on Tl-201 imaging. Baer et al. [30] studied 23 patients with angiographically proven coronary artery disease but without a previous infarction. The authors reported an overall sensitivity of 78% for the detection of coronary artery disease using dipyridamole and MRI.

Other studies have used dobutamine instead of vasodilator stress: Pennell et al. [31] compared dobutamine MRI with Tl-201 SPECT in 22 patients with coronary artery disease. Twenty-one of the patients showed ischemia on Tl-201 SPECT, with 20 (95%) exhibiting new wall motion abnormalities during dobutamine MRI. Baer et al. [32] compared Tc-99m-sestamibi SPECT with dobutamine MRI and reported comparative sensitivities for MRI and Tc-99m-sestamibi SPECT: 84% versus 87%.

Van Rugge et al., using quantitative analysis of dobutamine MRI data, demonstrated a sensitivity of 91% and a specificity of 80% [33]. An overview of the results of the available MRI studies detecting coronary artery disease is presented in Table 22.3. The data are consistent in showing a comparable sensitivity and specificity to radionuclide imaging.

Prognostic studies using MRI in patients with known or suspected coronary artery disease are not available. However, Wu et al. [34] have demonstrated that in pa-

TABLE 22.3 *Diagnostic Accuracy of MRI for the Detection of Coronary Artery Disease*

Study	No. Patients	Stressor	MPI Sens (%)	MRI Sens (%)
Pennell [29]	40	Dipy	—	62
Baer [30]	23	Dipy	—	78
Matheijssen [50]	10	Dipy	100	100
Pennell [31]	22	Dobut	95	91
Baer [32]	35	Dobut	87	84
Baer [51]	28	Dobut	—	85
Van Rugge [52]	37	Dobut	—	81
Van Rugge [33]	39	Dobut	—	91
Nagel [40]	208	Dobut	—	86

MPI, myocardial perfusion imaging; sens, sensitivity; Dipy, dipyridamole; Dobut, dobutamine.

Source: Adapted from Van der Wall and Bax [49].

tients with microvascular obstruction after acute myocardial infarction, as assessed by MRI, long-term prognosis was poor.

MRI Techniques to Assess Myocardial Viability

Various approaches with MRI have been proposed for the assessment of viability [35]. The earliest studies employed resting MRI and focused on the end-diastolic wall thickness (EDWT), systolic wall thickening (SWT), and signal intensity without contrast-enhancement (SI). Other studies have combined the information from resting MRI with the assessment of contractile reserve during dobutamine stimulation. More recent studies, employing contrast media, have evaluated perfusion on the tissue level. In the next paragraphs these different techniques are discussed.

Resting MRI and EDWT, SWT and SI

Earlier data [36] have already demonstrated that patients with chronic myocardial infarction frequently exhibit severely reduced EDWT and decreased SI in the infarct region, likely to represent scar tissue. Perrone-Filardi et al. [37] compared resting MRI with FDG PET and Tl-201 reinjection imaging in patients with chronic coronary artery disease and LV dysfunction. Their main conclusion was that the majority of the segments classified viable by FDG PET and Tl-201 reinjection also exhibited preserved EDWT and SWT at rest.

Baer et al. [38] compared MRI with FDG PET and showed that segments without SWT and EDWT < 5.5 mm were mainly nonviable on FDG PET. More recently, these authors [39] tested the predictive value of EDWT against outcome after revascularization and demonstrated that EDWT (cutoff level 5.5 mm) was 92% sensitive but only 56% specific in the prediction of improvement of function following revascularization. Therefore, EDWT < 5.5 mm is an excellent marker of scar tissue, but EDWT > 5.5 mm does not necessarily imply improvement of function postrevascularization.

Dobutamine MRI

Like dobutamine echocardiography, MRI during the infusion of low-dose dobutamine can be used to evaluate contractile reserve in dysfunctional myocardium. The lower dosages of dobutamine (10 μg/kg/min) are mainly used to detect contractile reserve (and hence viability), while the higher dosages (up to 40 μg/kg/min) are mainly used to detect ischemia (indicating coronary artery disease). Both approaches have been evaluated successfully with MRI. Nagel et al. [40] have demonstrated that high-dose dobutamine MRI had a sensitivity of 86% and a specificity of 86% to detect coronary artery disease as compared to coronary angiography. In patients with chronic coronary artery disease, Baer et al. [38,41] have compared dobutamine MRI with FDG PET and dobutamine echocardiography and demonstrated excellent agreement between these three approaches. Subsequently, these authors showed that dobutamine MRI could adequately predict improvement of regional LV function after revascularization; moreover, the diagnostic accuracy of dobutamine MRI was superior to that of resting MRI (using EDWT > 5.5 mm as "viability marker"). Another important observation from this study was that the extent of viable tissue predicted the magnitude of improvement of LVEF postrevascularization. In patients with acute myocardial infarction, contractile reserve on dobutamine MRI was also predictive of improvement of function [42,43]. The major advantages of dobutamine MRI over dobutamine stress echocardiography are the image quality and the possibility to quantify the extent and severity of the wall motion abnormalities. The addition of tagging to dobutamine MRI may even further enhance the diagnostic accuracy of the technique, since it enables distinction of responses to dobutamine by different myocardial layers [43].

Contrast media

The use of contrast agents in cardiac MRI has been studied for many years [44]. Very recently, Kim et al. have demonstrated the use of contrast-enhanced MRI for the detection of viability and subsequent prediction of improvement of function in 50 patients with chronic ischemic LV dysfunction [45]. Using this approach, hyperenhanced regions represent scar tissue, and with the high resolution of MRI it is possible to detect different stages of infarct transmurality. The results showed that the higher the transmurality, as evidenced by hyperenhancement, the lower the likelihood of recovery of function postrevascularization. In contrast, segments without hyperenhancement had a high likelihood of recovery. This approach may become very effective in the assessment of myocardial viability.

ELECTRON BEAM COMPUTED TOMOGRAPHY

Detection of Coronary Artery Disease

EBCT is a sensitive and reproducible method for the detection of coronary artery calcification. Contrast angiography can also be performed with current EBCT techniques. Due to rapid speed at which images can be required (50 ms), a study can be completed during single breathhold and requires no patient preparation. Coronary calcification is typically defined as having a density of > 130 Hounsfield units. The calcium burden in each major coronary artery is summed to generate a total coronary artery calcium score, which is directly related to the total atherosclerotic plaque burden present in the epicardial coronary arteries [46]. Strong relations have been reported between the extent of total plaque area and coronary artery calcification, and between the severity of calcification and the presence of a hemodynamically significant coronary artery stenosis [47]. However, the total calcium area may underestimate total plaque area, and the relationship between obstructive coronary artery disease and severity of calcification is still too imprecise to be used as a definite criterion for proceeding directly to coronary angiography.

Detection of Myocardial Ischemia

Comparison with nuclear imaging

A recent trial explored the complementary role of EBCT and stress myocardial perfusion SPECT for identifying both preclinical coronary artery disease and silent ischemia in a generally asymptomatic population with risk factors for developing coronary artery disease [48]. The purpose of this study was to identify (1) patients with preclinical coronary artery disease who might benefit from aggressive risk factor modification; and (2) patients who are at relatively higher short-term risk for cardiac events based on the presence of silent myocardial ischemia. Of the 3895 patients studied with EBCT, 411 patients underwent both EBCT and stress SPECT imaging. Of the patients with a low calcification score < 100, only 1% had an abnormal SPECT, whereas 46% of patients with a high score > 400 had an abnormal SPECT. Large ischemic defects (> 15% of the left ventricular circumference) were virtually confined to a score > 400. This study supports the role of EBCT as an initial screening test for identifying patients with varying degrees of coronary atherosclerosis. The authors emphasize the effectiveness of selectively combining SPECT with EBCT in patients with a score > 400 in order to identify those with silent ischemia or occult disease. Of course, the clinical utility of EBCT for detecting myocardial ischemia remains to be proven.

CONCLUSIONS

Among the different imaging modalities for detecting

myocardial ischemia, nuclear imaging offers by far the largest numbers of both diagnostic and prognostic data. Stress echocardiography has become the major counterplayer in the field because of its versatility and wide availability. Current data suggest that echocardiography provides roughly similar data as scintigraphic data, provided that these data are being handled by experts in the field. Still, there remain differences, mainly related to the ischemic cascade: nuclear imaging has a higher sensitivity for the detection of coronary artery disease and a normal scan is associated with a higher event-free survival-rate as compared a normal stress echo.

Major assets of SPECT imaging are its accuracy, reproducibility, and quantification. The introduction of gated SPECT will undoubtedly contribute to improving these assets. MRI, although unsurpassed in terms of resolution, is still clinically underused and has no substantial data on prognostics and cost-efficacy. Data on perfusion are still suboptimal but the functional consequences of myocardial ischemia can be visualized excellently. EBCT has the option of early detection of coronary artery disease but the inherent characteristics of the technique prevent the visualization of myocardial perfusion and thus ischemia. Furthermore, LV function cannot be studied during stress, precluding the detection of functional disturbances due to ischemia. It is hoped that all four techniques will advance over the next decade, as the early and accurate detection of coronary artery disease and its functional sequelae are of paramount interest to the individual patient suspected for coronary artery disaese.

REFERENCES

1. Secknus M, Marwick TH. Evolution of dobutamine echocardiography protocols and indications: safety and side effects in 3011 studies over 5 years. J Am Coll Cardiol 1997;29:1234.
2. Picano E, Marini C, Pirelli S, et al. Safety of intravenous high-dose dipyridamole echocardiography. Am J Cardiol 1992;70:252.
3. Zoghbi WA, Cheirif J, Kleiman NS, et al. Diagnosis of ischemic heart disease with adenosine echocardiography. J Am Coll Cardiol 1991;18:1271.
4. Marwick T, Willemart B, D'Hondt AM, et al. Selection of the optimal nonexercise stress for the evaluation of ischemic regional myocardial dysfunction and malperfusion. Comparison of dobutamine and adenosine using echocardiography and 99mTc-MIBI single photon emission computed tomography. Circulation 1993:87:345.
5. Marwick TH. Current status of stress echocardiography for diagnosis and prognostic assessment of coronary artery disease. Coron Artery Dis 1998;9:411.
6. Geleijnse ML, Fioretti PM, Roelandt JRTC. Methodology, feasibility, safety and diagnostic accuracy of dobutamine stress echocardiography. J Am Coll Cardiol 1997;30:595.
7. Nesto RW, Kowalchuk GJ. The ischemic cascade: temporal se-

quence of hemodynamic, electrocardiographic and symptomatic expressions of ischemia. Am J Cardiol 1987;57:23C.

8. Geleijnse ML, Elhendy A. Can stress echocardiography compete with perfusion scintigraphy in the detection of coronary artery disease and cardiac risk assessment? Eur J Echocardiogr 2000; 1:12.

9. Poldermans D, Fioretti PM, Boersma E, et al. Long-term prognostic value of dobutamine-atropine stress echocardiography in 1737 patients with known or suspected coronary artery disease. A single center experience. Circulation 1999;99:757.

10. Geleijnse ML, Elhendy A, Cornel JH, et al. Cardiac imaging for risk stratification with dobutamine-atropine stress-testing in patients with chest pain. Echocardiography, perfusion scintigraphy, or both? Circulation 1997;98:2679.

11. Olmos LO, Dakik H, Gordon R, et al. Long-term prognostic value of exercise echocardiography compared with exercise 201Tl, ECG, and clinical variables in patients evaluated for coronary artery disease. Circulation 1998;98:2679.

12. Brown KA. Do stress echocardiography and myocardial perfusion imaging have the same ability to identify the low-risk patient with known or suspected coronary artery disease? Am J Cardiol 1998;81:1050.

13. Ross J Jr. Assessment of ischemic regional myocardial dysfunction and its reversibility. Mechanism of myocardial "stunning." Circulation 1986;74:1186.

14. Elhendy A, Trocino G, Salustri A, et al. Low-dose dobutamine echocardiography and rest-redistribution thallium-201 tomography in the assessment of spontaneous recovery of left ventricular function after recent myocardial infarction. Am Heart J 1996;131:1088.

15. Gimple LW, Beller GA. Assessing prognosis after acute myocardial infarction in the thrombolytic era. J Nucl Cardiol 1994;1:198.

16. Van Daele M, McNeill AJ, Fioretti PM, et al. Prognostic value of dipyridamole sestamibi single-photon emission computed tomography and dipyridamole stress echocardiography for new cardiac events after an uncomplicated myocardial infarction. J Am Soc Echocardiogr 1994;7:370.

17. Picano E, Sicari R, Landi P, et al. Prognostic value of myocardial viability in medically treated patients with global left ventricular dysfunction early after an acute uncomplicated myocardial infarction. A dobutamine stress echocardiographic study. Circulation 1998;98:1078.

18. Huitink JM, Visser FC, Bax JJ, et al. Predictive value of planar 18F-fluorodeoxyglucose imaging for cardiac events in patients after acute myocardial infarction. Am J Cardiol 1998;81:1072.

19. Bax JJ, Poldermans D, Elhendy A, et al. Sensitivity, specificity and predictive accuracies of various non-invasive techniques for detecting hibernating myocardium. Curr Probl Cardiol 2001; 26:144.

20. Afridi I, Kleiman NS, Raizner AE, et al. Dobutamine echocardiography in myocardial hibernation. Optimal dose and accuracy in predicting recovery of ventricular function after coronary angioplasty. Circulation 1995;91:663.

21. Bax JJ, Poldermans D, Elhendy A, et al. Improvement of left ventricular ejection fraction, heart failure symptoms and prognosis after revascularization in patients with chronic coronary artery disease and viable myocardium detected by dobutamine stress echocardiography. J Am Coll Cardiol 1999;34:163.

22. Chaudhry FA, Tauke JT, Alessandrini RS, et al. Prognostic implications of myocardial contractile reserve in patients with coronary artery disease and left ventricular dysfunction. J Am Coll Cardiol 1999;34:730.

23. Senior R, Kaul S, Lahiri A. Myocardial viability on echocardio-

graphy predicts long-term survival after revascularization in patients with ischemic congestive heart failure. J Am Coll Cardiol 1999;33:1848.

24. Williams MJ, Odabashian J, Laurer MS, et al. Prognostic value of dobutamine echocardiography in patients with left ventricular dysfunction. J Am Coll Cardiol 1996;27:132.

25. Afridi I, Grayburn PA, Panza J, et al. Myocardial viability during dobutamine echocardiography predicts survival in patients with coronary artery disease and severe left ventricular systolic dysfunction. J Am Coll Cardiol 1998;32:921.

26. Meluzin J, Cerny J, Frelich M, et al. Prognostic value of the amount of dysfunctional but viable myocardium in revascularized patients with coronary artery disease and left ventricular dysfunction. J Am Coll Cardiol 1998;32:912.

27. Panza JA, Dilsizian V, Laurienzo JM, et al. Relation between thallium uptake and contractile response to dobutamine. Implications regarding myocardial viability in patients with chronic coronary artery disease and left ventricular dysfunction. Circulation 1995;91:990.

28. Cornel JH, Bax JJ, Elhendy A, et al. Agreement and disagreement between "metabolic viability" and "contractile reserve" in akinetic myocardium. J Nucl Cardiol 1999;6:383.

29. Pennell DJ, Underwood SR, Ell PJ, et al. Magnetic resonance imaging using dipyridamole; A comparison with thallium-201 emission tomography. Br Heart J 1990;64:362.

30. Baer FM, Smolarz K, Jungehülsing FM, et al. Feasibility of high-dose dipyridamole-magnetic resonance imaging for detection of coronary artery disease and comparison with coronary angiography. Am J Cardiol 1992;69:51.

31. Pennell DJ, Underwood SR, Manzara CC, et al. Magnetic resonance imaging during dobutamine stress in coronary artery disease. Am J Cardiol 1992;70:34.

32. Baer FM, Voth E, Theissen P, et al. Coronary artery disease: findings with GRE MR imaging and technetium-99m methoxy-isobutyl-isonitrile SPECT during simultaneous dobutamine stress. Radiology 1994;193:203.

33. Van Rugge FP, Van der Wall EE, Spanjersberg SJ, et al. Magnetic resonance imaging during dobutamine stress for detection and localization of coronary artery disease: quantitative wall motion analysis using a modification of the centerline method. Circulation 1994;90:127.

34. Wu KC, Zerhouni EA, Judd RM, et al. Prognostic significance of microvascular obstruction by magnetic resonance imaging in patients with acute myocardial infarction. Circulation 1998;97: 765.

35. Higgins CB. Prediction of myocardial viability by MRI. Circulation 1999;99:727.

36. McNamara MT, Higgins CB. Magnetic resonance imaging of chronic myocardial infarcts in man. AJR 1986;146:315.

37. Perrone-Filardi P, Bacharach SL, Dilsizian V, et al. Regional left ventricular wall thickening. Relation to regional uptake of 18Fluorodeoxyglucose and 201Tl in patients with chronic coronary artery disease and left ventricular dysfunction. Circulation 1992; 86:1125.

38. Baer FM, Voth E, Schneider CA, et al. Comparison of low-dose dobutamine-gradient-echo magnetic resonance imaging and positron emission tomography with [18F]fluorodeoxyglucose in patients with chronic coronary artery disease. A functional and morphological approach to the detection of residual myocardial viability. Circulation 1995;91:1006.

39. Baer FM, Theissen P, Schneider CA, et al. Dobutamine magnetic resonance imaging predicts contractile recovery of chronically dysfunctional myocardium after successful revascularization. J Am Coll Cardiol 1998;31:1040.

40. Nagel E, Lehmkuhl HB, Bocksch W, et al. Noninvasive diagnosis of ischemia-induced wall motion abnormalities with the use of high dose dobutamine stress MRI. Comparison with dobutamine stress echocardiography. Circulation 1999;99:763.

41. Baer FM, Voth E, LaRosee K, et al. Comparison of dobutamine transesophageal echocardiography and dobutamine magnetic resonanace imaging for detection of residual myocardial viability. Am J Cardiol 1996;78:415.

42. Dendale P, Franken PR, Waldman G, et al. Low-dosage dobutamine magnetic resonance imaging as an alternative to echocardiography in the detection of viable myocardium after acute infarction. Am Heart J 1995;130:134.

43. Geskin G, Kramer CM, Rogers WJ, et al. Quantitative assessment of myocardial viability after infarction by dobutamine magnetic resonance tagging. Circulation 1998;98:217.

44. Van der Wall EE, Vliegen HW, De Roos A, et al. Magnetic resonance imaging in coronary artery disease. Circulation 1995;92:2723.

45. Kim RJ, Wu E, Rafael A, et al. The use of contrast-enhanced magnetic resonance imaging to identify reversible myocardial dysfunction. N Engl J Med 2000;343:1445.

46. Rumberger JA, Sheedy PF, Breen JF, et al. Electron beam computed tomographic coronary calcium score cutpoints and severity of associated angiographic lumen stenosis. J Am Coll Cardiol 1997;29:1542.

47. Guerci AD, Spadar LA, Goodman KJ, et al. Comparison of electron beam computed tomography scanning and conventional risk factor assessment for the prediction of angiographic coronary artery disease. J Am Coll Cardiol 1998;32:673.

48. He Z-X, Hedrick TD, Pratt CM, et al. Severity of coronary artery calcification by electron beam computed tomography predicts silent ischemia. Circulation 2000;101:244.

49. Van der Wall EE, Bax JJ. Current clinical relevance of cardiovascular magnetic resonance and its relationship to nuclear cardiology. J Nucl Cardiol 1999;6:462.

50. Matheijssen NAA, Louwerenburg HW, Van Rugge FP, et al. Comparison of ultrafast dipyridamole magnetic resonance imaging with dipyridamole sestaMIBI SPECT for detection of perfusion abnormalities in patients with one-vessel coronary artery disease: assessment by quantitative model fitting. MRM 1996;35:221.

51. Baer FM, Voth E, Theissen P, et al. Gradient-echo magnetic resonance imaging during incremental dobutamine infusion for the localization of coronary artery stenoses. Eur Heart J 1994;15:218.

52. Van Rugge FP, Van der Wall EE, De Roos A, et al. Dobutamine stress magnetic resonance imaging for the detection of coronary artery disease. J Am Coll Cardiol 1993;22:431.

53. Brown KA, Rosman DR, Dave RM. Stress nuclear myocardial perfusion imaging versus stress echocardiography: prognostic comparisons. Progr Cardiovasc Dis 2000;43:231.

23 | Cost-effectiveness analysis in nuclear cardiology

LESLEE J. SHAW

DIAGNOSTIC COSTS FOR CARDIOVASCULAR DISEASE

Over the past few decades, there is an ever-increasing societal burden by the encumbered resources for health care. The continuing rise in health-care costs often exceeds that of inflation accounting for approximately 13% to 16% of our gross domestic product [1]. In the United States, recent estimates of the total expenditures for cardiovascular disease approach $300 billion annually [2]. This would include approximately 14% of costs for private payers and approximately one-third of all Medicare costs. For diagnostic testing, recent estimates by the American College of Cardiology (ACC) reveal that up to 50% of Medicare payments received by cardiologists are for a diagnosis of coronary disease. Furthermore, annual rates of exercise testing approach 12 million patients annually with half of testing being performed with cardiac imaging (including ultrasound, nuclear, magnetic resonance, and positron emission tomographic imaging). Figure 23.1 depicts recent data from the ACC on reimbursement for varying subspecialties within cardiology (including nuclear cardiology procedures) [2]. Since 1998, nuclear cardiology procedures encumber approximately 10% of Medicare reimbursement for cardiology subspecialty procedures. Current data suggest that cardiac imaging procedures are growing at a rate of approximately 10% annually. Due to recent changes in reimbursement, containing health-care costs in the hospital and hospital outpatient setting (e.g., Hospital Outpatient Prospective Payment System [HOPPS]), the largest growth sector has been in the freestanding outpatient facility.

Although regional variation exists on the growth of nuclear cardiology procedures, it appears that actual rates of increase have, in many cases, exceeded 10% annually. Several factors appear to be favoring the growth in nuclear cardiology procedures. These include an environment of positive contribution margins or re-imbursement for stress testing, measures of ventricular function, and regional myocardial perfusion interpretation for the physician as well as the technical component. The growth in interest in noninvasive cardiology has been further promoted by a declining job market for interventional cardiology. Furthermore, as evidence-based medicine is currently the mainstay upon which managed care and large health-care payers evaluate procedural validity, the vast array of published evidence in nuclear cardiology allows for a more supportive environment for growth in gated SPECT imaging. In addition, there has been tremendous criticism of the overuse of catheter-based procedures. In the area of diagnostic cardiac services, the recent angiographic guidelines estimated that referral to cardiac catheterization is inappropriate in nearly one-third of patients [3]. One of the banes of an overuse of diagnostic angiography is that it often leads to unnecessary revascularization (i.e., for "cosmetic" purposes) without a subsequent improvement in outcome. The overuse of catheterization has often led to high normal catheterization rates, in many cases approaching 50%. Thus, the potential exists that nuclear procedures may effectively act as a gatekeeper and reduce unnecessary catheterization. With percutaneous procedureas accounting for > 1% of all U.S. health-care expenditures, the use of nuclear imaging as a gatekeeper could have a profound impact upon containing medical resource utilization nationally.

DEVELOPING EVIDENCE-BASED PRACTICE PATTERNS

Historically, clinical decision making was based on the accumulation of a wide array of experiences. By definition, a skilled clinician would be one who was exposed to a wide range and diversity of clinical scenarios. This method of medical reasoning has been the basis for medical education. A major drawback with this type

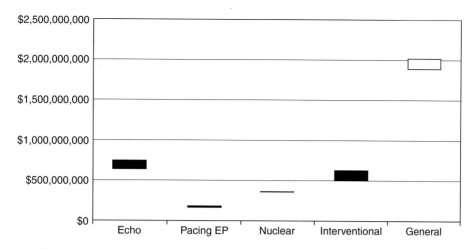

FIGURE 23.1 1998–2002 (estimates) of Medicare reimbursement for cardiology subspecialty procedures. Echo, echocardiography; Pacing EP, pacing electrophysiology. (Source: http://www.acc.org)

of reasoning is that recent untoward experiences weigh heavily in the physician's reasoning. For example, the most recent patient who had an adverse drug reaction would precipitate a more cautious approach to future patients by most physicians. Conversely, evidence-based medicine would advocate integrating patient outcome data from published, peer-reviewed literature with clinical reasoning and as a basis for establishing clinical pathways in varying disease states [4]. For nuclear cardiology, evidence-based medicine would require a threshold level of evidence to justify the added cost of any test (or add-on) in a patient's workup. This evidence would include large, multicenter, observational series as well as randomized trial data in sufficiently large and diverse patient populations. The new movement in evidence-based medicine is also being applied to the introduction of new technologies, in particular when comparative modalities exist.

Evidence-based medicine is increasingly driving clinical decisions for health-provider institutions and for individual physicians [5]. Evidence-based medicine involves taking into account the best available evidence regarding the effectiveness, risks, and cost of a medical procedure before implementing the procedure into clinical practice. The field arose after observations of wide variability across and within institutions with respect to the frequency, usage, and outcomes of specific procedures [6]. Also contributing to the development of evidence-based medicine was the Congressional Office of Technology Assessment's startling finding that only 10% to 20% of standard medical practices have been proven effective in controlled studies [5,6]. The ideal clinical testing indication, then, must be designed (1)

based on clinical evidence, rather than group opinion, expert testimony, or consensus; (2) to explicitly state the magnitude of testing and treatment options on pertinent health and economic outcomes; and (3) to contain both clinical care recommendations and estimated outcomes for the treatments of interest [5]. This chapter focuses on both the health-care policy issues related to nuclear cardiology use and on the ever-increasing supportive evidence that justifies its use in relation to other comparative modalities. This vast amount of evidence should then set higher standards for evidence dwarfing comparators and establishing quality guidelines for reimbursement and effective allocation of limited health-care resources.

ESTIMATING COST OF CARE

Our initial discussion begins with a brief definition of health-care cost and the methodologies applied to account for resource utilization.

Direct Medical Care Costs

The overall direct cost of treating coronary artery disease (CAD) in the United States is estimated to be $53.1 billion in 1996 and $71.5 billion by 2003 [7]. This staggering and increasing cost is the result of a sedentary and aging American population. The direct medical cost for treating one case of CAD-associated events is estimated to be $17,532 for a fatal acute myocardial infarction and $15,540 for a nonfatal acute myocardial infarction in 1996 [7].

Cost Components

Two components are considered when determining patient encumbered charges for episodic health care: hospital and physician costs. A combination of hospital bills (UB-92s), modeling, and chart review, as well as cost-charge ratios may be used to derive hospital costs. In addition, physician resource use is generated using resource-based relative values (RBRVS). Physician professional costs can be estimated using the RBRVS methodology. This process involves a number of steps. First, procedures as defined by current procedure terminology (CPT) codes, CPT modifiers, and physician charges hospitals may be obtained from hospitals with centralized billing. Next, RBRVS physician work relative value units (RVUs), practice cost RVUs, malpractice RVUs, and total RVUs from the Medicare Fee Schedule (MFS) are merged. It is important to use the latest MFS for obtaining RVUs given that the RBRVS in the most current MFS reflect the most up-to-date perspective on the level of physician inputs to CPT services and procedures. Two different conversion factors may be used to convert the service RVUs into cost estimates. The first is the Medicare national conversion factor for the latest year available (i.e., $36.61 for year 2000) [2]. A second conversion factor is a national conversion factor based on Blue Cross–Blue Shield (BCBS) or the Health Insurance Association of America (HIAA) data. The difference between these two cost estimates will provide an indication of the additional professional costs for private payers compared to Medicare.

Indirect Care Costs

Indirect costs for CAD include patient-related costs that are not directly billable including out-of-pocket expenses, travel time, out-of-work costs, and lost productivity (to name a few). The indirect costs for CAD have not been clearly identified, yet are thought to be considerable. For an average patient with a myocardial infarction, drug costs are estimated to be $278 per year [7]. This cost translates to a nationwide cost of $3.2 billion per year for medication alone [7]. Other home health costs and other medical durables costs account for approximately $1.5 billion in medical expenses [8,9]. These expenses do not take into consideration transportation, child care, and other nonmedical costs related to the patient's condition. This overall burden ranges from a conservative $1300 up to $5000 per year [10]. Early identification and diagnosis of CAD, through more accurate testing, may dramatically improve clinical outcomes and lower the cost of CAD throughout the entire health-care system.

Lost Corporate Performance

Lost corporate performance is difficult to quantify. Large self-insured employers, such as General Electric, are increasingly involved in managing the medical care of their employees, as it directly affects the productivity of the company. Companies are looking for a high value approach to patient management. Integrated care processes, an active commitment to prevention, and continuous research to improve the process are some of the elements now looked at by health-care purchasers.

It is estimated that the lost productivity through morbidity or fatality is as high as $46 billion for CAD alone [9]. This amount nearly equals the $47 billion cost of providing the care for treatment of CAD. Most employers would favor a meaningful change in the process of care that allows for more rapid diagnosis and quicker return of the patient to the working world. In the case of stress SPECT, greater accuracy and faster diagnosis in cardiac imaging will have a tangible impact on corporate performance, allowing patients to be treated more effectively and returned to work more quickly.

Consumer Satisfaction

Published studies clearly demonstrate a positive correlation between accurate and fast diagnosis, patient satisfaction, and effectiveness of health-care delivery [8]. In the outpatient radiology setting, studies show a direct increase in patient satisfaction correlated with appropriate management of the patient's workup, including a triage approach to ensure that the imaging modality is best suited to achieve the best diagnosis. This triage approach is also applicable to cardiac imaging. Once patients are appropriately triaged for nuclear imaging, the probability of redundant, repeated, or inconclusive tests can be greatly reduced based upon current evidence. The most common downstream test following an inconclusive stress SPECT is the more intrusive and costly cardiac catheterization. For this reason, tracking of inappropriate downstream catheterization (or false positive rates) may soon be used as a measure of nuclear laboratory performance. Other measures of patient satisfaction include the backlog or wait for scheduling a test and patient wait time in the laboratory.

Procedure and Supply Costs Methodology

The majority of hospitals use either internal cost accounting systems or Medicare's Cost-to-Charge ratio to derive cost information for medical procedures. Recently, we examined the cost of common diagnostic

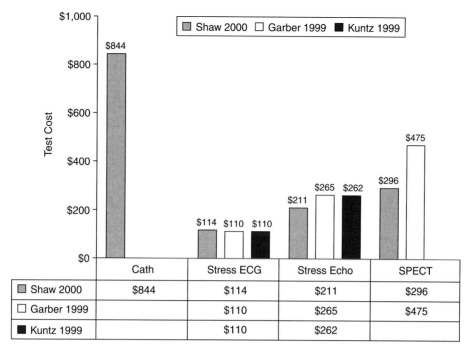

FIGURE 23.2 Weighted average costs from Premier Healthcare Organization institutions and published research [11]. Cath, cardiac catheterization; ECG, electrocardiogram; Echo, echocardiography; SPECT, stress single photon emission computed tomography.

tests from 210 owner-operated U.S. hospitals [11]. For each cardiac diagnostic test, in Figure 23.2, a weighted average was determined for each procedure cost by calculating an average for the entire data set for that procedure, subsequently calculating a 95% confidence interval and deriving upper and lower confidence limits [11]. Procedure costs were weighted by the total number of procedures to arrive at a final mean estimate. The resulting weighted average was then used as the cost of each procedure for a clinico-economic analysis [11]. Cost data for procedure for coronary arterial bypass graft and percutaneous transluminal coronary angioplasty can be derived from the full Medicare Medpar database and are adjusted nationally for severity, excluding any outlying data points. DRG 106 is utilized for coronary artery bypass graft (CABG) and DRG 112 for percutaneous transluminal coronary angioplasty (PTCA) [11]. Supply cost data for pharmacologic stress tests, such as dobutamine, are obtained from various contractual agreements and vary by volume or special pricing arrangements. For most cost analysis, the Red Book price is used as the average wholesale price for each drug, or each manufacturer provides radiopharmaceutical cost.

A major consideration in accounting cost is the per-

spective used in the analysis. For most analysis used for clinical research purposes, the societal perspective is taken. However, within health-care systems or practices, the perspective of the patient or hospital may be preferred.

CALCULATING COSTS

Diagnostic Algorithms Using Nuclear Cardiology

Within the current diagnostic workup of patients, let us examine the use of nuclear imaging as a gatekeeper to cardiac catheterization for patients with suspected cardiac ischemia. Color Figure 23.3 details routine patient workup for suspected cardiac ischemia that includes nuclear cardiology as well as other stress testing procedures [11]. Of particular note, this detailed algorithm provides insight into the estimation of the cost for each portion of a patient management strategy. At each juncture of the clinical workup, patients with low risk or normal test result default to lower cost management options (i.e., "watchful waiting" or risk factor modification versus high-cost cardiac catheterization). Prior research supports a low cardiac catheter-

PATIENT SCENARIO

Suspected Ischemic Heart Disease–Intermediate Probability of CAD/Stress SPECT/Catheterization

52-year old male referred for evaluation of chest pain. Patient smokes one pack per day and has hypertension. ER evaluation was performed and cardiology consult was obtained. A stress thallium was performed as the patient was of intermediate likelihood of CAD. The nuclear scan was positive for ischemia. Catheterization was performed and revealed a 60%–70% stenosis in proximal LAD. A stent was placed.

CARE PATH DIAGRAM

PROCEDURE

CODING/ACTUAL COST

Total = $6,760.90

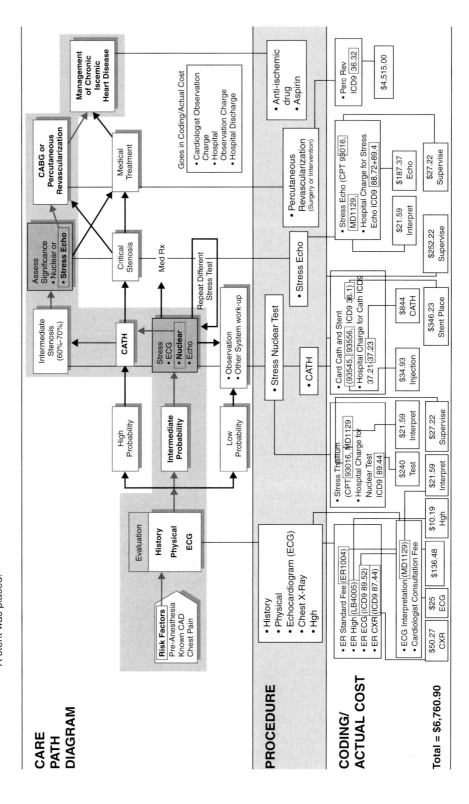

FIGURE 23.3 Clinical care pathway of a patient with suspected coronary artery disease. The patient has an intermediate probability of disease and undergoes stress SPECT imaging and cardiac catheterization. Cost accounting for the patient evaluation takes place by identifying each billable item on the patient's discharge or outpatient record. Cost is then accounted for by adding the tests utilized in the patient workup. ER, emergency room; CXR, chest X-ray; Card Cath, cardiac catheterization; Echo, echocardiogram; Perc Rev, percutaneous coronary revascularization. (Source: Premier Innovations Institute.)

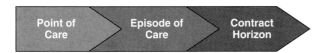

FIGURE 23.4 Major time periods for estimating cost. The point of care is defined as the time at which the clinician makes the decision to use one imaging modality. The episode of care is defined as the full care processes. The contract horizon is defined as the time for a renewal of a health-care plan (~2–3 years).

ization rate for patients with a normal nuclear scan (< 5%) [12,13]. Using this routine workup, stress nuclear imaging may provide a basis for cost efficiency and reduce inappropriate use of invasive procedures within the diagnostic workup of patients with suspected cardiac ischemia.

Cost care paths are used to simulate the clinical outcomes and economic costs of the care process, which are evaluated through three clinical periods (Source: Premier Innovations Institute, Figure 23.4):

Point of Care: defined as the time at which the clinician makes the decision to use one cardiac imaging modality versus another cardiac imaging modality.

Episode of Care: defined as the full care process described in each care path.

Contract Horizon: defined as the time for a renewal of a health-care plan (~2–3 years).

Economic Evidence on SPECT Imaging

Simple cost models

One of the simplest cost models is the cost to identify a particular outcome [13–17]. In 1994, Christian and colleagues defined the cost to identify left main or three-vessel CAD with stress SPECT imaging as excessive in patients with a normal resting electrocardiogram [15]. In an analysis of 5083 patients, the cost to identify cardiac death or myocardial infarction was $5179, but only $3652 if testing was limited to patients at intermediate likelihood of coronary disease [13]. By comparison, Christian et al. reported a cost of $20,550 to identify three-vessel or left main disease for patients with a normal rest ECG [15]. In the preoperative risk evaluation, the cost to avert an in-hospital event was reported to be more favorable for intermediate-risk patients with cardiac risk factors or for those of advanced age (i.e., > 70 years) [14]. Other examples of the cost to identify a cardiac death or myocardial infarction have been put forth [13,14,16]. A challenge to the use of these models is that there are no standards or thresholds for excess cost in diagnostic testing. Thus, the analysis requires subset analysis and comparisons in

varying patient cohorts: for example, costs in patients with a normal versus abnormal rest electrocardiogram (ECG), elderly versus younger patients, and intermediate versus low pretest risk patient subsets. Despite this limitation, one would expect that costs would rise with risk, such that, high-risk patients are also higher cost. Conversely, lower-risk patients should be lower cost. A modeling analysis may be constructed whereby expected cost (i.e., low to high risk) may be compared with actual costs to discern areas of excess spending or underuse of medical services.

Cost savings models

Cost savings, also termed cost minimization, defines lower cost strategies of equivalent choices (i.e., given similar outcomes between a test comparison). This latter requirement for a cost savings model is frequently overlooked in many analyses. For example, health-care administrators who identify tests by their upfront test cost only and not by their induced cost secondary to misclassification fail to encompass all of the costs associated with a particular test choice. As such, test comparisons should include some measure of diagnostic or prognostic test performance. One method for calculating the clinico-economic model of a diagnostic care path includes the use of the following formula where Cost (Loss) = Waste (FP) + Retest Cost (FN) [11]. Retest Cost (FN) is defined as false negative tests from the first testing pass multiplied by the test cost. Waste Cost (FP) is defined as false positive tests from the first testing pass multiplied by the cost of cardiac catheterization. Most recently, Shaw and colleagues compared cost of cardiac testing in 210 U.S. hospitals (N = 24,967) [11]. The episode of care for this analysis was 180-day costs for patients who underwent cardiac testing including stress nuclear, echocardiography, treadmill testing, as well as cardiac catheterization. From this data set (Fig. 23.5), the average cost to identify CAD ranged from $355 for gated SPECT with Tc-99m to $1320 for exercise electrocardiography. The rationale supporting lower costs for Tc-99m imaging is the recent introduction of gated imaging that allows for the assessment of global and regional ventricular function providing for ~30% improvement in test specificity (i.e., reduction in false positives). Higher costs for exercise electrocardiography relate to lower diagnostic accuracy including a diminished specificity.

Other examples of costs savings models have been published [12–16]. Berman et al. defined costs of using hierarchical testing strategies for patients with and without an abnormal rest electrocardiogram [12]. For

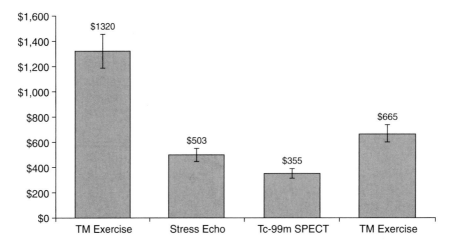

FIGURE 23.5 The average cost to identify coronary disease for intermediate pretest risk patients. TM Exercise, treadmill exercise; Echo, echocardiogram; SPECT, single photon emission computed tomography.

patients with a normal rest electrocardiogram, an exercise treadmill testing without imaging was associated with a 25% lower cost than that of direct catheterization [12]. For patients with an abnormal rest electrocardiogram, nuclear imaging followed by catheterization in patients with ischemia had 38% lower costs than direct catheterization [12]. A similar analysis was published from the Economics of Noninvasive Diagnosis Multicenter Study Group (END) that revealed cost savings from 30% to 41% when cardiac catheterization was limited to patients only

with provocative ischemia on their stress perfusion scan (Fig. 23.6) [18].

Patient selection for cardiac catheterization

One method of understanding cost models is to examine in more detail portions of the diagnostic workup (Fig. 23.6) [18]. Cost waste from SPECT imaging may be accounted from the false positive (i.e., unnecessary testing) and false negative (i.e., downstream admissions for acute coronary syndromes) test rates. A number of

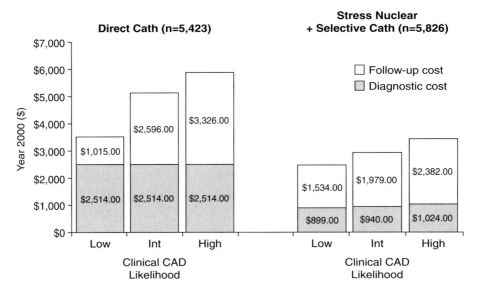

FIGURE 23.6 Results from the Economics of Noninvasive Multicenter Study Group of stable chest pain patients. Substantial cost savings were realized when cardiac catheterization was limited to patients with provocative ischemia: a 30% to 40% cost savings (inflation-adjusted to year 2000). Cath, cardiac catheterization; Int, intermediate; CAD, coronary artery disease.

prior reports have examined the advantages of using stress SPECT imaging as a gatekeeper for cardiac catheterization. In economic terms, this may be defined as the principle of selective resource use where stress SPECT imaging results further limit the decision to perform coronary angiography by excluding low-risk patients. Hachamovitch et al. was the first to report that when catheterization was limited to patients with a summed stress score > 8 or moderate-severe perfusion abnormalities, a 17% reduction in coronary angiography could be achieved [13].

The implications for developing diagnostic cost efficiency may be illustrated by identifying the total cost savings that could be accrued by stress SPECT imaging as an initial test of choice for stable chest pain patients when compared with an invasive, cardiac catheterization approach. This type of analysis was recently put forth by the END investigators [18]. From the recent guidelines for stable angina from the ACC/AHA/ACP-ASIM, stress cardiac imaging is the initial test of choice for patients with Canadian cardiovascular class I or II angina (i.e., mild-moderate chest pain) [19]. Based upon current guidelines, catheter-based intervention is highly indicated for patients with stable symptoms with a large area of ischemic myocardium subtending a significant coronary stenosis [3,19]. Despite the body of evidence, national practice patterns reveal a frequent use of direct catheterization. We compared the cost implications of using nuclear imaging as an initial diagnostic test and limiting cardiac catheterization only to patients with provocative ischemia. These results reveal a 30%–40% cost savings when provocative ischemia is a requisite prior to referral to catheterization (Fig. 23.6) [18]. Translating this evidence from seven hospitals to any hospital's population reveals that for every 1000 patients referred to cardiac catheterization, use of a stress SPECT scan could result in a savings ~$3 million. The primary benefit would be in excluding catheterization for patients who have normal perfusion results who would receive little therapeutic benefit from percutaneous intervention. Similar results have been reported in the Economics of Myocardial Perfusion Imaging in Europe (EMPIRE) study [20]. We are currently expanding on the evidence put forth in the END study into a disease management strategy that is being applied in the Clinical Outcomes of Revascularization and Aggressive Drug Evaluation (COURAGE) trial. The COURAGE trial is a 3260-patient, randomized, controlled trial of current maximal medical therapy versus medical therapy plus percutaneous coronary intervention in reducing cardiac death or myocardial infarction for patients with catheterization-defined coronary dis-

ease (excluding poor left ventricular dysfunction or three-vessel–left main CAD). In the COURAGE trial, nuclear imaging is being used to decide whether treated CAD patients should return to the angiographic suite. In patients with recurrent symptoms who are being treated medically or had PCI, if insufficient ischemia is documented on stress SPECT imaging, then continued medical management is warranted. Conversely, for those with recurrent symptoms and worsening ischemia, then reangiography and revascularization are considered appropriate.

COST-EFFECTIVENESS ANALYSIS

The term cost-effectiveness is often used to identify all forms of cost analysis. However, by definition, cost-effectiveness analysis attempts to conjoin both the costs encumbered by a therapy or test choice with the outcome advantages or disadvantages of those choices [21–30]. Cost-effectiveness analysis is used when comparing varying test techniques defined as the marginal cost difference of one test divided by outcome differences; namely, cost-effectiveness analyses compare the amount of resources consumed by a test in relation to its accrued benefits. The simple equation for incremental or marginal cost-effectiveness is $C_{Test\ \#1} - C_{Test\ \#2}/O_{Test\ \#1} - O_{Test\ \#2}$ where C is cost and O is outcome. For a test to be cost-effective, it must optimize either the cost or outcome portion of the equation. A dominant strategy results when both cost and outcomes are improved. Although the outcome differences can be one of any significant outcomes ranging from changes in symptoms to life years saved, the U.S. Public Health Service (PHS) has put forth standards that cost-effectiveness analysis should use the common metric of cost per life year saved [21–30]. This type of analysis appears to fit with therapeutic agents, it does not, however, appear to reflect the practical usage of a diagnostic test [21,22]. Diagnostic tests do not save lives per se but identify disease or risk. Subsequent therapies and decisions of the treating physician result in an improvement in patient quality and quantity of life years. As such, there is no accepted standard for cost-effectiveness of a diagnostic test. There are those, however, who have put forth incremental modeling strategies of cost-effectiveness that deal with the identification of disease or clinical outcome that more closely mirror actual test interpretation. For example, in Figure 23.7, the incremental cost-effectiveness of varying test choices is depicted [11]. In this example, test costs vary from diagnostic cost-effectiveness. Test costs increase with higher equipment and labor costs, such as positron emission tomography or mag-

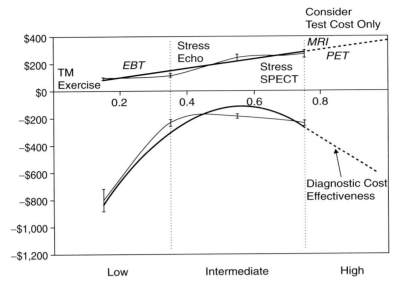

FIGURE 23.7 Incremental cost-effectiveness of noninvasive cardiac tests by pretest risk of coronary disease. Based upon work completed with the Premier Healthcare Organization, these results reveal that for low-risk patients, the use of electron beam tomography or treadmill exercise may be the more cost-effective strategy. For intermediate-risk patients, stress echocardiography and SPECT imaging provide dominant strategies and their use may be based on local epxertise. Higher-cost tests, such as magnetic resonance and positron emission tomography, have yet to have established vast cost-effectiveness data. TM Exercise, treadmill exercise; EBT, electron beam tomography; Echo, echocardiogram; SPECT, single photon emission computed tomography; MRI, magnetic resonance imaging; PET, positron emission tomography.

netic resonance imaging. However, improved sensitivity and specificity can lower overall diagnostic costs and result in dominant strategies or negative cost-effectiveness ratios.

These results coincide with one of the general tenets of cost-effectiveness where tests become more cost-effective concomitant to being more accurate in detecting disease or outcome risk. Another tenet is the high-risk cost-effectiveness model where treatment of higher-risk patients results in greater therapeutic benefit and improved cost-effectiveness ratios. For example, the model of high-risk cost-effectiveness was published for preoperative risk stratification prior to vascular surgery [14]. From this analysis, preoperative risk stratification including pharmacologic stress SPECT imaging was more cost-effective for symptomatic patients, those with an intermediate likelihood of coronary disease, and for those patients over age 70 years [14]. For each of these patient subsets, the cost-effectiveness ratios were < $50,000 per life year saved (the standard threshold for economic efficiency) [11,13,14,18,21,22]. Goldman et al. have published other reports on the cost-effectiveness of a variety of diagnostic tests in a review of economic evidence in cardiology (i.e., a league table of economic evidence)

[28]. Other reviews that include updated evidence on stress SPECT imaging reveal that stress myocardial perfusion imaging is cost-effective for various patient subsets including patients without a prior coronary diagnosis who are at intermediate risk, stable chest pain patients, and elderly patients [11,13,14,18,21,22]. For patients with a prior diagnosis, less economic extensive research has been published, however, current national guidelines support the use of nuclear cardiology techniques for more precise delineation of disease progression [3,19].

CONCLUSIONS

An ever-increasing body of evidence supports the fact that nuclear cardiology techniques are increasingly cost-effective for varying patient subsets. The assessment of myocardial perfusion and global and regional ventricular function as a clinically effective tool can result in cost-effective management of patients with suspected cardiac ischemia including intermediate likelihood patients, those with stable chest pain, and the elderly; also for preoperative risk stratification and for those after exercise treadmill testing.

REFERENCES

1. Smith S, Freeland M, Heffer S, et al. The next ten years of health spending. Health Affairs, 1998;17:128.

2. http:/www.acc.org

3. Scanlon PJ, Faxon DP, Audet AM, et al. ACC/AHA Guidelines for coronary angiography: a report of the American College of Cardiology / American Heart Association Task Force on practice guidelines. J Am Coll Cardiol 1999;33:1756.

4. Lonn E, Yusuf S. Evidence based cardiology: emerging approaches in preventing cardiovascular disease. Br Med J 1999; 318:1337.

5. Eddy DM. Clinical decision making: from theory to practice. A collection of essays from the Journal of the American Medical Association. Sudbury (MA): Jones and Bartlett Publishers; 1996.

6. Assessing the Efficacy and Safety of Medical Technologies. September 1978. NTIS order #PB-286929.

7. http://www.americanheart.org/statistics/index.html

8. Kangarloo H, Ho B, Lufkin RB, et al. Effect of conversion from a fee-for-service plan to a capitation reimbursement system on a circumscribed outpatient radiology practice of 20,000 persons. Health Policy and Practice 1996;201:79.

9. Direct costs were extrapolated from estimates for 1997 by Thomas A. Hodgson, chief economist and acting director, Division of Health and Utilization Analysis, OAEHP, CDC/NCHS. Estimates of indirect costs were made by Thomas J. Thom, statistician in the division of Epidemiology and Clinical Applications, NHLBJ.

10. Weintraub WS, Mauldin PD, Becker E, et al. A comparison of the costs of and quality of life after coronary angioplasty or coronary surgery for multivessel CAD. Results from the Emory Angioplasty Versus Surgery Trial (EAST). Circulation 1995;92:2831.

11. Shaw L, Muluagh S, Jacobson C, Golynsky L, Strittmatter D, Campbell P, Kiteman D, Ford JK, Guilloteau FR, Denham CR. Cost implications of diagnosing coronary disease. Eur Heart J 2000;21:477.

12. Berman DS, Hachamovitch R, Kiat H, et al. Incremental value of prognostic testing in patients with known or suspected ischemic heart disease. J Am Coll Cardiol 1995;26:639.

13. Hachamovitch R, Berman DS, Shaw LJ, et al. Incremental prognostic value of myocardial perfusion single photon emission computed tomography for the prediction of cardiac death: differential stratification for risk of cardiac death and myocardial infarction. Circulation 1998;97:535.

14. Shaw LJ, Hachamovitch R, Eisenstein E, et al. Cost implications for implementing a selective preoperative risk screening approach for peripheral vascular surgery patients. Am J Managed Care 1997;3:1817.

15. Christian TF, Miller TD, Bailey KR, et al. Exercise tomographic thallium-201 imaging in patients with severe coronary artery disease and normal electrocardiograms. Ann Intern Med 1994;121:825.

16. Shaw LJ, Miller DD, Romeis JC, et al. Prognostic value of noninvasive risk stratification and coronary revascularization in nonelderly and elderly patients referred for evaluation of clinically suspected coronary artery disease. J Am Geriatr Soc 1996;44:1190.

17. Berman D, Hachamovitch R, Lewin H, et al. Risk stratification in coronary artery disease: implications for stabilization and prevention. Am J Cardiol 1997;79:10.

18. Shaw LJ, Hachamovitch R, Berman DS, et al. The economic consequences of available diagnostic and prognostic strategies for the evaluation of stable angina patients: an observational assessment of the value of precatheterization ischemia. Economics of Noninvasive Diagnosis (END) Multicenter Study Group. J Am Coll Cardiol 1999;33:661.

19. Gibbons R, Chatterjee K, Daley J, et al. ACC/AHA/ACP-ASIM guidelines for the management of patients with chronic stable angina. J Am Coll Cardiol 1999;33:2092.

20. Underwood SR, Godman B, Salyani S, et al. Economics of myocardial perfusion imaging in Europe—The EMPIRE study. Eur Heart J 1999;20:157.

21. Garber AM, et al. Cost-effectiveness of alternative test strategies for the diagnosis of coronary artery disease. Ann Intern Med 1999;130:719.

22. Kuntz KM. Cost-effectiveness of diagnostic strategies for patients with chest pain. Ann Intern Med 1999;130:709.

23. Schwartz JS. Economics and cost effectiveness in evaluating the value of cardiovascular therapies. Comparative economic data regarding lipid-lowering drugs. Am Heart J 1999;137:S97.

24. Finkler S. Cost Accounting for Health Care Organizations: Concepts and Applications. Gaithersburg, MD: Aspen Publishers, 1994.

25. Laupacis A, Feeny D, Detsky AS, et al. How attractive does a new technology have to be to warrant adoption and utilization? Tentative guidelines for using clinical and economic evaluations. CMAJ 1992;146:473.

26. Weinstein MC, Stason WB. Cost-effectiveness of coronary artery bypass surgery. Circulation 1982; 66(5 Pt 2): III56.

27. Mark D. Medical economics and health policy issues for interventional cardiology. Textbook of Interventional Cardiology, 2nd edition. Philadelphia: W. B. Saunders, 1993.

28. Goldman L, Garber AM, Grover SA, et al. 27th Bethesda Conference: matching the intensity of risk factor management with the hazard for CAD events. Task Force 6. Cost effectiveness of assessment and management of risk factors. J Am Coll Cardiol 1996;27:1020.

29. Shaw LJ, Eisenstein EL, Hachamovitch R, et al. A primer of biostatistic and economic methods for diagnostic and prognostic modeling in nuclear cardiology: Part II . J Nucl Cardiol 1997; 4(1 Pt 1): 52.

30. Drummond MF, Jefferson TO. Guidelines for authors and peer reviewers of economic submissions to the BMJ. The BMJ Economic Evaluation Working Party. BMJ 1996;313:275.

24 | Interpreting and reporting nuclear studies

AMI E. ISKANDRIAN AND MARIO S. VERANI

There are several crucial steps for providing high-quality nuclear studies (Table 24.1). The American Society of Nuclear Cardiology (ASNC) guidelines are helpful and may be worth reviewing from time to time (see Chapter 25). In this chapter, we discuss the last two issues related to interpretation and reporting.

INTERPRETING SPECT PERFUSION STUDIES

As outlined in Table 24.2, start by knowing the patient. Find out the age, gender, height, weight, breast cup size, reason for the study, prior percutaneous transluminal coronary angioplasty (PTCA), prior coronary artery bypass graft (CABG), prior myocardial infarction (MI), risk factors, prior study, and medications. Did he or she have a prior study? What were the nonimaging stress performance results such as angina, ST shifts, blood pressure response, workload and maximal heart rate achieved. These are important to put the imaging results in perspective and to even the playing field when communicating the results to the treating physician. Remember to compare the current study with prior studies. This means you actually re-evaluate the old study and not just rely on the report. Avoid reading from hard copies or X-ray films; there is no substitute for reading directly from the computer, as you have the freedom to adjust and fine-tune the contrast, intensity, and color displays.

The reporting formats for single-photon emission computed tomography (SPECT) are summarized in Tables 24.3–8 and of RNA in Tables 24.9 and 24.10. The report should be informative and precise and should help rather than hinder patient care. We strongly oppose equivocal reports that use terms such as "probably," "possibly," or "borderline normal." You just have to put yourself on the receiving end and ask your-self, the million-dollar questions: Did this report help me in managing this patient? Will I send another patient to this laboratory? Remember you have to be consistent every time, as there is no room for compromise. This policy is good for your patient and is good for your business!

An example of a computer-generated report form used at the University of Alabama at Birmingham (UAB) is shown in Table 24.8.

INTERPRETING AND REPORTING

Please avoid jargon and ambiguities such as breast attenuation, as such terms may be meaningful to the imaging specialty but have no meaning or may be confusing to the primary care physician. Other popular but useless terms are "clinical correlation is required," "there is heterogeneity," "there is creep," "the perfusion is normal in the gray scale but abnormal in the color scale," "the defect is due to scar but ischemia cannot be excluded."

The conclusion part of the report should be clear and concise and should incorporate the perfusion as well as functional data. For the functional data from the gated SPECT images, use the cine display and look at motion in gray scale and thickening in color scale. Inspect both the slices and three-dimensional images. Look for changes in wall motion between rest and poststress images. Note if the endocardial border is completely depicted. Watch for flickering as a sign of poor ECG gating. Remember that gating may be poor even if there is no obvious flickering. An ECG strip may be of help. In atrial fibrillation, use the higher of the two EF numbers (rest versus poststress). In low–high dose or dual-isotope protocols, the high-dose or technetium tracer EF is more likely to be the correct one. In most patients the poststress EF is similar

TABLE 24.1 *Procedures Needed to Assure High-Quality Nuclear Cardiology Studies*

1. Selecting the appropriate test
2. Selecting the appropriate stress protocol
3. Selecting the appropriate imaging protocol
4. Maintaining up-to-date imaging systems
5. Interpreting with skill
6. Reporting results

TABLE 24.2 *Interpreting the SPECT Perfusion Images*

1. Know the patient: age, sex, weight, etc.
2. Review the rotating images: stress and rest
3. Review the slices
   a. Color and gray scales: short-axis, vertical-long axis, and horizontal-long axis
   b. Artifacts
   c. Alignment
   d. Scaling of both stress and rest
   e. Hot spots within and outside the heart
   f. Localized uptake in lungs, breast, axilla, mediastinum (Figs. 24.1 and 2)
   g. Subdiaphragmatic abnormality such as ascites, bowel, stomach, gall bladder, liver, and spleen size (Fig. 24.3)
4. Are the images normal or abnormal?
   a. If abnormal, where is the abnormality?
   b. How large and severe is the abnormality?
   c. Is it in one, two, or three vascular territories?
   d. What is the nature of the abnormality: fixed, reversible, or mixed?
   e. Is there LV dilatation, fixed, transient (or both)?
   f. Is there RV dilatation?
   g. Is the lung uptake increased? (Figs. 24.4).
   h. Is the image quality reasonable to make definitive conclusions?
5. Review the quantitative data and comparison to normal data base
6. Review both rest and stress gated SPECT data
7. Review attenuation/scatter/depth resolution corrected images if available
8. Compare to prior studies if available

TABLE 24.3 *How to Report a SPECT Study*

1. Provide protocol data
2. Provide a two-part report: descriptive and conclusion
3. Provide functional data
4. Avoid jargon
5. Avoid ambiguities
6. Be concise and quantitative

TABLE 24.4 *Protocol Data in Report*

1. Age	6. Type of stress
2. Sex	7. Type of protocol
3. Date of study	8. Type of tracer
4. Medical record number	9. Doses
5. Referring MD	

TABLE 24.5 *Report of Perfusion Data*

1. Is the perfusion normal or abnormal?
2. Where is the site(s) of the defect?
3. Is it mild, moderate, or severe?(degree of uptake reduction)
4. Is it small, moderate, or large? (extent of abnormality)
5. What percentage of LV myocardium is involved?
6. Is it reversible? How much? (completely, almost completely, partially reversible, or fixed)
7. In viability studies, remember a half empty glass is also half full! A fixed defect means viable myocardium unless it is very severe
8. Is there LV dilatation? (fixed, transient, both)
9. Is there RV dilatation?
10. Is there increased lung tracer uptake?
11. Are there extracardiac findings of importance?

TABLE 24.6 *Report of Gated SPECT*

1. Describe LV regional wall motion and thickening in the post-stress and rest images
2. Describe LV size
3. Indicate LVEF
4. Describe RV size and motion

TABLE 24.7 *Conclusions of Report*

1. Summarize study results "this conclusion is based on perfusion, function, and others"
2. Is there one-, two-, or three-vessel disease? Which?
3. Quantify the total defect size
4. Quantify the ischemic burden
5. Summarize LV/RV function

The UAB School of Medicine
Department of Medicine/Division of Cardiovascular Disease
Nuclear Cardiology
Myocardial Perfusion SPECT Study

Patient: Blue Rose | Age/Sex: 79, Male
Medical Record No: 99 999 99 | Date of Study: 07 24/02
Referring Physician: Brown, XY | Indication for Study: CHF
Attenuation Correction: No | Isotope/Protocol: MIBI: Lo stress/Hi stress
Stress Dose: 12 mCi | Rest Dose: 34 mCi
Height: 171 [cm] | Weight: 182 lbs.

Stress Test:

Type of stress: Adenosine | Chest Pain During Test: Yes
Baseline ECG: Normal | Rhythm: NSR
Resting HR: 62 bpm | Resting Systolic BP 120 mm Hg
Peak HR: 72 bpm | Peak Systolic BP: 104 mm Hg
Stress ECG Results: Negative

1. SPECT Perfusion (see Fig. 9.9, p. 153 for scores of stress/rest)

2. Gated SPECT Regional Wall Motion/Thickening (see Fig. 9.9, p 153 for scores)

3. Perfusion defect-size (example 30%)

4. Gated SPECT Global Ventricular Function:
   LVEF: Post-stress: 70%   Rest: 65%
   LV Size: normal [or mildly, moderately, severely enlarged]
   RV Size: normal [or mildly, moderately, severely enlarged]
   RV function: normal [or mildly, moderately or severely depressed]

5. Other findings:
   Transient ischemic dilatation (TID): No [or Yes]
   Lung-heart ratio (LHR): Normal [or abnormal]
   Post-stress stunning: Yes [or No]

6. ***Results and Conclusions*** (Examples)
The myocardial perfusion pattern is normal.
The LV size and wall motion/thickening are normal with EF of 70%. The RV function/size are normal.
or, if abnormal
There is a large area of ischemia, involving approximately 30% of the LV myocardium, consistent with three-vessel CAD. There is evidence of post-stress stunning with wall motion abnormality and a decrease of EF from 55% at rest to 37% post-stress. There is transient LV dilatation. The resting LV and RV functions and sizes are normal.

I have personally reviewed the ECG and images and interpreted the study and agree with the above report.

Ami E. Iskandrian, MD
Professor, and Director, Nuclear Cardiology

TABLE 24.9 *Items to Be Considered When Interpreting Gated Equilibrium RNA*

1. Labeling quality	6. Normalization
2. Counts	7. Gray vs color scale
3. ROI for EF calculations	8. LV size/wall motion
4. Background activity	9. LV diastolic indices
5. Time-activity curve (LV volume curve)	10. RV function
	11. Other findings

TABLE 24.10 *Items to Be Considered When Interpreting First-Pass RNA*

1. Position: supine/upright	11. Color vs gray scale
2. Projection: ant/RAO/LAO	12. Count-statistics
3. Injection: bolus integrity	13. Representative (summed) LV and RV beat
4. Frame rate	14. LV: wall motion/ regional ejection fraction index (REFI)
5. Bolus transit time	15. RV: wall motion/ regional ejection fraction (RVEF)
6. ROI: single or dual	16. Others
7. Background activity	
8. Beat selection	
9. Abnormal rhythm?	
10. 10-Cine vs static view of data	

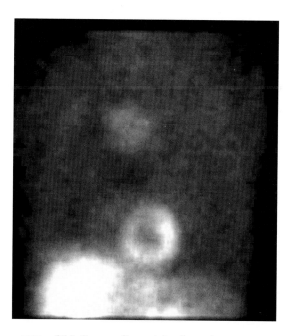

FIGURE 24.1 Extracardiac activity due to lung tumor.

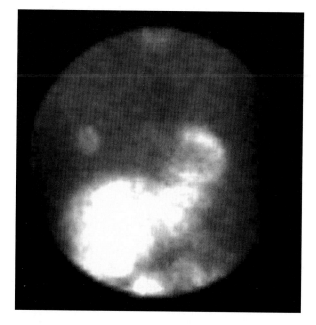

FIGURE 24.2 Extracardiac activity due to breast carcinoma.

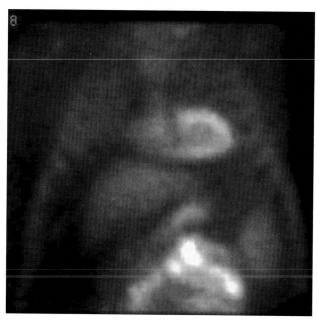

FIGURE 24.3 Liver cirrhosis with small liver and ascites.

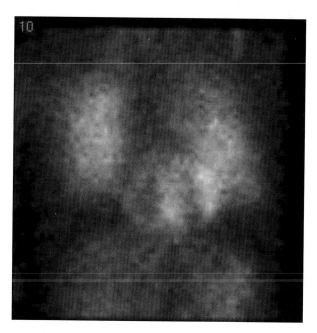

FIGURE 24.4 Increased lung uptake in a patient with multivessel CAD.

to the rest EF, but in some patients it is lower due to postischemic stunning. This finding is seen in roughly 15% of patients with CAD and often signifies severe ischemia. Be sure to make a comment on that in the report. If the poststress EF is higher than the rest EF, report the high number especially if it is the one obtained with the high dose.

In "viability" studies, the severity of defect is important. A mild-to-moderate fixed defect means the presence of viable myocardium and this should be clearly stated. Remember a glass that is half empty is also a glass that is half full. If you emphasize the empty part (fixed defect), the message on viability will be lost by the referring physician.

25 | ACC/AHA/ASNC guidelines and position papers

AMI E. ISKANDRIAN AND MARIO S. VERANI

A list of published guidelines and statements generated by the American Society of Nuclear Cardiology (ASNC) and by ACC/AHA is provided in Table 25.1. They can be downloaded from http://www.asnc.org and http://www.cardiosource.com

The scope of these guidelines varies considerably; some are of technical nature such as "how to do" and others are of clinical nature such as "when to do." It is likely that, on a regular basis, new guidelines will continue to appear and old ones will be revised as new information becomes available. The guidelines are simply that: "guidelines," and are therefore not indisputable. They are supposed to reflect mainstream opinion and are written by a panel of experts. Independent panels of experts review the initial drafts. The guidelines may conceivably reflect biases of the panel members and especially those of the more vocal members. For this reason, not everyone will agree with every statement in them. A case in point is the risk assessment after acute myocardial infarction. The guidelines put a great emphasis on treadmill exercise testing alone. The reality is that most cardiologists use an imaging modality and many prefer pharmacologic testing to exercise testing. It is also probably true that by the time a guideline is published, new information becomes available that is not included in the guideline. In general, the guidelines have proved useful as means for standardization and consistency. Third-party payers, for reimbursement purposes, have used some of these guidelines and they are often used in medicolegal cases. They are, as would be expected, especially useful to novice physicians.

TABLE 25.1 *Guidelines and Statements Published by the ASNC and ACC/AHA*

Year	Title	Source
1995	Clinical application of radionuclide angiography	J Nucl Cardiol 1995;2:551
	ACC/AHA Task Force Report. Guidelines for Clinical Use of Cardiac Radionuclide Imaging	J Am Coll Cardiol 1995;25:521
1996	Statement on mobile and remote-site provision of nuclear cardiology imaging services	J Nucl Cardiol 996;4:174
	Clinical relevance of a normal myocardial perfusion scintigraphic study	J Nucl Cardiol 1996;4:172
	Acute Myocardial Infarction: ACC/AHA Practice Guidelines for the Management of Patients with Perioperative Cardiovascular Evaluation for Non-cardiac Surgery	J Am Coll Cardiol 1996;28:1328 J Am Coll Cardiol 1996;27:910
1997	Design and implementation of a nuclear cardiology testing facility in a private-practice cardiology office setting	J Nucl Cardiol 1997;4:156
	ACC/AHA Guidelines for Exercise Testing	J Am Coll Cardiol 1997;30:260
1998	Non-perfusion application in nuclear cardiology: report of a task force of the American Society of Nuclear Cardiology Approved 1998	J Nucl Cardiol 1998;5:218
	Management of Patients with Valvular Heart Disease: ACC/AHA Practice Guidelines for Radiation Safety in the Practice of Cardiology: Expert Consensus Document Nuclear Cardiology Services: Policy Statement	J Am Coll Cardiol 1998;32:1486 J Am Coll Cardiol 1998;31:892 J Am Coll Cardiol 1998;31:720

(continued)

TABLE 25.1 *Guidelines and Statements Published by the ASNC and ACC/AHA (Continued)*

Year	Title	Source
1999	ASNC Position Statement on ECG-Gating of Myocardial Perfusion SPECT Scintigrams	J Nucl Cardiol 1999;6:470
	Wintergreen Panel Summaries, Part 1	J Nucl Cardiol 1999;6:93
	ACC/AHA/ACP-ASIM Guideline for the Management of Patients with Chronic Stable Angina	J Am Coll Cardiol 1999;33:2092
	Coronary Angiography: ACC/AHA Practice Guidelines	J Am Coll Cardiol 1999;33:1756
	Coronary Artery Bypass Graft Surgery (CABG): ACC/AHA Practice Guidelines for	J Am Coll Cardiol 1999;34:1262
	Assessment of Cardiovascular Risk by Use of Multiple-Risk-Factor Assessment Equations: Expert Consensus Document	J Am Coll Cardiol 1999;34:1348-59
	Imaging Guidelines for Nuclear Cardiology Procedures, Part 2	J Nucl Cardiol 1999;6:G48
2000	Credentials recommended for cardiologist seeking hospital privileges to perform nuclear cardiology procedures	Approved by board of directors, April 21, 2000
	American College of Cardiology/American Heart Association Clinical Competence Statement of Stress Testing	J Am Coll Cardiol 2000;36:1441
	Adult Cardiovascular Medicine (COCATS): Revised June 2000. Task Force #5: Training in Nuclear Cardiology	J Am Coll Cardiol 1995;25:1
	Management of Patients with Unstable Angina and Non-ST-Segment Elevation Myocardial Infarction: Practice Guidelines for	J Am Coll Cardiol 2000;36:970
2001	Updated imaging guidelines for nuclear cardiology procedures, Part 1	J Nucl Cardiol 2001;8:5
	Bar Harbor Invitation Meeting	J Nucl Cardiol 2001;8:224
	Percutaneous Coronary Intervention: ACC/AHA Guideline for (Revision of the 1993 PTCA Guidelines)	J Am Coll Cardiol 2001;37:2239i–lxvi

26 | Practical aspects of running a nuclear cardiology laboratory

MANUEL D. CERQUEIRA

Beyond the technical aspects of acquiring and interpreting images, the practice of nuclear cardiology requires compliance with federal and state regulations governing the use of radiation, documentation of competence or certification of the medical staff that is interpreting the images, and accreditation of the facilities and equipment where the studies are performed. Some of these requirements are mandatory, while others are voluntary but strongly recommended by professional medical societies to help promote quality in nuclear cardiology. In some cases these requirements may be used by payers of medical services as "gatekeepers"—some would say hurdles—to those providing diagnostic services. This chapter reviews the regulations, regulators, and organizations that address these practical aspects of nuclear cardiology. The major regulators are the Nuclear Regulatory Commission (NRC) and Agreement States. Physicians can be certified by the Certification Board of Nuclear Cardiology (CBNC). Finally, laboratories can be accredited by the Intersocietal Commission for the Accreditation of Nuclear Medicine Laboratories (ICANL). The background, rationale, existing regulations, and application procedures for each of these organizations are reviewed. The material presented is current but is subject to change, and the individual organizations should be contacted directly to obtain the most recent information. Web site addresses are provided when available.

PHYSICIAN TRAINING REQUIREMENTS FOR LICENSURE AS AUTHORIZED USER OF RADIOPHARMACEUTICALS FOR IMAGING AND LOCALIZATION STUDIES

The NRC licenses hospitals, private clinics, and individual physicians to possess and administer radioactive materials for medical purposes. The NRC directly regulates and monitors this privilege in the following 16 states: Alaska, Connecticut, Delaware, District of Columbia, Hawaii, Idaho, Indiana, Michigan, Missouri, Montana, New Jersey, South Dakota, Vermont, Virginia, West Virginia, and Wyoming. Through written agreements with the NRC, 31 states (i.e., Agreement States) have assumed regulatory authority for facilities using radioactive materials within their borders. In regulating such material, the basic radiation protection standards imposed by an Agreement State must be as strict as those of the NRC. Some Agreement States have imposed and enforced more stringent requirements than the NRC. As an example, Texas and Georgia require that the 200 hours of didactic training in radiation safety must be obtained in an Accreditation Council for Graduate Medical Education (ACGME) training program. This means that training received in programs outside of residency training, usually cardiologists taking radiation safety and basic science courses, do not meet the eligibility criteria in these states. Even if an applicant has had an NRC or Agreement State license in another state, these two states may not grant an authorized user license to such physicians. The three remaining states, Minnesota, Pennsylvania, and Wisconsin, are currently operating under NRC regulation, but they have sent the NRC letters of intent to become Agreement States.

These inconsistent laws across the United States makes it confusing for applicants, difficult for training programs, and limit the geographic mobility of physicians wishing to practice nuclear cardiology. Physicians in training or considering relocating their nuclear cardiology practice to a particular state or region need to contact the Agreement State office or the NRC region to obtain clarification on the exact requirements for licensure. Specific details including a directory with contact numbers and mailing addresses for each state can be found at http://www.hsrd.ornl.gov/nrc/asframe.htm. The NRC can be contacted at http://www.nrc.gov.

485

The current requirements for physicians seeking to become authorized users for performing imaging and localization studies using radioactive materials are defined in the United States Nuclear Regulatory Commission Rules and Regulations, Title 10, Chapter 1, Code of Federal Regulations-Energy Part 35 Medical Use of Byproduct Material Subpart J-Training and Experience Requirements 35.920, Training for Imaging and Localization Studies. Physicians wishing to perform radionuclide imaging studies limited to a single organ such as the heart may be expected to meet the same requirements as physicians applying for general nuclear medicine privileges. In such a case the total hourly didactic and clinical experience may be limited to cardiac imaging studies for those physicians wishing to practice only nuclear cardiology. Relevant regulations that are currently in place by the NRC are summarized in Tables 26.1–4.

There has been an extensive revision of Part 35 and the proposed Board Certification and training and experience eligibility requirements to become an authorized user are listed in Table 26.5. The NRC and Congress have approved these recommendations. They will be published in the Federal Registrar and be implemented in the NRC regulated states 6 months following publication. The Agreement States will have up to 3 years following publication to become compliant with the revised requirements or make alternative rule proposals to the NRC. Some states have already expressed to the NRC that the existing policies have worked properly and they have no intent to implement the new policies. Since the Agreement States are allowed to have stricter requirements than the NRC federal policy, the states may be allowed to maintain the existing training and experience requirements in the future despite the approved revisions at the federal level. The revised guidelines will not apply to physicians who have completed or already started training.

Given the uncertain implementation of the revised rules in NRC-regulated states and the lack of willingness of Agreement States to fully implement the changes, clarification should be obtained prior to starting a training program or seeking a license to use radioisotopes from the appropriate Agreement State or the NRC. Meeting the criteria outlined in Tables 26.1–4 is the greatest guarantee that applicants will be granted an authorized user license.

The NRC and Agreement States require that physicians seeking to become authorized radiopharmaceutical users through an individual license, such as would be required for an outpatient diagnostic facility or inclusion on an institutional license, meet at least one of the requirements listed in Table 26.1. The NRC accepts

TABLE 26.1 *Current Nuclear Regulatory Commission Physician Requirements for Authorization to Use Radiopharmaceuticals*

1. Board Certification
   a. Nuclear Medicine by the American Board of Nuclear Medicine
   b. Diagnostic Radiology by the American Board of Radiology; or
   c. Diagnostic Radiology or Radiology by the American Osteopathic Board of Radiology;
   d. Nuclear Medicine by the Royal College of Physicians and Surgeons of Canada; or
   e. American Osteopathic Board of Nuclear Medicine

OR Training and experience consisting of the following:

2. Didactic, practical and supervised experience
   a. Classroom and laboratory training (200 hours)
   b. Supervised work experience (500 hours)
   c. Supervised clinical experience (500 hours)

that individuals who are board certified by the listed boards meet all the hourly requirements listed in item 2 in Table 26.1 as a result of their training. This acceptance is based on the requirements of residency accreditation organizations that such training programs provide a minimum number of hours of training in the basics of radiation physics, radiopharmacy, and radiation safety as well as supervised radiation related experience. Board eligible physicians in these areas also meet the requirements on the basis of item 2 in Table 26.1. Such training and experience must have been completed within 5 years of the application for licensure. If training was completed longer than 5 years prior to applying, there must be clear documentation of related continuing medical education and clinical experience since completion of the training.

Since most cardiologists are not board certified in nuclear medicine or radiology, in order to obtain a license to use radiopharmaceuticals they must meet the hourly training and experience requirements as listed in item 2 of Table 26.1 and detailed in Tables 26.2–4. Table 26.2 lists the didactic classroom and laboratory training that is required and a summary list of the areas to be covered. Table 26.3, supervised work experience, and Table 26.4, supervised clinical experience,

TABLE 26.2 *Classroom and Laboratory Training (200 hours)*

1. Radiation physics and instrumentation
2. Radiation protection
3. Mathematics pertaining to the use and measurement of radioactivity
4. Radiopharmaceutical chemistry
5. Radiation biology

TABLE 26.3 *Supervised Work Experience (500 hours)*

1. Ordering, receiving, and unpacking radioactive materials safely and performing the related radiation surveys;
2. Calibrating dose calibrators and diagnostic instruments and performing checks for proper operation of survey meters;
3. Calculating and safely preparing patient or human research subject dosages;
4. Using administrative controls to prevent the misadministration of byproduct material;
5. Using procedures to contain spilled byproduct material safely and using proper decontamination procedures; and
6. Eluting technetium-99m from generator systems, measuring and testing the eluate for molybdenum-99 and alumina contamination, and processing the eluate with reagent kits to prepare technetium-99m labeled radiopharmaceuticals.

list the required areas of radiation safety and clinical patient contact. There is no consensus whether these two separate blocks of time can be accumulated concurrently or separately. If they can be done concurrently, this would make the total training and experience time requirement equal to 700 hours or approximately 4 months. If they must be done separately, this would require 1200 hours or approximately 6 months of total time to become an authorized user.

The most foolproof approach for trainees or physicians in practice is to accumulate a total of 1200 hours, as this will meet the eligibility requirements in any NRC or Agreement State under the old rules or the proposed revision listed in Table 26.5.

The major changes in Part 35, as listed in Table 26.5, address the issues of board certification and the number of hours. Under the new regulations, new certification boards will be able to apply and be recognized by the NRC so that physicians who have passed these boards will automatically qualify for authorized user licensure. The major requirement for the boards is that the minimum training and experience requirements for candidates meet the NRC criteria. The NRC has initiated an application process for boards, and the Certification Board of Nuclear Cardiology has submitted a

TABLE 26.4 *Supervised Clinical Experience (500 hours)*

1. Examining patients or human research subjects and reviewing their case histories to determine their suitability for radioisotopic diagnosis, limitations, or contraindications;
2. Selecting the suitable radiopharmaceuticals and calculating and measuring the dosages;
3. Administering dosages to patients and using syringe radiation shields;
4. Collaborating with the authorized user in the interpretation of radioisotope test results; and
5. Patient or human research subject follow-up.

request for recognition. It has met all the requirements and it is anticipated that it will be approved and thereby all physicians certified by the CBNC in the future will qualify for licensure by showing proof of certification.

Under the proposed revisions, individuals who are not certified by an approved board can apply on the basis of training and experience. As shown in Table 26.5, the requirements are for a total of 700 hours and there is no specific breakdown in terms of the number of classroom and didactic hours. The new regulations list only the content to be covered during the course of training. The signature of the authorized user who has served as the preceptor for the applicant will be accepted as proof that all of the necessary content has been presented and successfully mastered by the trainee. This puts a new responsibility on the preceptor to verify that the individual who has been trained is competent in all areas of radiation safety and the ability to conduct safe clinical studies that will protect patients, the public, and the staff working in the nuclear cardiology facility.

CERTIFICATION BOARD OF NUCLEAR CARDIOLOGY

The Certification Board of Nuclear Cardiology (CBNC) was founded in 1996 as the Certification Council of Nuclear Cardiology, but the name was changed in 1999 in order to meet the NRC Board requirements under the proposed revisions of Part 35. Part of the motivation to form CBNC was the recognition that nuclear cardiology is performed by cardiologists, radiologists, and nuclear medicine physicians. For some of these specialists nuclear cardiology is a very small part of their training and board examination in these specialties does not adequately test knowledge or expertise in nuclear cardiology. Poorly trained individuals provide poor-quality nuclear cardiology service and the whole field suffers. Letters of invitation were sent to professional medical societies whose members provided nuclear cardiology services to participate in the development of a certification body with representation and oversight

TABLE 26.5 *Proposed Revisions to NRC Physician Requirements for Authorization to Use Radiopharmaceuticals*

1. Certified by approved board

or

2. Training and experience
   a. Minimum of 700 hours
   b. Signature of authorized user preceptor

from all the participating organizations. For various reasons, some societies elected not to participate, and the American Society of Nuclear Cardiology and the American College of Cardiology are cosponsors of the CBNC.

The CBNC has tested 2405 physicians since the first examination was given to 609 applicants in October 1996. In 2000 there were 429 applicants. The average percentage passing the examination has been approximately 80% each year and there are 1909 diplomates of the CBNC. For further details contact http://www.cbnc.org.

The Purpose of Physician Certification

The purposes of the CBNC Certification Program are to establish the domain of the practice of nuclear cardiology for certification; to assess the level of knowledge demonstrated by specialists in a valid manner; to encourage professional growth; to enhance the quality of the practice of nuclear cardiology; to recognize individuals who meet the requirements set by CBNC; and to serve the public by encouraging quality patient care in the practice of nuclear cardiology. Some payers have required that physicians providing nuclear cardiology services be boarded by the CBNC.

Examination Development

A national survey of experts and practitioners in the field of nuclear cardiology was conducted in 1996 as part of a Practice Analysis process to define the knowledge areas appropriate for an examination. The data were collected from a cross section of outpatient and hospital-based specialists from all geographic areas within the United States and Canada. The responses were analyzed to develop the examination specifications and determine the content of the examination. This resulted in the definition of major content areas as well as subtopics for creating the examination questions.

The examination questions were developed by the CBNC Examination Committee, an expert panel of the CBNC, under the guidance of a test development organization and approved by the CBNC Board of Directors. The examination question pool is updated on a yearly basis to reflect current knowledge. Individual questions are modified or deleted based on statistical analysis of the examination.

The certification examination consists of 175–200 multiple-choice questions that must be answered in 4.5 hours. Each question contains four options or choices, only one of which is the correct or best answer. Some questions include interpretation of images presented on hard copy. The passing score for the examination was set by an independent national panel of peers representing the disciplines involved in the practice of nuclear cardiology and drawn from private practice and academia. The passing score is based on an expected level of knowledge and is not related to the distribution of scores obtained during a particular examination administration. Thus, in any given year, a candidate has the same chance of passing the examination whether the group taking the examination at that time tends to have high scores or low scores. In other words, each candidate is measured against a standard of knowledge, not against the performance of the other individuals taking the examination.

The first examination was given in October 1996, to 610 applicants. Subsequently 2405 physicians have taken it and there are currently 1909 diplomates of the CBNC. The passing rate has been approximately 80% for each of the 5 years in which it was administered. Certification is for a limited period of 10 years, after which those holding certificates dated October 26, 1997, or later will need to be recertified. There is no limit on the number of times that candidates may apply for and take the examination. However, if a candidate does not succeed in passing the examination after three attempts, he or she will be required to show proof of courses or seminars taken to remedy deficiencies.

Eligibility Requirements

Eligibility requirements for physicians taking the examination address medical licensure, board certification, and training and experience in providing nuclear cardiology services. They vary depending on the type of specialty training, when the training was completed, and whether the applicant resides in or out of the United States. General information is provided in the section that follows, but more specific details can be obtained from the CBNC web site, at http://www.cbnc.org or directly from the candidate bulletin.

Requirements for Candidates Residing in the United States

Requirement 1: licensure

Applicants must hold a current, unconditional, unrestricted license to practice medicine at the time of application and must provide a copy of the current license.

Requirement 2: board certification

Applicants must be physicians who, at the time of application, are board certified by a board that holds membership in either the American Board of Medical Specialties, or the Bureau of Osteopathic Specialists of the American Osteopathic Association.

Requirement 3: training/experience in the provision of nuclear cardiology services

All applicants who completed a cardiology fellowship or a radiology or nuclear medicine residency must submit a letter signed by a preceptor authorized user who meets the NRC requirements in Part 35.290 or 35.390 or equivalent Agreement State requirements stating that "your formal training in nuclear cardiology meets the Level 2 training requirements as outlined in the ACC/ASNC COCATS Guidelines. The letter must also state "you have achieved a level of competence sufficient to function independently as an authorized user for the medical uses authorized under NRC Part 35.200." The wording is very critical, as it meets the NRC requirements for boards applying for recognition for licensure without having to document training and experience requirements. The relevant revised COCATS Guidelines requirements for Level 2 training are contained in Appendix 1.

Applicants who completed a residency/fellowship in a specialty other than cardiology, nuclear medicine, or radiology must submit written verification, signed by a preceptor authorized user who meets the NRC requirements in Part 35.290 or 35.390 or equivalent Agreement State requirements, stating that "you have satisfactorily completed at least 700 hours of didactic training or work experience which includes radiation safety, interpretation of clinical cases and hands-on experience as outlined in the American College of Cardiology/American Society of Nuclear Cardiology COCATS Guidelines." The statement must also certify "you have achieved a level of competence sufficient to function independently as an authorized user for the medical uses authorized under NRC Part 35.200."

Eligibility Requirements for Candidates Residing outside the United States at the Time of Application

Requirement 1: licensure

Applicants must hold a current, unconditional, unrestricted license to practice medicine within their country at the time of application and must provide a copy of the current license.

Requirement 2: board certification

Applicants must submit evidence that they are board certified. If the country in which they practice does not cer-

tify the medical specialty, they must submit a letter stating this fact. In many countries, board certification similar to what exists in the United States is not available.

Requirement 3: training/experience in the provision of nuclear cardiology services

Applicants who have had formal training in nuclear cardiology, nuclear medicine, or radiology, must submit a statement from the training director stating that this training was equivalent to Level 2 training in nuclear cardiology as recommended in the American College of Cardiology/American Society of Nuclear Cardiology COCATS Training Guidelines.

If applicants have not received formal training in nuclear cardiology, nuclear medicine, or radiology and wish to qualify through experience, they must submit a statement from their division or laboratory head (for hospital or institution-based physicians) or a physician colleague (for nonhospital or non-institution-based physicians) that is written on organizational letterhead. This letter must state that training experience was equivalent to COCATS Level 2 training in nuclear cardiology.

INTERSOCIETAL COMMISSION FOR THE ACCREDITATION OF NUCLEAR MEDICINE LABORATORIES (ICANL)

It has long been recognized by the nuclear cardiology community that the quality of laboratories providing nuclear cardiology services is variable and that some may be poorly organized and have inferior equipment, and the reports provided to referring physicians are in some cases substandard. For this reason the Intersocietal Commission for the Accreditation of Nuclear Medicine Laboratories was organized as a nonprofit independent organization in November 1997. The mission of the organization was to ensure high-quality patient care and to promote health care by providing a mechanism to encourage and recognize the provision of quality nuclear cardiology services by a process of voluntary accreditation. Letters of invitation were sent to professional medical societies whose members provided nuclear cardiology services to participate in the development of essentials and standards for good quality practice and to establish an accreditation body with representation and oversight from all the participating organizations. Current sponsoring organizations include the American Society of Nuclear Cardiology, the American College of Cardiology, the Society of Nuclear Medicine, the Society of Nuclear Medicine Technologists Section, the American College of Nuclear Physicians, and the Academy of Molecular Imaging.

Members of the supporting organization completed the Essentials and Standards for Nuclear Cardiology in February 1998, and these were sent to the practicing nuclear cardiology community in the summer of 1998 for outside review. Modifications were made based on the responses and the accreditation process was pilot tested in the fall of 1998. Further modifications were made and the full program was implemented in the winter of 1998.

The accreditation process was to be applied to all nuclear medicine facilities. The first module to be developed was for nuclear cardiology. The American College of Nuclear Physicians and the Society of Nuclear Medicine had been conducting an on-site Laboratory Accreditation Program for a number of years and this program was merged into the ICANL process in the winter of 2001. As a result of the merger, it was elected to phase in a mandatory on-site visit as part of the ICANL process that could be performed by a physician, technologist, or physicist.

This section gives specific details on the Standards and Essentials that have been developed by the ICANL. The ICANL process helps to integrate the material previously presented on issues related to licensure, radiation safety, and physician certification.

General Process for Accreditation of Nuclear Cardiology Laboratories

The three broad components that are evaluated as part of the nuclear cardiology laboratory accreditation process include structure and organization, the process of testing, and outcome and quality assessment. For each of these areas, minimum standards have been established by the ICANL. In some cases these are absolute requirements that must be met for accreditation, while others are only recommendations. A nuclear cardiology laboratory being considered for accreditation, by definition, must consist of at least one gamma camera, a medical director, and usually a nuclear medicine technologist. It may be a single site, a conglomerate of sites, a mobile laboratory, or a combination of the above. There may be additional physicians, nuclear medicine technologists, and other professional and technical personnel. When more than one technical staff member is employed, a technical director, supervisor, chief technologist, or manager is responsible for supervision of the technical staff. The laboratory must be in compliance with the NRC regulations or in Agreement States with state regulations for medical diagnostic use of radioisotopes.

Facilities must purchase the Essentials and Standards made available by the ICANL. All the paperwork must be completed and submitted with copies of all required documentation and an application fee. Sites may apply for accreditation for myocardial perfusion imaging alone or for complete service, which includes equilibrium radionuclide angiography. Each applicant must submit recent clinical studies randomly selected by the ICANL. As an example, sites will be asked to submit the second case of the second Wednesday in June, the first case of the third Friday in June, etc. Laboratories applying for perfusion imaging alone will be asked to submit five SPECT perfusion studies and those applying for complete service must submit five additional randomly selected equilibrium radionuclide angiography cases. Sites must submit digital data of the selected case, hard copy of the cases, and the final stress and image interpretation reports.

The ICANL staff and two members of the ICANL board review completed applications. The clinical cases are reviewed on a workstation by the reviewer for the quality of the studies and accuracy of interpretation. The written reports from the site are examined and compared to the cases submitted. The two reviewers submit a written report and each laboratory is presented and discussed by a quorum of a panel consisting of half of the ICANL board. A formal vote is taken on accreditation. Sites may be accredited, deferred pending submission of additional material, or denied accreditation. A site visit may be requested if there are too many deficiencies. In the future, a site visit will be required for all laboratories. In cases where there is a tied vote by the review panel or an appeal is made by a site denied accreditation, the case is presented to a quorum consisting of the other half of the ICANL board that did not take part in the initial review.

Specifics of the Standards

The standards by which nuclear cardiology laboratories are evaluated for accreditation are reviewed in detail.

Structure and Organization

Standards have been established for personnel and supervision, nonimaging medical services, physical facilities, safety and confidentiality, and equipment and instrumentation.

Personnel and supervision

The essential personnel include a medical director, technical director, interoperating medical staff, nuclear medicine technologists, nonimaging personnel (nurses, ECG technologists, etc.), clerical personnel, and in some programs there may be physician and nuclear medicine technologist trainees. For each of these individuals there are specific requirements defined for training, licensure, responsibilities, supervision, and CME. Requirements and recommendations for Continuing Medical Education (CME), Basic Life Support (BLS), and Advanced Life Support (ACLS) apply to all personnel directly involved in imaging and performance of stress. In general all physician and technical personnel are required to have 15 hours of appropriate CME credit in nuclear cardiology every 3 years. Initial BLS and ACLS certification and recertification every 3 years is recommended for all physicians, technologists, nurses, and exercise physiologists working in the laboratory.

The medical director and the interpreting physician staff must be physicians licensed in the state and listed as authorized users on an NRC license or approved by an Agreement State regulatory body. The medical director and interpreting physician staff must meet one or more of the following training and experience requirements:

1. Certification in nuclear cardiology by the CBNC.
2. Board certified or board eligible within 2 years of finishing training in cardiology and completion of a minimum of a 4-month formal (Level 2 1995 ACC/ASNC COCATS Training Guidelines) training program in nuclear cardiology. This is mandatory for cardiologists who began their cardiology training in July 1995, or later.
3. Board certification in cardiology and training equivalent to Level 2 training, or at least 1 year of nuclear cardiology practice experience with independent interpretation of at least 600 nuclear cardiology studies. This requirement applies only to cardiologists who began their cardiology training before July 1995.
4. Board certified or board eligible within 2 years of finishing training in nuclear medicine.
5. Board certified or board eligible within 2 years of finishing training in radiology with at least 4 months of nuclear cardiology training.
6. Board certification in radiology and at least 1 year of nuclear cardiology practice experience with independent interpretation of at least 600 nuclear cardiology studies.

Members of the technical staff and nuclear medicine technologists must have appropriate credentials in nuclear medicine technology from the American Registry of Radiologic Technologist, Nuclear Medicine Technologist Certification Board, and/or state license. Non-

imaging support staff must have appropriate training for the roles they perform in the laboratory.

Physical facilities

The standards covered in this section include imaging procedure, interpretation, and storage areas. These standards are in place to ensure patient comfort, safety, and privacy. Although absolute room sizes are not listed, each application must be accompanied by a floor plan that clearly identifies space within the laboratory where these functions can be performed. Although the standards do not give absolute footage, the reviewer for the facility will make an assessment on whether all functions are provided and if they can realistically be performed in the space identified.

Imaging procedure areas. This standard covers the requirements for radioisotope handling, imaging, performing stress, and an area where patients and physicians can review the results of studies. Although a full service "hot lab" is not required for all nuclear cardiology laboratories, compliance with federal and state regulations demand clearly identified areas for radiopharmaceutical receipt, preparation, calibration, administration, storage, and disposal. Even if radioisotopes are purchased from a unit-dose pharmacy, many of these tasks still need to be performed in the facility and appropriate space needs to be available. However, much less space will be required, because the required tasks with unit dose are fewer. It is not mandated that a completely separate injection area be available.

The distance between the site of stress testing and the imaging room must be appropriate relative to the type of perfusion tracer that is being used. When using thallium-201 (Tl-201), the stress facility must be close to the imaging area to start patient imaging within 10 to at most 15 minutes following injection. If the Tc-99m agents or dual isotope are used, this distance is not critical. All areas must allow sufficient space for entry and holding of wheelchairs and stretchers.

Space for performing formal patient consults is not required, but there must be a designated area to review studies with patients, provide them with appropriate education, and, if necessary, to examine the patient.

Interpretation area. Laboratories are required to have an area designated for the processing, interpretation, and consultative review of the completed studies. This area should be sufficiently removed from direct patient imaging areas so that individuals involved in these functions are not exposed to radiation.

Storage areas. File space must be available for the storage of digital data, patient records, and final reports. Consensus has not been reached on how long such material must be kept available in the laboratory area. The minimum time is 1 year and after 2–3 years the relevance of imaging studies for making management decisions lessens. However, best practice nuclear cardiology requires comparison to prior studies and having old studies available is highly recommended. The practice of making hard copy and not storing digital data is not recommended, as this does not allow image reprocessing or manipulation when old studies need to be reviewed.

Safety and confidentiality

Covered in this section are patient safety, radiation safety, and patient confidentiality. It requires identification of individuals in the nuclear cardiology laboratory who will be responsible in case of problems, recommends training, and requires that strict and written procedures be in place to deal with each of these areas.

Patient safety standard. All procedures and examinations are performed under conditions that ensure patient safety. The medical director is responsible for patient care and safety policies in the nuclear cardiology laboratory.

For the day-to-day operation of the facility, the medical director or a designated member of the medical staff is responsible for the total care and safety of the patients while they are in the nuclear cardiology laboratory. Physicians, nurses, and technologists supervising or involved in stress procedures should be adequately trained in advanced life support. All medical and technical staff must be familiar with the procedure within the hospital, or in outpatient facilities, the community procedure required to mobilize resuscitation teams. All nuclear cardiology laboratories must have the appropriate equipment for resuscitation, and all electrical equipment should be routinely inspected and appropriate records kept.

Radiation safety. Laboratory operations must be in compliance with accepted NRC, state and institutional radiation safety standards for medical diagnostic use of radioisotopes.

Ultimately the medical director is responsible for maintaining all aspects of radiation safety in the nuclear cardiology laboratory. This responsibility may be delegated to the technical director, radiation safety officer, or health physics consultant when these individuals meet the training and experience requirements established by the NRC or Agreement State. All medical and technical staff and support personnel coming in contact with patients or working in areas where radioisotopes are administered should be monitored for radiation exposure according to federal or state guidelines. All medical and technical staff shall be trained and experienced in the receipt, preparation, calibration, administration, storage, disposal, and record keeping requirements of radioactive materials. All technical staff shall be trained and experienced in the safe handling practice for radioactive materials including containment and decontamination procedures for radioactive spills.

All personnel in the laboratory potentially exposed to or handling radioactive materials need to receive radiation safety instruction upon hire and thereafter on an annual basis. The radiopharmacy needs to have adequate equipment and shielding material to ensure safe receipt, preparation, storage, and disposal of radiopharmaceuticals and radioactive materials. This is a requirement even if material is received in unit doses.

Patient confidentiality. All patient records are kept in such a manner as to maintain confidentially. Requirements for confidentiality apply to all aspects of the operation of the laboratory. Thus, all hard copy and digital data, interpretation and review of studies, and conveyance of results to the patient and the referring physician must be done in such a manner that access to the information is limited to individuals with the appropriate authority. This responsibility to maintain patient confidentiality extends to all medical and technical staff and all nonimaging personnel.

Equipment and instrumentation

Equipment and instrumentation used in a nuclear cardiology laboratory will include at least the following: dose calibrator, imaging equipment, computers, exercise equipment, radiation monitoring devices, and resuscitation equipment. Equipment shall be routinely inspected and records kept on file.

Dose calibrator and radiation monitoring devices. Every laboratory is required to have a dose calibrator to verify the radiopharmaceutical dose prior to administration to patients. Ancillary radiation monitoring equipment shall be present in the laboratory as needed and in good working condition. This equipment must be checked and inventoried as per institutional or the Occupational Safety and Health Administration (OSHA) guidelines. Linearity and other performance characteristics must be verified by certified service providers and detailed written records kept on-site and available for NRC or state audit and review.

Nuclear imaging equipment. The gamma cameras and computer equipment used for patient imaging shall be in good working condition as verified by daily, weekly, monthly, and quarterly quality control. All equipment shall have detailed records of ongoing in-laboratory quality assessment and service records.

Stress and ECG equipment. The motorized treadmills, bicycles, and infusion pumps, used for administration of pharmaceuticals, require inspection and verification of accuracy and safety at regularly specified time intervals. Service and safety inspection records need to be kept on file. Electrocardiographic monitoring systems used in conjunction with stress testing need to be inspected at least annually.

Emergency equipment. Emergency resuscitation equipment needs to be present in the laboratory and in good working condition. This equipment must be checked and inventoried, and drugs updated/replaced as required by the institutional requirements and the minimum requirements of the Occupational Safety and Health Administration (OSHA) guidelines. Defibrillators need to be kept in working order and charged at all times.

PROCESS OF NUCLEAR CARDIOLOGY TESTING

Procedures

Protocols

The laboratory shall have written protocols describing details for all procedures to ensure standardized operation. The protocols shall be in compliance with accepted published guidelines for nuclear cardiology procedures and reviewed annually [1,2].

1. *Receipt, preparation, calibration, administration, storage and disposal of radiopharmaceuticals.* All aspects related to radiopharmaceuticals need to be defined, monitored, documented, and in compliance with NRC and Agreement State governing bodies.

2. *Imaging Procedure Protocols.* Although all possible radionuclide imaging procedures may not be performed in a particular laboratory, those that are performed should have written protocols. Written protocols for each type of imaging procedure must define all components of the examination. It is necessary to have equipment-specific protocols for procedures such that the unique aspects of each camera system and processing parameters are listed. It is not appropriate to just provide the manufacturer's suggested acquisition and processing parameters. These protocols need to describe in full:

    a. Appropriate clinical indications
    b. Patient identification
    c. Patient assessment (including status of pregnancy/breast feeding)
    d. Patient preparation
    e. Appropriate radiopharmaceutical dose(s)
    f. Camera/computer-specific acquisition protocols
    g. Camera/computer-specific processing protocols
    h. Camera/computer-specific display protocols

3. *Exercise and/or Pharmacologic Testing.* Exercise-specific protocols shall be in compliance with accepted published guidelines for exercise testing [3]. Recommendations for pharmacologic testing guidelines have been included in the ASNC guidelines [1,2]. All stress testing protocols must include the following:

    a. Description of graded protocols (e.g., Bruce, modified Bruce, Naughton, etc.)
    b. Specific infusion protocols and parameters, as appropriate for all the pharmacologic stress agents used in the laboratory
    c. Frequency and timing of assessing symptoms, heart rate, blood pressure, and electrocardiographic tracings
    d. Exercise and pharmacologic testing end points for injection and termination of exercise or drug infusion. Reaching 85% of the target heart rate alone is not an end point to inject the radiopharmaceutical or terminate stress.
    e. Radiopharmaceutical injection criteria
    f. Treatment of adverse effects
    g. Duration and components of poststress monitoring

4. *Quality Assessment of Imaging Equipment.* Routine assessment of basic parameters and calibration of imaging equipment will be performed according to approved written standards. If SPECT equipment is physically moved from site to site, either portable equipment moved within a facility or as part of a mobile system, it is recommended that the quality assurance steps listed above be performed after each move.

Test	Frequency
Energy peaking	Daily
Intrinsic or extrinsic uniformity	Daily

Intrinsic or extrinsic sensitivity	Weekly
Resolution and linearity	Weekly
Super high (30 million) count floods	Monthly, or per manufacturer's recommendations
Center of rotation	Monthly, or per manufacturer's recommendations
Preventive maintenance	Every 6 months, or per manufacturer's recommendations

5. *Quality Assessment of Nonimaging Equipment.* A policy shall exist for routine inspection and testing of all nonimaging equipment, such as dose calibrators and survey meters, and be in accordance with the NRC or state requirements. Some basic recommendations follow:

Equipment	Test	Frequency
Dose calibrator	Accuracy/constancy	Daily
Dose calibrator	Linearity	Quarterly
Dose calibrator, survey meter	Accuracy	Yearly

6. *Radiation Safety in the Radiopharmacy, Patient Areas, Stress and Imaging Laboratories.* Written protocols shall meet all NRC, state or, if applicable, radiation safety committee or radiation safety officer requirements. Specific protocols must be provided for the following in addition to all other mandated requirements:

Test	Frequency
Survey areas, trash, etc.	Daily
Wipe tests	Weekly

7. *Handling of Radioactive Spills.* Written protocols need to define the procedures to be followed for radioactive spills. These must address issues of confinement and decontamination procedures for the stress testing or imaging areas.

8. *Medical Emergency Procedures.* A protocol must be in place for handling any medical emergency that may arise in the nuclear cardiology laboratory during the stress or imaging procedure. It needs to specifically identify who is to be contacted, how to summon the CODE team, or for outpatient facilities, how to contact emergency transport systems (911).

Image Interpretation and Reporting

Examinations are interpreted and a final report provided by the medical director or members of the medical staff of the laboratory.

Images are preferably interpreted from computer screen display. Assessment of excessive patient motion and other potential causes for artifacts and assessment of wall motion and ventricular function must be assessed from cine display on computer screen. Total reliance on interpretation from X-ray film or hard copies is not recommended. The variability in quality of the final reports has been one of the major problems in the laboratory accreditation process, and templates have been suggested for the major type of reports that are generated [4].

1. Final interpretation of examinations shall include consideration of all available clinical and imaging information. This includes, but is not limited to:
   a. Radionuclide images
   b. Clinical information, clinical indication/question
   c. Stress data. Although a separate written report of the stress portion of the study is usually required, the nuclear report must contain sufficient detail of the stress portion to allow an assessment of the adequacy of stress.

2. The report will be typed or computer generated and will accurately reflect the content and results of the study. This includes, but is not limited to:
   a. The patient's name, gender, age, and identification number.
   b. The date of the examination.
   c. The clinical indications leading to the performance of the examination. There must be sufficient detail to support the ICD-9 codes submitted for billing the procedure.
   d. An adequate description of the test performed. The description will include the type of examination, the radiotracer dose, and the type of stress.
   e. An overview of the results of the examination including pertinent positive and negative findings. Where appropriate, this will include localization and quantification of abnormal findings, including stress ECG findings.
   f. The reasons for limited examinations, if applicable.
   g. A summary of the test findings.
   h. An overall succinct impression.

3. Retention of Records. All patient records will be maintained and accessible for the appropriate period of time as prescribed by state, institution, or other guidelines or other rules/regulations for retention.

OUTCOME AND QUALITY ASSESSMENT

Study Volume

The annual procedure volume must be sufficient to maintain proficiency in examination interpretation and performance.

It is recommended that a laboratory should perform a minimum of 300 nuclear cardiology patient studies annually in order for the technical and medical staff to maintain adequate skills. For full service laboratories, there should be a distribution between the various types of procedures performed that is proportional to the percentage of each performed in the facility over the course of 1 year.

Reports

All examinations performed in the laboratory must have a final interpretation by a qualified physician on the medical staff of the laboratory. This standard includes the need to interpret and communicate the results to the referring physician within 1 working day of completing the study. A final written report should be completed within 2 working days and sent to the referring physician.

Quality Assessment

The laboratory shall conduct internal quality assessment at regular time intervals. This standard applies to the following areas: equipment, technical quality of studies, and study interpretation. These programs most be performed on an ongoing basis and be adequately documented not only in terms of what was done but also in terms of corrective actions.

Equipment quality assessment

The laboratory shall maintain records of all routine quality assessment of equipment as described in prior sections. Records must also be maintained of service, scheduled maintenance, and repairs due to malfunction.

Technical quality assessment

Under the supervision of the technical director and the medical director, the laboratory shall have a defined quality assessment program that evaluates the ongoing technical quality of the procedures performed in the laboratory. This program should have predefined indicators of quality and predefined thresholds that indicate the need for corrective action. The laboratory should maintain minutes or reports of quality assessment evaluations and corrective actions taken.

1. Indicators may be: back-log for scheduled exam-

inations, late reporting, long patient waiting time, misadministrations, radioactive spills, adverse effects, poor quality of examinations, poor reproducibility of computer processing, etc.

2. Thresholds are determined for each indicator.

3. Corrective actions are measures taken to improve the operation of the laboratory.

Interpretive quality assessment

Under the supervision of the medical director, the laboratory shall have a defined quality assessment program that evaluates the ongoing quality of study interpretation. This program should have predefined indicators of quality and predefined thresholds that indicate the need for corrective action. The medical director should maintain minutes or reports as necessary of quality assessment evaluations and document, if applicable, corrective measures taken.

A quality assessment program may consist of:

1. Correlation of interpretation of studies with patient outcome, such as results of cardiac catheterization, angiography, or subsequent cardiac events.

2. Reproducibility of interpretation with previous interpretation, or with interpretation of the same study by other qualified interpreting physicians.

Patient and Referring Physician Satisfaction

The laboratory should have a mechanism in place to evaluate the satisfaction of the patient with the laboratory's services. This is routinely done with questionnaires for patients undergoing testing. Examples of the questionnaire used at each laboratory must be submitted.

The laboratory should have a mechanism in place to evaluate the satisfaction of the referring physicians with the laboratory's services.

REFERENCES

1. Port S. Imaging Guidelines for Nuclear Cardiology Procedures, Part 2. J Nucl Cardiol 1999;6:G49.
2. DePuey EGE. Updated imaging guidelines for nuclear cardiology procedures, part 1. J Nucl Cardiol 2001;8:G5.
3. ACC/AHA. Guidelines for Exercise Testing. J Am Coll Cardiol 1997;30:260.
4. Wackers FJ. Intersocietal Commission for the Accreditation of Nuclear Medicine Laboratories (ICANL) position statement on standardization and optimization of nuclear cardiology reports. J Nucl Cardiol 2000;7:397.

Appendix: Revised 2002 COCATS guidelines for level II training in nuclear cardiology

OVERVIEW OF NUCLEAR CARDIOLOGY TRAINING

Training in nuclear cardiology at all levels should provide an understanding of the indications for specific nuclear cardiology tests, the safe use of radionuclides, basics of instrumentation and image processing, methods of quality control, image interpretation, integration of risk factors, clinical symptoms and stress testing and the appropriate application of the resultant diagnostic information for clinical management. Training in nuclear cardiology is best acquired in Accreditation Council for Graduate Medical Education (ACGME) approved training programs in cardiology, nuclear medicine or radiology. An exception to this ACGME requirement is the didactic and laboratory training in radiation safety and radioisotope handling that may be provided by qualified physicians/scientists in a non-ACGME program when such a program is not available as part of the clinical ACGME training program. Didactic, clinical case experience and hands-on training hours require documentation in a logbook, having the trainee's name appear on the clinical report or other specific record. The hours need to be monitored and verified by the nuclear cardiology training preceptor.

SPECIALIZED TRAINING—LEVEL 2

(Minimum of 4 Months)

Fellows who wish to clinically practice the specialty of nuclear cardiology are required to have at least 4 months of training. This includes a minimum of 700 hours of didactic, clinical study interpretation, and hands-on clinical case and radiation safety training in nuclear cardiology. In training programs with a high volume of procedures, clinical experience may be acquired in as short a period as 4 months. In programs with a lower volume of procedures, a total of 6 months of clinical experience will be necessary to achieve Level 2 competency. The additional

training required of Level 2 trainees is to enhance clinical skills and to qualify to become an authorized user of radioactive materials in accordance with the regulations the Nuclear Regulatory Commission (NRC) and/or the Agreement States. Requirements do vary among the Agreement States; therefore those seeking licensure are advised to check the Agreement State/NRC internet web site at http://www.hsrd.ornl.gov/nrc/home.html.

Didactic

Lectures and self-study

The didactic training should include in-depth details of all nuclear cardiology procedures. This program may be scheduled over a 12- to 24-month period concurrent and integrated with other fellowship assignments.

Radiation safety

Classroom and laboratory training needs to include extensive review of radiation physics and instrumentation, radiation protection, mathematics pertaining to the use and measurement of radioactivity, chemistry of byproduct material for medical use, and radiation biology. There should be a thorough review of regulations dealing with radiation safety for the use of radiopharmaceuticals.

Interpretation of clinical cases

Fellows should participate in the interpretation of all nuclear cardiology imaging data for the 4–6 month training period. It is imperative that the fellows have experience in correlating catheterization/angiographic data with radionuclide-derived data in a minimum of 30 patients. A teaching conference in which the fellow presents the clinical material and nuclear cardiology results is an appropriate forum for such an experience. A total of 300 cases should be interpreted under preceptor supervision, either from direct patient studies or from a teaching file consisting of diverse types of procedures (see Table 1 below).

Hands-on experience in clinical cases

Fellows acquiring Level 2 training should have hands-on supervised experience in a minimum of 35 patients: 25 patients with myocardial perfusion imaging and 10 patients with radionuclide angiography. Such experience should include pretest patient evaluation, radiopharmaceutical preparation (including experience with relevant radionuclide generators), performance of the study, administration of the dosage, calibration and setup of the gamma camera, setup of the imaging computer, processing the data for display, interpretation of the studies, and generating clinical reports.

Work experience

This experience must be under the supervision of an authorized user who meets the NRC requirements of Part 35.290 or 35.390 or equivalent Agreement State requirements, and must include the following:

a. Ordering, receiving and unpacking radioactive materials safely and performing the related radiation surveys;

b. Calibrating instruments used to determine the activity of dosages and performing checks for proper operation of survey meters;

c. Calculating, measuring and safely preparing patient or human research subject dosages;

d. Using administrative controls to prevent a medical event involving the use of unsealed byproduct material;

e. Using procedures to safely contain spilled radioactive material and using proper decontamination procedures;

f. Administering dosages of radioactive drugs to patients or human research subjects; and

g. Eluting generator systems appropriate for preparation of radioactive drugs for imaging and localization studies, measuring and testing the eluate for radionuclide purity, and processing the eluate with reagent kits to prepare labeled radioactive drugs.

Additional experience

In addition, the training program for Level 2 training must provide experience in computer methods for analysis. This should include perfusion and functional data derived from thallium or technetium agents and ejection fraction and regional wall motion measurements from radionuclide angiographic studies.

Index

Page numbers followed by "cf" indicate color figures; numbers followed by "f" indicate figures; numbers followed by "t" indicate tables.